HEAD AND NECK IMAGING

HEAD AND NECK IMAGING

Editors

PETER M. SOM, M.D.

Professor of Radiology and Otolaryngology
Chief of Head and Neck Radiology Section, Department of Radiology
Mount Sinai Medical Center of City University of New York
New York, New York

R. THOMAS BERGERON, M.D.

Professor of Clinical Radiology, Department of Radiology
State University of New York Health Science Center at Brooklyn
Chairman and Attending Radiologist
Department of Radiology, Long Island College Hospital
Brooklyn, New York

Associate Editors

HUGH D. CURTIN, M.D.

Professor of Radiology and Otolaryngology
University of Pittsburgh School of Medicine
Director of Radiology, Eye and Ear Hospital
Pittsburgh, Pennsylvania

DEBORAH L. REEDE, M.D.

Associate Professor of Clinical Radiology
State University of New York Health Science Center at Brooklyn
Vice Chairman of Radiology, Attending Radiologist
Long Island College Hospital
Brooklyn, New York

SECOND EDITION

with 2495 illustrations

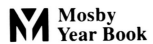
Mosby
Year Book

St. Louis   Baltimore   Boston   Chicago   London   Philadelphia   Sydney   Toronto

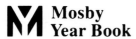

Mosby Year Book

Dedicated to Publishing Excellence

Editors: George Stamathis, Anne S. Patterson
Developmental Editor: Elaine Steinborn
Assistant Editor: Jo Salway
Production Editor: Cynthia A. Miller
Book and Cover Design: Gail Morey Hudson
Production: Ginny Douglas

SECOND EDITION

Mosby–Year Book, Inc.
11830 Westline Industrial Drive, St. Louis, Missouri 63146

Library of Congress Cataloging-in-Publication Data

Head and neck imaging / editors, Peter M. Som, R. Thomas Bergeron ;
   associate editors, Hugh D Curtin, Deborah L. Reede. — 2nd ed.
      p.   cm.
   Rev. ed. of: Head and neck imaging, excluding brain / edited
by R. Thomas Bergeron, Anne G. Osborn, Peter M. Som. 1984.
   Includes bibliographical references.
   Includes index.
   ISBN 0-8016-5524-2
   1. Head--Tomography.   2. Neck--Tomography.   I. Som, Peter M.
II. Bergeron, R. Thomas, 1931– .   III. Head and neck imaging,
excluding the brain.
   [DNLM: 1. Head--radiography.   2. Neck--radiography.
3. Tomography, X-Ray Computed.   WE   705 H43031]
RC936.H43   1991
617.5′107572--dc20
DNLM/DLC
for Library of Congress   90-6467
                                                                      CIP

C/MV/MV 9 8 7 6 5 4 3 2

Contributors

WILLIAM G. ARMINGTON, M.D.

Arcadia Radiology Associates
Arcadia, California

BRUCE S. BAUER, M.D.

Associate Professor, Department of Surgery
Northwestern University Medical School;
Chief, Division of Plastic Surgery
The Children's Memorial Hospital
Chicago, Illinois

R. THOMAS BERGERON, M.D.

Professor of Clinical Radiology, Department of Radiology
State University of New York Health Science Center at
Brooklyn; Chairman and Attending Radiologist
Department of Radiology, Long Island College Hospital
Brooklyn, New York

LARISSA T. BILANIUK, M.D.

Professor of Radiology
Hospital of the University of Pennsylvania
Philadelphia, Pennsylvania

IRA FRANKLIN BRAUN, M.D.

Associate Professor of Radiology
Director of Neuroradiology, Clinical Director of MRI
Department of Radiology
Virginia Commonwealth University/Medical College of
Virginia
Richmond, Virginia

RONALD E. BROADWELL, M.D.

Clinical Assistant, Department of Radiation Sciences
Resident Physician, Department of Radiology
Loma Linda University School of Medicine
Loma Linda, California

HUGH D. CURTIN, M.D.

Professor of Radiology and Otolaryngology
University of Pittsburgh School of Medicine;
Director of Radiology, Eye and Ear Hospital
Pittsburgh, Pennsylvania

WILLIAM PATRICK DILLON

Associate Professor Radiology and Neurology
Department of Neuroradiology
University of California Medical Center
San Francisco, California

H. RIC HARNSBERGER, M.D.

Associate Professor of Radiology
University of Utah
Salt Lake City, Utah

ANTON N. HASSO, M.D., F.A.C.R.

Professor of Radiology, Department of Radiation Sciences
Loma Linda University School of Medicine;
Director of Neuroradiology, Department of Radiology
Loma Linda University Medical Center
Loma Linda, California

ROY A. HOLLIDAY, M.D.

Assistant Professor of Radiology
New York University School of Medicine
New York, New York

RICHARD WIER KATZBERG, M.D., M.B.A.

Professor and Chairman, Department of Radiology
Oregon Health Science University
Portland, Oregon

DESMOND A. KERNAHAN, M.D.

Retired; Formerly Chief, Division of Plastic Surgery
The Children's Memorial Hospital
Chicago, Illinois

DAVID P.C. LIU, M.D.

Clinical Assistant Professor, Department of Radiology
State University of New York at Brooklyn;
Assistant Attending Physician, Department of Radiology
Long Island College Hospital
Brooklyn, New York

WILLIAM W.M. LO, M.D.

Clinical Professor of Radiology
University of Southern California;
Radiologist, St. Vincent Medical Center
Los Angeles, California

MAHMOOD F. MAFEE, M.D.

Professor of Radiology
Magnetic Resonance Imaging-Radiology
University of Illinois, College of Medicine;
Director, MRI Center;
Director, Radiology Section Eye and Ear Infirmary
Department of MRI, Radiology
University of Illinois Hospital
Chicago, Illinois

DAVID G. McLONE, M.D., Ph.D.

Professor of Surgery
Northwestern University Medical School;
Division Head, Pediatric Neurosurgery
Department of Surgery, Children's Memorial Hospital
Chicago, Illinois

LYN NADEL, M.D.

Assistant Professor of Radiology, Department of Radiology
Virginia Commonwealth University/Medical College of
Virginia; Attending Neuroradiologist
Department of Radiology
Medical College of Virginia Hospitals
Richmond, Virginia

THOMAS P. NAIDICH, M.D.

Clinical Professor of Radiology
University of Miami School of Medicine;
Director of Neuroradiology, Department of Radiology
Baptist Hospital of Miami
Miami, Florida

ROBIN E. OSBORN, D.O.

Neuroradiologist, University of California at San Diego;
Director of Neuroradiology, Department of Radiology
Naval Hospital
San Diego, California

DEBORAH L. REEDE, M.D.

Associate Professor of Clinical Radiology
State University of New York Health Science Center at
Brooklyn; Vice Chairman of Radiology, Attending Radiologist
Long Island College Hospital
Brooklyn, New York

CHARLES J. SCHATZ, M.D.

Associate Clinical Professor of Radiology and Otolaryngology
University of Southern California;
Director of Head and Neck Radiology
Cedars Sinai Medical Center
Los Angeles, California

WENDY R.K. SMOKER, M.D.

Associate Professor of Radiology
Radiology-Neuroradiology Section, University of Utah;
Clinical Director of MRI, University of Utah Hospitals
Salt Lake City, Utah

PETER M. SOM, M.D.

Professor of Radiology and Otolaryngology
Chief of Head and Neck Radiology Section
Department of Radiology, Mount Sinai
Medical Center of City University of New York
New York, New York

JOEL D. SWARTZ, M.D.

Associate Professor of Radiologic Sciences
Medical College of Pennsylvania
Philadelphia, Pennsylvania

ALFRED L. WEBER, M.D.

Professor of Radiology, Harvard Medical School;
Chief of Radiology, Massachusetts Eye and Ear Infirmary;
Radiologist, Massachusetts General Hospital
Boston, Massachusetts

PER-LENNART WESTESSON, D.D.S., Ph.D.

Associate Professor, Department of Clinical Dentistry,
Department of Radiology, Senior Research Associate,
Department of Orthodontics, Eastman Dental Center
University of Rochester
Rochester, New York

ZIBUTE G. ZAPARACKAS, M.D.

Associate Professor of Ophthalmology
Northwestern University/Children's Memorial Hospital
Chicago, Illinois

ROBERT A. ZIMMERMAN, M.D.

Professor of Radiology
University of Pennsylvania School of Medicine;
Section Chief, Pediatric Neuroradiology
Hospital of the University of Pennsylvania and
the Children's Hospital of Philadelphia
Philadelphia, Pennsylvania

This book is dedicated
to the memory of my father
Dr. Max L. Som.

PMS

Preface

Over the last decade, since work began on the first edition of this book, head and neck imaging has become firmly established in both the clinical and radiological communities. The rapid development and refinement of the field have resulted from several factors, including the continued improvement of computed tomography, the development and advancement of magnetic resonance imaging, the rich and inventive applications of these technologies to head and neck disease, the scientific and clinical maturation of those radiologists who were already established in the field, and the attraction of many additional physicians to this subspecialty. Interest in this discipline is now shared by radiologists trained either in classical neuroradiology or body imaging and by clinicians and surgeons from a variety of other specialties. To reflect all of these changes, this book has been completely revised from the first edition.

The editors of HEAD AND NECK IMAGING have gathered contributors who are nationally and internationally renowned as experts and who are acknowledged for their independent work, creativity, and teaching ability in each area of the field. This group was given the task of creating a reference text for head and neck imaging that both includes the established techniques and emphasizes the present state of the art and how it is applied in modern clinical management. The contributors' enthusiastic response as well as the strong support of the publisher have resulted in this present edition.

The entire subject of head and neck imaging is critically addressed in this book. Each chapter is a thorough examination of a topic, with discussion of the pertinent embryology, anatomy, and pathology. As a result, the book can be used by the newly interested practitioner to develop skills in the field, or it can be utilized as a current reference for the more experienced physician interested in head and neck imaging. The book also offers extensive bibliographies for each chapter and emphasizes clinical and pathological correlations.

Peter M. Som
R. Thomas Bergeron

Preface to the first edition

The introduction of computed tomography (CT) and the subsequent spectacular refinement of x-ray imaging technology over the past decade have revolutionized the workup of patients with head and neck disease. Although these afflictions have always existed in abundance, radiologists have been able to attend only a few of them, reflecting tacit acknowledgment of the limited benefits this specialty had to offer. Technologic advancement has changed that. As a consequence, an enormous reservoir of once elusive pathology has suddenly become susceptible to the probing inquiry of modern invention. But even the most dedicated radiologist has discovered himself ill-equipped to address the challenge of contemporary head and neck radiology. For the most part he finds himself insecure in his understanding of basic anatomy, unaware of pathology, uncertain of clinical course, and unprepared to advise on the preferred imaging technique to best demonstrate suspected disease.

The imaging modalities that are now available—and CT is pre-eminent among them—provide more visual information than many radiologists know how to use. All of the intellectual resources of even the best of interpreters are challenged regularly by this extraordinary technology. In many ways the goal of this book is to make the interpreter as good as his images.

The editors and contributors in this work have approached their task with certain goals in mind: to familiarize the newcomer in the field with developmental anatomy when it is important in understanding anomalies and developmental variants; to stress surgical anatomy when those landmarks are the best way to communicate the location and extent of disease; to relate pathologic anatomy with recognizable clinical disease states; to refine approaches to differential diagnoses based not only on radiologic criteria but also on clinical nuances; and ultimately to give direction on the method of diagnostic approach, leading to the most efficient method of arriving at the most likely diagnosis with the greatest degree of certainty.

This book is meant to serve as a teaching resource for the newly interested as well as a source of in-depth information for the more sophisticated reader. There is a strong emphasis on anatomy; however, it has been placed in the context of relevance to the interpretation of images and to the understanding of progression of disease.

The more traditional imaging modalities have not been neglected or ignored because they have not always been replaced by newer ones. These conventional techniques are presented and their place in the evaluation of patients with head and neck disease is emphasized.

The editors give public thanks to their distinguished contributors, many of whom are unchallenged experts in their particular field of endeavor. Their excellent work has helped this book become a reality. Each of the editors also carries a debt to many associates and fellow workers who have helped bring this work to fruition, and we express our thanks to them.

R. Thomas Bergeron
Anne G. Osborn
Peter M. Som

Contents

Head and Neck Imaging

1 Embryology and Congenital Lesions of the Midface

THOMAS P. NAIDICH
ROBIN E. OSBORN
BRUCE S. BAUER
DAVID G. MCLONE
DESMOND A. KERNAHAN
ZIBUTE G. ZAPARACKAS

BASIC EMBRYOLOGY OF THE FACE, EYE, AND CORPUS CALLOSUM

The embryogenesis of the midface and upper lip, the optic nerve and globe, and the corpus callosum share many spatial, temporal, and histologic features, which appear to explain the frequency of concurrent anomalies of these structures.

Face

The face has a dual embryonic origin.[1] The median facial structures, bone and soft tissue, derive from the frontonasal prominence. The lateral facial structures, bone and soft tissue, arise from the branchial arches. For this reason, anomalies tend to affect either median or lateral structures separately and/or their lines of junction.

The major features of the face develop in the fourth to eighth week of gestation by growth, migration, and merging of a number of processes bordering the stomo-deum, which is a slitlike invagination of the ectoderm that marks the location of the mouth.[2] At 4 weeks of gestation (Fig. 1-1, A), the stomodeum is bordered superiorly by the unpaired, median frontal prominence; laterally by the paired maxillary processes; and inferiorly by the paired mandibular processes. The frontal prominence is composed of surface ectoderm and a thin layer of mesenchyme overlying the developing forebrain. This mesenchyme derives principally from neural crest cells,[3] not mesoderm per se. The maxillary and the mandibular processes derive from the first branchial arch. The nasal placodes form paired epithelial thickenings near the lateral margins of the overhanging frontal prominence.

By 5 weeks of gestation (Fig. 1-1, B and C), horseshoe-shaped elevations have appeared around the nasal placodes, so the placodes seem recessed beneath the surface. These recesses are called the *nasal pits*. The medial limbs of the horseshoes are designated the *nasomedial processes*, while the lateral limbs of the horseshoes are designated the *nasolateral processes*. The nasomedial processes are longer than the nasolateral processes. The lowermost portions of the nasomedial limbs are designated the *globular processes*.[4] At this time, the nasomedial and the nasolateral processes lie adjacent to, but appear separated from, the now larger maxillary processes. The mandibular arches have enlarged. These merge together during the fifth week to form the lower lip and underlying structures.

During the sixth week (Fig. 1-1, D and E), the nasomedial processes increase in size and become displaced toward each other by marked enlargement of the two maxillary processes lateral to them. They merge with the frontal prominence to form the frontonasal prominence. From this key frontonasal prominence will come the nasal bones, frontal bones, cartilaginous nasal capsule, central one third of the upper lip, central one

1

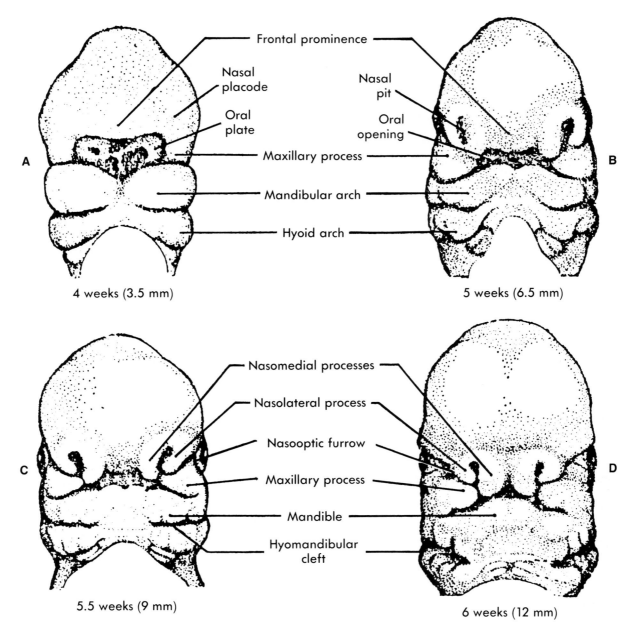

Fig. 1-1   A-F, Embryogenesis of face from 4 to 8 weeks of gestation. (From Patten BM: The normal development of the facial region. In Pruzansky S: Congenital anomalies of the face and associated structures, Springfield, Ill, 1985, Charles C Thomas, Publisher.)

third of superior alveolar ridge including the incisors, and primary palate. At each side, a groove called the nasooptic furrow extends from the medial canthus of the orbit toward the developing nose along the line between the nasolateral and the maxillary processes. The nasolacrymal duct will develop along this line. It is not known whether the deep portion of the furrow becomes the nasolacrymal duct or whether a separate epithelial tube grows down from the orbit to the nasal cavity along the course of the furrow.[2] By the seventh week,

the nasolateral processes merge with the maxillary processes to complete the ala nasi of each side. The nasomedial processes still remain ununited.

By the eighth week (Fig. 1-1, F), the upper lip is formed by the merging of each nasomedial process with the ipsilateral maxillary process, followed by the merging of the two nasomedial processes in the midline. This merging completes formation of the columella and the philtrum (Fig. 1-1, E). Merging of the maxillary and mandibular processes forms the cheeks and the corners

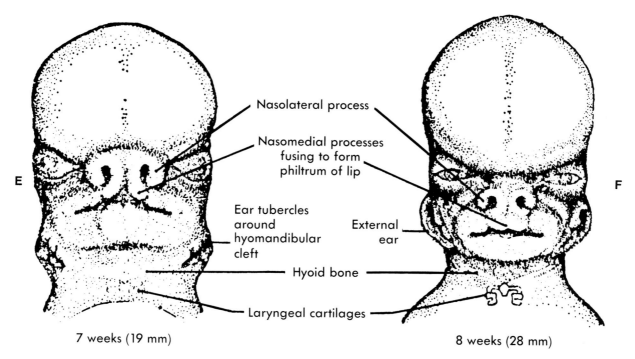

E — 7 weeks (19 mm)

F — 8 weeks (28 mm)

Nasolateral process

Nasomedial processes fusing to form philtrum of lip

Ear tubercles around hyomandibular cleft

External ear

Hyoid bone

Laryngeal cartilages

Fig. 1-1, cont'd   For legend see opposite page.

of the mouth. During this time, descent of the nose and medial migration of the orbits above the nose are also observed.

The frontonasal process (including the merged nasomedial processes) may be considered to constitute an *intermaxillary segment*. The superficial portion of this segment, termed the *prolabium*, forms the medial portion of the upper lip. The deeper gnathogingival segment will develop into the premaxillary portion of the upper jaw containing the four upper incisors. The palatal component will form a triangular midline wedge of palate designated the *primary palate*. This becomes continuous with the rostral-most portion of the nasal septum.

The maxillary processes form the lateral portions of the upper jaw and contribute all of the upper teeth behind the incisors. During the 6th to 8th week, the maxillary processes also give rise medially to paired palatal shelves. Initially these shelves curve ventrally alongside the tongue (Fig 1-2, *A* and *B*). When growth of the mandible permits descent of the tongue, these shelves swing medially, toward each other above the tongue (Fig. 1-2, *C* and *D*). The shelves then merge (1) with each other in the midline and (2) with the primary palate anteriorly to form the definitive palate (Fig. 1-2, *E* and *F*). That portion of the definitive palate contributed by the maxillary processes is designated the *secondary palate*. The secondary palate is far larger than the primary palate. The lines of fusion of the palate appear Y-shaped. The incisive foramina lie at the midpoint of the

Y, marking the junction between the V-shaped primary palate anteriorly and the paired halves of the secondary palate more posteriorly. While the palate is forming, the nasal septum grows downward and fuses with its cephalic surface.

Formation of the Mouth, Nostrils, and Posterior Choanae. The ectoderm overlying the early forebrain extends into the stomodeum. At this site, it lies adjacent to the developing foregut. The junctional zone between the surface ectoderm and the subjacent endoderm is called the *buccopharyngeal membrane*.

The line of attachment of the buccopharyngeal membrane corresponds to Waldeyer's throat ring connecting the nasopharyngeal adenoids, the palatine tonsils, and the lingual tonsils.[5] Dissolution of the buccopharyngeal membrane in the early somite stage permits communication between the mouth and the foregut regions. The position of Waldeyer's ring in the postnatal human, deep to a well-developed mouth, indicates the extent to which formation of the face arises by the thickening of the tissue external to the original surface level, represented by the stomodeum.

By a similar thickening of surrounding surface tissue, the nasal pits become progressively recessed. The ectoderm overlying the nasal pits fuses with the ectoderm overlying the stomodeum to form the bucconasal (oronasal) membrane. Eventual disappearance of this membrane establishes communication between the nose and the upper part of the stomodeal cavity. The external openings of the nasal pits are designated the *nostrils*

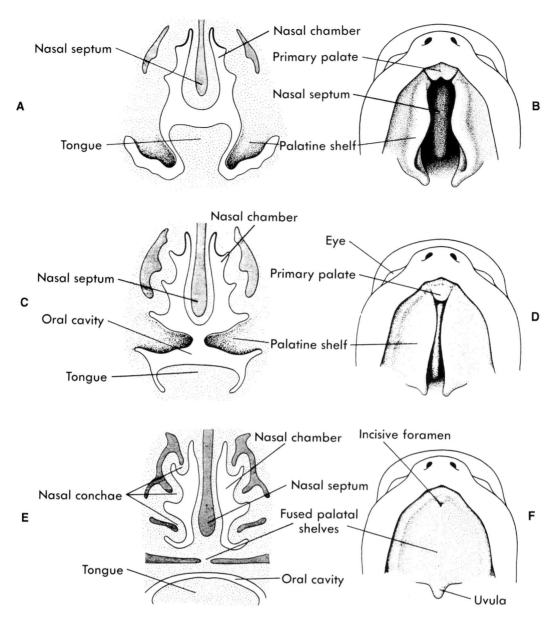

Fig. 1-2   A-F, Embryogenesis of the palate from 6½ to 10 weeks of gestation. (From Langman J: Medical embryology; human development, normal and abnormal, ed 2, Baltimore, 1969, Williams and Wilkins.)

(external nares). The new, more dorsal openings into the stomodeal cavity are called the *posterior nares,* or *primitive choanae.* The paired nostrils and primitive choanae gradually become separated by the developing nasal septum. By the middle of the second month of gestation, the secondary palate subdivides the more rostral portion of the original stomodeal chamber into separate nasal and oral cavities. The palatal shelves elongate the nasal cavities, so that the new posterior openings—the *secondary,* or *permanent, choanae*—now are located at the junction of the nasal cavity and nasopharynx.

The fusion of the palatal processes of the maxillary swellings with the septum occurs along the anterior or ventral three quarters of the nasal septum by the ninth week. Thus the left and right nasal chambers become separated about the same time as the nasal chambers separate from the oral cavity. Posteriorly or dorsally, the palatal shelves fail to fuse with the nasal septum and instead form the *soft palate.*[5-9] Development of the nasal cavity is complete by the second month of fetal life. From the second to sixth month of prenatal life, the nostrils are closed by epithelial plugs that then recannalize to reestablish a patent nasal cavity.[5]

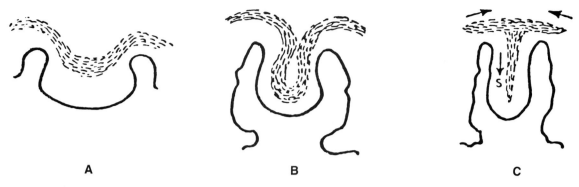

Fig. 1-3 Embryogenesis of nasal septum. Diagramatic representation of coronal section of the frontonasal process above the stomodeum (proposed theory). **A,** Early embryo. Dashed lines represent cartilage. **B,** Folding of frontonasal process narrows its transverse dimension and begins formation of the nasal septum. **C,** Continued medial migration further reduces the transverse dimension and merges the originally bilaminar folded cartilage to a single layer.

The exact origin and development of the nasal septum are poorly understood. It is known that the septum is originally thicker and then narrows progressively. The septum may arise by fusion of the mesenchymal cores of the nasomedial and frontal processes to form the frontonasal processes. The core would then gradually thin out, atrophy, and disappear. Badrawy, however, suggests that the narrowing of the frontonasal process could arise by an inward folding of the cartilage of the nasofrontal prominence (Fig. 1-3). This action would simultaneously cause approximation of the sides of the nose, deepening of the nasal fossae, and creation of the intervening septum.[10]

At the sixth fetal week, the nasal capsule consists of one continuum of hyaline cartilage. The lower part of the nasal capsule ossifies in membrane from various centers outside the perichondrium. The membranous bone of the vomer is ossified at birth.[11] The upper part of the nasal capsule, like the neighboring base of the cranium, ossifies in cartilage. At birth the ethmoidal plate is still cartilage; it commences to ossify postnatally *(vide infra)*. The anterior portion of the cartilaginous nasal septum is never enclosed by bone. The hyaline cartilage grows and persists as the cartilaginous part of the septum and the cartilage of the external nose. More posteriorly, the original cartilage of the septum remains sandwiched for a time between two laminae of membranous bone before it finally atrophies and disappears.[11] Processes develop along the lateral nasal walls, which eventually give rise to the turbinates.

During the fifth and sixth weeks of gestation, the earliest evidence of the cranium is found when several dense mesenchymal masses migrate to regions that correspond to the primitive ethmoid, auditory, nasal, and optic centers. The first evidence of intracartilaginous skull formation arises in the basisphenoid, basiocciput, and around the auditory vesicles. The developing brain is enveloped by a membranous cranium. The primitive cranial foramina remain when the developing cranial membrane grows around the cranial nerves. At this time, the sides and roof of the calvarium are a connective tissue capsule in which membranous bones are destined to appear.[6,12-14]

At about the second fetal month, fusion of the mesenchymous elements occurs, followed by cartilage formation. This action results in the formation of the primitive base of the cranium. Cartilage also forms around the auditory and olfactory primary centers. Initially, these cartilage centers are widely separated from that of the primitive base of the cranium. However, by the day 45 of gestation, the auditory capsule has fused with the basal cartilage. Concurrently, a broad, thin cartilage plate grows anteriorly from the lateral aspects of the occipital cartilage around the lower portion of the brain to form the early foramen magnum.[12,13]

The entire fused cartilaginous area is called the *chondrocranium*. Within it, various ossification centers appear, and from them, the chondrocranium is almost entirely converted into bone. The chondrocranium is continuous with the remaining cranial vault; consequently, some of the skull bones are of both cartilaginous and intramembranous origin. The bones of the cranial vault, face, and vomer are entirely of intramembranous origin with ossification occurring directly in the membrane; more specifically, they are the parietal, frontal, nasal, lacrimal, zygomatic, vomer, inferior concha, maxilla, and palatal bones. Bones formed chiefly in cartilage, but partly in membrane, are the occipital, sphenoid, and temporal bones. The ethmoid bone is the only craniofacial bone to be entirely of cartilaginous origin.[6,12-14]

Eye

During the fourth week of gestation, the optic vesicle begins to invaginate to form the optic cup. This invagination extends along the inferolateral border of the optic cup and the optic stalk to form the fetal choroidal fissure. The lips of the fissure begin to close together during the sixth week but then do fuse together, obliterating the choroidal fissure by the end of the seventh week.[15] The fissure begins to close near the equator of the future globe and continues to close in two directions, both proximally and distally. The anterior end of the optic cup forms the pupil. Defective closure of the anterior end of the ocular choroidal fissure bordering the pupil produces colobomas of the iris (and, perhaps, adjacent choroid). Defective closure of the midportion of the fissure produces colobomas of the choroid. Defective closure of the fissure where the cup joins the optic stalk (future optic nerve) produces papillary and peripapillary colobomas and pits of the optic disc.[2,15-18] Large papillary colobomas are associated with microphthalmos.

During the fifth week of gestation, mesenchyme invades the then-open choroidal fissure and contributes to the formation of the hyaloid vasculature, which nourishes the developing eye. The developing hyaloid artery enters the choroidal fissure along the optic stalk and then becomes enclosed within the globe and the optic nerve as the choroidal fissure closes. The hyaloid artery grows anteriorly to reach the posterior surface of the developing lens where it ramifies on its posterior surface. Glial cells derived from Bergmeister's papilla proliferate to form the sheath of the hyaloid artery. This artery and sheath later undergo regression. By term, the portion of the hyaloid artery within the globe has atrophied almost completely. The residual anteriormost segment forms a characteristic, clinically insignificant opacity on the posterior surface of the lens: the Mittendorf dot. The residual portion of the hyaloid artery within the optic nerve forms the central artery of the retina. Atrophy of Bergmeister's papilla forms the physiologic optic cup. Incomplete regression of the hyaloid vessels and their sheath may be associated with remnant vessels in the persistent primary vitreous of the posterior chamber and with proliferation of fibroglial tissue just anterior to the papilla. Excess regression of the artery and sheath may produce a deepened physiologic cup; this process has been proposed as another mechanism for the development of papillary colobomas.[2,15-19] The diverse anomalies of the papilla discussed here may be designated generically as optic nerve dysplasia.

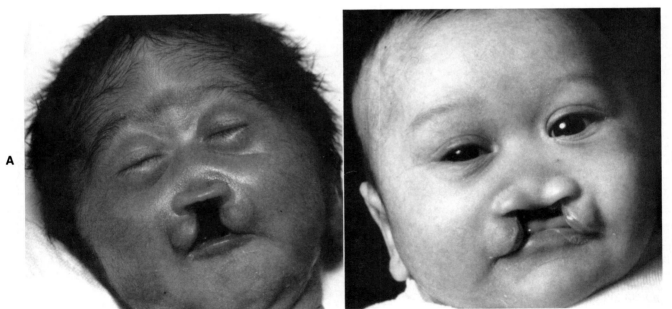

Fig. 1-4   Absence of intermaxillary segment with hypotelorism in two patients. **A,** Severe holoprosencephaly. **B,** Holoprosencephaly not detectable by axial computed tomography. In each case, the maxillary processes formed normal lateral thirds of the upper lips. Midline rectangular defects indicate the site of deficient intermaxillary segment with absent prolabium, incisors and primary palate. There was consequent cleft of secondary palate.

Corpus Callosum

The nature and sequences of events leading to the formation of the corpus callosum are poorly understood. It is widely accepted, however, that the corpus callosum forms by a series of stages during the period from 3 weeks of gestation (closure of the anterior neuropore) to approximately 8 weeks of gestation. The anterior commissure may be recognized at about 7 to 8 weeks, the hippocampal commissure slightly thereafter, and the earliest definite corpus callosal fibers by the tenth week of gestation. The genu and splenium are recognizable by 20 weeks of gestation and have adult shape (not size) by 22 weeks. More detailed discussions of the corpus callosum and septum pellucidum are offered elsewhere.[20,21]

COMMON FACIAL CLEFTS

Failure of the proper development of the frontonasal process and/or failure of its merging with adjacent processes results in a coherent series of malformations. Thus, insufficiency of the frontonasal process may result in absence of the intermaxillary segment with a roughly rectangular defect in the middle one third of the upper lip, absence of the incisors, absence of the primary palate with a cleft in the secondary palate, and hypotelorism. The resultant facies is one common manifestation of holoprosencephaly (Fig. 1-4).

Failure of the nasomedial processes to merge with the maxillary processes on one or both sides produces the typical unilateral or bilateral *common (lateral) cleft lip* (Figs. 1-5 and 1-6). Posterior extension of the cleft between the primary and secondary palates and then further backward between the left and right halves of the secondary palate produces the typical unilateral or bilateral *common (lateral) cleft palate*. Because the two processes fail to merge, they may grow discordantly resulting in malposition of the premaxillary segment. Widened nostril, depressed ala nasi, and anomalous nasal septum commonly concur.

Failure to merge the nasolateral process with the maxillary process results in an oblique cleft extending from the inner canthus to the nose. This cleft may occur in association with bilateral common cleft lip and palate (Fig. 1-7).

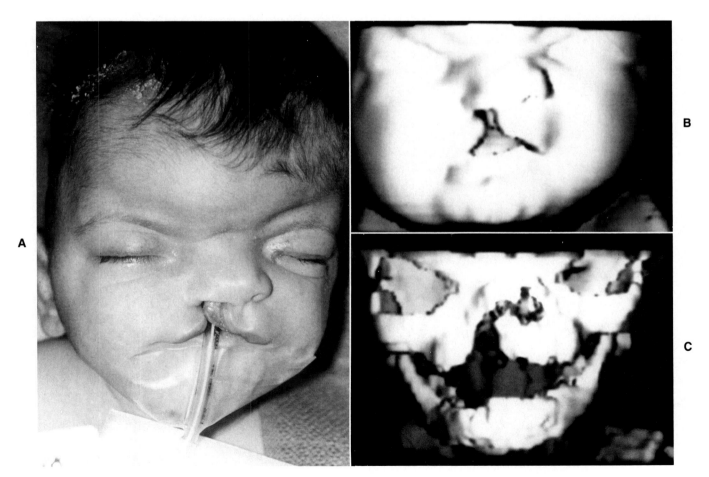

Fig. 1-5   Unilateral common cleft lip and palate in 4-day-old girl. **A,** Facies. **B,** Skin surface 3DCT **C,** Bone surface 3DCT.   *Continued.*

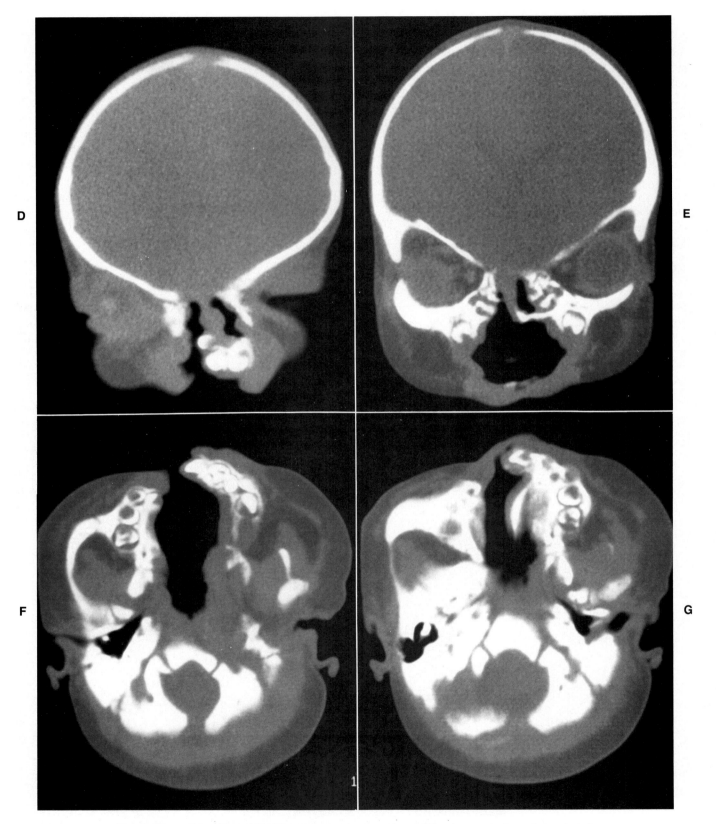

Fig. 1-5, cont'd   **D** and **E,** Direct coronal noncontrast CTs demonstrate unilateral cleft lip and palate with attachment of the nasal septum toward the contralateral palatal shelf. **F** and **G,** Axial noncontast CT. There is discordant growth of the two maxillae, union of one palatal shelf to the bony septum and deviation of the septum to the intact side.

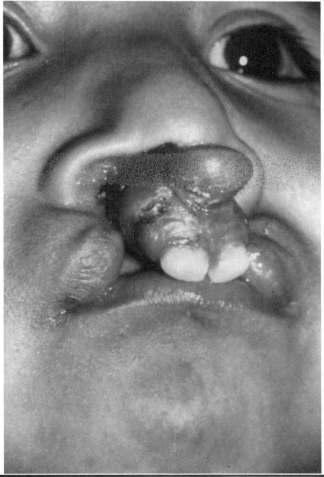

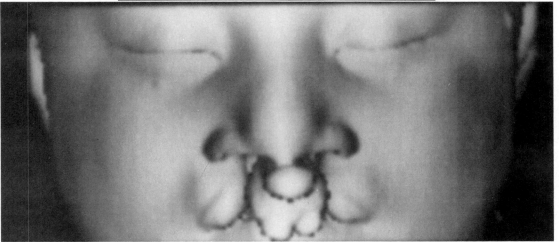

Fig. 1-6   Bilateral common cleft lip and cleft palate with discordant growth of the inter-maxillary segment in 4-year-old boy. **A,** Patient facies. Skin surface 3DCT in **B,** frontal and **C,** lateral views. Bone surface 3-dimensional CT in **D,** oblique and **E,** lateral views. Normal canthi, alae nasi, and lateral thirds of the lip and jaw indicate normal formation and merging of the maxillary and nasolateral processes. The abortive prolabium, central incisors, and central third of the superior alveolar ridge are supported on the vomer, well anterior to expected position, because failure to merge led to discordant growth of the maxillary and intermaxillary segments.   *Continued.*

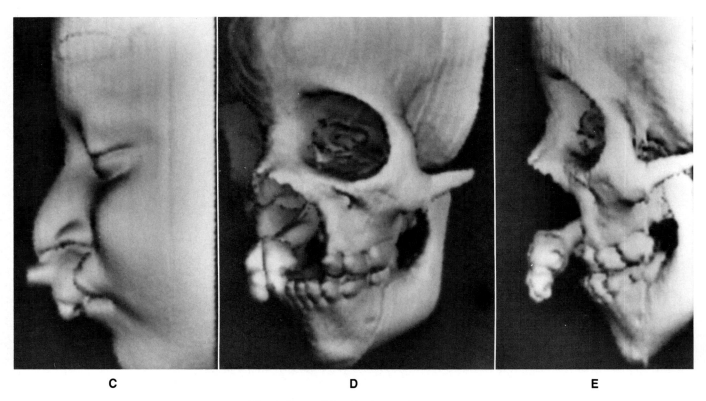

C   D   E

Fig. 1-6, cont'd   For legend see p. 9.

Failure to merge the maxillary with the mandibular process, unilaterally or bilaterally, results in a transverse facial cleft, also designated as Wolf mouth or macrostomia (Fig. 1-8).

Failure of the two nasomedial processes to merge in the midline produces the rarer *true midline cleft lip.* Posterior extension of this cleft may result in a cleft superior alveolar ridge, diastasis of the medial incisors, double frenulum of the upper lip, and a cleft primary palate. Such a cleft palate may continue posteriorly as a midline cleft of the secondary palate or uvula (see following discussion of midline cleft lip).

In some patients, bands of amnion constrict the amniotic cavity. They mold the developing embryo, sometimes pressing deeply into tissue to amputate digits or produce long linear scars that may contain amnion at birth. Such bands can lead to nonanatomic facial clefts and encephaloceles (Fig. 1-9).

MIDLINE CLEFT LIP AND MEDIAN CLEFT FACE SYNDROME

The diverse midline craniofacial dysraphisms fall naturally into two groups: an inferior group (A), in which the clefting primarily involves the upper lip (with or without the nose), and a superior group (B), in which the clefting primarily affects the nose (with or without the forehead and upper lip). Group A is associated with basal encephaloceles, i.e., sphenoidal, sphenoethmoidal, and ethmoidal encephaloceles; with callosal agenesis (rarely lipoma) and with optic nerve dysplasias such as optic pits, colobomata, megalopapilla, persistent hyperplastic primary vitreous with hyaloid artery and morning glory syndrome. Group B consists of those patients with the median cleft face syndrome. This group is characterized by hypertelorism, a broad nasal root, and a median cleft nose, (with or without median cleft upper lip, median cleft premaxilla, and cranium bifidum occultum frontalis).[22,23] Group B patients manifest an increased incidence of frontonasal and intraorbital encephaloceles, anophthalmos/microphthalmos and callosal lipomas (less frequently, callosal agenesis). Group B has only a weak association with basal encephaloceles or with optic nerve dysplasia.

Group A (Inferior Group)

True clefting of the *upper* lip is typically associated with *hyper*telorism and is a clear stigma of the likely concurrence of basal encephalocele, callosal agenesis or lipoma, and any of the diverse forms of optic nerve dysplasia (Fig. 1-10). The labial defect observed varies from a small notch, to a vertical linear cleft, to a small triangular deficiency of the midline upper lip vermillion

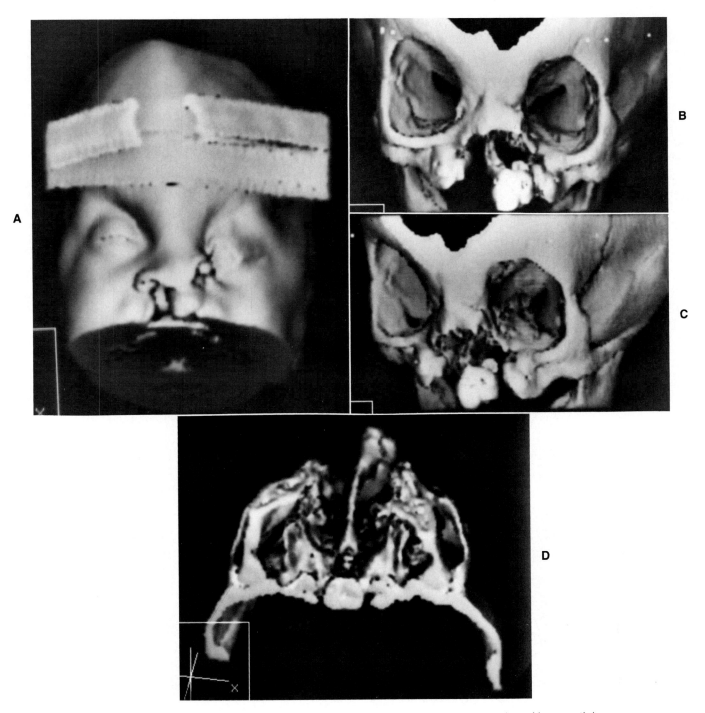

Fig. 1-7   Substantially asymmetrical bilateral common cleft lip and palate. Note partial clefting along the nasooptic furrow. **A,** 3-dimensional CT of air-soft tissue surface displays the wide right cleft lip, the incomplete merging of the left lip and distortion of the prolabium, the nostrils and the alae nasi. The left orbit is asymmetrically lower than the right with lower palpebral fissure. **B-D,** 3-dimensional CTs of the bone surface show the wide cleft of the superior alveolar ridge on the right, substantial deviation of the vomer and the central incisors to the left, narrow left cleft superior alveolar ridge seen best in oblique view **(C)** and deficiency in the orbital floor anteromedially.

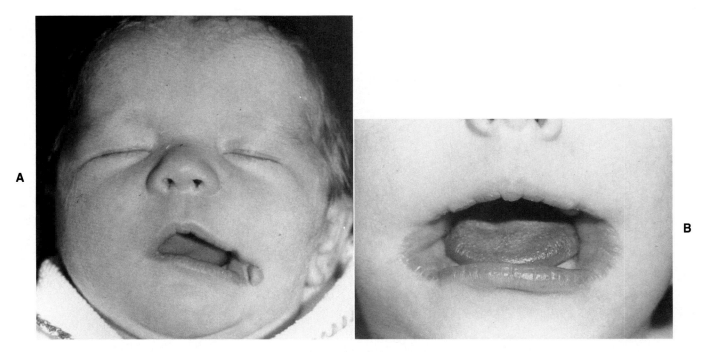

Fig. 1-8 Transverse facial cleft and macrostomia as shown in patient facies. **A,** Unilateral, infant girl. **B,** Bilateral, 8-month-old boy with callosal agenesis and bilateral cortical blindness. (Reprinted from Bauer BS, Wilkes GH, and Kernahan DA: Incorporation of the W-plasty in repair of macrostomia, Plast Reconstr Surg, 31:507, 1963.

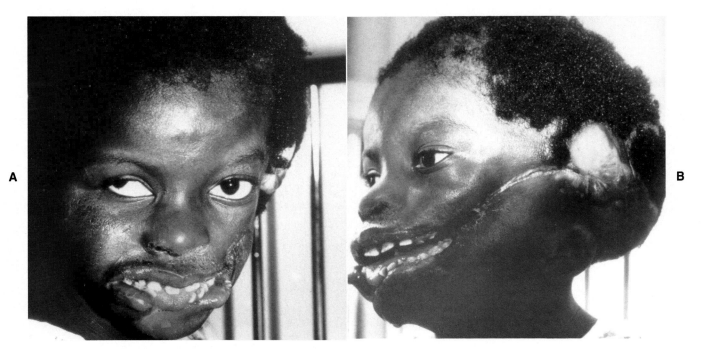

Fig. 1-9 Non-anatomic clefts occurring with syndrome of amnionic bands in 12-year-old mentally retarded girl. **A** and **B,** Patient facies. A long thin band-like scar extends across the scalp and face from the temporoparietal region through cheek and corner of mouth to lower lip. The large posterior zone of atrophic skin and absent hair is associated with a bulge that displaces the ear inferiorly. This is the site of a temporoparietal encephalocele. On CT the alveolar ridge showed notching and separation of teeth where it was crossed by the band.

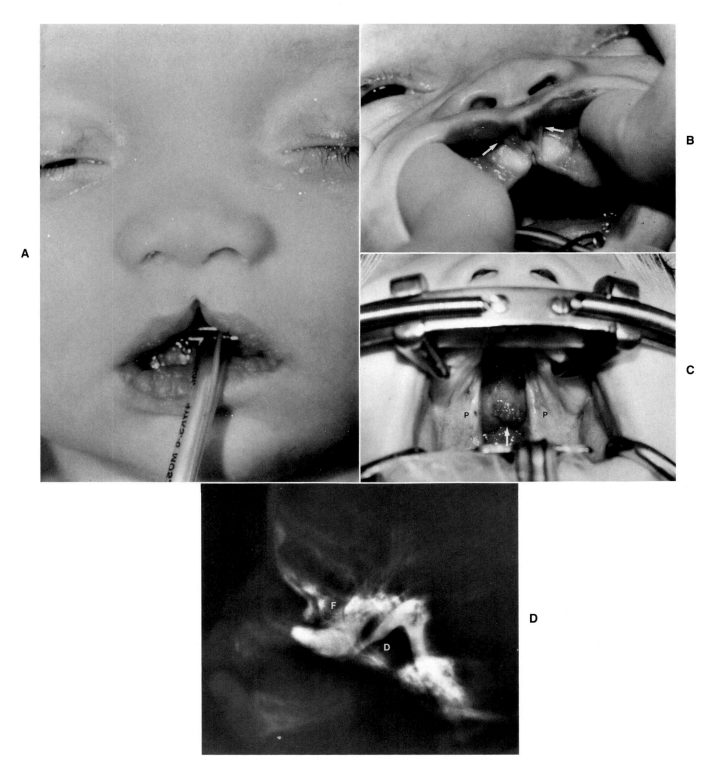

Fig. 1-10   True midline cleft lip and palate with hypertelorism and callosal agenesis. Patient facies. **A,** Incomplete cleft of upper lip vermillion and philtrum, hypertelorism, and normal nose. **B,** Diastasis of the incisors and cleft superior alveolar ridge with double frenula *(arrows)*, one frenulum to each half ridge. **C,** Cleft secondary palate with wide separation of the palatal shelves *(P,P,)* exposing to view inferior surface of a large transsphenoidal encephalocele *(arrow)*. This protruded below the cleft palate into the oral cavity when the patient cried. **D,** Left lateral exposure of a positive contrast cisternogram/ventriculogram displaying the characteristic "boot-of-Italy" shape of transsphenoidal encephaloceles and their characteristic position immediately anterior to the dorsum sellae *(D)*. The sac is the third ventricle, its containing wall of hypothalamus, pituitary stalk and pituitary gland and the associated "suprasellar" cisterns. Frontal lobe *(F)* protrudes into the large defect anteriorly.

Table 1-1 Anomalies associated with 30 basal encephaloceles*

Anomaly	Manifestation	Number	%
Encephalocele site†	Sphenoidal	18	60.0
	Sphenoethmoidal	10	33.3
	Ethmoidal	2	0.7
	Hypothalamus, third ventricle and/or pituitary in cephalocele	15	50.0
Endocrine dysfunction	Hypothalmic/pituitary	6	20.0
	Diabetes insipidus with normal anterior pituitary	1	0.3
Corpus callosum	Agenesis	12(+1?)	40.0(43.0?)
Facial anomalies	Median cleft lip but not nose	15	50.0
	Median cleft lip plus median cleft nose	4	13.3
	"Fissure lip"‡[89]	1	0.3
	"Harelip"‡[102]	1	0.3
	Cleft palate‡ (of any type)	14	47.0
Eye anomalies	Hypertelorism	22	73.0
	Optic nerve dysplasia§	12	40.0
	Persistent fetal ocular vasculature	1	0.3
	Microphthalmos	2	0.7
Other pathology	Absent optic chiasm	1	0.3
	Absent chiasm and tracts	1	0.3
	Polymicrogyria	1	0.3
	Preauricular skin tags	1	0.3
	Hypospadias, chordee, lumbar dimple plus hemangioma	1	0.3

*Includes data from references 22(patient 13), 28, 29(case 1), 30, 31(case 3), 32, 33(cases 1 and 2), 34, 35(cases 1 and 2), 36(case 7), 37, 38, 39, 40, 41, 42, 43, 44, 45(cases 1-5), 46, 47, 48, 49. Series with no contributory data on eye or on facial changes excluded (32, 44).
†In many cases, this is the best guess from the limited data available.
‡In these cases, the exact nature of the cleft is uncertain.
§Any of the spectrum: optic pit, optic coloboma, megalopapilla, morning glory disc.

(with or without the philtrum) with absence of the labial tubercle. This defect is designated *true midline cleft upper lip*. Rarely this defect may also occur as an isolated finding or as part of the orofacial digital syndromes I and II.[24,25]

Median cleft lip is a rare anomaly. In Fogh-Andersen's[26] series of 3988 craniofacial clefts collected over 30 years, median clefts of the upper lip were observed in only 15 cases (0.38%). Five (0.13%) were true median cleft lips (as considered here); three more (0.08%) were true median cleft lips occurring as part of the orofacial digital syndrome, and seven (0.17%) were pseudomedian cleft lips. An additional four cases (0.10%) were cases of median cleft nose.

Basal encephaloceles are also rare anomalies, estimated to constitute 1.2% of all encephaloceles (Fig. 1-11).[27] Table 1-1 summarizes the findings in a total of 30 cases collected from the literature and personal material. In this series, 50% manifested midline cleft lip (but not nose), an additional 13% manifested midline cleft lip plus nose, 40% to 43% manifested callosal agenesis, and 40% manifested optic nerve dysplasia (i.e., any of the spectrum of optic pit, optic/perioptic coloboma, morning glory disc and/or megalopapilla). Since the reports are incomplete in many cases, the true concurrence of these anomalies is likely to be even higher.

To date, no report details the true incidence of encephalocele, callosal agenesis, and facial clefting in patients with optic nerve dysplasias[50-53]; however, Beyer et al[54] found one sphenoidal encephalocele in eight patients with ten morning glory discs, a single series incidence of 10% to 15%.

Lipoma of the corpus callosum is observed in approximately 0.06% of all patients in both in vivo and necropsy studies.[51] Agenesis of the corpus callosum is present in 35% to 50% of such cases.[55] Lipoma may be

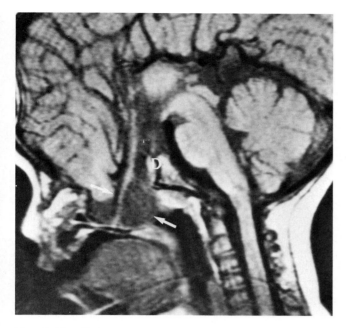

Fig. 1-11 Sphenoethmoidal encephalocele with callosal agenesis in 4-year-old boy. Midline sagittal T₁-weighted spin echo magne tic resonance image (TR/TE = 600/25) discloses absence of the corpus callosum, dehiscence in the skull base immediately anterior to the dorsum sellae *(D)* extending into the ethmoid bone, and downward herniation of the third ventricle *(arrows)* and its walls. (Courtesy of Robert A Zimmerman, MD, Philadelphia.)

associated with midline subcutaneous lipomas, with cranium bifidum, and with frontonasal encephaloceles.[22,56,57]

Group B (Superior Group)

Median cleft face syndrome (also called *frontonasal dysplasia*) is a rare form of dysraphism that affects the midface (Fig. 1-12). The characteristic physical findings in median cleft face syndrome include hypertelorism, cranium bifidum occultum frontalis, widow's peak hairline, and midline clefting of the nose (may involve upper lip, premaxilla, and palate).[22,23,58-60] There may also be common clefts of the upper lip and palate, primary telecanthus, ocular colobomas, microphthalmia, and notching of the alae nasae. Hypertelorism is present in all cases of median cleft face syndrome and is the one obligatory finding.[23] The next most constant finding is true midline bony clefting of the nose. The other facial deformities may be present, or not, in varying degree.

The types of facial clefting seen in this syndrome have been classified differently by different authors.[22,23,60] DeMyer classified the median cleft face syndrome into

Table 1-2 DeMyer classification

Facies	Characteristics
I	Hypertelorism
	Median complete cleft nose
	Absence, hypoplasia, or median clefting of upper lip and premaxilla
	Cranium bifidum
II	Hypertelorism
	Median cleft nose
	A. Nose completely cleft
	B. Cleft nose with divided nasal septum
	C. Slight hypertelorism
	No median cleft of upper lip, premaxilla or palate
	Cranium bifidum present or not
III	Hypertelorism
	Median cleft nose and upper lip with or without median cleft premaxilla
	No median cleft palate
	No cranium bifidum
IV	Hypertelorism
	Median cleft nose
	No median cleft of upper lip, premaxilla or palate
	No cranium bifidum

From DeMyer W: Neurology 17:961, 1967.

Table 1-3 Sedano classification*

Facies	Characteristics
A	Hypertelorism
	Broad nasal root
	Median nasal groove with absence of nasal tip
	No true clefting of the facial midline
	Anterior cranium bifidum present or not
B	Hypertelorism
	Broad nasal root
	Deep median facial groove or true cleft of the nose or nose plus the upper lip
	Cleft palate present or not
	Anterior cranium bifidum present or not
C	Hypertelorism
	Broad nasal root
	Nasal alar notching (unilateral or bilateral)
	Anterior cranium bifidum present or not
D	B + C

From Sedano HO et al: J Pediatr 76:906, 1970.
*Anterior cranium bifidum may be present or not in all four facies, A through D.

four classic facies that represent the most frequently encountered combinations of the major and minor defects (Table 1-2).[1] Sedano[23] proposed an alternate classification of median cleft face syndrome (Table 1-3). These systems differ, in part, in the importance attributed to notching of the alae nasae. In our opinion, the Sedano classification appears to correlate best with the intracranial pathology and is the most useful system (Table 1-4). Tessier proposed another system for classi-

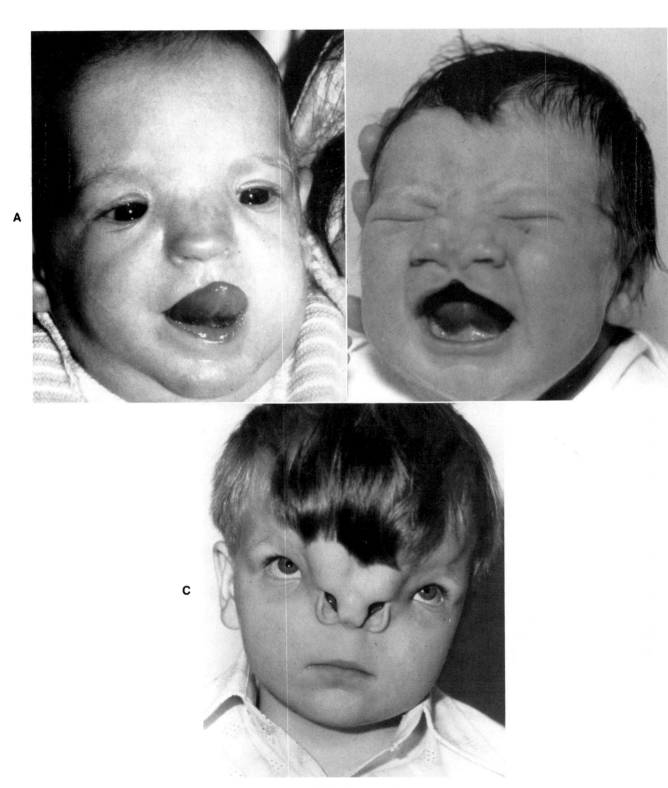

Fig. 1-12 Median Cleft Face Syndrome: Typical Facies. **A,** Sedano Facies Type A in 3-month-old boy. **B,** Sedano Facies Type B in 4-day-old boy. **C,** Sedano Facies Type D in 3½-year-old boy. (From Naidich TP et al: J Comput Assist Tomogr 12:57, 1988.)

Table 1-4 Correlation of Sedano and DeMyer classifications

Sedano classification	Corresponding DeMyer classification (per Sedano[23])	Corresponding DeMyer classification (observed in this series)
Type A	IV	IIB, IV
Type B	IA,* IIB, III	I, IIA, IIB
Type C	IIC	—
Type D	IA,* IB, IIA	I, IIA, IIC

*Patients who would be classified into DeMyer's Group IA may be classified as either Sedano facies type B or Sedano facies type D.[23]

fying the craniofacial skeletal clefts and their associated soft tissue counterparts.[60] In his system the clefts most frequently associated with the median cleft face syndrome are found along the Tessier number 0 to 14 and 1 to 13 meridians. Some patients with median cleft face syndrome appear to have a furrowing of their nose rather than a "clefting." Such cases support Badrawy's theory that the nasal septum forms as a folding of the frontonasal process with subsequent resorption and thinning, since improper folding and resorption could lead to the facies observed.

Nearly all cases of median cleft face syndrome occur sporadically with no evidence for a genetic basis.[3] Only a few familial cases have been reported.[22,58,61,62] An unexpectedly high 12% to 18% of patients with median cleft face syndrome are the products of twin gestation,[22,58,61] but the other twin is usually normal.

Focal neurologic deficits are not reported with median cleft face syndrome[22,23,61,63-71] and do not appear to form a part of the disease. These patients have variable intellectual development. Patient IQ does not appear to be related to the severity of facial clefting.

Median cleft face syndrome has been found to coexist with a variety of other syndromes or syndrome-like sequences, including the Goldenhar-Gorlin syndrome (oculoauricular-vertebral dysplasia), characterized by hypoplasia of the soft tissue and bony structures of the face resulting in (1) ocular anomalies such as upper lid colobomas, epibulbar dermoids and lipomas, microphthalmia, and anophthalmia; (2) auricular anomalies such as deformity, hypoplasia, or aplasia of the external ear, preauricular skin tags and preauricular sinuses; and (3) vertebral anomalies such as block vertebra, hemivertebra, spina bifida, and associated rib anomalies (Fig. 1-13).[72-74]

In one review of 11 cases of median cleft face syndrome, there were 3 type A facies, 4 type B, 4 type D, and no type C. Hypertelorism and broad nasal root were found in 100% (by definition), true midline bony cleft of the nose in 8 of 11 (all cases except type A facies), median cleft upper lip in 3 of 11, common cleft

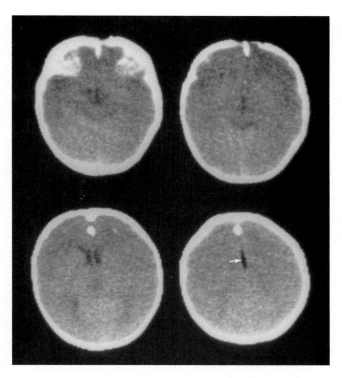

Fig. 1-13 Median cleft face syndrome with concurrent Goldenhar syndrome. Noncontrast axial CT sections demonstrate bilateral paramedian cranium bifidum, calcified falx, and midline interhemispheric lipoma *(white arrow)*. (From Naidich TP et al: J Comput Assist Tomogr 12:57, 1988.)

lip in 3 of 11, common cleft palate in 3 of 11, cranium bifidum in 6 of 11, calcified falx in 6 of 11, interhemispheric lipoma in 5 of 11, Goldenhar-Gorlin-syndrome in 2 of 11 and twinning in 2 of 11 patients.[58]

The imaging features of median cleft face syndrome include hypertelorism, cranium bifidum, facial clefting, and intracranial calcifications, related to either interhemispheric lipoma and/or calcification of the anterior aspect of the falx (Fig. 1-14).[59,75] The calcification of the falx produces a thick frontal crest. The crest is found most commonly when a lipoma is present but may be present without associated lipoma.[59]

NORMAL DEVELOPMENT OF THE NASAL SEPTUM AND FRONTONASAL JUNCTION

The normal nasal septum and skull base form in a predictable fashion. Knowledge of this pattern is necessary for interpreting imaging studies of this region without serious error. In brief, the cartilage of the nasal capsule is the foundation of the upper part of the face (Figs. 1-15 and 1-16).[76] The bony elements of the facial skeleton appear around it and replace it, in part (Figs. 1-17 and 1-18). The lateral masses of the ethmoid form by enchondral ossification of the nasal capsule. The frontal processes of the maxillary bones, premaxillary bone, nasal bones, lacrimal bones, and palatine bones all form in membrane in close relationship with the roof and lateral walls of the cartilaginous nasal capsule.[76] The vomer develops in membrane in relation to the perichondrium of the septal process.[76] Eventually, nearly all the nasal capsule becomes ossified or atrophied. All that remains of the cartilage of the nasal capsule in adults is the anterior part of the nasal septum and the alar cartilages that surround the nostrils.

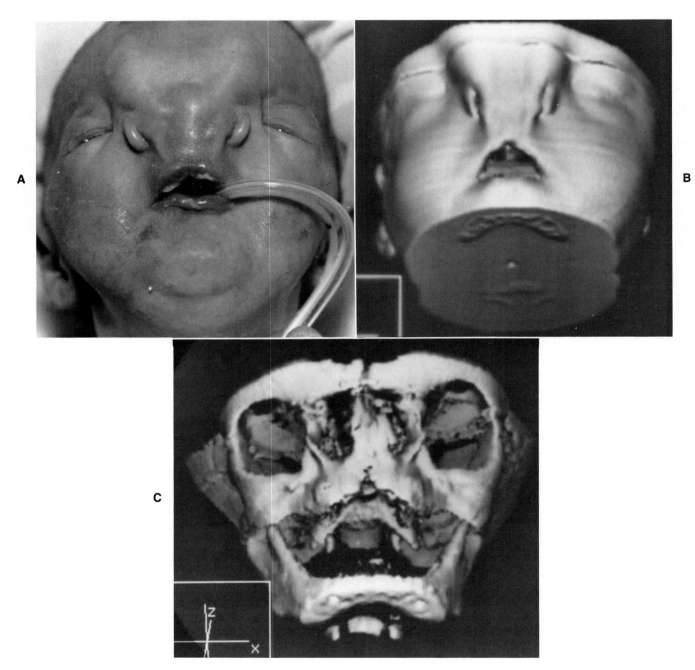

Fig. 1-14 Median cleft face syndrome with nasal dermal sinus and interhemispheric lipoma in 3½-month-old girl. **A,** Sedano Facies Type D with a midline notch in the upper lip and a tiny midline ostium from the nasal dermal sinus. **B,** 3-dimensional CT of the skin surface and **C,** the facial skeleton emphasize the hypertelorism, the median notching in the upper lip and superior alveolar ridge, the thick bony midline and the lateral position of the nasal passages. (From Naidich TP et al: J Comput Assist Tomogr 12:57, 1988.)

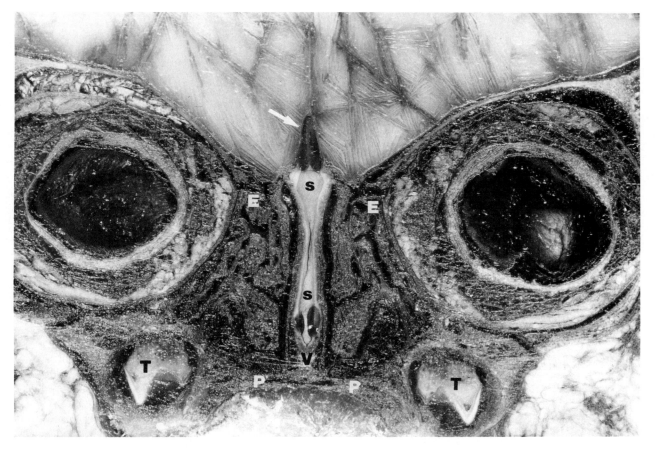

Fig. 1-15 Coronal cryomicrotome section through the nasal cavity of a full term stillborn at the level of the optic globes. The lateral ethmoid centers *(E, E)*, the midline vomer *(V)*, and the palatal shelves *(P, P)* of the maxillae are well ossified. The unossified septal cartilage *(S)* slots into the vomerine groove in the upper surface of the Y-shaped vomer. The crista galli *(arrow)* is beginning to ossify forming a pointed "cap". The cribriform plates have not ossified. Note the normal position of the floor of the anterior fossa with respect to the two orbits and optic globes. *T*, Unerupted teeth.

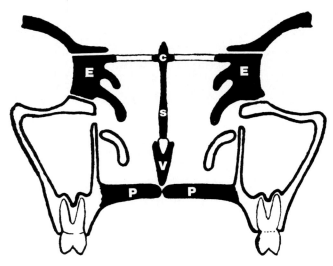

Fig. 1-16 Diagrammatic representation of the pattern of ossification around the nasal cavity. The ossified crista *(C)* and septal cartilage *(S)* form a "cristal" cross that is isolated from the lateral ethmoid centers *(E)* by the unossified cribriform plates and from the vomer *(V)* by the sphenoidal tail. Although the maxillae are ossified, only the palatal shelves *(P)* have been inked in to emphasize their relationships to the vomer. (Modified from Scott JH: Br Dent J 95:37, 1953.)

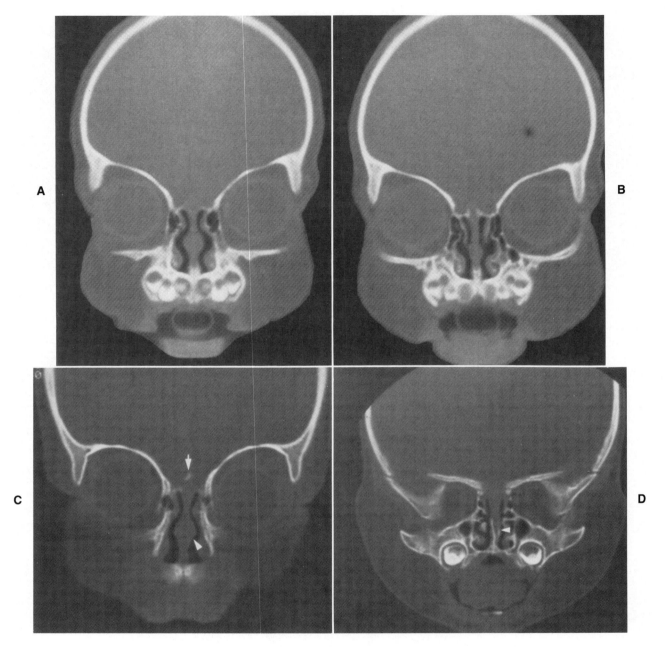

Fig. 1-17   Normal patterns of ossification of the nasal capsule as shown by direct coronal CTs in progressively older patients. **A** and **B,** 4-month old girl. The lateral ethmoid centers and a small segment of vomer are ossified. The midline septal cartilage is entirely unossified. **C** and **D,** 5-month-old boy. The lateral ethmoid centers, the palatal shelves, the vomer, and the tip *(white arrow)* of the crista galli are ossified. The widened midportion of the septum *(white arrowhead in **C**)* is designated the septal diamond. The two sides of the vomerine groove give the posterior septum a "bilaminar" appearance *(white arrowhead in **D**).* **E,** 8-month-old boy. Anteriorly, the crista galli is *in*completely ossified forming a hollow cap. **F,** Further posteriorly the crista and the cribriform plates have ossified together, roofing over the nasal cavity. The perpendicular plate of ethmoid is beginning to ossify as a bilaminar plate. The Y-shaped vomer is larger. **G,** 9-month-old girl. The ossified perpendicular plate has enlarged and extended inferiorly toward the septal diamond. The ossified crista resembles a hollow diamond. In both **H,** a 12-year-old girl, and **I,** a 17-year old boy, the ossified perpendicular plate reaches the top of the septal diamond where it widens into a knob or it forks. **J,** 11-month-old boy. The nasal septum frequently buckles at the septal diamond.

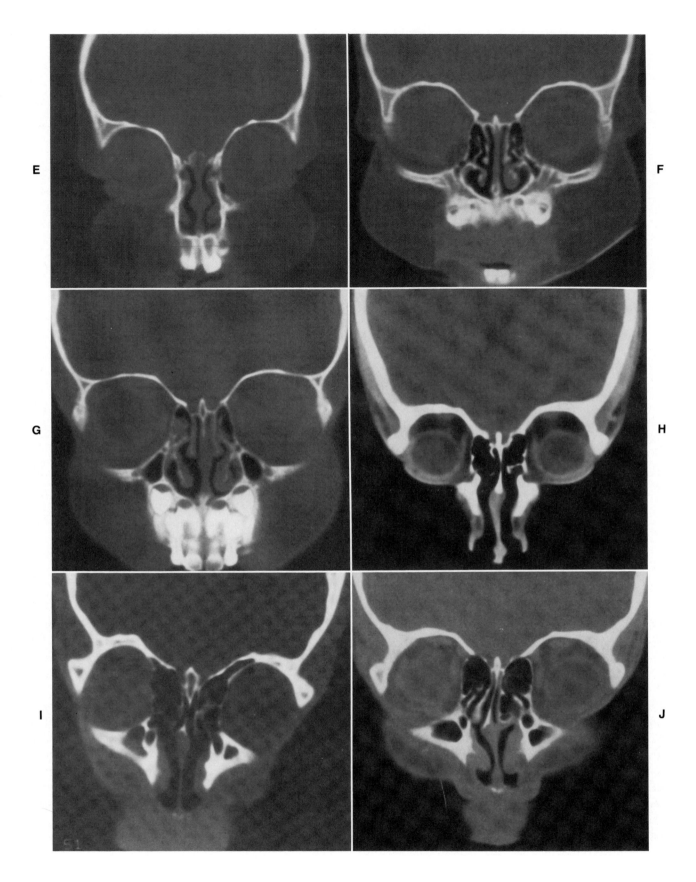

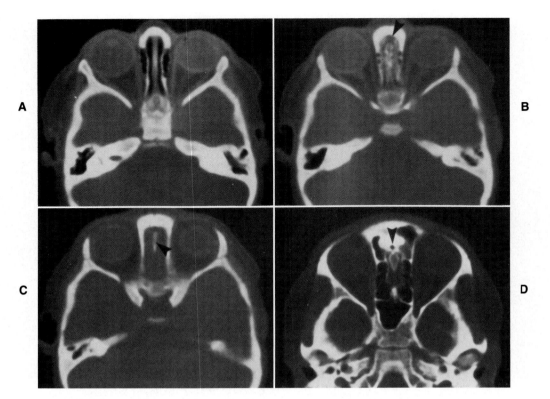

Fig. 1-18 Normal pattern of ossification as shown on axial noncontrast CTs. In the 11-month old girl shown in **A** through **C,** serial axial images display the following: **A,** The normal, thin nasal septum with faint parallel ossifications representing the vomer. **B,** The normal midline defect *(black arrowhead)* anterior to the normal, parallel ossification within the closing cribriform plates and crista. **C,** The upper portion of the crista *(arrowhead)* with a small fossa anterior to it. Comparing these images with the coronal sections in Fig. 1-19 aids understanding of the way in which the parallel ossifications arise. **D,** 12-year-old boy. The foramen cecum *(black arrowhead)* is a well-defined ostium situated just anterior to the diamond shaped ossified crista galli.

More specifically, the midline septal cartilage is directly continuous with the cartilaginous skull base. At birth, the skull base has three major ossification centers: the *basioccipital* center, the *basisphenoid* center, and the *presphenoid* center. The septal cartilage has not yet ossified. The lateral masses of the ethmoid have ossified, forming paired paramedian bones, but the cribriform plate is still cartilaginous or fibrous.[76] At birth, therefore, the entire midline of the face may be a lucent stripe of cartilage situated between the paired ossifications in the lateral masses of the ethmoids. This lucent midline can simulate a midline cleft on imaging studies. The septal cartilage extends along the midline from the nares to the presphenoid bone.[76] Anteriorly and inferiorly the septal cartilage attaches to the premaxillary bone by fibrous tissue.[76] Posteriorly the septal cartilage is continuous with the cartilage of the cranial base. Inferiorly, the lower edge of the septal carti-

lage is slotted into a U- or V-shaped groove that runs along the entire upper edge of the vomer (Fig. 1-19 and see Fig. 1-16).[76] This groove is designated the *vomerine groove* and should not be mistaken for a midline cleft in the septum.

At about the time of birth or during the first year, a fourth, *mesethmoid* center appears in the septal cartilage anterior to the cranial base. This center will form the perpendicular plate of the ethmoid.[76] The residual portion of still-unossified septal cartilage that extends posterosuperiorly toward the cranial base between the perpendicular plate and the vomer is designated the *sphenoidal tail* of the septal cartilage.[76]

Initially, the ossifying perpendicular plate is separated from the rest of the facial skeleton by (1) the unossified cartilage or fibrous tissue of the cribriform plates and (2) the sphenoidal tail (see Figs. 1-15, 1-16, and 1-19). About the third to sixth year, the lateral

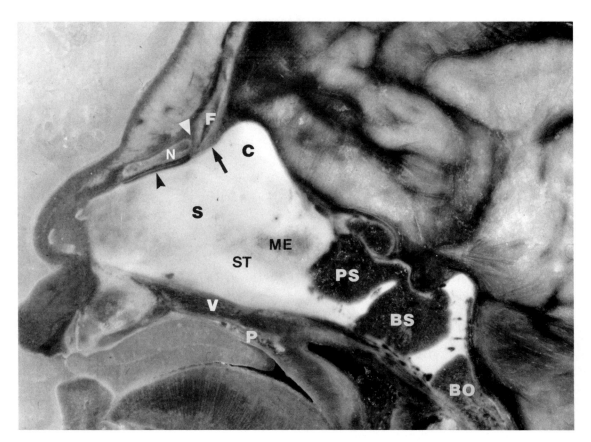

Fig. 1-19 Midsagittal cryomicrotome section of a full term newborn demonstrates the normal relationships, at birth, among the ossified frontal bone *(F)*; the ossified nasal bone *(N)*; the nasofrontal suture *(white arrowhead)*; and the cartilaginous nasal capsule *(large white structure)* that forms the yet unossified nasal septum *(S)* and crista galli *(C)*. The ossified hard palate *(P)* and ossified vomer *(V)* lie below the septal cartilage. Note the direct line from the prenasal space *(black arrowhead)* through the foramen cecum *(black arrow)* to the normal depression or "fossa" just anterior to the crista galli. The midline septal cartilage is directly continuous with the cartilaginous skull base. The basioccipital *(BO)*, the basisphenoidal *(BS)*, and the presphenoidal *(PS)* ossification centers are well formed. The mesethmoidal *(ME)* ossification center is just beginning to form. When the vomer and mesethmoid enlarge, the residual cartilage between them is designated the sphenoidal tail *(ST)*.

masses of the ethmoid and the perpendicular plate of the ethmoid become united across the roof of the nasal cavity by ossification of the cribriform plate.[76,77]

Somewhat later, the perpendicular plate unites with the vomer below.[76] As the two bones approach, the vomerine groove may become converted into a vomerine tunnel. It should not be mistaken for a bony canal around a dermal sinus or cephalocele.

Growth of the septal cartilage continues for a short period after craniofacial union is complete, which probably explains the common deflection of the nasal septum away from the midline.[76]

Because the appearance of the nasal septum varies with patient age, one must interpret computed tomog-

raphy (CT) "evidence" of midline defects and sinus tracts carefully. Review of the CT appearance of the midline anterior fossa and nasal septum in 100 children age 2 days to 18 years revealed the following normal patterns (see Figs. 1-17 and 1-18)[78]:

1. The lateral ethmoid centers were ossified in all subjects.
2. No midline ossifications of the anterior fossa or septum were present in 14% of patients less than 1 year of age.
3. The cribriform plate was not ossified in patients under 2 months of age. It could be ossified from 2 to 8 months of age. It was fused across the midline from 8 months onward. This ossification oc-

curred earlier than is stated in the literature.[76]

4. The tip of the crista could be ossified from 2 days onward. It was invariably ossified from 2½ years onward.

5. The crista plus the cribriform plate formed a $\wedge$-ossification with no ossification of the perpendicular plate in patients from 2 months to 5 months of age.

6. The ossified crista, cribriform plate, and perpendicular plate could form a bony "cristal cross" from 4 months onward. These ossifications invariably formed a cross from 11 months onward.

7. A zone of unossified tissue was seen within the crista in 60% of those with a cristal cross. Such ostia could be present at any age from 4 months onward.

8. The perpendicular plate of the ethmoid could be ossified as a single plate in patients aged 11 months to 18 years. It was ossified in the vast majority of patients older than 2 years.

9. The perpendicular plate ossified as 2 parallel laminae in 15% of patients.

10. The nasal septum was widest at the midpoint of its vertical dimension in nearly all subjects of all ages. This widening was designated the septal diamond.

11. The ossified perpendicular plate widened inferiorly or split to form an inverted Y at the septal diamond in 30% of patients, all older than 6 years.

12. The ossified perpendicular plate reached as far inferiorly as the septal diamond in 32% of all patients, 92% after age 6, and 100% after age 13.

13. The ossified vomer exhibited a V- or Y-shaped superior border in 80% of patients at any age. The vomerine ossification appeared as a single point anteriorly and a V or Y posteriorly in 21%. In 8%, it was seen only as a single point.

In a *normal* situation, then, one may expect to see no ossification in the midline of children under 1 year of age, an unossified zone within 60% of the cristal crosses, a "bilaminar" perpendicular plate of ethmoid in 15%, and a V- or Y-shaped upper surface of the vomer in at least 80% of patients (Figs. 1-17 and 1-18). These should not be overinterpreted as indications of pathologic condition.

In the early embryo, the developing frontal bones are separated from the developing nasal bones by a small fontanelle called the *fonticulus nasofrontalis*.[79] The nasal bones are separated from the subjacent cartilaginous nasal capsule by the prenasal space (Fig. 1-20). This space extends from the base of the brain to the nasal tip.[80] Midline diverticula of dura normally project *anteriorly* into the fonticulus nasofrontalis and *antero-inferiorly* into the prenasal space. These diverticula

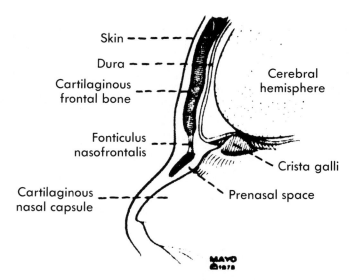

Fig. 1-20   Diagrammatic representation of the normal embryonic relationships among the dura, fonticulus nasofrontalis, prenasal space and surrounding structures. (From Gorenstein A et al: Arch Otolaryngol 106:536, 1980. Copyright © Mayo Clinic.)

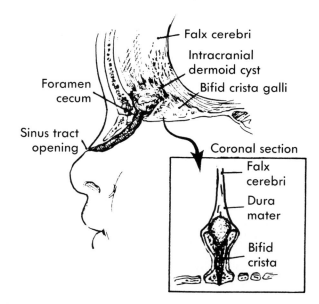

Fig. 1-21   Diagrammatic representation of a "typical" nasal dermal sinus and cyst traversing the prenasal space and the enlarged foramen cecum to form a mass anterior to and within a grooved, "bifid" crista galli. *Insert:* The anatomic relationships of the leaves of the falx to the sides of the crista galli direct upward extension of the mass into the *inter*dural space between the leaves of the falx. (From Gorenstein A et al: Arch Otolaryngol 106:536, 1980. Copyright © Mayo Clinic.)

may touch the ectoderm. Normally, the diverticula regress before the closure of the bone plates of the anterior skull base. The fonticulus nasofrontalis is closed by the nasal processes of the frontal bone to make the frontonasal suture.[79] The prenasal space becomes obliterated.[81] The cartilaginous nasal capsule develops into the upper lateral nasal cartilages[79] and the ethmoid bone, including the crista galli, cribriform plates, and perpendicular plate of the septum. The two leaves of the falx insert into the crista galli, one leaf passing to each side of the crista.

At the skull base, the frontal and ethmoid bones close together around a strand of dura, leaving a small ostium designated the foramen cecum. Normally this transmits a small vein. This foramen is easily seen at the bottom of a small depression that lies just in front of the crista galli. Whether the foramen is situated exactly at the fronto-ethmoidal junction or between the nasal processes of the frontal bones[79] is not certain.

If the diverticula of dura become adherent to the superficial ectoderm, they may not regress normally. Instead, they may pull ectoderm with them as they retreat, creating an (ecto)dermal tract that extends from the glabella through a canal at the nasofrontal suture to the crista galli or beyond the crista to the interdural space between the two leaves of the falx.[79,82,83] A similar persistent tract may pass from the external surface of the nose, under or through the nasal bones, and ascend through the prenasal space to enter the cranial cavity at the foramen cecum just anterior to the crista galli (Fig. 1-21). Such a tract would be associated with a widened foramen cecum, distortion and grooving of the crista galli, and extension into the interdural space between the two leaves of the falx. Depending on the precise histology of the portions of the tract that persist, these tracts could develop into superficial glabellar and nasal pits, fully patent glabellar and nasal dermal sinuses, and/or one or several (epi)dermoid cysts and/or fibrous

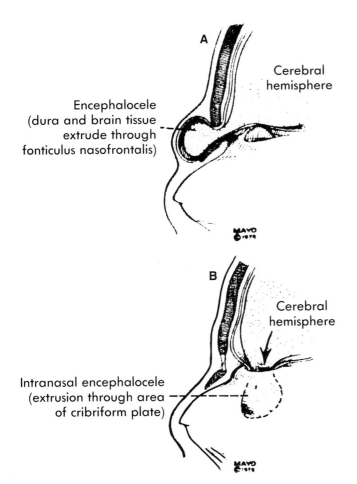

Fig. 1-22 Schematic representation of the origin of **A,** extranasal (glabellar) cephaloceles and, **B,** intranasal transethmoidal cephaloceles. (From Gorenstein A et al: Arch Otolaryngol 106:536, 1980. Copyright © Mayo Clinic.)

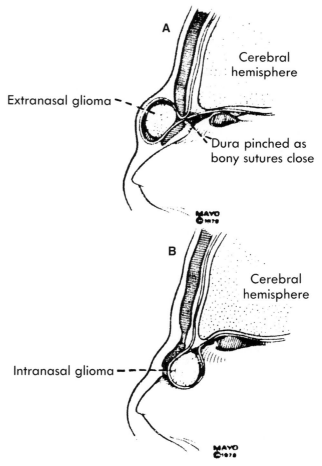

Fig. 1-23 Schematic representation of the origin of, **A,** extranasal gliomas and, **B,** nasal gliomas. (From Gorenstein A et al: Arch Otolaryngol 106:536, 1980. Copyright © Mayo Clinic.)

cords—exactly as the analogous remnants of the vitelline duct and neurenteric canal do. Rarely, the sinus tracts, cysts, and cords may extend into or become adherent to the brain itself.[84]

Nasal cephaloceles and gliomas may arise by an analogous mechanism. If the same dural diverticula were to persist as patent communications that contained leptomeninges, cerebrospinal fluid (CSF) and neural tissue, they would constitute glabellar and nasal meningoencephaloceles (Fig. 1-22). Were such developing meningoencephaloceles to become pinched off and (nearly) isolated from the cranial cavity by subsequent constriction of the dura and bone, they would then constitute heterotopic foci of meninges and neural tissue at the glabella and nose. These benign nonneoplastic heterotopias are given the dreadful name of glabellar and nasal gliomas (Fig. 1-23).

NASAL DERMAL SINUSES AND DERMOIDS

Dermoids of the skull occur at diverse locations believed to be related to the sites of closure of the neural tube, the sites of diverticulation of the cerebral hemispheres, and the lines of closure of the cranial sutures. In Pannell's series of 94 dermoids of the skull, 43% were midline, 45% were frontotemporal, and 13% were parietal.[85] The midline dermoids affected the anterior fontanelle (25), glabella (1), nasion (2), vertex (1), and occipital/suboccipital region (11). The frontotemporal dermoids affected the sphenofrontal (15), frontozygomatic (16), and sphenosquamosal (11) sutures. The parietal dermoids affected the squamosal (8), coronal (1), lambdoid (1), and parietomastoid (2) sutures.

A nasal dermal sinus is a thin epithelial-lined tube that arises at an external ostium situated along the midline of the nose and that extends deeply for a variable distance, sometimes reaching the intradural intracranial space. A nasal dermal cyst is a midline epithelial-lined cyst that arises along the expected course of the dermal sinus. It may exist as an isolated mass, or it may coexist with a dermal sinus (Fig. 1-24). Histologically, nasal dermal sinuses may be true dermoids containing skin adnexae or pure epidermoids devoid of such adnexae.[86] Dermoids and epidermoids are equally common. However, dermoid cysts and sinuses are found more commonly along the bridge of the nose. Pure epidermoids are more common at the glabella-nasion and have a sevenfold increased incidence of associated infection.[86]

Nasal dermal sinuses and cysts constitute 3.7% to 12.6% of all dermal cysts of the head and neck and 1.1% of all such cysts throughout the body.[79] They may be detected at any age, but most appear early (mean age 3 years).[87] There is no sex predilection.[79,87,88] Most cases arise sporadically, though kindreds with nasal dermal sinus have been reported.[89,90]

The lesions may appear at any site from the glabella downward along the bridge (dorsum) of the nose to the base of the columella. Approximately 56% of lesions appear as midline cysts, the other 44% as midline sinus ostia. The external ostium of the sinus lies at the glabella-nasion in 29%, the bridge of the nose in 21%, the nasal tip in 21%, and the base of the columella in 29%.[87] Rarely, multiple sinus ostia are present, or sinuses and cysts coexist at both the glabella and nasal bridge.[79]

Nasal (epi)dermoid *cysts* are usually found in one of three areas: in the midline just superior to the nasal tip, at the junction of the upper and lower lateral cartilages, or in the medial canthal area. Glabellar cysts external to the frontal bone are less common. The cysts may be soft and discrete or indurated. They may erode through the overlying skin to form secondary pits.

Clinically, these lesions appear as midline pits or fenestra, occasionally containing sparse wiry hairs (Fig. 1-25); as intermittent discharge of sebaceous material and/or pus; as intermittent inflammation; as increasing size of the mass with variable degrees of broadening of the nasal root and bridge; as intermittent episodes of meningitis, or as a behavioral change secondary to a frontal lobe abscess. At times the ostium is tiny and undetectable until pressure is applied against the adjacent tissue to express cheesy material from the ostium.[79]

The deep extension of nasal dermal sinuses and cysts is variable. They can be shallow pits that end blindly in the superficial tissues. They can wander extensively intracranially and extracranially.[79] In Bradley's review of 67 children with nasal dermoids,[86] the lesion was confined to the skin in 61% and extended deeply to invade the nasal bones in 10%. The lesion extended into the septal cartilage in 10%, the nasal bones and cartilage in 6%, and the cribriform plate in 12%. Rare sinuses traverse the entire anteroposterior extent of the nasal septum to end at the basisphenoid where they attach to the dura just anterior to the sella.[79] The frequency of intracranial extension has been found to vary widely from 57% to 0%.[80]

Intracranial extension can be associated with cysts and sinuses at any site. Sinuses at the base of the columella are least likely to extend intracranially. Thus in Pensler's series,[87] each of four sinuses situated at the base of the columella passed directly to the nasal spine of the maxilla, with no intracranial extension. However, Mühlbauer and Dittmar[89] reported a similar sinus that ascended to end in the ethmoid air cells; it did not enter the cranial cavity.

True intracranial extension of (epi)dermoid usually affects the epidural space of the anterior fossa near the crista galli and may continue deeper, between the two leaves of the falx as an interdural mass.[87] Rarely the lesions also extend into brain.[84] An additional 31% of cases have intracranial extension of a fibrous cord de-

Text continued on p. 32.

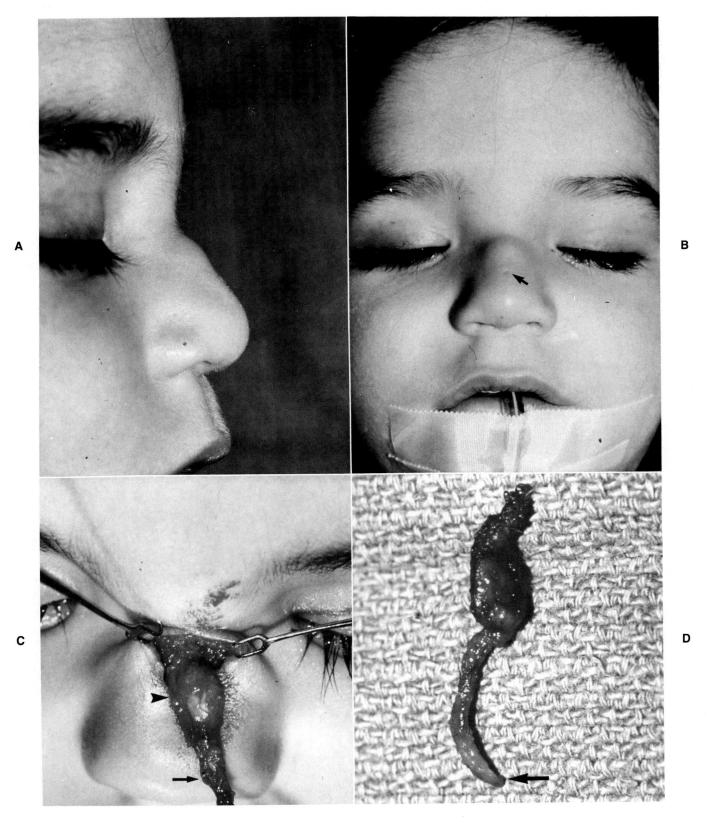

Fig. 1-24 Nasal dermal sinus in 10-month-old boy with increasing swelling of the nose. **A** and **B,** Swelling and a pinpoint ostium *(arrow)* on the dorsum of the nose. **C,** Surgical dissection traces the sinus tract *(black arrow)* inward from the ostium to a well-defined ovoid dermoid cyst *(black arrowhead)* within the septum. The cyst reached just to the cribriform plate. **D,** Operative specimen demonstrates the proportions and contours of the dermal sinus and cyst. Arrow indicates the superficial cutaneous end of the tract.

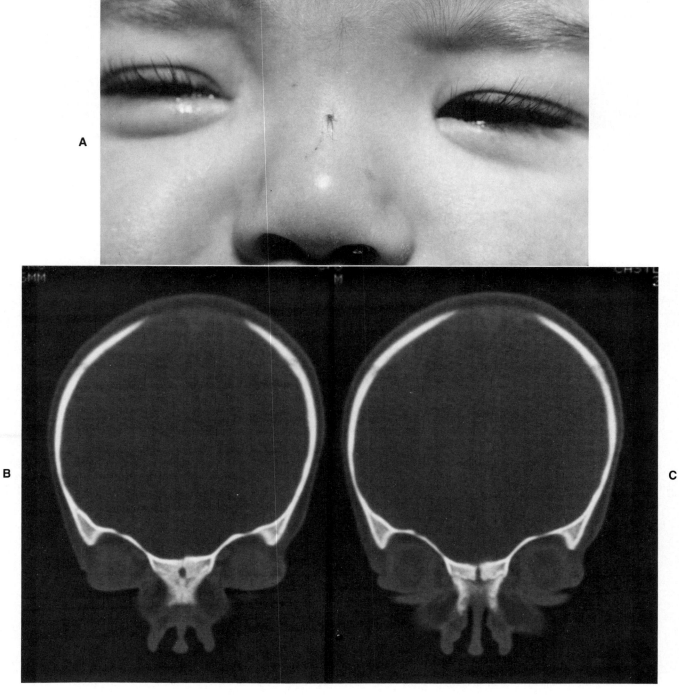

Fig. 1-25   Nasal dermal sinus with intracranial extension in 1-year-old girl with clinically evident sinus. **A,** A small tuft of hairs protrudes from a midline dermal sinus on the dorsum of the nose. **B** and **C,** Direct coronal CT. A well-marginated canal penetrates between the nasal process of the frontal bones.

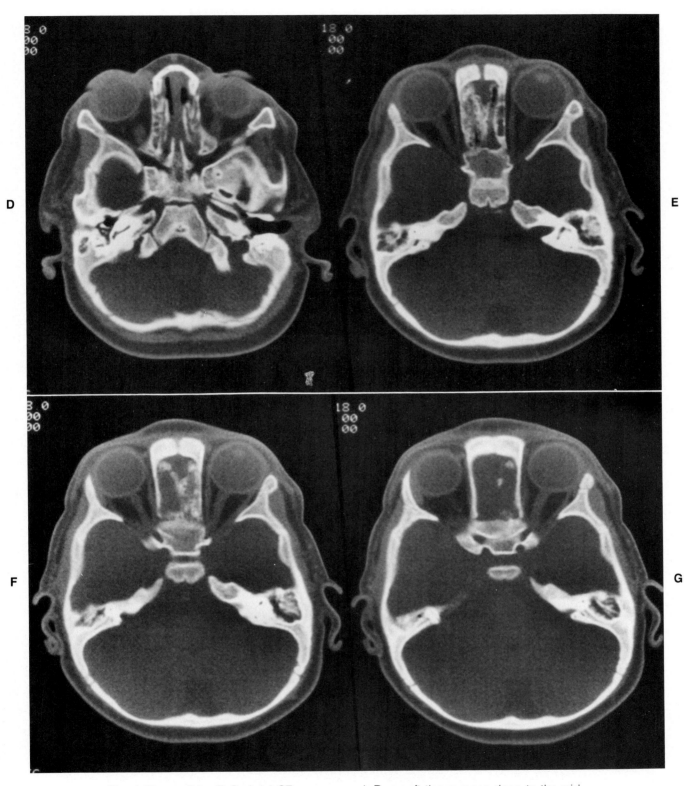

Fig. 1-25, cont'd   D-G, Axial CT scans reveal, **D,** a soft tissue mass deep to the widened nasal bridge; **E,** the bony canal leading to the widened nasal septum, and **F** and **G,** the large foramen cecum and bifid crista galli. At surgery the dermal sinus tract and extranasal dermoid were traced upward through the foramen cecum into a 2 to 3 cm intracranial dermoid. This extended intradurally but did not attach to brain. A second "arm" of the intranasal dermoid passed posteriorly toward the sphenoid bone.

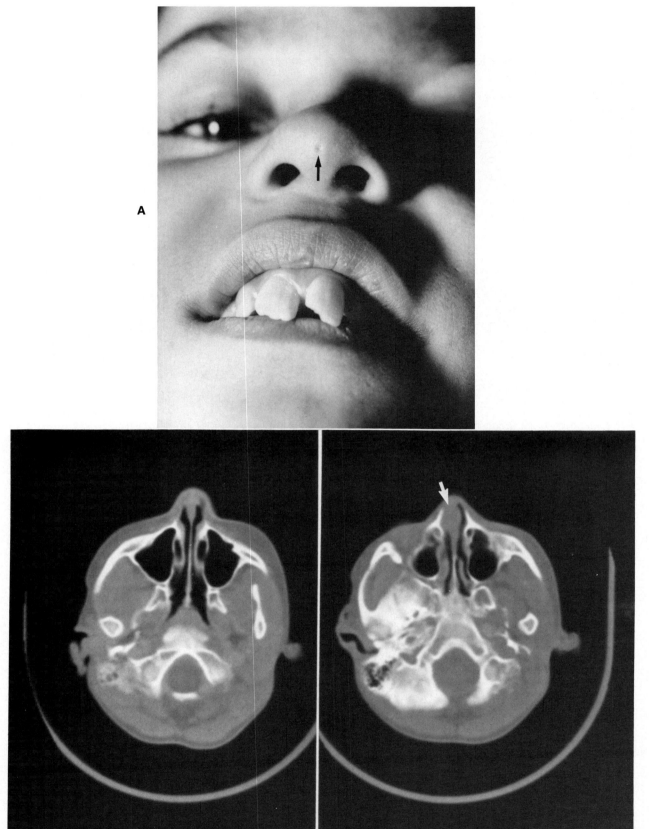

Fig. 1-26 Nasal dermal sinus, intranasal dermoid, intracranial dermoid, and multilocular cerebral abscesses in 10-year-old boy. **A,** Dermal sinus *(arrow)* at the nasal tip. **B-E,** Serial axial CTs demonstrate molding of the nasal bones by an intranasal mass, **B,** *(white arrow)* and a bony canal **D** and **E,** *(black arrows)* through the nasal septum into the skull base.

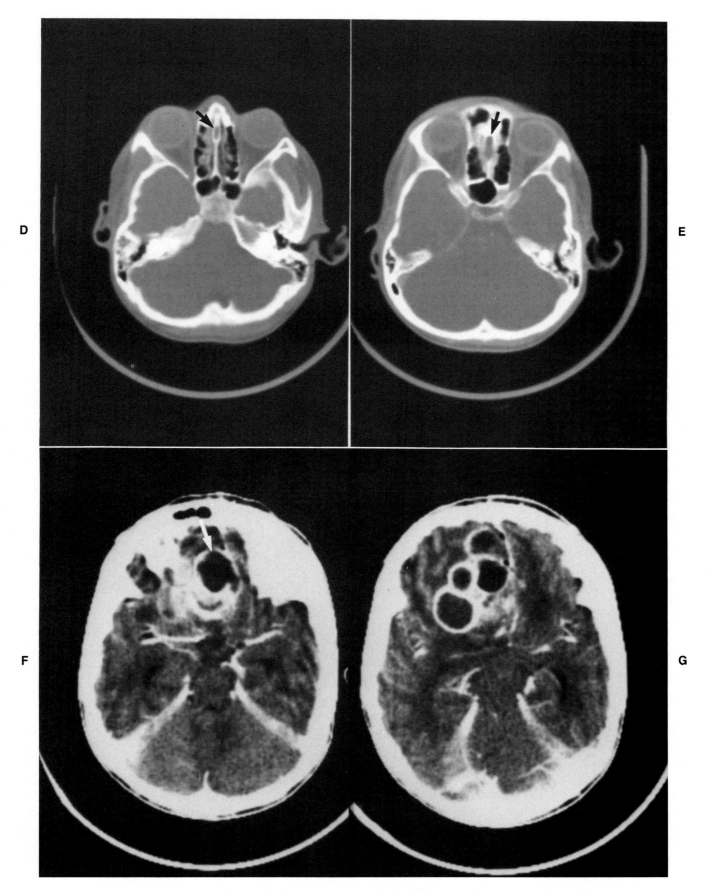

Fig. 1-26, cont'd   F and **G,** Contrast-enhanced axial CT scans demonstrate the multi-locular right frontal abscesses extending upward from the skull base. The very lucent right paramedian cyst *(arrow)* is the intracranial dermoid itself.

Continued.

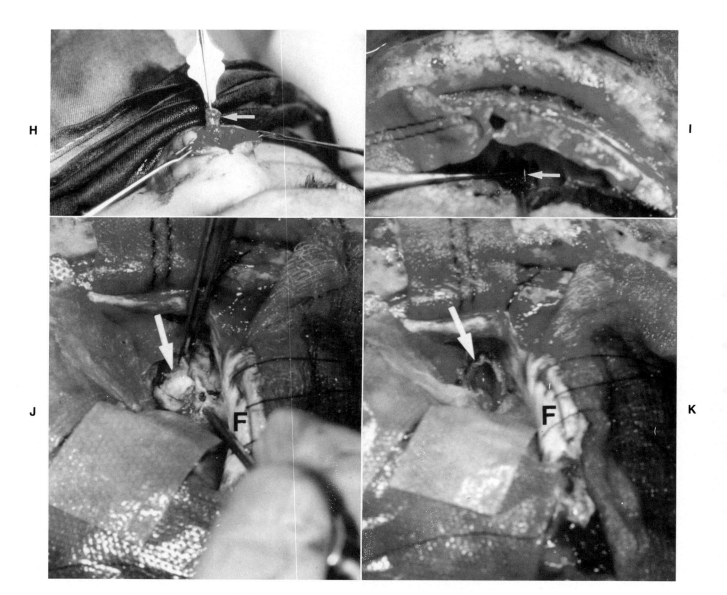

Fig. 1-26, cont'd **H-K,** At surgery, a probe was passed through the dissected dermal sinus tract *(white arrow in **H**)* into the extradural intracranial space *(white arrow in **I**)*. Dissection downward along the falx *(F)* revealed the intradural dermoid *(white arrow in **J**)* that was debrided to display the cyst wall *(white arrow in **K**)*.

void of (epi)dermoid elements.[87] At present, intracranial extension of a fibrous cord is not considered significant and has not been associated with sequelae on follow-up examinations.[87]

Nasal dermal sinuses are resected for cosmetic reasons, to avoid or treat the complications of local infection, and to prevent or treat secondary meningitis and cerebral abscess (Fig. 1-26). Late development of squamous cell carcinoma is a theoretical rationale for resection, but such carcinoma has not been observed with nasal dermal sinuses to date.

In patients with dermal sinuses and cysts, CT suc-

cessfully displays the course of the tract and any sequelae of infection. The ostium and tract usually appear as an isodense fibrous channel or as a lucent dermoid channel that extends inward for a variable distance. Bony canals indicate the course of the sinus through the nasal bones, ossified nasal septum, and skull base. An uncomplicated dermoid cyst appears as a well-defined lucency with an isodense capsule (Fig. 1-27). Swelling and edema around the cyst suggest secondary inflammation (Fig. 1-28).[91] The intracranial ends of dermoid cysts typically lie in a hollowed-out gully along the anterior surface of a thickened enlarged crista.[79] This hol-

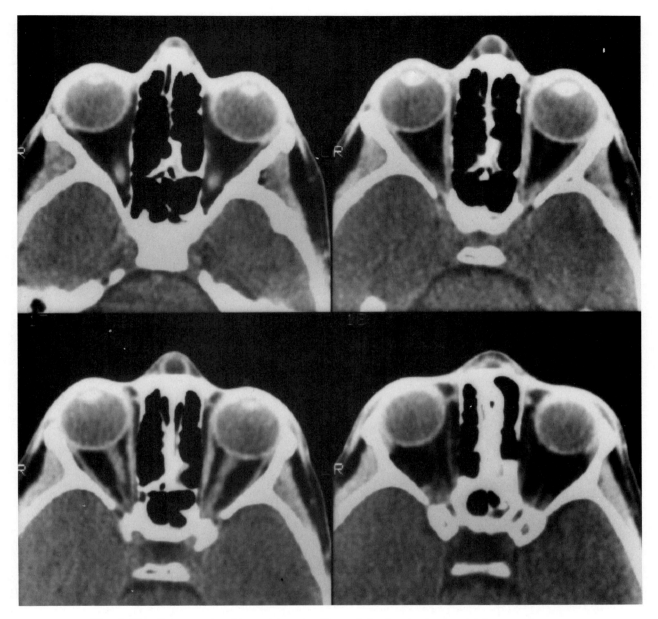

Fig. 1-27 Extranasal epidermoid cyst with no infection in 4-year-old boy as demonstrated by axial noncontrast CTs. The well-defined isodense cyst wall and lucent center are clearly separable from adjoining soft tissues. The nasal bones are flattened. No intracranial component is present.

low gives a false impression of a "bifid" crista.[79] The intracranial portion of the dermoid may be lucent or dense.

Unfortunately, the only sure proof of an intracranial extension is the actual demonstration of an intracranial mass. CT demonstration of an enlarged foramen cecum and distorted crista galli is suggestive, but not proof, of an intracranial extension. Foraminal enlargement and distortion of the crista seem to form part of this malformation and may be present (1) with intracranial extension, (2) without intracranial extension, or (3) with intracranial extension of a *fibrous* cord rather than a dermoid.[47] To avoid unnecessary craniotomies, therefore, surgical studies[79,87] suggest that the best approach is to dissect the extracranial portion of the tract along its entire length from the superficial ostium to the *extra*cranial surface of the enlarged foramen cecum. The tract is then severed, and the severed end is sent for pathology. If the cephalic end has dermal elements, the dissection is then extended intracranially. If no dermal el-

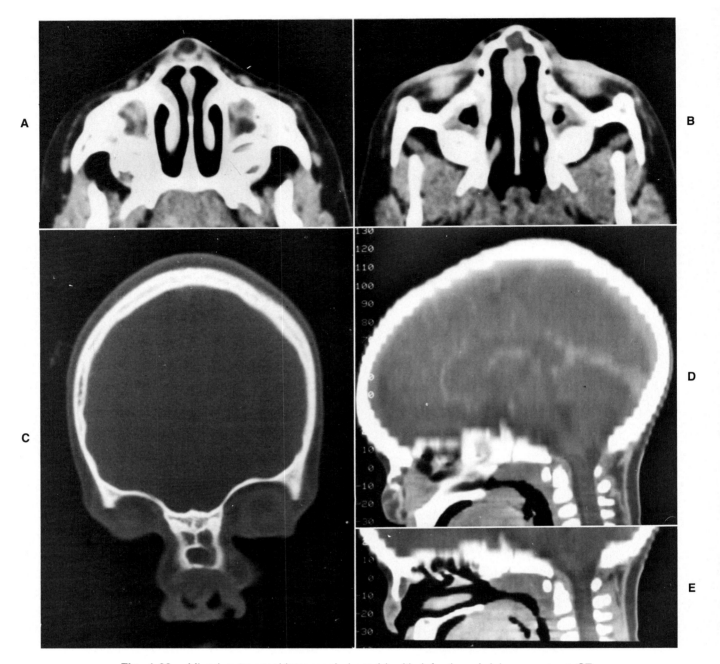

Fig. 1-28 Mixed extranasal-intranasal dermoid with infection. Axial noncontrast CTs demonstrate, **A,** extranasal and, **B,** intranasal mass, scalloped erosion of the nasal bones, and edema of the fat planes surrounding the cyst. **C,** Direct coronal and, **D** and **E,** reformatted sagittal contrast-enhanced CTs show the broadening and erosion of the nasal bridge and the relationship of the extranasal and intranasal portions of the dermoid cyst.

ements are found and if no mass was shown by CT, the procedure is concluded at that point.

NASAL GLIOMAS

Nasal gliomas are benign masses of glial tissue of congenital origin that occur intranasally and/or extranasally at or near the root of the nose. They may or may not be connected to the brain by a pedicle of glial tissue. By definition, they do not contain any CSF-filled space that is connected with either the ventricles or the subarachnoid space of the head.[92]

Nasal gliomas and cephaloceles form a spectrum of

related diseases (see Figs. 1-20 to 1-23). Characteristic encephaloceles contain ependyma-lined ventricles filled with CSF. Prototypical nasal gliomas consist of solid masses of glial tissue, which are entirely separate from the brain.[92] Transitional forms include solid lesions with *microscopic* ependyma-lined canals, solid lesions intimately attached to the brain by glial pedicles with no ependyma-lined spaces, and solid lesions attached to the dura by fibrous bands with no glial pedicles.[92] Analysis of cases reveals that the presence or absence of a pedicle and *thin* ependyma-lined channel is not helpful in making surgically and radiologically useful distinctions among these lesions. Thus the medically significant differential diagnosis between nasal gliomas and encephaloceles depends on the presence (encephalocele) or absence (nasal glioma) of communication between the intracranial CSF and any fluid spaces within or surrounding the mass.[93] Indeed, nasal gliomas remain connected with intracranial structures in 15% of cases, usually through a defect in or near to the cribriform plate.[83]

Nasal gliomas are uncommon lesions, with perhaps 100 cases now reported. They occur sporadically with no familial tendency[83] and no sex predilection.[83] They are rarely associated with other congenital malformations of the brain or body.

Nasal gliomas are subdivided into extranasal (60%), intranasal (30%), and mixed (10%) forms (Fig. 1-29).[83] The *extra*nasal gliomas lie external to the nasal bones and nasal cavities. Most frequently these occur at the bridge of the nose, to the left or right of the midline, but, curiously, not in the midline itself. Extranasal gliomas may also be found near the inner canthus; at the junction of the bony and cartilaginous portions of the nose; or between the frontal, nasal, ethmoid, and lacrimal bones.

*Intra*nasal gliomas lie within the nasal or nasopharyngeal cavities, within the mouth, or, rarely, within the pterygopalatine fossa (Fig. 1-30). In mixed nasal gliomas, the extranasal and intranasal components communicate via a defect in the nasal bones or around the lateral edges of the nasal bones. Rarely, the two portions communicate through defects in the orbital plate of the frontal bone or the frontal sinus. When *extra*nasal gliomas lie to *both* sides of the nasal bridge, the two components communicate with each other via a defect in the nasal bones, constituting a mixed nasal glioma.[93]

Clinically, extranasal gliomas usually appear in early infancy or childhood as firm, slightly elastic, reddish to bluish, skin-covered masses. Capillary telangiectasias may cover the lesion. They exhibit no pulsations, do not increase in size with Valsalva maneuver (crying), and do not pulsate or swell following compression of the ipsilateral jugular vein (negative Fürstenburg sign).[83,92,94,95] These lesions usually grow slowly in proportion to adjacent tissue but may grow more or less rapidly.[83] They can cause severe deformity by displacing the nasal skeleton, the adjoining maxilla, and the orbital walls.[83] Hypertelorism may result.

*Intra*nasal gliomas usually appear as large, firm, poly-

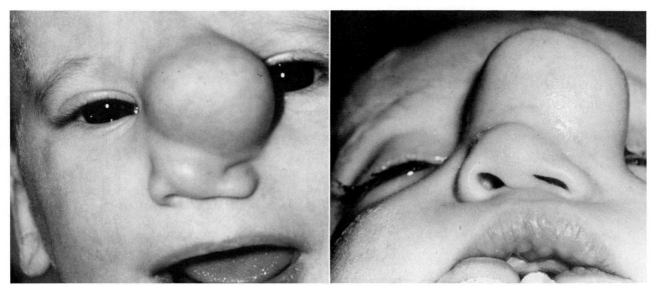

Fig. 1-29 Mixed extranasal-intranasal glioma in 8-month-old boy with nasal mass that was present at birth and grew in proportion with the child. **A** and **B,** Two views of the face demonstrate a 3 × 3 cm firm left paramedian subcutaneous mass that displaces the septal and alar cartilage, narrowing the nostril. The mass did not pulsate or change size with crying. *Continued.*

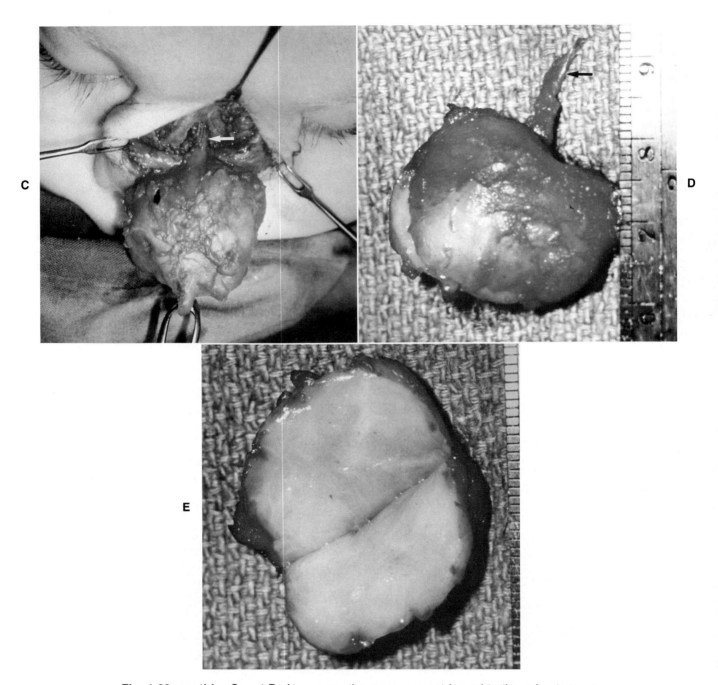

Fig. 1-29, cont'd **C** and **D,** At surgery, the mass was not bound to the subcutaneous tissue. It lay nearly entirely external to the nasal bones, to the left of midline. A narrow stalk *(arrows)* passed directly through the left nasal bone and extended upward to the left cribriform plate. **E,** Bisecting the specimen revealed a homogeneous mass of smooth grayish-white shiny tissue. Histological examination revealed brain and fibrous tissue consistent with nasal glioma.

poid submucosal masses that may extend inferiorly toward or nearly to the nostril.[83,95] They commonly attach to the turbinates and lie medial to the middle turbinate, between the middle turbinate and the nasal septum.[83] Rarely, they attach to the septum itself.

These intranasal masses expand the nasal fossa, widen the nasal bridge, and deviate the septum contralaterally. Obstruction of the nasal passage may lead to respiratory distress, especially in infants. Blockage of the nasolacrimal duct may cause epiphora on the affected

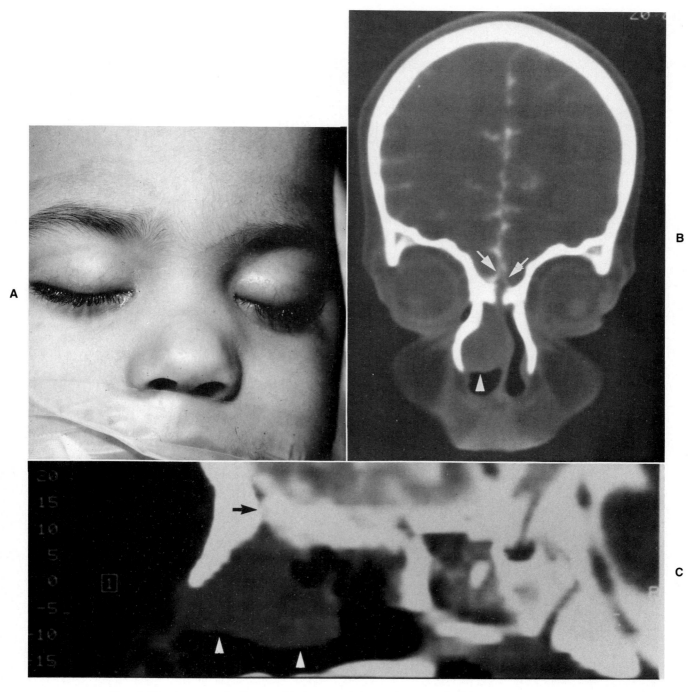

Fig. 1-30 Intranasal glioma with intracranial attachments. **A,** Widening of the nasal bridge and the left nostril (present prior to intubation). **B** and **C,** Water-soluble positive contrast cisternography. Direct coronal and reformatted sagittal CT sections demonstrate a large left unilateral intranasal mass *(arrowheads)* that deviates the nasal septum rightward, bows the left nasal bone outward, and extends superiorly through a widened foramen cecum *(black arrow)* into the interdural space *(white arrows)* between the leaves of the falx. Opacified CSF outlines the intracranial portion of the mass but does not extend extracranially into or around the intranasal portion of the mass. **D** and **E,** Frontal intraoperative photographs oriented like **A** and **B.** In **D,** the scalp *(S)* has been reflected over the orbits *(O, O).* Keyhole resection of the frontonasal junction exposes the frontal dura *(D, D)* and nasal cavity, bounded by remnant frontal bone *(F, F)* at the supraorbital ridges and remnant nasal bone *(N, N)* laterally. The frontal dura of each side is reflected inward in the midline *(white arrowhead)* to form the falx. The interdural space (white arrows) is widened inferiorly. In **E,** further dissection frees the interdural portion *(between forceps)* of the nasal glioma and proves it is directly continuous with the intranasal portion *(white arrowhead)* of the mass.

Continued.

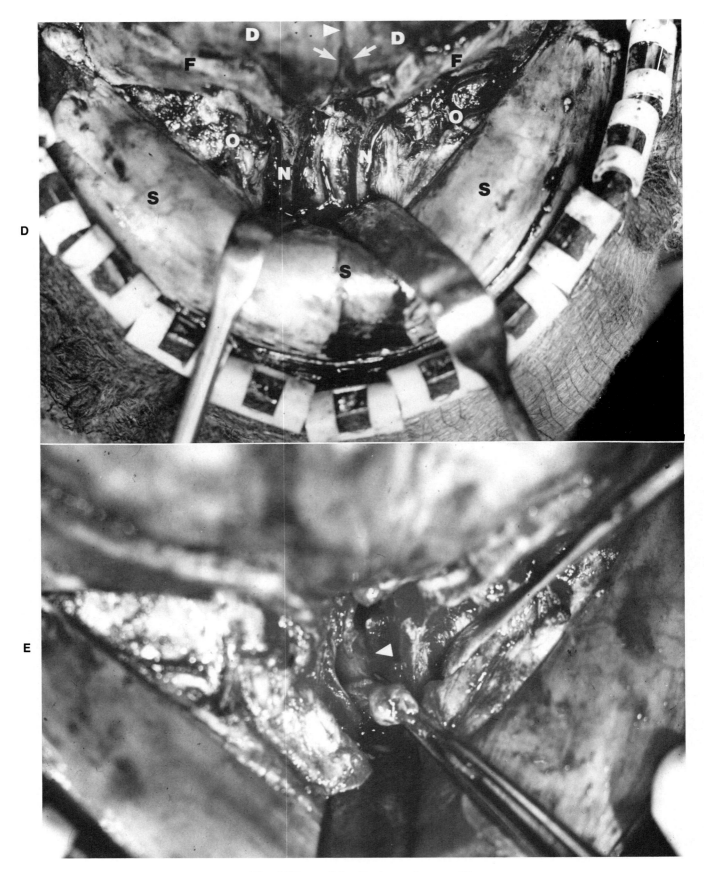

Fig. 1-30, cont'd For legend see p. 37.

side. CSF rhinorrhea, meningitis, or epistaxis may be the presenting complaint.

Intranasal gliomas are commonly confused with inflammatory polyps. However, nasal gliomas usually have a firmer consistency[92] and appear less translucent than inflammatory polyps.[96] Intranasal gliomas typically lie medial to the middle turbinate, whereas inflammatory polyps typically lie inferolateral to the middle turbinate. Only posterior ethmoid polyps project into the same space as the nasal glioma. Most important, nasal gliomas usually occur in infancy, whereas ordinary nasal polyps are almost unheard of under 5 years of age.[97]

Pathologically, nasal gliomas resemble reactive gliosis rather than neoplasia.[97] No invasion of surrounding tissue has ever been observed; no metastases have been reported.[98] Thus they are classified as heterotopias, not neoplasias.

Histologic studies show that the nasal glioma consists of small or large aggregates of fibrous or gemistocytic astrocytes. The cells may be multinuclear, but they exhibit no mitotic figures and no bizarre nuclear forms.[95] Fibrous connective tissue enwraps the blood vessels and extends outward to form collagenous septa that partially subdivide the mass.[95] Prominent zones of granulation tissue may be present.[95] The lesion is usually not encapsulated.[83] However, astrocytic processes, fibroblasts, and collagen may form a loose or dense connective tissue capsule.[95] Extranasal gliomas are then surrounded by dermis with dermal appendages.[83] Intranasal gliomas are surrounded by minor salivary glands, fibrovascular tissue, and nasal mucosa.[83]

Only 10% of reported nasal gliomas contain neurons.[95] This lack of neurons in 90% has been attributed to insufficient supply of oxygen to support them or to failure of neurons to differentiate from the embryonic neuroectoderm within the isolated glioma.[95]

Imaging studies display the nasal glioma as an isodense soft tissue mass that deforms the nasal fossa with or without evidence of extension through the glabella, nasal bones, cribriform plate, or foramen cecum (Fig. 1-30). Calcification may be present in rare cases.[92] Routine CT studies usually fail to differentiate between nasal glioma and encephalocele, unless the communicating CSF space is very large. It is often necessary to rule on the presence or absence of CSF communication by magnetic resonance (MR) or by positive contrast CT cisternography to achieve a correct differential diagnosis.

CEPHALOCELES

Cephaloceles are congenital herniations of intracranial contents through a cranial defect. When the herniation contains brain, it is a meningoencephalocele. If the herniation contains only meninges, it is a cranial meningocele. Cephaloceles are classified by the site of

---

CLASSIFICATION OF CEPHALOCELES

I. Occipital cephaloceles
   A. Cervico-occipital (continuous with cervical rachischisis)
   B. Low occipital (involving foramen magnum)
   C. High occipital (above intact rim of foramen magnum)
II. Cephaloceles of the cranial vault
   A. Temporal
   B. Posterior fontanelle
   C. Interparietal
   D. Anterior fontanelle
   E. Interfrontal
III. Frontoethmoidal cephaloceles (*sincipital cephaloceles*)
   A. Nasofrontal
   B. Nasoethmoidal
   C. Nasoorbital
IV. Basal cephaloceles
   A. Transethmoidal
   B. Sphenoethmoidal
   C. Transsphenoidal
   D. Frontosphenoidal
V. Cephaloceles associated with cranioschisis
   A. Cranial-upper facial cleft
   B. Basal-lower facial cleft
   C. Acrania and anencephaly

Modified from Suwanwela C and Suwanwela N: J Neurosurg 36:201, 1972.

---

the cranial defect through which the brain and meninges protrude (see box).[99,100] The size of the fluid spaces does not determine patient prognosis.

Cephaloceles situated in the anterior part of the skull are often designated *sincipital* cephaloceles[97] and include the frontoethmoidal cephaloceles and the interfrontal subtype of cranial cephaloceles.[97] Basal cephaloceles include intranasal, nasopharyngeal, and posterior orbital cephaloceles classified as transethmoidal, sphenoethmoidal, transsphenoidal, and frontosphenoidal cephaloceles. The fundamental difference between sincipital and basal cephaloceles is that sincipital cephaloceles always appear as external masses along the nose, orbital margin, or forehead; whereas basal cephaloceles are not visible externally, unless they grow large enough to protrude secondarily through the nostril or mouth.[77]

Cephaloceles are common lesions, with an incidence of 1 per 4000 live births.[101] Overall, occipital cephaloceles are the most frequent type (67% to 80%). Sincipital cephaloceles (15%) and basal cephaloceles (10%) are less common.[101] The occipital and the sincipital cephaloceles appear to be distinctly different diseases. Occipital cephaloceles are linked with neural tube defects such as myelomeningocele; sincipital cephaloceles are not.[102] Occipital cephaloceles are the most frequent

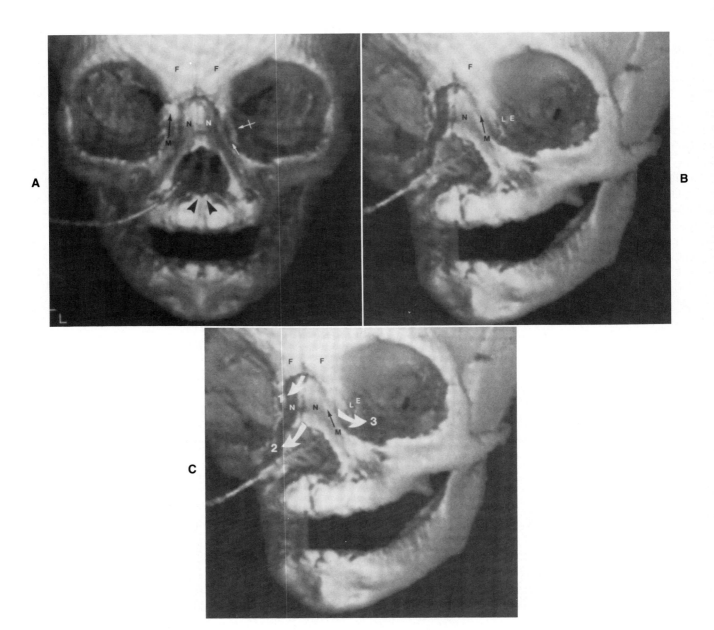

Fig. 1-31 Normal facial skeleton of a 4-month, 4-week-old boy showing pathways for the frontoethmoidal cephaloceles. **A** and **B,** Reformatted 3-dimensional CT images display the contours and relationships of the individual bones of the skull and face, plus the intervening sutures: ethmoid bone or lamina papyracea *(E);* frontal bone *(F);* lacrimal bone *(L);* frontal process of the maxilla *(M);* and nasal bone *(N).* Note the interfrontal, internasal, frontonasal, and frontomaxillary sutures; the nasal spines *(arrowheads)* of the maxillae; and the lacrimal sac fossa *(arrow).* The anterior crest of the lacrimal sac fossa is formed by the frontal process of maxilla and the posterior crest *(crossed white arrow)* by the lacrimal bone. Cartilaginous structures are not displayed by this technique. **C,** The sites through which the 3 subtypes of the frontoethmoidal cephaloceles protrude are indicated by the 3 numbered arrows: *(1),* Nasofrontal cephalocele. The facial end of the canal lies between the frontal and nasal bones. The frontal bones form the superior margin of the defect. The nasal bones, frontal processes of the maxillae and nasal cartilage form the inferior margin of the defect. *(2),* Nasoethmoidal cephalocele. The facial end of the canal lies between the nasal bones and the nasal cartilage. The nasal bones and the frontal processes of the maxillae form the superior margin of the defect. The nasal cartilage and nasal septum form the inferior margin of the defect. *(3),* Nasoorbital cephalocele. The facial end of the canal lies in the medial wall of the orbit. The frontal process of maxilla forms the anterior margin of the defect. The lacrimal bone and lamina papyracea of the ethmoid form the posterior wall of the defect.

type among people of European descent, while sincipital cephaloceles are the most frequent type among Malaysians and certain other South-East Asian groups. Thus, among Australian aborigines (nearly) all cephaloceles are sincipital, whereas among Australians of European descent 67% are occipital and 2% are sincipital.[102]

Frontoethmoidal cephaloceles are characterized by a cranial defect at the junction of the frontal and ethmoid bones.[100] In 90%, the intracranial end of the defect is a single midline ostium that corresponds to the foramen cecum. In 10%, an intact midline bridge of bone divides the defect into bilateral paired ostia situated at the anterior ends of the cribriform plates.

The frontoethmoidal cephaloceles are subdivided into three types in accord with the position of the *facial end* of the cranial defect (Fig. 1-31).[100] In the nasofrontal form (50% to 61%), the facial end of the defect lies between the frontal and the nasal bones so the ostium presents at the nasion between deformed orbits (Figs. 1-32 and 1-33).[103,104] Specifically, in this type the frontal bones are displaced superiorly. The nasal bones, frontal processes of maxillae, and nasal cartilage are all displaced inferiorly, away from the frontal bone, but retain a normal relationship to each other. The ethmoid bone is displaced inferiorly, so that the midline portion of the anterior fossa is very deep and the crista projects into the defect from its inferior rim. The anterior portions of the medial orbital walls are displaced laterally.

The bone canal is short because the intracranial (frontoethmoidal) and the extracranial (nasofrontal) ends of the defect lie close together.[100]

The associated soft tissue mass lies at the glabella or nasal root.[100] The mass may be small (1 to 2 cm) or larger than the infant's head. Most of the nasofrontal cephaloceles are firm solid masses and exhibit no transmitted pulsations. Some are cystic, compressible, pulsatile and increase in size with Valsalva maneuver (crying).[100] The mass usually grows as the child grows. Cystic masses may increase in size disproportionately rapidly as CSF pools within the sac. The cephalocele may be covered by intact skin, thin skin that ruptures to leak CSF, or no skin at all, exposing brain to the environment. The falx frequently extends into the sac, partially subdividing it. The herniated brain may be well preserved with recognizable gyri and sulci that converge toward the hernia ostium, or the herniated brain may be reduced to a mass of distorted gliotic tissue. Typically the brain is not adherent to the base of the sac at the ostium, but it may be adherent to the meninges at the dome of the sac (60%).[103]

The tips of the frontal lobes usually protrude into the defect, symmetrically or asymmetrically. The olfactory bulbs may herniate with the brain; the olfactory tracts are stretched. The optic nerves enter the skull normally but may then recurve sharply anteriorly toward the hernia orifice. The internal carotid arteries course with

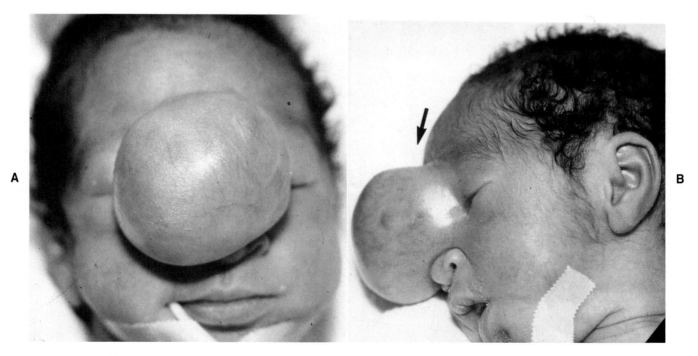

Fig. 1-32   Nasofrontal form of frontoethmoidal cephalocele in newborn girl. **A** and **B,** Frontal and lateral views of the face. A large skin-covered midline mass protrudes between the two orbits, overlies the nasal bones and nasal cartilage and compresses the nostrils. Arrow indicates the angle of observation for the surgical photographs.

Continued.

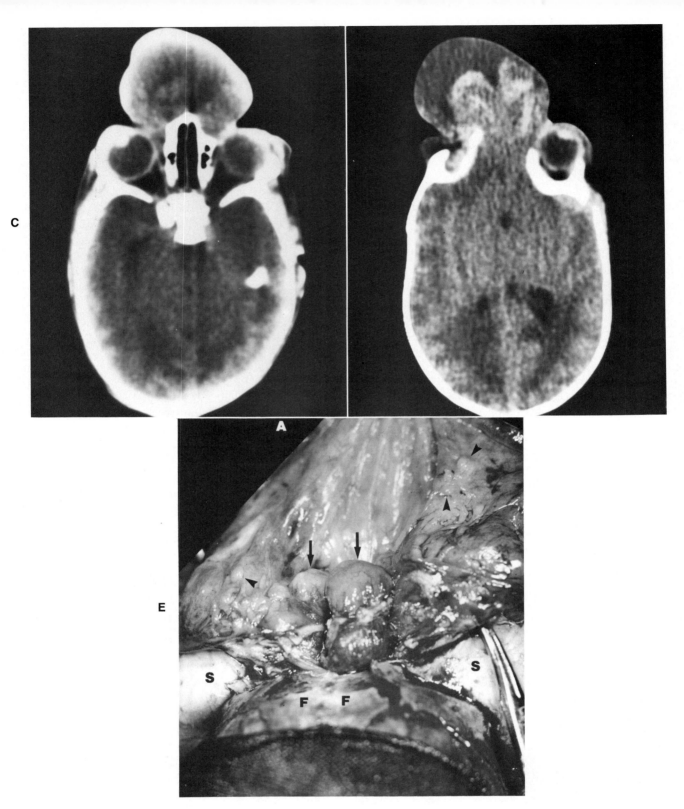

Fig. 1-32, cont'd   C, Noncontrast CT and **D,** Contrast enhanced CT on 2 different days, oriented as in, **E,** the following surgical specimen. The ostium of the cephalocele lies above the ethmoid and nasal bones but below the frontal bones, so the lesion is a frontonasal type of frontoethmoidal cephalocele. The mass is predominantly cystic. The inferior portions of both frontal lobes protrude directly into the sac to different degrees, greater on the left. **E,** Surgical photograph. Anterior, *(A),* view of the frontal bone *(F)* after reflection of the scalp *(S)* anteriorly and opening of the upper wall of the cephalocele to expose its contents. Most of the sac was filled by CSF. Portions of both frontal lobes *(arrows)* protrude into the sac, separated by the interhemispheric fissure. Multiple glial nodules *(black arrowheads)* stud the meninges that form the inner lining of the sac.

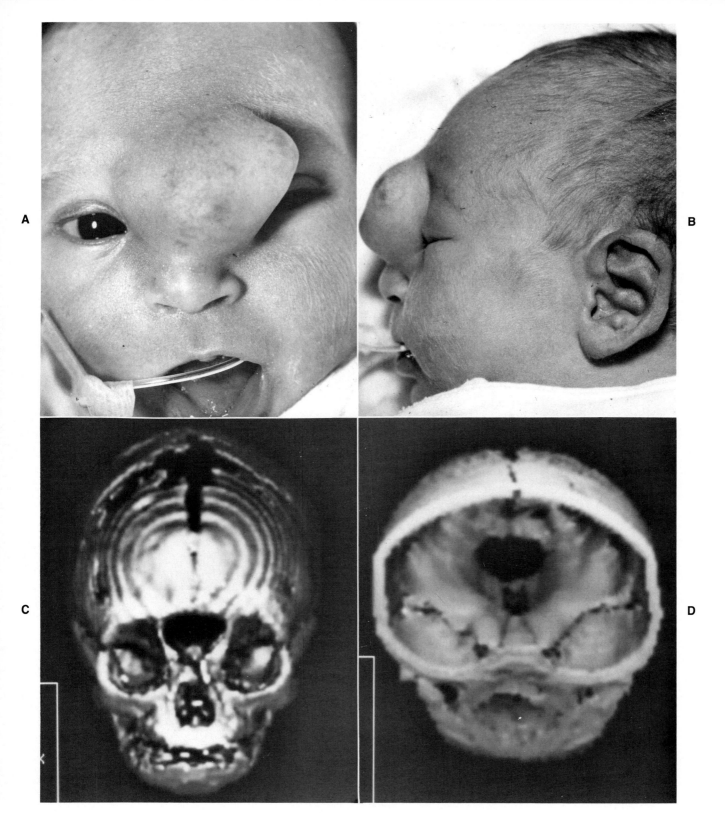

Fig. 1-33   Nasofrontal form of frontoethmoidal cephalocele in one-week-old girl. **A** and **B,** Lobulated 3 × 3 cm skin-covered mass that protrudes between the orbits over the nasal bones and nasal cartilage. 3-dimensional CT of bone surface viewed from, **C,** anterior and, **D,** posterior (intracranial) show the characteristic deformities of the frontal bones superolateral to the ostium and the characteristic position of the nasofrontal sutures, nasal bones and crista galli inferior to the ostium.   *Continued.*

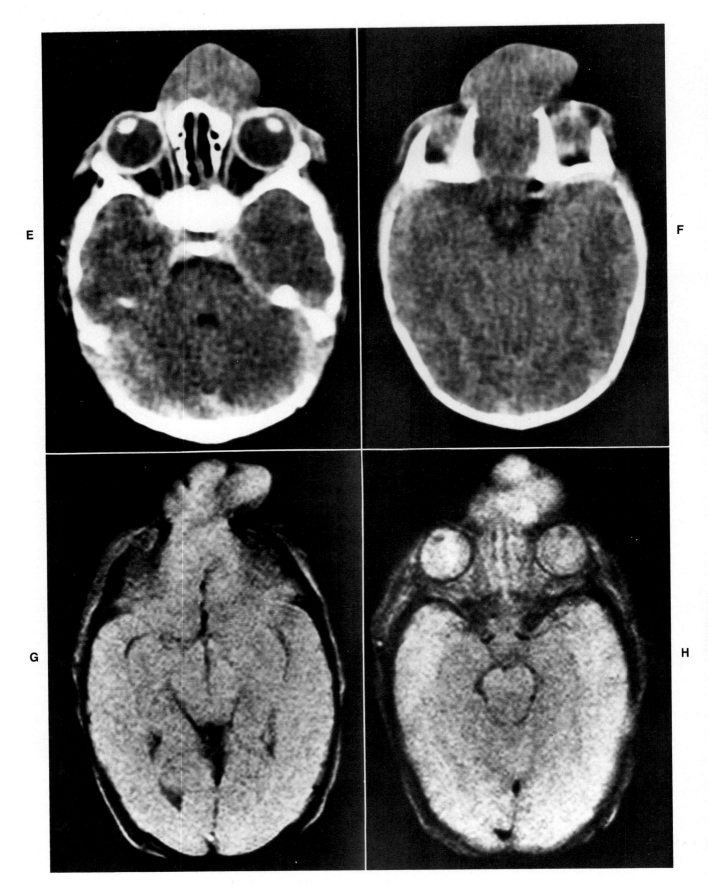

Fig. 1-33, cont'd For legend see opposite page.

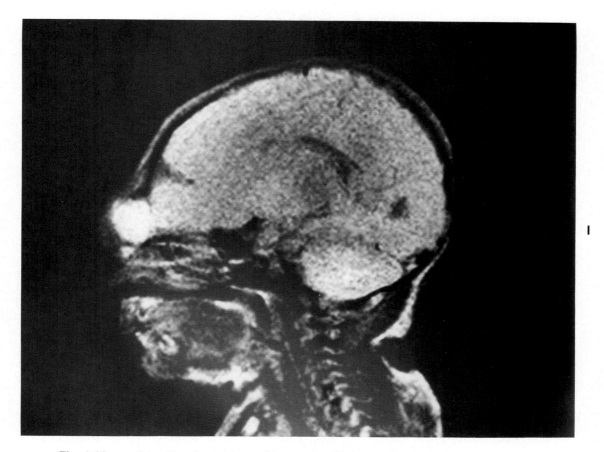

I

Fig. 1-33, cont'd   Nasofrontal form of frontoethmoidal cephalocele in one-week-old girl. **E** and **F,** Axial noncontrast CTs. Portions of both frontal lobes *(arrows)* protrude anteriorly through a defect in the frontal bones to form a lobulated mass anterior to the nasal bones. Since the superior margin of the ostium is frontal bone while the inferior margin is nasal bones, this is a nasofrontal cephalocele. Note the larger size of the defect on the left and the crista galli at the floor of the intracranial end of the canal. At surgery, the superior margin of the ostium was formed by frontal bones. The sac contained distorted, lobulated neural tissue that protruded through the defect and a small dermoid at the tip of the mass. The whole lesion was resected. Histological examination revealed that the sac contents were glial tissue containing numerous blood vessels. **G** and **H,** Axial and **I,** sagittal spin echo MRI (TR/TE = 2000/50) demonstrate the direct continuity of frontal lobe through the defect into the encephalocele sac.

the optic nerves. The anterior communicating artery may lie near the ostium. Concurrent anomalies such as holoprosencephaly and hydrocephalus may be present.

In the nasoethmoidal form (30% to 33%) of frontoethmoidal cephaloceles, the facial end of the defect lies between the nasal bones and the nasal cartilage, so the ostium is situated at the widened *dorsum* of the nose (Fig. 1-34). Specifically, in the nasoethmoidal form, the nasal bones and the frontal processes of the maxillae remain attached to the frontal bones above the sac, forming the anterosuperior wall of the canal. The nasal cartilage, nasal septum, and ethmoid bone are displaced posteroinferiorly, forming the posteroinferior wall of the canal. The crista projects upward into the canal from the depths of the floor. The medial walls of the or-

bit form the lateral borders of the defect and may be bony or membranous. In this group, because the canal is long, a greater distance exists between the intracranial (frontoethmoid) and extracranial (nasoethmoid) ends of the defect.

Clinically, nasoethmoidal cephaloceles are similar to nasofrontal cephaloceles except that the defect and soft tissue mass lie more inferiorly along the dorsum of the nose and often extend to the inner canthus (see Fig. 1-34). Cystic swellings may be present on both sides of the nose. Hydrocephalus is common. In Suwanwela's series, one of three patients had concurrent agenesis of the corpus callosum with an interhemispheric cyst.[97,100]

Harverson et al[105] detailed the radiologic differences between the nasofrontal and nasoethmoidal cephaloce-

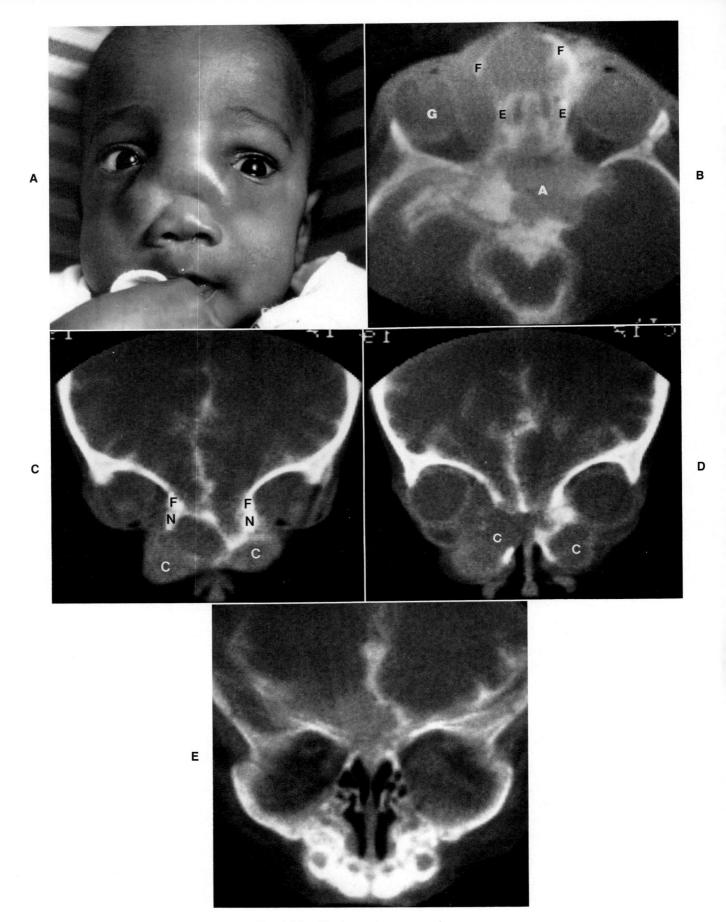

Fig. 1-34 For legend see opposite page.

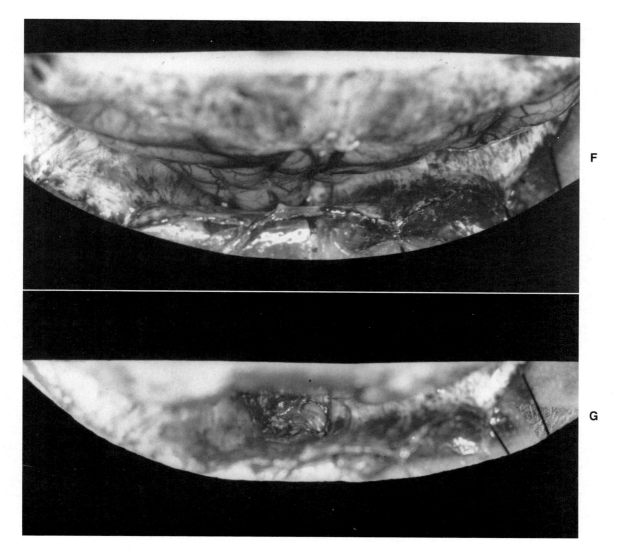

F

G

Fig. 1-34, cont'd   Combined nasoethmoidal and nasoorbital form of frontoethmoidal cephalocele in 5½-month-old boy with complete agenesis of the corpus callosum. **A,** Patient facies reveal hypertelorism, bulging at the glabella, and cystic swellings at the inner canthi and nasolabial folds bilaterally. Water-soluble positive contrast CT cisternograms are also shown. **B,** Axial CT demonstrates separation of the frontal *(F)* and ethmoidal *(E)* bones by the encephalocele. The lesion bulges into the orbit displacing the muscle cone and globe *(G)* laterally. Large noncommunicating suprasellar arachnoid cyst *(A)*. **C-E,** Direct coronal CTs demonstrate normal relationship of the frontal *(F)* and nasal *(N)* bones ruling out the nasofrontal form of cephalocele. The facial end of the defect lies between the nasal bone and the nasal cartilage, so this is a nasoethmoidal form of frontoethmoidal cephalocele. The frontal process of maxilla is also separated from the ethmoid bone, so this lesion has a component of nasoorbital cephalocele. The left globe is deviated and compressed by the cephalocele and associated cysts. In **B,** the right cyst *(C)* lies anterior to maxilla, causing the visible swelling. The interhemispheric fissure deviates far to one side. **F** and **G,** At surgery the falx attached to the roof of the left orbit. The contralateral right frontal lobe extended into the midline and then herniated inferiorly. When this was retracted, a bluish cyst could be observed beneath the frontal lobe extending into the orbit. Following resection of all cysts, one could look from the intracranial space through the ostium to observe nasal mucosa posteromedially and orbital fat anteriolaterally.

les. In the nasofrontal form the defect in the frontal bone is V-shaped. The superior aspects of the medial orbital walls are bowed and displaced laterally. The nasal bones remain attached to the cribriform plate at the lower margin of the ostium. Thus the cribriform plate and nasal bones are seen to lie unusually low between the orbits. A large gap exists between the frontal and ethmoidal bones. The soft tissue mass lies directly in front of the bone defect, usually in the midline, and it is often spherical. Conversely in the nasoethmoidal form, the bone defect is usually circular and is situated between the orbits, causing increased interorbital distance. The nasal bones remain attached to the frontal bones along the upper margins of the ostium. The cribriform plate lies at a normal height with respect to the orbits. The soft tissue mass lies to one side of the midline, beside the nasal cartilage. It may be bilateral.[105]

In the nasoorbital form of frontoethmoidal cephalocele (6% to 10%), the facial end of the defect lies at the medial wall of the orbit, so the ostium shows at the inner canthus and nasolabial folds. Specifically, the frontal process of the maxilla is separated from the lacrimal and ethmoid bones. The abnormal frontal process of the maxilla forms the anterior margin of the defect. The lacrimal bone and lamina papyracea of the ethmoid form the posterior edge of the defect.[100] The frontal bones, nasal bones, and nasal cartilage retain their normal relationship to one another. In this type, the intracranial (frontoethmoid) and extracranial (medial orbital) ends of the defect are widely separated, so the canal is very long.

Patients with nasoorbital cephalocele may have cystic soft tissue masses at the nasolabial folds between the nose and the lower eyelid. These masses may contain nubbins of brain.[100]

Suwanwela and Hongsaprabhas[97] reviewed the clinical findings in 25 patients with frontoethmoidal cephaloceles. Microcephaly was present in 24%, unilateral or bilateral microphthalmos in 16%, hydrocephalus in 12%, and seizures in 4%. Mental retardation was present in 43% of those old enough to test. CSF leakage and continuous bleeding from the exposed brain were major problems in those cephaloceles that lacked a skin cover or in which the thin skin cover ruptured. Rappoport et al[103] found significant associated congenital anomalies such as microphthalmos, mental retardation, and syndactyly with appendicular constriction bands in 33% of these patients. In one patient with a large frontoethmoidal cephalocele, an arachnoid cyst overlying the right frontal lobe communicated with the external sac.

The anterior basal cephaloceles tend to occur in patients with more generalized cranio-facial-cerebral dysraphism manifested in part as a midline cleft upper lip, optic nerve dysplasias, and callosal dysgenesis.[19,106]

There are two major types, transethmoidal and transsphenoidal cephaloceles. The transethmoidal defects lie anteriorly, either along the midline or along the cribriform plate and do not involve the sella turcica. The hernia sac extends inferiorly into the sinuses or the nasal cavity and typically contains portions of the frontal lobes and olfactory apparatus.

The transsphenoidal cephaloceles extend downward through a defect in the floor of the sella turcica to reach the nasal cavity (see Fig. 1-11). If the palate is cleft, they may also extend further inferiorly into the oral cavity. The posterior margin of these defects is always the dorsum sellae. The lateral walls are the cavernous sinuses and the widely separated halves of the sphenoid bone. The anterior extent is very variable. The defect may involve the sella only, sella plus planum, or the sphenoid plus part of the posterior ethmoid bone. The latter form is sometimes designated *sphenoethmoidal cephalocele*.

Transsphenoidal cephaloceles typically contain the pituitary gland and the hypothalamus, the anterior recesses of the third ventricle, and the optic apparatus. Symptoms vary. In neonates and infants, the intranasal/pharyngeal soft tissue mass usually causes a runny nose, nasal obstruction, mouth breathing, or snoring. Frequently, these symptoms are ignored.[107] If noted, the intranasal lesions then discovered may be mistaken for nasal polyps exactly as is true for nasal gliomas.[81,108] If the early signs are not appreciated, the basal cephaloceles may not be detected until adulthood, when they tend to appear as visual disturbance, pituitary-hypothalamic dysfunction, or CSF rhinorrhea.[107]

Clinical diagnosis of basal cephalocele is achieved most easily by appreciating that cleft hypertelorism, median cleft upper lip with or without cleft nose, and optic nerve dysplasias are highly significant stigmata. They suggest the presence of basal cephaloceles, especially the transsphenoidal cephaloceles (see Table 1-2).[19,57]

REFERENCES

1. DeMyer W: Median facial malformations and their implications for brain malformations, Birth Defects (Orig Article Ser) 11:155, 1975.
2. Patten BM: The normal development of the facial region. In Pruzansky S, editor: Congenital anomalies of the face and associated structures, Springfield, Ill, 1985, Charles C Thomas, Publisher.
3. Johnston MC, Hassell JR, and Brown KS: The embryology of cleft lip and cleft palate, Clin Plast Surg 2:195, 1975.
4. Kawamoto HK Jr: The kaleidoscopic world of rare craniofacial clefts: order out of chaos (Tessier classification), Clin Plast Surg 3:529, 1976.
5. Davies J: Embryology and anatomy of the face, palate, nose and paranasal sinuses. In Paparella MM and Shumrick DA, editors: Otolaryngology, vol 1, Philadelphia, 1973, WB Saunders Co.
6. Arey LB: Developmental anatomy, Philadelphia, 1962, WB Saunders Co.
7. Corliss CE: Patten's human embryology, New York, 1976, McGraw-Hill, Inc.

8. Moore KL: The developing human, Philadelphia, 1977, WB Saunders Co.

9. Wilson DB: Embryonic development of the head and neck. III: the face, Head Neck Surg 2:145, 1979.

10. Badrawy R: Midline congenital anomalies of the nose, J Laryngol Otol 81:419, 1967.

11. Last RJ: Anatomy regional and applied, ed 6, London, 1978, Churchill-Livingstone, Inc, p 398.

12. Etter LE: Atlas of roentgen anatomy of the skull, rev ed 3, Springfield, Ill, 1970, Charles C Thomas, Publisher.

13. Henderson SG and Sherman LS: The roentgen anatomy of the skull in the newborn infant, Radiology 2:107, 1946.

14. Streeter GL: Developmental horizons in human embryo, 1948. In Paparella MM and Shumrick DA, editors: Otolaryngology, vol 1, Philadelphia, 1973, WB Saunders Co.

15. Langman J: Medical embryology: human development, normal and abnormal, ed 2, Baltimore, 1969, Williams & Wilkins.

16. Apple DJ, Rabb MF, and Walsh PM: Congenital anomalies of the optic disc, Surv Ophthal 27:3, 1982.

17. Steinkuller PG: The morning glory disk anomaly: case report and literature review, J Pediatr Ophthal Strabismus 17:81, 1980.

18. Yanoff M and Fine BS: Ocular pathology: a text and atlas, ed 2, Philadelphia, 1982, Harper & Row Publishers, Inc, p 608.

19. Naidich TP et al: Midline craniofacial dysraphism: midline cleft upper lip, basal encephalocele, callosal agenesis, and optic nerve dysplasia, Concepts Pediatr Neurosurg 4:186, 1977.

20. Probst FP: Congenital defects of the corpus callosum: morphology and encephalographic appearances, Acta Radiol (suppl) 331:1, 1973.

21. Rakic P and Yakovlev P: Development of the corpus callosum and cavum septi in man, J Comp Neurol 132:45, 1968.

22. DeMyer W: The median cleft face syndrome: differential diagnosis of cranium bifidum occultum, hypertelorism, and median cleft nose, lip and palate, Neurology 17:961, 1967.

23. Sedano HO et al: Frontonasal dysplasia, J Pediatr 76:906, 1970.

24. Gorlin RJ, Anderson VW, and Scott CR: Hypertrophied frenuli, oligophrenia, familial trembling and anomalies of the hand; report of four cases in one family and a forme fruste in another, N Engl J Med 264:486, 1961.

25. Townes PL, Wood BP, and McDonald JV: Further heterogeneity of the oral-facial-digital syndromes, Am J Dis Child 130:548, 1976.

26. Fogh-Anderson P: Rare clefts of the face, Acta Chir Scand 129:275, 1965.

27. Ingraham RD and Matson DD: Spina bifida and cranium bifidum. IV. An unusual nasopharyngeal encephalocele, N Engl J Med 228:815, 1943.

28. Avanzini G and Crivelli G: A case of sphenopharyngeal encephalocele, Acta Neurochir 22:205, 1970.

29. Baraton J et al: The neuroradiological examination of endocrine disorders of central origin in the child (precocious puberty, hypopituitarism), Pediatr Radiol 4:69, 1976.

30. Byrd SE et al: Computed tomography in the evaluation of encephaloceles in infants and children, J Comput Assist Tomogr 2:81, 1978.

31. Corbett JJ et al: Cavitary developmental defects of the optic disc: visual loss associated with optic pits and colobomas, Arch Neurol 37:210, 1980.

32. Danoff D, Serbu J, and French LA: Encephalocoele extending into the sphenoid sinus, J Neurosurg 24:684, 1966.

33. Ellyn F, Khatir AH, and Singh SP: Hypothalamic-pituitary functions in patients with transsphenoidal encephalocele and midfacial anomalies, J Clin Endocr Metab 51:854, 1980.

34. Exner A: Über basale Cephalocelen, Dt Z Chir 908:23, 1907.

35. Goldhammer Y and Smith JL: Optic nerve anomalies in basal encephalocele, Arch Opthal 93:115, 1975.

36. Jacob JB: Les Ménigo-encéphalocèles antérieures de la base du crane, Maroc Méd 40:73, 1961.

37. Koenig SB, Naidich TP, and Lissner G: The morning glory syndrome associated with sphenoidal encephalocele, Ophthalmology 89:1368, 1982.

38. Larsen JL and Bassoe HH: Transsphenoidal meningocele with hypothalamic insufficiency, Neuroradiology 18:205, 1979.

39. Lewin ML and Shuster MM: Transpalatal correction of basilar meningocele with cleft palate, Arch Surg 90:687, 1965.

40. Lichtenberg G: Congenital tumour of the mouth involving the brain and connected with other malformations, Trans London Soc Pathol 18:250, 1867.

41. Manelfe C et al: Transsphenoidal encephalocele associated with agenesis of corpus callosum: value of metrizamide computed cisternography, J Comput Assist Tomogr 2:356, 1978.

42. Modesti LM, Glasauer FE, and Terplan KL: Sphenoethmoidal encephalocele: a case report with review of the literature, Child's Brain 3:140, 1977.

43. Oldfield MC: An encephalocele associated with hypertelorism and cleft palate, Brit J Surg 25:747, 1938.

44. Pinto RS et al: Neuroradiology basal anterior fossa (transethmoidal) encephaloceles, Radiology 117:79, 1975.

45. Pollock JA, Newton TH, and Hoyt WF: Trans-sphenoidal and transethmoidal encephaloceles: a review of clinical and roentgen features in 8 cases, Radiology 90:442, 1968.

46. Sadeh M et al: Basal encephalocele associated with suprasellar epidermoid cyst, Arch Neurol 39:250, 1982.

47. Sakoda K et al: Sphenoethmoidal meningoencephalocele associated with agenesis of corpus callosum and median cleft lip and palate: case report, J Neurosurg 51:397, 1979.

48. Van Nouhuys JM and Bruyn GW: Nasopharyngeal transsphenoidal encephalocele, crater-like hole in the optic disc and agenesis of the corpus callosum: pneumo-encephalographic visualization in a case, Psychiatria Neur Neurochir 67:243, 1964.

49. Weise GM, Kempe LG, and Hammon WM: Transsphenoidal meningohydroencephalocele: case report, J Neurosurg 37:475, 1972.

50. Collier M and Adias L: Les anomalies congénitales des dimensions papillaires, Cliniq Ophtal 2:1, 1960.

51. Kindler P: Morning glory syndrome: unusual congenital optic disk anomaly, Am J Ophthal 69:376, 1970.

52. Krause U: Three cases of the morning glory syndrome, Acta Ophthal 50:188, 1972.

53. Malbran JL and Maria-Roveda J: Megalopapila, Archos Oftal B Aires 26:331, 1951.

54. Beyer WB, Quencer RM, and Osher RH: Morning glory syndrome: a functional analysis including fluorescein angiography, ultrasonography, and computerized tomography, Ophthalmology 89:1362, 1982.

55. Yock DH Jr: Choroid plexus lipomas associated with lipoma of the corpus callosum, J Comput Assist Tomogr 4:678, 1980.

56. Suemitsu T et al: Lipoma of the corpus callosum: report of a case and review of the literature, Child's Brain 5:476, 1979.

57. Zee CS et al: Lipomas of the corpus callosum associated with frontal dysraphism, J Comput Assist Tomogr 5:201, 1981.

58. Naidich TP et al: Median cleft face syndrome: MR and CT data from 11 children, J Comput Assist Tomogr 12:57, 1988.

59. Pascual-Castroviejo I, Pascual-Pascual SI, and Perez-Higueras A: Fronto-nasal dysplasia and lipoma of the corpus callosum, Euro J Pediatr 144:66, 1985.

60. Tessier P: Anatomical classification of facial, craniofacial, and lateral facial clefts, J Maxillofacial Surg 4:69, 1976.

61. Cohen MM et al: Frontonasal dysplasia (median cleft face syndrome): comments on etiology and pathogenesis, Birth Defects 7:117, 1971.

62. Warkany J, Bofinger MK, and Benton C: Median facial cleft

syndrome in half-sisters: dilemmas in genetic counseling, Teratology 8:273, 1973.

63. Bakken AF and Aabyholm G: Frontonasal dysplasia: possible hereditary connection with other congenital defects, Clin Genet 10:214, 1976.

64. Fontaine G et al: La dysplasie frontonasale, J Genet Hum 31:351, 1983.

65. Fragoso R et al: Frontonasal dysplasia in the Klippel-Feil syndrome: a new associated malformation, Clin Genet 22:270, 1982.

66. Francois J et al: Agenesis of the corpus callosum in the median facial cleft syndrome and associated ocular malformations, Am J Ophthalmol 76:241, 1973.

67. Fuenmayor HM: The spectrum of frontonasal dysplasia in an inbred pedigree, Clin Genet 17:137, 1980.

68. Hori A: A brain with two hypophyses in median cleft face syndrome, Acta Neuropathol 59:150, 1983.

69. Ide CH and Holt JE: Median cleft face syndrome associated with orbital hypertelorism and polysyndactyly, Eye Ear Nose Throat Monthly 54:37, 1975.

70. Kinsey JA and Streeten BW: Ocular abnormalities in the median cleft face syndrome, Am J Ophthalmol 83:261, 1977.

71. Roizenblatt J, Wajntal A, and Diament AJ: Median cleft face syndrome or frontonasal dysplasia: a case report with associated kidney malformation, J Pediatr Ophthalmol Strabis 16:16, 1979.

72. Aleksic S et al: Intracranial lipomas, hydrocephalus, and other CNS anomalies in oculoaricularvertebral dysplasia (Goldenhar-Gorlin syndrome), Child's Brain 11:285, 1984.

73. Gorlin RJ, Pindborg JJ, and Cohen MM Jr: Syndromes of the head and neck, New York, 1964, McGraw-Hill Co, p 10.

74. Shokeir MHK: The Goldenhar syndrome: a natural history, Birth Defects 13:67, 1977.

75. Kurlander GJ, DeMyer W, and Campbell JA: Roentgenology of the median cleft face syndrome, Radiology 88:473, 1967.

76. Scott JH: The cartilage of the nasal septum (a contribution to the study of facial growth), Br Dent J 95:37, 1953.

77. Mood GF: Congenital anterior herniations of brain, Ann Otol Rhinol Laryngol 47:391, 1938.

78. Naidich TP, Takahashi S, and Towbin RB: Normal patterns of ossification of the skull base: ages 0-16 years. Paper presented at the 71st Scientific Assembly and Annual Meeting, Radiological Society of North America, Chicago, Nov 19, 1985.

79. Sessions RB: Nasal dermal sinuses—new concepts and explanations, II. Laryngoscope 92:(suppl 29), 1982.

80. McQuown SA, Smith JD, and Gallo AE Jr: Intracranial extension of asal dermoids, Neurosurgery 12:531, 1983.

81. Choudhury AR and Taylor JC: Primary intranasal encephalocele: report of four cases, J Neurosurg 57:552, 1982.

82. Chaudhari AB et al: Congenital inclusion cyst of the subgaleal space, J Neurosurg 56:540, 1982.

83. Gorenstein A et al: Nasal gliomas, Arch Otolaryngol 106:536, 1980.

84. Card GG: Pathologic quiz, Arch Otolaryngol 104:301, 1978.

85. Pannell BW et al: Dermoid cysts of the anterior fontanelle, Neurosurgery 10:317, 1982.

86. Bradley PK: Nasal dermoids in children, Int J Pediatr Otorhinolaryngol 3:63, 1981.

87. Pensler JM, Bauer BS, and Naidich TP: Craniofacial dermoids, Plast Reconstr Surg 82:953, 1988.

88. Griffith BH: Frontonasal tumors: their diagnosis and management, Plast Reconstr Surg 57:692, 1976.

89. Mühlbauer WD and Dittmar W: Hereditary median dermoid cysts of the nose, Br J Plast Surg 29:334, 1976.

90. Plewes JL and Jacobson I: Familial frontonasal dermoid cysts: report of four cases, J Neurosurg 34:683, 1971.

91. Johnson GF and Weisman PA: Radiological features of dermoid cysts of the nose, Radiology 82:1016, 1964.

92. Black BK and Smith DE: Nasal glioma: two cases with recurrence, Arch Neurol Psychiatr 64:614, 1950.

93. Walker EA Jr and Resler DR: Nasal glioma, Laryngoscope 73:93, 1963.

94. Christianson HB: Nasal glioma: report of a case, Arch Derm 93:68, 1966.

95. Smith KR Jr et al: Nasal gliomas: a report of five cases with electron microscopy of one, J Neurosurg 20:968, 1963.

96. Witrak PJ, Davis PC, and Hoffman JC Jr: Sinus pericranii: a case report, Pediatr Radiol 16:55, 1986.

97. Suwanwela C and Hongsaprabhas C: Fronto-ethmoidal encephalomeningocele, J Neurosurg 25:172, 1966.

98. Kurzer A, Arbelaez N, and Cassiano G: Gliomas of the face: case report, Plast Reconstr Surg 69:678, 1982.

99. Finerman WB and Pick EI: Intranasal encephalo-meningocele, Ann Otol Rhinol Laryngol 62:114, 1953.

100. Suwanwela C and Suwanwela N: A morphological classification of sincipital encephalomeningoceles, J Neurosurg 36:201, 1972.

101. Blumenfeld R and Skolnik EM: Intranasal encephaloceles, Arch Otolaryng 82:527, 1965.

102. Simpson DA, David DJ, and White J: Cephaloceles: treatment, outcome and antenatal diagnosis, Neurosurgery 15:14, 1984.

103. Rappoport RL II, Dunn RC, and Alhady F: Anterior encephalocele, J Neurosurg 54:213, 1981.

104. Wakisaka S et al: Sinus pericranii, Surg Neurol 19:291, 1983.

105. Harverson G, Bailey IC, and Kiryabwire JWM: The radiological diagnosis of anterior encephalocoeles, Clin Radiol 25:317, 1974.

106. Cohen MM Jr and Lemire RJ: Syndromes with cephaloceles, Teratology 26:161, 1982.

107. Yokota A et al: Anterior basal encephalocele of the neonatal and infantile period, Neurosurgery 19:468, 1986.

108. Schmidt PH and Luyendijk W: Intranasal meningoencephalocele, Arch Otolaryngol 99:401, 1974.

2 Sinonasal Cavity

PETER M. SOM

SECTION ONE
INTRODUCTION TO THE SINONASAL CAVITY

ANATOMY AND PHYSIOLOGY

The external nose has an overall pyramidal shape.[1-4] The upper or cranial portion of the nose that joins the forehead is called the root. The lower or caudal free margin is known as the apex or tip. The upper midline margin that is supported by the nasal bones is called the bridge, and the more caudal midline, slightly curved ridge is referred to as the dorsum. The lateral nasal margins or sides have expanded, rounded lower aspects called the alae, which unite with the upper lip at the nasolabial sulcus. The caudal aspect of the mid-line nasal septum along with the nasal alae form the boundaries of the nostrils or nares, which are the external openings of the nose that provide entrance into the nasal fossa or nasal vault. The lower aspect of the nasal septum that borders the nostrils and merges with the nasolabial sulcus is called the columella (Fig. 2-1).

The two nasal bones are usually narrower and thicker on their cranial margins and wider and thinner on their caudal aspects. The medial articular surfaces are broader than the lateral margins. The posterior aspects of the nasal bones in the midline project backward and downward to form a small crest that contributes to the nasal septum. It articulates with the nasal process of the frontal bone, the perpendicular plate of the ethmoid bone and the septal cartilage of the nose (Fig. 2-2). Rarely, the nasal bones can be fused in the midline or absent and replaced by an elongated frontal process of the maxilla. The nasal bones can also very infrequently be multiple.

In the dried skull, the osseous opening of the nose is called the pyriform aperture. The lateral nasal cartilages attach to the upper edges of this aperture. There are five major nasal cartilages that form the main support of the lateral and lower nose. There are two lateral or upper nasal cartilages; two greater alar or lower nasal cartilages; and a median, septal or quadrangular cartilage. Frequently, the lateral nasal and septal cartilages are fused into a single cartilage, the nasoseptal cartilage. There are also a variable number of minor cartilages, which include two or three lesser alar cartilages and one or more accessory cartilages (Fig. 2-3). The alar cartilages are formed from elastic cartilage, while the remaining nasal cartilages are formed from hyaline cartilage. Both the bony bridge of the nose and the portion of the nasal dorsum formed by the lateral nasal cartilages have an intrinsic physical strength because they are supported in the midline by their fused opposite and thus form an archlike system. These structures are additionally supported in the midline by the septal cartilage. The greater alar cartilages have slender medial crura and broader lateral crura. The lateral crura are curved plates that form the boundaries of the lateral aspects of the nostrils. In supporting the alae of the nose, the greater alar cartilages are assisted by the lesser alar cartilages. The medial crura run together and join to form the mobile portion of the nasal septum and the support of the columella.[1-5]

The nasal cavities or nasal fossae are separated in the midline by the nasal septum. Each cavity is roughly pear-shaped, being narrow above and wide below (Fig.

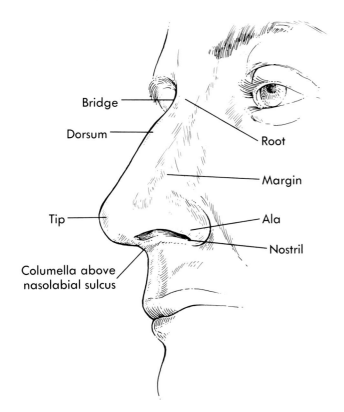

Fig. 2-1   Left anterior oblique view of nose.

Bridge

Dorsum

Root

Margin

Tip

Ala

Nostril

Columella above nasolabial sulcus

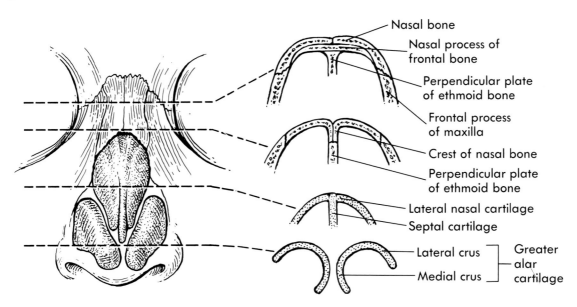

Nasal bone

Nasal process of frontal bone

Perpendicular plate of ethmoid bone

Frontal process of maxilla

Crest of nasal bone

Perpendicular plate of ethmoid bone

Lateral nasal cartilage

Septal cartilage

Lateral crus ⎤ Greater

Medial crus ⎦ alar cartilage

Fig. 2-2   Frontal view of nose with cross-sectional diagrams at various levels. (Modified from Anatomy for Surgeons, vol 1, The head and neck. New York, 1954, Harper and Brothers.)

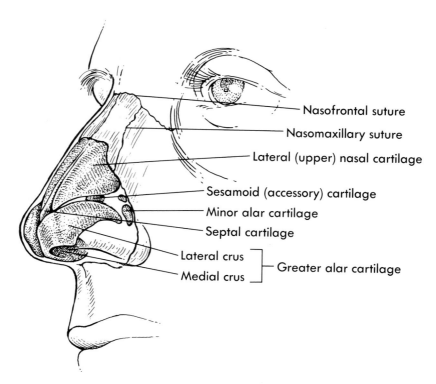

Nasofrontal suture

Nasomaxillary suture

Lateral (upper) nasal cartilage

Sesamoid (accessory) cartilage

Minor alar cartilage

Septal cartilage

Lateral crus ⎤
         ⎬ Greater alar cartilage
Medial crus ⎦

Fig. 2-3   Left anterior oblique view of nasal skeleton.

2-4). The roof is formed by the thin cribriform plate of the ethmoid. It is only 5 mm across at its widest posterior margin. The floor is formed by the hard palate. Anteriorly, the hard palate is formed by the palatine processes of the maxillae (anterior two-thirds of the hard palate) and posteriorly by the horizontal portions of the palatine bones (posterior one-third of the hard palate) (Fig. 2-5).

The anterior portion of the nasal fossa that corresponds to the alar region of the nose is called the vestibule. It is lined with skin that contains hairs and sebaceous glands. Along the nasal septum there is no line of demarcation between the vestibule and the remaining nasal fossa. However, along the lateral wall, there is a ridge, the limen vestibuli, that corresponds to the lower margin of the lateral nasal cartilage and marks the line of change from the skin of the vestibule into the mucous membrane of the remaining nasal fossa (Fig. 2-6).

The mucosa of the nasal fossa is a reddish, vascular, pseudostratified columnar ciliated epithelium that contains both serous and mucous glands (Schneiderian membrane). In the upper margins of the nasal fossa, in a region bounded laterally by the superior nasal concha with the lateral nasal wall above this level and medially by a corresponding portion of the nasal septum, there is a yellowish, less vascular, nonciliated epithelium that is the olfactory mucosa. It contains the bipolar olfactory nerve fibers that transform the physical and chemical stimuli into a nerve impulse, which is then transmitted

cranially via nerve fibers through the cribriform plate into the olfactory bulbs.[1-4] This mucosa secretes a lipo-lipid material that spreads evenly over the surface of the olfactory epithelium, keeping it moist. This is physiologically an important function since either odor or fragrance can be perceived only if the substance is in a solution. With a dried olfactory mucosa, therefore, there is no perception of smell.[2] Because there is no ciliary action on the olfactory mucosa, a person must sniff in order to bring the particulate material, via the olfactory recess, to this mucosa.

The mucosa lining the paranasal sinuses is very similar to that of the nonolfactory portion of the nasal fossa except it is less vascular, thinner, and more loosely attached to the bone.

The nose functions in breathing, warming, moisturizing, and cleaning the inspired air. The serous, watery secretions moisten the inspired air; it is estimated that about 2 L of water are produced daily by the serous glands, half of which is used to humidify the inspired air.[6] In addition, a surface film of mucus traps particulate matter. There is a coordinated ciliary action of the nasal mucosa that propels mucus backward and downward into the nasopharynx at the rate of about 1 cm per minute. This movement of mucus is also affected by gravity and traction that result from swallowing. It has been estimated that three-fourths of the bacteria entering the nose are trapped by the mucus and that this nasal mucous blanket is renewed about every 10 minutes.[6]

The major portion of the nasal septum is formed by

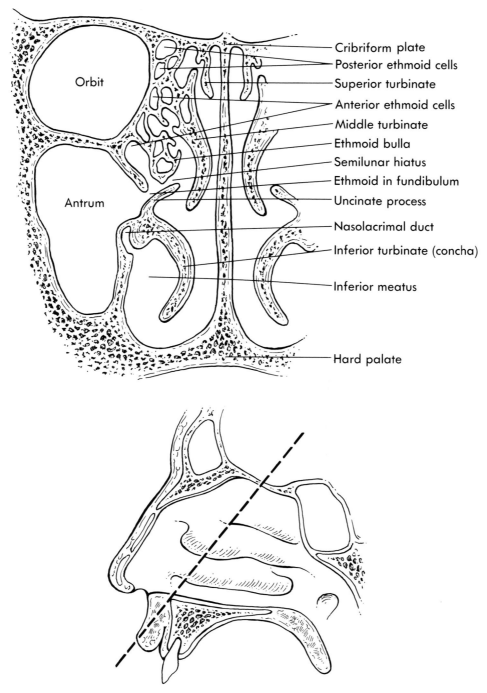

Cribriform plate
Posterior ethmoid cells
Superior turbinate
Anterior ethmoid cells
Middle turbinate
Ethmoid bulla
Semilunar hiatus
Ethmoid in fundibulum
Uncinate process
Nasolacrimal duct
Inferior turbinate (concha)
Inferior meatus
Hard palate

Orbit

Antrum

Fig. 2-4   Composite oblique section through the nasal fossae structures in a plane depicted in the smaller diagram. Some of the more important landmarks are identified.

the perpendicular plate of the ethmoid bone posteriorly and the septal cartilage anteriorly. The vomer completes the posteroinferior portion of the septum. The medial crura of the greater alar cartilages form the anteroinferior septal margin, or mobile septum. Nasal crests from the maxilla and palatine bones complete the inferior nasal septal margin (see Fig. 2-5). The proportionate size of the septal cartilage and the perpendicu-

lar plate of the ethmoid bone will vary from patient to patient. The septum provides the major support for the dorsum of the nose and the region below this, extending to the tip. Damage to the septal cartilage can result in a depressed, "saddle nose" deformity.

The septal cartilage has an unusual mobile articulation with the surrounding bones. The thin edge of the cartilage fits into a groove on the edge of the receiving

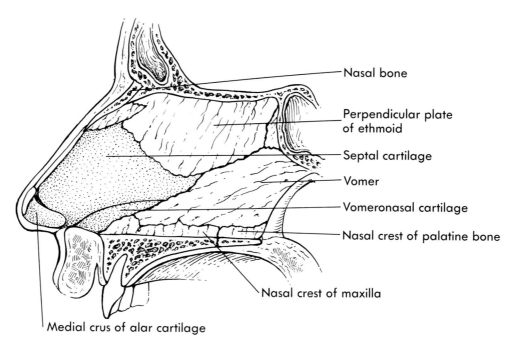

Nasal bone

Perpendicular plate of ethmoid

Septal cartilage

Vomer

Vomeronasal cartilage

Nasal crest of palatine bone

Nasal crest of maxilla

Medial crus of alar cartilage

Fig. 2-5   Diagram of lateral view of the nasal septum.

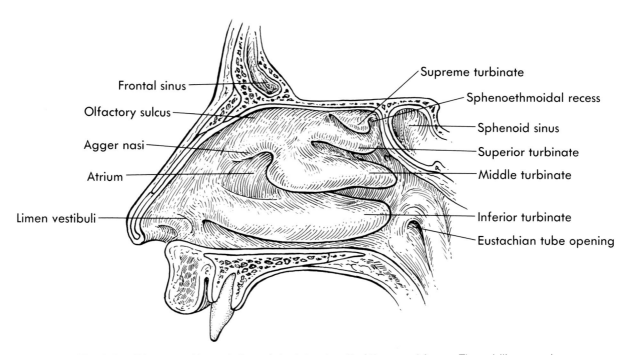

Frontal sinus

Olfactory sulcus

Agger nasi

Atrium

Limen vestibuli

Supreme turbinate

Sphenoethmoidal recess

Sphenoid sinus

Superior turbinate

Middle turbinate

Inferior turbinate

Eustachian tube opening

Fig. 2-6   Diagram of lateral view of the lateral wall of the nasal fossa. The midline nasal septum has been removed.

bones. Only connective tissue stabilizes this junction. This allows a mobility that minimizes the chance of fracture and allows considerable septal deviation without dislocation.

When compared to the medial septal wall, the lateral nasal wall is complex. The paranasal sinuses open into it, and three or four nasal turbinates or conchae project from it. These conchae are delicate, scroll-like projections of bone that are named, respectively, from below to upward, as inferior, middle, superior, and supreme turbinates. These structures become smaller as they ascend the nasal cavity.

The air space beneath and lateral to each concha is called the meatus. The inferior meatus thus lies beneath and lateral to the inferior turbinate. The middle and superior meati have similar relationships to their respective conchae (see Fig. 2-4). The supreme concha is present only in 60% of patients; the supreme meatus is usually only a small furrow beneath it.[1]

The dominant structures of the lateral nasal wall are the inferior and middle turbinates, which start anteriorly in a coronal plane at approximately the level of the forehead and extend posteriorly to the level of the back of the hard palate. At about half the distance between the anterior tip of the middle turbinate and the dorsum of the nose, on the lateral nasal wall, is a small bony projection, the agger nasi. It marks the location of the most anterior ethmoid or agger nasi cells. Above this, there is a narrow sulcus, the olfactory sulcus, that leads to the cribriform plate or roof of the nasal vault. Below and behind the agger nasi is a small depression, the atrium, which leads into the middle meatus proper. The superior concha starts anteriorly at about the mid-

portion of the middle concha and ends at about the same level posteriorly as both the inferior and middle turbinates. Just above the superior concha and behind, lying in front of the anterior wall of the sphenoid sinus is the sphenoethmoidal recess. The ostium of the sphenoid sinus usually opens into this space. The posterior tips of the superior and middle turbinates point directly to the anterior lip of the sphenopalatine foramen in the lateral nasal wall (see Fig. 2-5).

The inferior turbinate is an independent bone which is covered by a thick mucous membrane that contains a dense venous plexus, large vascular spaces and erectile tissue. The nasolacrimal duct is the only major ostium to open into the inferior meatus. This ostium usually lies high and anteriorly in the lateral nasal wall under the attachment of the inferior turbinate, approximately 2 cm posterior to the nostril. When the nasolacrimal duct opening is high in the inferior meatus, it tends to be wide. When it is located lower in the lateral nasal wall it tends to be slitlike. As it runs obliquely through the mucosa, it is protected by a fold of this mucous membrane known as the plica lacrimalis or valve of Hasner.

The middle turbinate is part of the ethmoid bone and like the inferior concha is also covered with some erectile tissue and a thick, vascular mucous membrane. The line of attachment of the middle turbinate is somewhat complex. Anteriorly it attaches superiorly to the lateral margin of the cribriform plate. About 1 cm posterior to the anterior tip of the turbinate, the line of attachment of the middle concha tilts laterally toward the lateral nasal fossa wall (medial portion of ethmoid labyrinth). This lateral line of attachment then gradually arches

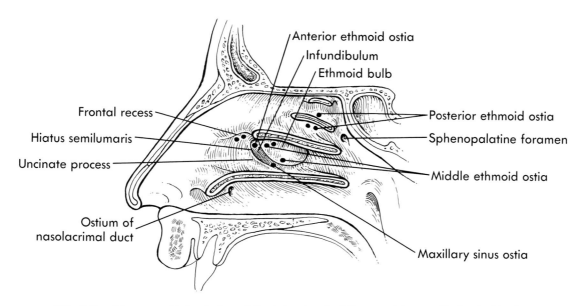

Fig. 2-7   Diagram of lateral view of the lateral wall of the nasal fossa with the turbinates removed. The most constant locations of the sinus ostia are indicated.

backward and downward along the lateral nasal fossa. The middle turbinate overhangs the important and somewhat complicated middle meatus. The highest part of the middle meatus is anterior and is known as the frontal recess. The nasofrontal duct draining the frontal sinus opens directly into this recess about 50% of the time, with some of the anterior ethmoid cells also opening separately into the recess. In the other 50% of cases, the frontonasal duct drains directly into the ethmoid cells, which in turn drain into the frontal recess. The middle meatus continues downward and backward as a slightly curved, semicircular slit, the hiatus semilunaris. It is into this slit that most of the remaining ethmoid cells and the maxillary sinus drain. It is delineated above by the ethmoidal bulla and below by the uncinate process of the ethmoid. The ethmoid bulla is a rounded bulge of the lateral nasal wall of the middle meatus, lying just beneath the attachment of the middle turbinate. The bulla represents the bony medial wall of the anterior and middle ethmoid cells, most of which open directly on or above the bulla (Fig. 2-7 and see Fig. 2-4).

The uncinate process of the ethmoid is a thin, slitlike projection of bone extending upward from the line of attachment of the inferior turbinate. The uncinate process has a variable height ranging from being absent to 22 mm. The average height is about 5 mm. Since the hiatus semilunaris is the space between the undersurface of the bulla and the top of the uncinate process, the width of the hiatus will vary inversely with the height of the uncinate process. Thus a tall uncinate process will create a narrow, slitlike hiatus semilunaris. Rarely, the overhanging ethmoid bulla can touch the uncinate process and effectively block the hiatus semilunaris. Normally, the greatest width of the hiatus is 3 mm (see Figs. 2-4 and 2-7).[1-4]

The ethmoidal infundibulum is a lateral and downwardly directed space that extends from the hiatus semilunaris. Its medial wall is the uncinate process, and the lateral infundibular wall is either partially or entirely membranous. The major ostium to open into the infundibulum is that of the maxillary sinus. This usually is situated in the posterior portion of the infundibulum. Alternately, this anatomy can be visualized from the maxillary sinus. The antral ostium is high on the medial sinus wall, and it does not open directly into the nasal fossa. Rather it opens into a narrow channel, the ethmoidal infundibulum, which in turn communicates with the nasal fossa via the hiatus semilunaris. This channel is about 5 mm in length. In nearly 40% of patients, accessory antral ostia also open into the infundibulum, as do some of the anterior ethmoid cells and the majority of the middle ethmoid cells.[1-4] The anterior aspect of the infundibulum usually is continuous with the frontal recess and the ostium of the frontal sinus (see Figs. 2-4 and 2-7).

From a clinical perspective, a high uncinate process and a deep, narrow ethmoidal infundibulum can render access to the antral ostium difficult or impossible; this situation occurs nearly half of the time. The region of the uncinate process, ethmoidal infundibulum, maxillary sinus ostium, middle turbinate, frontal recess, and the bulla ethmoidalis is referred to as the ostiomeatal complex.

Most of the posterior ethmoid cells drain into the superior meatus, and a posterior cell drains into the supreme meatus in three-fourths of the patients with supreme turbinates.

The teleologic explanation for the division of the nasal fossa by the nasal septum is that one nasal chamber can rest while the other carries on the functions of the nose.[4] This alternation of nasal function is referred to as a nasal cycle and is present in about 80% of patients. In such a normal nose, one side of the nasal fossa opens with production of serous and mucous secretions while the opposite airway closes with almost complete cessation of such activity. The passage of respiratory air is carried on almost entirely through the open nasal chamber. As the functioning side pours out serous and mucous secretion, the ipsilateral mucosa shrinks; concurrently there is shunting of blood to the opposite, highly vascular mucosa primarily over the inferior and middle turbinates. The nonfunctioning side retains secretions and becomes vascularly congested and engorged. The total nasal resistance or conductance tends to remain constant throughout the cycle. This nasal cycle is most common in the second through fourth decades of life and gradually decreases with progressive age.

The cycle varies from 30 minutes to 7 hours. The effect of gravity on the pooling of blood in the excessively vascular tissues over the turbinates is commonly demonstrated by the observation that in many patients, when they lie on one side, the dependent nasal chamber becomes progressively obstructed over a 15- to 20-minute period. When the patient turns to the opposite side, the clogged nasal fossa opens and the dependent chamber becomes congested in 10 to 15 minutes.[5]

Because there is both a superficial mucosal vascular plexis and a deep erectile vascular zone, there are four major responses that the nasal tissue can give depending on the nature of the inspired air: (1) Hyperemia of surface vessels and filling of the erectile, cavernous tissue in response to cold, dry air; (2) ischemia of the surface vessels and shrinkage of the erectile, cavernous tissue in response to warm, moist air; (3) ischemia of the surface vessels and filling of the erectile, cavernous tissue in response to warm air of average relative humidity; and (4) hyperemia of the surface vessels and shrinkage of the erectile, cavernous tissue in response to superficial irritation.[2]

The motor supply to the nasal respiratory muscles (the procerus, the nasalis, the depressor septi nasi) is mediated through the seventh cranial nerve. The integration of their contraction with the respiratory cycle is carried to the seventh cranial nerve via the tenth cranial nerve. The physiologically important control of the circulation and secretomotor function to the normal airway is mediated by the autonomic system, primarily via the sphenopalatine ganglion. Sympathetic stimulation results in a pale, dry, shrunken mucosa, while parasympathetic stimulation causes a hypersecreting, hyperemic, swollen mucosa. Pain, temperature, and touch are mediated by branches of the first division of the fifth cranial nerve.[6,7]

The vascular and nerve supplies of the nasal fossa almost anatomically coincide. One difference is that the nerves tend to pass out of the nose while the arteries are reinforced by vessels that pass into the nose.[2] The lymphatic drainage follows the veins rather than the arteries. The lymphatics of the anterior half of the nose drain across the face to enter into the submandibular lymph nodes. The lymphatics of the posterior half of the nose and nasopharynx drain into the retropharyngeal and internal jugular chain of nodes.

The venous drainage of the nose is into the anterior facial vein, then via the common facial vein to the internal jugular vein. The anterior facial vein also communicates with the ophthalmic veins, which drain either directly or via the pterygoid venous plexus into the cavernous sinus. Thus, infection of the nose may rapidly spread into the cavernous sinus.[6]

The vascular anatomy of the nasal fossa is complex, involving both external and internal carotid arterial supply. Of the five arteries that supply the mucoperiosteum of the nasal cavity, the sphenopalatine artery is the most important.[8]

The sphenopalatine artery originates from the third, or pterygopalatine, segment of the maxillary artery. Prior to its exit from the pterygopalatine fossa, the sphenopalatine artery occasionally gives rise to a posterior nasal branch. More commonly, it first exits from the superomedial aspect of the pterygopalatine fossa by way of the sphenopalatine foramen. The sphenopalatine artery then enters the nasal fossa behind and slightly above the middle concha.

The sphenopalatine artery has two major groups of branches: the posterior lateral nasal branches and the posterior septal branches. The posterior lateral nasal arteries ramify over the nasal conchae, first giving off branches that supply the inferior turbinate and then giving rise to superior branches that supply the middle and superior turbinates. These lateral nasal branches also assist in supplying the maxillary, ethmoid, and sphenoid sinuses.

After giving origin to the posterior lateral nasal branches, the main trunk of the sphenopalatine artery continues medially along the roof of the nasal cavity. When it reaches the nasal septum, the sphenopalatine

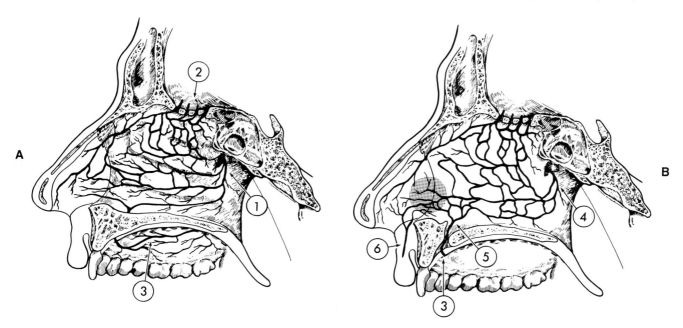

Fig. 2-8 Diagrams in lateral view of the vascular supply of the **A,** lateral nasal wall and **B,** The nasal septum. *1,* The posterior lateral nasal branches of the sphenopalatine artery; *2,* the anterior and posterior ethmoidal arteries; *3,* the greater palatine artery; *4,* the posterior septal branches of the sphenopalatine artery; *5,* the nasopalatine artery; and *6,* the septal branch of the superior labial artery. The area of Kiesselbach's plexus is in dots on **B**. (From Osborn AG: AJR 130:89, 1978. Copyright 1978, American Roentgen Ray Society.)

artery gives off its medial branches, the posterior septal arteries. These branches course anteriorly along the nasal septum. The most inferior of these branches becomes the nasopalatine artery. This vessel runs through the incisive canal to become continuous with the greater palatine artery (Fig. 2-8).

The anterior and posterior ethmoid arteries originate from the ophthalmic artery and send numerous small branches through the cribriform plate to anastomose with nasal branches of the sphenopalatine artery. This rich anastomotic network provides an important potential collateral pathway between the internal and external carotid circulations.

There are two other arteries that also provide some blood supply to the nasal fossa. The terminal branch of the greater palatine artery enters the incisive foramen, where it anastomoses with the nasopalatine artery (a septal branch of the sphenopalatine artery). The final artery supplying the nasal fossa is the septal branch of the superior labial artery. It originates from the facial artery and supplies the medial wall of the nasal vestibule.

Little's or Kiesselbach's area is a localized region of the anteroinferior nasal septum (see Fig. 2-8). It is supplied by branches of the facial, sphenopalatine and greater palatine arteries. This is often referred to as Kiesselbach's plexus and is the site of 90% of the cases of epistaxis.[1]

THE PARANASAL SINUSES

All of the paranasal sinuses originate as evaginations from the nasal fossae.[9] As such, they are lined by a mucosa similar to that found in the nasal cavity. It is a pseudostratified columnar ciliated epithelium that contains both mucous and serous glands.

Frontal Sinus

The frontal sinuses arise from one of several outgrowths originating in the region of the frontal recess of the nose. They are, in effect, displaced anterior ethmoid cells.[9,10] Because the frontal sinus develops from a variable site along the lateral nasal fossa, this sinus will, depending on its precise site of origin, drain via a nasofrontal duct into the frontal recess or more posteriorly directly into the anterior infundibulum. Less often, the frontal sinus will drain directly into the anterior ethmoid cells, which in turn open into the infundibulum or on the bulla ethmoidalis. The frontal sinuses are the only paranasal sinuses to be absent at birth, and they start to develop only after the second year of life.[11] The development is quite variable. They both fail to develop in only 4% of the population. On the average, by the age of 4 years the cranial extent of the frontal sinus reaches half the height of the orbit, extending just above the top of the most anterior ethmoid cells. By

the age of 8 years, the top of the frontal sinuses is at the level of the orbital roof, and by the age of 10 years, the sinuses extend into the vertical portion of the frontal bone. The final adult proportions are reached only after puberty.[1,11]

Because of the variable site of development of the frontal sinuses, the ethmoidal infundibulum acts as a channel for carrying the secretions (and infection) from the frontal sinus to some anterior ethmoid cells and the maxillary sinus only approximately 50% of the time. It is only in the patient whose nasofrontal duct opens directly in the frontal recess or above the infundibulum (85% of cases) that the frontal sinus is accessible to intranasal cannulation.

Factors implicated as influencing frontal sinus growth include a relationship between the cessation of frontal lobe growth and the development of the frontal sinus. Frontal lobe expansion normally ceases its anterior growth by age 7 years, at which time the inner frontal table stops its forward migration. Any further development of the frontal bone occurs secondary to anterior growth of the outer frontal table and sinus pneumatization. In the Dyke-Davidoff-Masson syndrome with underdevelopment of a hemicerebrum and in cases of early childhood damage to the frontal lobe, the ipsilateral frontal sinus is abnormally enlarged.[12,13] A direct relationship between the mechanical stresses of mastication and frontal sinus enlargement has been demonstrated, and a similar direct relationship with growth hormone also exists.[13,14]

In some patients a frontal bulla develops. This is an upward displacement of the frontal sinus floor caused either by encroachment from the opposite frontal sinus or more frequently by an underlying ethmoid cell. This bulla may influence frontal sinus drainage, and it has been implicated as a cause of chronic frontal sinusitis in some patients.[1]

Each frontal sinus is usually a single cavity, although duplication has been reported.[1] Usually the frontal sinuses are asymmetric in size. The larger one can cross the midsagittal plane so that a midline incision may inadvertently enter this sinus when the surgeon is attempting to enter the opposite smaller sinus.[1] The frontal sinus can pneumatize both the vertical and the horizontal (orbital) plates of the frontal bone. The former lies between the anterior and posterior cortical plates of the frontal bone, while the horizontal extension lies between the roof of the orbit and the floor of the anterior cranial fossa. The deepest area of the vertical portion of the sinus is near the midline, at the level of the supraorbital ridge.[15] The bone is thin here, and the sinus is best approached for a trephination at this level. This thin floor also permits the controlled fracture necessary in creating an osteoplastic flap of the frontal sinus.[15] The normal sinus borders tend to be serpentine or scalloped, and intrasinus septa may extend into the sinus from one-half to one-third the height of the sinus cavity. These are better developed in the larger sinuses, and the hypoplastic frontal sinuses may have only a single concave margin without any septation (see Fig. 2-10, B).

The intersinus septum is usually in the midline at the base or lower portion of the sinus. It may then deviate far to one side depending on the differential growth rates of the frontal sinuses (see Fig. 2-10, B). Although the septum is almost always complete, focal areas of acquired or congenital dehiscence can occur, which allow intercommunication between the two frontal sinuses or herniation of the mucosa of one sinus into the contralateral sinus.[9] The normal well-developed frontal sinus will abut the superomedial orbital margin, but it will not encroach on the orbit and remodel it. Any flattening of this orbital margin should suggest the presence of an expanding frontal sinus process (mucocele).

There is a rich venous plexus (Breschet's canals) that communicates both with the diploic veins and the dural spaces. The main arterial supply is via the supraorbital artery and the sinus lymphatics drain across the face to the submandibular lymph nodes.

Ethmoid Complex

The ethmoid sinuses begin formation in the fifth fetal month, when numerous separate evaginations arise from the nasal cavity. There is a great variation in the openings of these cells because they arise from diverticula that are situated above, on, or below the ethmoid bulla, any portion of the middle meatus, the frontal recess, or the superior meatus or above and behind the superior nasal concha.[1] These cells are present at birth and continue to grow and honeycomb the ethmoid bone either until late puberty or until the sinus walls reach a layer of compact bone. The adult ethmoid has 3 to 18 cells, and these cells are grouped as anterior, middle, or posterior, according to the location of their ostia.[15] The ethmoid complex averages $3.3 \times 2.7 \times 1.4$ cm in size, and the number and size of the ethmoid cells are inversely related. In general, the posterior cells are both larger and fewer than the anterior cells.

The ostia of the ethmoid sinuses are the smallest ones of any paranasal sinus. They measure only 1 to 2 mm in diameter.[15] The anterior ethmoid cells have smaller ostia than the posterior cells, a factor probably contributing to the higher incidence of anterior ethmoid mucoceles.[15]

The fetal support of the middle and superior turbinates is a partition of bone, the basal lamella, that continues from the base of the turbinates laterally through the mass of ethmoid cells to attach to the medial side of the lamina papyracea. In the case of the middle conchae, the basal lamella only extends from its more posterior portion where it is attached to the lateral nasal wall. No basal lamella is present along the anterior portion of the middle turbinate where it attaches to the lateral cribriform plate. The basal lamella for the superior turbinate is along the most posterior aspect of the lateral nasal vault. These two lamella thus divide the ethmoid cells into anterior, posterior, and postreme groups. In the adult, the lamella is not a straight dividing plate because the developing air cells have pushed and distorted the original straight partition that was present in the fetal ethmoid bone.[15] Usually in the adult, the actual lamellar bone cannot be distinguished from the adjacent ethmoid septa.

Most anatomists divide the ethmoid cells into anterior, middle, and posterior groups. The three groups are not sharply delineated from one another, however, and the anterior and middle groups are occasionally combined into a single "anterior" group. The anterior ethmoid sinuses are separated from the medial orbital wall by the lacrimal bone. The posterior ethmoid sinuses are separated from the orbits by the lamina papyracea.[16]

The anterior group, which can have up to 11 cells, opens into the ethmoidal infundibulum or into the hiatus semilunaris. The middle group opens into the middle meatus above the hiatus semilunaris, and the posterior group opens by one or more ostia into the superior meatus.[6,16]

Each ethmoidal labyrinth lies between the orbit and the upper nasal fossa. The left and right groups of ethmoid cells are connected in the midline by the cribriform plate (nasal roof) of the ethmoid bone. The crista galli extends from the midline upward into the floor of the anterior cranial fossa. The perpendicular plate of the ethmoid bone extends downward from the cribriform plate to help form the nasal septum. The medial wall of each ethmoid labyrinth is formed by a thin lamella of bone from which arise the middle, superior, and supreme turbinates (anteriorly, the attachment of the middle turbinate is at the lateral margin of the cribriform plate). The lateral ethmoid labyrinthian wall is formed anteriorly by the overlying lacrimal bone, while posteriorly it is formed by the thin lamina papyracea, which separates the ethmoid cells from the orbit. The lateral caudal margin of the ethmoid cell complex articulates with the maxilla forming the ethmoidomaxillary plate.

The roof of the ethmoid complex is formed by a medial extension of the orbital plate of the frontal bone, which projects to articulate with the cribriform plate. This is often referred to as the fovea ethmoidalis. The ethmoidal vessels and nerves pass into the ethmoid complex via the anterior and posterior ethmoidal canals. The upper portion of these canals is formed by the frontal bone, while the lower margins are formed by the ethmoid bone. Thus, a line connecting these canals identifies the frontoethmoid junction and is just below the dural line.

The anterior and middle ethmoid sinuses are supplied by the anterior ethmoidal nerve and vessels, and the lymphatics drain into the submandibular lymph nodes. The most anterior ethmoid cells, the agger nasi cells, are present in 90% of people and are situated anterior to the frontonasal duct. Rarely, the posterior ethmoid cells are supplied by the posterior ethmoidal nerve and vessels, and the posterior lymph drains into the retropharyngeal lymph nodes. Rarely, the posterior cells grow backward into the body of the sphenoid bone and essentially replace the sphenoid sinus, which compensates by being rudimentary. The ethmoid cells can pneumatize the middle turbinate (concha bullosa) (4% to 12%) and rarely the superior conchae or uncinate process.[15,17] The proximity of the posterior ethmoid cells to the orbital apex, optic canal, and optic nerve can give rise to loss of vision as a complication of surgery on these sinuses.

Sphenoid Sinus

The sphenoid sinuses emerge in the fourth fetal month as evaginations from the posterior nasal capsule into the sphenoid bone. This occurs just above a small crescent-shaped ridge of bone, the sphenoidal conchae, that projects from the undersurface of the body of the sphenoid bone. These conchae grow forward, fusing with the posterior ethmoid labyrinth. Complete absence of the sphenoid sinus is rare. The degree of pneumatization, however, varies considerably. The sinus starts its major growth in the third year of life and by age 10 to 12 years, the sinus usually has obtained its adult configuration.[10] The lack of any sinus pneumatization by the age of 10 years should suggest the possibility of "occult" sphenoid pathology.[18] The average sinus measures $2 \times 2 \times 1.5$ mm, and the posterior limit of the sinus is variable. In 60% of pneumatized sinuses, they extend posteriorly to the anterior sella wall and extend beyond this to lie under the sella floor. In 40% of the sinuses, they extend only to the anterior wall of the sella turcica. In less than 1% of cases, the sphenoid sinuses do not develop posteriorly enough to reach the anterior sella wall. In this latter group of patients, the thick bony posterior sinus wall is a contraindication to transsphenoidal hypophysectomy.[19]

The sphenoidal sinus septum is usually in the midline anteriorly, aligned with the nasal septum. However, from this point it can deviate far to one side, creating two unequal sinus cavities. With the exception of the sinus roof, the other sinus walls are of variable thickness depending on the degree of pneumatization. Even in poorly developed sinuses, the roof is thin, of-ten measuring only 1 mm. This wall is thus consistently vulnerable to perforation during surgery.

The anatomic relationships of the sphenoidal sinus are important because of the symptoms that can arise from disease in the sinus as well as the complications that can arise during surgery. From anteriorly to posteriorly, the sinus roof is in relationship to the floor of the anterior cranial fossa, the optic chiasm, and the sella turcica. The lateral wall is related to the orbital apex, the optic canal, the optic nerve, the cavernous sinus, and the internal carotid artery. Posteriorly are situated the clivus, prepontine cistern, pons, and basilar artery. The sinus floor is the roof of the nasopharynx, and the anterior sinus wall is the back of the nasal fossa. In well-pneumatized sinuses, ridges may project into the lateral sinus wall corresponding to the carotid artery and maxillary nerve and into the sinus floor corresponding to the vidian nerve canal.[20] Regions of bony dehiscence also have been reported.

In 48% of people, there are lateral recesses from the main sinus cavity that extend into the greater sphenoid wing as it forms the floor of the middle cranial fossa and the posterior orbital wall, the lesser sphenoid wing, or the pterygoid process. There is great variability between the degree of pneumatization on the left and right sides. The pterygoid process is pneumatized in 25% of cases and is extensively pneumatized in 8%.[21]

The normal drainage of each sphenoid sinus in the erect posture is entirely through ciliary action since the ostium is typically located 1.5 cm above the sinus floor. The ostium is usually 2 to 3 mm in diameter and 2 to 5 mm from the midline. Sinus septa occur, and they can interfere with gravity drainage of the sinus when tilting the head.

The sphenoid sinus receives its nerve supply from the posterior ethmoidal nerve. Its blood supply is from the maxillary artery, and the lymphatics drain into the retropharyngeal lymph nodes.[2]

Maxillary Sinus

The maxillary sinus is the first of the paranasal sinuses to form. At approximately the seventieth day of gestation, after each nasal fossa and its turbinates are already established, a small ridge develops just above the inferior turbinate that marks the future uncinate process. Shortly after this, an evagination starts just above this ridge and enlarges laterally from the nasal cavity. By birth, a rudimentary sinus approximately $7 \times 4 \times 4$ mm is present with its longest dimension in the anteroposterior axis.[13] The developing maxillary sinus initially lies medial to the orbit. The growth rate of the maxillary sinus has been estimated to be 2 mm vertically and 3 mm anteroposteriorly each year.[22] By the end of the first year, the lateral margin of the sinus extends under the medial portion of the orbit. The sinus reaches the infraorbital canal by the second year and passes infero-laterally to it during the third and fourth years. By the ninth year the lateral sinus margin extends to the malar bone. Lateral growth ceases at the fifteenth year.

In infancy, the maxillary sinus floor lies at the level of the middle meatus. By the eighth to ninth year the si-nus floor is near the level of the nasal fossa floor.[23] From this point there is considerable variation in the further growth of the lower recess of the sinus. If, in fact, the sinus continues to grow downward, it reaches the actual plane of the hard palate by age 12 years.

The final descent of the sinus, signaling the cessation of sinus growth, does not end until the third molar has erupted. In 20% of adults the most dependent portion of the maxillary sinus is above the nasal cavity floor; it lies at the same level in 15% of adults and below this level in 65% of adults.[23] The mean dimensions of the adult maxillary sinus are 34 mm deep, 33 mm high, and 23 mm wide. The average volume of the adult maxillary sinus is 14.75 ml.

Grossly, the maxillary sinuses tend to develop sym-metrically with only minor variations being common. Unilateral hypoplasia and bilateral hypoplasia occur, re-spectively, in 1.7% and 7.2% of people.[24] Hypoplasia of the maxilla will result from trauma, infection, surgical intervention, or irradiation that occurs during the de-velopment of this bone. These conditions can damage the maxillary growth center and produce a small maxilla and thus a hypoplastic sinus. Underdevelopment also occurs in first and second branchial arch anomalies such as Treacher Collins' syndrome and mandibulofacial dy-sostosis and in thalessemia major, where the demand for marrow prohibits sinus pneumatization.

The maxillary sinus lies within the body of the maxil-lary bone. Behind the orbital rims, each sinus roof, or orbital floor, slants obliquely upward so that the highest point of the sinus is in the posteromedial portion, lying directly beneath the orbital apex. The groove and canal for the maxillary nerve lie in the middle third of the si-nus roof. The medial antral wall is the inferolateral wall of the nasal cavity. The curved posterolateral wall sepa-rates the sinus from the infratemporal fossa. The ante-rior sinus wall is the facial surface of the maxilla, perfo-rated about 1 cm below the orbital rim by the infraor-bital foramen. Each sinus has four recesses: the zygo-matic recess, extending into the malar eminence or body of the zygoma; the palatine recess, small and vari-able and extending into the hard palate; the tuberosity recess, extending downward above and behind the third upper molar; and the alveolar recess, extending into the alveolar process of the maxilla.

The floor of the sinus is lowest near the second pre-molar and first molar teeth and usually lies 3 to 5 mm below the nasal floor. The roots of the three molar teeth often form conical elevations that project into the sinus floor. Less often, the roots of the premolar and, rarely, the canine teeth project into the antrum. Occa-sionally there is dehiscent bone over the tooth roots, and this results in only sinus mucosa covering these roots and separating them from the main sinus cavity.[15] The lower expansion of the antrum is intimately related to dentition, for when a tooth erupts, the space vacated by it becomes pneumatized, thus expanding the sinus lumen.

For the maxillary sinus, as well as for all of the other paranasal sinuses, the ostium is always located at the site of the initial embryonic evagination from the nasal chamber. In the case of the antrum, the ostium is on the highest part of the medial wall and is approximately 4 mm in diameter. It does not open directly into the nasal fossa, but rather into the ethmoidal infundibulum, which via the hiatus semilunaris opens into the nasal cavity. The channel of the infundibulum is approxi-mately 5 mm long and is directed upward and medially into the nasal fossa. The sinus ostial location dictates that sinus drainage in the erect position is accomplished by cilial action. A narrow infundibulum can further in-terfere with sinus drainage, as can intraantral septation that can compartmentalize portions of the maxillary si-nus. These uncommon septa usually divide the antrum into anterior and posterior sections, each of which may drain via accessory ostia into the nasal fossa. Rarely, a horizontal septum can divide the antrum into superior and inferior or medial and lateral portions.

In the adult skull, the medial wall of the maxillary bone has a large hole, the maxillary hiatus, that exposes the interior of the maxillary sinus. This hole is covered, in part, by portions of four bones. The perpendicular plate of the palatine bone lies posteriorly, while the lac-rimal bone is situated anterosuperiorly. The inferior turbinate covers the inferior portion of the maxillary hi-atus, and resting above the line of attachment of this turbinate is the uncinate process of the ethmoid bone. The remaining central portion of the maxillary hiatus is covered, respectively, by the nasal and sinus mucous membranes, in which are situated the infundibulum and maxillary ostium. This membranous area is impor-tant in efforts to irrigate the antrum. When the natural maxillary ostium cannot be clinically located, primarily because of a large uncinate process, the thin membra-nous area of the middle meatus can be penetrated.[15]

The nerve supply to the antrum is via branches of the second division of the trigeminal nerve; namely, the su-perior alveolar nerves (posterior, middle, anterior), the anterior palatine nerve, and the infraorbital nerve. Of these, the posterior superior alveolar nerve pierces the posterior antral wall and runs forward and downward in a small canal to supply the molar teeth. The lymphatics of the main sinus drain into the lateral retropharyngeal and internal jugular nodes, while those of the lateral portion of the antrum drain into the submandibular nodes.

REFERENCES

1. Hollinshead WH: The nose and paranasal sinuses. In Anatomy for surgeons, vol 1, The head and neck, New York, 1954, Hoeber-Harper Book, pp 229-281.
2. Last RJ: Anatomy regional and applied, ed 6, London, 1978, Churchill Livingstone, Inc, pp 398-406.
3. Goss CM, editor: Gray's anatomy of the human body, ed 27, Philadelphia, 1963, Lea & Febiger, pp 1167-1176.
4. Williams HL: Nasal physiology. In Paparella MM and Shumrick DA: Otolaryngology, vol 1, Basic science and related disciplines, Philadelphia, 1973, WB Saunders Co, pp 329-346.
5. Zinreich SJ, Kennedy DW, Kuman AJ, et al.: MR imaging of normal nasal cycle: comparison with sinus pathology, J Comput Assist Tomogr 12:1014, 1988.
6. Paff GH: Anatomy of the head and neck, Philadelphia, 1973, WB Saunders Co, pp 183-203.
7. Fried R: The hyperventilation syndrome: research and clinical treatment, Baltimore, 1987, The Johns Hopkins University Press.
8. Osborn AG: The nasal arteries, AJR 130:89, 1978.
9. Schaeffer JP: The embryology, development and anatomy of the nose, paranasal sinuses, nasolacrimal passageways and olfactory organs in man, Philadelphia, 1920, P. Blakiston's Son & Co.
10. Van Alyea OE: Nasal sinuses: anatomic and clinical consideration, Baltimore, 1942, Williams & Wilkins.
11. Dodd GD and Jing BS: Radiology of the nose, paranasal sinuses and nasopharynx, Baltimore, 1977, Williams and Wilkins.
12. Enlow DH: Handbook of facial growth, Philadelphia, 1975, WB Saunders Co, pp 120-121.
13. Shapiro R and Schorr S: A consideration of the systemic factors that influence frontal sinus pneumatization, Invest Radiol 15:191, 1980.
14. Clementine C, editor: Gray's anatomy of the human body, ed 30, Philadelphia, 1985, Lea & Febiger, p 299.
15. Ritter RN: The paranasal sinuses: anatomy and surgical technique, ed 2, St. Louis, 1978, The CV Mosby Co.
16. Goss CM, editor: Gray's anatomy of the human body, ed 27, Philadelphia, 1963, Lea & Febiger.
17. Zinreich SJ, Mattox DE, Kennedy DW, et al.: Concha bullosa: CT evaluation, J Comput Assist Tomogr 12:778, 1988.
18. Fujioka M and Yound LW: The sphenoidal sinuses: radiographic pattern of normal development and abnormal findings in infants and children, Radiology 129:133, 1978.
19. Yanagisawa E and Smith AW: Normal radiographic anatomy of the paranasal sinuses, Otolaryngol Clin North Am 6(2):429, 1973.
20. Pandolfo I, Gaeta M, Blandino A, et al.: The radiology of the pterygoid canal: normal and pathologic findings, AJNR 8:479, 1987.
21. Etter LE: Atlas of roentgen anatomy of the skull, Springfield, Ill, 1955, Charles C Thomas, Publisher.
22. Proetz AW: Essays on the applied physiology of the nose, ed. 2, St. Louis, 1953, Annals Publishing Co.
23. Alberti PW: Applied surgical anatomy of the maxillary sinus, Otolaryngol Clin North Am 9(1):3, 1976.
24. Karmody CS, Carter B, and Vincent ME: Developmental anomalies of the maxillary sinus, Trans Am Acad Ophthalmol Otolaryngol 84(4, Part 1):723, 1977.

SECTION TWO
IMAGING

RADIOGRAPHIC TECHNIQUE
Plain Films

Although numerous radiographic views are available for the plain film evaluation of the paranasal sinuses, only four of these projections are normally employed in the routine examination. These consist of two frontal projections, the Caldwell view and the Waters view, a base (submentovertex) view, and a lateral view. Supplemental studies occasionally may be employed. These include the oblique projection (Rhese view), other craniocaudal angulations of the frontal projection (transorbital, posteroanterior projections), Towne views, the Granger view, and the modified Waters view.[1,2]

The paranasal sinus radiographic examination should include a lateral film with a horizontal beam, taken either as a cross-table lateral film or with the patient erect. This allows any free fluid present to be clearly identified as an air-fluid level. If instead the film is taken with an overhead beam with the patient prone or supine, with the head turned to the side, the fluid will layer out along the dependent wall and no air-fluid level will be demonstrated.

Horizontal Beam 5 Degrees Off-Lateral View

With the patient's head in a lateral position relative to the cassette, the nose is then rotated 5 degrees toward the cassette from the true lateral position. If the patient is seated, the cassette is usually placed in the vertical position. If lying down, the patient is placed in either the semiprone or the prone position, and the cassette is positioned horizontally. The central ray enters perpendicular to the cassette and is centered at the outer canthus of the eye in the middle of the film. The orbitomeatal line is parallel to the base of the film (Fig. 2-9). The purpose of using the 5 degree off-lateral view rather than the true lateral view is to rotate the poste-

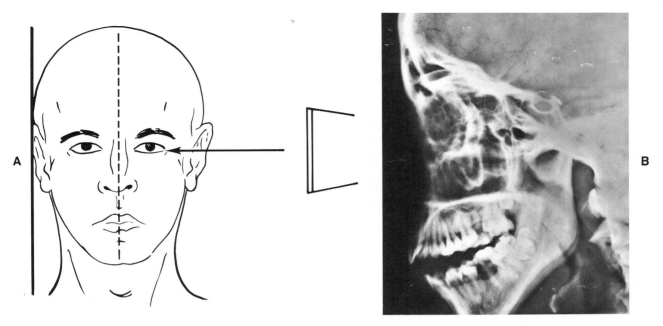

Fig. 2-9   Lateral view. **A,** Positioning diagram. **B,** Sample radiograph.

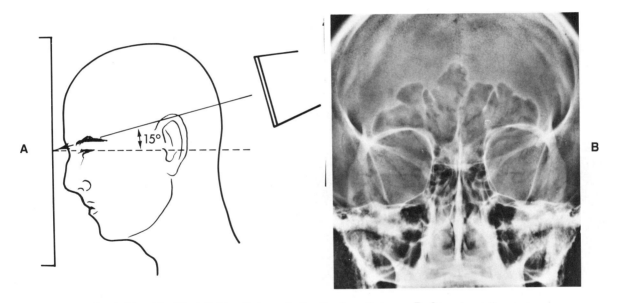

Fig. 2-10   Modified Caldwell view. **A,** Positioning diagram. **B,** Sample radiograph.

rior walls of the maxillary antra slightly so that they do not superimpose on one another in this projection. This permits evaluation of the integrity of the bony margins of the posterior aspect of the maxillary antra individually.

Modified Caldwell View

The patient is positioned directly facing the cassette in either the sitting or the prone position. The midsag-

ittal plane is perpendicular to the film. The orbito-meatal line is perpendicular to the cassette, and the central ray is angled 15 degrees caudally as it enters the posterior skull. The central ray also serves as the centering point of the skull on the cassette. Properly positioned, this view projects the petrous pyramids in the lower third of the orbits (Fig. 2-10). The Caldwell view is the best projection for examining the frontal and ethmoid sinuses in the frontal projection.

Modified Waters View

The patient is positioned facing the cassette in either the erect or the prone position. The orbitomeatal line is angled 37 degrees to the plane of the cassette. The central ray is centered on the film perpendicular to the cassette, emerging at the anterior nasal spine of the patient (Fig. 2-11, *A*).

Variations in the positioning angle may be required to give the "perfect" Waters view. On one hand, if the head is not extended sufficiently, the petrous pyramids will be projected over the maxillary sinuses, thereby obscuring sinus detail. On the other hand, if the head is hyperextended, the maxillary sinuses become distorted and foreshortened, thus obscuring sinus disease. The "perfect" Waters view has the petrous pyramids projected just below the floor of the sinus cavities. This is the best single view for evaluation of the maxillary antra in the frontal projection. Another variation is to use the Mahoney modification with the mouth open.[2] The open-mouth Waters view normally allows good visualization of the lower posterior sphenoid sinus margins (Figs. 2-11, *B* and *C*).

Modified Base (Submentovertical or Submentovertex) View

The modified base view was described by Schuller and Pfeiffer.[2] The reference line used is the infraorbital line, which runs from the infraorbital margin to the

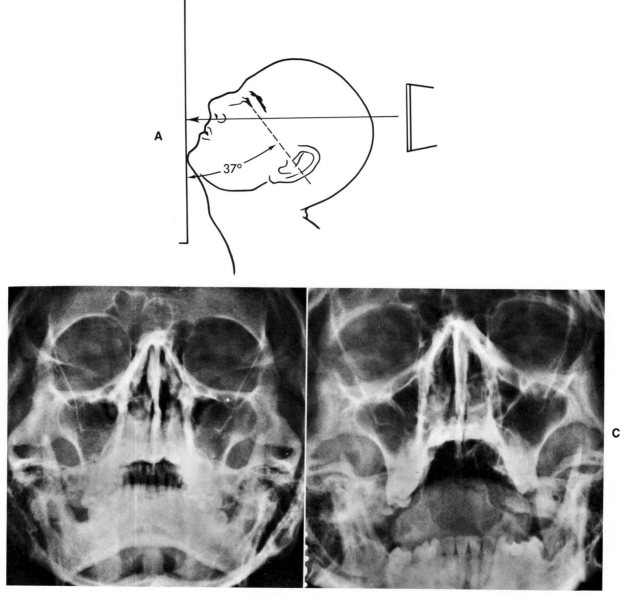

Fig. 2-11   Modified Waters view. **A,** Positioning diagram. **B,** Sample closed mouth radiograph. **C,** Sample open mouth radiograph.

center of the external auditory meatus. The goal of the positioning is to have the infraorbitomeatal line parallel to the film plane. This projection is considerably easier to obtain in either the sitting (erect) or the prone position. Patients with cervical or thoracic degenerative disease, those with a short neck, or those who are obese will have difficulty extending the head sufficiently if the examination is attempted with the patient supine. The central ray is directed perpendicular to the infraorbitomeatal line and centered ¾ inch anteriorly to the plane of the external auditory meatus (Fig. 2-12). A modification, with the centering 1½ inches in front of the external auditory meatus, has also been suggested.

A variation of the traditional submentovertex view is the Welin or overangulated base view. The view results in an average angle of 120 degrees open posteriorly between the infraorbitomeatal line and the cassette. This overangulation is accomplished by tilting the cassette top toward the patient with the patient's head fully extended in the modified base projection. The central ray is directed to the level of the frontal sinus. This position is a useful adjunct view for evaluation of the anterior and posterior walls of the frontal sinuses (Fig. 2-13). It is also a good view for evaluating the lateral, and to a lesser extent, medial walls of the maxillary antra. The sphenoid and ethmoid sinuses, with the nasal cavity superimposed, are thrown into relief with this projection.

Rhese or Oblique View

The Rhese view is excellent for study of the posterior ethmoid air cells, which are otherwise obscured by superimposition of the anterior cells in the frontal views. Superimposition of the anterior right and left ethmoid cells in the Rhese view, however, tends to limit its use-

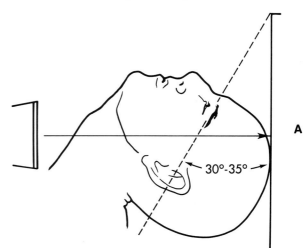

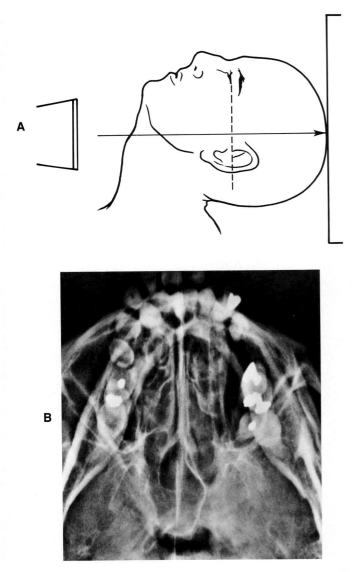

Fig. 2-12   Modified base view. **A,** Positioning diagram. **B,** Sample radiograph.

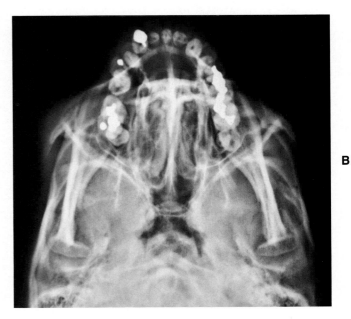

Fig. 2-13   Overangulated base view. **A,** Positioning diagram. **B,** Sample radiograph.

fulness in paranasal sinus examination. Correct positioning will have the optic canal placed just off the midorbit in the lower outer quadrant. Each side is taken separately and then compared. The patient is placed in either a seated erect position or the prone position. Then the median sagittal plane of the body is centered to the midline of the cassette. With the orbit centered in the portion of the cassette to be used, the flexion of the head is adjusted so that the canthomeatal line is perpendicular to the film. The patient's head is rotated so that the median sagittal plane forms an angle of 53 degrees with the plane of the film. The central ray enters the skull posteriorly at an angle of 15 degrees with the canthomeatal line and emerges at the midorbit

(Fig. 2-14).[2] Short of sectional imaging, the oblique views, coupled with a Caldwell view, provide the least obscured images of the ethmoid cells.

Nasal Bone Lateral View

The patient is usually placed in a semiprone position, with the body rotated so that the median sagittal plane

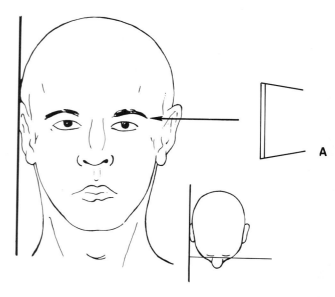

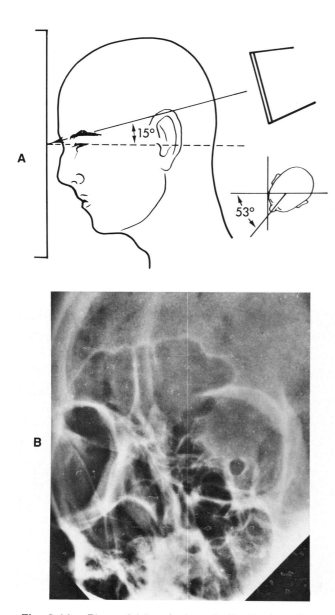

Fig. 2-14 Rhese (oblique) view. **A,** Positioning diagram. **B,** Sample radiograph.

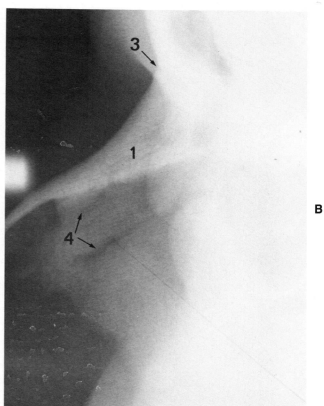

Fig. 2-15 Lateral nasal bone view. **A,** Positioning diagram. **B,** Sample radiograph.

of the head is horizontal and parallel to the plane of the table top. The interpupillary line is also perpendicular to this plane. The flexion of the head should be such that the orbitomeatal line is parallel with the transverse axis at the table top. The jaw should be supported with a sandbag to prevent rotation. The film is placed under the frontonasal region and centered at the nasion. The focal-film distance should be 36 inches (Fig. 2-15).

Nasal Bone Axial View

The success of this projection depends on either having the patient hold the occlusal film correctly between the front teeth or placing the larger film cassette under the patient's chin so that the plane of the film is at right angles to the glabelloalveolar line. The central ray should be directed along this line at right angles to the plane of the film (Fig. 2-16).

SECTIONAL IMAGING TECHNIQUES
Computed Tomography

The sinonasal cavities are well suited for investigation by computed tomography (CT). Because the imager is as interested in soft tissue disease as in bony changes, each scan should be photographed at an appropriate

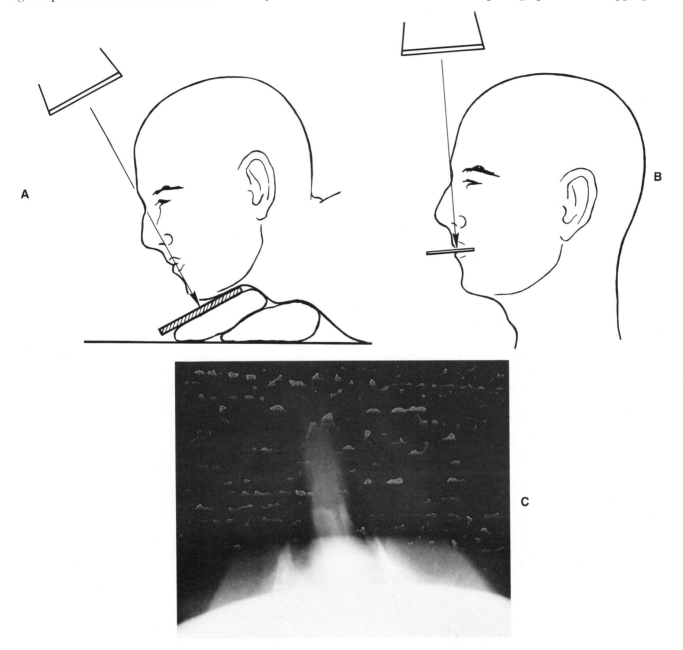

Fig. 2-16 Axial nasal bone view. **A,** Positioning diagram with film under chin. **B,** Positioning diagram with film in teeth. **C,** Sample radiograph.

window level to optimize both subtle soft tissue differences in attenuation and fine bony detail. Unfortunately, there is no one combination of window and center (level) settings that accomplishes both of these aims. The soft tissues are best shown at narrow windows that allow easy discrimination between attenuation values of muscle, fat, tumor, and the like and prompt detection of any enhancement differences on postcontrast CT scans. These soft tissue settings range in window values from around 150 to 400 HU. Conversely, the bony detail is best seen at wide window settings. These bone window settings are in the range of 2000 to 4000 HU, with the higher windows providing the finer bony resolution. In addition to being able to evaluate the gross architectural structure of the bone, these wide windows also allow the most accurate evaluation of air–soft tissue interfaces. The algorithms in use in virtually every CT device have difficulty in handling the abrupt transition from very low (air) and very high (bone) attenuation regions. This is especially noticeable when the devices are set at narrow window parameters. In this circumstance the air spaces and bone appear slightly larger than when they are viewed at wide window settings; the more accurate appearance correlates with the wide window settings. This same phenomenon creates volume averaging errors within air and bone at narrow window settings. Thus, small soft tissue masses will be obscured by any surrounding air, and focal areas of bone erosion may not be seen at narrow window settings. It is at the wide window settings that the air–soft tissue interface as well as focal bony changes are most accurately visualized.

The basic CT scanning protocol should include all of the paranasal sinuses, hard palate, and maxillary teeth. This scan volume also will include the skull base, orbits, and nasopharynx. Thus, all of the areas that contribute to the majority of sinonasal cavity pathology will be included in the study.

The study is performed with the patient supine. The preferred scan plane is the inferior orbitomeatal (IOM) plane, and that can be easily ascertained from a lateral scout film (i.e., the gantry angle). In addition, the top of the frontal sinuses and the maxillary teeth can be localized easily from the scout film; these define the upper and lower limits of the examination. The routine study should be obtained with 5 mm thick contiguous scans throughout the scan volume. Narrower slice thicknesses are usually not necessary unless a specific region of interest is present, in which instance a few thin sections (1.5 to 2.0 mm) can be obtained through this area.

In the IOM plane, there are three critical bony regions that are essentially parallel to the scan plane: the floor of the anterior cranial fossa, portions of the orbital floor, and the hard palate. Since knowledge of extension of disease across these bony planes is critical for the surgeon in determining some surgical procedures (i.e., antral tumor growing into the orbit, nasoethmoid or sphenoid tumors growing into the anterior cranial fossa), when imaging of these bony planes is essential, *coronal scans also should be obtained*. Additionally, if the CT scan is being performed to evaluate the osteomeatal complex, coronal scans also must be performed.

Because most adult patients have dental amalgams or metal bridges that cause considerable degradation of the CT images, direct 90-degree coronal scans (to the IOM plane) are of little diagnostic value. In addition, many patients cannot sufficiently extend their necks (because of pain, vertigo, arthritis, or others) in either the supine or prone position to obtain such 90-degree coronal studies. In general, a scan plane is chosen that extends from a caudad margin just anterior to the dental fillings to a cephalad point just posterior to the study area (i.e., orbit, sphenoid). These coronal studies are routinely obtained as 5 mm thick contiguous slices. However, if the examination is being performed to evaluate the osteomeatal complex, thin slices (1.5 mm) should be obtained. Similarly, if there is a localized area of interest in the coronal study, slices thinner than 5 mm can be taken through this area.[3,4]

Whenever possible, postcontrast studies should be obtained, since differential contrast enhancement may help accurately localize both normal and pathologic structures. This is especially evident when trying to distinguish whether a nasal mass extends into an adjacent sinus or if there is any intracranial extension of disease. Contrast media can be administered by two methods. The first uses one of the commercially available concentrated drip contrast materials. The examination is started when a third to a half of this contrast material has run into the patient. This technique will give good postcontrast scans (especially with the newer, faster CT scanners), provided the examination is completed while the contrast medium is still running. However, there is a waiting time for the initial contrast material "to load" the patient. This in turn delays patient put-through on the machine. A modification of this technique is to give an initial "loading dose" of 20 to 50 ml of regular contrast material and then run in the concentrated drip. This allows scanning to begin immediately and provides a longer interval over which the study can be done with the drip still running.

Magnetic Resonance Imaging (MRI)

MRI offers several advantages over CT in that there is no radiation as an inherent part of the examination and at present there is no consistent need for contrast material. Even if gadolinium DTPA is used, it has virtually no associated incidence of adverse reactions. In addition, multiplanar image acquisition is attainable while the patient lies supine. The soft tissue definition is superior to that of CT, and although bone cannot be directly imaged, invasion of bone marrow spaces and gross bone erosion can be identified.[5,6] However, fine bone alterations are not well seen on MRI and are far better demonstrated on CT. The basic MRI examination should be performed in the transverse (axial) plane with scan slices no thicker than 5 mm. A narrow interslice distance (1 mm) is suggested, and a spin echo long TR (time to repetition) and short and long TEs (time to echo) should be used to produce a proton density weighted image (PDWI, also called a mixed or balanced image because it has both T_1 and T_2 information variably present in it) and a T_2 weighted image (T_2 WI). Coronal scans can then be obtained, these being easily localized off the transverse studies. If the pathology is best demonstrated on the transverse T_2 WIs, then coronal T_2 studies should also be obtained. The TR can, to some degree, be varied to help limit the total duration of the MRI study. In addition, with a longer TR, more spin echo scan slices can be obtained on a single scan sequence. These variables can be used to obtain optimal MRI parameters. Usually the TR will vary from 1800 to 3000 msec while the TE will vary from 20 to 35 msec for the first echo and 75 to 120 msec for the second echo, depending on the magnet size and the manufacturer. T_1 weighted images (T_1 WIs) will provide the clearest anatomic detail, and these studies can be obtained whenever such detail is needed. Usually the TR will be 300 to 450 msec and the TE will be 20 to 35 msec. Sagittal scans have the greatest application near the midline, detailing the roof of the nasal fossae, ethmoid complex, sphenoid roof, and palatal region. Sagittal scans can also nicely demonstrate the orbital roof and floor in specific cases. One of the greatest challenges for the imager is to tailor the examination to each patient so that all of the necessary information is accumulated without unduly lengthening the MRI examination and thereby limiting the patient put-through.

If gadolinium (Gd) DTPA is used, T_1W scans are obtained in order to evaluate any T_1 relaxation time shortening. These scans can be obtained immediately after injection of the gadolinium or up to 30 minutes after this injection. This time interval allows the MRI to be done without significantly reducing any enhancement effect.

PLAIN FILM AND SECTIONAL IMAGING ANATOMY

Despite the most careful and meticulous attention to technical detail, plain film examinations have substantial limitations. Even if interpreted by a knowledgeable radiologist, soft tissue disease and bone destruction, if present, will be underestimated consistently. Because of comparatively low cost, availability, low radiation dose, and ease of the examination, plain film studies are still the most frequent initial study. It behooves the radiologist, therefore, to become fluent in the language of plain film sinonasal anatomy in order to then move with ease and assurance through the visual thicket of normal radiographic anatomy and it variants. Facility in this regard must be achieved before mastery in the analysis of the pathologic case is possible. The role of the radiologist in evaluating disease in the sinonasal cavities is heightened when one considers that the clinician has direct observation of only a small portion of the volume of interest: the middle and lower nasal fossae. Clearly, radiography provides the most thorough noninvasive evaluation of the nasal cavity and paranasal sinuses.

This section addresses the normal sinonasal anatomy as seen on plain films, multidirectional tomography, CT and MRI scans. The common denominator leading to the successful interpretation of all of these examinations is the anatomy itself, and once this is learned, its depiction as rendered by any specific modality will be clear and easily approached. Technology per se is irrelevant, as long as it meets the final test of delineation of structure.

The normal sinonasal anatomy will be presented in two sections. The first discusses the normal anatomy as seen on plain films and contains a presentation of anatomic variants and potential problems that are created by overlying soft tissue structures and bones.[7-12] The second section presents sectional (tomographic) anatomy[13-18] and is illustrated with CT and MR images.

Plain Film Anatomy

The Frontal Sinuses. The vertical portion of the frontal bone—and thus the main portion of the frontal sinuses—is best visualized in the Caldwell and Waters projections (see Figs. 2-10 and 2-11). On occasion, the Rhese view can better display some of the sinus contours, particularly in the smaller sinuses (see Fig. 2-14). The anterior and posterior sinus walls are best evaluated in the lateral and base (submentovertex) views (Fig. 2-17 and see Fig. 2-9). However, in these projections, only those portions of the sinus walls parallel to the incident beam (perpendicular to the film plane) are visualized. The adjacent curvilinear surfaces are obliquely oriented to the incident x-ray beam and only contribute to the perceived density of the adjacent calvarium. Thus, on the lateral view, only the midsagittal anterior and midsagittal posterior frontal sinus tables are visualized; while on the base view (depending on the angulation and the particular curvature of the skull), it is usually the caudal portions of the sinus walls that are identified. It is important to remember that only these limited areas of the frontal sinus anterior and

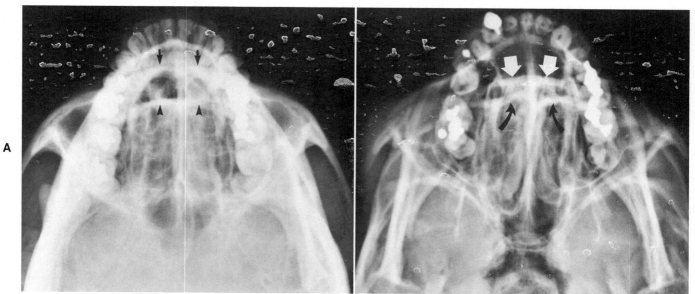

Fig. 2-17 **A,** Base view, slightly underpenetrated. This projection nicely displays the zygomatic arches and the anterior *(arrows)* and posterior *(arrowheads)* frontal sinus walls, which are projected over the teeth and palate. **B,** Overangulated base view with the anterior table of the frontal sinus *(large arrows)* and the posterior table *(curved arrows)* projected over the palate and nasal structures.

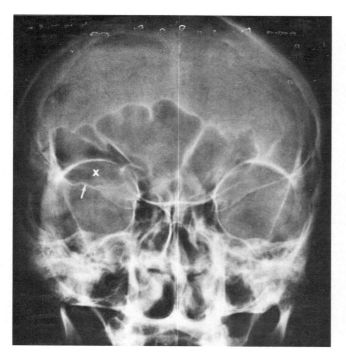

Fig. 2-18 Caldwell view shows well developed frontal sinuses. On the right side, the sinus pneumatizes the roof of the orbit. This is seen as air *(x)* contained within a thin white sinus margin *(arrow)* that is projected through the orbit.

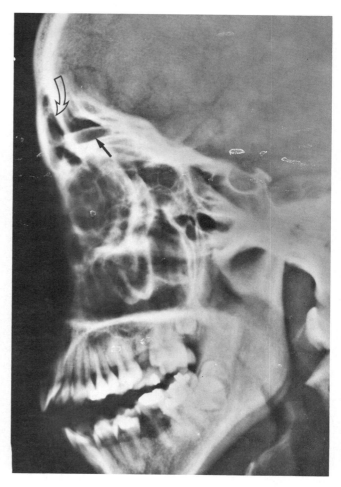

Fig. 2-19 Lateral view shows frontal sinus to extend anteriorly and vertically into the frontal bone *(curved open arrow)* as well as posteriorly and horizontally into the orbital roof *(arrow)*.

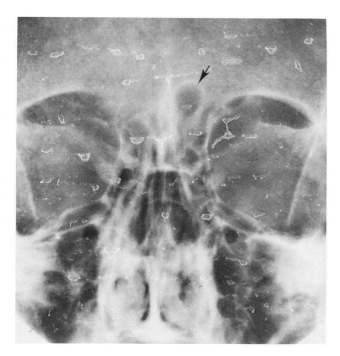

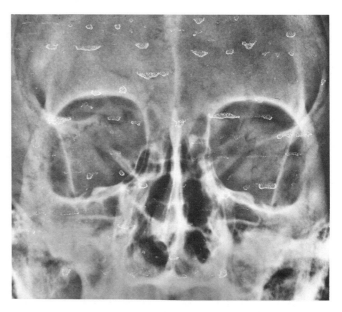

Fig. 2-21   Caldwell view shows bilateral hypoplastic frontal sinuses.

Fig. 2-20   Caldwell view shows aplastic right frontal sinus and hypoplastic left frontal sinus *(arrow)*. Note the smooth rounded contour of the hypoplastic sinus.

posterior walls are seen routinely on these projections. One may not assume that the entire sinus table is normal simply because it appears intact on the lateral or base views. This is especially true in suspected fractures of the posterior table or if an erosion of this bone is in question. Sectional imaging will clarify the issue.

The horizontal portion of the frontal sinus is best seen in Caldwell and lateral views (Fig. 2-18 and see Fig. 2-17). The depth of this recess can be best assessed by evaluating the posterior extent of pneumatization in the bony roof of the orbit as seen in either lateral or Waters projections (Fig. 2-19).

Because the frontal sinuses develop independently from one another on either side from anterior ethmoid cells, asymmetry is the rule. Differential sinus growth is responsible for displacement of the intersinus septum to one side. However, this septum is usually near the midline at its inferior extreme, near the level of the glabella (see Figs. 2-10 and 2-18). If the intersinus septum is displaced far to one side at this lower margin, an expansile process such as a mucocele within a frontal sinus should be suspected.

Unilateral or bilateral aplasia or hypoplasia occurs. The smaller sinuses usually consist of a single centrally concave recess (Figs. 2-20 and 2-21). Because of their small size, there is little sinus air compared to the amount of overlying bone, and these sinuses almost always appear somewhat "clouded" on plain films, even if disease free. As such, they are difficult to evaluate.

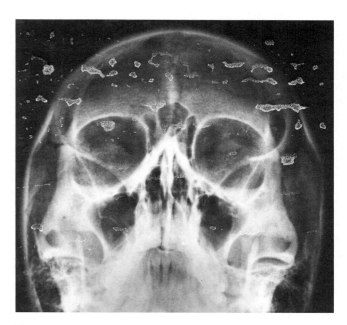

Fig. 2-22   Waters view shows hypoplastic frontal sinuses and small central sinus cell, a not uncommon finding. This view should be considered as a complimentary view to the Caldwell projection for evaluating the frontal sinuses.

Rhese and Waters views may help to evaluate these small sinuses (Fig. 2-22).

The normally developed frontal sinus is always less dense than the adjacent frontal bone. The frontal bone, as part of the calvarium, is composed of cortical bone, forming both its inner and outer tables. Interposed between the two is its middle table, or diploic space. The

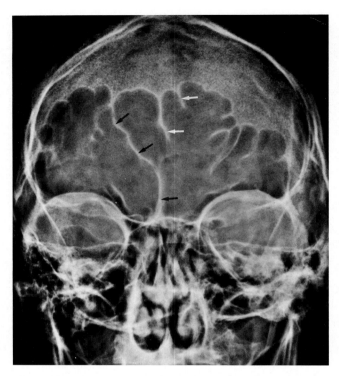

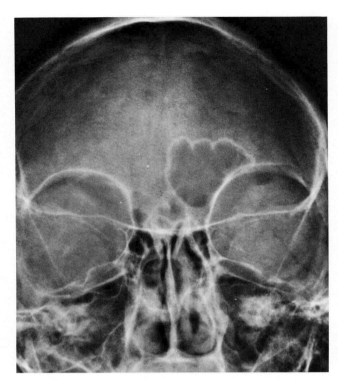

Fig. 2-23 Caldwell view shows well developed frontal sinus. Note the scalloped contour and the septations that project into the sinus cavity (white arrows). The intersinus septum is to the right of midline cranially, but is near the midline caudally (black arrows). Despite the large size of the frontal sinuses, the orbital contours remain normal and are not encroached upon.

Fig. 2-24 Caldwell view shows left frontal sinus to be moderately well developed while right frontal sinus is hypoplastic.

diploic space is made up of a bony lattice-work that is less dense than cortical bone, but osseous nonetheless. Frontal sinus development proceeds by invagination of an air-containing mucosal sac into the diploic space, thus displacing the osseous lattice-work otherwise sandwiched between the inner and outer tables of the skull. Therefore, despite the cortical nature of the bone comprising their inner and outer walls, the sinuses invariably appear less dense than the adjacent frontal bone. In general, the density of the normal frontal sinus is comparable to that of the superior orbital fissure as seen on the Caldwell view.

The larger sinuses have scalloped margins with septations that can project well into the sinus cavity (Fig. 2-23 and see Fig. 2-10). If this scalloping is lost and instead a smoothly ovoid shape is seen, an expansile process such as a mucocele should be considered. It is the slow progressive erosion of the septa and the bone between the scallops that creates this smooth appearance in a well-developed sinus in the presence of an expansile process.

No matter how large the frontal sinuses grow, they will never violate the orbital contour (see Fig. 2-23). If there is a downward and lateral flattening of the super

omedial orbital rim, a mucocele should again be suspected.

The normal superomedial orbital margin can often appear unsharp on Caldwell or Waters views. This is because this area curves not only from medial to lateral in the orbital rim, but also from vertical to horizontal as the bone of the forehead region merges into the bone of the orbital roof. Usually a repeat Caldwell view at a slightly different angulation or a Rhese view will allow this orbital margin to be visualized intact so that erosion is not suspected erroneously.

The margins of each frontal sinus are outlined by a thin (1 mm) dense rim, the mucoperiosteal (white) line, which separates the sinus from the adjacent frontal bone (see Figs. 2-10 and 2-23). If this line is not visualized, it could be because of active infection, which is common, or bone destruction from tumor, which is rare. In active inflammatory disease, there is increased vascularity, which results in increased mobilization of calcium and a loss of the mucoperiosteal white line. In chronic infection, the thin, sharp, white line becomes replaced by an unsharp, thick zone of sclerosis or reactive bone. This thickened white zone indicates only that the frontal sinus was exposed to previous chronic infection and does not necessarily imply that there is currently active infection in the sinus.

In the Caldwell view, the lambdoidal perisutural

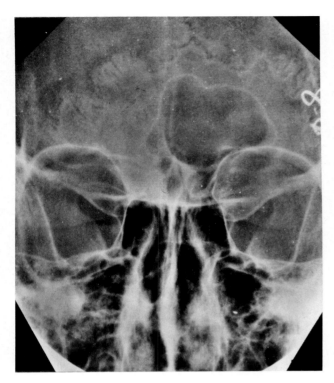

Fig. 2-25 Caldwell view shows moderately well developed left frontal sinus. The right frontal sinus is aplastic. The perisutural sclerosis of the lambdoid suture projected over the frontal area may mimic a clouded sinus contour.

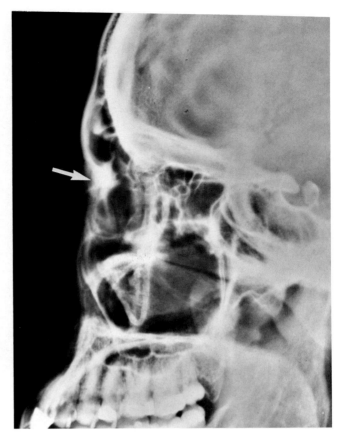

Fig. 2-26 Lateral view shows normal bone density near the anterior base of the frontal sinuses *(arrow)*. This "pseudoosteoma" is not seen on either the Caldwell or Waters views.

sclerosis of the occiput, a normal finding, can be projected over the region of the frontal sinus and mimic a chronically thickened reactive margin of an opacified sinus (Figs. 2-24 and 2-25). Comparison of the Caldwell film to Waters or Rhese views permits correct interpretation.

On occasion, it may be difficult to distinguish between a completely clouded (opacified) frontal sinus and an absent (aplastic) sinus. With good quality films, some frontal sinus margin can almost always be identified, albeit poorly, on at least one of the plain films in the sinus series. If no such margin is seen, an aplastic sinus is the probable diagnosis. Sectional imaging will resolve any remaining issue.

On the lateral view there usually is a bone density area seen at the base of the frontal sinuses anteriorly, near the nasion (Fig. 2-26). This represents the overlapping lower bony sinus walls and the superomedial orbital margins. The nasofrontal suture is usually just anteriorly situated. The dense bony area should not be confused with an osteoma. When seen from the front (Caldwell and Waters views), no osteoma is visualized and the bone in this region appears normal. Occasionally on the lateral view, small bony ridges also can be seen projecting from the anterior or posterior sinus walls. These are the sinus septa seen from the side.

The Ethmoid Sinuses. The ethmoid sinuses are best

evaluated in the routine sinus examination on the Caldwell view. However, in every plain film projection some ethmoid cells are superimposed on others. This reflects the fact that the ethmoid sinuses are not a single sinus cavity, as are the other paranasal sinuses, but rather are formed by 3 to 18 cells that are packed into the ethmoid bone. This superimposition can lead to confusion on the plain film examination when the patient has symptoms referable to these cells and yet the ethmoid sinuses appear normal. This situation arises because an isolated group of cells can be totally opacified, while all of the adjacent cells remain normal. The air in these normal cells tends to nullify the plain film "clouding" of the infected cells, and the net effect is often very unimpressive. In this clinical circumstance, sectional imaging may be necessary.

On the Caldwell view, the normal density of the ethmoid sinuses can be judged by comparing it to the air density around the inferior turbinate of the nasal fossae. This reflects the fact that the ethmoid sinuses and the nasal fossae are of approximately the same anteroposterior depth, and thus the density of the air volume should be about the same.

The thin lamina papyracea forms the lateral boundary

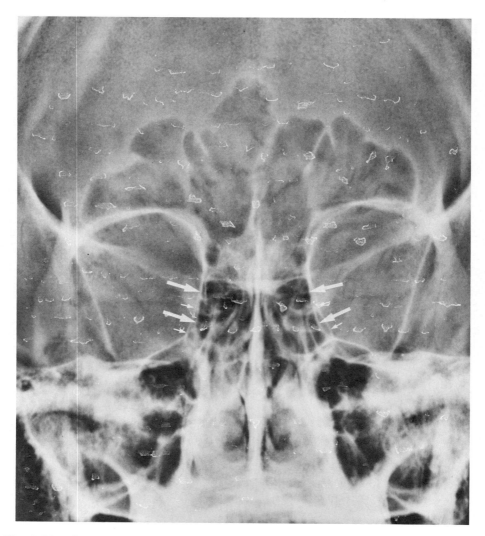

Fig. 2-27   Caldwell view shows posterior ethmoid lamina papyracea *(small arrows)* to be lateral to the more anterior lamina papyracea *(large arrows).* The medial orbital wall extends obliquely between them, and this appearance results from the conical shape of the orbit. Also note the horizontally oriented normal ethmoid septa.

of the ethmoid bone, separating it from the orbit. This medial orbital wall is oriented obliquely to an antero-posterior incident beam. Thus, the majority of this oblique, thin bony plate is not visualized on routine plain film studies. The straight or slightly concave lateral line that appears to form the medial orbital wall on a Caldwell view is, in reality, only the posterior ethmoid margin near the sphenoid bone. The anterior margin abutting the lacrimal bone is more medially placed and often is poorly seen (Fig. 2-27). It can be best localized by following the outline of the orbital rim from the superior aspect around to the superomedial margin and then caudally to the medial contour.

On the Waters view, only the most anterior ethmoid cells can be visualized, with the lacrimal bone separating them from the orbit (Fig. 2-28). The middle and

posterior ethmoid cells are hidden from view by the nasal fossae structures. Similarly, the lateral and base views have so many overlapping structures that only gross localization of an ethmoid process can be achieved. On the base view, the palate, nasal septum, turbinates, and anterior calvarium overlay the ethmoids, while on the lateral view, the lateral orbital margins and even the frontal processes of the maxilla may project as vague dense zones overlying the ethmoid cells (Fig. 2-29 and see Figs. 2-12 and 2-19). These should not be misinterpreted as sites of pathology. Although some isolation of the posterior ethmoid cells can be obtained on a Rhese view, some overlapping of ethmoid cells still occurs. Sectional imaging is indicated for proper mapping.

On the Caldwell view, a small indentation or groove

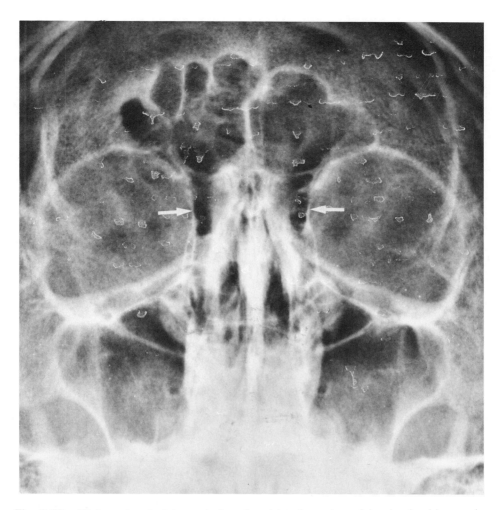

Fig. 2-28 Waters view isolates anterior ethmoid cells and overlying lacrimal bones *(ar-rows).*

is often seen along the upper medial orbital wall. This is the anterior ethmoidal canal, and it transmits the vessels of the same name along with the nasociliary nerve (Fig. 2-30). Since the canal is formed from the ethmoid bone *below* and the frontal bone *above*, it represents the level of the floor of the anterior cranial fossa. Less often seen on plain films are the posterior ethmoidal canals, which transmit the posterior ethmoidal nerve and vessels. (A line drawn between these anterior and posterior canals when the surgeon has exposed the medial orbital bony wall will thus identify the level just below the dura.)

The ethmoidomaxillary plate is the posteroinferior boundary between the ethmoid and maxillary bones. It is best seen in the Caldwell view and is a useful plain film landmark for localizing the spread of tumors (Fig. 2-31).

Supraorbital ethmoid cells are ethmoid sinus extensions into the orbital plate of the frontal bone. Unlike the frontal sinuses, the supraorbital ethmoid cells tend to be symmetric. If such a cell is present on one side, it

should be present on the opposite side. If one of these supraorbital cells is not seen, opacification or destruction should be suspected. Sectional imaging performed in the coronal plane will resolve any questionable case.

On the Caldwell view, the supraorbital ethmoid cells appear as slightly curvilinear lucent zones in the superomedial orbital roof (Fig. 2-32). Their posterior extent is best evaluated on either a Waters or a lateral view. It is important to ascertain whether a pathologic process is in a supraorbital ethmoid sinus or in the frontal sinus, since the surgical approaches to these sinuses differ greatly.

The Maxillary Sinuses. The maxillary sinuses are best evaluated in the Waters view. Unlike the frontal and sphenoid sinuses, the maxillary sinuses tend to be symmetric in size and configuration with only minor variations being common. When some degree of hypoplasia is present, the roof of the smaller antrum has a greater downward slant on its lateral margin than does the larger sinus (Fig. 2-33). On plain films this may simulate a blowout type orbital floor fracture (Fig. 2-34).

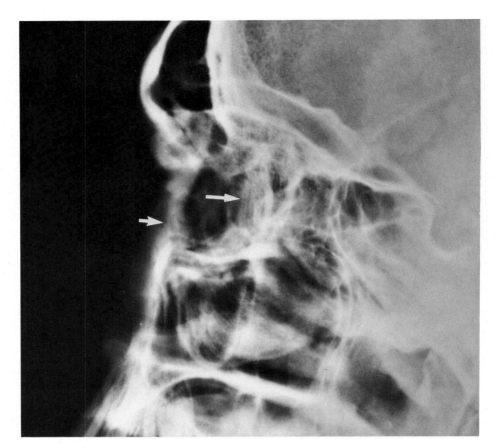

Fig. 2-29   Lateral view shows frontal process of the maxilla *(small arrow)* and lateral orbital rims *(large arrow)* to be projected over the ethmoid cells.

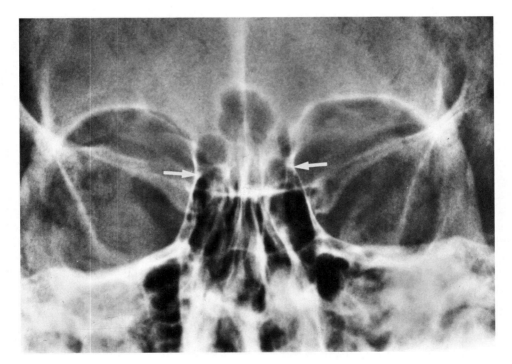

Fig. 2-30   Caldwell view demonstrates medial indentations in the lamina papyracea *(arrows)* that represent the anterior ethmoidal canals. These canals mark the level of the floor of the anterior cranial fossa.

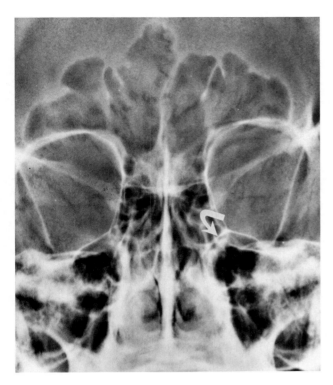

Fig. 2-31 Caldwell view shows ethmoidomaxillary plate *(curved arrow)*. This is the boundary between the postero-inferior ethmoid bone and the maxillary bone.

However, in the hypoplastic sinus, there usually is an identifiably thicker lateral bony sinus wall that results from the poorer than normal pneumatization of the maxilla. Although this may be misdiagnosed as thickened sinus mucosa, this confusion is not likely to be made by the radiologist who is aware of the appearance of a hypoplastic antrum.

A small sinus can also occur from diseases of the sinus wall that cause bone expansion with resultant encroachment into the antral cavity (Fig. 2-35). These include fibrous dysplasia, giant cell tumors, brown tumors, and Paget's disease. In these cases at least one dimension of the original sinus may be identified as being fully developed, and the "bony changes" can be visualized bulging into the sinus as well as being formed by abnormally textured bone. These changes differentiate these conditions from a simple hypoplastic antrum. Often sectional imaging may be necessary to resolve difficult cases.

Similarly, conditions that cause arrest in the growth of the maxilla will result in a hypoplastic antrum. These conditions include severe infection, trauma, tumor, irradiation, and congenital first arch syndromes.

The most lateral extension of the maxillary sinus is the zygomatic recess. This portion of the sinus hollows out the body of the zygoma, and when compared to the

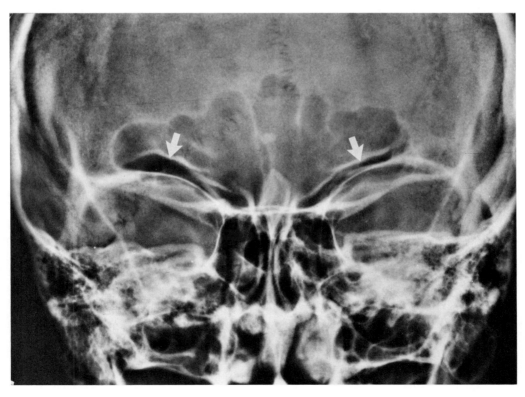

Fig. 2-32 Caldwell view shows curvilinear collection of air *(arrows)* just above each orbital margin. The reason these areas appear so dark is that the air in these supraorbital ethmoid cells is projected over the air in the frontal sinuses.

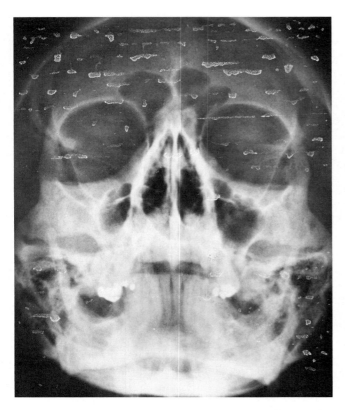

Fig. 2-33 Waters view shows right maxillary sinus to be smaller than the left. This hypoplasia is noted by the thicker lateral bony wall and the more exaggerated downward slant of its roof when compared to the left side. Also note that there is a suggestion of mucosal thickening in this normal hypoplastic right antrum due to its smaller sinus cavity and thicker sinus walls when compared to the left side.

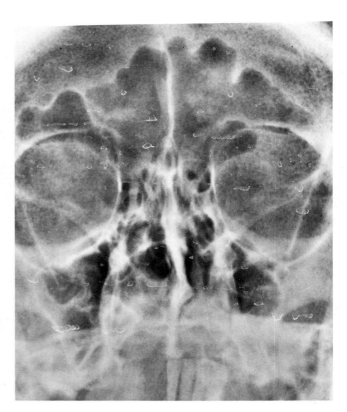

Fig. 2-34 Waters view shows hypoplastic antrum on the left side as noted by the downward slant of the sinus roof and the slightly thicker lateral sinus wall when compared to the right side. This patient had been hit in the left eye and this film was initially misinterpreted in the emergency room as a blow-out fracture.

main antral cavity, it has less air and more surrounding bone. Because of this, the recess usually appears "clouded" on a Waters view, and this is often misinterpreted as representing mucosal thickening (see Figs. 2-22 and 2-28). True mucosal changes extend along the adjacent lower lateral antral wall, and it is there that such mucosal disease should be evaluated.

On the lateral view, the anterior and posterior walls of the zygomatic recesses are seen as two overlapping Vs projected over the main maxillary sinuses. These should be evaluated routinely to assess the possibility of early bone destruction in these recesses (Fig. 2-36).

On the lateral view, the cranial continuation of the posterior wall of the zygomatic recess is also the most anterior margin of the temporal fossa and represents that portion of the greater sphenoid wing that forms the oblique orbital line on the Waters and Caldwell views (Fig. 2-37).

The infratemporal maxillary sinus wall is a sigmoid-shaped, curved posterolateral surface. It is poorly seen on the Caldwell and Waters views. The most lateral ex-

tent (the back of the zygomatic recess) and the most medial margin (the anterior wall of the pterygopalatine fossa) can be identified on the lateral view (see Fig. 2-37). The base view provides the best visualization of the curved nature of this wall as well as an enface projection of portions of the pterygopalatine fossa and pterygoid plates (Figs. 2-38 and 2-39).

The medial wall of the maxillary sinus is best seen on the Caldwell view. Unfortunately, the overlying nasal structures anteriorly and the sphenoid sinuses and skull base structures posteriorly obscure most detail. Only the inferior turbinates and the lower medial antral wall are identified consistently (Fig. 2-40). The clinically important ostiomeatal complex can be visualized well only on coronal sectional imaging (see Fig. 2-39).

Slight asymmetry, minimal rotation, and the physiologic nasal cycle can all contribute to making one nasal turbinate larger than the other. This asymmetry should not be overdiagnosed as pathological. On the lateral view, the posterior tips of the inferior conchae are often seen projecting over the posterior antra, and they

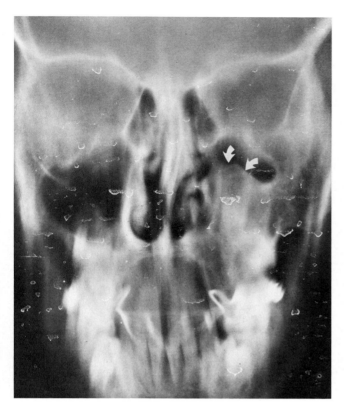

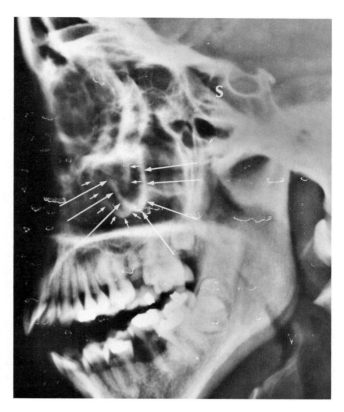

Fig. 2-35   Coronal tomogram of patient with ossifying fibroma of the lateral wall and floor of the left antrum. The arrows indicate the elevation of the floor of the sinus by this expansile mass. This may simulate the findings of a hypoplastic sinus, but it has a distinctly different appearance (compare to Figs. 2-33 and 2-34).

Fig. 2-36   Lateral view has large arrows pointing to the zygomatic recess of one maxillary sinus and small arrows outlining the opposite zygomatic recess. These recesses are routinely seen on lateral views as overlapping *Vs*. The air around them is air in the main maxillary sinus cavities, which are located nearer the midline. The *S* is in the sphenoid sinus with its posterior and superior limits well seen on this lateral film.

should not be confused with a pathologic mass. Also on the lateral view, air trapped under or above the inferior turbinate can produce a linear lucency that may mimic a fracture (Fig. 2-41).

Little consistent detail about the middle turbinates can be obtained from plain film studies, and sectional imaging is necessary to provide accurate information.

The anterior antral wall is not well seen on any view. Both the lateral and the overangulated base views reveal only limited portions of this wall (see Fig. 2-39).

The lateral view best delineates the inferior extension of the maxillary sinus and its relationship to the hard palate and teeth roots (Fig. 2-42). The sinus cortex of this alveolar recess can be elevated normally by unerupted molar teeth. Although this is well seen on the lateral view, it can simulate an air-fluid level or a localized mass on a Waters view. This is especially notable in older children and teenagers.

The antral roof, or orbital floor, is flattest and lowest anterolaterally. It is also highest and most angulated (oblique) posteromedially. The majority of the midpor-

tion of the antral roof is seen almost tangentially on a Caldwell view, and thus this large surface is usually seen as a single line in this projection. A second smaller, more slanted line is seen superomedially on the Caldwell view, which represents a portion of the orbital apex floor; a notch at the lateral aspect of this latter line identifies the site of the infraorbital groove (Fig. 2-43).

On the lateral view, the orbital floor is usually seen as two separate lines: one anteriorly, near the level of the inferior orbital rim, represents the lowest and flattest area of the floor; the second, located higher and more posteriorly, represents the orbital apex region. The slanting floor joining these two areas is not visualized on the lateral view (Fig. 2-42).

The Waters projection gives a better view of the inferior orbital rim. However, much of the orbital floor is seen obliquely en face, and small fractures, depressions, or erosions may not be detected. Three roughly parallel lines are seen near the inferior orbital margin in the Waters view. The most superior of these is the

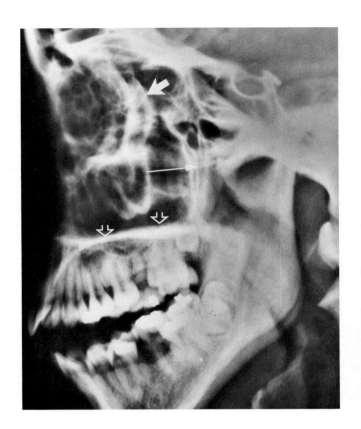

Fig. 2-37 Lateral view has long arrows pointing to one posterior antral wall, which also forms the anterior margin of the pterygomaxillary fissure near the midline. The short arrow indicates the upward continuation of the posterior portion of one *"V"* that forms the zygomatic recess of one antrum (see Fig. 2-36). The short arrow points to the bone just behind the orbit, which forms the anterior border of the temporal fossa. Open arrows indicate the upper flat nasal fossa surface of the hard palate. The lower oral surface is slightly concave downward in configuration.

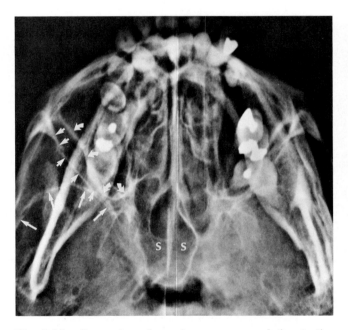

Fig. 2-38 Base view shows large arrows pointing to the curved anterior margin of the right middle cranial fossa (greater sphenoid wing). The small, straight arrows indicate the straighter posterior wall of the right orbit. The lateral margin is formed by the zygoma, the medial portion by the greater sphenoid wing. The curved arrows outline the "sigmoid" shaped posterior wall of the maxillary sinus. Each sphenoid sinus cavity *(S)* is well seen.

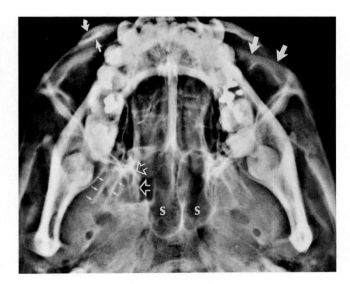

Fig. 2-39 Base view has open arrows pointing to the medial pterygoid plate. Because the lateral pterygoid plate curves laterally as it descends from the skull base, the two small arrows point to the line of the lateral pterygoid plate near the skull base, while the three small arrows indicate the lateral pterygoid plate near the level of the hard palate. The large arrows point to the anterior wall of the left zygoma and maxilla. The frontal bone's anterior table *(curved arrow)* and posterior table *(small straight arrow)* are also indicated on the right side. Each sphenoid sinus cavity *(S)* is well seen.

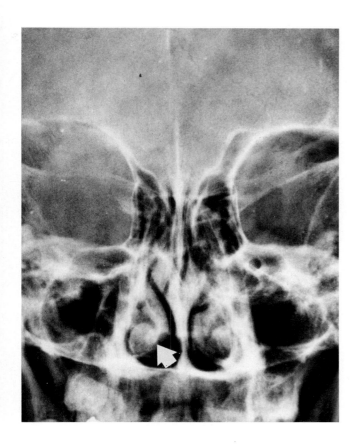

Fig. 2-40 Caldwell view has arrow indicating the right inferior turbinate. Only the inferior turbinates and portions of the middle turbinates are routinely seen on plain films. As long as a thin zone of air can be identified outlining the inferior turbinate, this turbinate is probably not pathologically enlarged.

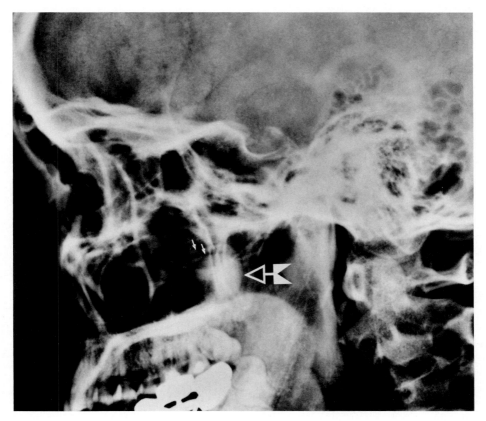

Fig. 2-41 Lateral view has large arrow pointing to posterior tip of normal inferior turbinate. Normal air just above turbinates *(small arrows)* may mimic a fracture line.

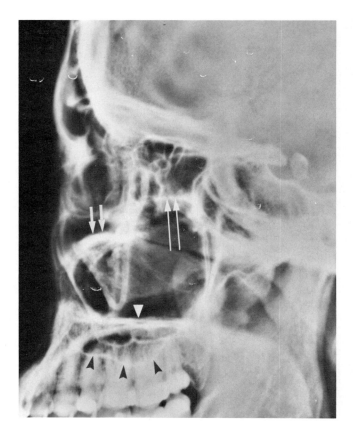

Fig. 2-42   Lateral view demonstrates maxillary sinus extension *(black arrowheads)* below the level of the hard palate *(white arrowhead)*. The smaller arrows point to the anterior, lateral, and inferior orbital floor on one side, while the *longer arrows* point to the posterior, medial, and superior orbital floor near the orbital apex.

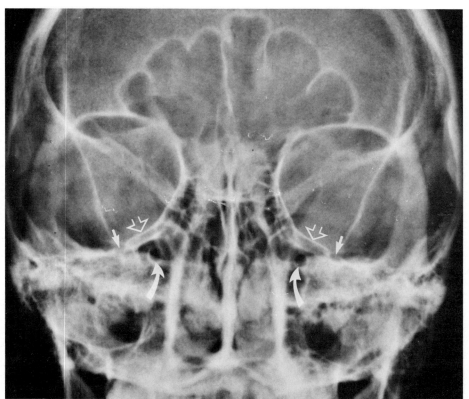

Fig. 2-43   Caldwell view has open arrowheads indicating posteromedial orbital floors. The straight arrows point to posterior margin of infraorbital canals. The curved arrows point to each foramen rotundum.

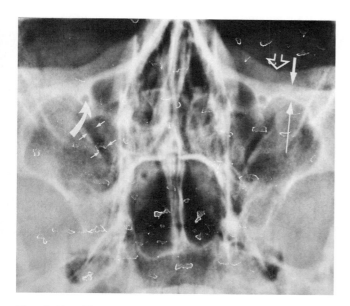

Fig. 2-44 Waters view has curved arrow pointing to infraorbital foramen. The open arrow indicates soft tissue line over inferior orbital rim. The short arrow points to the bony inferior orbital rim, while the long arrow indicates the lowest point of the orbital floor, which is about 1 cm posterior to the orbital rim. The small arrows outline the margins of the superior orbital fissure projected through the right antrum.

soft tissue skin margin overlying the inferior orbital rim. The middle line is the actual bony inferior orbital rim, and the lowest line is the roof of the antrum located about 1 cm behind the rim, the lowest point of the orbital floor. About 1 cm below the middle third of the inferior orbital rim, the infraorbital foramen is seen. It transmits the second division of the trigeminal nerve to the cheek and nasal region (Fig. 2-44).

On the Waters view, a small lucency can occasionally be seen in the lateral antral wall. This is the canal for the posterior superior alveolar nerve and should not be confused with a fracture (Fig. 2-45).

On the Caldwell view, the foramen rotundum is projected through the superomedial portion of the antrum (Fig. 2-46 and see Fig. 2-43). The superior orbital fissure is easily identified and normally has a slightly concave lateral appearance (see Figs. 2-44 and 2-46). If the superior orbital fissure is followed inferiorly and slightly laterally, it points to the foramen rotundum. The maxillary nerve (V_2) runs through this foramen, crosses the pterygopalatine fossa and retromaxillary fissure, enters the infraorbital fissure, exits via the infraorbital canal, and supplies the cheek and nasal regions.

The two foramina rotunda are usually symmetric in size and configuration. The superior orbital fissures, on the other hand, need not be as symmetric. The most important observation is that the two bony rims of this

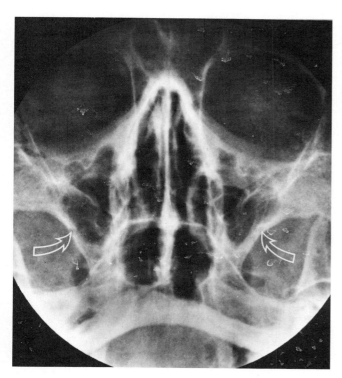

Fig. 2-45 Waters view with arrows indicating the canals for the posterior, superior alveolar nerves.

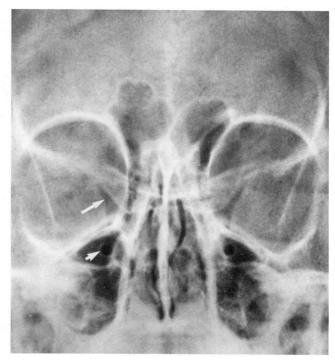

Fig. 2-46 Caldwell view shows superior orbital fissure *(large arrow)* and foramen rotundum *(short arrow),* which is at the lower lateral margin of the superior orbital fissure.

fissure are sharply defined with a good thin cortex. These fissures are narrower superolaterally and wider inferomedially. It is through this wider area that the veins and nerves traverse the fissure (Fig. 2-47 and see Fig. 2-46). On the Waters view, the lower portions of the superior orbital fissures are projected through the upper medial antra. These can simulate either a fracture of the inferior orbital rim or a septum of the antral roof (see Figs. 2-44 and 2-47).

The infraorbital fissure can sometimes be seen on the Waters view as a pair of parallel thin cortical lines that are oriented anteroposteriorly. Their course and parallel, rather than divergent, configuration will distinguish them from the posteriorly located superior orbital fissure.

The inferior orbital fissure is poorly seen on the routine sinus views and can be best evaluated on the Towne view (Fig. 2-48).

The oblique orbital lines (linea innominata) are seen in both the Waters and the Caldwell views. They represent the most anterior portions of the medial temporal fossa and usually are made up by the greater sphenoid wings. At the lower margin of each innominate line, a sharp medial turn is seen, indicating the lower margin of the temporal fossa and the beginning of the infratemporal fossa. Occasionally this line can be seen to continue medially and then bend downward, now outlining the lateral pterygoid plate (Figs. 2-49 and 2-50).

The superior bony margin of the middle cranial fossa is a concave posterior ridge that is formed medially by the lesser sphenoid wing and laterally by the posterior edge of the orbital plate of the frontal bone. The curved margin can be seen projected through the orbit and upper antrum on the Waters view (see Figs. 2-49 and 2-50).

The body of the zygoma and the zygomatic arches are well seen in the Waters and base views (see Figs. 2-17 and 2-50). Alternate views for this arch are the underpenetrated base view and the "jug handle" or oblique zygomatic projection. The posterior portions of the arch are best seen on a Towne view. The zygomaticotemporal suture in the zygomatic arch is an obliquely oriented line that can be seen routinely and should not be confused with a fracture.

Occasionally, the zygomaticofacial canal can be seen in the lateral body of the zygoma. It transmits the zygomaticofacial nerve.

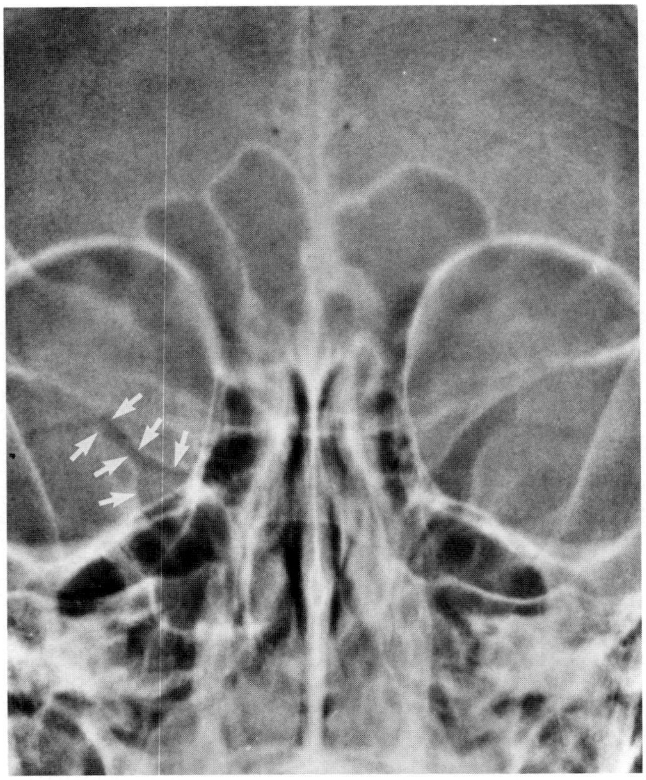

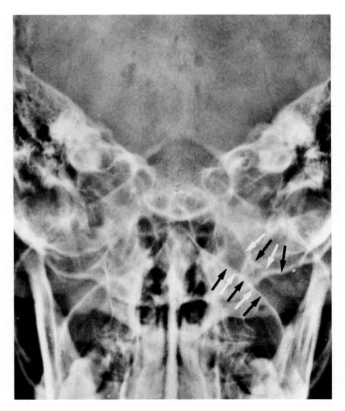

Fig. 2-47 Caldwell view with arrows outlining margins of the superior orbital fissure. The lower margins of this fissure are projected through the orbital floor and the antrum (see Fig. 2-44). The nerves and veins that traverse the superior orbital fissure all pass through the larger medial portion of the fissure.

Fig. 2-48 Towne's view with arrows outlining margins of the inferior orbital fissure. The superior line is formed by the sphenoid bone, while the inferior line is formed by the maxilla.

On the Waters view, the soft tissue shadow of the upper lip can often be seen traversing the lower antrum. This shadow usually extends lateral to the lower maxillary sinus margin. Similarly, a mustache also can produce such a shadow. These soft tissue densities should not be confused with true retention cysts of the lower antrum, which unlike the above shadows can be identified as cysts on a lateral view. Similarly, the nasal alae can mimic cysts of the medial antral wall in the Waters view (Fig. 2-51 and see Fig. 2-49).

Soft tissue swelling of the cheek can mimic clouding of the antrum on a Waters view. This usually can be identified by elevation of the superior skin line over the inferior orbital rim. However, sectional imaging may be necessary in some cases to isolate the maxillary sinus from the overlying swollen skin and subcutaneous tissues.

In the lateral view, the coronoid processes of the mandible project over the inferoposterior maxillary sinuses. This is especially noted if the mouth is closed. If these coronoid processes are blunt or rounded, they may simulate retention cysts (Fig. 2-52). If the coronoid processes are sharply pointed, they may simulate a fractured bone segment or an unerupted tooth.

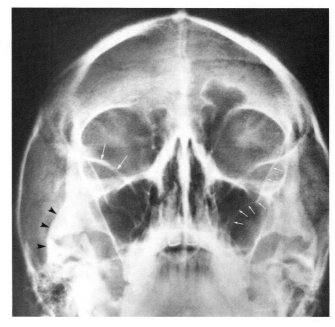

Fig. 2-50 Waters view with smaller arrows outlining the left oblique orbital line and its inferior extension to the infratemporal fossa and finally the lateral pterygoid plate (see Fig. 2-49). The larger arrows point to the upper anterior margin of the right middle cranial fossa. The arrowheads outline the right zygomatic arch.

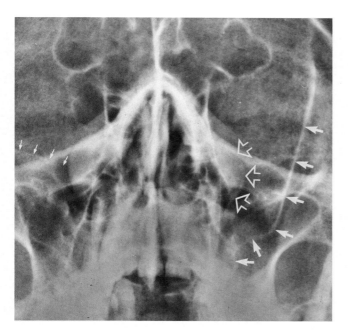

Fig. 2-49 Waters view has arrows pointing to left oblique orbital line. At its lower margin the line bends medially at the level of the infratemporal fossa. The line then bends downwards at the level of the lateral pterygoid plate. The small, white arrows point to the upper rim of the right middle cranial fossa. The open arrows indicate the left nasal margin, which can mimic a cyst or polyp in the medial antrum.

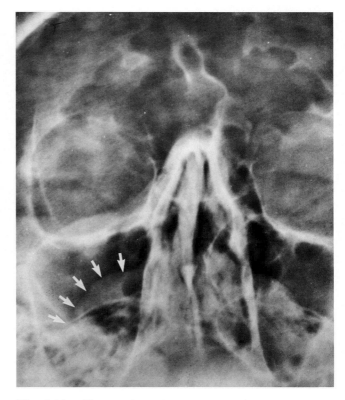

Fig. 2-51 Waters view with arrows outlining the shadow of the upper lip, which is projected over the lower maxillary sinus.

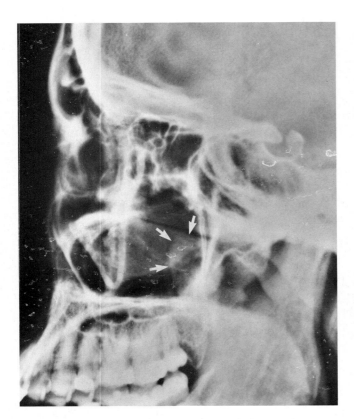

Fig. 2-52 Lateral view with arrows pointing to the coronoid process of the mandible, which is projected over the lower, posterior antrum in the closed mouth view.

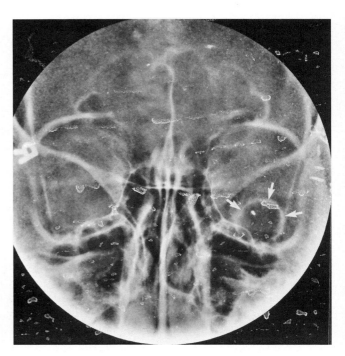

Fig. 2-53 Caldwell view with white arrows outlining a lateral sphenoid sinus recess that extends into the greater wing of the sphenoid bone as it forms the posterior orbital wall. Note that the lower medial aspect of the recess does not have a thin white mucoperiosteal line around it because it is at this point that the recess communicates with the main sphenoid sinus cavity.

The Sphenoid Sinuses. The sphenoid sinuses are probably the most difficult sinuses to evaluate by routine films because they are buried deep in the skull base, surrounded by the facial bones, nasal cavity structures, and occiput on the frontal views and the mastoids and lateral skull base structures on the lateral view. The sphenoid sinuses are extremely variable in their configuration. About half of the population has only a central sinus cavity while the other half has, in addition, lateral recesses. These recesses can extend into the greater wings of the sphenoid, lesser wings, and pterygoid processes.

The central or main sphenoid sinus is best evaluated on the lateral, base, and open mouth Waters views (see Figs. 2-11, 2-36, 2-38, and 2-39). The sinus roof (planum sphenoidale), the sella floor (lamina dura), and the posterior development of the sinus cavity are all well seen on the lateral view; the floor and anterior sinus walls, however, are partially obscured by the overlapping lateral skull base. The base view provides a means of evaluating the sinus depth and lateral extension. The open mouth Waters view allows evaluation of the lower posterior sinus wall as it is projected through the mouth.

The sinus extensions into the greater wing of the sphenoid wing can go up into the posterior orbital wall and down into the floor of the middle cranial fossa. These are seen best on the Caldwell and Waters views. On the Caldwell view, a "lytic" area with a thin cortical white line outlining its contour will be visualized through the lower lateral orbit (Figs. 2-53 and 2-54). The lower, medial portion of the marginal white line is never visualized, because it is at this margin that this sphenoid recess communicates with the main sinus cavity. On the Waters views, the lateral sphenoid sinus recesses in the floor of the middle cranial fossae are projected through the maxillary sinuses. They have a variable shape depending on the configuration of the recess. They can appear as "dog ears" or simulate compartments of the maxillary sinus (Fig. 2-55). Regardless of their shape, they always join the central sphenoid sinus medially, and when normal, are always rimmed by a thin white cortical line.

Pterygoid pneumatization results in a triangular lucency in the pterygoid plates in the lateral view and a round or oval lucency in the pterygoid process in the base view (Fig. 2-56). These recesses are again outlined by a thin white cortical line. The appearances of all of these recesses are classic, and having learned them, the interpreter will not confuse these normal variants with pathologic processes.

Special attention should be addressed toward evalu-

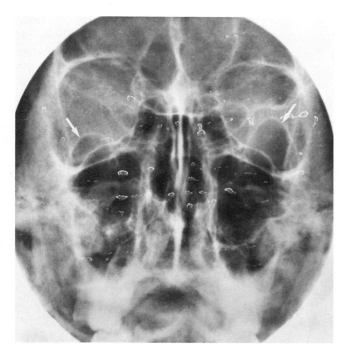

Fig. 2-54 Caldwell view shows lateral sphenoid sinus pneumatization of the greater sphenoid wings as they form the posterior orbital walls *(arrows)*. They are limited on all but their inferomedial margins (where they join the main sinus cavity) by the thin white mucoperiosteal line of the sinus margin.

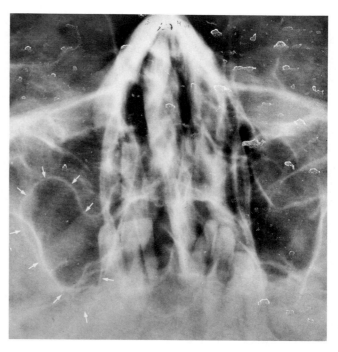

Fig. 2-55 Waters view shows lateral recesses of sphenoid sinuses extending into the greater sphenoid wings in the floor of the middle cranial fossa. The arrows outline the right recess projected through the maxillary sinus. There is also a recess on the left side.

ating the posterior extent of the main sphenoid sinus cavity as it relates to the anterior sella wall, since this may have surgical implications. If more than 1 or 2 mm of bone remain between the posterior margin of the pneumatized sinus and the anterior sella wall, a transsphenoidal hypophysectomy will usually be avoided by most surgeons. This situation obtains in less than 1 percent of the cases. This relationship is most easily seen in the lateral view.

Associated Structures Surrounding the Paranasal Sinuses. There are a number of important structures that surround the paranasal sinuses and project over them on the plain film examinations.

On the lateral view, the anterior walls of the middle cranial fossa are seen as paired curvilinear lines that project over the sphenoid sinus cavities and merge posteroinferiorly with the bone density of the skull base. The planum sphenoidale is clearly identified as a straight bony line. Less well seen is the cribriform plate that continues anteriorly from the planum sphenoidale. However, a line drawn connecting the nasion and anterior planum will very closely approximate the level of the cribriform plate. The fovea ethmoidalis (ethmoid sinus roofs) lie just lateral to and above the cribriform plates. They usually can be identified as slightly concave, downward, thin bony lines positioned just above

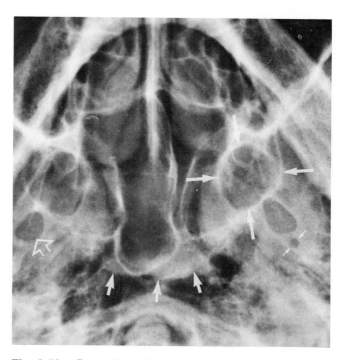

Fig. 2-56 Base view with large arrows outlining pneumatized pterygoid process. The small arrows point to the foramen spinosum and the open arrow indicates the right foramen ovale. The medium white arrows outline the posterior margin of the tongue.

the plane of the cribriform plates. The orbital roofs are situated higher and more laterally than the fovea ethmoidalis. Thus, one can roughly localize a lytic process on a lateral film by evaluating which of these lines is eroded. The more superior the line, the more lateral the process (Fig. 2-57).

The midline crista galli is best seen on the Caldwell view. This intracranial structure rests on the midline upper surface of cribriform plates (Fig. 2-58).

The bony nasal septum is not seen optimally on any plain film projection, but is best evaluated on the Caldwell view. Only gross deviation of the bony septum can be appreciated. The cartilaginous septum is poorly seen on plain films and can be well visualized only on sectional imaging.

In the lateral view, the anterior nasal spine usually has a sharply triangular appearance. The film must often be "bright lighted" to properly evaluate the spine. Destruction of the anterior nasal spine should raise the question of prior surgery or trauma. Midfacial anomalies, Hansen's disease (leprosy), and carcinomas can also result in nonvisualization of this spine.

The hard palate is best evaluated in the lateral view. Its upper nasal surface is flat and usually has a clear cortical margin. The lower oral surface is slightly concave downward, also with a good cortical margin (see Fig. 2-37).

In the base view, three pairs of lines are consistently seen. The most posterior of these is concave posteriorly and represents the greater wings of the sphenoid bone as they form the anterior margin of the middle cranial fossae. Each of the second pair of lines is a relatively straight anterior line that is obliquely oriented to the midsagittal plane. It is comprised medially by the sphenoid bone as it forms the posterior orbital wall, and laterally by the orbital surface of the zygoma. The suture between these bones often can be identified clearly. Medially these two paired sphenoid lines join at the pterygoid processes. The third pair is a sigmoid (S-

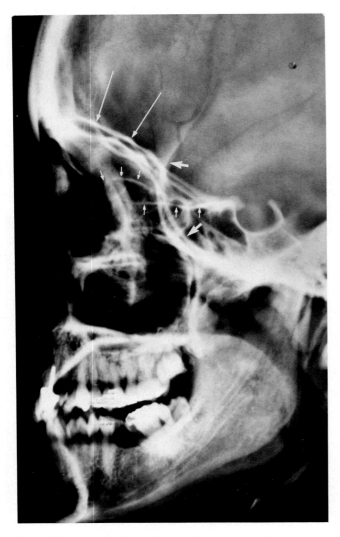

Fig. 2-57   Lateral view with small arrows pointing upward indicating the planum sphenoidale in the midline. The small arrows pointing downward outline the roof of the ethmoid sinuses (fovea ethmoidalis). The long arrows indicate the laterally positioned roofs of the orbit. The short arrows outline the curved anterior margins of the middle cranial fossa.

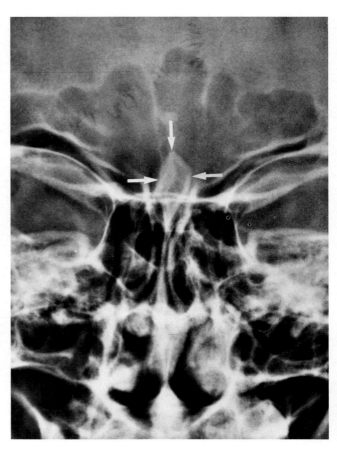

Fig. 2-58   Caldwell view with arrows indicating the crista galli, which rests atop the roof of the nasal cavity.

shaped) line that represents the infratemporal or posterolateral antral wall. Depending on the angulation used to make the base view, the sigmoid line can be anterior to, overlapping and crossing, or posterior to the orbital lines (see Figs. 2-38 and 2-39).

In the base view, the pterygoid fossa is seen as a V-shaped space with its apex placed anteriorly. The medial pterygoid plate is seen as a single thin bony line. However, the lateral pterygoid plate is seen as two separate thin bony lines. The lateral line represents the most caudal end of the lateral pterygoid plate as it lies at the level of the hard palate. The central line (or medial line of the lateral pterygoid plate) represents this plate near the skull base. The presence of two lines representing a single lateral plate arises because this plate has a curved, laterally tilted configuration (best appreciated on a frontal tomogram). This anatomy results in the main body of this plate being oblique to a craniocaudally directed incident beam, with only the upper and lower bony margins being directly "on end" to the beam. Occasionally, the hamulus of the medial

pterygoid plate can be seen on the base view. The pterygoid fossa is thus the space, open posteriorly, between the medial and central pterygoid lines near the skull base and between the medial and lateral lines near the hard palate.

In the base view, the frontal bone casts two transverse lines across the anterior portion of the ethmoid and maxillary sinuses. These lines correspond to the anterior and posterior cortical tables of the frontal bone. In addition, the anterior surface of the body of the zygoma and the anterior wall of the maxilla cast a transverse line across the anterolateral skull contour. The relationship of the frontal table lines to the zygomaticomaxillary lines depends on the angulation used in the base view (Fig. 2-59 and see Figs. 2-38 and 2-39). In the more markedly angulated base view, the lacrimal canals can also be seen projected through the medial antral walls and hard palate.

The nasopharyngeal soft tissues should be carefully and routinely examined because disease can spread from this area into the sinonasal cavities and vice versa.

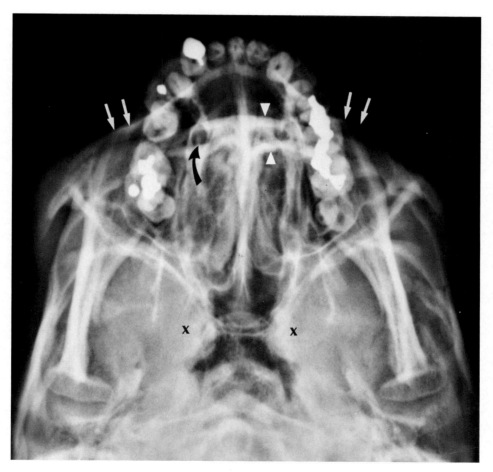

Fig. 2-59 Base view with *arrows* indicating the anterior wall margin of the maxilla and zygoma. The curved arrow points to the nasolacrimal duct, which in this film is projected over frontal bone's anterior and posterior margins *(arrowheads)*. The soft tissue shadows of the palatine tonsils *(X)* can also be seen.

This evaluation is best accomplished on the lateral view. The presence of a soft tissue fullness in the roof and uppermost posterior wall of the nasopharynx may indicate adenoidal tissue, lymphoma, nasopharyngeal carcinoma, or other disease states. If an adenoidal mass abuts on the upper surface of the soft palate, it may account for respiratory related symptoms, and thus, obliteration of the nasal airway should also be noted in the radiologist's report.

On the base view, the uvula and posterior surface of the soft palate as well as the back of the tongue can cast transverse shadows across the skull base. In particular the tongue base can often be visualized extending transversely across the sphenoid sinuses. This should not be confused with sinus clouding and should be correlated with the lateral and open mouth Waters views.

On the base view, the air in the nasopharynx and oropharynx is seen routinely as a lucent zone projected over the central skull base. The degree of tube angulation and neck extension will determine if this air shadow primarily represents the nasopharynx or the oropharynx. Thus a rectangular shadow with its greatest width extending from side to side suggests the nasopharynx, while a more square-shaped shadow suggests the oropharynx. On the routine base view, fullness in the region of the palatine tonsils can produce lateral soft tissue masses that overlie the posterior nasal fossae (see Fig. 2-55).

On the lateral view, the pinna of the ear occasionally can be projected over the sphenoid sinus and nasopharynx. This may simulate a mass and is usually seen in slightly underpenetrated films. It can be identified as an artifact by tracing out the entire ear.

The nasal bones are best evaluated in the lateral view (see Fig. 2-15). The nasofrontal suture is identified easily at the level of the nasion. The nasomaxillary sutures often can also be seen. There are no normal sutures or bone segments that routinely involve the midline nasal bones. Thus, normally there should be no lucent lines that extend across the midline nasal bones. Any such line or lines must suggest the diagnosis of a fracture. Usually radiolucent lines can be seen roughly paralleling the plane of the midline nasal bones. These are the normal grooves for the nasociliary nerves and vessels and should not be confused with fractures. Medial depression of the nasal bones is best evaluated in the occlusal (axial) and Waters views. Attention also should be paid to the anterior nasal spine, since it may be avulsed in trauma or destroyed by granulomatous disease or tumor.

In a patient with recent nasal trauma, clinical examination will diagnose whether or not a fracture is present. The examiner places thumb and index finger on either side of the bridge of the nose and gently rocks the fingers from side to side. In cases of fracture, the patient will have exquisite local pain. In cases of hemorrhage and edema (deforming the nasal contour) without fracture, the patient will be only slightly tender. Thus, the x-ray request slip for nasal films should actually read: "Nasal fracture, please evaluate for the number of fractures and any displacement." The radiologist's report should include a comment on the number and location of the fractures and whether there is depression or elevation of the fracture segments.

Tomographic Imaging Anatomy

Because on even the best quality plain films the radiologist consistently will underestimate the extent and presence of soft tissue disease and bone erosion, whenever fine mapping of disease is required, some form of tomographic examination is indicated. Three modalities can provide this information with varying degrees of success. Prior to the early 1970s, multidirectional tomography was the traditional tomographic tool. It provides "larger than life" fine bone detail and gross assessment (albeit more refined than on plain films) of soft tissue masses. Blurring artifacts and volume averaging shadows contribute to interpretation problems, but ease of positioning readily allows direct coronal studies to be obtained. Dental fillings provide no degrading artifacts. Lateral (sagittal) studies can be obtained easily; base (axial-transverse) projections, however, are difficult for the patient because positioning is uncomfortable.

High resolution CT scanning provides excellent bone detail and accurate soft tissue mapping. Although fine detail, thin section scanning can eliminate most problems with volume averaging, image degradation from dental fillings may occur. "Modified" angulated (off axial) scans are necessary to circumvent metallic dental restorations. The traditional scan plane, as well as the most comfortable scan position for the patient, is the axial projection. Direct 90 degree coronal scans are usually unobtainable because of inability to hyperextend the neck adequately. Modified coronal scans are usually obtained in a plane somewhere between the superior orbitomeatal (SOM) and true coronal planes. This can be accomplished with the patient positioned either prone or supine. Alternately, thin section axial scans can be obtained and then 90 degree coronal, paraaxial, or sagittal scans can be reconstructed. Unfortunately, for the most part, these reconstructed scans lack the refined detail of directly obtained studies. Although direct sagittal scans can be obtained, they require a table modification and a cooperative patient, and they consume extra examination time. Although soft tissue structures can be well seen on noncontrast examinations, postcontrast scans offer additional information about the degree of tissue enhancement and possible differential enhancement between normal and abnormal tissues. The CT examination is readily available throughout the country, and some consideration must be given to contrast reactions and radiation dose.

MRI provides a means of obtaining direct coronal, transverse, and sagittal scans. There is minimal image degradation from dental fillings. In general the examination time is longer than for a comparable high resolution CT study. Because of this, motion artifact may play a more pronounced role in MRI than it does in CT. New fast scan software is reducing the MRI time to now be competitive with CT; however, at present, these fast scan films do not have as high a resolution as the longer scanning techniques. Because of the machine design, claustrophobia causes up to 10% of patients to reject the MRI examination. Soft tissues are more clearly imaged than by CT, and without the need for intravenous contrast agents, most disease processes can be accurately localized with some degree of tissue specificity (i.e., infection vs tumor vs hemorrhage). Unfortunately, bone is only identified by an absence of MR signal and, at times, confusion may arise with other sources of absent signal (i.e., air, dystrophic calcification, scar, flowing blood). In general, bone is more accurately assessed by CT, where it is directly visualized. With MRI, there is no need to consider radiation effects; however, the cost of the MRI study is usually greater than that of a CT study, and the MRI scanners, in general, are less available than CT scanners. MRI cannot be performed on patients with pacemakers, and pregnancy or the presence of intracranial vascular clips currently are also considered relative contraindications to MRI.

Since the anatomy is the one common denominator regardless of which modality is used to study it, the basic clinically relevant anatomy will be presented as it appears in a combination of studies from these three modalities. The anatomy will be described in idealized planes.

Coronal Tomographic Anatomy, Starting Anteriorly and Extending Posteriorly (Figs. 2-60 to 2-79).[13-18] Far anteriorly, the alar and septal nasal cartilages are seen. Behind these, the frontal processes of the maxillary bones form curved arches that extend from the lateral maxillae to the more medial nasal bones. Depending on

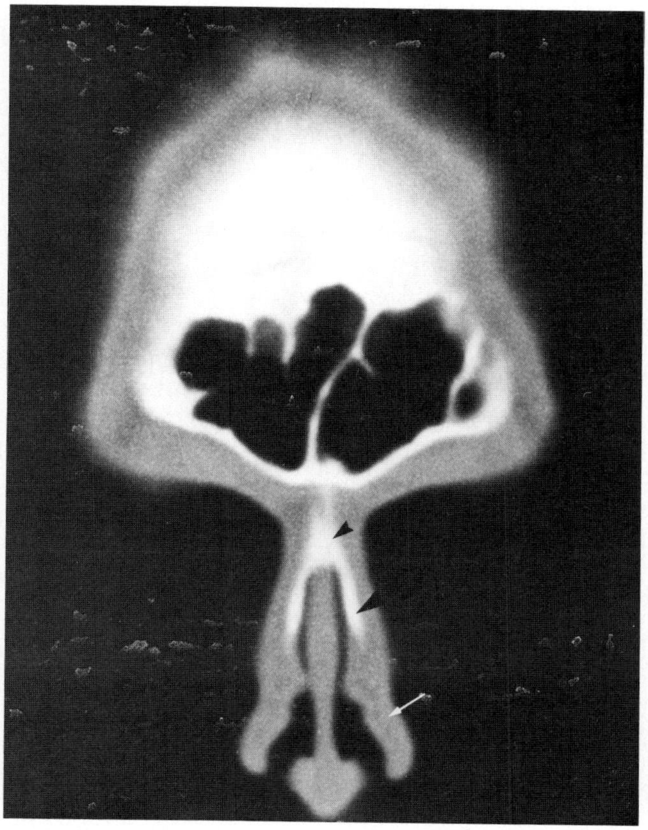

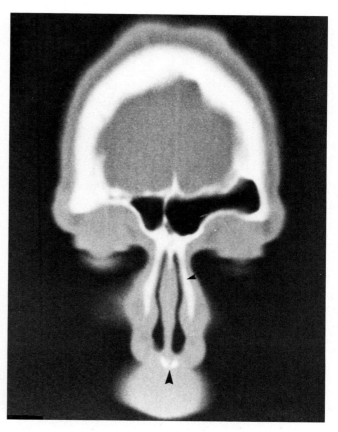

Fig. 2-60 Coronal CT scan. The small arrowhead indicates nasal bones. The large arrowhead points to the frontal process of the maxilla. The arrow points to the nasal alar and the cartilaginous nasal septum is in the midline. The frontal sinus is clearly seen with the intersinus septum and the normal scalloped sinus margins.

Fig. 2-61 Coronal CT scan. The small arrow indicates the frontal process of the maxilla, the large arrowhead points to the nasal spine. The anterior cranial fossa is seen surrounded by the frontal bones. Extension of the frontal sinus into the orbital roof is seen on the left side.

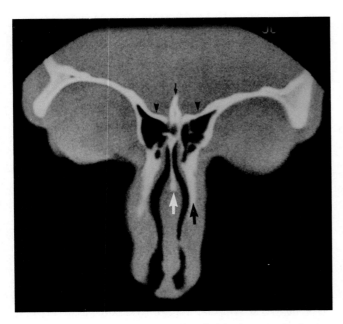

Fig. 2-62 Coronal CT scan. Small, black arrow indicates the crista galli. The arrowheads point to the fovea ethmoidalis. The white arrow indicates the perpendicular plate of the ethmoid bone with the cartilaginous nasal septum caudal to it. The black arrow points to the frontal process of the maxilla. Anterior ethmoid cells are also seen.

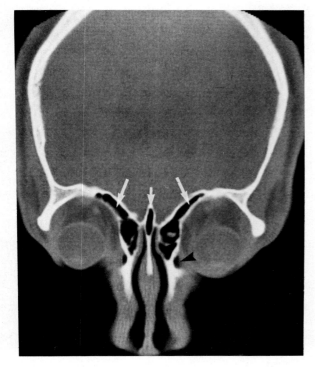

Fig. 2-63 Coronal CT scan. Long arrows point to the supraorbital extension of the ethmoid sinuses. The short arrow indicates a pneumatized crista galli. The beginning of the lacrimal fossa is indicated by the arrowhead.

the precise angulation of the coronal plane, the anterior nasal spine and premaxilla also may be visualized. About 1 cm behind the anterior premaxilla is the incisive foramen. This foramen extends cranially as two separate incisive canals that open on either side of the base of the nasal septum. These canals transmit the terminal branches of the sphenopalatine arteries and their anastomoses with the greater palatine arteries. The canals also transmit the nasopalatine nerves. The nasal septum is formed anteriorly to posteriorly by the medial crura of the alar cartilages, the septal cartilage, the perpendicular plate of the ethmoid bone, and the vomer; while below, the nasal crests of the maxilla and palatine bones contribute to the base of the septum.

The anterior tips of the inferior conchae and the inferior meati start to come into the coronal plane. The lower medial antral wall is clearly seen as it forms the lateral wall of the inferior meatus. Portions of the anterior maxillary wall and the most medial antrum also may be visualized. The base of the nasal bones near the frontonasal and frontomaxillary sutures come into the plane of view, as may the most anterior portion of the frontal bone and the base of the frontal sinuses. The superomedial orbital rims also can be seen. The supraorbital notch, which transmits the supraorbital artery and nerve, is visualized.

The lower bony nasal septum is formed by the vomer, while the upper portion is formed by the perpendicular plate of the ethmoid bone. The posterior margin of the septal cartilage fills in the gap between these bones. The agger nasi cells may be seen superiorly along the lateral wall of the nasal vault. The nasal atrium is the anterolateral nasal space below and medial to the agger nasi. The olfactory recess, the narrow channellike space on either side of the upper nasal septum, is seen. The anterior cribriform plates lie above these recesses. Medial to the supraorbital notch (or foramen) is the frontal notch, which transmits the frontal artery and the frontal nerve.

The medial wall of the lacrimal fossa is seen as a groove in the medial orbital wall. The lacrimal fossa is seen anterior to the nasolacrimal canal in the medial antral wall. This reflects the anatomy of the nasolacrimal canal, which runs downward and posteriorly at about a 20 degree angle with the coronal plane. The normal space (separation) in the medial orbital floor for the lacrimal fossa and sac should not be confused with a focal site of erosion. Portions of the medial orbital floor also start to come into the scan plane.

The lower opening of the nasolacrimal canal can be seen in the medial antral wall under the inferior turbinate (inferior meatus). The medial wall of the nasolacrimal canal is formed superiorly by the lacrimal bone and inferiorly by the lacrimal process of the inferior tur-

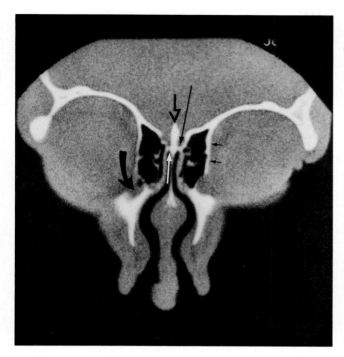

Fig. 2-64   Coronal CT scan. Open arrow points to the crista galli, and the long thin arrow points to the cribriform plate, which lies between the crista galli and the fovea ethmoidalis. The white arrow lies over the olfactory recess of the nasal fossa and points to the bottom of the cribriform plate. The two small arrows indicate the lamina papyracea. The curved arrow points to the lacrimal fossa.

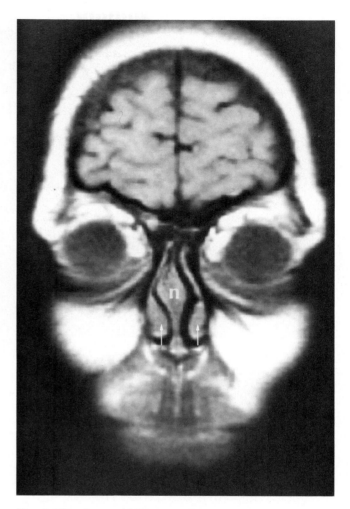

Fig. 2-65   Coronal MRI scan. Cartilaginous nasal septum *(n)* is seen in the midline with middle tubrinates on either side *(arrows)*. Olfactory recesses of nasal fossa lie between the middle turbinates and the nasal septum. The air of the nasal fossa and the bone of the floor of the anterior cranial fossa merge into a region of signal void, decreasing detail when compared to CT. The fat of the subcutaneous regions of the cheeks is seen as high signal beneath each orbit.

binate. The lateral wall is formed entirely by the maxilla. The thin lacrimal bone forms the anterior medial orbital wall, which overlies the anterior ethmoid cells. The lacrimal bone has a slightly concave lateral configuration. The ethmoid lamina papyracea, which lies just behind the lacrimal bone, tends to have a straighter configuration.

The upper, posterior frontal sinus wall may be seen. The middle portions of both the superior and inferior orbital rims are now visualized. The anterior tips of the middle turbinates come into the scan plane. Anteriorly, the attachment of the middle turbinate is along the lateral margin of the cribriform plate and is a useful means of localizing the level of the nasal roof (on more posterior scans, the attachment of the middle concha will tilt laterally). The anterior portion of the middle meatus is seen lateral to the middle concha. The infraorbital foramen and canal are seen in the middle third of the orbital floor.

While the anterior cranial fossa is seen in the midline, the lower and lateral portions of the frontal sinuses are still in the scan plane. More of the lateral orbital rim is visualized. The medial orbital wall is now formed by the lamina papyracea of the ethmoid bone, and the

orbital configuration is circular. A lateral crest of the nasal septum is seen occasionally at the line of junction between the perpendicular plate of the ethmoid bone and the vomer.

The ethmoid infundibulum is identified in the scan plane. The ethmoid bulla—and ethmoid cells—is above the infundibulum; the uncinate process of the ethmoid bone forms the lower medial wall of the infundibulum. The uncinate process rests on the junction of the inferior concha with the medial wall of the maxilla. The maxillary sinus opens into the lower lateral portion of the infundibulum, while the upper medial aspect of the infundibulum opens via the hiatus semilunaris into the middle meatus. A portion of the medial

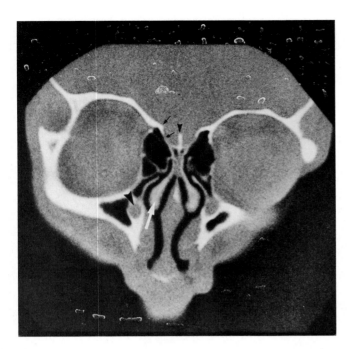

Fig. 2-66 Coronal CT scan. Small arrows point to the fovea ethmoidalis. The posterior thin margin of the cribriform plate is indicated in the midline by the small arrowhead. The arrow points to the middle turbinate. The large arrowhead points to the nasalacrimal duct and the anterior portion of the maxillary sinus is seen just lateral to it.

antral wall in this region is formed entirely by mucosa. This membranous portion is C-shaped with the top of the C above the attachment of the inferior turbinate and the bottom of the C below this level. The back of the C is posterior to the uncinate process. The crista galli is seen as a biconvex bone (often pneumatized) that rests on the midline cribriform plates. If supraorbital ethmoid cells are present, they can be seen extending into the orbital roof. The main maxillary sinus cavity is seen with its zygomatic and alveolar recesses. If there are ethmoid air cells pneumatizing the middle turbinate, they will be seen. More of the orbital rim is seen, with only the lateral orbital wall being incomplete in the scan plane.

The roof of the orbit has bony ridges on its cranial aspect. These reflect in a general way the impressions of the gyri of the base of the frontal lobes. The attachment of the middle turbinate remains along the lateral edge of the cribriform plate. The lateral orbital rims are finally complete, and the zygomaticofrontal sutures are well seen. The small zygomaticotemporal canal may be seen in the body of the zygoma directed horizontally.

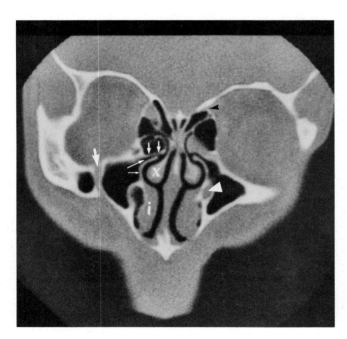

Fig. 2-67 Coronal CT scan. The two small arrows rest in the ethmoid sinuses and are pointing to the bulla ethmoidalis. The single small arrow points to the uncinate process, while the larger arrow above it lies in the infundibulum. *X* lies on the middle turbinate and *i* lies on the inferior turbinate. The large arrowhead indicates the nasolacrimal duct. The larger arrow points to the infraorbital canal. The small arrowhead points to the ethmoidal canal.

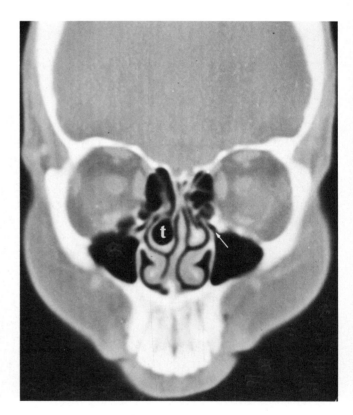

Fig. 2-68 Coronal CT scan. The *t* lies in the air space of a pneumatized right middle turbinate (concha bullosa). The osteomeatal complex is again seen on the left side as in Fig. 2-67. The arrow points to the infundibulum.

Also noted is the narrowing of the posterior crista galli. Thus, in the midline the cribriform plates lie at a lower level than the roofs of the ethmoid sinuses, which are situated on either side of the nasal roof. More laterally, the orbital roofs lie higher than the fovea ethmoidalis.

The palatine spines are seen on the oral surface of the hard palate. Lateral to the spines are the palatine grooves in which run the palatine vessels and nerves. The posterior edge of the crista galli comes into view. Near this level, the anterior ethmoidal canals are seen. They transmit the anterior ethmoidal nerves and vessels. The lower margins of these canals are formed by the ethmoid bones, while the upper margins are formed by the frontal bones. The zygomatic arch is well seen and its upper surface serves as the line of attachment for the fascia of the temporalis muscle. Between the lateral skull surface and the zygomatic arch is the space of the lower portion of the temporal fossa, while below and medially is the infratemporal fossa. The lateral orbital wall inferiorly starts to become incomplete. This is the beginning of the inferior orbital fissure, which is angled at about 45 degrees (open anteriorly)

with the midsagittal plane. This fissure is narrowest in its midportion and widens both at its medial and lateral margins. The orbital configuration slowly becomes more triangular in shape because the medial orbital floor elevates and the lower lamina papyracea tilts laterally, as the larger posterior ethmoid cells are encountered. The beginning of the superior turbinate is seen. The attachment of the middle turbinate has started to migrate toward the lateral nasal wall (medial surface of the ethmoid bone).

The shape of the maxillary sinus is becoming an oval with the long axis in the craniocaudal plane. The greater palatine foramen can be seen at the lateral junction of the hard palate and the maxillary alveolus. The anterior surface of this canal is formed by the maxilla, the posterior surface by the palatine bone. Thus, posterior to this plane, the hard palate is formed by the horizontal plates of the palatine bone. This is roughly the posterior third of the hard palate. Most of the medial antral wall is now formed by the vertical plate of the palatine bone.

The posterior ethmoidal canals come into the scan

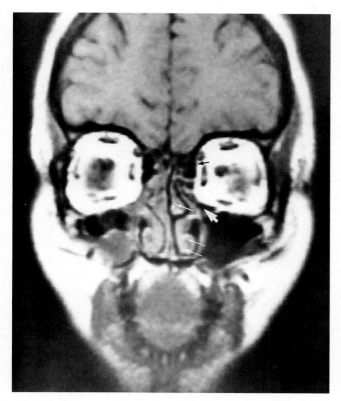

Fig. 2-69   Coronal MRI scan. The air in the left ethmoid sinuses is indistinguishable from the lamina papyracea, which is indicated by the small arrow. The middle *(single arrow)* and inferior *(two arrows)* turbinates are seen as is the nasal septum. The anterior osteomeatal complex is seen on the left side. The large arrow points to the infundibulum. Inflammatory disease is present in the right ethmoid, antrum, middle turbinate, and osteomeatal complex.

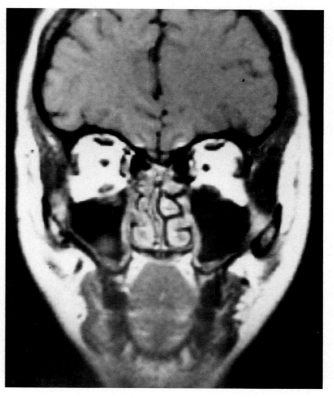

Fig. 2-70   Coronal MRI scan. The configuration of the maxillary sinuses is becoming broader in the craniocaudal axis. The actual bone in the floor and medial wall of the orbit is not seen against the air in these sinuses. The middle and inferior turbinates are again seen as in Fig. 2-69.

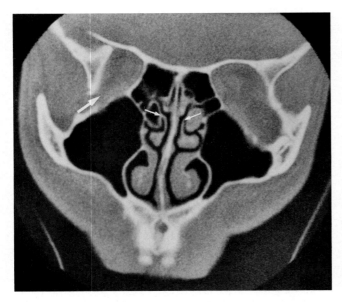

Fig. 2-71   Coronal CT scan. The attachment of the middle turbinates is now lateral to the ethmoid sinuses *(arrows)* rather than to the lateral edges of the cribriform plates as in Figs. 2-65 to 2-69. The large arrow points to the inferior orbital fissure.

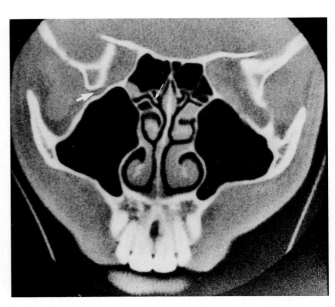

Fig. 2-72   Coronal CT scan. Small arrow points to superior turbinate. Larger arrow points to inferior orbital fissure leading into the apex of the orbit. The configuration of the maxillary sinus is now broader in the craniocaudal axis than it is in the medial-to-lateral axis.

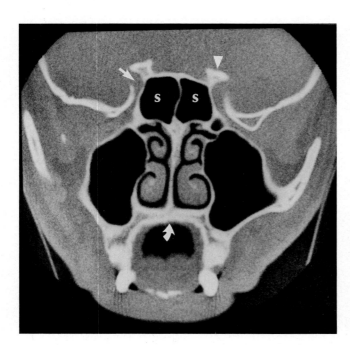

Fig. 2-73   Coronal CT scan. The anterior portions of the sphenoid sinuses *(S)* are seen. The arrow points to the optic canal, which is immediately lateral to the sphenoid sinus. The anterior clinoid process is just above the canal *(arrowhead)*. Portions of the superior orbital fissure are seen just caudal to the optic canals. The curved arrow indicates the oral surface of the hard palate.

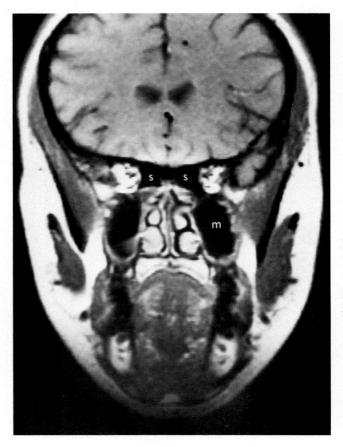

Fig. 2-74   Coronal MRI scan. The anterior sphenoid sinuses *(S)* are seen. The maxillary sinus *(m)* is oblong, with the greatest length in the craniocaudal axis.

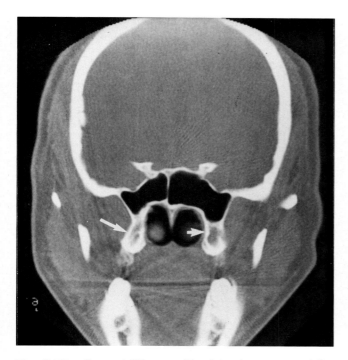

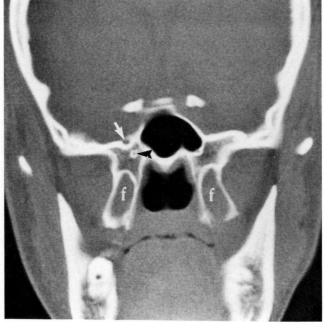

Fig. 2-75   Coronal CT scan. The lateral recesses of the sphenoid sinus into the floor of the middle cranial fossa and pterygoid processes is seen. The large arrow points to the lateral pterygoid plate. The small arrow points to the medial pterygoid plate.

Fig. 2-76   Coronal CT scan. The foramen rotundum is seen on the right *(arrow)*. The vidian or pterygoid canal is also seen on the right side *(arrowhead)*. The pterygoid fossa *(f)* is seen between the medial and lateral pterygoid plates.

plane. Near this level, the anterior margin of the middle cranial fossa and the posterior orbital wall merge as the greater sphenoid wing. The lower segment of the pterygopalatine canal is seen extending upward from the greater palatine foramen toward the pterygopalatine fossa. The most posterior medial wall of the antrum is still formed by the vertical portion of the palatine bone.

The olfactory recess on either side of the nasal septum widens into the sphenoethmoidal recess. This marks the junction between the ethmoid and sphenoid bones. The sphenoid sinus ostia open into these recesses. The posterior edge of the vomer joins the undersurface of the sphenoid bone at the sphenoid rostrum, a prominent triangular ridge on the underbody of the sphenoid bone that forms this articulation. Laterally, the coronoid process of the mandible is seen.

The pterygopalatine fossa is a small space directly behind the maxilla and in front of the pterygoid process of the sphenoid bone. In direct continuity with it is the cranial portion of the pterygopalatine canal inferiorly (which communicates with the mouth) and the sphenopalatine canal medially (which communicates with the nasal fossa). Laterally lies the infratemporal fossa, while above is the inferior orbital fissure, which, in turn, opens into the orbit. Within 5 mm posteriorly, the in-

tracranial communications with the pterygopalatine fossa come into view. These are from medially outward and caudally upward: the pterygoid (vidian) canal, the foramen rotundum, and (via the orbit) the superior orbital fissure. (The most important contents of the pterygopalatine fossa are the sphenopalatine ganglion, the maxillary nerve, and the maxillary artery.) The anterior portion of the main sphenoid sinus cavity is in the scan plane. The intersinus septum is in the midline anteriorly, but posteriorly may be angulated sharply to one side. (This creates two unequal sized sinuses, and once the scan plane moves posterior to such an angled septum, it will appear as if there were only one sphenoid sinus.) The pterygoid plates come into view. The medial plate is almost vertically oriented. The lateral plate is tilted so that its lower end is lateral. The pterygoid fossa lies between these plates. The medial (internal) pterygoid muscle arises from the medial side of the lateral pterygoid plate within the pterygoid fossa, while the lateral (external) pterygoid muscle arises from the lateral side of the lateral plate.

The superior orbital fissure and the optic canal come into the scan plane. The optic canal may cause an indentation on the upper lateral sphenoid sinus wall. (This proximity of the orbital apex to the sphenoid sinus is important clinically, for it relates sphenoid sinus dis-

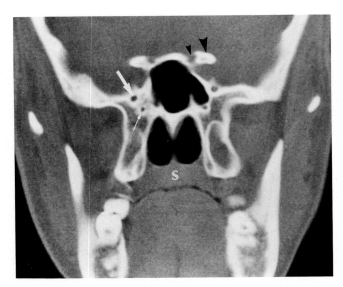

Fig. 2-77   Coronal CT scan. The small arrowhead indicates the optic canal, the large arrowhead points to the anterior clinoid process. The larger arrow points to the foramen rotundum. The smaller arrow indicates the vidian or pterygoid canal. Note that the left pterygoid canal abutts the floor of the sphenoid sinus. The soft palate *(S)* is indicated.

ease to orbital symptoms.) The foramen rotu[n]... also cause an indentation in the lower latera[l]... sinus wall. The smaller pterygoid canal is s... medially to the foramen rotundum, and this ... may cause an indentation in the sphenoid ... The planum sphenoidale, or sinus roof, ha... visualized since the main sphenoid sinus ... view. The recesses of the sphenoid sinus int... goid processes and the greater and lesse... wings are all well seen. The laterally curve[d]... the lower medial pterygoid plate is in the ... The tendon of the tensor veli palatine m... around this hamulus.

As the cavernous sinuses are entered, a... pression is seen on the upper, lateral sph[enoid]... wall. Directly below the medial margin of ... ous sinus, a small bony septum often is see... into the sphenoid sinus. (When these septa... the surgeon can stay medial to or betwee[n]... the cavernous sinuses will not inadverte... tered.) The roof of the sphenoid sinus is n... (lamina dura) of the sella turcica. Benea... floor is the roof of the nasopharynx.

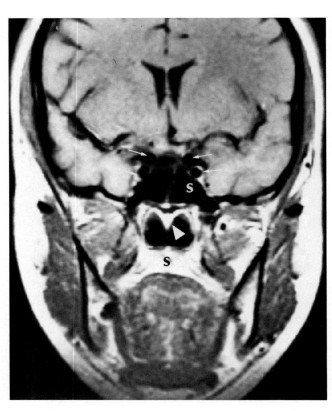

Fig. 2-78   Coronal MRI scan. The carvernous sinus vessels *(arrows)* are seen. The sphenoid sinus *(white S)* and its recesses are also seen, but they are not as clearly defined as on CT. The soft palate *(black S)* is also seen, as is the mucosa over the roof of the posterior nasal fossa *(arrowhead)*.

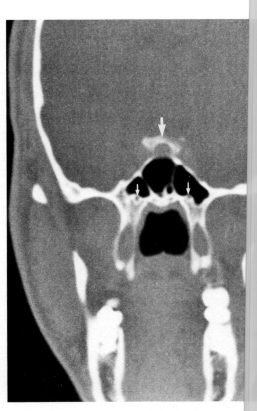

Fig. 2-79   Coronal CT scan. The dorsum s... by the large arrow. The pterygoid canals ar... into the floor of the sphenoid sinuses *(sma...* posterior edges of the pterygoid plates are ...

sverse) Tomographic Anatomy, Starting
xtending Cranially (Figs. 2-80 to 2-108).
eolar ridge is seen. There is some nor-
he bony margin caused by the tooth
l aspects of this section, the infe-
recesses of the maxillary sinuses can be
pneumatizing the alveolar ridges and surrounding
he tooth roots. The incisive foramen lies behind the
central incisor teeth in the midline. It opens cranially
into the two incisive canals, which are on either side of
the base of the nasal septum. They transmit the terminal branches of the sphenopalatine arteries and the nasopalatine nerves. The hamulus of the medial pterygoid
plate may be seen. It is around this bony prominence
that the tendon of the tensor veli palatini muscle
passes. Posteriorly, the ramus of the mandible is visualized with the mandibular canal in its medial side. This
canal transmits the inferior alveolar vessels and nerve
(sensory branch of the mandibular nerve V₂).

There is more extensive pneumatization of the maxillary alveolus, and several incomplete septa can be seen
dividing the alveolar recesses of the antra. The hard
palate is visualized and the oral surface slopes downward at its periphery to meet the inner aspect of the alveolar ridge. Because of this concavity in the axial
plane, the lateral margins of the hard palate often appear thinner than the midline. When the main body of

the hard palate is seen, the intermaxillary suture can be
identified in the midline. Anteriorly, the maxillary alveolar ridge is seen as a bony prominence that will enlarge into the anterior nasal spine on more cranial
scans. The palatine grooves on the oral surface of the
hard palate may be identified on either side of the midline. The pterygoid plates are seen, and the pyramidal
process of the palatine bone forms the lowest portion of
the anterior pterygoid fossa, which is located between
the medial and lateral pterygoid plates.

The septa in the alveolar recesses have disappeared,
and the lower portions of the main maxillary sinuses are
entered. Anteriorly, the anterior nasal spine is seen.
The base of the nasal septum is visualized in the midline, and on either side of the septum anteriorly, the
incisive canals may be seen. More posteriorly, the
greater palatine foramen may be visualized just anterior
to the pterygoid fossa. This foramen connects the pterygopalatine canal with the more cranial pterygopalatine
fossa. The canal transmits the anterior palatine nerve
and the descending palatine artery. Occasionally the
lesser palatine foramen may be identified. It also extends to the pterygopalatine fossa and opens just posterior to the greater palatine foramen. The lesser palatine
foramen transmits the posterior palatine nerve.

The lower nasal cavities are fully in view. The inferior turbinates are seen, as are the inferior meati lying

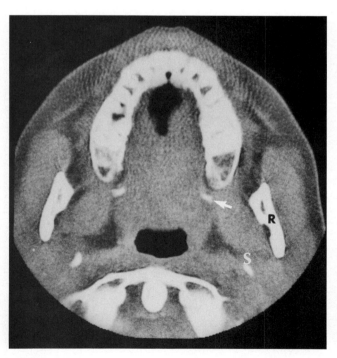

Fig. 2-80 Axial CT scan. The maxillary alveolus is seen
with the roots of the upper teeth imbedded in the alveolus.
The arrow indicates the hamulus of the pterygoid plate. The
styloid process *(arrow)* and the ramus of the mandible *(R)*
are seen. The medial pterygoid muscle runs between the
pterygoid fossa and the medial aspect of the ramus.

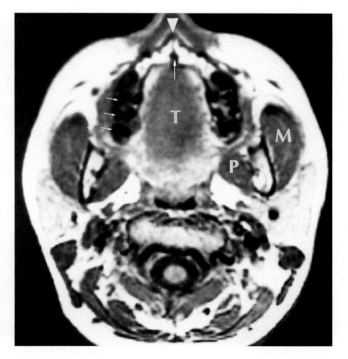

Fig. 2-81 Axial MRI scan. The roots of the teeth *(small ar-*
rows) can be seen as signal voids in the maxillary alveolus.
The incisive foramen *(larger arrow)* is seen just behind the
anterior nasal spine *(arrowhead).* The upper surface of the
tongue *(T)* is seen in the mouth. The pterygoid *(P)* and
masseter *(M)* muscles are also well seen.

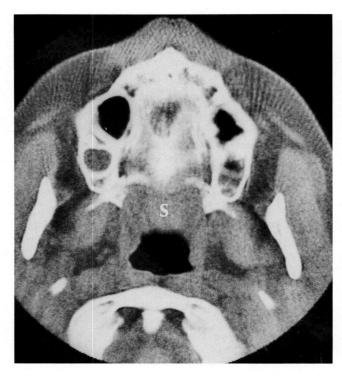

Fig. 2-82 Axial CT scan. The inferior recesses of the maxillary sinuses are seen extending down into the cranial aspect of the maxillary alveolus. Small septations are also commonly seen and these rarely extend up into the main sinus proper. The soft palate *(S)* is seen posterior to the hard palate.

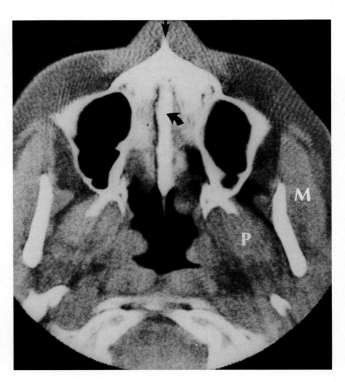

Fig. 2-83 Axial CT scan through the lowermost portion of the nasal cavity. The curved arrow indicates the lower nasal septum abutting the top of the hard palate. The lower portions of the maxillary sinuses are seen extending below the level of the hard palate. The medial pterygoid *(P)* and masseter *(M)* muscles are well seen as is the lowermost nasopharynx, which begins at the level of the hard palate.

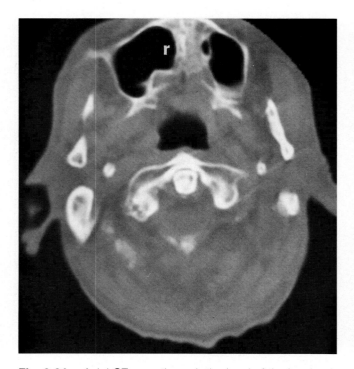

Fig. 2-84 Axial CT scan through the level of the hard palate shows a palatal recess of the right maxillary sinus *(r)* extending into the hard palate.

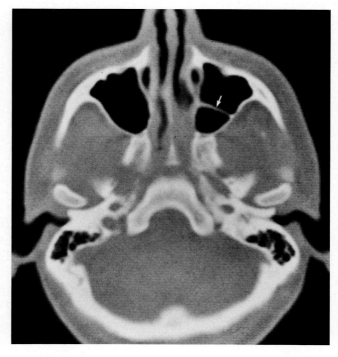

Fig. 2-85 Axial CT scan shows an antral septum *(arrow)*, which divides the left maxillary sinus into a separate anterior and posterior compartment, each of which drains into the nasal fossa.

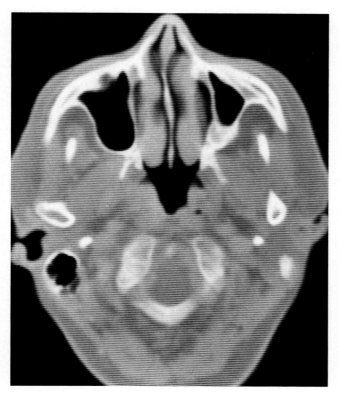

Fig. 2-86 Axial CT scan with a hypoplastic left maxilla and maxillary sinus. The thicker bone along the anterior and posterior sinus walls and the smaller air cavity when compared to the normal right side accounts for the impression of haziness or mucosal thickening in the hypoplastic sinus on plain films.

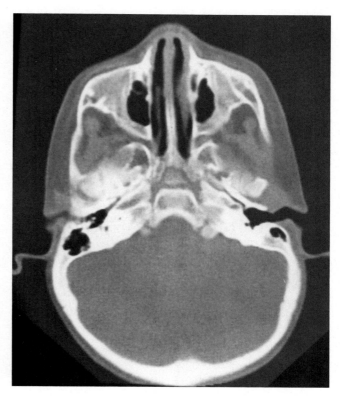

Fig. 2-87 Axial CT scan on a normal child about 2 years old. The developing maxillary sinuses have only partially pneumatized the maxilla. This, in a similar manner to Fig. 2-86, accounts for the apparent clouding on plain films of many such small sinuses.

just lateral to each inferior turbinate. The medial walls of the maxillary sinuses are partially bone and partially membrane. This membranous area forms a C shape, which is closed posteriorly and bridges the posterior attachment of the inferior turbinate. Posteriorly, the coronoid process and the neck of the mandible are seen separated by the mandibular notch.

The anterior wall of the maxillary sinus has a slightly concave anterior configuration. This is the canine fossa, and it lies cranial to the lateral incisor and canine teeth and caudal to the infraorbital canal. The caninus muscle arises from this fossa. Behind the maxillary sinuses, but anterior to the medial pterygoid plates, the pterygopalatine and lesser palatine canals may be identified. The infratemporal fossa fat is seen abutting the curved posterolateral antral walls. There is a thinning in this curved sinus wall that corresponds to the canal for the posterior superior alveolar nerve. This should not be confused with a site of bone erosion. The body and anterior arches of the zygoma are seen.

The pterygopalatine fossa is seen just behind the medial posterior aspect of the maxillary sinus, immediately anterior to the pterygoid process of the sphenoid bone.

The anterior medial bony boundary of the fossa is formed by the palatine bone and the sphenopalatine foramen. This foramen may be seen connecting the nasal fossa with the pterygopalatine fossa. Within the pterygopalatine fossa are the sphenopalatine ganglion, portions of the maxillary nerve, and the internal maxillary artery. These structures are supported by fat, which fills the majority of the fossa. Posteriorly, the pterygoid (Vidian) canal and the foramen rotundum may be seen in the skull base, extending into the middle cranial fossa. The middle turbinates and middle meati are seen. The posterior tip of the middle choncha points to the level of the sphenopalatine foramen. The infraorbital foramen may create a focal indentation or defect in the anterior antral wall. This occurs about 1 cm below the inferior orbital rim. The nasolacrimal canal is seen in the medial antral wall. Because the nasolacrimal canal runs upward and forward at about a 20 degree angle to the coronal plane, this canal is seen more anteriorly placed in the medial antral wall on the more cranial scans. Posteriorly, the nasal septum thickens as the alae of the vomer articulate with the rostrum of the sphenoid bone.

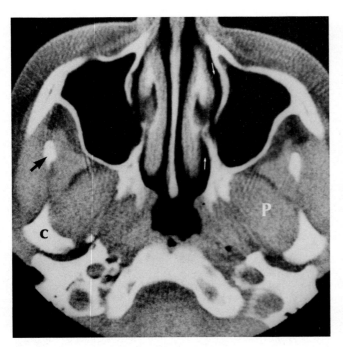

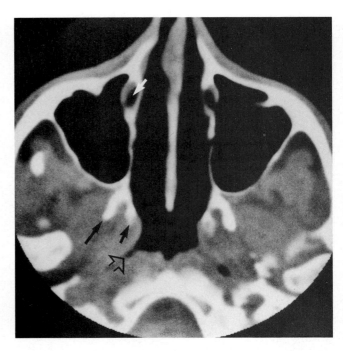

Fig. 2-88 Axial CT scan through the midmaxillary sinuses. The inferior turbinates are seen and the air space lateral and below them *(small arrows)* is the inferior meatus. The coronoid process of the mandable is seen *(arrow)* with the space of the mandibular notch directly behind it and the mandibular condyle *(c)* behind that. The lateral pterygoid muscle *(P)* is also seen extending from the lateral pterygoid plate to the mandibular condyle.

Fig. 2-89 Axial CT scan shows the nasal septum in the midline. The white arrow indicates the nasolacrimal duct. The long, black arrow points to the lateral pterygoid plate and the short, black arrow points to the medial pterygoid plate. The open arrow points to the lateral nasopharyngeal recess and the fossa of Rosenmuller.

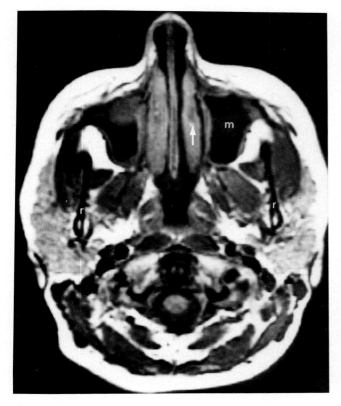

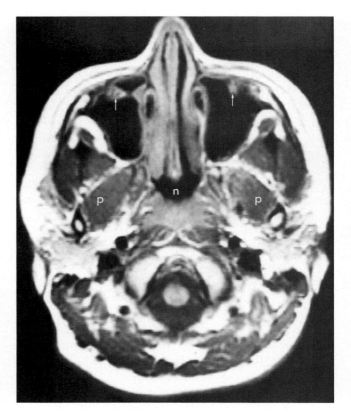

Fig. 2-90 Axial MRI scan shows the maxillary sinuses *(m)* and the inferior turbinates *(arrow)*. The masseter and pterygoid muscles are seen on either side of the ramus of the mandible *(r)*.

Fig. 2-91 Axial MRI scan shows lowermost anterior portion of orbit, seen in the anterior antrum *(arrows)*. The nasopharynx *(n)* and lateral pterygoid muscles *(p)* are also seen.

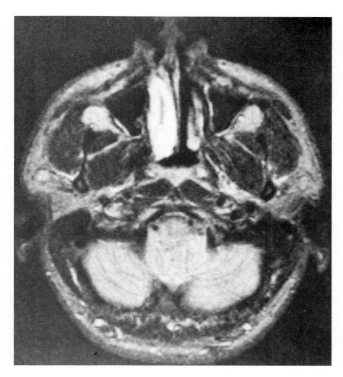

Fig. 2-92 Axial MRI scan. This T$_2$W study shows a high signal intensity in the right inferior turbinate, which is also apparently enlarged. This is a normal turbinate experiencing the normal nasal cycle.

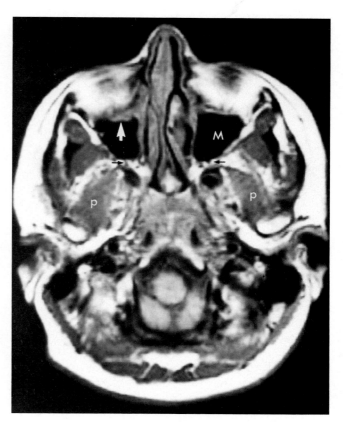

Fig. 2-93 Axial MRI scan through the upper portion of the maxillary sinuses *(m)*. More of the orbital content is seen anteriorly *(arrows)*. The pterygopalatine fossae *(small arrows)* are also well seen as are the lateral pterygoid muscles *(p)*.

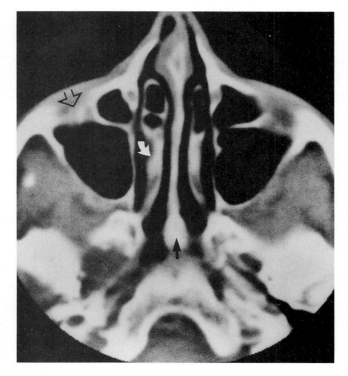

Fig. 2-94 Axial CT scan with open arrow indicating the beginning of the anterior orbit. Curved arrow rests in the middle meatus and points to the partially pneumatized middle turbinate. Arrow points to the rostrum of the sphenoid and the posterior nasal septum.

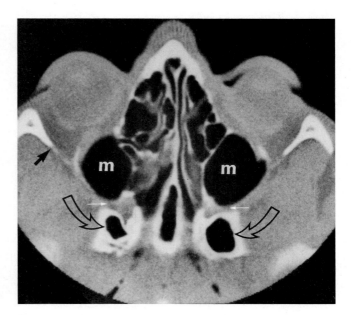

Fig. 2-95 Axial CT scan with curved arrows pointing to the pneumatized pterygoid processes of the sphenoid bone. There is also some pneumatization of the rostrum of the sphenoid lying between the pterygoid processes. Small arrows indicate the pterygopalatine fossae. Upper portions of the maxillary sinuses *(m)* are seen. Large arrow points to the zygomaticosphenoid suture.

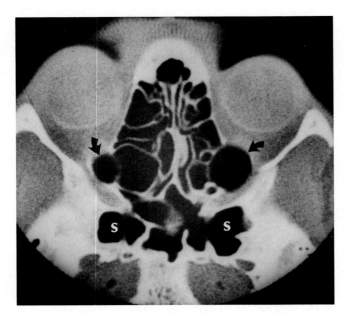

Fig. 2-96 Axial CT scan. Curved arrows indicate cranial recesses of the maxillary sinuses near the apex of the orbit. The air cells medial to these are ethmoid sinus cells. The sphenoid sinus *(s)* has small lateral recesses.

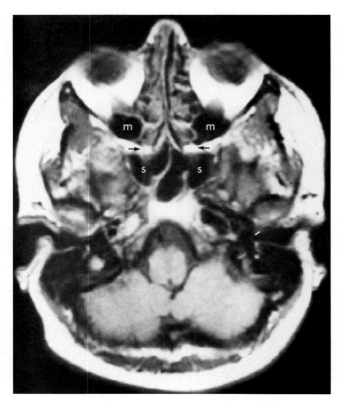

Fig. 2-97 Axial MRI scan. Upper recesses of the maxillary sinuses *(m)* are seen in the apex of the orbits. The sphenoid sinus *(s)* is also seen. Upper portion of the pterygopalatine fossa is indicated by small arrows.

The flattest and most caudal portion of the orbital floor is seen lying anterolaterally in the orbit. Because the inferior orbital rim is concave upward, this bony rim is seen first in the midline, and then on more cranial scans it is identified on either side of a central area of orbital soft tissues. This central region widens progressively on more cranial scans until the main orbital plane is entered. The lacrimal sac fossa is seen along the anteromedial orbital margin, slightly more cranial than the level of the flattest portion of the orbital floor. It is identified when the lateral bony margin of the nasolacrimal canal opens toward the orbit. The anterior crest is formed by the lacrimal bone. The lowermost ethmoid cells are seen, and the posterior lateral attachment of the middle turbinate is identified. The middle meatus is just lateral to the turbinate; however, in the axial plane the detailed anatomy of the hiatus semilunaris, infundibulum, and uncinate process cannot be well seen. These are better identified in the coronal plane. The sphenoid sinus bases come into the scan plane. Any pneumatization of the pterygoid processes already will have been identified. The intersphenoid sinus septum is usually in the midline anteriorly. It then may veer sharply to one side, creating two unequal sized sinuses.

The posterior and highest recesses of the maxillary sinuses are seen in the posteromedial orbital floor. These recesses appear as round or ovoid air spaces with a thin bony wall separating them from the orbital contents, and they should not be confused with the ethmoid sinus cells. The main ethmoid complex is entered. From anteriorly to posteriorly the bones forming a line from the nose to the back of the medial orbital wall are the nasal bone, the frontal process of the maxilla, the lacrimal bone, the lamina papyracea of the ethmoid bone, and the sphenoid bone. Of these bones, the lamina papyracea is the only one that may normally have focal dehiscences. Thus, before an erosion in this bone is diagnosed, comparison to the opposite lamina papyracea should be made. If sphenoid sinus recesses are present in the posterior orbital wall and floor of the middle cranial fossa (greater wing of the sphenoid), they will be seen. The posterior sphenoid sinus wall is identified, and on either side is an indentation made by the carotid sulcus. Just cranial to this area, the floor of the sella turcica is seen. Anteriorly will be the tuberculum and the planum sphenoidale. (An enlarged sella turcica will descend into the sphenoid sinus and may be mistaken for a primary intrasphenoid sinus process. Coronal or sagittal scans will resolve any issue.)

On either side of the nasal septum the nasal cavity has become a narrow slit called the olfactory recess. Portions of the cribriform plates and fovea ethmoidalis may be seen. The intracranial surface of the cribriform

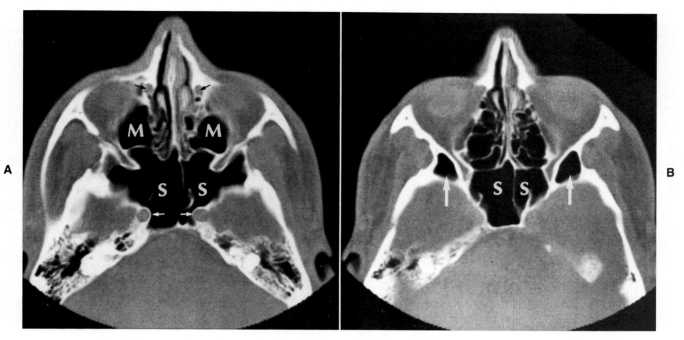

Fig. 2-98   A, Axial CT scan shows the sphenoid sinuses *(s)* with lateral recesses in the greater wings of the sphenoid bone as they form the floor of the middle cranial fossae. Upper recesses of the maxillary sinuses *(M)* are also seen. The indentations of the carotid arteries into the main sphenoid sinus cavities are shown by white arrows. Black arrows point to the nasolacrimal ducts. **B,** Axial CT scan more cranial than **A** shows the continuation of the lateral recesses into the greater sphenoid wings as they form the posterior orbital walls *(arrows).* Although they appear separate from the main sphenoid sinus cavities *(S)* on this scan, these are in reality recesses of the sinus.

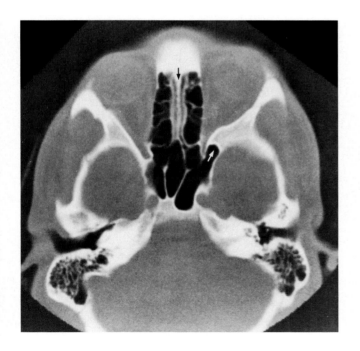

Fig. 2-99   Axial CT scan through the upper ethmoid sinuses. The nasal septum *(black arrow)* is seen in the midline and the air of the olfactory recesses is on either side of the septum. The ethmoid sinuses are lateral to these olfactory recesses. The sphenoid sinus has a recess into the left posterior orbital wall *(white arrow).*

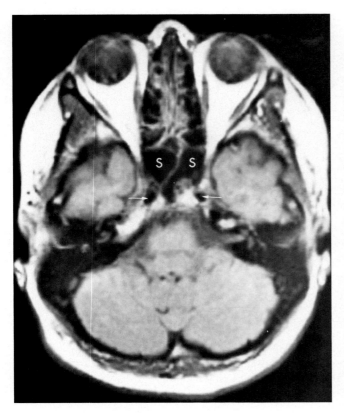

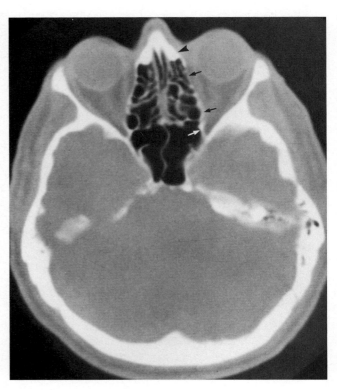

Fig. 2-100   Axial MRI scan through the ethmoid sinuses. The sphenoid sinuses *(S)* are seen as are the carotid arteries *(arrows).* Although the lamina papyracea is not seen, the clear distinction of the ethmoid complex from the orbital contents indicates that the bone is intact.

Fig. 2-101   Axial CT scan. The medial orbital wall is made up of the lacrimal bone *(arrowhead),* the lamina papyracea *(black arrows)* and the sphenoid sinus *(white arrow).*

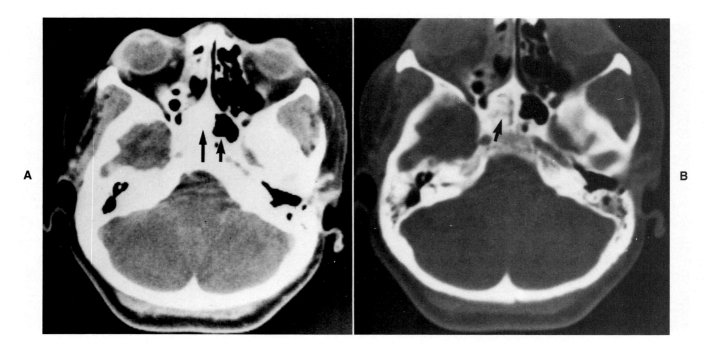

Fig. 2-102   **A,** Axial CT scan at narrow window-setting shows a small left sphenoid sinus *(short arrow)* and an apparent aplastic right sphenoid sinus *(long arrows).* **B,** Axial CT scan same level as **A** at wide window-setting shows an osteoma obliterating the right sphenoid sinus cavity *(arrow).*

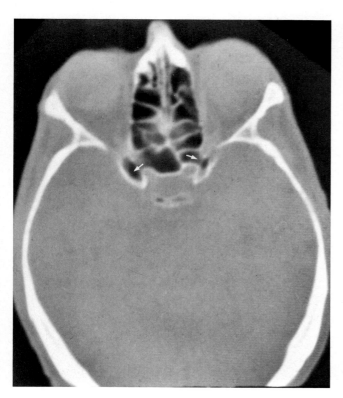

Fig. 2-103   Axial CT scan reveals extensions of the sphenoid sinuses into the anterior clinoid processes *(arrows)*.

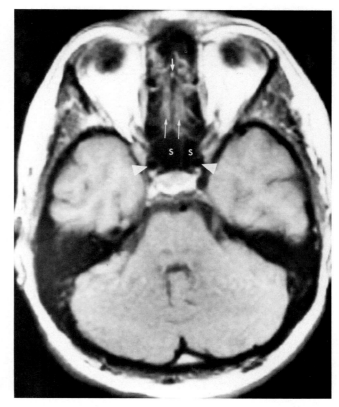

Fig. 2-104   Axial MRI scan through the upper ethmoid sinuses. The crista galli *(small arrow)* is seen. Soft tissues on either side are the normal sinodural tissues of the midline floor of the anterior cranial fossa *(longer arrows)*. The sphenoid sinuses *(S)* and carotid arteries *(arrowheads)* are also seen.

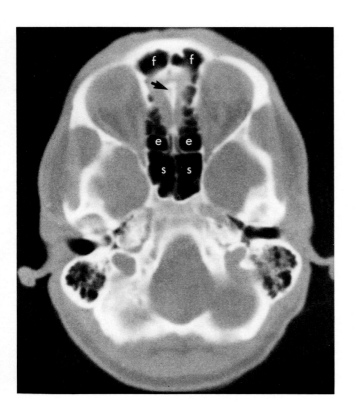

Fig. 2-105   Axial CT scan with arrow pointing to the crista galli. Soft tissues around the crista galli are the normal sinodural tissues of the midline floor of the anterior cranial fossa. The bases of the frontal sinuses *(f)* are seen anteriorly while the upper ethmoid *(e)* and sphenoid sinuses *(s)* are seen posteriorly.

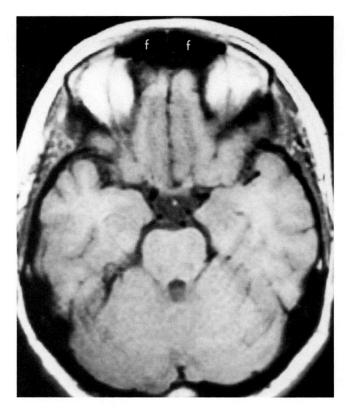

Fig. 2-106 Axial MRI scan through the lower frontal sinuses *(f)*. The uppermost portions of the orbit are seen as are the midline structures of the anterior cranial fossa.

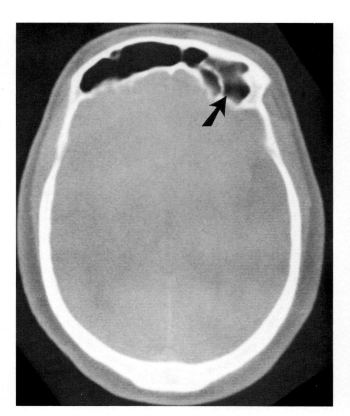

Fig. 2-107 Axial CT scan shows extension of the left frontal sinus into the roof of the left orbit *(arrow)*.

Fig. 2-108 Axial CT scan shows the frontal sinuses. The septations and scalloped sinus margins are well seen. The posterior and anterior sinus walls are also best evaluated in this axial plane.

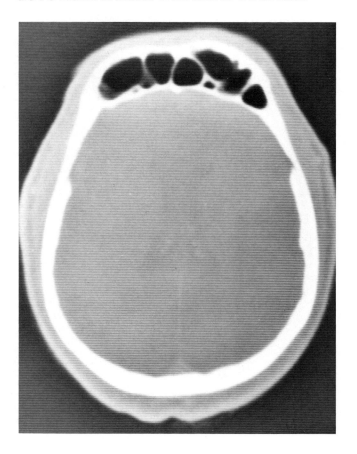

plates is identified by the presence of the crista galli. (The midline base of the anterior cranial fossa structures often create a pseudomass behind the crista galli. This can be resolved as a "fake" on coronal scans.) The base of the frontal sinuses and any supraorbital ethmoid cell or frontal sinus pneumatization of the orbital roof will be seen at this level.

The anterior and posterior frontal sinus walls are well seen. The intersinus septum and small septae from the sinus walls can be identified. The anterior cranial fossa structures can also be well seen. Since there is independent growth of the left and right frontal sinuses, one may be well developed while the other is aplastic. On CT, wide windows may be necessary to distinguish an aplastic or hypoplastic sinus from a completely clouded, normally developed sinus.

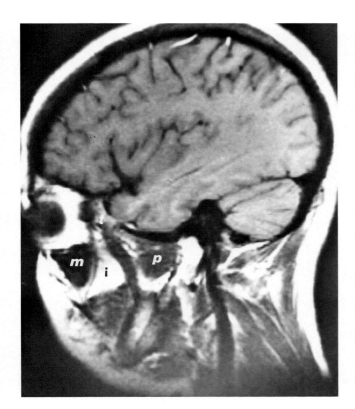

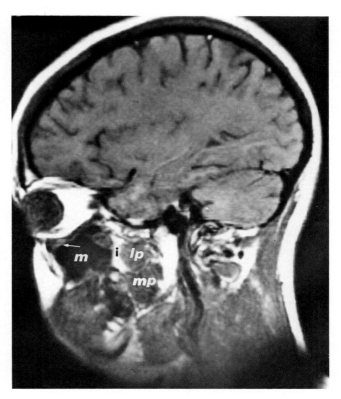

Fig. 2-109   Sagittal MRI scan shows the air and bone of the zygomatic recess of the maxillary sinus *(m)*. Directly behind it is the fat of the infratemporal fossa *(i)*. Above this is the anterior margin of the temporal fossa *(t)*. The lateral pterygoid muscle *(p)* is seen just deep to the ramus of the mandible.

Fig. 2-110   Sagittal MRI scan shows the mid portion of the maxillary sinus *(m)*. A portion of the infratemporal nerve *(arrow)* is seen in the roof of the sinus. Behind the sinus is the fat of the infratemporal fossa *(i)* and the lateral pterygoid *(lp)* and medial pterygoid *(mp)* muscles.

Sagittal Tomographic Anatomy, Starting Laterally and Extending Medially (Figs. 2-109 to 2-114). The body of the zygoma is seen at the lower margin of the lateral orbital rim. A small channel may be seen in the lateral orbital wall (zygomaticotemporal canal) and in the zygomatic body (zygomaticofacial canal). The frontozygomatic suture may also be seen. The roof of the orbit and the anterior wall of the middle cranial fossa are visualized; the open space below and posterior to the orbit is the infratemporal fossa.

Depending on the size of the sinus, the lateral extent of the maxillary sinus can be seen in the body of the zygoma (zygomatic recess). The sphenozygomatic suture in the posterolateral orbital wall may be seen. The lateral one-third of this wall is formed by the zygoma, while the medial two-thirds is formed by the sphenoid bone. The lateral aspect of the frontal sinus may also be seen provided this sinus is sufficiently well developed. The plane of the mandibular condyle, coronoid process, and upper mandibular ramus is visualized with the corresponding articular eminence and glenoid fossa of the temporomandibular joint.

The lower margin of the sphenozygomatic suture starts to widen into the anterolateral aspect of the inferior orbital fissure. This fissure separates the lateral orbital wall from the orbital floor. The fissure is about 2 cm long, and its anterior end is 2 cm behind the orbital rim. The inferior orbital fissure is narrowest in its midpoint and wider both anterolaterally and posteromedially. It is at the level of the lateral margin of the inferior orbital fissure that the temporal fossa becomes the infratemporal fossa. The zygomaticosphenoid and zygomaticomaxillary sutures are near this plane.

The infraorbital canal runs in the middle third of the orbital floor. It extends from the inferior orbital fissure posteriorly to the anterior maxilla. This canal runs parallel to the orbital floor except in its most anterior portion where it turns downward to exit in the infraorbital foramen, which is about 1 cm below the inferior orbital rim. The configuration of the antrum is now rectangular. Behind the antrum, the medial aspect of the infratemporal fossa begins to narrow into the sphenomaxillary (retromaxillary) fissure, which in turn will open more medially into the pterygopalatine fossa. At the level of the medial aspect of the sphenomaxillary fissure, the foramen spinosum can be seen in the floor of

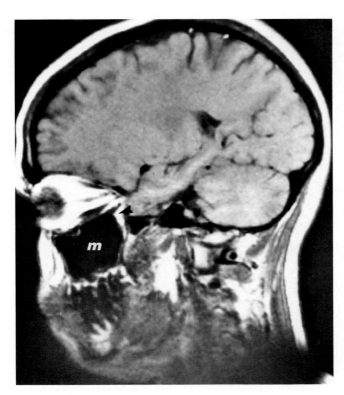

Fig. 2-111 Sagittal MRI scan shows the most medial and largest portion of the maxillary sinus *(m)*. The maxillary teeth in the maxillary alveolus are seen directly below the sinus. The infratemporal fossa has narrowed and is now near the pterygopalatine fossa *(arrowhead)*, which is just below the apex of the orbit.

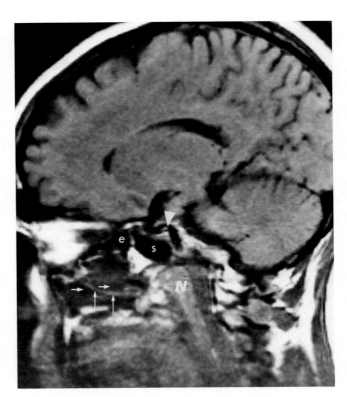

Fig. 2-112 Sagittal MRI scan in a plane just medial to the medial antral wall. Air is seen in the inferior and middle meatus *(short arrows)* separated by the attachment of the inferior turbinate *(two vertical arrows)*. The posterior ethmoid cells *(e)* and sphenoid sinus *(s)* are seen. The carotid artery is just above and behind the sphenoid sinus *(arrowhead)*. The lateral aspect of the nasopharyngeal mucosa *(N)* and the constrictor musculature are also seen.

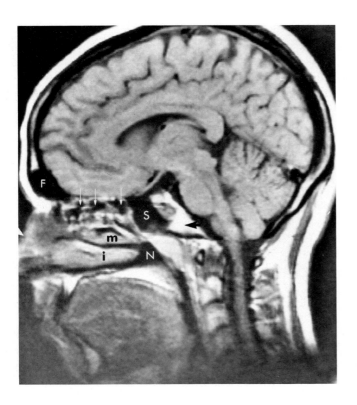

Fig. 2-113 Sagittal MRI scan shows the inferior *(i)* and the middle *(m)* turbinates outlined by air in the nasal fossa. The lateral cartilages of the nose *(arrowhead)* are seen anteriorly. Posteriorly is the nasopharynx *(N)*. The sphenoid *(s)* and frontal *(F)* sinus cavities are seen, as are scattered anterior and middle ethmoid cells *(arrows)*. Marrow is present in the clivus *(large arrow)*.

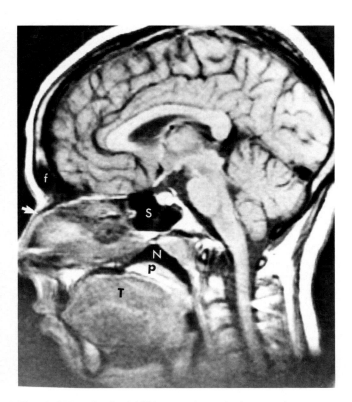

Fig. 2-114 Sagittal MRI scan through the nasal septum. The nasal bones *(arrow)* are seen anteriorly. The lateral portion of the frontal sinus *(f)* is also seen. The sphenoid sinus *(s)* is seen posteriorly. Air is seen in the nasopharynx *(N)* just above the soft palate *(p),* and the tongue musculature *(T)* is also visualized.

the middle cranial fossa connecting the cranial cavity with the infratemporal fossa.

The roof of the orbit (frontal bone) is now separated from the posterior orbital wall (greater sphenoid wing) by the superior orbital fissure. The slight anterior concavity of the anterior maxillary sinus wall defines the margins of the canine fossa. The frontal sinus now has a tall triangular configuration just above the orbit. The relationship to the anterior cranial fossa (posterior table) and the forehead (anterior table) are well seen.

At about the level of the lateral pterygoid plate, the pterygopalatine fossa is entered. This fossa connects superiorly with the inferior orbital fissure. Just posterior to the pterygopalatine fossa is the horizontally oriented foramen rotundum. More posteriorly in the scan plane, the foramen ovale is seen in the floor of the middle cranial fossa; and even more posteriorly, the impression of the Gasserian ganglion on the anterior petrous tip is visualized. The wider medial portion of the superior orbital fissure is seen. The maxillary sinus is at its largest size medially, and some posterolateral ethmoid cells may be seen at the level of the posterior antral roof (orbital floor).

The lacrimal sac fossa and portions of the nasolacri-

nal canal can be seen. This canal is directed downward and posteriorly. Portions of the lateral nasal wall come into the scan plane. These include the attachment of the inferior turbinate, the infundibulum, the hiatus semilunaris, and the posterior attachment of the middle turbinate. The superior orbital fissure is near its widest portion, and the anterior clinoid process may be seen just above this fissure. The pterygopalatine canal can be seen extending down from the pterygopalatine fossa. Some of the ethmoid cells may be in the scan plane. Those just above the hiatus semilunaris are the cells of the ethmoid bulla. The lateral extent of the sphenoid sinus may also be visualized.

The sphenopalatine foramen is seen connecting the nasal cavity with the laterally positioned pterygopalatine fossa. The small pterygoid (vidian) canal may be seen connecting the posterior pterygopalatine fossa with the floor of the middle cranial fossa. The floor of the frontal sinus is no longer complete because the nasofrontal duct is present. This duct usually drains into the frontal recess, which is the most anterior, superior portion of the middle meatus. The inferior, middle, and superior turbinates come into the plane of the scan. The sphenoid sinus is well visualized, and the impression of the carotid artery along its upper, posterolateral margin can be seen. The optic canal can be visualized directly under the anterior clinoid process.

The agger nasi ethmoid cells may be seen as the most anterior medial ethmoid cells, lying just anterior to the middle turbinate. The undersurface of the sphenoid sinus is actually covered by the vaginal processes of the medial pterygoid plates and the alae of the vomer. The openings of the anterior and posterior ethmoidal canals may be visualized in the floor of the anterior cranial fossa. The posterior clinoid process may also be seen.

The cribriform plate of the ethmoid bone (nasal roof) is faintly seen. The sphenoethmoidal recess is the area of the nasal cavity just behind the superior turbinate. The ostium of the sphenoid sinus drains into this recess. The roof of the sphenoid sinus (planum sphenoidale) lies directly behind the cribriform plate. At the posterior aspect of the planum sphenoidale can be seen respectively from anteriorly to posteriorly the limbus, the chiasmatic sulcus, the tuberculum sellae, the lamina dura (anterior wall and floor) of the sella, and the dorsum sellae.

The nasofrontal suture and the midline portions of the nasal bones can be seen. The crista galli is visualized just above the cribriform plate. Portions of the nasal septum are seen. The hard palate, premaxilla, and anterior nasal spine are in the scan plane. The incisive canal above and the incisive foramen below are seen in the most anterior hard palate. The incisive canal marks the junction between the premaxillary and postmaxillary portions of the maxilla. Posteriorly, the ala of the vomer articulates with the rostrum of the sphenoid.

REFERENCES

1. Dodd GD and Jing BS: Radiology of the nose, paranasal sinuses and nasopharynx, Baltimore, 1977, Williams and Wilkins.
2. Merrill V: Atlas of roentgenographic positions, ed 3, St. Louis, 1967, The CV Mosby Co.
3. Mancuso AA and Hanafee WN: Computed tomography and magnetic resonance imaging of the head and neck, ed 2, Baltimore, 1985, Williams and Wilkins, pp 1-19.
4. Som P: Paranasal sinuses and pterygopalatine fossa. In Carter BL, editor: Computed tomography of the head and neck, New York, 1985, Churchill Livingstone, Inc, pp 101-130.
5. Brant-Zawadzki M and Norman D: Magnetic resonance imaging of the central nervous system, New York, 1987, Raven Press, Inc.
6. Lloyd GAS, Lund VJ, Phelps PD, et al.: Magnetic resonance imaging in the evaluation of nose and paranasal sinus disease, Br J Radiol 60:957, 1987.
7. Yanagisawa E and Smith HW: Radiographic anatomy of the paranasal sinuses IV, Caldwell view, Arch Otolaryngol 87:311, 1968.
8. Yanagisawa E and Smith HW: Normal radiographic anatomy of the paranasal sinuses, Otolaryngol Clin North Am 6(2):429, 1973.
9. Yanagisawa E and Smith HW: Radiology of the normal maxillary sinus and related structures, Otolaryngol Clin North Am 9(1):55, 1976.
10. Yanagisawa E and Smith HW, and Merrell RA: Radiographic anatomy of the paranasal sinuses III, Submentovertical view, Arch Otolaryngol 87:299, 1968.
11. Yanagisawa E, Smith HW, and Thaler S: Radiographic anatomy of the paranasal sinuses II, Lateral view, Arch Otolaryngol 87:196, 1968.
12. Zizmor J and Noyek A: Radiology of the nose and paranasal sinuses. In Paparella MM and Shumrick DA: Otolaryngology, vol 1, Philadelphia, 1973, WB Saunders Co, pp 1043-1095.
13. Potter GD: Sectional anatomy and tomography of the head, New York, 1971, Grune & Stratton, Inc.
14. Gambarelli J, Guérinel G, Chevrot L, et al.: Computerized axial tomography: an anatomic atlas of serial sections of the human body, anatomy-radiology-scanner, Berlin, 1977, Springer-Verlag.
15. Ferner H, editor: Pernkopf's Atlas of topographical and applied human anatomy, vol 1, Head and neck, Baltimore, 1980, Urban and Schwarzenberg, Inc.
16. Schatz CJ and Becken TS: Normal and CT anatomy of the paranasal sinuses, Radiol Clin North Am 22:107, 1984.
17. Terrier F, Weber W, Ruenfenacht D, et al.: Anatomy of the ethmoid: CT, endoscopic and macroscopic, AJNR 6:77, 1985.
18. Daniels DL, Rauschning W, Lovas J, et al.: Pterygopalatine fossa: computed tomography studies, Radiology 149:511, 1983.

SECTION THREE
NONNEOPLASTIC DISORDERS

INFLAMMATORY CONDITIONS
Acute Viral and Bacterial Rhinosinusitis

The "cold" is the most common malady involving the upper respiratory tract. The clinical manifestations of this viral infection usually persist only 2 to 3 days, and the evoked inflammatory changes are completely reversible. The most commonly implicated viruses are rhinoviruses, parainfluenza and influenza viruses, adenoviruses, and respiratory syncytial virus.[1] The typical cold remains primarily a viral rhinitis with no significant sinusitis. If the sinonasal cavities are examined radiographically, the paranasal sinuses are usually normal, while there may be mucosal thickening of the nasal fossae and swelling of the turbinates. If this swollen mucosa happens to cause obstruction of a sinus ostium (most commonly the maxillary sinus), the oxygen tension within the sinus changes and the normal bacterial flora becomes altered. This results in an acute bacterial sinusitis. Because of the possibility of nasal fossa contamination, the accurate determination of the pathogens responsible for a bacterial sinusitis requires either direct sinus puncture or open surgical biopsy.[2] The most commonly implicated pathogens from such studies are *Streptococcus pneumoniae* (pneumococcus), *Haemophilus influenzae*, and a β-hemolytic streptococcus. Rarely, *Staphylococcus aureus* and *Pseudomonas* infections can occur.[3] Pathogenic anaerobes are rare in acute sinusitis. However, in cases of chronic sinusitis with persistently low intrasinus oxygen tensions, anaerobes predominate. These include peptostreptococci, *Bacteroides* sp., and fusobacteria.[4,5] In the case of the maxillary sinus, it is estimated that 10% to 20% of the infections are secondary to dental infection or are the result of a complication of a tooth extraction.[6]

If the sinus ostial obstruction is transient, the bacterial sinusitis usually will resolve with conservative treatment within 4 to 7 days. The onset of such a secondary or superinfection complicating a viral rhinitis is evidenced clinically when the virally induced watery nasal discharge changes to a mucopurulent exudate. Bacterial sinusitis is also associated with pain that is usually localized over the affected sinus. By comparison, headache is estimated to occur in only 3% of patients with sinusitis, and in these cases it usually is either a frontal headache secondary to a frontal sinusitis or a suboccipital headache secondary to sphenoid sinusitis.[7] Somewhat unexplainably, bone remodelling or destruction does not usually cause pain unless an associated infection is present.

Acute bacterial sinusitis, being the result of sinus ostial obstruction, is in effect a sinus-by-sinus-event, depending in part on what is causing the ostial obstruction. Thus, a unilateral nasal mass often will result in a unilateral pansinusitis. The frontal sinus blockage either may be caused by direct obstruction of its nasal drainage or the result of obstruction of anterior ethmoid cells in those cases in which the frontal sinus drains directly into these sinuses. Although a pansinusitis can occur in acute bacterial disease, most often there is unilateral or isolated sinus involvement. Even when both antra are affected, one is usually more severely afflicted than the other. Thus, in general, asymmetric sinusitis is a hallmark of bacterial disease.

Chronic sinusitis results from either persistent acute inflammation or repeated episodes of acute or subacute sinusitis. Chronic disease can result in an atrophic, sclerosing, or hypertrophic polypoid mucosa. These varied mucosal changes can coexist with one another and with areas of acute inflammation of either an infectious or allergic etiology. Because chronically inflamed and scarred mucosa loses some of its ciliary function, it becomes less resistent to infection. Thus, a vicious cycle of infection and reinfection is often present in patients with chronic sinusitis. The bony sinus walls around a chronically infected sinus often become thickened and sclerotic. This reactive bony change can be found with all chronic inflammations whether they are of bacterial, fungal, or granulomatous etiology.

By comparison to bacterial sinusitis, *allergic sinusitis* tends to symmetrically involve the nasal fossae and paranasal sinuses. This probably reflects the underlying systemic nature of this process. Another helpful distinguishing factor between allergic and bacterial sinusitis is the presence of nasal polyposis. Nasal polyps are common in allergic patients, while they are uncommon in patients with routine bacterial sinusitis. In addition, most allergic polyps are multiple, whereas most inflammatory polyps are solitary.

Nearly 10% of the population has allergic rhinitis and sinusitis. The most common form is seasonal pollinosis, and the prevalent form in North America is ragweed allergy. Spores, molds, and mites are also important antigens.[8] Allergic reactions are manifestations of type I immunologic disorders, which reflect an IgE reagin-antibody reaction with a resulting release of mediators that produce symptoms of sneezing, nasal obstruction, and watery rhinorrhea. Profuse secretions associated with nasal obstruction can result in some retained secretions and eventual infection.[8] Thus, the coexistence of bacterial and allergic sinusitis is not uncommon. The resulting hypertrophic, thickened, and redundant allergic sinus mucosa is often referred to as hypertrophic polypoid mucosa, which is less capable than normal mucosa of resisting subsequent infections.

Rarely, in the maxillary sinus, this hypertrophic mucosa can be so redundant that it prolapses into the nasal fossa and simulates an antrochoanal polyp.[9]

In the pediatric patient, sinus opacification and mucosal thickening have a questionable correlation with the presence of active infection. This is particularly true in children under 2 years, in whom tears, retained normal secretions, and normal redundant or loose mucosa may account for these radiographic findings.[10-12] In all patients, such paranasal sinus findings should always be very carefully evaluated in light of the clinical setting before a diagnosis of active infection is made. In addition, one should not apply the adjectives *acute* or *chronic* to the diagnosis of sinusitis in a patient based only on the findings of a single examination. This approach can, in most cases, be fraught with difficulty. For example, on a single radiographic study the presence of mucosal thickening may represent one of several clinical situations: mucosal disease in a patient who had a normal sinus several days earlier represents new, active acute disease; contrariwise, a sinus with mucosal thickening that several days earlier was completely opacified represents either resolving acute or subacute disease. Lastly, mucosal thickening that is unchanged and persistent on serial examinations may represent allergic inflammation or scarred, noninfected mucosa. Thus, unless clinical correlation and comparison to recent prior examinations can be made, the radiologist should only report "mucosal thickening." (Even if chronic reactively thickened bone is identified around a sinus cavity, there may not be any active disease present in the sinus, and any thickened soft tissue may represent fibrosis.) Only when an air-fluid level is present in a patient with signs and symptoms compatible with acute bacterial sinusitis, should the radiologist confidently diagnose "acute sinusitis."

Persistent sinusitis in a pediatric patient may indicate the presence of cystic fibrosis (mucoviscidosis). Because of persistent nasal obstruction and sinusitis, the frontal sinuses in these children are often hypoplastic. Additional conditions to consider in children with repeated episodes of sinusitis include immune deficiency syndromes, AIDS, allergic sinusitis, and unusual allergies such as aspirin intolerance. Lastly, the presentation of a "nasal polyp" in the first few years of life should raise the suspicion of an encephalocele.[13]

Radiology and Sectional Imaging of Abnormal Sinus Mucosa

Normal sinus mucosa is so thin that it is not seen on plain films, tomograms, CT scans, or MR images. On all of these studies, the sinus air appears to abut di-

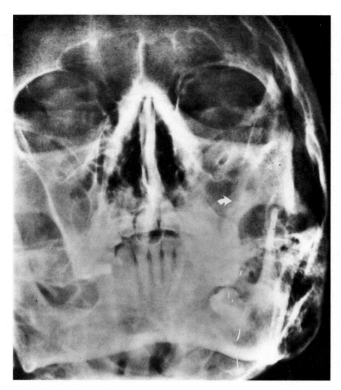

Fig. 2-115 Waters view shows "clouded" right maxillary sinus. Distinct mucosal thickening is not identified. The left antrum is also "hazy," but there is a definite area of mucosa thickening seen along the lateral sinus wall *(arrow)*. Sinusitis.

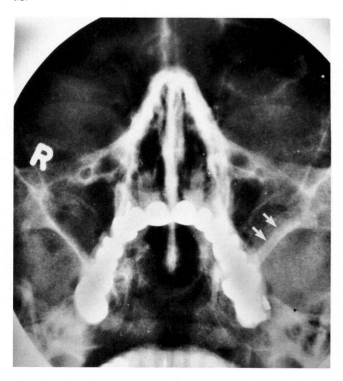

Fig. 2-116 Waters view shows minimal mucosal thickening *(arrows)* in the left maxillary sinus. This uniform mucosal thickening parallels the sinus wall contour.

rectly against the bony sinus walls. Thus, it is a relatively simple task to evaluate whether or not the sinus mucosa (mucoperiostium) is normal. If no soft tissue density is seen separating the sinus air and bony wall, this mucosa is normal. This evaluation is more easily and thoroughly performed on CT and MRI than on plain films or complex motion tomograms.

There are a number of pathologic conditions that can cause the sinus mucosa to become sufficiently thick to be identified. The differential diagnosis includes fibrosis, noninfected inflammation (e.g., allergy, chemical irritation), infection, tumor, or a combination thereof. In general, the sensitivity and specificity of analyzing these changes is greater on sectional imaging studies than it is on plain films. On plain films, the earliest sign of thickened mucosa is often a hazy or vaguely "clouded" appearance of the involved sinus. In these cases, a thickened mucosal margin per se may not be identified. If one can be certain that this appearance is not the result of technical factors (the entire film looks hazy, there is overlying swelling of the soft tissues of the cheek, etc.), then this sinus is abnormal. Commonly, this appearance results from the combination of retained secretions and minimal mucosal thickening (Fig. 2-115). Once the mucosa is thick enough to be distinctly identifiable as such, it usually appears as a uniform soft tissue density zone that separates the sinus air from the bone (Figs. 2-116 to 2-119). This type of change is usually easily identified in the frontal sinuses and along the lower lateral walls of the maxillary sinuses. Because the zygomatic recess of the antrum has less air and thicker surrounding bone than the main sinus cavity, this recess always appears slightly clouded when compared to the main sinus on routine films (see Figs. 2-22 and 2-28). This should not be misinterpreted as representing mucosal thickening. If the mucosa is evaluated along the lower lateral sinus wall, this interpretive error should not occur.

Hypoplasia of the maxillary sinus may cause this sinus to appear diseased on plain film studies (see Figs. 2-33 and 2-34). Although in most cases the greater downward angulation of the lateral aspect of the orbital floor (antral roof), the larger ipsilateral orbit, and often the larger superior orbital fissure allow antral hypoplasia to be diagnosed on routine sinus films, precise evaluation of the mucosa within this hypoplastic sinus may be impossible. These problems can be resolved easily by sectional imaging in the axial plane, where the cheek, antral walls, and sinus mucosa are all well seen and easily separated from one another.[14,15]

In recent years, endoscopic nasal surgery has enjoyed increasing currency. The premise of this approach is that there is ostiomeatal obstruction of the antrum and that the surgical creation of an inferior meatal antral window to promote antral drainage is only par-

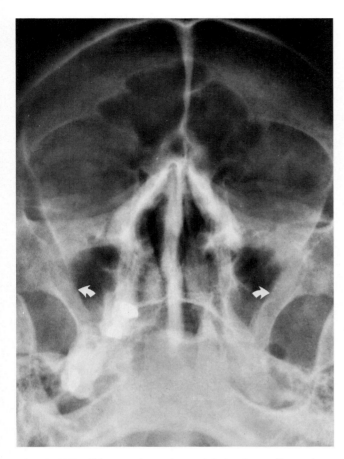

Fig. 2-117 Waters view shows bilateral maxillary sinus mucosal thickening *(arrows)*. Sinusitis.

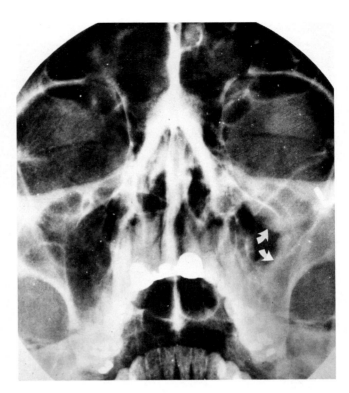

Fig. 2-118 Waters view shows mucosal thickening *(arrows)* in the left antrum. As the mucosa becomes progressively thickened, it heaps up into polypoid masses. Sinusitis.

tially effective. This is because the normal mucociliary clearance is directed toward the natural maxillary sinus ostium along the upper medial antral wall. The ostiomeatal complex is best imaged on thin section coronal CT scans (see Figs. 2-67 to 2-69). When the imager investigates this area, the region of the infundibulum, hiatus semilunaris, and bulla ethmoidalis, in particular, must be carefully evaluated for the presence of even mild degrees of mucosal thickening that may cause ostial obstruction. This must be noted carefully so that the endoscopic surgeon knows prior to surgery precisely what disease to anticipate.[16,17]

The unique anatomy of the ethmoid complex can also lead to underdiagnosis on plain films. This is consequent to the fact that the individual ethmoid sinus cavities are numerous, closely packed together, and small in size when compared to the other sinuses. Because of this, the increased density associated with mucosal thickening in an isolated group of ethmoidal cells may be almost completely nullified by air-containing surrounding cells and the adjacent sphenoid sinus.

The sensitivity of a plain film examination of the ethmoid sinuses may be increased by paying close attention to the intrasinus septa. Poorly seen septa may be-

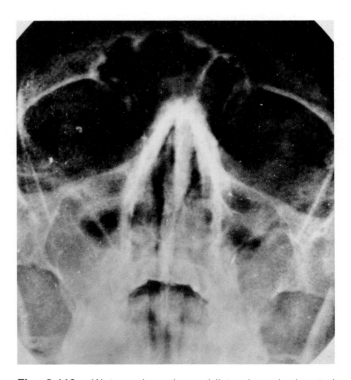

Fig. 2-119 Waters view shows bilateral marked antral mucosal thickening. Sinusitis.

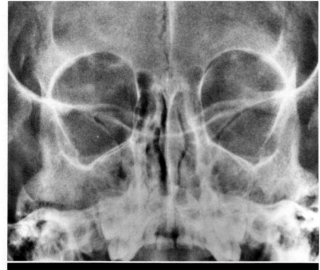

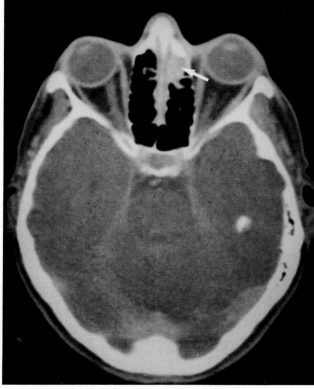

Fig. 2-120   **A,** Waters view shows opacification of the left hypoplastic frontal sinus and ethmoid sinuses (compare to normal right side). The maxillary sinuses are also almost totally opacified. Sinusitis. **B,** Axial CT scan on patient with normal plain films. There is localized inflammatory disease in the left anterior ethmoid cells *(arrow).* The middle and posterior left ethmoid sinuses and the left sphenoid sinus are normal and are air filled. This air negates the soft tissue density of the localized disease, and frontal plain films may appear normal.

tray the presence of mucosal thickening, fluid (Fig. 2-120), or both. Definitive diagnosis of minimal, or focal, ethmoid cell disease usually requires sectional imaging. The lack of visualization of these ethmoid septa with no obvious soft tissue mass may also result from pneumosinus dilatans, mucocele, or previous ethmoidectomy.

In the sphenoid sinuses, minimal mucosal thickening is usually not identifiable on plain films because these sinuses are partially obscured by many overlapping bone and soft tissue structures.

The degree of soft tissue thickening in the paranasal sinuses can vary from 1 to 2 mm to a hypertrophic polypoid type that fills the entire sinus cavity. In fact, the ratio of mucosa to fluid is variable, and the totally opacified inflammatory sinus cavity can vary from being primarily filled with retained secretions and only a minimally thickened mucosa (i.e., mucocele) to being almost entirely filled with redundant mucosa with only a small amount of secretions.

When active infection has been present for several days, the associated increased vascularity results in an increased mobilization of calcium, and this in turn results in a "washing out" of the thin mucoperiosteal white line. This is most evident in the frontal sinus.

Conversely, when inflammation has been present for many months or years, a thickened, dense reactive bone develops in the sinus wall, or around the sinus in the adjacent frontal bone in the case of the frontal sinus (Figs. 2-121 and 2-122). In the maxillary sinus, the thickened, sclerotic bone may result in a smaller sinus cavity, a finding well seen on CT scans. In addition, if focal decalcification of the antral walls occurs in inflammatory disease, it is most likely to affect the medial wall and least likely to involve the posterior or infratemporal antral wall.[18]

In the sphenoid sinus, chronic infection may result in a thickened, sclerotic bony reaction around the involved sinus and along the sphenoid sinus septum (Fig. 2-123). Patients with sphenoid sinusitis may present with suboccipital pain or headaches. Rarely, cavernous sinus thrombophlebitis and thrombosis can develop as a complication of sphenoid sinusitis. Eventually, signs and symptoms of meningismus and meningitis can occur. In any such patient, a scan performed to evaluate the brain should always include the skull base and paranasal sinuses.

Osteomyelitis of the bones of the face and sinonasal cavities is an unusual event. In spite of antibiotics, however, occasional focal sites of osteomyelitis occur. The involved bone has a mottled, irregular appearance on plain films and CT (Fig. 2-124). There may be sequestra, and the adjacent bone is often thickened and sclerotic, reflecting a reactive change to chronic infection. Such mottled areas with sequestra should be care-

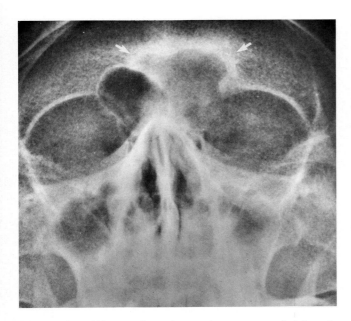

Fig. 2-121 Waters view shows dense zone of sclerosis around the left frontal sinus *(arrows)*. The sinus is clouded and mucosal thickening is present in both maxillary sinuses. Chronic frontal sinusitis and acute antral sinusitis.

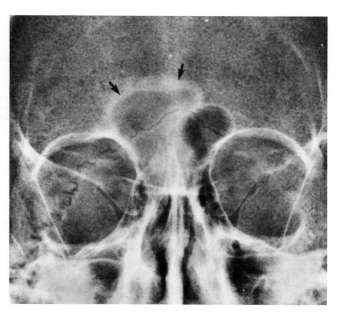

Fig. 2-122 Caldwell view shows a zone of reactive sclerosis around the right frontal sinus *(arrows)*. The sinus clouding could be due to acute or chronic infection or fibrosis. Minimal clouding is also present in the right posterior ethmoid sinuses. Chronic sinusitis.

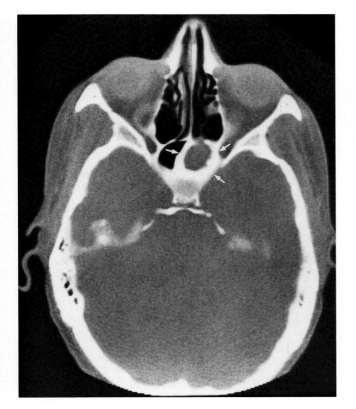

Fig. 2-123 Axial CT scan shows an opacified left sphenoid sinus with reactive, sclerotic thickening of the sphenoid intersinus septum and the walls of the left sphenoid sinus *(arrows)*. Chronic sinusitis.

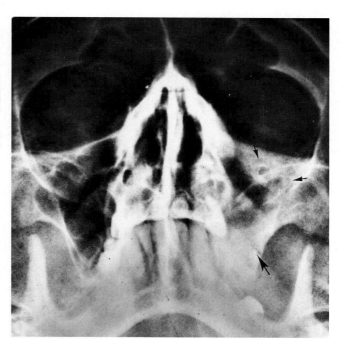

Fig. 2-124 Waters view shows thickened, sclerotic bone along the walls of the left maxillary sinus *(arrows)*. Focal lucencies within the bone represent sites of erosion. Osteomyelitis secondary to mucormycosis.

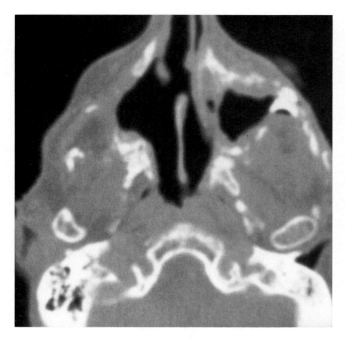

Fig. 2-125 Axial CT scan shows extensive sclerosis and fragmentation of the facial bones. Some of the osseous structures have been extruded as sequestra. Radiation osteitis.

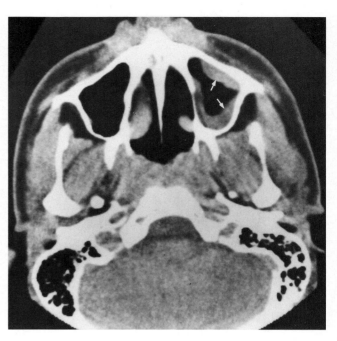

Fig. 2-126 Axial CT scan shows areas of smooth mucosal thickening *(arrows)* in the left maxillary sinus, which are typical of either fibrosis or inflammation.

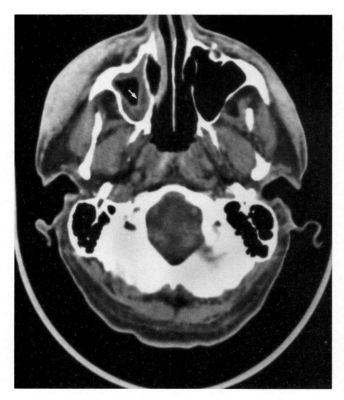

Fig. 2-127 Axial postcontrast CT scan shows smooth mucosal thickening in the right antrum with a thin zone of minimal enhancement at the mucosal surface *(arrow).* Active inflammation. Silicone has been injected into the face as part of a plastic surgery procedure.

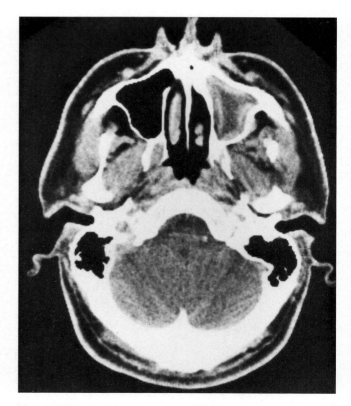

Fig. 2-128 Axial postcontrast CT scan shows enhancement of the mucosal surface in the left maxillary sinus. Between the enhancing mucosa and the bony sinus wall is a thin zone of nonenhancing submucosal edema. Within the central sinus cavity (outlined by the enhancing mucosa) is entrapped mucoid secretions. Active inflammation.

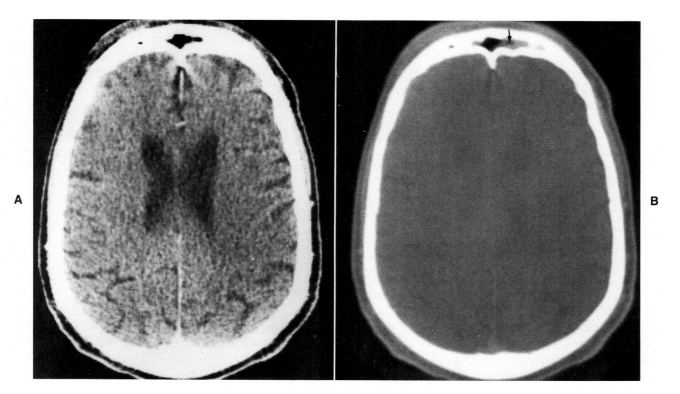

Fig. 2-129   **A,** Axial CT scan viewed at "soft tissue" window setting shows an apparently well aerated frontal sinus. **B,** Axial CT scan, same image as **A,** viewed at "bone" window setting shows inflammatory mucosal thickening in the left frontal sinus *(arrow).*

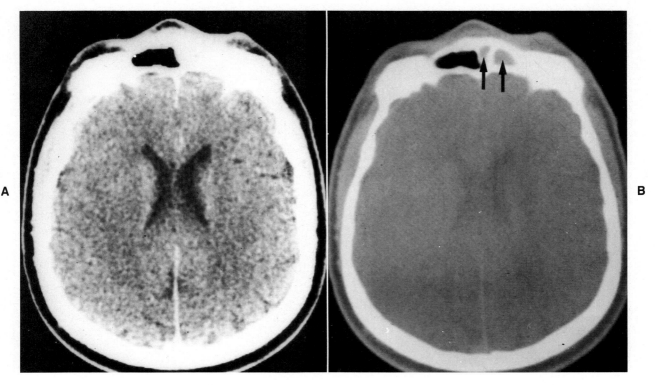

Fig. 2-130   **A,** Axial CT scan viewed at "soft tissue" window setting reveals a normal right frontal sinus and an apparent aplastic left frontal sinus. **B,** Axial CT scan, same image as **A,** viewed at "bone" window setting shows opacification *(arrows)* of a left frontal sinus. Sinusitis.

fully looked for, since they may be responsible for chronic pain.

More commonly, osteomyelitis may be seen associated with posttraumatic or iatrogenic conditions. This may be most evident in the osteoplastic flap procedure for frontal sinus surgery, where a poorly vascularized bone flap over a sinus that was chronically infected may lead to osteomyelitis of the flap. This is a recognized complication of this procedure.

A related condition is postirradiation osteitis. Rarely seen today in the facial bones because of megavoltage equipment and improved radiation treatment planning, radiation osteitis is probably most commonly encountered in the mandible, usually in patients irradiated for carcinomas of the tongue and floor of the mouth. In the paranasal sinuses, typically in patients irradiated for antral carcinomas, the first manifestation may be the development of a swollen, inflamed area over the zygoma and maxilla that may initially suggest the presence of tumor recurrence. Eventually a bone sequestrum is extruded, and there is temporary improvement; the area resolves until another sequestrum is extruded. At this point the diagnosis of radiation osteitis is clinically established. It is not uncommon in these patients to find that they were irradiated 10 to 20 years before, with

the patient being disease and symptom free until the osteitis became manifest. On CT, the involved facial bones appear shattered, fragmented, and sclerotic (Fig. 2-125). Superficial sequestra should be identified and localized.

When evaluating mucosal thickening on postcontrast CT scans, if the thickened mucosa does not enhance, it is probably not actively infected and usually is either edematous (chemical, allergy) or fibrosed (Fig. 2-126). Active infection usually has a thin zone of surface mucosal enhancement with submucosal edema (Fig. 2-127). If these changes are sufficient to cause retained sinus secretions, the sinus often has the appearance of roughly concentric rings; i.e., an outer bony dense ring, a low mucoid attenuation (10 to 18 HUs) submucosal ring, a thin infected mucosal enhancing ring, and a central zone of entrapped mucoid secretions (Fig. 2-128). Although most minimal to moderate mucosal thickening gives a fairly uniformly thick soft tissue zone on sectional imaging, the thicker, more redundant mucosa can appear almost nodular or "wavelike." In these instances, all of the sinus walls tend to be uniformly involved, a finding that is unlike the focal nodularity usually seen with tumors.

In all cases, the sinuses should be viewed at wide

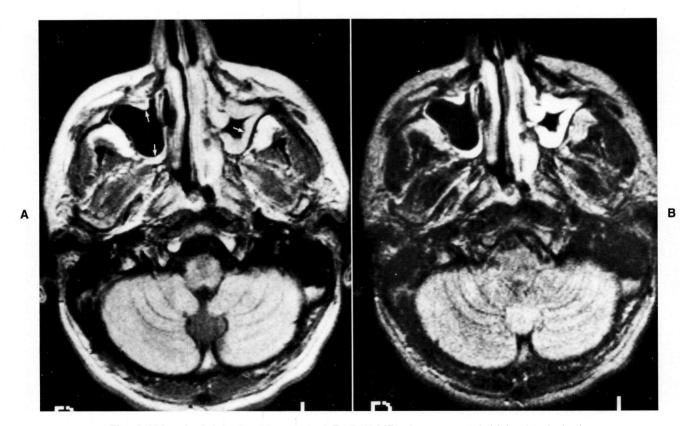

Fig. 2-131 **A,** Axial mixed image and **B,** T$_2$W MRI show mucosal thickening in both maxillary sinuses *(arrows).* The changes are more pronounced on the left side. On **A** the mucosa has an intermediate signal intensity where as on **B** it has a high signal intensity. Sinusitis.

window settings so that sinus disease is not obscured and falsely interpreted as an aplastic sinus (Figs. 2-129 and 2-130).

On MRI, the thickened, inflamed mucosa typically has a low signal intensity on T_1-weighted images (WIs), an intermediate intensity signal on PD WIs, and a high intensity signal on the T_2 WIs (Figs. 2-131 to 2-134). These changes reflect the high water and specific protein content of the inflamed tissues. The intensely long T_2 signal is helpful in differentiating inflamed tissues from almost all sinonasal tumors, which have intermediate intensity T_2-weighted signals.

By comparison, fibrosis gives a low to intermediate signal intensity on all imaging sequences. This is useful in differentiating it from inflammation on the T_2 WIs. However, since both tumor and scar may give low to intermediate intensity signals on T_2 WIs, they cannot at present be confidently differentiated by MRI.

Swelling of one nasal turbinate, especially in the absence of concurrent paranasal sinus disease, most probably reflects the normal nasal cycle. On postcontrast CT scans, this turbinate will enhance while on MR scans it will give low signal intensity on T_1 WIs, intermediate signal intensity on PD WIs, and high signal intensity on T_2 WIs (Fig. 2-135). This can be easily misinterpreted

as representing infection. Clinical correlation can help resolve any issue.[19]

Nasal turbinate swelling may also represent an allergy to contrast material on postcontrast CT scans. This is particularly easy to diagnose if on an initial noncontrast scan, the turbinates appeared normal.[20]

On rare occasions, mucosal thickening in the nasal fossae and paranasal sinuses can be seen in patients with concurrent orbital pseudotumor. These mucosal changes may be noninfectious and consistent with pseudotumor.[21] The association of the orbital and sinonasal disease may suggest this diagnosis; however, more commonly, orbital pseudotumor is found as either an isolated finding or associated with routine unrelated sinonasal inflammatory disease.

Air-Fluid Levels

Most air-fluid levels occur in the maxillary sinuses and result from acute bacterial sinusitis. However, it is likely that less than half of those who have this affliction actually have an air-fluid level. Nonetheless, bacterial sinusitis clearly is the most common cause of a paranasal sinus air-fluid level (Figs. 2-136 to 2-139).

The next most common cause is sinus lavage in the treatment of acute bacterial sinusitis. Warm saline is

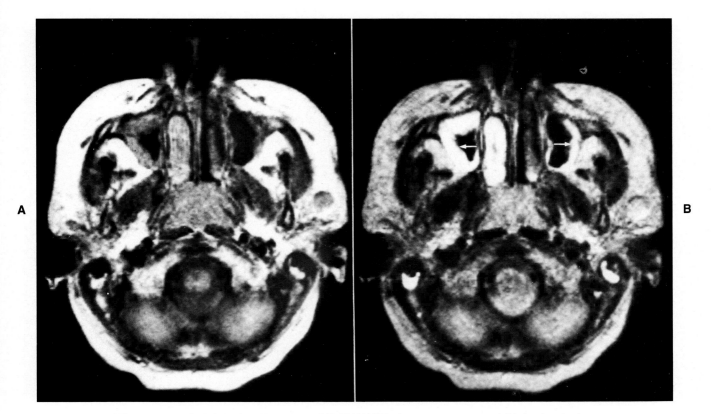

Fig. 2-132 **A,** Axial mixed image and **B,** T_2W MRI show some mucosal thickening in the right antrum in **A** with intermediate signal intensity. The left sinus appears normal. However, on **B** bilateral sinusitis is seen *(arrows)* with high T_2W signal intensity.

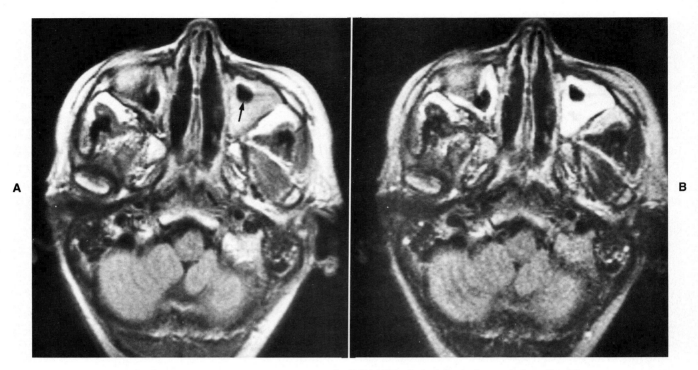

Fig. 2-133 **A,** Axial mixed image and **B,** T$_2$W MRI show bilateral antral sinusitis. The area of signal void *(arrow)* in the left antrum is the remaining air in this sinus. The sinusitis has an intermediate signal intensity in **A** and a high signal intensity in **B.**

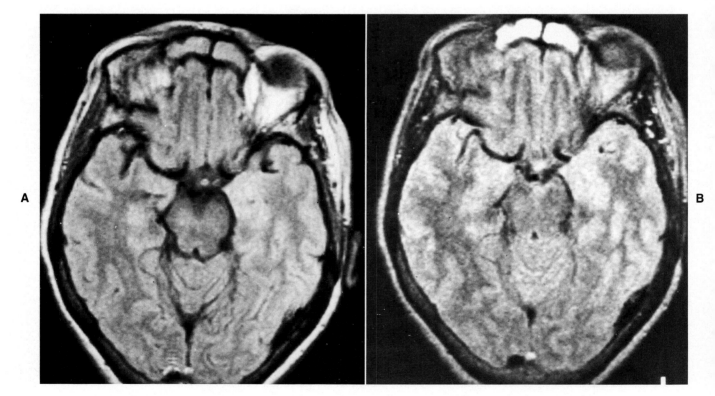

Fig. 2-134 **A,** Axial mixed image and **B,** T$_2$W MRI scan show opacification of both frontal sinuses with sinusitis and obstructed secretions that have intermediate, **A,** and high, **B,** signal intensities.

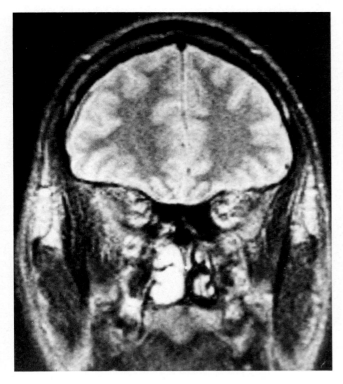

Fig. 2-135   Coronal T₂W MRI scan shows enlargement with high signal intensity of the right middle and inferior turbinates. This is part of the normal nasal cycle, and these were otherwise normal turbinates.

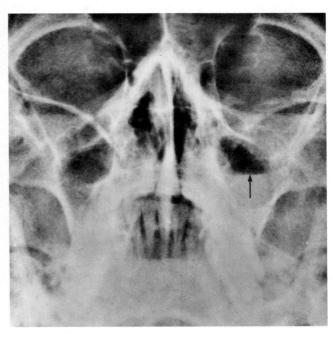

Fig. 2-136   Waters view shows left maxillary sinus air-fluid level *(arrow)* with minimal mucosal thickening. The remaining sinuses are normal. Acute bacterial sinusitis.

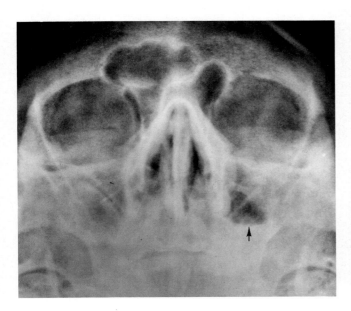

Fig. 2-137   Waters view shows left maxillary sinus air-fluid level with antral mucosal thickening. There is also right antral mucosal thickening and haziness. Active bacterial sinusitis.

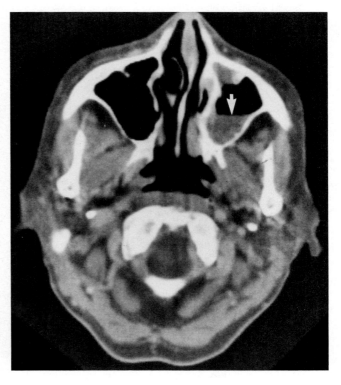

Fig. 2-138   Axial CT scan shows left maxillary sinus air-fluid level *(arrow)*. Minimal mucosal thickening is also present in the anterior left antrum. Right maxillary sinus is normal. Acute bacterial sinusitis.

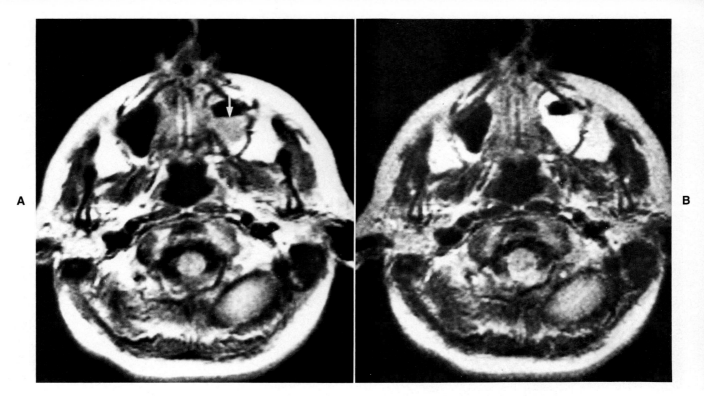

Fig. 2-139 **A,** Axial T₁W and **B,** T₂W MRI scans show left maxillary sinus air-fluid level *(arrow)*. The fluid has low-to-intermediate signal intensity in **A** and high signal intensity in **B.** Also seen on **B** is some mucosal thickening in the anterior left antrum and the posterior right antrum. Acute bacterial sinusitis.

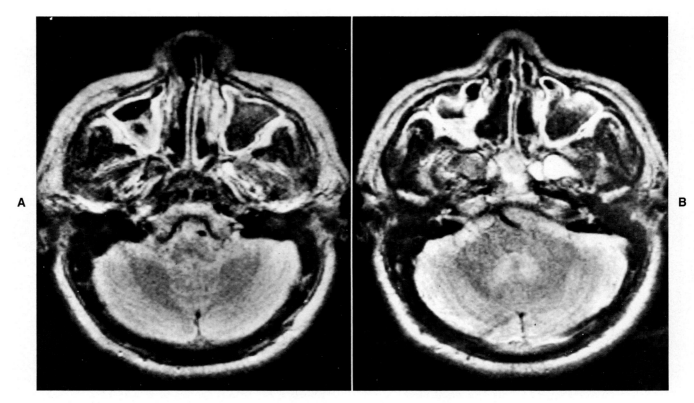

Fig. 2-140 **A,** Axial mixed and **B,** T₂W MRI scans show material with a low signal intensity on both images filling the left antrum (fresh blood). Both maxillary sinuses are lined by a thin layer of material that has high signal intensity on both images (chronic mucosal thickening). There is also an air-fluid level in the right antrum which has mixed signal intensity in **A** and high signal in **B** (sinus secretions and fresh blood).

flushed into the sinus (almost exclusively the maxillary sinus) in order to wash out debris and promote drainage. This saline takes at least 2 to 4 days to empty from the sinus. Thus, if a follow-up film is taken within 4 days of such a lavage, the radiologist will not know if the fluid within the sinus is retained saline or reaccumulated inflammatory secretions. To avoid this problem, follow-up studies should not be obtained until at least 5 to 7 days after an antral lavage.

A mucosal tear or rent can occur with trauma

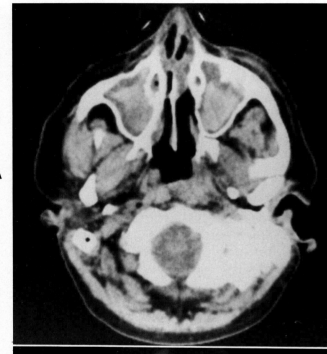

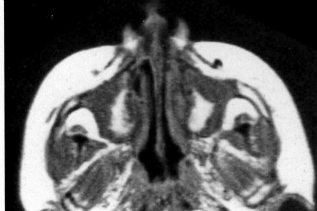

Fig. 2-141 **A,** Axial CT scan and **B,** T₁W MRI scan. In **A** there are central areas of increased attenuation in both maxillary sinuses that are separated from the sinus walls by a thin zone of low attenuation (mucoid) material. This picture is consistent with dried sinus secretions, polyps, mycetoma and hemorrhage. In **B** the central areas of the antra have high T₁W signal intensity with surrounding low signal intensity material. Old hemorrhage with inflammation.

whether or not there is an associated sinus wall fracture. The resulting air-fluid level (secretions and blood) usually indicates such a mucosal tear in light of an appropriate trauma history. However, the coincidence of an acute sinusitis in a patient who then has trauma may confuse the radiologist. On CT scans, the intrasinus blood is denser than mucosal edema and inflammatory secretions; while on MRI T_1 WIs and PD WIs, fresh blood has a low signal intensity, and intrasinus blood (after 24 to 48 hours) will give a high signal intensity. By comparison, acute inflammatory related tissues give only a low to intermediate intensity signal on T_1 WI and PD WIs (Figs. 2-140 and 2-141). Thus, sectional imaging can be used to resolve questionable cases of sinus hemorrhage.[21-23]

In patients who have sustained severe trauma, and especially those with loss of consciousness, treatment usually involves placement of a nasotracheal or nasogastric tube, or both, and bed rest in a supine position. These factors combine to interfere with normal sinus drainage, and within 24 hours, air-fluid levels can be seen in any or all of the paranasal sinuses.[11] After several days the sinuses may become completely filled with secretions, and films will reveal an apparent pansinusitis. These sinus opacifications usually clear within a few days after the nasal tubes are removed and the patient has started to vary his head position.

Barotrauma is a disorder that affects aviators, parachutists, divers, and caisson workers. It most often is associated with an upper respiratory infection (34%), accompanied by swelling of the mucosa around the sinus ostium; this anatomic substrate prevents rapid pressure equilibration across this ostium. Mucosal and submucosal hemorrhage occurs, usually associated with pain over the involved sinus. Epistaxis is the second most common symptom. The frontal sinus is involved in 68% of the cases, the ethmoid sinus in 16%, and the maxillary sinus in 8%. On plain film studies, mucosal thickening can be detected in the frontal sinuses (24%), the ethmoid sinuses (15% to 19%), and in the antrum (74% to 80%); however, an air-fluid level (present in 12% of cases) is seen only in the maxillary sinus.[24]

Hemorrhage can also result from bleeding disorders such as Von Willebrand's disease in which bleeding tends to occur at mucosal surfaces. Hemophilia, on the other hand, tends to involve internal bleeding and is not associated with sinus air-fluid levels. Coagulation disorders and acute leukemia may also produce air-fluid levels, and rarely, chemically induced sinusitis can produce an air-fluid level. Chromates as well as other industrial pollutants have been implicated in such cases. Despite the rhinitis and rhinorrhea associated with allergy, few air-fluid levels are seen in allergic patients.

The significance of an air-fluid level varies depending on the paranasal sinus involved. In the frontal sinuses, an air-fluid level usually means acute bacterial sinusitis

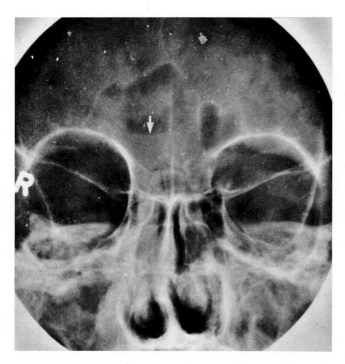

Fig. 2-142 Caldwell view shows soft tissue clouding of both frontal sinus and the right ethmoid sinuses. There is also a right frontal sinus air-fluid level *(arrow)*. Acute bacterial sinusitis.

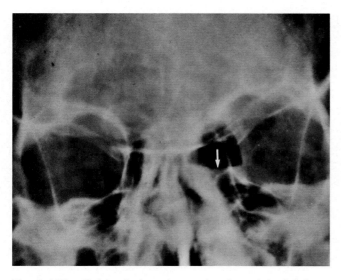

Fig. 2-143 Caldwell view shows clouding of the left frontal sinus. The left ethmoid complex is widened and there is an air-fluid level *(arrow)*. Ruptured left ethmoid mucopyocele.

(Fig. 2-142). Because of the rich venous emissary network that exists between the frontal sinus mucosa and the dural spaces of the adjacent anterior cranial fossa, intracranial complication of frontal sinusitis can occur readily, often within 48 to 72 hours.[25] The presence of frontal sinus air-fluid levels in patients with clinical sinusitis calls for immediate alerting of the clinician, since these patients require prompt, vigorous treatment, often including intravenous antibiotics. Failure of clinical resolution within another 24 to 48 hours after the onset of treatment usually mandates trephination.

An ethmoid sinus air-fluid level is rare and usually not associated with either trauma or acute infection. However, if an ethmoid mucocele ruptures and partially drains into the nasal fossa, an air-fluid level may result in what is invariably a mucopyocele. This unusual happening, therefore, is the most common cause of an ethmoid air-fluid level (Fig. 2-143).

As has been stated earlier, in the sphenoid sinus an air-fluid level may mean the presence of acute sinusitis or nasal cavity obstruction. As well, in a patient who has been unconscious for several days, an air-fluid level may only indicate poor drainage of this sinus in the supine position, since its ostium is on the anterior sinus wall. In a traumatized patient, a sphenoid sinus air-fluid level may also mean the presence of either hemorrhage or cerebrospinal fluid (CSF) from a skull base fracture. Most often these fractures do not involve the sphenoid sinus walls, but rather the floor of the anterior cranial fossa or the mastoid portion of the temporal bone. In the case of basal anterior cranial fractures, since the dura is firmly attached to the bones of the anterior cranial fossa floor, any fracture of these bones is likely to cause a rent in the dura itself. Ultimately, this may cause CSF rhinorrhea.[26]

With the patient supine, CSF escapes through the rent and drains back into the sphenoethmoidal recess; from there some of the CSF drains into the sphenoid sinus; some drains into the nasal cavity. In the case of a temporal bone fracture with an intact tympanic membrane, the CSF drains into the hypotympanum of the middle ear, then escapes via the eustacian tube into the upper nasopharynx and nasal fossa, and then into the sphenoid sinus. Thus, via this route, CSF rhinorrhea may reflect a temporal bone fracture.

An antral air-fluid level most often indicates the presence of acute bacterial sinusitis or recent antral lavage, but may also indicate trauma or sinus obstruction caused by nasal tubes or a mass.

Cysts and Polyps

The most common local complications of inflammatory sinusitis are polyps and cysts. Of these, the most prevalent is the mucous retention cyst, which is found on routine plain film examinations in about 10% of patients.[27] The mucous retention cyst results from the obstruction of a seromucinous gland. The wall of the resulting cyst is the epithelium of the duct and gland itself.[28] Although by strict pathologic criteria this qualifies a retention cyst to be called a "mucocele," the radiographic and clinical findings are so different between mucoceles and retention cysts that pathologists now recognize these two entities as clearly distinct.

Mucous retention cysts can occur in any paranasal sinus along any wall. The commonest location is in the maxillary sinus.

Serous retention cysts result from the accumulation of serous fluid in the submucosal layer of the mucosa. Thus, the wall of this cyst is the mucosa of the sinus distinguishing it from the mucous retention cyst. These cysts tend to occur in the base of the maxillary sinuses.

Polyps result from a local upheaval of mucosa, not unlike the serous cyst. The pathogenesis also remains unclear, although allergy, atopy, infection, and vasomotor impairment have been proposed as etiologic factors.[29] Increase in polyp size results largely from intercellular accumulation of fluid; the presence of collagen synthesis within the stroma appears to represent an attempt of the stroma to limit growth of the polyp. Paranasal sinus and nasal polyps appear to be the same polyp histologically, just located in different places.

There is no reliable pathologic marker to distinguish inflammatory from allergic polyps (i.e., polyps associated with infection and polyps associated with allergy), so this may be done best by evaluating the number of sinuses involved and symmetry of the paranasal sinus disease. Inflammatory and allergic polyps rarely bleed and appear to be little damaged by either manipulation or compression. Fibrosis and neovascularization of polyps (especially nasal polyps) can result in a lesion that is pathologically indistinguishable from an angiofibroma. However, because of anatomic location (nasal vs nasopharynx) and the angiographic and sectional imaging appearance (these polyps are poorly vascularized and there is no extension into the pterygopalatine fossa), these lesions can be identified by the radiologist as distinct.[30]

The intrasinus polyp and the retention cyst cannot be differentiated clearly either on plain films or sectional imaging, including MRI. However, this is of little consequence since both are common benign entities.

On plain films and CT scans, these lesions are homogeneous soft tissue masses with smooth outwardly convex borders (Figs. 2-144 to 2-153). Multiple or single lesions may be present, and most are small and clearly do not fill the entire sinus cavity. If a cyst occurs in the antral roof of a patient with a history of recent trauma, the plain film examination may simulate a blow-out fracture (see Fig. 2-147). However, coronal imaging will demonstrate an intact orbital floor with the cyst or

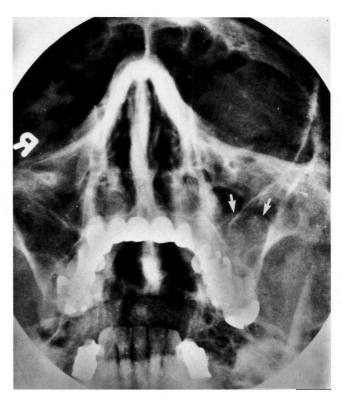

Fig. 2-144 Waters view shows solitary, typical left antral retention cyst or polyp *(arrows)*. This cyst has a smooth outwardly convex contour. The remaining antrum and the other sinuses are normal.

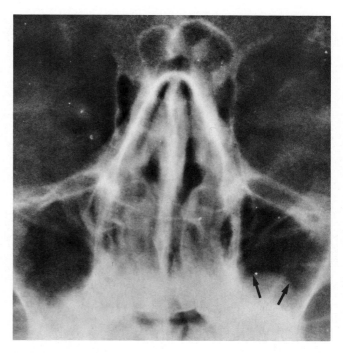

Fig. 2-145 Waters view shows left maxillary sinus retention cyst or polyp in the inferior portion of the sinus *(arrows)*. There is minimal inflammatory type mucosal thickening in both antra.

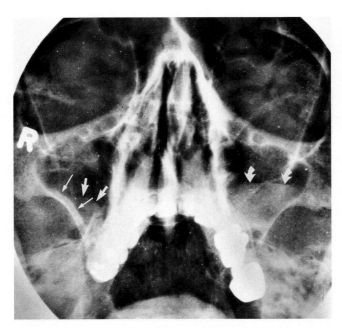

Fig. 2-146 Waters view shows a large "flat" retention cyst *(curved arrows)* in the left antrum. This can simulate an air-fluid level if careful attention is not paid to its slightly convex upper surface. There is minimal mucosal thickening in the right antrum *(thin arrows)* and another small retention cyst is present in the lower right maxillary sinus *(arrows)*.

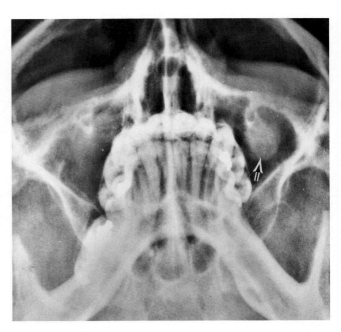

Fig. 2-147 Waters view shows retention cyst *(arrow)* in the roof of the left antrum.

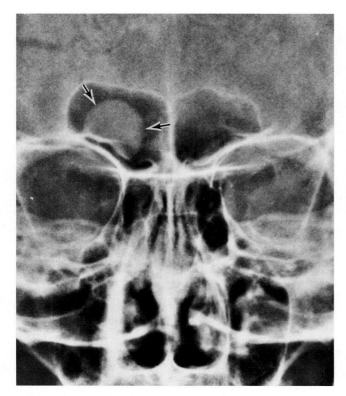

Fig. 2-148 Caldwell view shows retention *(arrows)* in the right frontal sinus. Note that this sinus is otherwise normal.

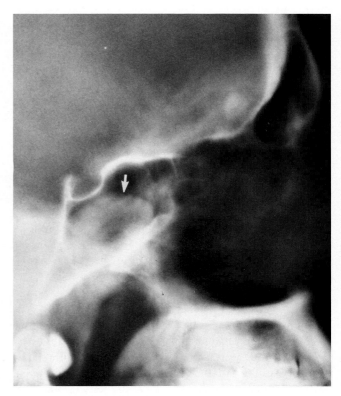

Fig. 2-149 Lateral view shows solitary retention cyst *(arrow)* in the sphenoid sinus.

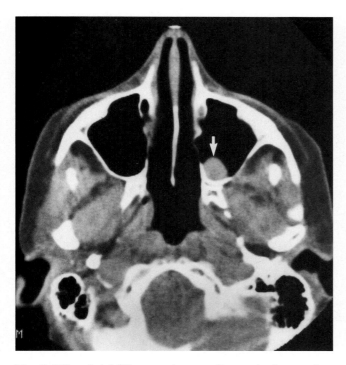

Fig. 2-150 Axial CT scan shows solitary retention cyst or polyp *(arrow)* in the posterior recess of the left antrum.

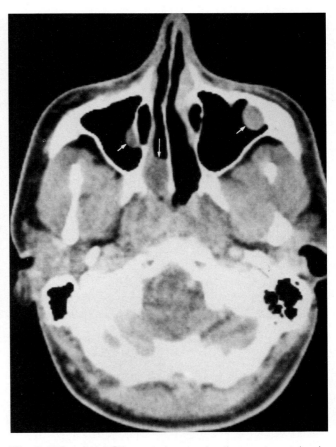

Fig. 2-151 Axial CT scan shows retention cyst or polyp in the left and right maxillary sinuses *(small arrows)*. There also is a small polyp *(arrow)* in the posterior right nasal fossa.

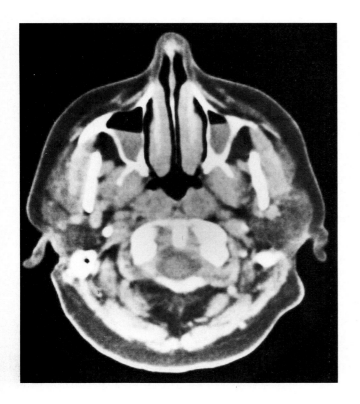

Fig. 2-152 Axial CT scan shows solitary retention cyst in each maxillary sinus. These cysts may simulate air-fluid levels if their upper slightly convex contour and its nonparallel relationship to the plane of the floor are not noted.

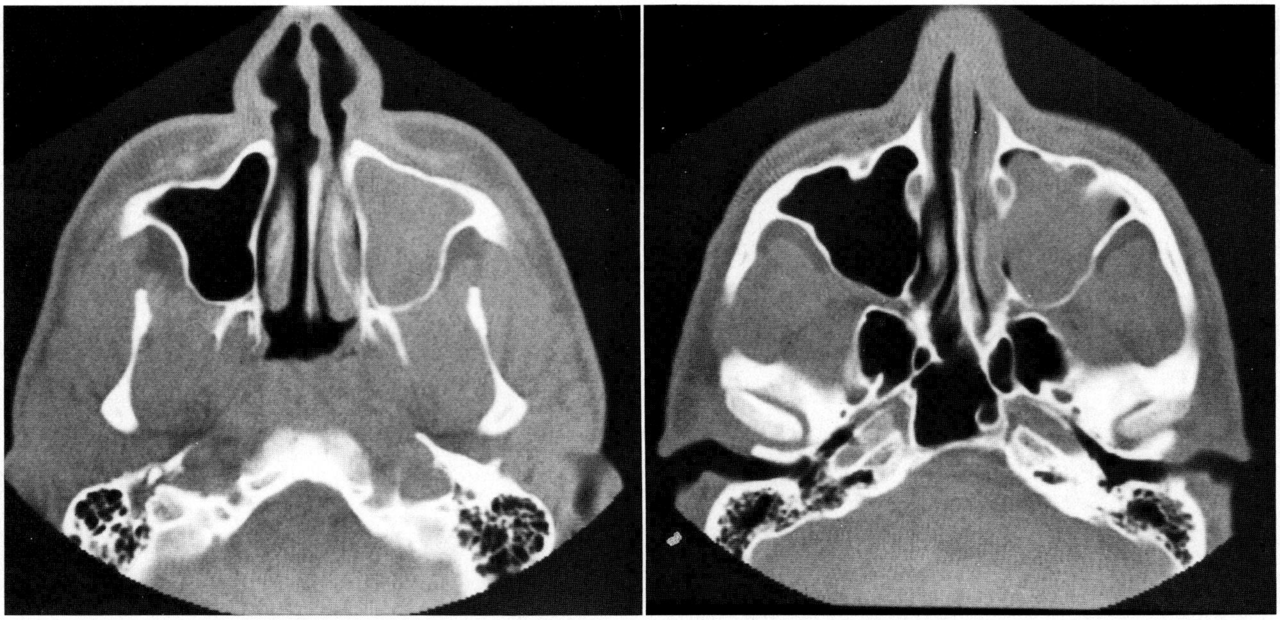

Fig. 2-153 Axial CT scans in **A,** the midplane and **B,** upper portions of the left maxillary sinus. In **A** the sinus appears to be opacified. However, in **B** air can be seen outlining the upper surface of a large retention cyst or polyp.

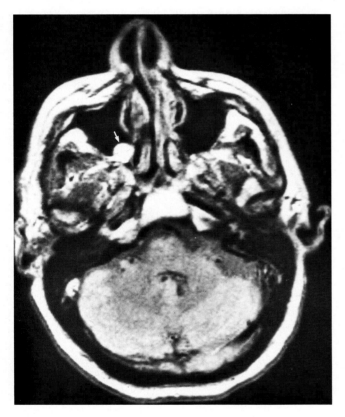

Fig. 2-154 Axial mixed image MRI scan shows small retention cyst *(arrow)* in the right antrum. This cyst has a high signal intensity reflecting either a high protein content and/or an element of T_2 contribution.

polyp in the antral mucosa. On the Water's view, a prominent infraorbital canal (with its attendant soft tissue contents) can mimic a cyst in the roof of the antrum. Similarly, the nasal alae can simulate a medial wall antral cyst (see Figs. 2-49 and 2-51), while unerupted teeth or the lips or a moustache can simulate a cyst on the floor of the maxillary sinus. The coronoid process of the mandible can simulate a cyst on the posterior floor of the antrum on a lateral plain film taken with the patient's mouth closed (see Fig. 2-52).

When a cyst becomes moderately large (i.e., about half of the volume of the antrum), it starts to behave like a water-filled thin balloon in that its upper surface flattens out, somewhat resembling an air-fluid level (see Fig. 2-107). However, careful evaluation will reveal a slightly convex upper border, and on sectional imaging, the convex polypoid appearance is even better seen along the upper and lower portions of the lesion. A true air-fluid level results in the fluid level being present throughout the involved sinus. Additionally, the planar surface of the fluid will directly reflect gravity in every head position.

On MRI, these cysts or polyps usually have characteristics similar to those of mucosal inflammation, again reflecting the high water and low specific protein content. Thus, they tend to have low to intermediate intensity signals on T_1 WIs and PD WIs and high signal intensities on T_2 WIs. If the protein content of the cyst fluid increases because of infection or the passage of time, the T_1-weighted and PD weighted signal inten-

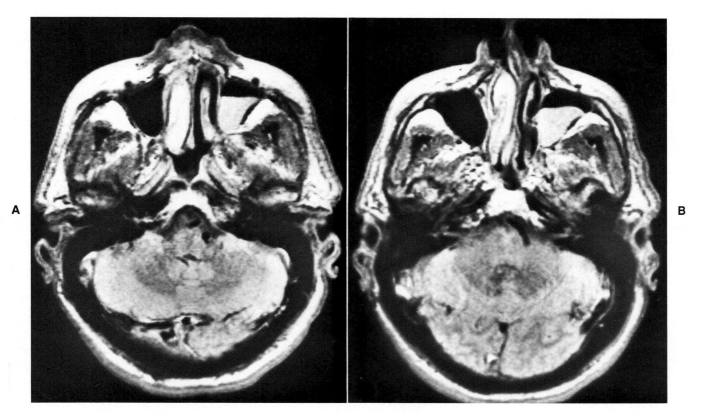

Fig. 2-155   Axial mixed MRIs **A,** low in the antrum and **B,** higher in the antrum show retention cyst in the left antrum. If the contour of the upper surface is not clearly noted on all scans, this cyst could be mistaken for an air-fluid level.

sities become high, reflecting the shortening of the T_1 relaxation time (Figs. 2-154 to 2-157).

These lesions are usually asymptomatic and constitute incidental findings on radiographic studies. However, if the cyst or polyp becomes large enough to fill the sinus cavity, the lesion can obstruct sinus drainage and cause symptoms. Rarely, these lesions can remodel the sinus walls to cause some expansion of the sinus cavity. But in most cases some small pockets of remaining sinus air can be identified overlying a part of the convex margin of the lesion on sectional imaging (Fig. 2-153). This distinguishes such a cyst from a mucocele, although when a cyst is this large, the distinction is more of intellectual interest than clinical significance.

On occasion, an antral polyp may expand sufficiently to prolapse through the sinus ostium and present as a "nasal" polyp. Antrochoanal polyps thus represent 4% to 6% of all nasal polyps. Most are unilateral, solitary lesions; interestingly, however, bilateral antral inflammatory disease is found in 30% to 40% of cases. Almost 8% of these patients have other nasal polyps, and 15% to 40% of patients have a history of allergy.[31-33] These latter statistics have prompted the suggestion that there is an etiologic relationship to allergy, but this has not been borne out.

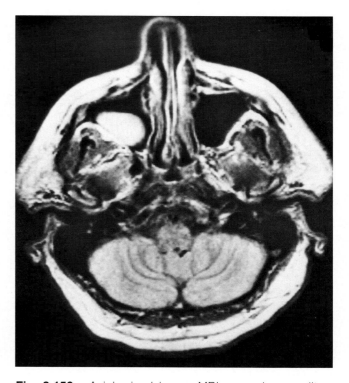

Fig. 2-156   Axial mixed image MRI scan shows solitary retention cyst or polyp with an intermediate signal intensity filling about half of the right antrum.

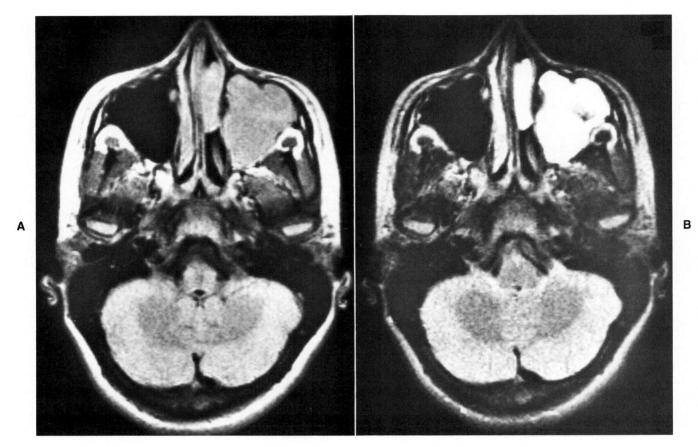

Fig. 2-157 A, Axial mixed image and **B,** T₂W MRI scans show multiple polyps or cysts filling the left maxillary sinus. These lesions have the typical intermediate, **A,** and high, **B,** signal intensities usually found with cysts and polyps.

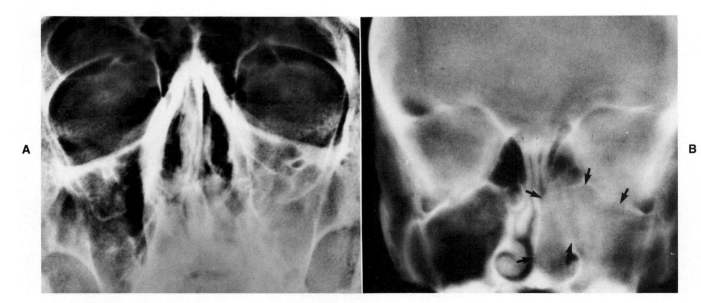

Fig. 2-158 A, Waters view and **B,** coronal multidirectional tomogram on patient with an opacified left antrum. On **B** a soft tissue mass is seen filling the maxillary sinus, widening the infundibulum and prolapsing into the left nasal fossa *(arrows)*. Antrochoanal polyp.

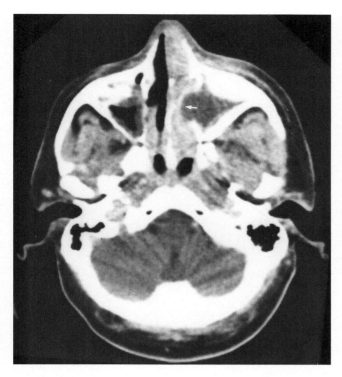

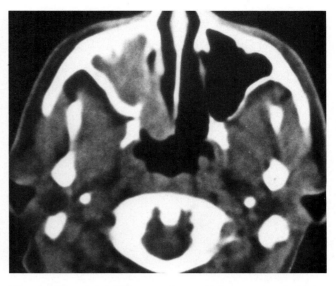

Fig. 2-160   Axial CT scan shows right antral soft tissue mass that has prolapsed into the posterior right nasal fossa. Antrochoanal polyp.

Fig. 2-159   Axial postcontrast CT scan shows low attenuation (mucoid secretion) mass in the left maxillary sinus that is bulging into the left nasal fossa *(arrow)*. There are inflammatory mucosal changes seen in both nasal fossae and in the right antrum. Left antrochoanal polyp.

Conversely, most antrochoanal polyps occur in teenagers and young adults. If such a polyp is surgically snared in the nasal fossa like a nasal polyp, without regard to its antral stalk, 20% to 30% of the cases will recur, usually within two years of the incomplete excision.[33] These polyps are properly treated via a Caldwell-Luc approach.

When small, antrochoanal polyps appear as a soft tissue mass that completely fills one maxillary sinus. There is widening of the infundibular region and slight extrusion of the antral mass into the lateral wall of the nasal fossa. At this stage, it can be confused with hypertrophic polypoid antral mucosa that may also extend through the sinus ostium. As the polyp continues to grow, it fills the ipsilateral nasal fossa and extends back into the nasopharynx. Rarely, it may grow sufficiently to hang down into the oropharynx. Although the medial antral wall may be destroyed eventually, the remaining antral walls are rarely remodelled. Although this can be a difficult diagnosis on plain films, it is misdiagnosed rarely on sectional imaging. This latter technique renders easy the distinction between the inferior turbinates and a choanal mass.

On CT, most of these polyps have a mucoid (10 to 18 HUs) attenuation, although if the mucosal surface is

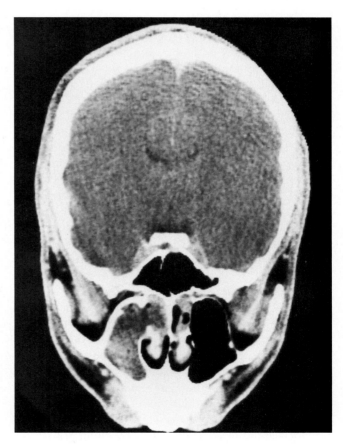

Fig. 2-161   Coronal CT scan shows right antral mass that is bulging into the right nasal fossa. Antrochoanal polyp.

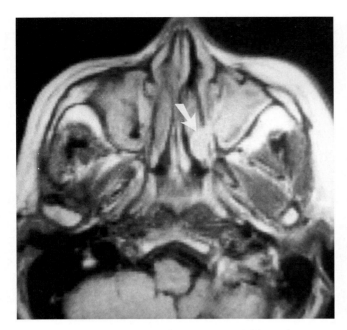

Fig. 2-162 Axial mixed image MRI scan shows inflammatory changes in both maxillary sinuses. On the left side, a polypoid mass *(arrow)* is seen extending into the nasal fossa. Antrochoanal polyp.

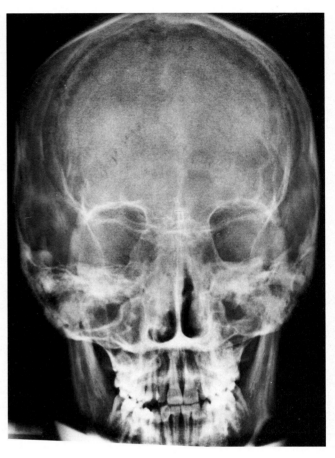

Fig. 2-163 Caldwell view shows opacification of frontal and ethmoid sinuses with hypertelorism. There is also disease in the upper left nasal fossa and almost the entire right nasal fossa. Polyposis.

primarily imaged, some enhancement may be present. Their MRI characteristics again usually reflect their high water and low protein content. Thus, they tend to have low to intermediate intensity signals on T_1 WIs and PD WIs and high signal intensity on T_2 WIs (Figs. 2-158 to 2-162).

Nasal polyps are most often associated with allergy and when found in this clinical setting are usually numerous rather than solitary. Histologically, there are a number of secondary changes that can occur with these polyps. These include infarction, surface ulceration, mucoid liquification, stromal cell atypia, metaplasia of the surface epithelium, and the very rare development of carcinoma in these metaplastic cells. The importance of stromal atypia lies in its potential misinterpretation as a malignancy because of its microscopic resemblance to a sarcoma.[29,31]

Polyps are the most common expansile lesions in the nasal cavity. Although they usually are small and cause little deformity, if left unattended in the presence of progression, they can become highly deforming. Eventually they may remodel, disrupt, and destroy the central facial region. They can destroy the medial antral walls, can cause hypertelorism, and can break through intracranially either via the roof of the nasal cavity and ethmoid complex or via the sphenoid sinus. This degree of marked destruction is usually found only in patients living in medically underserved areas.

Although surgery is the treatment of choice for large

polyps, in allergic patients, desensitization has in some cases shown dramatic results in reducing the number and size of these polyps.[33]

Etiology. Polyps have been associated not only with allergy, but with vasomotor rhinitis, infectious rhinosinusitis, diabetes mellitus, cystic fibrosis, aspirin intolerance, and nickel exposure.[33] In vasomotor rhinitis, an instability of the autonomic nervous system has been implicated as the underlying problem. Nasal congestion, watery discharge, and eventually nasal polyps can be found as responses to emotional stress, endocrine imbalance, atmospheric pressure changes, and irritants, as well as in reaction to medications.[34]

Infectious rhinosinusitis is caused by a variety of agents that produce an acute and chronic inflammation with secondary polyp formation. These patients commonly have a secretory IgA deficiency.[35]

There is evidence to suggest a relationship between nasal polyps and diabetes mellitus. In order to develop these polyps, there must be a local irritant (allergy, infection) and fluctuating glucose levels.[36]

Between 10% and 20% of children with cystic fibrosis

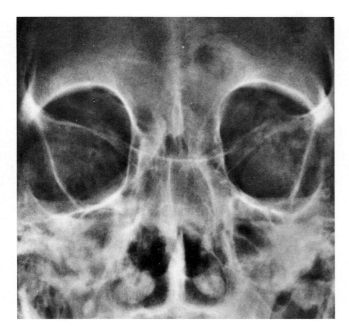

Fig. 2-164 Caldwell view shows opacification and mucosal disease in all of the paranasal sinuses and both mid and upper nasal fossae. This is a slight hypertelorism. Polyposis.

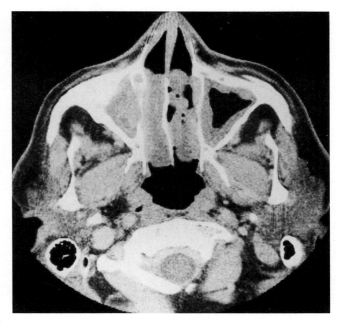

Fig. 2-165 Axial CT scan shows multiple bilateral nasal polyps with inflammatory mucosal thickening in the left antrum and opacification of the right antrum. Polyposis and sinusitis.

have nasal polyps. In general, nasal polyps in children are uncommon, and 29% of such polyps in children are associated with cystic fibrosis. Thus the presence of chronic sinusitis and nasal polyps in a child must always bring to mind the diagnosis of cystic fibrosis.[37,38]

Aspirin intolerance may be a systemic disease rather than a simple allergic response. It is classically characterized by intolerance to aspirin, nasal polyps, and bronchial asthma. About 20% of patients with nasal polyps have asthma, and conversely about 30% of asthmatic patients have polyps.[37,39]

Nickel workers who have worked 10 years or more in the nickel refining process have a 4% incidence of nasal polyps and an increased risk for developing carcinomas in the lung, nasal fossa, and larynx.[40]

Radiographically, the polyps are often seen on plain films only as a vague increased soft tissue density within the nasal fossa (Figs. 2-163 and 2-164). On sectional imaging, they usually can be identified as discrete single or multiple broad-based soft tissue masses. On CT the majority of the polyps tend to have a mucoid attenuation (10 to 18 HUs) with mucosal enhancement occasionally seen at the polyp's surface. However, those polyps that have had sufficient time to develop stromal collagen and fibrous tissue tend to have a higher attenuation (20 to 35 HUs) (Figs. 2-165 to 2-170). On MRI, typically the dominant feature is the high water and low protein content that gives the pol-

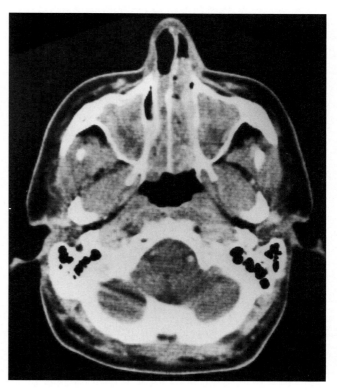

Fig. 2-166 Axial CT scan shows bilateral nasal fossa polypoid masses and bilateral antral opacification. Polyposis and sinusitis.

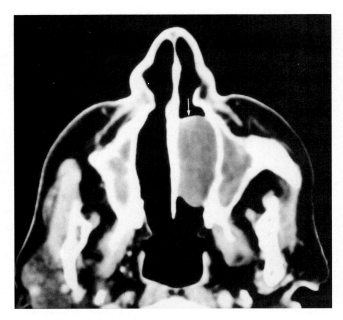

Fig. 2-167 Axial CT scan shows solitary mucoid attenuation left nasal mass *(arrow)*. There is also inflammatory disease in both antra. Polyp and sinusitis.

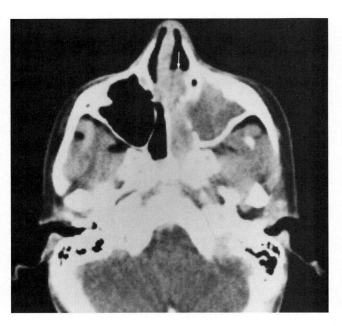

Fig. 2-168 Axial postcontrast CT scan shows minimally enhancing left nasal fossa mass *(arrow)*. The mass obstructs the left antrum, which is opacified. Polyp and sinus obstruction.

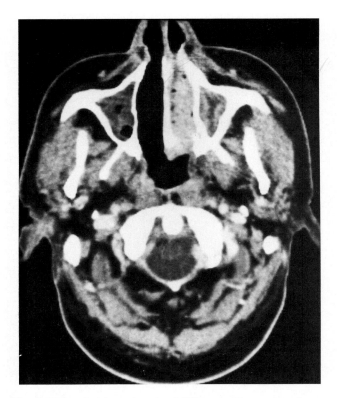

Fig. 2-169 Axial postcontrast CT scan shows an enhancing left nasal fossa mass. There is active inflammation (mucosal enhancement) in the left antrum and mucoid secretions in the right antrum. Polyp and sinusitis.

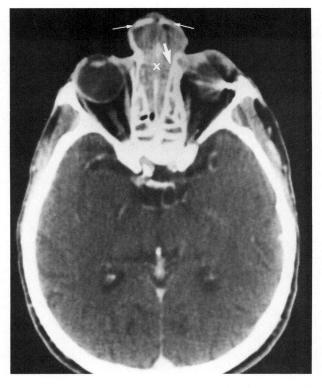

Fig. 2-170 Axial postcontrast CT scan shows bilateral nasal masses that have displaced the nasal bones anteriorly *(small arrows)* and eroded part of the nasal septum *(x)*. The upper nasal fossae are also widened and the medial aspect of the ethmoid sinuses have been displaced laterally *(arrow)*.

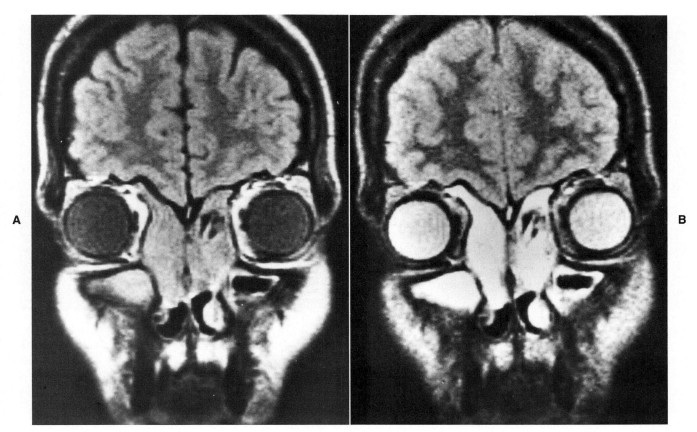

Fig. 2-171   A, Coronal mixed image and **B,** T$_2$W MRI scans show bilateral nasoethmoid expansile masses causing hypertelorism. These masses have the same signal intensities as the mucosal thickening in the left antrum and the material in the right antrum; namely an intermediate signal intensity in **A** and a high signal intensity in **B.** Polyposis and sinusitis.

yps a low to intermediate signal intensity on T$_1$ WIs and PD WIs and high signal intensity on T$_2$ WIs (Fig. 2-171). If the polyps have been present for a long time, they may have different MRI appearances (see p. 142).

When there are multiple polyps crowded within the nasal vault, they can form an overall conglomerate mass that may be difficult, if not impossible, to distinguish from a tumor. This is especially true of bulky lesions, such as inverting papillomas and lymphomas, that tend to remodel the surrounding bone. However, there are two appearances of sinonasal polyps, if present, that allow their diagnosis to be established firmly on CT studies.

The first of these is the ethmoid polypoid mucocele in which there is either unilateral or bilateral involvement of the ethmoid labyrinth, which is characterized by widening of the ethmoid complex with little, if any, destruction of the delicate ethmoid septa.[41,42] The individual ethmoid cells are filled with polypoid mucosa and entrapped mucoid secretions. By comparison, a solid mass (polyp or tumor) will destroy these septa,

and in this circumstance it is impossible to distinguish a benign lesion from a low grade malignant process. The preservation of ethmoidal septa as seen in polypoid mucoceles, therefore, unequivocally signifies the presence of benign disease (Figs. 2-172 to 2-174).

The second circumstance in which there is a unique CT appearance of benign disease is characterized by the presence of either a unilateral or bilateral expansile sinonasal mass within which are cascading, looping, or curvilinear soft tissue polypoid lesions in a background matrix of mucoid attenuation (10 to 18 HUs) secretions. For the most part, the polypoid masses are separated from the adjacent bones by a thin zone of mucoid material and this distinguishes the CT appearance from that of tumors, which abut the bone directly as they either remodel or destroy it (Figs. 2-175 to 2-177). This unique CT appearance is seen in about 20% of patients with nasal polypoid masses and, when present, indicates benign disease.

This latter CT appearance can also be caused by mycetomas (usually from aspergillosis) (see Figs. 2-178 and 2-179). The CT appearance of a central antral density

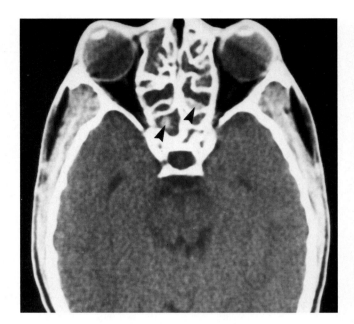

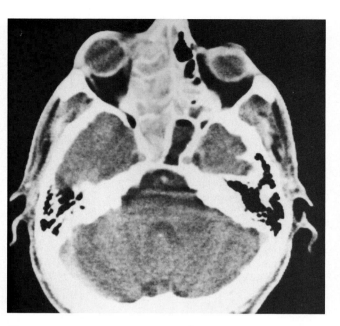

Fig. 2-172 Axial CT scan shows opacification of ethmoid sinuses with widening of the anterior and middle ethmoid complex. The lamina papyracea remain intact. Several discrete polyps *(arrowheads)* are seen within the mucoid secretions filling the ethmoid cells. The delicate intercellular septa are intact. Polypoid mucocele.

Fig. 2-173 Axial postcontrast CT scan shows widening and opacification of entire right ethmoid complex and posterior left ethmoid cells. The right sphenoid sinus is also involved, while the left sphenoid sinus has mucoid attenuation secretions. The intercellular ethmoid septa are intact. Polypoid mucocele.

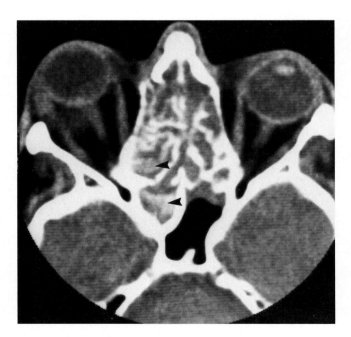

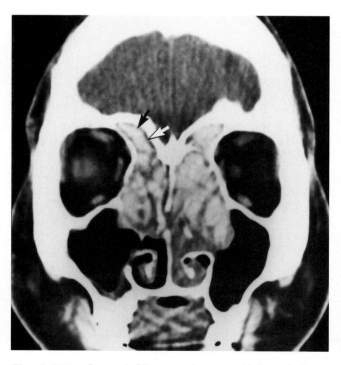

Fig. 2-174 Axial CT scan shows opacification with some expansion of the ethmoid complex. Several discrete polyps are seen *(arrowheads)* in the right sphenoid sinus and the ethmoid sinuses. The intercellular ethmoid septa are virtually intact. Polypoid mucocele.

Fig. 2-175 Coronal CT scan shows multiple soft tissue masses in the ethmoid sinuses and nasal fossa bilaterally. The polypoid masses are separated from the bone by a thin zone of mucoid attenuation material *(arrows)*. The polyps are also imbedded within a matrix of this mucoid material. Polyposis.

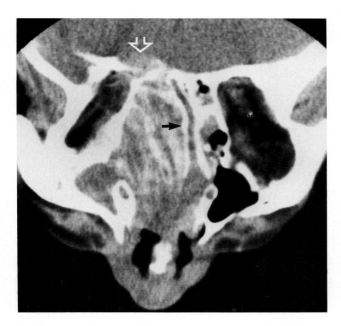

Fig. 2-176 Coronal CT scan shows expansile right na-soethmoid mass that has displaced the nasal septum to the left *(arrow)*. The mass has also focally broken into the floor of the anterior cranial fossa *(open arrow)*. Within the mass are discrete polypoid densities embedded within a mucoid matrix. Polyposis.

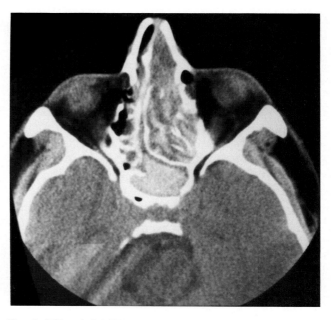

Fig. 2-177 Axial CT scan shows soft tissue mass (polyp) in the sphenoid sinus that is for the most part separated from the bone by a zone of mucoid attenuation. There is an expansile left nasoethmoid process that has discrete poly-poid soft tissue masses seen within a mucoid matrix. Poly-posis.

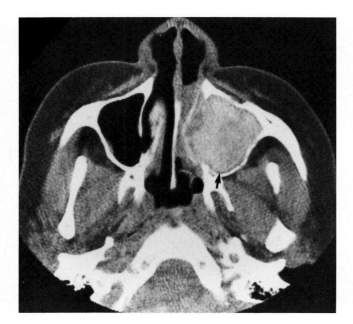

Fig. 2-178 Axial CT scan shows soft tissue mass in the left antrum, which is separated from the sinus wall by a thin zone of mucoid attenuation material *(arrow)*. There is some remodelling of the medial antral wall. Aspergilloma.

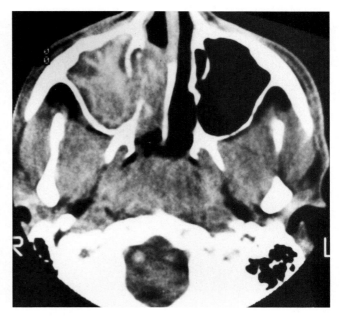

Fig. 2-179 Axial CT scan shows stellate soft tissue mass in the right antrum and nasal fossa. The mass is separated from the bone by a thin zone of mucoid attenuation mate-rial. There is focal destruction of the medial antral wall. As-pergilloma.

separated from the sinus wall by a zone of lower attenuation can also be seen in cases of intrasinus hemorrhage (see Fig. 2-141) and rarely with densely inspissated intrasinus secretions with surrounding mucosal edema.[43] Although a specific diagnosis may not always be possible on CT, this appearance reliably indicates that the soft tissue mass is not a tumor.[29]

As already mentioned, the MRI characteristics of polyps are typically those of a low to intermediate intensity signal on T_1 WIs and PD WIs and a high intensity signal on T_2 WIs. However, when polyps have had sufficient time to erode through the floor of the anterior skull base, they have a different MRI appearance. Because of their chronicity, there has been time for a variable concentration of the mucous protein and a variable degree of resorption of the free water in the sinonasal fluids that comprise much of the polyps and the related areas of entrapped mucous secretions.[44] These factors, in turn, cause variable degrees of T_1 and T_2 relaxation time shortening. This results in low, intermediate, and high signal intensities on all imaging sequences, and it is this nonhomogeneity that distinguishes these lesions from tumors. In very proteinaceous collections there can be so much T_1 and T_2 shortening that signal voids are seen on the MRI scans (Figs. 2-40 and 2-180 to 2-183).

Mycetomas, on the other hand, have very few mobile protons and thus, have low signal intensity on all imaging sequences. Any inflammatory reaction around the mycetoma will have the typical MRI characteristics of

infections or polyps (Fig. 2-184).[45] An intrasinus hemorrhage initially will have a low signal intensity on all imaging sequences; but when the blood is oxidized to methemoglobin, it has a high signal intensity on T_1 WIs and PD WIs and an intermediate signal intensity on T_2 WIs (see Figs. 2-140 and 2-141). Thus by using MRI, these lesions can be distinguished in almost all cases.[46,47]

Fungal Diseases

The radiographic characteristics of fungal disease vary from being nonspecific to highly suggestive of fungal infection. In the early stages of infection, a nonspe-

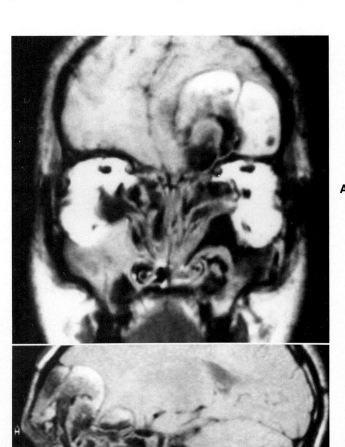

Fig. 2-181 **A,** Coronal and **B,** sagittal T_1W MRI scans show multiple sinonasal polypoid masses that have broken into the medial aspect of each orbit as well as intracranially. These are areas of high, intermediate, and low signal intensity throughout the lesion. There are also areas of signal void. Polyposis.

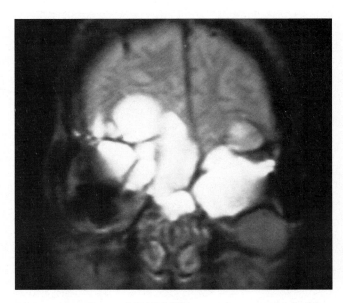

Fig. 2-180 Coronal T_2W MRI scan shows multiple bilateral polypoid masses extending intracranially from the ethmoid and frontal sinuses. These masses had high signal intensity on both T_1W and T_2W scans. Polyposis.

cific mucosal inflammation may be present either in the nasal fossa or a paranasal sinus (Figs. 2-185 and 2-186). Most often either the maxillary sinus or ethmoid sinuses are involved. Occasionally the sphenoid sinus is affected as the only involved paranasal sinus, this occurring most commonly with aspergilloma. The frontal sinuses are only rarely involved in fungal disease.[48] Air-fluid levels are very uncommon, and when present suggest a nonfungal bacterial infection. The surrounding bone may become reactive, thickened, and sclerotic or eroded or remodelled. Most often, it is the combination of these bone changes that suggests either an unusual infection or fungal disease.[49] The associated soft tissue disease is often found both in the nasal fossa and the paranasal sinuses, and in the case of the maxillary sinus, the nasal disease may act as a bridge to disease extension into the cheek (Fig. 2-187). The more common form of antral bacterial sinusitis rarely extends into the soft tissues of the cheek and face, and whenever this unusual combination of involvement is seen, an aggressive infection or fungal disease should be suspected.[50] When a mycetoma is very dense, intrasinus concretions can be seen on plain films and, when present, are highly suggestive of fungal disease.[51,52]

A variety of fungal diseases have been reported to involve the sinonasal cavities. These include aspergillosis,

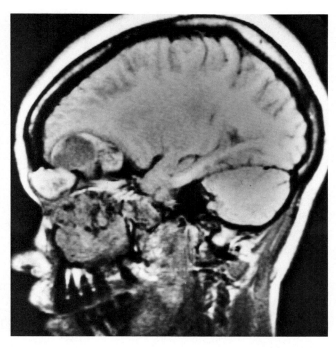

Fig. 2-182 Sagittal T₁W MRI scan shows multiple polypoid masses filling the nasal cavity, ethmoid and maxillary sinuses and breaking into the floor of the anterior cranial fossa. There are areas of high, intermediate, and low signal intensity scattered throughout the process. Polyposis.

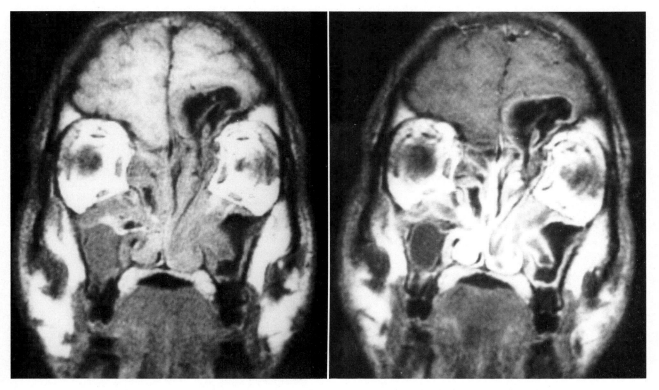

Fig. 2-183 Coronal T₁W MRI scans without **A,** Gd-DTPA and **B,** post Gd-DTPA. There are polypoid masses in the nasal cavity and the maxillary and ethmoid sinuses, which have broken intracranially. There are areas of high, intermediate, and low signal intensity. In **B** the mucosal surfaces of the polyps become bright. Polyposis.

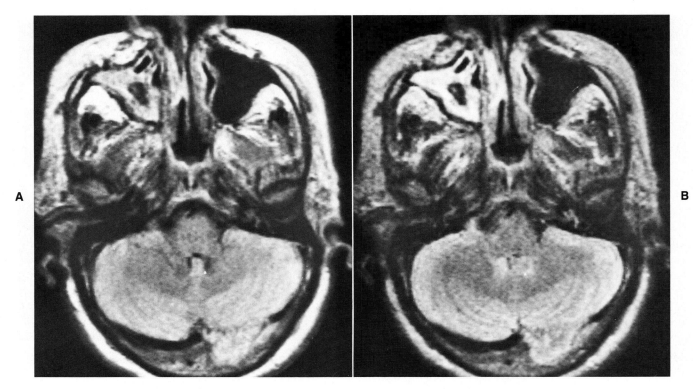

Fig. 2-184 **A,** Axial mixed image and **B,** T_2W MRI scans show inflammatory-type mucosal thickening (**A** is intermediate and **B** is high signal intensity) in the right maxillary sinus. In the center of the sinus is an ovoid mass with low signal intensity. This is a mycetoma with surrounding inflammation.

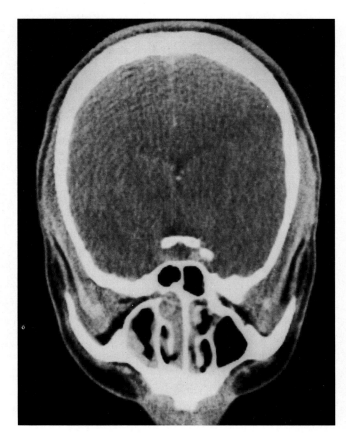

Fig. 2-185 Coronal CT scan shows nonspecific mucosal thickening in nasal fossae and right maxillary sinus. Mucormycosis.

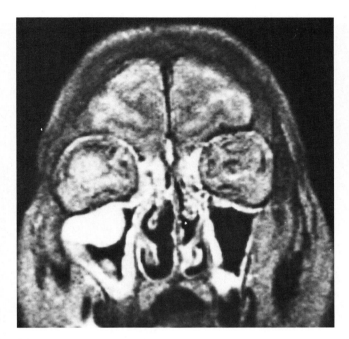

Fig. 2-186   Coronal T$_2$W MRI scan shows high signal intensity mucosal thickening in nasal fossae and the ethmoid and maxillary sinuses. This is a nonspecific inflammatory picture. Aspergillosis.

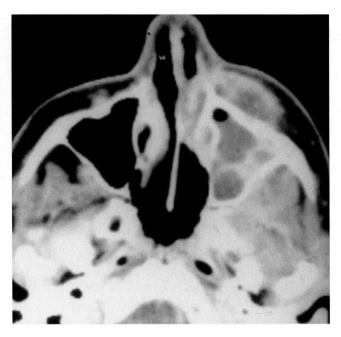

Fig. 2-187   Axial postcontrast CT scan shows inflammatory disease in the left antrum, left nasal fossa, and left cheek. This is an unusual distribution of disease for routine bacterial disease. Aspergilosis.

mucormycosis, candidiasis, histoplasmosis, cryptococcosis, coccidioidomycosis, myospherulosis, North American blastomycosis, and rhinosporidiosis.[53] Of these, the first three are the most commonly encountered and are nongranuloma producing while the last two produce granulomas.

Nongranuloma Producing Fungal Diseases. *Rhinocerebral mucormycosis* (also, phycomycosis or zygomycosis) is a disease caused by several genera of the fungi of the class Zygomycetes (formerly Phycomycetes) and the family Mucoraceae. The genera in order of decreasing frequency are *Rhizopus*, *Mucor*, and *Absidia*. The disease becomes established when a suitably predisposed host (50% to 75% of patients having poorly controlled diabetes mellitus) inhales the spores, which are ubiquitous in nature and part of the normal respiratory flora. The organism is highly invasive and tends to spread rapidly from the nasal fossa to the paranasal sinuses. It invades blood vessels, causing endothelial damage that initiates thrombosis, ischemic and hemorrhagic infarction, and, finally, purulent inflammation. From these sinuses eventually there is invasion of the orbits and cavernous sinuses via the ophthalmic vessels. Invasion of the base of the brain is an end stage event. The entire progression of the disease can occur in only a few days.

Besides affecting diabetic patients who have ketoacidosis, the disease occurs in patients with hematologic malignancies (e.g., acute leukemia); chronic renal failure and acidosis; malnutrition; cancer; cirrhosis; and prolonged antibiotic, steroid, or cytotoxic drug therapy. Clinically, black crusting, necrotic tissue is seen over the turbinates, septum, and palate. In immunosuppressed patients, focal ischemic areas may be found instead of the more typical black crusts. In the cases occurring in nondiabetic patients, pulmonary and disseminated infections are more common. Among survivors there is a high incidence of blindness, cranial nerve palsies, and hemiparesis. The best available therapy is adequate surgical debridement and systemic intravenous therapy with amphotericin B.[53]

Aspergillosis infection is caused by the fungus *Aspergillus*, a member of the Ascomycetes class. It is an ubiquitous organism, frequently found in soil, decaying food, fruits, and plants. The spores are also common contaminants of the respiratory tract and the external auditory canal. *A. fumigatus* accounts for nearly 90% of the infections; however, *A. flavus* and *A. niger* can also cause infections. Involvement of the paranasal sinuses is uncommon, except in the Sudan, where it may be endemic.[53-55] Paranasal sinus disease usually occurs in otherwise healthy patients, and there is no relationship between the paranasal sinus infection and pulmonary aspergillosis, which occurs most often in debilitated patients. *Aspergillus* sinusitis represents colonization of one of the paranasal sinuses, usually the maxillary sinus, with the growth of a mat of tangled hyphae (aspergilloma or mycetoma). The sphenoid and ethmoid sinuses may also be involved either alone or in combination with the antrum. The frontal sinuses are rarely affected.[56] Symptoms vary greatly from none to chronic nasal discharge, which may be foul smelling. Pain can be localized to the involved sinus. The clinical hallmark is a chronic sinusitis that fails to respond to antibiotic therapy.[53] The infection can invade bone and may at times suggest the presence of a carcinoma. When aspergillus sinusitis occurs in immunosuppressed patients, it may be highly invasive and result in the destruction of the sinuses within a few days.[57] Aspergillosis causes a small vessel thrombosis and ischemic and hemorrhagic infarction similar to that of mucormycosis. Treatment is usually surgical extirpation and adjuvant antifungal chemotherapy. An allergic form of aspergillus sinusitis can also occur. These patients usually have asthma, recurrent nasal polyps, and pansinusitis. The treatment is wide local debridement, adequate sinus aeration, and postoperative systemic steroids.[58]

Petrillidium boydii (formerly called *Allescheria boydii*) is the current nomenclature for this fungus of the Ascomycetes family. It is a ubiquitous organism in nature, most commonly found in rural areas. It has been isolated from soil, poultry, cattle manure, and polluted waters. Only rarely is disease reported in humans, and most of these cases are in immunosuppressed patients. However, this disease can occur in otherwise normal patients. As in aspergillosis, this disease may be either saprophytic or invasive. *P. boydii* has been reported to involve the maxillary, ethmoid, and sphenoid sinuses. The present treatment of choice is miconazole with surgical debridement if necessary.[59,60]

The yeasts of the genus *Candida* are part of the normal mucocutaneous flora. However, under certain circumstances they may produce either a minor or a life threatening disease. Minor infections may result as overgrowths in patients on antibiotic therapy. The more severe *Candida* infections occur almost exclusively in patients with compromised immune systems. Today, candidiasis represents the most common and lethal of the opportunistic fungal infections among immunocompromised patients.[53] Most infections are caused by *Candida albicans*, but *C. tropicalis, C. stellatoidea,* and *C. krusei* may also cause disease. When the paranasal sinuses are affected, it is usually in otherwise healthy patients who have been on broad-spectrum antibiotics. The maxillary sinuses are almost exclusively involved, and orbital and intracranial complications are rare. Infections can also occur after maxillary trauma. The treatment of choice for the sinus disease is antral lavage with topical nystatin.[61]

Histoplasmosis capsulatum is an inhabitant of soil, and human infection results from inhalation of infested air. Most infestations result in pulmonary disease and regional lymph node spread. However, rarely there can be involvement of the nasal mucous membranes resulting in edema and nasal obstruction. Even more rarely, pansinusitis can occur. The current treatment of choice is amphotericin B.[53]

Cryptococcosis neoformans is a true yeast pathogen that is the major organism responsible for causing fungal meningoencephalitis in otherwise normal and in immunocompromised patients. The organism is found in soil; avian species, especially pigeons, act as animal reservoirs.[53] Sinonasal disease is uncommon and identical to that of histoplasmosis. The treatment is the same as for histoplasmosis.

Coccidioidomycosis is a disease caused by the dimorphic fungus *Coccidioides immitis*. The pathogenesis and clinical manifestation of the disease are almost identical to that of histoplasmosis.

Myospherulosis is not a fungal disease, but rather an iatrogenic pseudomycotic condition that is caused by the interaction of red blood cells with petrolatum, lanolin, or traumatized human adipose tissue.[53] Large sporangium-like sacs filled with spherules are produced and are often mistaken for a fungus. The disease was first recognized as skin lesions in East Africans; however, in the United States the disease has involved the nose, paranasal sinuses, and middle ear. In these patients, there was always prior surgery (i.e., Caldwell-Luc procedure), and the surgical defect was packed with gauze impregnated with petrolatum. The importance of this disease is to recognize it as an innocuous iatrogenic process so that it is not confused with a true fungal disease and given unwarranted therapy.

Granuloma Producing Diseases

There are a variety of diseases that produce granulomatous changes in the sinonasal cavities. A brief description of each will be presented, followed by some general comments about their imaging characteristics.

Actinomycosis is a noncontagious, suppurative or granulomatous disease that is characterized by a slowly spreading cellulitis of the soft tissues of the neck. Only rarely does this disease involve the paranasal sinuses, and in those cases it is usually by extension of the infection, which normally is localized to the mandible. The most common precursor for this disease is poor dentition with an apical abscess. *Actinomyces israelii* (rarely, *A. eriksonii*) is the primary causative agent. *A. israelii* is a normal constituent of the human mouth flora, and this infection is endogenous in origin. *A. israelii* is an anaerobic, gram-positive, filamentous bacterium (not a fungus). As with other anaerobes, it grows best in devitalized tissue with a low oxygen tension. Sulfur granules form when *Actinomyces* become connected by a protein-polysacchride substance, and this reaction is a response to tissue inflammation. The histologic hallmark is a nest of filamentous bacteria that are basophilic and gram-positive, but not acid fast. This latter property is helpful in distinguishing it from *Nocardia asteroides*, which may otherwise be very similar to *A. israelii*. There are some biochemical reactions that also can be used to distinguish these two branching bacteria. If untreated, *A. israelii* infection may spread to the thoracic or abdominal viscera either by direct extension or by hematogenous dissemination. Central nervous system involvement is rare. Therapy is high doses of penicillin G, to which virtually all anaerobic mouth bacteria are highly sensitive.

Nocardia asteroides is clinically and radiographically indistinguishable from actinomycosis infection and can only be differentiated, albeit at times with difficulty, in the laboratory.[53,62]

Tuberculosis is caused by *Mycobacterium tuberculosis*, which is a strict aerobe and stains acid-fast. The disease has a worldwide distribution; and even though the overall incidence has declined in the past 50 years, it is still not a rare disease.[63] Whenever the paranasal sinuses are involved, it is almost always secondary to a pulmonary infection. The sinus disease may be nonspecific; however, when bone involvement occurs, the dominant symptom is pain. The treatment is prolonged antituberculous chemotherapy.

Syphilis is a worldwide disease that has been on a rise in incidence since the 1980s.[64] The disease is caused by *Treponema pallidum*. The lesion of the primary stage of syphilis is the chancre, and it has been reported in the nose and mouth.[53,65] It appears as a papule that erodes and becomes ulcerated with indurated margins. The gumma represents a destructive, painful, granulomatous process, which most likely represents a hypersensitivity reaction to *T. pallidum* and represents the progression of the secondary stage of the disease to the tertiary phase. It tends to develop in intramembranous bones such as the scalp, face, nose, nasal septum, and paranasal sinuses.[53,65,66] The treatment of choice remains penicillin.

Congenital syphilis may develop if transplacental infection occurs after the fourth fetal month and within 2 years of the time of the acquired maternal infection.[66] The primary manifestations are in the mucocutaneous tissues and bones; and in the head and neck the stigmata include frontal bossing (of Parrot), small maxilla, high palatal arch, Hutchinson's triad (Hutchinson incisors), interstitial keratitis, eighth nerve deafness, saddle nose, and mulberry molars.[67] The spirochete causes a periostitis that interferes with bone development.

Rhinoscleroma is a chronic inflammatory process that primarily involves the nose and nasopharynx, causing indurated nonulcerative inflammatory nodules. The disease is caused by *Klebsiella rhinoscleromatis*, a gram-negative bacterium. The disease is unusual in the United States and mainly occurs in Eastern Europe,

the Middle East, and Latin America.[53] The disease usually begins in the first to third decade of life with a mucopurulent nasal discharge. This progresses through a florid chronic inflammatory stage to finally reach a fibrotic stage, at which time atrophy of the nasal turbinates may be present.[68] The treatment of choice is surgical excision to open the airway and long-term antibiotic therapy, usually with tetracycline.[53]

South American blastomycosis (paracoccidioidomycosis) is caused by the dimorphic fungus *Blastomyces brasiliensis*. It produces painful, destructive granulomas of the nasal cavity and, rarely, involves the paranasal sinuses.[5] The disease is unusual in North America and occurs primarily in Central and South America, especially in Brazil. The primary treatment is with amphotericin B, which cures over 90% of the cases.[69]

North American blastomycosis is caused by *Blastomyces dermatitidis* and almost exclusively involves the larynx, where it can mimic carcinoma clinically. This disease primarily occurs in North America. The primary treatment choice is with amphotericin B.[53]

Leprosy is a chronic granulomatous disease caused by the pleomorphic acid fast bacterium *Mycobacterium leprae*. The disease occurs in almost all tropical and warm temperate regions, including Japan and Korea. It is endemic in several states of the United States. The changes in the sinonasal cavities are those of nonspecific chronic sinusitis and rhinitis. Later changes resemble those of a chronic granulomatous disease. A characteristic finding is progressive erosion of the anterior nasal spine. If previous surgery, trauma, and congenital maxillonasal dysplasia are not applicable to the patient, this finding is pathognomonic of leprosy (Fig. 2-188). The treatment of choice remains the long-term administration of sulfone derivatives (dapsone).[69]

Rhinosporidiosis is caused by the fungus *Rhinospiridum seebri*.[70] The disease is prevalent in India, Sri Lanka, and Brazil. It is rare in the United States. The fungus causes a chronic infection of the nose and nasopharynx, resulting in polypoid masses that cause obstruction of the nasal fossae and may be confused with neoplasms, especially cylindrical cell papilloma.[53] Commonly the disease afflicts the larynx, eyes, and ears. The nasal polyps are sessile, soft, pinkish, and usually unilateral; and they may diminish aeration in the paranasal sinuses. The treatment of choice is surgical excision or electrocautery.

Yaws is a tropical infection caused by the spirochete *Treponema pertenue*. Uncommonly, the late stages of the disease produce granulomas in the mucous membranes of the sinonasal cavities. These granulomas produce severe ulcerations of the nasal region (gangosa) and proliferative exostoses along the medial wall of the maxillary sinus (goundou). The treatment is penicillin.

Glanders, or farcy, is an infectious disease caused by

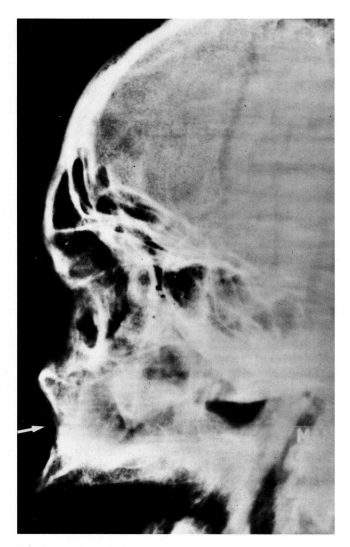

Fig. 2-188 Lateral view shows erosion of anterior nasal spine *(arrow)*. There is also soft tissue disease in the maxillary sinuses and nasal fossa. Leprosy.

the bacterium *Pseudomonas mallei*. The disease in humans is commonly contracted by contact with horses, mules, or donkeys. In humans the disease is characterized either by an acute fulminant febrile illness that may lead to death or a chronic indolent granulomatous disease. Farcy refers to the nodular abscesses found in the skin, lymphatics, and subcutaneous tissues.[69] The nasal manifestations of glanders are a nasal cellulitis and necrosis that produce septal perforations. The treatment is with sulfonamides.

American mucocutaneous leishmaniasis, or espundia, is caused by the parasites *Leishmaniasis mexicana* and *L. braziliensis*. The disease is endemic to Central and South America. After initial primary cutaneous sores, metastatic lesions develop in the nose and mouth that are painful, multilating erosions that can secondarily involve the sinuses.[69,71] Scarring may eventually constrict the nose or mouth, producing gross deformities that in-

terfere with swallowing. The majority of the oronasal diseases are caused by *L. braziliensis*, and the treatment of this established oronasal disease is with amphotericin B.

Wegeners granulomatosis is a disease whose central pathology is a necrotizing granulomatous vasculitis that usually first affects the upper and lower respiratory tracts, but eventually causes a disseminated small vessel vasculitis in kidneys and other organs. Although the disease may have a localized or limited form, usually there is a progression to the systemic form. The initial disease may present as a chronic nonspecific inflammatory process of the nose and sinuses and may remain as such for 1 to 2 years. Usually the nasal septum is first affected. The process becomes diffuse, and septal ulceration and perforations may result in a "saddle nose" deformity. Secondary bacterial infections complicate the clinical and imaging pictures. The disease may be autoimmune (collagen/vascular) related, and the treatment of choice is cyclophosphamide, steroids, and possibly other cytotoxic drugs. Long-term remissions have been achieved; however, it is impossible to predict how long a remission will last.[69,72]

Idiopathic (lethal) midline granuloma is a disease characterized by chronic necrotizing inflammations of the nose, sinuses, midline facial tissues, and upper airways. The lungs, kidneys, and other organs are uninvolved. The histopathology is nonspecific and reveals acute and chronic inflammation with or without granulomas. Because local irradiation of 5000 rads has achieved some long-term remissions, the word lethal is now omitted from the name. Some pathologists object to the entire name of lethal midline granuloma since the disease is not always lethal, is not always in the midline, and does not always have granulomas. The disease may be a lymphoma related process.[72,73]

Sarcoidosis is a systemic, multisystem granulomatous disease of unknown etiology that is characterized by noncaseating epithelial granulomas. These granulomas may, however, also be found in tuberculosis, leprosy, and berylliosis.[74] Sarcoid has a predilection for the Scandinavian countries and for the rural Southeastern United States. It is most common in black females with a median age of 25 years. Nasal sarcoid occurs in 3% to 20% of the patients with systemic sarcoidosis. When it occurs, there are multiple small granulomas of the nasal septum and turbinates. There may be nasal discharge, obstruction, and epistaxis. Polypoid degeneration of the nasal fossa mucosa may occur, but the paranasal sinuses are rarely affected. Rarely, sharply defined, lytic bone lesions may occur in the calvarium and facial skeleton. Steroid therapy may suppress the inflammatory reaction and provide symptomatic improvement, but fibrous organization of the granulomas may lead to organ dysfunction.[53,75]

Exposure to *beryllium* may result in chronic granulo-

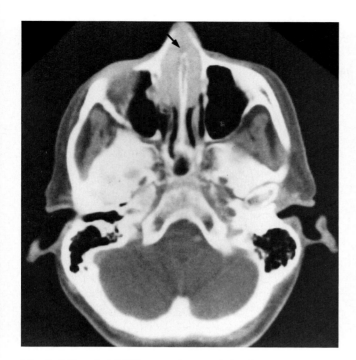

Fig. 2-189 Axial CT scan shows minimally enhancing bilateral nasal fossa mass that has caused erosion *(arrow)* of the anterior nasal septum. Wegeners.

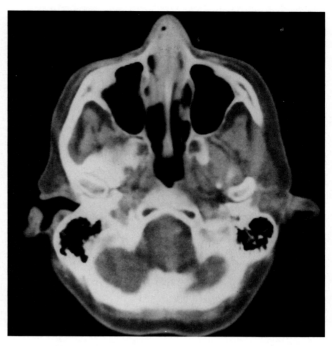

Fig. 2-190 Axial CT scan shows anterior nasal septal mass with erosion of the anterior nasal septum. Wegeners.

mas of the nasal fossa. These granulomas may be indistinguishable from those of tuberculosis, leprosy, and sarcoidosis.[71]

Chromate salts have been implicated in causing nonspecific granulomas of the nasal cavity. Involvement of the paranasal sinuses is a late and unusual event.

Cocaine abuse has become a major worldwide drug problem. Cocaine causes a necrotizing vasculitis and subsequent granuloma of the nasal septum, which, with prolonged exposure, usually results in septal erosion. A nonspecific mucosal inflammation may also occur in the nasal fossa.

The granulomatous diseases that involve the sinonasal cavities can be classified according to the presumed cause of the granuloma:

1. Granulomas caused by infectious disease: actinomycosis, nocardia, tuberculosis, syphilis, rhinoscleroma, South American blastomycosis, leprosy, rhinosporidiosis, yaws, glanders, American mucocutaneous leishmaniasis.
2. Granulomas caused by either autoimmune or collagen vascular related disease: Wegener's granulomatosis.
3. Granulomas caused by lymphoma related disease: midline granuloma.
4. Granulomas caused by idiopathic process: sarcoidosis.
5. Granulomas caused by exposure to chronic irritants: beryllium, chromate salts, cocaine.

As a group the granulomatous diseases that affect the sinonasal cavities all first exhibit nasal cavity involve-

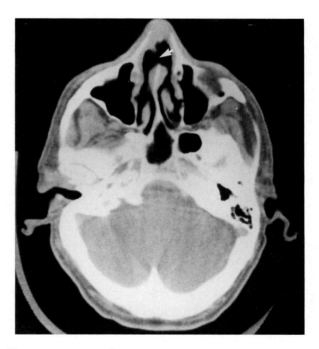

Fig. 2-191 Axial CT scan shows nodular soft tissue thickening of the nasal septum with an erosion *(arrow)* of the septum. Cocaine granuloma.

ment that can vary from a nonspecific inflammatory type reaction with mucosal thickening and nasal secretions to a localized soft tissue mass. The nasal septum may be focally thickened by a bulky soft tissue mass. Septal erosions may be present. The paranasal sinuses usually are involved only after the nasal fossa, and the maxillary and ethmoid sinuses are most often affected. Uncommonly, the sphenoid sinuses are involved, and the frontal sinuses are almost always spared. When the sinuses are involved, there is usually nonspecific inflammatory mucosal thickening; air-fluid levels are rare. The bones of the nasal vault and affected paranasal sinuses may be thickened and sclerotic, reflecting the chronic nature of the inflammatory reaction. Sinus obliteration by reactive bone may occur.[76,77] Similarly, there may be areas of bone erosion reflecting either an osteomyelitic process or necrosis from a granuloma. If the nasal disease becomes a bulky soft tissue mass, there may, in addition, be remodelling of the adjacent bones (Figs. 2-189 to 2-191).[68]

Mucoceles

Mucoceles are the most common expansile lesions of any paranasal sinus. They are defined pathologically as being formed by a cuboidal epithelium that surrounds mucoid secretions. Using these pathologic criteria, both mucoceles and mucous retention cysts fulfill this definition equally well.[41] However, the clinical and radiographic differences between these entities are so clearly defined that pathologists have agreed to distinguish between them.[78]

Classically, a retention cyst is a spherical mucoid filled cyst that develops when a mucous gland of the sinus mucosa becomes obstructed. The cyst wall is the epithelium of the duct; these are common, usually incidental findings, identified in 10% of people. Although they can occur in any sinus, they are most common in the antrum and rarely expand the sinus cavity or remodel the sinus bony walls.

By comparison, a mucocele develops from the obstruction of a sinus ostium or a compartment of a septated sinus. The wall of the lesion is the sinus mucosa, and the sinus cavity is expanded as the bony walls are remodelled. Mucoceles occur primarily in the frontal sinuses (60% to 65%), but they also are found in the ethmoid sinuses (20% to 25%), maxillary sinuses (10%), and the sphenoid sinuses (1% to 2%).[79-82] In those few cases where a retention cyst becomes so large that it completely fills the sinus cavity, distinction from an early mucocele that has not yet remodelled the sinus walls is impossible and of no clinical significance, since the surgical treatment of both is identical.

The classical mucocele is a noninfected lesion that presents with signs and symptoms that result from the mass itself: i.e., proptosis, bossing of the forehead, a mass in the superomedial orbit, inability to breath through the nose (one or both sides), and a change in voice quality (nasal sound), etc. Pain is rare and when noted indicates the presence of an infected mucocele or a pyocele (mucopyocele).

The sinus cavity expansion is the result of a dynamic process that consists of pressure necrosis that causes a slow erosion of the inner sinus bony wall while the outer periostium responds by producing new bone. In this way, the sinus wall is remodelled and the sinus cavity slowly expands.

Plain Films. On plain films, frontal sinus mucoceles first appear as slight clouding of the involved sinus or portion of the sinus. The normal contour scalloping of the average and well-developed frontal sinus becomes smooth, presenting an ovoid or rounded appearance. The normal thin mucoperiosteal white line becomes poorly seen, and if chronic sinusitis was present prior to the development of the mucocele, a zone of dense reactive bone may surround the sinus.

As the mucocele erodes the sinus contour in the vertical plate of the frontal bone, it also slowly erodes the anterior and posterior frontal sinus tables. This results in a loss of bone density on frontal plain films that more than compensates for the soft tissue density of the mucoid secretions. Thus, a frontal sinus mucocele tends to maintain a radiodensity that is equal to or slightly less than the normal soft tissue density of sinusitis, and if an expansile frontal sinus mass is seen that is denser than the adjacent frontal bone, the imager should consider a fibroosseous lesion rather than a mucocele. It is only in the few huge mucoceles that erode most of the posterior sinus table, that the plain film presentation is a radiolucent frontal sinus (Figs. 2-192 to 2-196).

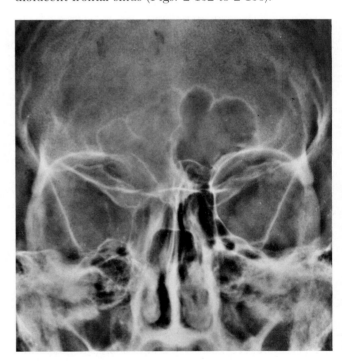

Fig. 2-192   Caldwell view shows clouding of right frontal sinus and right ethmoid sinuses. There is thinning or erosion of the right superomedial orbital rim. Sinusitis and right frontal sinus mucocele.

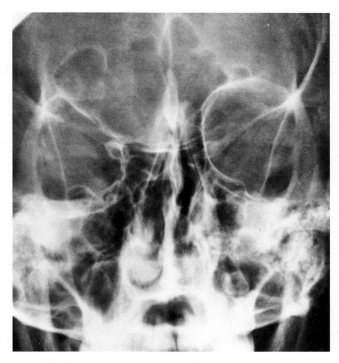

Fig. 2-193 Caldwell view shows slight haziness in right frontal sinus and flattening of right superomedial orbital rim. The intersinus septum is also displaced to the left side. Right frontal sinus mucocele.

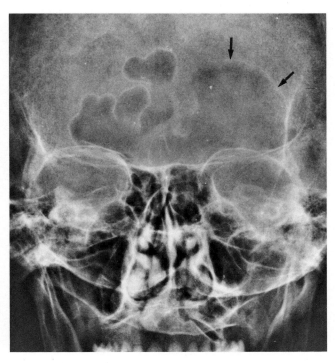

Fig. 2-194 Caldwell view shows loss of normal sinus scalloping *(arrows)* and portions of the white line in the left frontal sinus. Left frontal sinus mucocele.

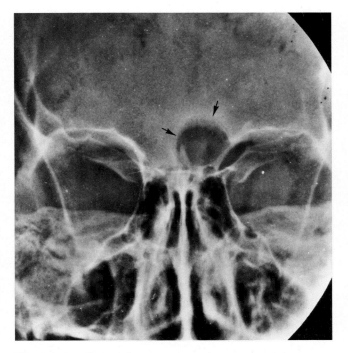

Fig. 2-195 Caldwell view shows left hypoplastic sinus that has lost the normal thin white line, has a vague zone of surrounding sclerosis *(arrows),* and is smoothly concave. There is also erosion of the left superomedial orbital rim. Frontal sinus mucocele.

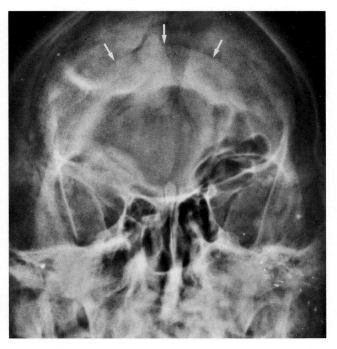

Fig. 2-196 Caldwell view shows smoothly contoured, enlarged frontal sinus. There is a surrounding zone of sclerosis, and only the lateralmost portion of the left frontal sinus appears normal. There is erosion of the right superior and superomedial orbital rim, and a mound of soft tissue is seen above the mass *(arrows).* Frontal sinus mucocele elevating the forehead and causing right proptosis.

In a hypoplastic frontal sinus, there is usually only a single, smooth, centrally concave sinus border. The normally present scalloped margins of larger sinuses are not present for assessment of possible erosion. However, whether the sinus is small or large, the normal frontal sinus will never violate the orbital contour. Any downward and outward displacement of the superomedial orbital rim should be considered presumptive evidence of a frontal sinus mucocele until proved otherwise (see Figs. 2-192, 2-193, and 2-196).

Similarly, since the base of the frontal intersinus septum is normally in the midline, displacement of this portion of the septum to one side should suggest to the radiologist that a frontal sinus mucocele is present (see Fig. 2-193).

Because only the midline segments of the anterior and posterior frontal sinus tables are seen on a lateral plain film, significant erosion of these tables *off the midline* can occur and remain undetected on plain films. Specifically, any posterior intracranial extension of a mucocele through the eroded posterior table off the midline is invisible on plain films. Since the absence of an intact posterior frontal sinus wall is of importance to the surgeon, preoperative sectional imaging of a suspected frontal sinus mucocele should *always* be performed. At times, even large, clinically silent intracranial extension of a mucocele can be discovered.

In addition to extending upward into the vertical plate of the frontal bone, mucoceles can extend posteriorly into the horizontal plate (orbital roof) of the frontal bone. Once in this area, a mucocele can extend both cranially into the floor of the anterior cranial fossa and caudally into the orbital roof. If such an extension is not appreciated by the surgeon at the time of surgery (usually performed for the more obvious vertical plate disease), complications from this orbital roof mucocele may require not only a second operation, but also an intracranial approach.

If such frontal sinus surgery was performed without preoperative sectional imaging, and if there is any retrospective suggestion on plain film studies that horizontal recess disease is present, a postoperative scan should be obtained in order to resolve the issue and provide a baseline study to which any further examinations can be compared.

Ethmoid mucoceles usually arise in the anterior rather than the posterior ethmoid cells.[83] This presumably reflects the fact that the anterior ethmoid ostia are the smallest of any in the paranasal sinuses.[84] The viscosity of mucus also plays an etiologic role, and this may explain why ethmoid mucoceles are most common in patients with mucoviscidosis.[85]

The typical ethmoid mucocele is an expansile lesion that thins and remodels the lamina papyracea, bowing it into the orbit. As a result, the eye is laterally displaced. Although such a mass is obvious clinically, it may be very difficult to diagnose on plain films and tomograms (Fig. 2-197). In part, this is because the obliquely oriented lamina papyracea is seen poorly on frontal films and partly because the ethmoid cells in front of or behind the mucocele may be normal; their

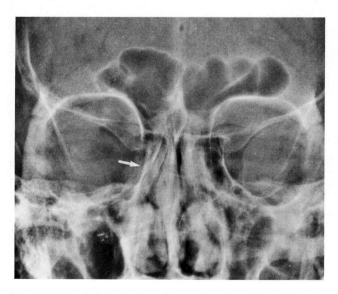

Fig. 2-197 Caldwell view shows clouding of the right ethmoid sinuses with thinning or destruction of the lower right lamina papyracea *(arrow)*. Ethmoid sinus mucocele.

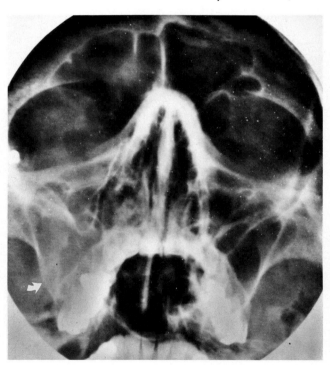

Fig. 2-198 Waters view shows opacified right maxillary sinus with thinning of lower lateral sinus wall *(arrow)* and some expansion of the sinus cavity. Maxillary sinus mucocele.

air density can partially nullify the soft tissue density of the mucocele. If an air-fluid level is seen in the ethmoid complex, this usually indicates the presence of an ethmoid mucocele that has ruptured, draining some of its contents into the nasal cavity and adjacent ethmoid. In these cases, a mucopyocele is usually present at the time of discovery (see Fig. 2-143).[86]

Ethmoid mucoceles also can arise in supraorbital ethmoid cells. These are best demonstrated on Caldwell films or coronal images. The obstructing process that leads to the development of these mucoceles is usually an infection or a polyp in the lower portion of the supraorbital cell. These mucoceles typically erode through the orbital roof and displace the globe inferiorly.

The entire ethmoid complex, either unilaterally or bilaterally, can be involved by polypoid mucoceles. The sectional imaging characteristics are the preservation of most of the ethmoid septa in an opacified, expanded ethmoid complex. When this constellation of findings is seen, the radiologist can be assured that tumor is not present.

The typical antral mucocele totally opacifies the antrum and expands the sinus cavity (Fig. 2-198). At an early stage one cannot differentiate a transiently obstructed sinus that is filled with mucoid secretion from a similar sinus that will remain obstructed and proceed into a mucocele. It is only after sinus expansion that a definitive diagnosis can be made. If the growth of the antral mucocele remains unchecked, eventually the outer maxillary periostium can no longer produce new bone, and frank bone destruction results. In these instances, plain film distinction from tumors may be difficult (Fig. 2-199). If the orbital floor is elevated, the patient may experience diplopia. Rarely, if the mucocele

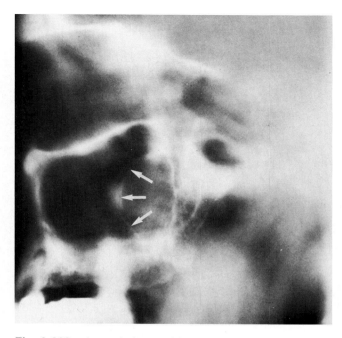

Fig. 2-200   Lateral view multidirectional tomogram shows an expanded compartment *(arrows)* in the posterior portion of the maxillary sinus. Mucocele of a sinus compartment.

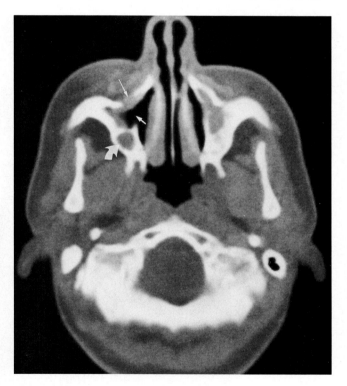

Fig. 2-201   Axial CT scan shows patient who has had a prior right Caldwell-Luc procedure. The surgical defect is seen in the anterior sinus wall *(arrow),* and there has been an antrostomy *(small arrow).* There is a localized, opacified compartment in the posterior sinus *(curved arrow)* that contained a mucocele that was overlooked at the first surgery. Inflammatory tissue is present in the left antrum. Mucocele of a sinus compartment.

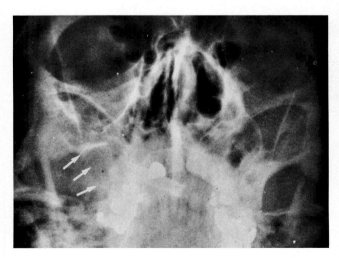

Fig. 2-199   Waters view shows opacification of right maxillary sinus with erosion of the lateral wall *(arrows).* This could be a carcinoma, but was an antral mucocele.

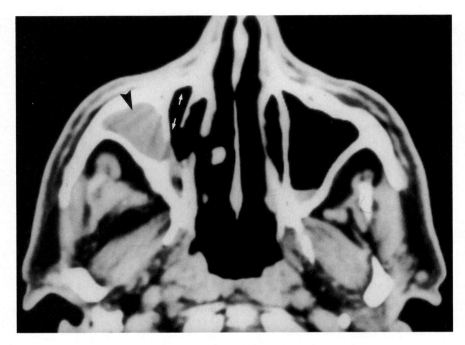

Fig. 2-202 Axial CT scan on patient after a right Caldwell-Luc procedure. There is an expansile mass *(arrowhead)* in the lateral portion of the sinus. The medial portion of the sinus *(small arrows)* is aerated. Postoperative mucocele.

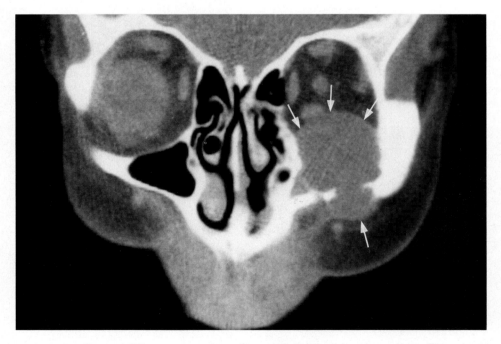

Fig. 2-203 Coronal CT scan on patient after a left Caldwell-Luc procedure. There is an expansile mass that has broken into the left orbit and the cheek *(arrows)*. Postoperative mucocele.

spontaneously collapses after the orbital floor is thinned, the globe may descend causing enophthalmos and diplopia. In an antrum that has been compartmentalized by a septum, a mucocele can develop within only one of these sinus sections. This may have significant clinical implications if this mucocele is in a posterior compartment; this region usually eludes the surgeon when the sinus is explored by a Caldwell-Luc approach. In such cases, the radiologist may be the only physician to detect this "hidden" mucocele and direct the surgeon to it (Figs. 2-200 and 2-201).[87]

In the patient who has had a prior Caldwell-Luc procedure, a fibrous septum may develop between the lateral margins of the anterior sinus wall bony surgical defect and the posterior sinus wall. This septum often is initiated by the development of synechia that progressively form a solid fibrous wall. This septum obstructs the sinus drainage from the lateral portion of the sinus, while the sinus cavity medial to the septum drains normally. Thus, the classical findings in such a patient are an expansile mass in the lateral maxillary sinus. When large enough, it may extend into the body of the zygoma and present in the cheek as a soft tissue mass, or it may extend into the lateral, inferior orbit (Figs. 2-202 and 2-203).

Sphenoid sinus mucoceles are the least common of the paranasal sinus mucoceles; however, because of their proximity to the optic nerves, they have the highest rate of complications resulting from their surgical correction. Most sphenoid mucoceles expand anterolaterally into the posterior ethmoids and the orbital apex. Less commonly, expansion may occur upward into the sella turcica and cavernous sinuses or downward into the nasopharynx and posterior nares. Intracranial extension in rare cases can even result in areas of brain necrosis.[88,89] Rarely, they may extend into the sphenoid sinus recesses in the greater wings and the pterygoid processes.[90]

If sufficiently large, sphenoid sinus mucoceles may cause optic canal and orbital apex syndromes. The critical role of the radiologist is to accurately localize the relationship of the optic nerve to the mass. From this information, the surgeon will know where to direct the instruments during decompression. Blindness is the major serious postoperative complication.

Multiple mucoceles have been reported to arise after facial fractures and in patients with severe allergies. The allergic patient with aspirin intolerance seems to be particularly prone to develop multiple mucoceles.[91]

Sectional Imaging. On CT scans a mucocele usually appears as an expanded sinus cavity that is filled with a fairly homogeneous material of mucoid attenuation (10 to 18 HUs). In a few cases the mucocele secretions may be particularly viscid and proteinatious, and the attenuation may be in the 20 to 40 HU range. The exact rea-

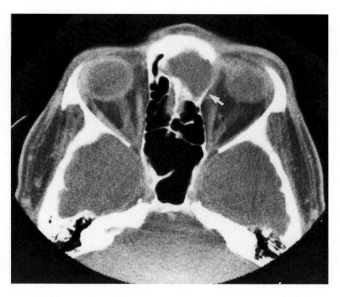

Fig. 2-204   Axial CT scan shows expansile left frontal sinus mass that is bulging into upper left orbit. The bone is primarily remodelled *(arrow)* rather than being destroyed. Mucocele.

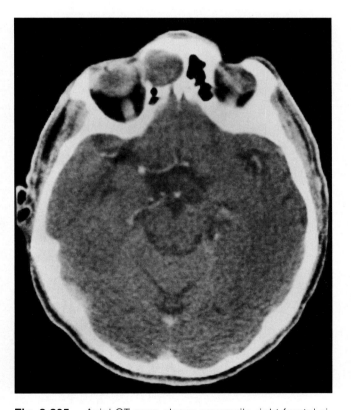

Fig. 2-205   Axial CT scan shows expansile right frontal sinus mass that has extended down into right superomedial orbit. Mucocele.

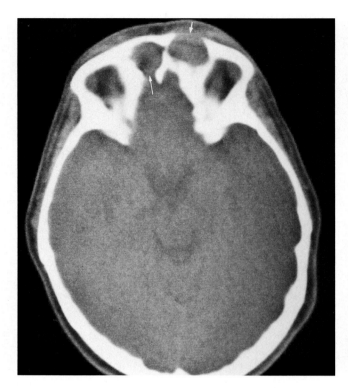

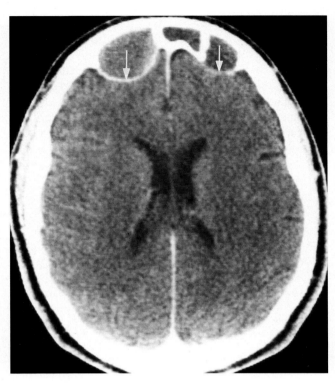

Fig. 2-206   Axial CT scan shows expansile mass in both the left and right frontal sinuses. The left mass has broken through the anterior sinus wall *(small arrow)* and the right-sided mass has broken through the posterior sinus wall *(arrow).* Bilateral frontal sinus mucoceles.

Fig. 2-207   Axial CT scan shows bilateral frontal sinus expansile masses. Each mass has thinned and remodelled the posterior sinus wall *(arrows)* and extended intracranially. The posterior sinus wall appeared intact on the plain film studies. Bilateral frontal sinus mucoceles.

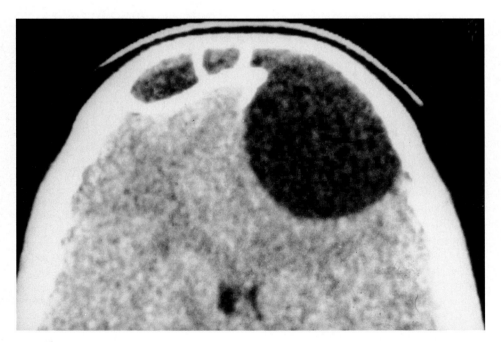

Fig. 2-208   Axial CT scan shows large "mucoid" attenuation mass in the left frontal sinus that has extended intracranially. A smaller mucocele that extended down into the orbit is present on the right side. Mucoceles.

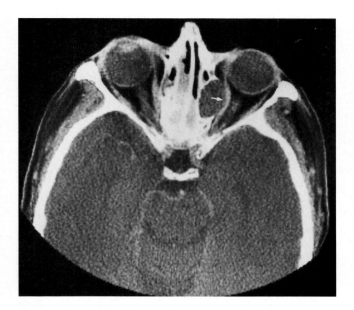

Fig. 2-209 Axial CT scan shows expansile left ethmoid sinus mass that has extended into the orbit and displaces the medial rectus muscle *(arrow)*. Ethmoid sinus mucocele.

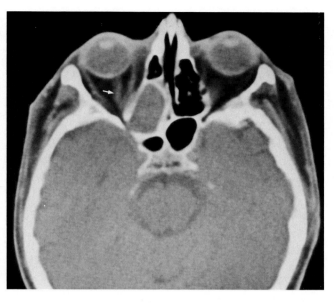

Fig. 2-210 Axial CT scan shows right posterior ethmoid expansile mass that compresses the orbital apex structures and laterally displaces the optic nerve *(arrow)*. Posterior ethmoid mucocele.

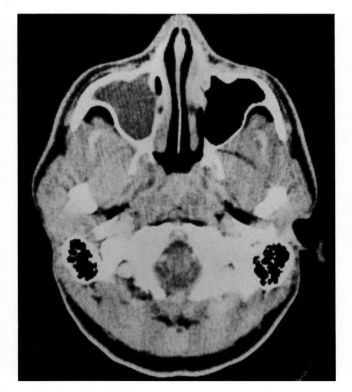

Fig. 2-211 Axial CT scan shows totally opacified right maxillary sinus. The sinus walls are normal. Without any remodelling of the sinus walls this obstructed sinus should not be diagnosed as a mucocele. Once remodelling occurs, it can be called an antral mucocele.

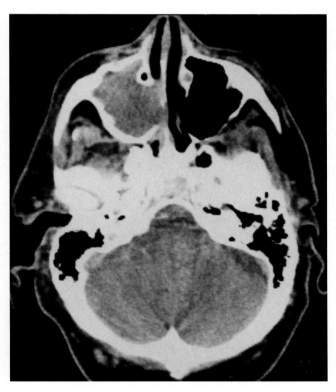

Fig. 2-212 Axial CT scan shows expansile right maxillary sinus mass that bulges into the right nasal fossa. Antral mucocele.

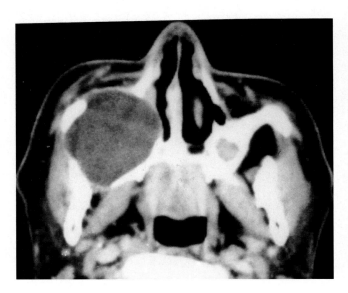

Fig. 2-213 Axial CT scan shows large expansile mucoid attenuation right antral mass. Portions of the antral wall are thinned or not seen. Antral mucocele.

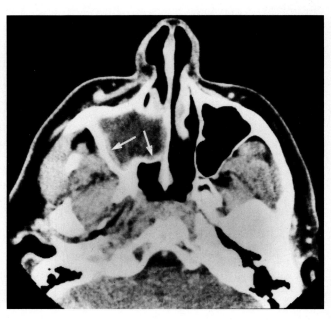

Fig. 2-214 Axial postcontrast CT scan shows expansile right antral mucoid attenuation mass that has a thin enhancing rim *(arrows)*. Antral mucopyocele.

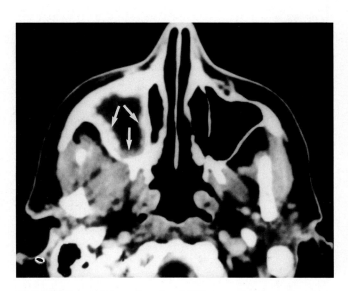

Fig. 2-215 Axial postcontrast CT scan shows mucoid attenuation right antral mass. There is a thin enhancing zone around the mucoid material *(arrows)*. Antral mucopyocele.

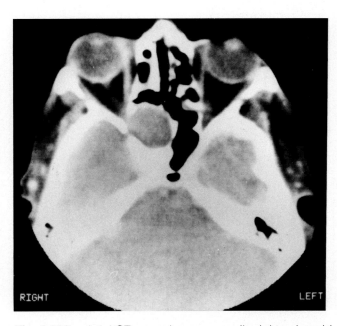

Fig. 2-216 Axial CT scan shows expansile right sphenoid sinus mass that encroaches on the orbital apex. Sphenoid mucocele.

son why some patients have this increased attenuation, and in rare cases apparent enhancement, is unclear. However, most mucoceles have an attenuation in the mucoid range less than that of muscle.[92] The sinus walls are remodelled and may be either of almost normal thickness, thinned, or eroded. In these latter cases, the sinus mucosa and the maxillary periostium are all that confine the mucous secretions (Figs. 2-204 to 2-216).

If a mucopyocele is present, the sinus mucosa surrounding the central mucous secretions is seen as a thin zone of enhancement just inside the bony sinus walls. This signifies the presence of the inflamed mucosa and establishes the diagnosis of an infected mucocele (see Figs. 2-214 and 2-215).[40]

On MRI, the signal intensities are dominated initially by the high water content of the mucous secretions (about 95% water). Thus, there usually is a low signal intensity on T_1 WIs, an intermediate signal intensity on PD WIs, and a high signal intensity on T_2 WIs. However, if the mucocele has been present for a long time (presumably on the order of many months), the T_1- and proton density-weighted signal intensities become higher. The primary causes appear to be a concentration of the proteinatious secretions, a slow resorption of water through the mucosa, and an increased viscosity of these secretions. This T_1 relaxation time shortening probably can be used as a rough scale of how long the mucocele has been present. A long T_1 signifies a recent lesion, an intermediate T_1 indicates a lesion of many months duration, while a short T_1 suggests a lesion of a much longer duration. This time scale is only a suggested guideline and may be altered once statistically relevant data are collected. One of the clinical problems in obtaining these data is establishing the precise time of the initial development of a mucocele, since it often is present for long periods before symptoms arise. The T_2 signal remains high in most of these lesions. However, when enough free water is resorbed from the mucocele and the protein concentration reaches about 25% to 35%, first the T_2W signal intensity and then the T_1W signal intensity become low.[44] Thus, mucoceles can have the following progressive MRI appearances: low T_1, high T_2; intermediate T_1, high T_2; high T_1, high T_2; intermediate-to-high T_1, low T_2; low T_1, low T_2 (Figs. 2-217 to 2-223).[44] If a mucopyocele is present, the infection appears to cause increased viscosity with a resulting shortening of the T_1 signal.

Cholesteatoma

In addition to mucoceles, there are several other entities that can enlarge an entire sinus cavity or a localized portion thereof. An epidermoid, or cholesteatoma, is a cystic mass with a stratified squamous epithelial wall and a central cavity filled with keratin. In the frontal bone they probably arise from a congenital rest or as

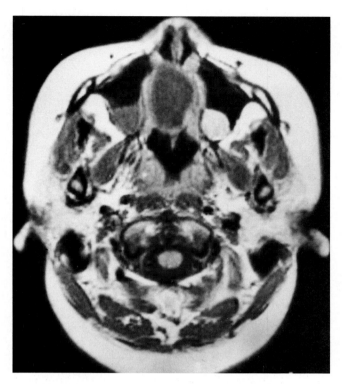

Fig. 2-217 Axial T_1W MRI scan shows expansile process that arose in a pneumatized middle turbinate (concha bullosa). This mucocele has a low T_1W signal intensity and also had a high T_2W signal intensity. Also present is a small retention cyst in the posterior recess of each antrum. On the right side the cyst has low T_1W signal intensity, while on the left side the cyst has an intermediate signal intensity.

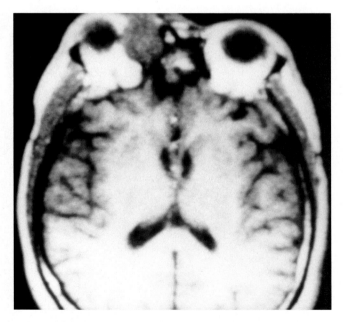

Fig. 2-218 Axial T_1W MRI scan shows low-to-intermediate signal intensity mass *(arrowhead)* in the superomedial right orbit. This mass extended down from the right frontal sinus and had a high signal intensity on T_2W images. Frontal sinus mucocele.

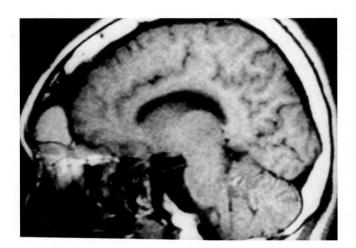

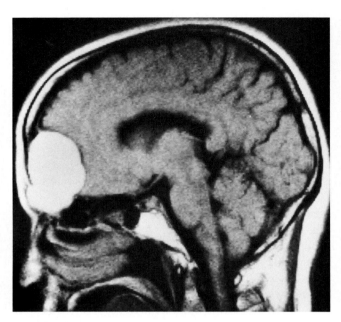

Fig. 2-219 Sagittal T₁W MRI scan shows expansile frontal sinus mass with an intermediate signal intensity. This mass had a high T₂W signal intensity. Frontal sinus mucocele.

Fig. 2-220 Sagittal T₁W MRI scan shows expansile frontal sinus mass with high signal intensity. Mucocele.

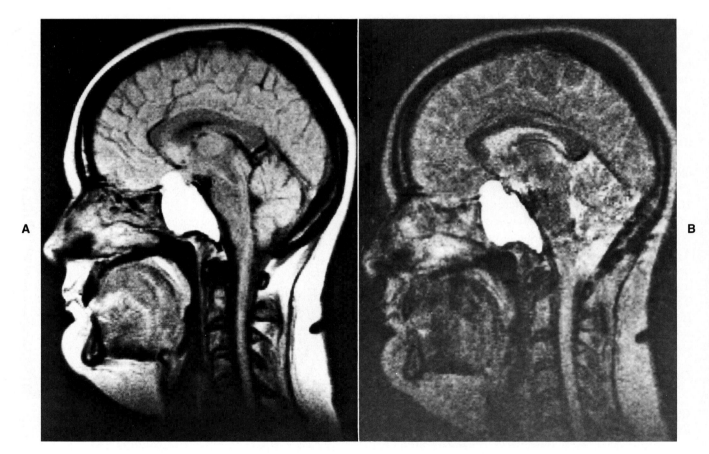

Fig. 2-221 **A,** Sagittal T₁W and **B,** T₂W MRI scans show expansile sphenoid sinus mass that has high signal intensity on both sequences. Mucocele.

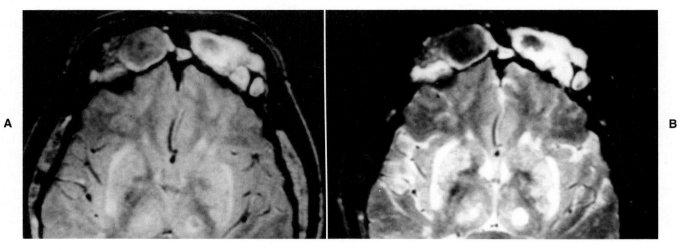

Fig. 2-222 **A,** Axial T₁W and **B,** T₂W MRI scans show bilateral expansile frontal sinus masses. On the right side the mass has low-to-intermediate T₁W and low T₂W signal intensities. On the left side the mass has high signal intensity on both T₁W and T₂W scans. Frontal sinus mucoceles.

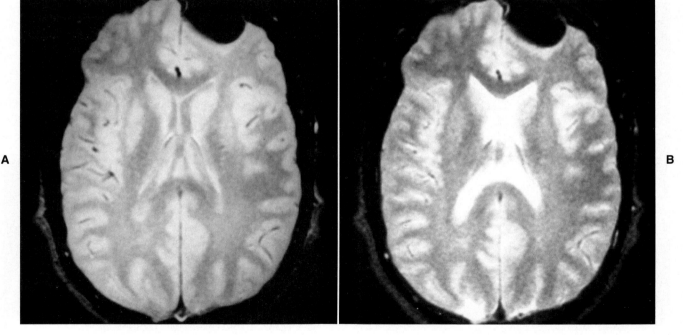

Fig. 2-223 **A,** Axial mixed image and **B,** T₂W MRI scans show expansile mass in the left frontal sinus that has signal void on both scans. This was a mucocele with dried, dessicated secretions.

a post–traumatic implant. They may develop either in the diploe or, less frequently, the outer table of the skull. On plain films the net effect of the bone loss secondary to the expansile process and the increased density secondary to the deposition of the keratin material with displacement of air within the sinus results in a lucent appearing lesion when compared to the adjacent normal frontal bone. The margins are slightly scalloped, and there is a thin, uniform white line that identifies the lesion's contour. These latter two findings help to differentiate a cholesteatoma from a mucocele (Fig. 2-224). Such confusion may occur if a cholesteatoma arises within or adjacent to the frontal sinus.[93,94]

Rarely, a cholesteatoma may occur within a paranasal sinus, usually the maxillary antrum, as a result of squamous metaplasia of the sinus mucosa, presumably secondary to chronic sinusitis. In the antrum, invasion of buccal epithelium via an oroantral fistula has also been proposed as a possible etiology.[94] A type of cholesteatoma or pseudocholesteatoma may also result within a chronically infected sinus after the active infection subsides. The breakdown products of the purulent exudate may contain cholesterol products and appear as cholesteatomatous debris.[95,96]

On CT, a cholesteatoma is an expansile lesion that has soft tissue, mucoidlike attenuation (usually 10 to 25 HUs) and may be indistinguishable from a mucocele. On MRI, the fatty components of the cholesterol usually result in a high signal intensity on T_1 WIs and PD WIs and an intermediate intensity signal on T_2 WI.[97,98]

Enlarged Aerated Sinuses

A paranasal sinus may be enlarged with normal sinus mucosa and either be normally aerated or hyperaerated. This unusual situation is the result of one of the entities referred to as *hypersinus, pneumosinus dilatans,* or *pneumocele.* Part of the confusion arises from a lack of certainty as to how large a sinus may be before it should be called abnormal, and part from the lack of a pathologically confirmed etiology for these processes.

A study of plain films on 100 normal patients judged a sinus to be abnormally large if it exceeded in size 99% of the normal population.[99,100] Taking into account magnification factors for films taken on a Franklin Head Unit (3.4%) and a standard 40 inch focal distance Caldwell view (10.3%), if a line drawn from the base of the crista galli to a point of maximum distance along the perimeter of the sinus exceeds 74.4 mm (head unit) or 79.3 mm (PA skull film), the sinus is larger than 99% of normal frontal sinuses and may be referred to as a hypersinus. This term refers to a larger than normal sinus that does not expand the normal contours of the bone in which the sinus is located (Fig. 2-225 and see Fig. 2-23).

The term *pneumosinus dilatans* refers to an aerated sinus that is abnormally expanded (either the entire sinus or a portion of the sinus) and whose walls, although intact and of normal thickness, have been outwardly displaced (remodelled) from their normal boundaries.

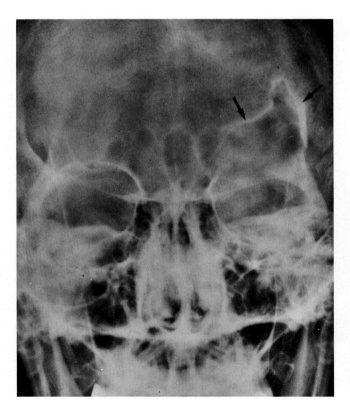

Fig. 2-224 Caldwell view shows lesion in the left frontal bone that has depressed the left superior orbital rim. The lesion has a well-defined scalloped, sclerotic rim *(arrows),* and the mass abuts the frontal sinuses. Cholesteatoma.

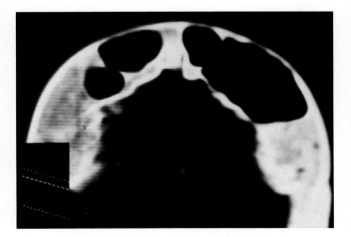

Fig. 2-225 Axial CT scan shows large frontal sinuses in patient with dense cortical-type calvarium and hyperostosis frontalis interna. Despite the size of these sinuses, there is no deformity of the forehead. This sinus measured as a hypersinus on a Caldwell view.

This causes frontal bossing, diplopia, a nasal mass, etc., depending on which sinus is involved and which portion of this sinus is expanded. Accordingly, it is this extension of the sinus beyond the normal bony boundaries that differentiates pneumosinus dilatans from hypersinus. If the entire sinus is not involved, the remaining sinus dimensions are usually normal (Fig. 2-226).

Pneumocele refers to an aerated sinus with either focal or generalized sinus cavity enlargement and thinning of the bony sinus walls. It is this latter feature that differentiates pneumosinus dilatans from a pneumocele (Figs. 2-227 to 2-229). This distinction has been developed in the clinical literature where the integrity, or lack of integrity, of the sinus wall was observed. Although a "valve" theory has been suggested as an etiology for the delayed pressure equilibration that apparently occurs in pneumoceles, no such valve has been demonstrated physiologically.

At present, there is no clear understanding of the factors that either influence the development of normal sinuses or signal the normal cessation of sinus growth. Consequently, the etiology of excessive sinus aeration and growth that produces hypersinus, pneumosinus dilatans, and pneumocele is unclear.[100] The pneumocele's growth can be arrested by creating a surgical window (i.e., antrostomy, ethmoidectomy, sphenoid-sinusotomy) to allow rapid pressure equilibration. The cosmetic deformity that may result from either a pneumosinus dilatans or a pneumocele can be dealt with surgically, if necessary, by collapsing the sinus.

In the sphenoid sinus, the planum sphenoidale may be bowed cranially by an overlying meningioma.[101,102] This may simulate a pneumosinus dilatans. However, only the roof of the sphenoid sinus is involved by the

presence of a tumor and a CT or MRI scan will demonstrate the lesion. Additionally, the bone is usually thickened if related to the presence of an overlying tumor.

Complications of Inflammatory Paranasal Sinus Disease Affecting Adjacent Areas

In the present antibiotic era, most acute paranasal sinus infections are successfully treated. It is only in a few cases that surgical intervention is required to help

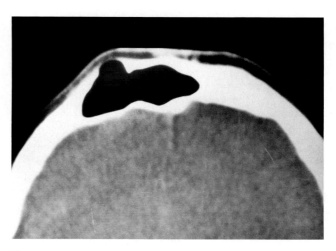

Fig. 2-227   Axial CT scan shows normal sized right frontal sinus that has focally thinned the anterior sinus wall to cause a bulge in the forehead. Pneumocele.

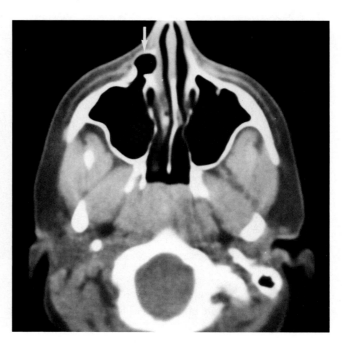

Fig. 2-228   Axial CT scan shows focal anterior enlargement of the right maxillary sinus *(arrow)* that has thinned the sinus wall and caused a mass in the cheek. Pneumocele.

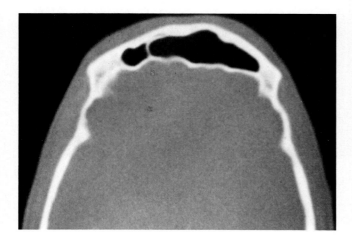

Fig. 2-226   Axial CT scan shows enlarged left frontal sinus that has not thinned the bone of either the anterior or posterior sinus walls. However, the anterior wall has been bowed forward causing a bulge in the forehead. Pneumosinus dilatans.

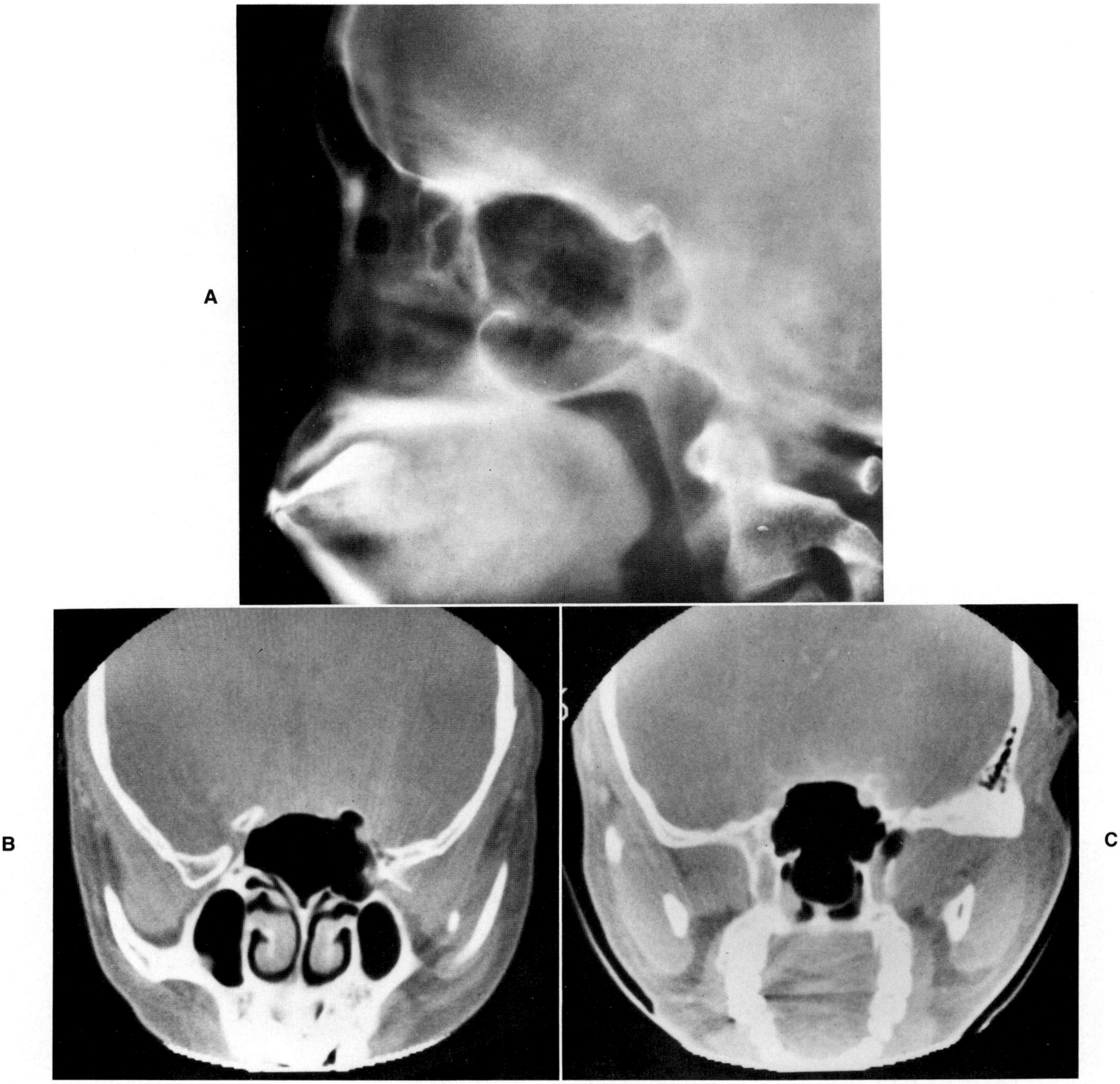

Fig. 2-229   A, Lateral multidirectional tomogram shows expanded sphenoid sinus that has thinned all of the bony sinus walls. The sinus floor is displaced downward so that it rests on the top of the soft palate. Coronal CT scans through **B,** anterior and **C,** posterior sphenoid sinus show the thinned sinus wall bone and the extension of the sinus into a pneumatized and expanded left anterior clinoid process. Pneumocele.

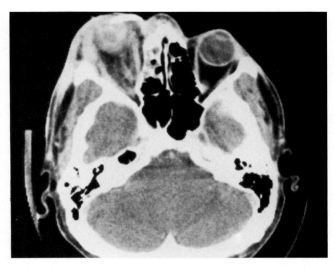

Fig. 2-230 Axial CT scan shows clouding of the right anterior ethmoid sinuses and proptosis of the right eye, increased attenuation of the right orbital fat, thickening of the right extraocular muscles, and preseptal soft tissue thickening. Ethmoid sinusitis and orbital cellulitis.

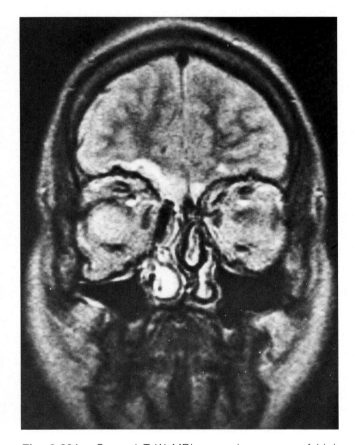

Fig. 2-231 Coronal T$_2$W MRI scan shows area of high signal just above the right orbit and in the base of the midline anterior cranial fossa. Cerebritis in a patient medically treated for frontal sinusitis.

control an acute infection. However, a delay in initiating proper treatment, organisms resistant to the chosen antibiotics, and incomplete treatment regimens all can allow an initially localized infection to spread to adjacent regions.[103,104]

About 3% of patients with paranasal sinusitis will experience some related orbital or preseptal inflammatory disease. These various complications include retention edema of the eyelids, preseptal cellulitis, preseptal abscess, orbital cellulitis, subperiosteal orbital abscess, orbital abscess, and cavernous sinus thrombosis (Fig. 2-230).[103,105] Such orbital complications are discussed in Chapter 10 on the orbit. In addition, 15% to 20% of the cases of retrobulbar neuritis are secondary to posterior ethmoid and sphenoid sinusitis, and in some of these cases the neuritis can apparently occur without other manifestations of orbital inflammatory disease.[80,106]

The ethmoid sinuses are clearly the most often implicated as the source of infection for orbital complications. The thin lamina papyracea and the anterior and posterior valveless ethmoidal veins allow rapid access of infection into the orbit.[107] When implicated as a source of orbital infection, in descending order of frequency, the remaining paranasal sinuses are the sphenoid, frontal, and maxillary.

Intracranial complications of sinusitis also occur infrequently, and these include meningitis, epidural abscess, subdural abscess, cerebritis, and cerebral abscess (Fig. 2-231).[108] Only 3% of intracranial abscesses originate from sinonasal cavity disease, and only 3% of headaches are reported to result from sinusitis.[103]

Intracranial spread of inflammatory disease in the paranasal sinuses most often stems from frontal sinusitis. As has been stated, this is because of the rich emissary network (Bechet's plexus) that connects the posterior sinus mucosa with the meninges; acting as a source for intracranial inflammatory disease, in decreasing order of frequency, the remaining paranasal sinuses are the sphenoid, ethmoid, and maxillary.

Osteomyelitis is also a complication of sinusitis and is most often encountered today in patients who have chronic, incompletely treated sinusitis or fungal disease. Less commonly, it can occur in patients who were previously irradiated in the facial area. The dominant clinical finding is persistent pain; and the radiographic manifestations include focal rarefaction of bone, sequestrum formation, reactive thickening of the bone, bony sclerosis, and ultimately fragmentation of the bone. Over the frontal sinus, a subgaleal abscess can form secondary to sinusitis. This occurs via osteothrombophlebitis and may or may not be associated from frank osteomyelitis. This subgaleal abscess is also called a Pott's puffy tumor.[109]

No matter whether the complications are intracranial

or intraorbital, they are more likely to occur in patients with acute sinusitis rather than in cases of chronic inflammatory disease. Only the osseous complications are more common in chronic infections.

Opacified Maxillary Sinus

When a patient presents with signs and symptoms of rhinitis and sinusitis, they often seek the advice of an otolaryngologist. Most of these specialists prefer to obtain a plain film examination of the paranasal sinuses to map the disease and provide a graphic means of following its response to treatment. On these initial films the sinus most often affected is the maxillary sinus, and frequently this sinus is totally opacified, presumably as a result of polypoid mucosal thickening and retained secretions.[110] The clinician most often will treat these patients with decongestants, antihistamines, nasal sprays, and antibiotics. Within 3 to 7 days, the presenting symptoms usually have abated, and the assumption is that the opacified sinus has also cleared. However, if follow-up sinus films are obtained on these now asymptomatic patients, the antrum remains opacified in 20% of cases, while in 80% of the people, some resolution of the sinusitis is noted by the radiographic observation of the presence of sinus aeration.[111]

The reason the antrum remains opacified, despite the resolution of the patient's symptoms, is that there is an underlying process in the sinus that causes periodic obstruction of the sinus ostium. This in turn causes the bacterial sinusitis that produces the patient's symptoms. If the underlying problem is not resolved, the patient will continue to have repeated episodes of antral sinusitis. This cycle will only be broken if the underlying disease in the antrum is identified and cured. To identify the 20% of patients who have such an underlying problem, a follow-up plain film examination should be obtained 1 to 3 weeks after the initiation of therapy. If the sinus remains opacified, either a CT scan or an MRI scan of the sinonasal cavities should be obtained in order to diagnose the clinically "occult" underlying sinus pathology. The lesions to consider as causes of intermittent obstruction include nasal polyps, an antrochoanal polyp, one or more large retention cysts or polyps, a mucocele, or a tumor. Each of these lesions is discussed in detail in this chapter.

FOREIGN BODIES

A great variety of foreign bodies have been reported in the sinonasal cavities. Some are made of plastic materials (e.g., beads, etc.) or other nonradiopaque materials (e.g., gauze, etc.) that cannot be visualized on plain films, while others are radiodense (i.e., metallic, etc.) and can be localized easily on routine radiographic examinations (Fig. 2-232). If a foreign body is present for a sufficiently long time, it may act as a nidus and be-

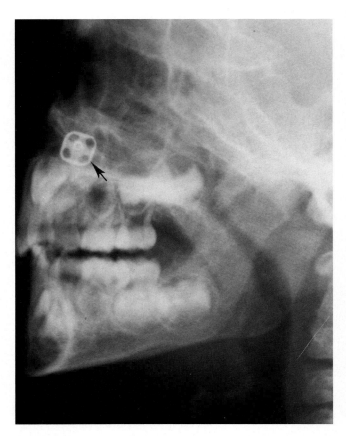

Fig. 2-232 Lateral view shows metallic snap foreign body in the nose *(arrow).*

come encrusted with mineral salts. As such, these calcified masses are referred to either as rhinoliths or sinoliths depending on whether they are respectively located in the nasal fossa or a paranasal sinus.[112,113]

REFERENCES

1. Potsic WP and Wetmore RF: Pediatric rhinology. In Goldman JL, editor: The principles and practice of rhinology, New York, 1987, John Wiley & Sons, Inc, pp 801-845.
2. Carpenter JL and Artenstein MS: Use of diagnostic microbiologic facilities in the diagnosis of head and neck infections, Otolaryngol Clin North Am 9:611, 1976.
3. Fried MP, Relly JH, and Strome M: Pseudomonas rhinosinusitis, Laryngoscope 94:192, 1984.
4. Evans FO, Sydnor JB, Moore WEC, et al.: Sinusitis of the maxillary antrum, N Engl J Med 293:735, 1976.
5. Frederick J and Braude AI: Anaerobic infection of the paranasal sinuses, N Engl J Med 290:135, 1974.
6. Van Alyea OE: Nasal sinuses: anatomic and clinical considerations, Baltimore, 1942, Williams & Wilkins.
7. Batsakis JG: Tumors of the head and neck: clinical and pathological considerations, ed 2, Baltimore, 1979, Williams & Wilkins.
8. Stahl RH: Allergic disorders of the nose and paranasal sinuses, Otolaryngol Clin North Am 7:703, 1974.
9. Nino-Murcia M, Rao VM, Mikaelian DO, et al.: Acute sinusitis mimicking antrochoanal polyp, AJNR 7:513, 1986.
10. Towbin R and Bunbar JS: The paranasal sinuses in childhood, Radiographics 2:253, 1982.

11. Odita JC, Akamaguna AI, Ogisi FO, et al.: Pneumatization of the maxillary sinus in normal and symptomatic children, Pediatr Radiol 16:365, 1986.

12. Glasier CM, Ascher DP, and Williams KD: Incidental paranasal sinus abnormalities on CT of children: clinical correlation, AJNR 7:861, 1986.

13. Shugar JMA: Embryology of the nose and paranasal sinuses and resultant deformities. In Goldman JL, editor: The principles and practice of rhinology, New York, 1987, John Wiley & Sons, Inc, pp 113-131.

14. Bassoiouny A, Newlands WJ, Ali H, et al.: Maxillary sinus hypoplasia and superior orbital fissure asymmetry, Laryngoscope 92:441, 1982.

15. Modic MT, Weinstein MA, Berlin AJ, et al.: Maxillary sinus hypoplasia visualized with computed tomography, Radiology 135:383, 1980.

16. Kennedy DW, Zinreich SJ, Shaalan H, et al.: Endoscopic middle meatal antrostomy: theory, technique and patency, Laryngoscope Suppl 43, 94(8, II Part 3):1, 1987.

17. Zinreich SJ, Kennedy DW, Rosenbaum AE, et al.: Paranasal sinuses: CT imaging requirements for endoscopic surgery, Radiology 163:769, 1987.

18. Silver AJ, Baredes S, Bello JA, et al.: The opacified maxillary sinus: CT findings in chronic sinusitis and malignant tumor, Radiology 163:205, 1987.

19. Kennedy DW, Zinreich SJ, Kumar AJ, et al.: Physiologic mucosal changes within the nose and ethmoid sinus: imaging of the nasal cycle by MRI, Laryngoscope 98:928, 1988.

20. Brock JG, Schabel SI, and Curry N: CT diagnosis of contrast reaction, J Comput Tomogr 5:63, 1981.

21. Eshaghian J and Anderson RL: Sinus involvement in inflammatory orbital pseudotumor, Arch Ophthalmol 99:627, 1981.

22. Som PM, Shugar JMA, Troy KM, et al.: The use of MR and CT in the management of a patient with intrasinus hemorrhage, Arch Otolaryngol 114:200, 1988.

23. Zimmerman RA, Bilaniuk LT, Hackney DB, et al.: Paranasal sinus hemorrhage: evaluation with MR imaging, Radiology 162:499, 1987.

24. Fagan P, McKenzie B, and Edmonds C: Sinus barotrauma in divers, Ann Otol Rhinol Laryngol 85:61, 1976.

25. Remmier D and Boles R: Intracranial complications of frontal sinusitis, Laryngoscope 90:1814, 1980.

26. Tamakawa Y and Hanafee WN: Cerebrospinal fluid rhinorrhea: significance of an air-fluid level in the sphenoid sinus, Radiology 135:101, 1980.

27. Fascenelli FW: Maxillary sinus abnormalities: radiographic evidence in an asymptomatic population, Arch Otol Laryngol 90:190, 1969.

28. Zizmor J and Noyek AM: Inflammatory diseases of the paranasal sinuses, Otolaryngol Clin North Am 6:459, 1973.

29. Som PM, Sacher M, Lawson W, et al.: CT appearance distinguishing benign nasal polyps from malignancies, J Comput Assist Tomogr 11:129, 1987.

30. Som PM, Cohen BA, Sacher M, et al.: The angiomatous polyp and the angiofibroma: two different lesions, Radiology 144:329, 1982.

31. Batsakis JG: The pathology of head and neck tumors: nasal cavity and paranasal sinuses, part 5. Head Neck Surg 2:410, 1980.

32. Smith CJ, Echevarria R, and McLelland CA: Pseudosarcomatous changes in antrochoanal polyps, Arch Otolaryngol 99:228, 1974.

33. Barnes L, Verbin RS, and Gnepp DR: Diseases of the nose, paranasal sinuses and nasopharynx. In Barnes L, editor: Surgical pathology of the head and neck, vol 1, New York, 1985, Marcel Dekker, Inc, pp 403-451.

34. Austen KF: Diseases of Immediate Type Hypersensitivity. In Thorn GW, Adams RD, Braunwald E, et al., editors: Harrison's principles of internal medicine, ed 8, New York, 1977, McGraw-Hill, Inc, pp 391-396.

35. Ballenger JJ: Diseases of the nose, throat and ear, ed 12, Philadelphia, 1977, Lea & Febiger, Inc, pp 105-114, 155-167.

36. Smith MP: Dysfunction of carbohydrate metabolism as an element in the set of factors resulting in the polysaccharide nose and nasal polyps (the polysaccharide nose), Laryngoscope 81:636, 1971.

37. Schramm VL, Jr and Effron MZ: Nasal polyps in children, Laryngoscope 90:1488, 1980.

38. Jaffe BF, Strome M, Khaw KT, et al.: Nasal polypectomy and sinus surgery for cystic fibrosis: a 10 year review, Otolaryngol Clin North Am 10:81, 1977.

39. Moloney JR: Nasal polyps, nasal polypectomy, asthma and aspirin sensitivity: their association in 445 cases of nasal polyps, J Laryngol Otol 91:837, 1977.

40. Torjussen W: Rhinoscopical findings in nickel workers, with special emphasis on the influence of nickel exposure and smoking habits, Acta Otolaryngol (Stockh) 88:279, 1979.

41. Som PM and Shugar JMA: The CT classification of ethmoid mucoceles, J Comput Assist Tomogr 4:199, 1980.

42. Jacobs M and Som PM: The ethmoidal "polypoid mucocele," J Comput Assist Tomogr 6:721, 1982.

43. Naul LG, Hise JH, and Ruff T: CT of inspissated mucous in chronic sinusitis, AJNR 8:574, 1987.

44. Som PM, Dillon WP, Fullerton GD, et al.: Chronically obstructed sinonasal secretions: observations on T_1 and T_2 shortening, Radiology 172:515, 1989.

45. Zinreich SJ, Kennedy DW, Malat J, et al.: Fungal sinusitis: diagnosis with CT and MR imaging, Radiology 169:439, 1988.

46. Som PM, Shugar JMA, Troy KM, et al.: Use of magnetic resonance and computed tomography in the management of a patient with intrasinus hemorrhage, Arch Otolaryngol 114:200, 1988.

47. Zimmerman RA, Bilaniuk LT, Hackney DB, et al.: Paranasal sinus hemorrhage: evaluation with MR imaging, Radiology 162:499, 1987.

48. Romett JL and Newman RK: Aspergillosis of the nose and paranasal sinuses, Laryngoscope 92:764, 1982.

49. Centeno RS, Bentson JR, and Mancuso AA: CT scanning in rhinocerebral mucormycosis and aspergillosis, Radiology 140:383, 1981.

50. Shugar JMA, Som PM, Robbins A, et al.: Maxillary sinusitis as a cause of cheek swelling, Arch Otolaryngol 108:507, 1982.

51. Kopp W, Fotter R, Steiner H, et al.: Aspergillosis of the paranasal sinuses, Radiology 156:715, 1985.

52. Stammberger J, Jakse A, and Beaufort F: Aspergillosis of the paranasal sinuses: x-ray diagnosis, histopathology and clinical aspects, Ann Otol Rhinol Laryngol 93:251, 1984.

53. Myerowitz RL, Guggenheimer J, and Barnes L: Infectious diseases of the head and neck. In Barnes L, editor: Surgical pathology of the head and neck, vol 2, New York, 1985, Marcel Dekker, Inc, pp 1771-1822.

54. Veress B, Malik OA, Tayeb AAE, et al.: Further observations on the primary paranasal aspergillus granuloma in the Sudan: a morphological study of 46 cases, Am J Trop Med Hyg 22:765, 1973.

55. Milosev B, Mahgoub ES, Abdel O, et al.: Primary aspergilloma of paranasal sinuses in the Sudan, Br J Surg 56:132, 1969.

56. Stevens MH: Aspergillosis of the frontal sinus, Arch Otolaryngol 104:153, 1978.

57. McGill TJ, Simpson G, and Healy GR: Fulminant aspergillosis of the nose and paranasal sinuses: a new clinical entity, Laryngoscope 90:748, 1980.

58. Waxman JE, Spector JG, Sale SR, et al.: Allergic aspergillus si-

nusitis: concepts in diagnosis and treatment of a new clinical entity, Laryngoscope 97:261, 1987.

59. Mader JT, Ream RS, and Heath PW: *Petriellidium boydii (Allescheria boydii)* sphenoidal sinusitis, JAMA 239:2368, 1978.

60. Travis LB, Roberts GD, and Wilson WR: Clinical significance of *pseudallescheria boydii:* a review of 10 years experience, Mayo Clin Proc 60:531, 1985.

61. Chapnick JS and Bach MC: Bacterial and fungal infections of the maxillary sinus, Otolaryngol Clin North Am 9:43, 1976.

62. Richtsmeier WJ and Johns ME: Actinomycosis of the head and neck. In Batsakis J and Savory J, editor: Critical review in clinical laboratory sciences, vol 11, 1979, CRC Press, pp 175-202.

63. MacGregor RR: A year's experience with tuberculosis in a private urban teaching hospital in the post-sanatorium era, Am J Med 58:221, 1975.

64. Centers for Disease Control: Annual Summary 1980, Morbidity-Mortality Weekly Report 19:3, 1981.

65. McNulty JS and Fassett RL: Syphilis: an otolaryngologic perspective, Laryngoscope 91:889, 1981.

66. Olansky S: Syphilis rediscovered. In Disease-a-month, Chicago, 1967, Year Book Medical Publishers, pp 1-30.

67. Fiumara NJ and Lessell S: Manifestations of late congenital syphilis: an analysis of 271 patients, Arch Dermatol 102:78, 1970.

68. Becker TS, Shum TK, Waller TS, et al.: Radiological aspects of rhinoscleroma, Radiology 141:433, 1981.

69. Beeson PB and McDermott W: Textbook of medicine, ed 14, Philadelphia, 1975, WB Saunders Co, pp 164-539.

70. Lasser A and Smith HW: Rhinosporidiosis, Arch Otolaryngol 102:308, 1974.

71. Harrison TR: Harrison's principles of internal medicine, ed 9, New York, 1980, McGraw-Hill, Inc.

72. Fauci AS and Wolff SM: Wegener's granulomatosis and related diseases, Disease of the Month 23:1, 1977.

73. Harrison DFN: Midline destructive granuloma: fact or fiction? Laryngoscope 97:1049, 1987.

74. Gordon WW, Cohn AW, Greenberg SD, et al.: Nasal sarcoidosis, Arch Otolaryngol 102:11, 1976.

75. Mailland AAJ and Geopfert H: Nasal and paranasal sarcoidosis, Arch Otolaryngol 104:197, 1978.

76. Green WH: Mucormycosis infection of the craniofacial structure, AJR 101:802, 1967.

77. Paling MR, Roberts RL, and Fauci AS: Paranasal sinus obliteration in Wegener granulomatosis, Radiology 144:539, 1982.

78. Hyams V: Personal communication, AFIP 1980.

79. De Juan EE, Green WR, and Iliff NT: Allergic periorbital mycopyocele in children, Am J Ophthalmol 96:299, 1983.

80. Finn DG, Hudson NR, and Baylin G: Unilateral polyposis and mucoceles in children, Laryngoscope 91:1444, 1981.

81. Zizmor J and Noyek AM: Cysts, benign tumors and malignant tumors of the paranasal sinuses, Otolaryngol Clin North Am 6:487, 1973.

82. Rogers JH, Fredrickson JM, Noyek AM: Management of cysts, benign tumors and bony dysplasia of the maxillary sinus, Otolaryngol Clin North Am 9:2330, 1976.

83. Lloyd DM, Bartram CI, and Stanley P: Ethmoid mucoceles, Br J Radiol 47:646, 1974.

84. Ritter FN: The paranasal sinuses: anatomy and surgical technique, St. Louis, 1973, The CV Mosby Co.

85. Canalis RF, Zajtchuck JT, and Jenkins HA: Ethmoid mucoceles, Arch Otolaryngol 104:286, 1978.

86. Zizmor J, Noyek AM, and Chapnik JS: Mucocele of the paranasal sinuses, Can J Otolaryngol 3(suppl), 1974.

87. Som P, Sacher M, Lanzieri CF, et al.: The hidden antral compartment, Radiology 152:463, 1984.

88. Close LG and O'Connor WE: Sphenoethmoidal mucoceles with intracranial extension, Otolaryngol Head Neck Surg 91:350, 1983.

89. Osborn AG, Johnson L, and Roberts TS: Sphenoidal mucoceles with intracranial extension, J Comput Assist Tomogr 3:335, 1979.

90. Chui MC, Briant TDR, Gray T, et al.: Computed tomography of sphenoid sinus mucocele, J Otolaryngol 12:263, 1983.

91. Price HI, Batnitzky S, Karlin CA, et al.: Multiple paranasal sinus mucoceles, J Comput Assist Tomogr 5:122, 1981.

92. Perugini S, Pasquini U, Menichelli F, et al.: Mucoceles in the paranasal sinus involving the orbit: CT signs in 43 cases, Neuroradiology 23:133, 1982.

93. Zizmor J and Noyek A: Radiology of the nose and paranasal sinuses. In Paparella MM and Shumrick DA: Otolaryngology, vol 1, Philadelphia, 1973, WB Saunders Co.

94. Taveras JM and Wood EH: Diagnostic Neuroradiology, Baltimore, 1964, Williams & Wilkins, pp 141-142.

95. Dodd GD and Jing B-S: Radiology of the nose, paranasal sinuses and nasopharynx, Baltimore, 1977, Williams & Wilkins, pp 131-133.

96. Verbin RS and Barnes L: Cysts and cyst-like lesions of the oral cavity, jaws and neck. In Barnes L, editor: Surgical pathology of the head and neck, vol 2, New York, 1985, Marcel Dekker, Inc, pp 1278-1281.

97. Koenig H, Lenz M, and Sauter R: Temporal bone region: high resolution MR imaging using surface coils, Radiology 159:191, 1986.

98. Latack JT, Kartush JM, Kemink JL, et al.: Epidermoidomas of the cerebellopontine angle and temporal bone: CT and MR aspects, Radiology 157:361, 1985.

99. Urken ML, Som PM, Lawson W, et al.: The abnormally large frontal sinus I: a practical method for its determination based upon an analysis of 100 normal patients, Laryngoscope 97:602, 1987.

100. Urken ML, Som PM, Lawson W, et al.: Abnormally large frontal sinuses II: nomenclature, pathology and symptoms, Laryngoscope 97:606, 1987.

101. Lombardi G: Radiology in neuro-ophthalmology, Baltimore, 1967, Williams & Wilkins.

102. Leonardi M and Fabris G: Pneumosinus dilatans: sign closely related to meningioma of the planum sphenoidale, Ann Radiol (French) 19:803, 1976.

103. Kutnick SL and Kerth JD: Acute sinusitis and otitis: their complications and surgical treatment, Otolaryngol Clin North Am 689, 1976.

104. Carter BL, Bankoff MS, Fisk JD: Computed tomographic detection of sinusitis responsible for intracranial and extracranial infections, Radiology 147:739, 1983.

105. Zimmerman RA and Bilaniuk LT: CT of orbital infection and its cerebral complications, Am J Roentgenol 134:45, 1980.

106. Rothstein J, Maisel RH, Berlinger NT, et al.: Relationship of optic neuritis to disease of the paranasal sinus, Laryngoscope 94:1501, 1984.

107. Bilaniuk LT and Zimmerman RA: Computer assisted tomography: sinus lesions with orbital involvement, Head Neck Surg 2:293, 1980.

108. Kaufman DM, Litman N, and Miller MH: Sinusitis: induced subdural empyema, Neurology 33:123, 1983.

109. Williams HL: Infections and granulomas of the nasal airways and paranasal sinuses. In Paparella MM and Shumrick DA: Otolaryngology, vol 3, Head and neck, Philadelphia, 1973, WB Saunders Co, pp 27-32.

110. Kay NJ, Setia RN, and Stone J: Relevance of conventional radiography in indicating maxillary antral lavage, Ann Otol Rhinol Laryngol 93:37, 1984.

111. Eichel BS: The medical and surgical approach in management of the unilateral opacified antrum, Laryngoscope 87:737, 1977.

112. Price HI, Batnitzky S, Karlin LA, et al.: Giant nasal rhinolith, AJNR 2:371, 1981.

113. RSNA case of the day: case IV, Rhinolith, Radiology 146:251, 1983.

SECTION FOUR
TUMORS AND TUMORLIKE CONDITIONS

Carcinomas of the nasal cavity and paranasal sinuses are rare, comprising only 0.2% to 0.8% of all malignancies[1,2] and just 3% of all tumors that arise in the head and neck.[2] Despite their statistically small incidence, sinonasal tumors are feared because of their poor prognosis. The grave outlook of these patients stems from the frequent advanced stage of the tumor at the time of diagnosis and the reluctance of surgeons to pursue aggressive treatment for fear of creating either an undesirable cosmetic deformity, a prolonged morbidity, or gross dysfunction. Furthermore, the complex, compact anatomy of the region often limits the extent of surgical resection and may lead to unwanted complications of radiation therapy that result from the difficulties of placing adequate treatment fields.[3,4]

Because many sinonasal tumors are accompanied by chronic inflammatory disease, the underlying tumor is easily overlooked. Pain usually does not accompany tumors alone, but rather signifies the presence of infection; if coexistent infection is not present, the patient may have relatively advanced tumor growth. The common presenting complaints include diplopia, decreasing vision, nasal stuffiness, epistaxis, and a facial mass. Patients with antral and ethmoidal cancers have an average delay of 6 months between the first onset of symptoms and the establishment of a final diagnosis.[3]

As imaging technology has improved, superior tumor mapping and staging have provided for more accurate information that permits more realistic treatment planning with regard to cure vs. palliation.[5] Surgical techniques have also improved, and with detailed tumor mapping one may attain better tumor extirpation with less morbidity and deformity. More accurate placement of radiation fields can also be attained.

To provide the tumor mapping necessary to make a decision about operability and curability, the radiologist must be aware of the critical areas of potential tumor extension that will alter a surgical or treatment approach. These areas include any tumor extension into the floor of the anterior and middle intracranial fossae, the pterygopalatine fossae, the orbits, and the palate.[6] In addition, because of the proximity of the various paranasal sinuses to one another and their free communication via the nasal fossae, tumors may spread with ease from one sinus to another. Thus the radiologist must detail the precise sinus involvement, remembering that tumor mapping may not only alter the surgical approach, but the radiation treatment plan as well.

Nodal metastasis from sinonasal carcinomas is one of the gravest prognostic signs. Although the primary draining lymph nodes of the paranasal sinuses and nasal vault are the retropharyngeal nodes, these nodes or the lymphatics leading to them are frequently obliterated in many adults by the repeated infections occurring during youth. Because of this, the secondary nodes, the upper internal jugular and submandibular groups, are the nodes most often involved by tumor. These occur in about 15% of patients and usually signify tumor extension to the skin, alveolar buccal sulcus, or pterygoid musculature.[4] Since these areas are all well demonstrated by sectional imaging techniques, the radiologist must be thorough and precise in reporting tumor extension.

Distinguishing the tumor from adjacent inflammatory disease remains one of the major problems faced by the radiologist in tumor mapping. Although inherent differential CT attenuation values may allow some distinction to be made, a more accurate differentiation usually can be achieved on postcontrast CT scans. Even in these cases, overlapping of tumor and inflammatory attenuation values often raises serious doubts as to where the actual tumor margin is located. It is in this regard that T_2-weighted MRI scans have great application. Because inflammatory reactions and secretions are dominated on MRI by their high water content, they have high T_2-weighted signal intensities. By comparison, virtually all (about 95%) of the sinonasal tumors are highly cellular neoplasms and have an intermediate-intensity signal on T_2-weighted studies (Fig. 2-233).[7,8] It is usually only the glandular-type, minor salivary gland tumors and the uncommon cystic-type schwannomas that have sufficient water content to produce high T_2-weighted signal intensities. Thus it is only when a glandular or cystic tumor is found through biopsy that the radiologist must be aware that this T_2-weighted signal intensity distinction between tumor and infection may not be accurate.

When tumors are small, they may not yet involve the adjacent bones of the paranasal sinuses or nasal vault. It is at this early stage that tumors often elude detection by both the clinician and radiologist, and, unfortunately, it is at this stage that they may be the most curable.[4] However, unless bone involvement is detected, it may not be possible to diagnose a malignancy. When the tumor becomes large enough to affect the adjacent bone, the type of bone involvement may suggest a particular histologic tumor group. The concept that the radiographic pattern of bone destruction can be related to tumor growth is not new. However, it was not until the CT era that the radiologist could achieve highly detailed bone resolution in multiple planes. This resolu-

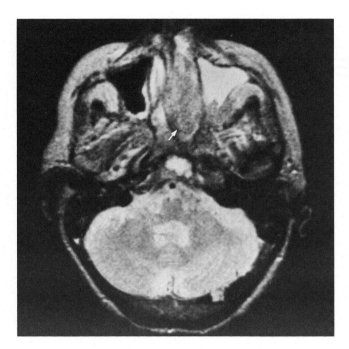

Fig. 2-233 Axial T₂W MRI scan shows polypoid mass in the left nasal cavity *(arrow)* with a low-to-intermediate signal intensity. The adjacent left maxillary sinus is obstructed with material that has a high signal intensity. Such a clear distinction of this nasal tumor and the obstructed sinus secretion was not possible on a CT scan. Inverted papilloma.

tion allowed the imager to distinguish aggressive bone destruction from bone remodeling.[9-11]

If the bone is aggressively destroyed so that small fragments are all that remain of the sinus wall or nasal vault, the most likely tumor is a squamous cell carcinoma (Figs. 2-234 and 2-235). Metastases from primary sites such as the lung and breast are also in this group of tumors, as are a few of the sarcomas and rare lesions such as fibrous histiocytomas. Most sinonasal sarcomas remodel bone rather than aggressively destroy it. This pattern of remodeling is also found with mucoceles, polyps, inverting papillomas, and rarer lesions such as minor salivary gland tumors, extramedullary plasmacytomas, lymphomas, esthesioneuroblastomas, and hemangiopericytomas (Figs. 2-236 and 2-237). Although in any given case, any tumor may have either an aggressively destructive appearance or primarily a remodeling pattern, most tumors tend to fall into one of these two groups. The radiologist can use this pattern of bone involvement to question some histologic diagnoses. For example, if a patient appears with a unilateral polypoid nasal mass, a biopsy report of "histiocytic lymphoma," and imaging studies that reveal a predominantly aggressive pattern of bone destruction rather than the bone remodeling characteristic of lymphoma, the radiologist should question the discrepancy and ask to obtain a sec-

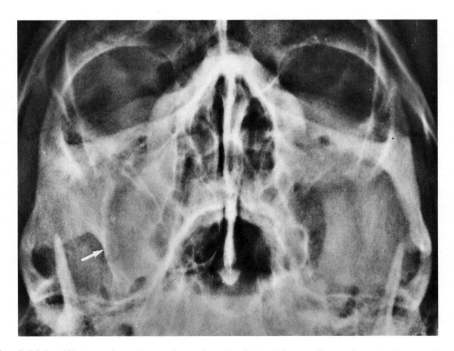

Fig. 2-234 Waters view shows lateral wall of the left maxillary sinus to be totally destroyed. The right lateral antral wall *(arrow)* is intact. This is an example of aggressive bone destruction. Left antral squamous cell carcinoma.

ond biopsy specimen for electron microscopy and histochemical testing. In this example, the final diagnosis is more likely to be an anaplastic carcinoma. Thus, in addition to accurate tumor mapping, the radiologist should pay careful attention to how the bone is involved by the soft tissue mass. This may alter a presumed diagnosis.

Some lesions are incorrectly diagnosed with light microscopy. They may be so highly undifferentiated that their histologic appearances are similar, confusing even the best pathologists. The lesions can be distinguished in almost all cases, however, by the use of electron microscopy and histochemical testing. Tumors that are most often confused histologically include anaplastic carcinoma, histiocytic lymphoma, embryonal rhabdomyosarcoma, extramedullary plasmacytoma, melanosarcoma, esthesioneuroblastoma, and Ewing's sarcoma. Because of this, many institutions routinely perform electron microscopic and histochemical testing on all small-cell, undifferentiated tumors.

It is unknown why some tumors are biologically aggressive and others are not. Some form of homeostatic patient immune mechanism appears to limit tumor growth for a variable period of time, sometimes many years. In addition to tumor biology, the critical anatomic location of the neoplasm has prognostic signifi-

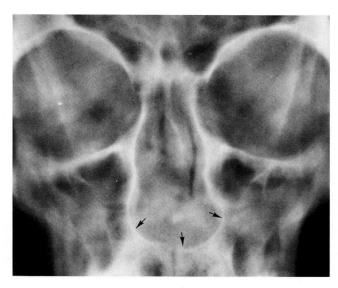

Fig. 2-236   Coronal multidirectional tomogram shows expansile mass in the lower nasal cavity. The nasal vault and palate have been remodelled *(arrows)* rather than aggressively destroyed. Histocytic lymphoma.

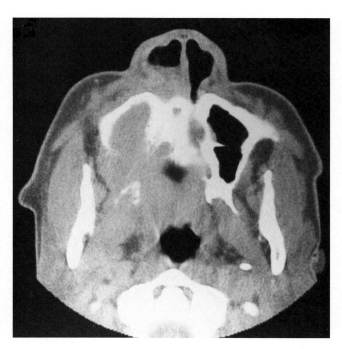

Fig. 2-235   Axial CT scan shows highly destructive lesion of the right maxillary sinus, palate, and pterygoid plates. Squamous cell carcinoma.

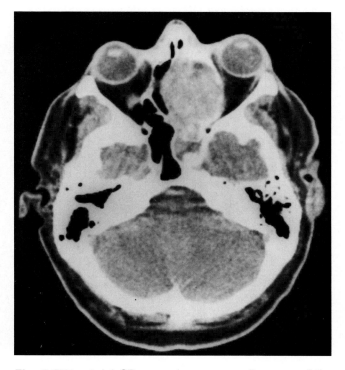

Fig. 2-237   Axial CT scan shows expansile mass of the left ethmoid sinuses. The lamina papyracea has been remodelled over the tumor's lateral margin. The nasal septum has been displaced by the lesion's medial margin. Minor salivary gland tumor.

cance. Thus a lesion confined to the antrum generally has a better prognosis than one located in the pterygopalatine fossa or central skull base. However, certain tumors seem to have a high inherent level of biologic aggressiveness, regardless of their location and relatively benign appearance on imaging. For example, a nasal fossa melanosarcoma usually has a "benign" polypoid imaging appearance, yet a 5-year survival prognosis of only one fifth that of a comparable squamous cell carcinoma. Once a malignancy is confirmed by biopsy, the radiologist should not use the pattern of tumor bone involvement to suggest a prognosis. Whatever the manner by which patients with sinonasal tumors die of their disease, the lethal propensity of certain tumors is poorly understood. In most instances, it is clearly unrelated to the manner by which the tumor destroys or remodels bone. On the other hand, the bone involvement can be used as a radiographic marker of a characteristic tumor growth pattern that most sinonasal neoplasms respect.

In addition to noting the pattern of bone involvement, any alteration of bone density also should be described, since sclerotic bone reactions are uncommon with sinonasal tumors. Most often, dense bone in the facial skeleton reflects the presence of chronic inflammation and is usually found with chronic bacterial sinusitis. However, if coupled with areas of focal bone erosion or remodeling, these bone changes should suggest a more aggressive infection, such as fungal or granulomatous disease. Although uncommon, frank osteomyelitis in the sinonasal cavities does occur and usually appears as mixed areas of bone rarefaction and sclerosis, often with sequestra. Radiation osteitis also can produce a sclerotic bone; however, in these patients extensive fragmentation of bone is common. Actual sclerotic (blastic) tumor bone in the sinonasal region is rare, but has been associated with anaplastic carcinomas, lymphoepitheliomas and osteosarcomas. The dense bone of fibrous dysplasia and ossifying fibroma is usually identifiable as such. The bone changes of Paget's disease may be indistinguishable from those of blastic metastatic prostate cancer. Blastic metastases from breast carcinoma can occur, usually with areas of lysis. Dense bone may be found as a reaction to meningiomas.

Tumoral calcifications are uncommon in the sinonasal cavities. They have been reported with osteoblastomas, osteochondromas, chondromas, and chondrosarcomas. Focal calcifications have been associated with inverting papillomas, esthesioneuroblastomas, and aspergillosis.

PAPILLOMA

The mucosa of the nasal fossae and paranasal sinuses is of ectodermal origin. During maturation the mucosa differentiates into ciliated columnar epithelium and into the mucous Bowman's glands. This unique mucosa may give rise to three distinct histomorphologic papillomas that are essentially not found in other areas of the body. These are individually referred to as the *fungiform, inverted,* and *cylindric cell* papillomas. Collectively, they are often called *schneiderian papillomas.*[1,2] These papillomas are not believed to be associated with allergy, chronic infection, smoking, or other noxious environmental agents, since the papillomas are almost invariably unilateral in location. Similarly, their rarity in children suggests against a viral etiology.[12-14]

Schneiderian papillomas are uncommon, representing only 0.4% to 4.7% of all sinonasal tumors. Nasal polyps are between 25 and 50 times more common than papillomas.[2]

Fungiform papillomas (septal, squamous, or exophytic papillomas) make up 50% of all schneiderian papillomas. Fungiform papillomas usually arise in males between the ages of 20 to 50 years, and 95% arise on the nasal septum. They may be solitary (75%), unilateral (96%), have a warty or verrucous appearance, and are not considered to be premalignant.[2,12,15]

Inverted papillomas (endophytic papillomas) represent 47% of schneiderian papillomas and most commonly occur in males between the ages of 40 to 70 years. The tumors characteristically arise from the lateral nasal wall, near the middle turbinate, and extend into the sinuses secondarily. Generally, this secondary

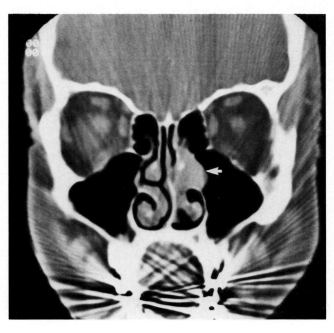

Fig. 2-238 Coronal CT scan shows small polypoid mass in left nasal fossa *(arrow).* There is no associated bone destruction. Inverted papilloma.

extension involves the maxillary and ethmoidal sinuses, but cases of lesion spread into the sphenoid and frontal sinuses have been documented.[2,12] On rare occasions, an isolated inverted papilloma may arise within a sinus without any nasal involvement.[2,12] About 8% of inverted papillomas arise from the medial septal wall and fewer than 4% occur bilaterally. The most common presenting symptoms are nasal obstruction, epistaxis, and anosmia. Secondary sinusitis and tumor extension into the sinuses and orbits can cause pain, purulent nasal discharge, proptosis, diplopia, and a nasal vocal quality.

Microscopically, these lesions have a hyperplastic zone of basement membrane–enclosed epithelium that grows endophytically into the stroma, which may undermine the polyp stalk. Because of this, localized surgery that does not remove sufficient mucosa from around the base or stalk of the polyp has been met with high recurrence rates that vary from 27% to 73%.[2] The lateral rhinotomy with en bloc resection of the lateral nasal wall and mucosa is the preferred procedure for all but the smallest localized lesions. Using a more extensive surgical approach has dropped recurrence rates to 0% to 14%, with most relapses occurring within 2 years of surgery.[2,12]

The reported rate of malignancies associated with inverted papillomas ranges from 3% to 24% (average 13%). The vast majority appeared concurrently with an inverted papilloma or in a patient with a history of inverted papilloma. It is rare for a malignancy to develop within an inverted papilloma. Although most reported cases are of squamous cell carcinomas, other tumors have been reported, including verrucous, mucoepidermoid, spindle cell, clear cell, and adenocarcinomas.[2]

The *cylindric cell papillomas* represent only 3% of the schneiderian papillomas. They have many similarities to inverted papillomas, including an affinity for the lateral nasal wall, age of onset, and predominance in males. Microscopically, both inverted and exophytic growth patterns exist. In the typical case, numerous small intraepithelial cysts are filled with mucin and neutrophils. This finding occasionally causes confusion with rhinosporidiosis; however, in this fungal disease the organisms are not limited to the epithelium and also occur within the stroma of the polypoid mass.[2]

The radiographic findings for all of these papillomas can vary from a small nasal polypoid mass to an expansile nasal mass that has remodeled the nasal vault and extended into the sinuses, causing secondary obstructive sinusitis.[16] Occasional calcifications can be seen within the polypoid tumors.[17] The nasal septum remains intact, but may be bowed by the mass to the opposite wall of the nasal vault (Figs. 2-233 and 2-238 to 2-240).

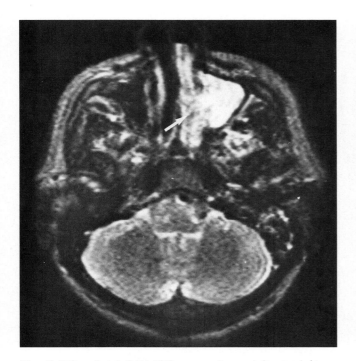

Fig. 2-239 Axial T$_2$W MRI scan shows left nasal fossa polypoid mass with intermediate signal intensity *(arrow)*. The mass obstructs, but does not fill, the maxillary sinus, which is filled with inflammatory secretions with high signal intensity. Inverted papilloma.

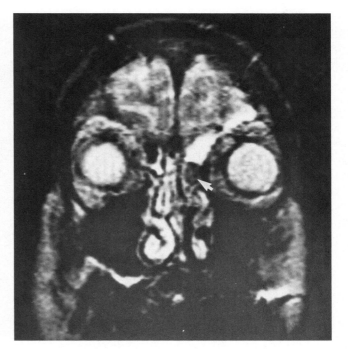

Fig. 2-240 Coronal T$_2$W MRI scan shows small low signal intensity mass in the left upper nasal fossa and ethmoid sinus *(arrow)*. Obstructed inflammatory secretions with high signal intensity are present in a left supraorbital ethmoid cell. Inverted papilloma.

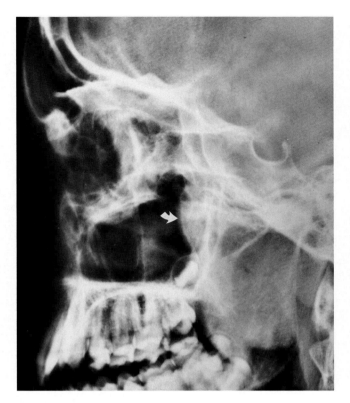

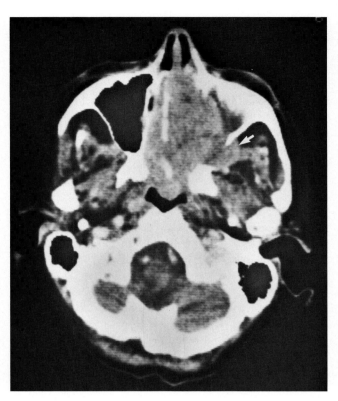

Fig. 2-241 Lateral view shows large nasopharyngeal mass that has displaced the posterior antral wall anteriorly *(arrow)*. The mass also extends into the sphenoid sinuses. Angiofibroma.

Fig. 2-242 Axial postcontrast CT scan shows left nasopharyngeal and nasal fossa enhancing mass that has widened the left pterygopalatine fossa and extended into the left infratemporal fossa *(arrow)*. Angiofibroma.

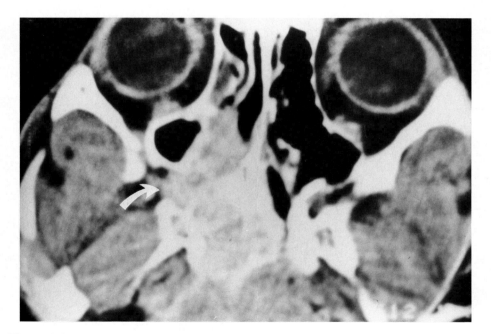

Fig. 2-243 Axial postcontrast CT scan shows enhancing nasopharyngeal mass that has extended into the right pterygopalatine fossa *(arrow)* and sphenoid sinus. Anteriorly there is minimal extension into the right nasal fossa. Angiofibroma.

ANGIOFIBROMA

The nasopharyngeal angiofibroma (juvenile angiofibroma) is an uncommon, highly vascular, nonencapsulated, polypoid mass that is histologically benign, but locally aggressive. It represents 0.05% of all head and neck neoplasms and is almost exclusively a lesion of males.[2] However, a few cases have been documented in females, and it has been suggested that when such a diagnosis is made, the patient should have sex chromosome studies to confirm that she is a female and not a mosiac.[18] Similarly, the more common nasal polyp or a fibrosed antrochoanal polyp must be excluded from the diagnosis.

The typical patient is a male between 10 and 18 years of age, although the tumor has been reported in other age groups.[2] The presenting symptoms include nasal obstruction, epistaxis, facial deformity, proptosis, nasal voice, sinusitis, nasal discharge, serous otitis media, headache, and anosmia.[2] Almost all angiofibromas have a nasopharyngeal origin near the pterygopalatine fossa and sphenopalatine foramen. Although the lesion may grow to fill the entire nasopharynx, its growth is not symmetric, and one side is always the primary site of involvement. Extension into the pterygopalatine fossa occurs in 89% of the cases and results in widening of this fossa with resultant anterior bowing of the posterior ipsilateral antral wall.[19] Although other slow-growing lesions have been reported to widen the pterygopalatine fossa in a similar fashion (e.g., lymphomas, lymphoepitheliomas, neuromas, and fibrous histiocytomas), 99% of the time the antral bowing is caused by nasopharyngeal angiofibromas.[20] In 61% of the patients, the sphenoid sinus is involved via tumor growth through the roof of the nasopharynx. Angiofibromas also spread into the maxillary sinuses in 43% of patients and into the ethmoid cells in 35%.[19] Intracranial extension occurs in 5% to 20% of cases and primarily involves the middle cranial fossa.[2] Most often this extension progresses from the pterygopalatine fossa into the orbit (through the inferior orbital fissure) and then intracranially through the superior orbital fissure. Direct intracranial extension from the sphenoid or ethmoid sinuses is uncommon. Because of the tumor's extreme vascularity, a biopsy should not be done in an outpatient or office facility. Sectional imaging and angiography can be used to establish the diagnosis.[21]

Plain film findings of angiofibromas include a soft tissue nasopharyngeal mass, widening of the pterygopalatine fossa with anterior bowing of the posterior antral wall, and opacification of the sphenoidal sinus (Fig. 2-241). A polypoid nasal mass may cloud the ipsilateral ethmoid and maxillary sinuses. If the superior orbital fissure is widened, intracranial extension will be present.

The postcontrast CT scans reveal an enhancing mass with the anatomic distribution described above (Figs. 2-242 and 2-243). Any intraorbital or intracranial extension is much better visualized on CT scans than on plain films. On postcontrast CT scans, the imaging must be done while contrast material is flowing freely. If scanning is delayed, the rich vascular tumor network washes out the contrast medium. Dynamic scanning also identifies the highly vascular nature of these tumors.[22] MRI reveals a mass of intermediate signal intensity on T_1-, proton density-, and T_2-weighted sequences, with multiple-flow void channels representing the major tumor vessels (Fig. 2-244).[23]

The primary task of the imager is to map the lesion for the surgeon and, in particular, document any intracranial spread into the cavernous sinuses, optic chiasm, and pituitary gland, since these sites are not considered resectable.

Angiography demonstrates that the major feeding vessels are the internal maxillary artery and ascending pharyngeal artery on the dominant side (Fig. 2-245). Additionally, cross-circulation from contralateral branches of the external carotid artery and occasionally feeding branches from the internal carotid arteries are found. When these latter branches are visualized, intracranial tumor extension is almost always present. Subselective angiography is usually necessary to identify all of the feeding vessels. Preoperative embolization of the external carotid artery nutrient branches greatly reduces the blood loss at surgery.[2]

The treatment of choice is surgery; unresectable intracranial disease, if present, can be irradiated. Control rates of 78% using a dose of 30 to 35 Gy rads have been reported, and an additional 15% of the cases can be controlled by a second course of radiotherapy.[24] Although the radiation effect on tumor vascularity causes some shrinkage, the fibrous tumor component remains unchanged.[2]

Experts disagree over the effect of estrogen therapy on angiofibromas. Although some cases of decreased tumor size and vascularity have been reported after estrogen therapy, this response is not achieved in most patients.[2] Similarly, the role of chemotherapy remains unclear.

ANGIOMATOUS POLYP

The angiomatous polyp is a fibrous nasal polyp with numerous vessels that arise, presumably, in response to minor trauma.[25] The clinical importance of this lesion is that histologically it can be confused with a nasopharyngeal angiofibroma.[19] Several points differentiate these two lesions:

1. The angiomatous polyp is located primarily in the nasal fossa and not in the nasopharynx.

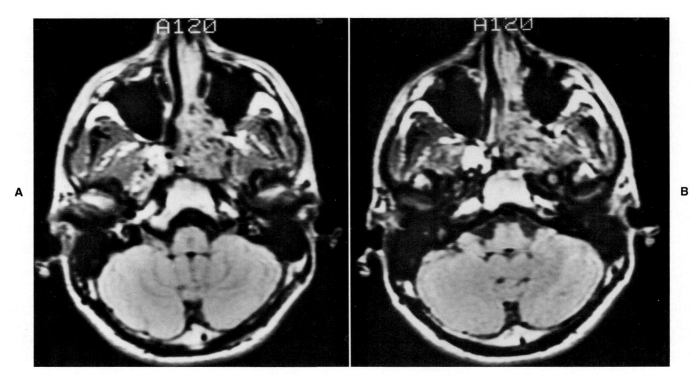

Fig. 2-244   Axial T₁W MR scans through **A,** the upper nasopharynx and **B,** the skull base show a nasopharyngeal and nasal fossa mass that extends through the left ptery-gopalatine fossa into the infratemporal fossa. The mass has low-to-intermediate signal intensity and multiple areas of signal (flow) void. Angiofibroma.

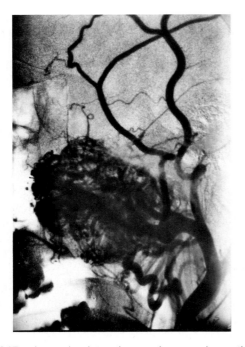

Fig. 2-245   Lateral subtraction angiogram shows the typical, highly vascular tumor appearance of an angiofibroma.

2. The polyp does not extend into the pterygopalatine fossa, and only rarely does it protrude into the sphenoid sinuses. In these cases the tumor enters the sinus through the anterior wall and not the sinus floor, as with angiofibromas.
3. These polyps do not extend intracranially.
4. The polyps have only a few demonstrable feeding vessels on angiography compared with the rich vascular supply of the angiofibroma.
5. On CT scans the angiomatous polyp does not enhance as well as the angiofibroma.
6. Vascular flow void channels are not seen on MRI.
7. These polyps are easily "shelled out" surgically as with a routine nasal polyp, whereas the nasopharyngeal angiofibroma is difficult to remove from its primary attachment site.
8. Angiography and embolization are not necessary in patients with angiomatous polyps (Fig. 2-246).

Thus, since the pathologist may confuse these lesions, the radiologist may be the first physician to identify the tumor and thereby render unnecessary further diagnostic procedures.

SQUAMOUS CELL CARCINOMA

When the distribution of sinonasal carcinomas is analyzed, 25% to 58% of the tumors arise in the antrum;

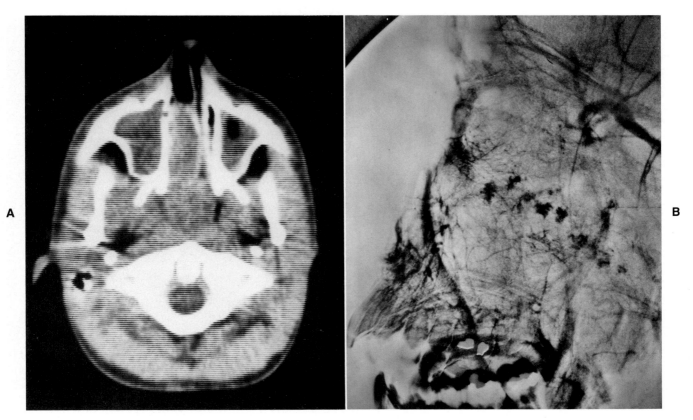

Fig. 2-246   A, Axial CT scan shows a right nasopharyngeal and nasal fossa mass that displaces the nasal septum to the left. The mass does not extend into the pterygopalatine fossa or the sphenoid sinus. A biopsy was read as an angiofibroma. **B,** A lateral subtraction angiogram shows only focal areas of increased vascularity without the typical vascular appearance of an angiofibroma. Angiomatous polyp.

however, the maxillary sinus is involved either directly or by extension in at least 80% of all patients. The nasal cavity is the site of origin in 25% to 35% of cases, the ethmoid complex in 10%, and the sphenoid and frontal sinuses account for only 1%.[1,2]

The incidence of *squamous cell carcinoma of the nose* has an epidemiologic relationship with nickel exposure. Workers exposed to nickel have a 40 to 250 times greater chance of developing this cancer.[2,26] Workers involved in the production of chromium, mustard gas, isopropyl alcohol, and radium are also at risk for developing carcinomas of the paranasal sinuses. Squamous cell carcinomas of the nose may have a 25- to 32-year latency period and usually arise on the middle turbinate. Some 15% to 20% of the patients have a history of chronic sinusitis and polyposis; however, it is unclear whether a cause-and-effect relationship exists.[2] Patients with inverted and cylindric cell papillomas, patients who have been treated with radiation and chemotherapy,[2] and patients with rhinoscleroma of the nasal cavity also may be at risk for developing a nasal carcinoma.[27]

Carcinomas of the nose occur primarily in males be-

tween 55 and 65 years of age. Most are low-grade tumors arising on the nasal septum near the mucocutaneous junction. The degree of differentiation appears to have no bearing on prognosis.[28]

The treatment may be surgery, radiation, or both. Local recurrences are found in 20% to 50% of the cases, and about 80% of these develop within the first year. Only 15% develop nodal metastases and only 10% have distant metastases. The overall 5-year survival rate is 62% and 15% of patients with a nasal carcinoma also have a metachronous or synchronous tumor, 40% of which occur in the head and neck and 60% of which occur below the clavicles in the lungs, gastrointestinal tract, and breasts.[2]

Because of their prevalence among sinonasal malignancies, carcinomas of the maxillary sinus have been studied with regard to correlating their specific location within the sinus, as well as patient prognosis. Attempts at such classifications have been deemed important in planning therapy and in comparing the treatment results of various medical centers. Initially the antrum was divided into an infrastructure and a suprastructure; however, this classification was soon modified into an

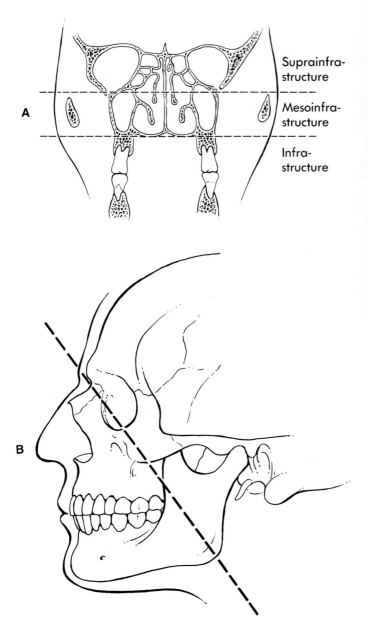

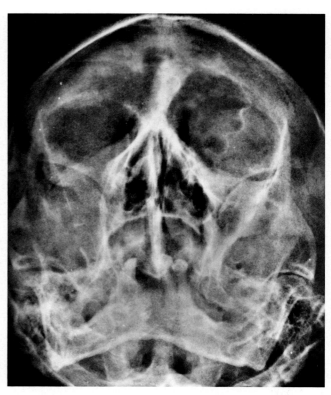

Fig. 2-248 Waters view shows almost complete destruction of right maxilla. Only a portion of the medial antral wall appears intact. The right zygomatic arch also remains intact. Squamous cell carcinoma.

Fig. 2-247 **A,** Diagram of coronal view of the sinonasal cavities. The lines divide the maxillary sinuses into suprainfrastructure, mesoinfrastructure, and infrastructure portions. Tumors limited to and below the mesoinfrastructure usually can be resected by a partial or total maxillectomy without an orbital exenteration. **B,** Diagram of lateral view of skull with Ohngren's line drawn. Tumors anterior to this line tend to have a better prognosis.

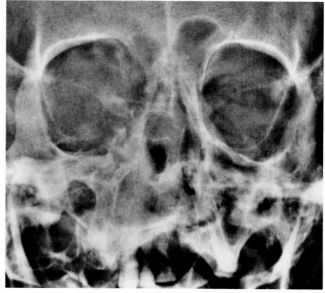

Fig. 2-249 Caldwell view shows clouding of right ethmoid and maxillary sinuses with destruction of the right lamina papyracea and a portion of the floor of the right orbit. Squamous cell carcinoma.

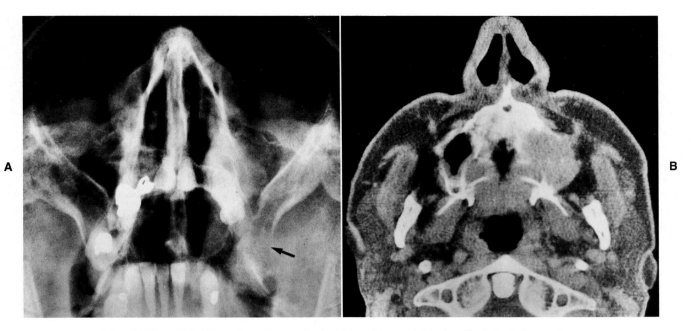

Fig. 2-250   A, Waters view shows destruction of lower lateral wall of the left maxillary sinus *(arrow).* **B,** Axial CT scan shows an aggressively destructive lesion of the lower antrum and palate. Squamous cell carcinoma.

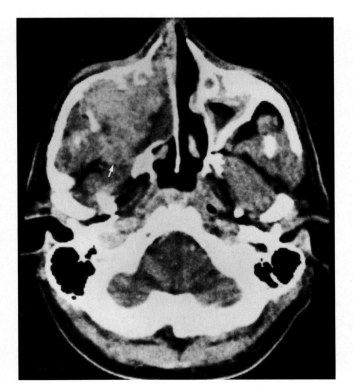

Fig. 2-251   Axial postcontrast CT scan shows homogeneous mass in right antrum that has destroyed the medial and lateral walls of the sinus and extended into the infratemporal fossa *(arrow).* Squamous cell carcinoma.

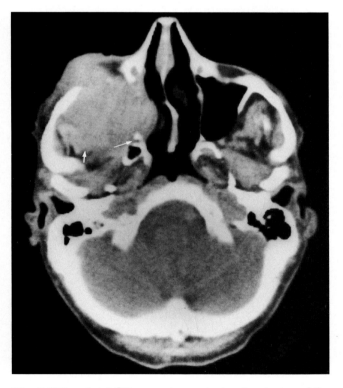

Fig. 2-252   Axial CT scan shows destructive lesion of the right antrum that has eroded all of the sinus walls and extended into the infratemporal fossa *(small arrows)* and the pterygopalatine fossa *(thin arrow).* Squamous cell carcinoma.

infrastructure, mesostructure, and suprastructure, with the lines of division being drawn on a coronal view of the sinuses through the antral floor and the antral roof (Fig. 2-247).[29] Using this system, tumors limited to the mesostructure and infrastructure require a partial or total maxillectomy, whereas tumors that involve the suprastructure require a total maxillectomy and orbital exenteration.

Ohngren divided the antrum into posterosuperior and anteroinferior segments by a line drawn on a lateral view of the face from the medial canthus to the angle of the mandible (Fig. 2-248). He suggested that tumors limited to the anteroinferior segment had a better prognosis.[29]

It was not until the early 1960s that the TNM system was first applied to antral cancers, and in 1976 The American Joint Committee on Cancer developed a TNM system based on Ohngren's line.[29]

Harrison[30] has criticized the TNM classification because it does not correspond to the clinical experience with these tumors. He suggested that a T_1 tumor is limited to the antral mucosa without bone erosion and without regard to Ohngren's line, since clinically it is often impossible to evaluate a tumor with regard to this line. A T_2 tumor has bone erosion, but no extension beyond the bone, and a T_3 tumor has extension to the orbit, ethmoid complex, or facial skin. Finally, a T_4 tumor extends to the nasopharynx, sphenoidal sinus, cribriform plate, or pterygopalatine fossa.

Antral carcinomas are almost twice as common in men as in women, and nearly 95% occur in patients over age 40 years.[2,31] Although the contrast medium Thorotrast is the only clearly established etiologic factor for carcinoma of the maxillary sinus, chronic sinusitis, polyposis, acute trauma, and chronic draining oroantral fistulas also may be causative factors.[2] When the tumors are small, they often are misdiagnosed as chronic sinusitis, nasal polyposis, lacrimal duct obstruction, tic douloureux, or cranial arteritis. By the time of the diagnosis, between 40% and 60% of patients have facial asymmetry, a tumor bulge in the oral cavity, and tumor extension in the nasal cavity. At least one of these findings is present in almost 90% of cases.[32] The treatment of choice appears to be surgery combined with radiation. Despite controversy in the literature, it appears that survival rates are about the same for either preoperative or postoperative radiation. Postoperative radiation has fewer complications, however.[2] The 5-year survival rate varies from 20% to almost 40%, with mean figures ranging from 25% to 30%.[33] The main cause of failure is local recurrence, and 75% of these occur within 5 months of initial treatment. Orbital exenteration is only performed if tumor involvement of the orbital periosteum has been documented at the time of surgery; criteria to discourage curative surgery include skull base destruction, a tumor in the pterygopalatine fossa, tumor extension into the nasopharynx, regional or generalized metastases, advanced patient age, poor general patient health, and the patient's refusal to accept treatment.[2,34]

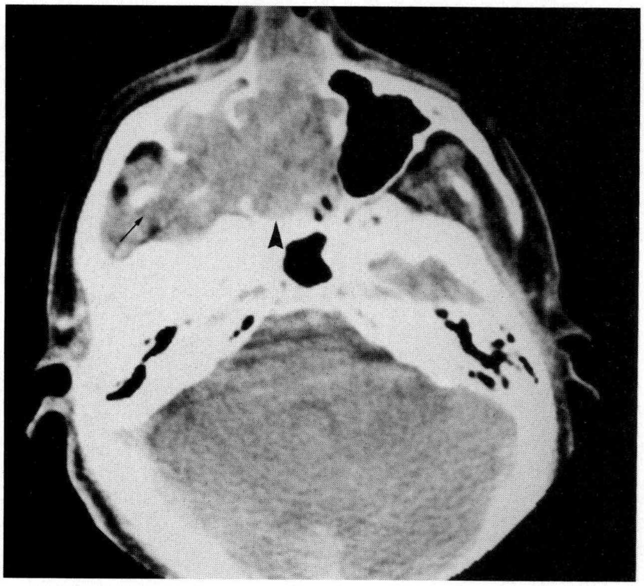

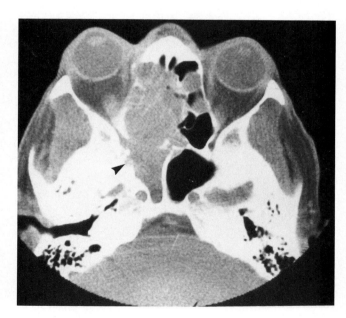

Fig. 2-253 Axial CT scan shows destructive lesion of the nasal cavity and right antrum that has extended into the infratemporal fossa *(arrow)* and the pterygopalatine fossa and eroded the skull base *(arrowhead)*. Squamous cell carcinoma.

Fig. 2-254 Axial CT scan shows destructive lesion of the right ethmoid sinus that has extended into the nasal fossa and the sphenoid sinus. There is focal erosion of the skull base *(arrowhead)*. Squamous cell carcinoma.

Although more than 100 cases of primary frontal sinus carcinoma have been reported, it is still a rare entity. The presenting symptoms are similar to those of acute frontal sinusitis, with patients having pain and swelling over the frontal sinus. However, in patients with frontal sinus carcinoma the frontal bone erodes rapidly and few patients survive more than 2 years.[4]

Primary sphenoid sinus carcinoma is rare. It is often difficult to distinguish such a tumor from a posterior ethmoid or nasal fossa carcinoma that has spread back into the sphenoid sinuses. As with frontal sinus carcinomas, few of these patients survive longer than 1 or 2 years.

It is the anaplastic form of carcinoma that can be confused histologically with embryonal rhabdomyosarcoma, melanoma, histiocytic lymphoma, esthesioneuroblastoma, and extramedullary plasmacytoma.[35]

On plain films, all patients have a soft tissue mass in the sinus cavity, and 70% to 90% have evidence of bone destruction.[32,36] The main reason to perform sectional imaging on these patients is to better visualize the extent of spread beyond the sinus cavity. The carcinomas enhance little, if at all, on contrast CT scans, and on MRI they have an intermediate-intensity signal with a fairly homogeneous internal architecture on T_1 WIs, PD WIs and T_2 WIs Uncommonly, localized areas of hemorrhage (high T_1W and T_2W signal intensities) or focal sites of necrosis (low T_1W and high T_2W signal intensities) can be seen (Figs. 2-234 and 2-248 to 2-258). The primary feature of these carcinomas is their strong tendency to aggressively destroy bone irrespective of whether the tumor is a highly differentiated squamous cell carcinoma or an undifferentiated carcinoma. Although bone remodeling can occur, it is uncommon. Usually the area of bone destruction is substantial compared with the size of the soft tissue tumor mass.

GLANDULAR TUMORS

Approximately 10% of all sinonasal tumors are of glandular origin.[2] These include all tumors categorized pathologically as specific minor salivary gland lesions (e.g., adenoid cystic carcinomas, mucoepidermoid carcinomas, acinous cell carcinomas, and benign and malignant pleomorphic adenomas), as well as malignancies grouped pathologically as adenocarcinomas. As a whole, glandular tumors vary from uniformly cellular tumors to highly pleomorphic lesions. The minor salivary gland tumors can arise anywhere within the sinonasal cavities, but most commonly they develop in the palate and then extend into the nasal fossae and paranasal sinuses.

Adenoid cystic carcinomas (cylindromas) account for about 35% of minor salivary gland tumors.[37] Of the primary sinonasal lesions, 47% arise in the maxillary sinuses, 32% involve the nasal fossae, 7% reside in the ethmoidal sinuses, 3% in the sphenoidal sinuses, and 2% in the frontal sinuses.[2] Adenoid cystic carcinomas usually arise in white persons between 30 and 60 years of age, although these neoplasms have been reported in an age range of 4 days to 86 years. Symptoms last an

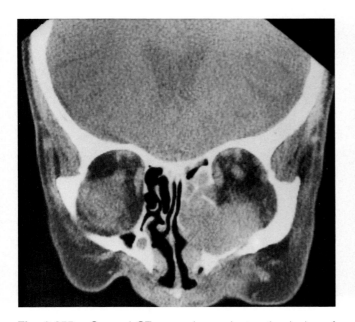

Fig. 2-255 Coronal CT scan shows destructive lesion of the left ethmoid sinus that has extended into the orbit. Squamous cell carcinoma.

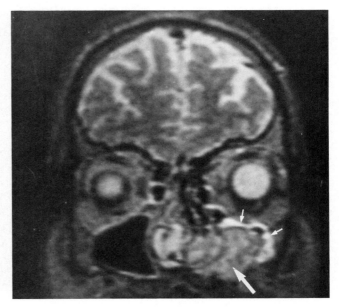

Fig. 2-256 Coronal T_2W MRI scan shows low-to-intermediate signal intensity mass that involves the left antrum and lower nasal fossa *(arrow)*. Inflammatory secretions with high signal intensity outline the upper and lateral margins of the antral portion of the tumor *(small arrows)*. Squamous cell carcinoma.

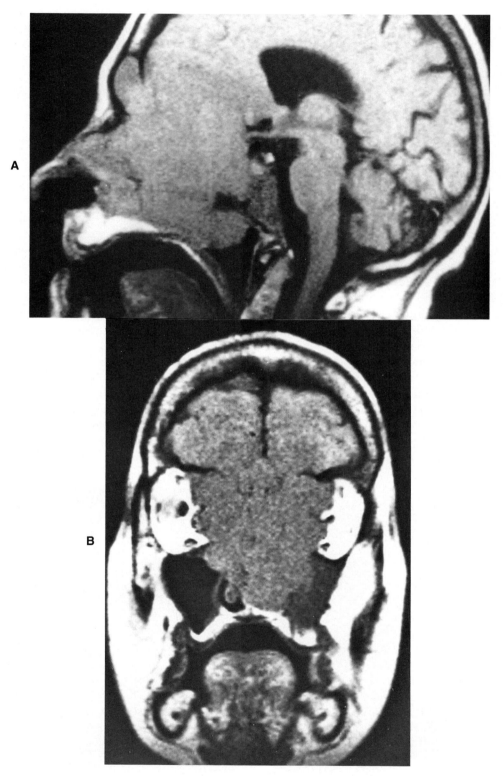

Fig. 2-257 **A,** Sagittal and **B,** coronal T_1W MRI scans show large homogeneous destructive lesion of the nasal fossa with a low-to-intermediate signal intensity. The tumor has eroded the central floor of the anterior cranial fossa, extended into the brain, both orbits, both ethmoids, and both antra. Squamous cell carcinoma.

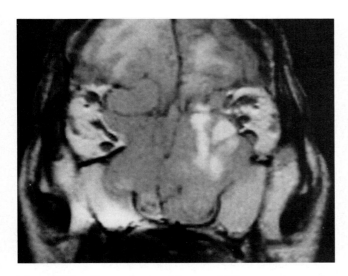

Fig. 2-258 Coronal mixed image MRI scan shows destructive lesion of the nasal cavity and both maxillary and ethmoid sinuses. The tumor invades both orbits and the anterior cranial fossa. The lesion has a homogeneous intermediate signal intensity except for several well defined areas of high signal intensity (hemorrhage). Squamous cell carcinoma.

average of 5 years and relate to the mass effect of the tumor. A dull pain signals perineural tumor invasion. Perineural spread is characteristic of this tumor, but it can occur with large areas of apparently normal intervening nerve. Because of this, the presence of "clean" surgical margins has little prognostic significance. The local postsurgical recurrence rate is 62% within 1 year and 67% to 93% within 5 years.[2]

Adenoid cystic carcinomas may recur 10 to 20 years after their initial treatment. As a result, 5-year survival data may give an erroneous indication of the absolute survival rate.[38] Some authorities have stated that no matter how long these patients have a disease-free interval, these patients will eventually die of adenoid cystic carcinoma. The disease-free interval for tumors without a solid or basaloid pattern appears to be longer than that for tumors with this pattern. The worst prognosis is for antral tumors, with 46% of patients being alive at 5 years, but only 15% having no evidence of disease.[2] About half of the sinonasal tumors have distant metastases, primarily to the lungs, brain, cervical lymph nodes, and bone.[2] Wide surgical excision is the treatment of choice, and, although adenoid cystic carcinomas are radiosensitive, they are not curable with radiation therapy. Despite the fact that survival may not be affected by radiation treatment, better local tumor control may be achieved if postoperative radiation is given.

A small number of glandular carcinomas cannot be placed into familiar histologic patterns. These tumors often resemble adenocarcinomas of the colon and are often referred to nonspecifically as *adenocarcinomas*. They occur primarily in males (75% to 90% of cases) between 55 and 60 years of age. The tumors are especially common in workers in the hardwood and shoe industries and in people using certain carcinogenic snuffs, particularly Bantus.[39,40] Most adenocarcinomas arise in the ethmoid sinuses and around the middle turbinates. Actual metastasis from a colonic carcinoma must always be considered in the differential diagnosis, but such an event is rare, with only 6% of all metastases to the sinonasal cavities coming from primary gastrointestinal tract tumors. The most common tumors that metastasize to the head and neck are tumors of the kidney, lung, breast, testis, and gastrointestinal tract.[2]

The clinical course of adenocarcinomas is similar to that of adenoid cystic carcinomas, with most deaths occurring within 3 years of diagnosis. Adenocarcinomas may have a lower tendency to metastasize to the cervical lymph nodes; however, adenocarcinomas have a predilection toward intracranial metastasis.[41]

Mucoepidermoid carcinomas rank third in frequency among sinonasal malignancies of the minor salivary glands, behind adenoid cystic carcinomas and adenocarcinomas. Most of these tumors involve the antrum and nasal cavity. Although they have the same histologic grading as the major salivary gland tumors, almost all minor salivary gland mucoepidermoid carcinomas are of the high-grade or intermediate-grade variety.[42] The biologic activity of these lesions resembles that of the adenocarcinomas.

Benign mixed tumors of the sinonasal cavities are rare, with most lesions occurring within the nasal fossa. Usually they arise from the nasal septum, although one fifth of the cases originate from the lateral nasal wall. The second most common site of origin is the maxillary sinus. Overall, pleomorphic adenomas are statistically the third most common minor salivary gland neoplasms. In order of decreasing frequency they include adenoid cystic carcinoma, adenocarcinoma, pleomorphic adenoma, mucoepidermoid carcinoma, undifferentiated carcinoma, acinous cell carcinoma, carcinoma expleomorphic adenoma, and oncocytoma.[42] Intranasal and paranasal pleomorphic tumors have a greater cellularity than their major salivary gland counterparts, and often the minor salivary gland lesions consist almost entirely of epithelial cells with little or no stroma.[43]

Wide surgical excision usually prevents recurrences; however, recurrence of the tumor may be delayed well beyond the traditional 5-year period.[3]

Typically, these lesions remodel bone. On CT scans the less cellular tumors may appear nonhomogeneous because of cystic degeneration, necrosis, or serous and mucous collections.[41] The highly cellular tumor tends to have a homogeneous appearance. On MRI these tumors have an intermediate signal intensity on T_1 WIs

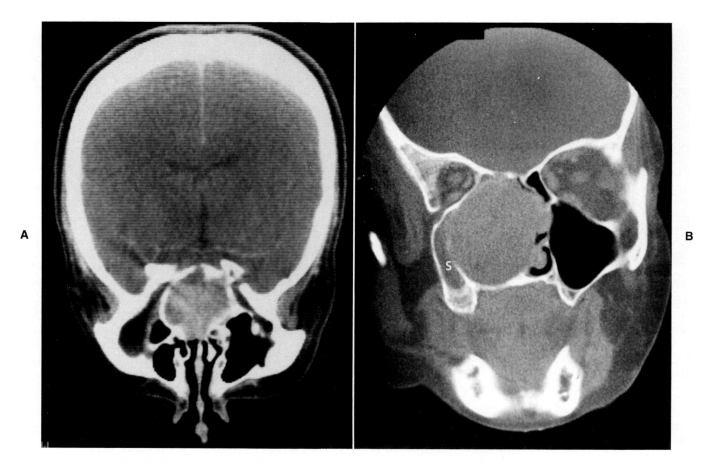

Fig. 2-259 **A,** Coronal CT scan shows nonhomogeneous expansile mass in the posterior nasal cavity, ethmoid sinuses, and sphenoid sinuses. The mass has remodelled the bone around it. Low-grade mucopidermoid carcinoma. **B,** Coronal CT scan shows expansile right nasal fossa and ethmoid sinus mass. The lesion has remodelled most of the surrounding bone, and it has obstructed what remains of the right maxillary sinus *(S)*. Minor salivary gland tumor.

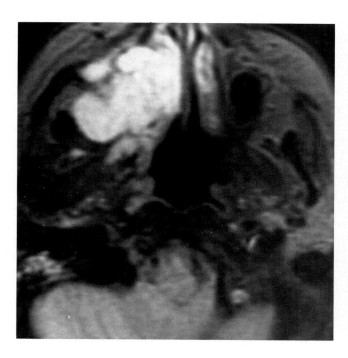

Fig. 2-260 Axial T$_2$W MRI scan shows expansile mass in right maxillary sinus that extends into the infratemporal fossa. The tumor has a high signal intensity. Low grade mucoepidermoid carcinoma.

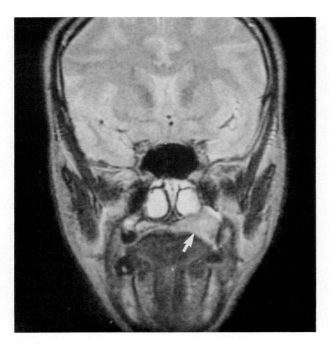

Fig. 2-261 Coronal mixed image MRI scan shows expansile and destructive mass in the left palate and lower left antrum *(arrow)*. This mass had intermediate signal intensity on mixed and T₂W MRI scans. Minor salivary gland high grade mucoepidermoid carcinoma.

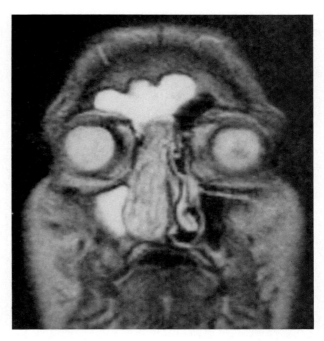

Fig. 2-262 Coronal T₂W MRI scans show expansile right nasoethmoid mass that extends into the base of the right frontal sinus. The lesion obstructs the right frontal and right maxillary sinuses. Adenocarcinoma.

and PD WIs. The T_2 signal intensity depends on the cellularity of the neoplasm. The highly cellular type tends to have an intermediate signal on T_2 WIs, whereas the stromal or less cellular variety has a bright signal on T_2 WIs (Figs. 2-259 to 2-262).

MALIGNANT MELANOMA

Sinonasal melanomas arise from melanocytes that have migrated during embryologic development from the neural crest to the mucosa of the nose and sinuses.[2] These tumors represent less than 3.6% of sinonasal neoplasms. Less than 2.5% of all malignant melanomas occur in the sinonasal cavities. These melanomas are two or three times more common in the nose than in the sinuses and most frequently arise from the nasal septum.[44,45] Occasionally, they develop about the inferior and middle turbinates; when in the paranasal sinuses, the antrum is the site of origin in 80% percent of the cases. Only a few cases develop in the ethmoid sinuses, and the frontal and sphenoid sinuses are virtually never involved as primary sites.[2,44,46] Sinonasal melanomas generally develop in patients 50 to 70 years of age. The most common complaints are nasal obstruction and epistaxis, with pain occurring as an initial complaint in only 7% to 16% of patients.[44,46] Between 10% and 30% of these melanomas are amelanotic lesions, and they may be multicentric in origin. Wide local sur-

gical excision with or without postoperative radiation is the treatment of choice.

Only 8% to 18% of patients with sinonasal melanomas have positive neck nodes, and between 55% and 65% of all melanoma patients have a local recurrence or metastases within the first year after surgery. Metastases tend to affect the lungs, lymph nodes, brain, adrenal glands, liver, and skin. Treatment of the recurrences yields surprisingly good results.[2] The 5-year survival rate averages 11% (ranging from 6% to 15%). Nasal melanomas have a better prognosis than those originating in the paranasal sinuses.[44] The average survival time of these patients is only 2 to 3 years, and the 10-year survival rate is 0.5%.[47]

Histologically, some melanomas resemble anaplastic carcinoma, histiocytic lymphoma, embryonal rhabdomyosarcoma, esthesioneuroblastoma, and extramedullary plasmacytoma.[35]

Melanomas tend to remodel bone, although elements of frank bone erosion also may be present. Because of their rich vascular network, melanomas enhance well on postcontrast CT scans, and their MRI appearance is that of a homogeneous mass of intermediate signal intensity on all imaging sequences. A few of the melanotic melanomas may have high T_1-weighted signal intensities because of the presence of paramagnetic melanin (Figs. 2-263 to 2-265).

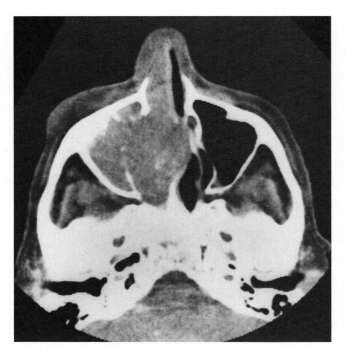

Fig. 2-263   Axial CT scan shows expansile right nasal fossa mass that obstructs the right antrum. Malignant melanoma.

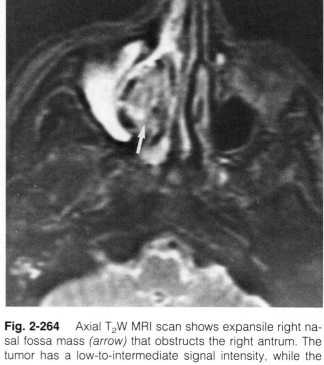

Fig. 2-264   Axial T₂W MRI scan shows expansile right nasal fossa mass *(arrow)* that obstructs the right antrum. The tumor has a low-to-intermediate signal intensity, while the obstructed secretions have a high signal intensity. Malignant melanoma.

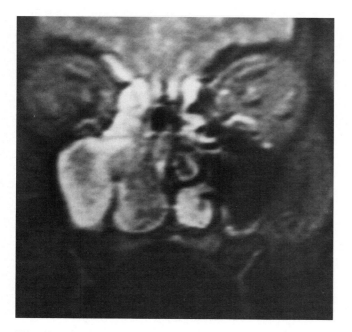

Fig. 2-265   Coronal T₂W MRI scan shows expansile low signal intensity mass in the right nasal fossa. The ethmoid sinuses are filled with obstructed secretions with high signal intensity. The right antrum is filled with obstructed secretions, which surround an extension of the tumor. Malignant melanoma.

NEUROGENIC NEOPLASMS

One of the difficulties in discussing neurogenic neoplasms (peripheral nerve tumors) is the confusing terminology that has arisen in the literature, with many names representing the same lesion. Controversy also has arisen on whether nerve sheath tumors arise from Schwann cells or neuroectodermal perineural cells.[48] Today most investigators use the term *Schwann cell* to describe both of these cells. It is accepted that a schwannoma, neuroma, neurinoma, neurilemoma, and perineural fibroblastoma all refer to the same tumor.[1]

A *traumatic neuroma* is not a true neoplasm, but a reparative pseudotumor that occurs after disruption of a peripheral nerve. If the proximal portion of the nerve cannot reestablish contact with the distal portion, the proliferating Schwann cells and axons grow haphazardly and form a traumatic neuroma. Excision with approximation of the nerve endings is the treatment of choice.[48]

A *neuroma (schwannoma)* is a benign, encapsulated, slowly growing nerve sheath tumor that occurs in patients 30 to 60 years of age. It is two to four times more common in women. Between 25% and 45% of these neuromas occur in the head and neck, with the most common site being the side of the neck. Only about 65 cases of neuromas have been reported in the sinonasal

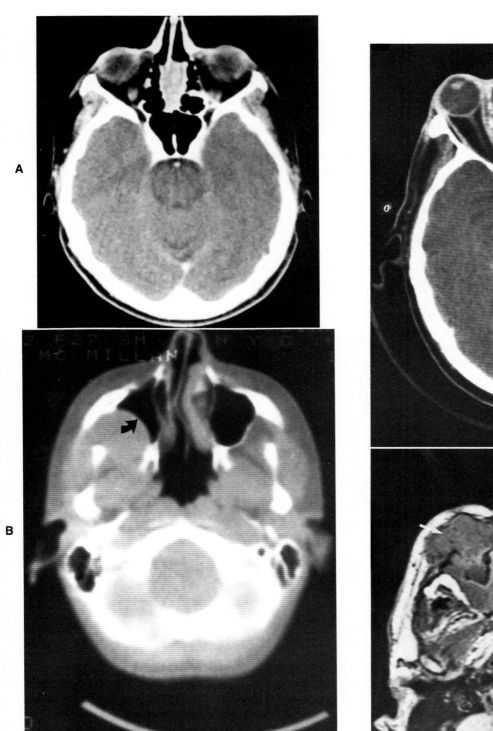

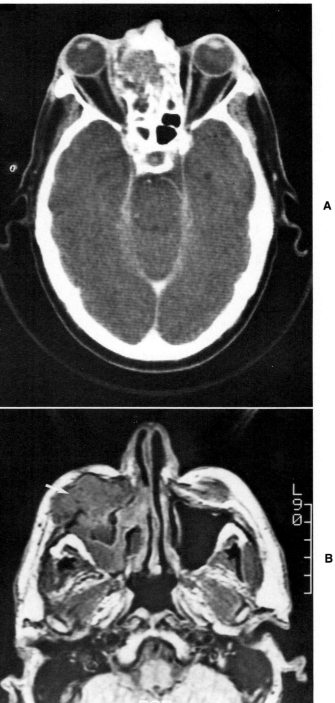

Fig. 2-266   A, Axial CT scan shows expansile, slightly nonhomogeneous, upper nasal cavity mass. Schwannoma. **B,** Axial CT scan shows expansile mass of the right infratemporal fossa, which bows the posterior antral wall anteriorly *(arrow).* Schwannoma of infratemporal fossa.

Fig. 2-267   A, Axial CT scan shows expansile right anterior ethmoid mass that erodes the lamina papyracea and bulges into the right orbit. Malignant schwannoma. **B,** Axial T$_1$W MRI scan reveals destructive lesion originating in the roof of the right antrum *(arrow).* The mass has a low signal intensity. Malignant schwannoma of V$_2$.

cavities, and most of these occur in the nasal fossa, maxillary sinuses, and ethmoidal sinuses.[1,48] The most common complaint is a painless mass. Neuromas rarely, if ever, undergo malignant change. At surgery, the nerve of origin may be identified stretched over the tumor. In these cases the surgeon may be able to extirpate the lesion while preserving the nerve. In neurofibromas the nerve is an integral part of the tumor and must be sacrified to excise the lesion.[48]

Neuromas can be of two major histologic types: the Antoni A, characterized by a compact arrangement of elongated spindled cells, or the Antoni B, characterized by a loose myxoid stroma with few spindled cells. This variation is reflected in their CT appearance, which ranges from a variably enhancing homogeneous ovoid mass to a primarily cystic lesion. About one third of the cases enhance more than muscle on postcontrast CT scans, one third have attenuation values of muscles, and one third are primarily cystic.[49] The enhancement occurs presumably because of extravascular extravasation of the contrast material into a poorly vascularized tumor matrix. Because of poor vascularity, the contrast medium is not rapidly dissipated within the vascular system. The MRI characteristics of neuromas are those of an intermediate signal intensity on T_1 WIs and PD WIs. The T_2 WIs vary according to whether the lesion is highly cellular (intermediate intensity) or cystic and stromal (nonhomogeneous high intensity). All neuromas are bone-remodeling lesions, and any site of aggressive bone destruction should raise the possibility of a malignancy rather than a neuroma (Figs. 2-266 and 2-267).

The *neurofibroma* is a benign, fairly well-circumscribed, but nonencapsulated nerve sheath tumor. Although it may occur as a solitary lesion, the finding of such a lesion, especially in a young patient, may herald the onset of other tumors with neurofibromatosis (von Recklinghausen's disease). Multiple neurofibromas, however, may also occur without the development of neurofibromatosis.[49] Approximately 8% (5% to 15%) of these tumors may have malignant degeneration.[50,51] The clinical appearance of a plexiform neurofibroma is considered to be a sign of neurofibromatosis, whether or not any other signs of the disease are present. This tumor usually remains within the confines of the perineurium and resembles a "giant nerve," "bag of worms," or a "string of beads."[48]

Neurofibromatosis is a hamartomatous disorder that is transmitted as an autosomal dominant trait with variable penetrance. It includes the presence of café au lait spots, multiple neurofibromas, and characteristic bone lesions.[52]

Neurofibromas can have a variable CT appearance, depending in part on the degree of cystic degeneration and fatty replacement present within the lesion. On postcontrast CT scans these tumors may have a variably enhancing homogeneous appearance, contain multiple cystic areas, or have a predominantly fatty attenuation. The degree of fatty replacement within some neurofibromas is far more extensive than that ever seen in neuromas and may at times cause the radiologist to suggest the diagnosis of a lipoma. Neurofibromas remodel bone and do not cause aggressive bone destruction. If bone has been destroyed, the possibility of a malignant degeneration should be considered.

A malignant schwannoma is a neuroectodermal sarcoma that is the malignant counterpart of a neurofibroma. Although it can occur as an isolated lesion, 25% to 50% are associated with neurofibromatosis. They occur primarily in patients 28 to 34 years of age. Only 9% to 14% of malignant schwannomas are found in the head and neck; the cranial nerves, large cervical nerves, sympathetic chain, and inferior alveolar nerve are the most commonly involved nerves. Symptoms include an enlarging mass, occasional pain, paresthesia, muscle weakness, and atrophy.[48]

Because Schwann cells can produce collagen and have a spindle shape, some malignant schwannomas are confused histologically with fibrosarcomas. However, electron microscopy reveals a basement membrane in the malignant schwannoma and no basement membrane in the fibrosarcoma.[48]

Malignant schwannomas associated with neurofibromatosis behave more aggressively than isolated lesions. The 5-year survival rates are 15% to 30% with neurofibromatosis and 27% to 75% without it. This difference is attributed to the fact that the tumors occurring with neurofibromatosis are pleomorphic. In addition, tumors that exceed 7 cm in size, have more than six mitoses per 10 high-power fields, and are located near the central body axis have a poorer prognosis. Local recurrences and hematogenous pulmonary metastases are common, whereas lymph node metastases are rare.[53]

Granular cell tumors (myoblastomas) are uncommon lesions that appear primarily in the skin of the nose, eyelids, forehead, scalp, and neck. They also may develop in the lips, floor of the mouth, palate, pharynx, larynx, and trachea. Most occur in patients 35 to 40 years old and, with the exception of the larynx, are twice as common in females. Treatment is excision; many incompletely excised lesions have failed to recur. Most granular cell tumors reach a size of 1 to 5 cm and are composed of polyhedral cells with acidophilic granular cytoplasm and round to oval nuclei. They may appear to "invade" nerves, but this is not a sign of a malignancy. No mitoses and necrosis are seen.[48] Rarely, a malignant granular cell tumor that appears to develop from a benign granular cell lesion is encountered. The malignancy can be diagnosed microscopically by frequent mitoses, necrosis, pleomorphic nuclei, and occasional spindle-shaped cells.[54]

TUMORS OF THE SYMPATHETIC NERVOUS SYSTEM

These tumors almost never involve the sinonasal cavities. They have been reported in the head and neck and most commonly arise in the cervical sympathetic chain as a neck mass or in the orbit, eyelids, tongue, pharynx, and larynx. Sometimes painful, lesions of the sympathetic nervous system may be associated with Horner's syndrome and vagal dysfunction.[48]

The neural plate's central portion invaginates in early embryogenesis to form the neural tube from which the brain, spine, and peripheral nerves develop. The lateral portions of the neural plates are not incorporated into the neural tube and instead form the left and right neural crests from which the sympathetic and parasympathetic systems develop.

The neural crest cells from which the sympathetic system develops are called *sympathogonia*. They normally differentiate into neuroblasts, which then mature into ganglion cells. If the cells fail to differentiate beyond the sympathogonia-neuroblast stage, the resulting lesion is called a *neuroblastoma*. If the tumor partially differentiates into mature ganglion cells, it is called a *ganglioneuroblastoma*. A tumor composed entirely of mature neural elements is called a *ganglioneuroma*. The more immature neuroblastoma is the most malignant of sympathetic nervous system lesions. The ganglioneuroblastoma is not as malignant, and the ganglioneuroma is benign.[48]

Olfactory Neuroblastoma

Olfactory neuroblastoma (esthesioneuroblastoma) is an uncommon tumor of neural crest origin that arises from the olfactory mucosa. The incidence peaks once in the 11- to 20-year age group (16.8% of all tumors) and again in the 50- to 60-year age group (22.8% of all tumors); however, the age of these patients ranges from 3 to 88 years.[48,55] This polypoid tumor may be soft or firm and may bleed profusely on biopsy. The three histologic subcategories, include the neuroblastoma with pseudorosettes (20% of cases), the neuroepithelioma with true rosettes (40% of cases), and the neurocytoma with sheets of cells, but no rosettes or pseudorosettes (40% of cases). It is this last variety that is most often confused with anaplastic carcinoma, histiocytic lymphoma, melanoma, extramedullary plasmacytoma, and embryonal rhabdomyosarcoma.[35] However, electron microscopy and histochemical testing can differentiate these lesions. The term olfactory neuroblastoma is currently preferred and refers to all histologic patterns. The staging system of Kadish, Goodman, and Wine refers to patients with disease confined to the nasal cavity as stage A, those with disease in the nasal cavity and one or more paranasal sinuses as stage B, and those with disease extending beyond the nasal cavity and paranasal sinuses as stage C.[56] Using this system, 30% of the patients are classified in stage A, 42% in stage B, and 28% in stage C. The respective 5-year survival rates are 75%, 68%, and 41.2%.[55,56] If surgical removal of the cribriform plate, dura, and olfactory bulb is reserved for only those patients with gross intracranial disease on imaging (stage C), and only an extended lateral rhinotomy is performed for stages A and B, the recurrence rates stay near 50%, and metastases will occur in 20% to 30% of patients.[48] However, if a craniofacial resection is performed as the initial procedure on all patients, initial results have suggested that cure rates may be above 90%. This approach takes into account the microscopic presence of intracranial tumor that can occur with an intact and normal-appearing cribriform plate.[57] Olfactory neuroblastomas are almost always unilateral and only in highly neglected cases do they appear as a bilateral nasal fossae mass. The role of imaging in these patients is to map the tumor so as to precisely anticipate surgical boundaries. On CT scans olfactory neuroblastomas are homogeneous, enhancing masses that remodel bone. They commonly extend into the ipsilateral ethmoid and maxillary sinuses and only

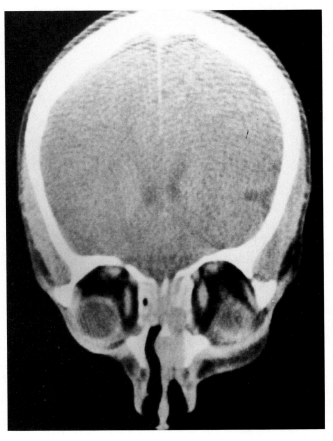

Fig. 2-268 Coronal CT scan shows mildly enhancing left nasal cavity and ethmoid sinus mass. There is some destruction of the upper nasal septum and possibly the cribriform plate. Esthesioneuroblastoma.

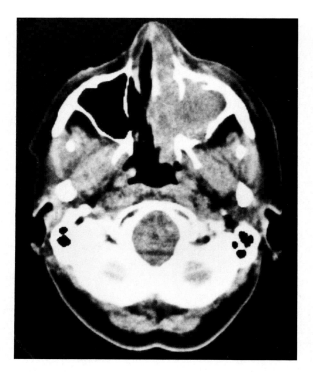

Fig. 2-269 Axial CT scan shows minimally enhancing expansile left nasal fossa mass that extends into the left antrum. Esthesioneuroblastoma.

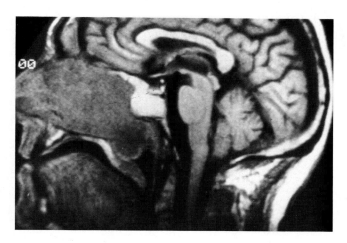

Fig. 2-270 Sagittal T₁W MRI scan shows large nasoethmoid mass with a low-to-intermediate signal intensity that erodes the floor of the anterior cranial fossa and obstructs the sphenoid sinus (high signal intensity). Esthesioneuroblastoma.

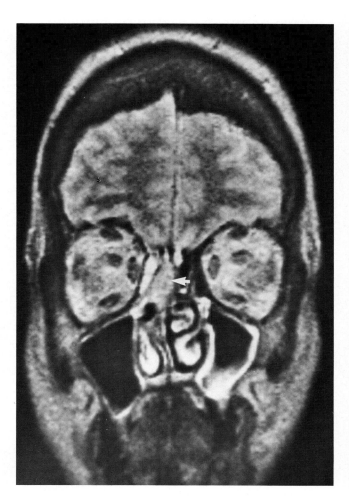

Fig. 2-271 Coronal T₂W MRI scan shows small right nasoethmoid mass (arrow) with inflammatory changes in the lateral right ethmoids and both maxillary sinuses (high signal intensity). Esthesioneuroblastoma.

rarely involve the sphenoid sinuses. Calcifications can occur within the tumor mass.[58] On MRI these tumors have an intermediate signal intensity on all imaging sequences (Figs. 2-268 to 2-271).

Melanotic Neuroectodermal Tumor of Infancy

The rare melanotic neuroectodermal tumor occurs 92% of the time in patients under 1 year of age. It is a rapidly growing, soft tissue mass that may invade bone.

However, despite this aggressive appearance, it is essentially benign, requiring local excision with curettage as treatment. Recurrences develop in only 15% of patients, and only two or three malignant cases have been reported, with metastases to lymph nodes, liver, bones, adrenal glands, and soft tissues.[48,59] The anterior maxilla is the most common site, accounting for 71% of all cases.

TUMORS OF THE PARAGANGLIOMA NERVOUS SYSTEM

Paragangliomas do not arise as primary lesions in the sinonasal cavities; however, large glomus jugulare tumors can involve the sphenoid and ethmoid sinuses secondarily. These lesions are discussed elsewhere in this book.

MENINGIOMA

Meningiomas are benign, slowly growing tumors that arise from clusters of meningocytes at the tips of the

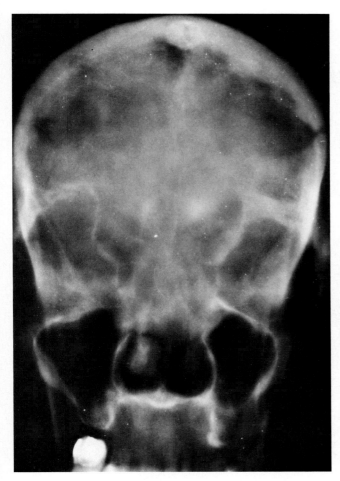

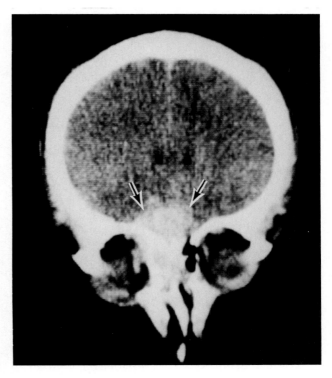

Fig. 2-273 Coronal postcontrast CT scan shows enhancing mass in the floor of the anterior cranial fossa *(arrows)* that extend into the ethmoid sinuses and nasal fossa. Intracranial meningioma extending extracranially.

Fig. 2-272 Coronal multidirectional tomogram shows mass that has extended into the nasal cavity and ethmoid sinuses by laterally displacing the bones of the orbital wall and ethmoid lamina papyracea. There are scattered calcifications within the mass. Intracranial meningioma extending extracranially.

arachnoid villi, usually in relationship to the major dural sinuses. They comprise 13% to 18% of all primary intracranial tumors and are two to four times more common in females, with a peak incidence occurring near 45 years of age.[48] These tumors can extend or arise outside of the neuroaxis; however, this is uncommon. Less than 1% of meningiomas arise as primary lesions outside of the brain or spine. Of all the meningiomas that occur outside of this neuroaxis, about one third are extensions from an intracranial or intraspinous lesion.[60,61] Most of these extraneuroaxis meningiomas occur in the head and neck and have been reported in the bones of the skull, orbit, nose, paranasal sinuses, oral cavity, middle ear, skin of the scalp, and cervical soft tissues.[48] In addition to being either a primary extracranial meningioma or an extension of an intracranial meningioma, such a lesion outside of the neuroaxis could represent a metastasis from an intracranial meningioma.[62]

The imaging characteristics of these sinonasal lesions show an enhancing mass that remodels bone. Most lesions lie in the nasal vault, and adjacent sclerotic, reactive bone may be a dominant feature. If the tumor has spread from the intracranial cavity, the remodeling of the skull base into the sinonasal cavities will be seen on coronal images. On MRI these tumors have intermediate signal intensities on all imaging sequences. Vascular flow voids have not been observed consistently in meningiomas (Figs. 2-272 to 2-274).

CHORDOMA

Chordomas are slow-growing, dysotogenetic tumors that arise from embryonic notochord remnants. They probably represent about 1% of all malignant bone tumors.[63] The vast majority occur in the skull base (clivus) and in the sacrococcygeal region. Rarely, chordomas have been reported in the maxilla and mandible.[64] In these cases, the tumor is presumed to arise in notochordal remnants that separated from the main notochord during the extreme mesodermal movements of the face that take place in early embryogenesis. These ectopic rests can be located in the paranasal sinuses.[64,65]

On postcontrast CT scans the classic chordoma is a minimally enhancing, destructive lesion that has areas of dystrophic calcification and residual bone fragments.

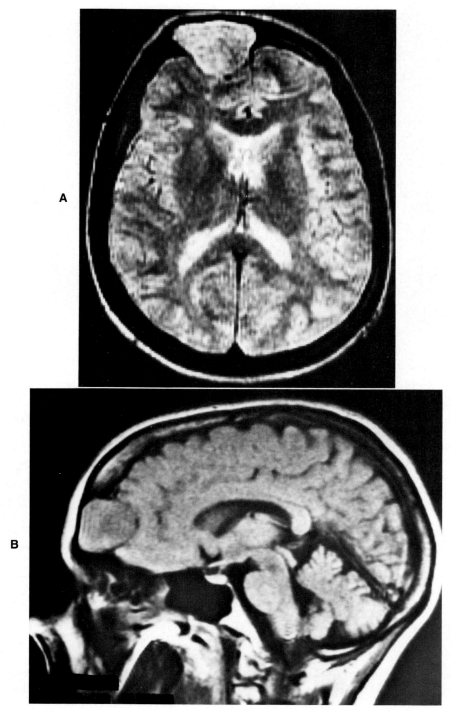

Fig. 2-274 **A,** Axial T$_2$W and **B,** sagittal T$_1$W images show expansile mass in the right frontal sinus that extends intracranially. The mass has low-to-intermediate signal intensity in **A** and high signal intensity in **B.** Frontal sinus meningioma.

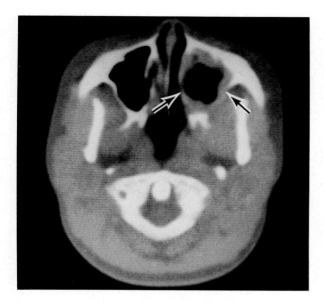

Fig. 2-275   Axial CT scan performed after surgical drainage of presumed mucocele shows thinning or destruction of the medial and posterior antral walls *(arrows)* with fairly uniform soft tissue thickening lining the antrum. Chordoma of antrum.

The only reported case in the maxillary sinus was scanned after aspiration and mimicked a mucocele (Fig. 2-275).[64] On MRI chordomas are extremely variable in their appearance, and they can have anywhere from a low to high signal intensity on any of the sequences.[66]

MESODERMAL TUMORS AND TUMORLIKE LESIONS

The true incidence of soft tissue tumors, especially the frequency of benign compared to malignant lesions, is nearly impossible to determine because many benign tumors such as lipomas and hemangiomas never undergo biopsy. However, sarcomas are malignant and ultimately require excision.[67] Sarcomas represent less than 1% of the total cancers reported in the United States. In children under age 16 these tumors represent 7% to 11% of all malignancies.[68] Of the total number of sarcomas, 10% to 15% occur in the head and neck.[69]

LYMPHOMAS

Among the sinonasal sarcomas, up to 80% are lymphomas, which may represent as much as 8% of all paranasal sinus malignancies.[1,70] The malignant lymphomas can be subdivided into non-Hodgkin's lymphomas, which represent about 75% of all cases, and Hodgkin's lymphomas.[71] Many classifications have been applied to non-Hodgkin's lymphomas. Of these, the Rappaport classification has achieved wide acceptance and is used by most investigators in the United States. This classification divides non-Hodgkin's lym-

phomas into the following types: lymphocytic, well differentiated; lymphocytic, poorly differentiated; mixed cell; histiocytic; and undifferentiated. Each of these groups can be further subdivided into either a nodular or diffuse type.

Between 2.2% and 6.5% of all lymphomas occur in the sinonasal cavities, and they represent a distinct group of the soft tissue malignancies in several ways.[72] Lymphomas have an equal sex distribution, whereas other sarcomas are more common in females. Lymphoma patients have only a 15% association with preexisting nasal polyposis and sinusitis, whereas other sarcoma patients have a high association. Lymphomas are the only soft tissue malignancies that are considered radiocurable. The remaining sarcomas as a group are not radiosensitive, and surgery and chemotherapy are currently the preferred modes of therapy.[70]

In the head and neck, only squamous cell carcinoma is a more common malignancy than non-Hodgkin's lymphoma.[73] About 40% of non-Hodgkin's lymphomas arise in extranodal sites. In the sinonasal cavities, these lymphomas can occur with or without associated nodal disease in the neck or elsewhere.[72] Evidence suggests that the presence of adenopathy with extranodal lymphoma may reduce the 5-year survival rate by 50%.[1] After treatment, overall the 5-year survival rates are 50% to 70%. Chemotherapy is emerging as the initial treatment modality for extranodal sinonasal lymphoma, with radiation being used in cases of incomplete tumor response.

In the nasal cavity and paranasal sinuses, the most common type of non-Hodgkin's lymphoma is the histiocytic lymphoma. It is this type of lymphoma that can be confused histologically with anaplastic carcinoma, melanoma, extramedullary plasmacytoma, esthesioneuroblastoma, and embryonal rhabdomyosarcoma.[35]

In the sinonasal cavities lymphomas tend to be bulky soft tissue masses that enhance to a moderate degree. These tumors also tend to remodel bone and occasionally erode bone.[74,75] Most often, the disease is located in the nasal fossae and maxillary sinuses. Less often, lymphoma is found in the ethmoid sinuses and only rarely in the sphenoid and frontal sinuses. On MRI it has an intermediate-intensity signal on all imaging sequences (Figs. 2-276 to 2-278).

Burkitt's lymphoma, a member of the non-Hodgkin's lymphomas, has distinct epidemiologic, clinical, and pathologic features. It occurs predominantly in children and is endemic in Central Africa, where it is the most common childhood malignancy and may be etiologically related to the Epstein-Barr virus. Nonendemic Burkitt's lymphoma is rare, occurs primarily in North America, and is not associated with the Epstein-Barr virus. Although this disease can involve head and neck structures such as the jaws, orbits, meninges, extradu-

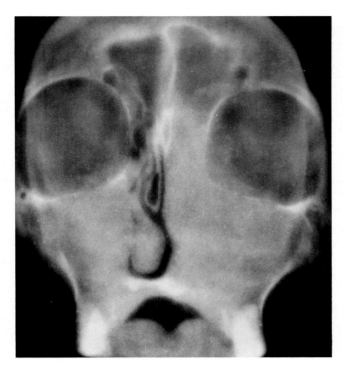

Fig. 2-276 Coronal multidirectional tomogram shows expansile, homogeneous mass in the ethmoid sinuses, maxillary sinuses and the left nasal fossa. The surrounding bone is intact. Histiocytic lymphoma.

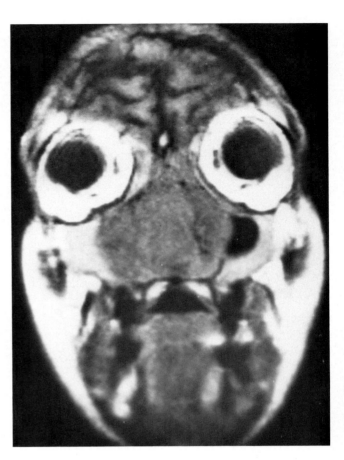

Fig. 2-278 Coronal T₁W MRI scan shows expansile bilateral nasal cavity mass that extends into the ethmoid and maxillary sinuses. The mass has a low-to-intermediate signal intensity. Histiocytic lymphoma.

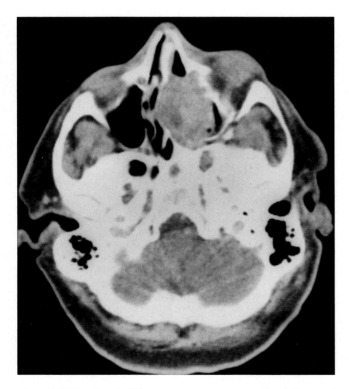

Fig. 2-277 Axial CT scan shows expansile left nasal fossa mass that extends into the left maxillary and ethmoid sinuses and up to the skull base. Histocytic lymphoma.

ral spaces, nasopharynx, and lymph nodes, it does not involve primarily the sinonasal cavities.[76]

Leukemia can be defined as an uncontrolled, malignant proliferation of blood cells and their precursors in the blood or bone marrow. The leukemias are generally classified according to the structure of the leukemic cells. They can be classified further into myeloid (non-lymphocytic) and lymphocytic categories, each of which can be subclassified into acute and chronic forms.[76] Rarely do primary leukemic infiltrates penetrate the sinonasal cavities. Instead, most patients with leukemia have involvement of the nose and paranasal cavities secondary to life-threatening infections and hemorrhage.

GRANULOCYTIC SARCOMA

Granulocytic sarcoma, or chloroma, is a rare localized malignant tumor composed of immature myeloid elements. The alternate term *chloroma* describes the green color of these lesions caused by the cytoplasmic enzyme myeloperoxidase. Granulocytic sarcoma occurs in only 3% of patients with acute and chronic myeloid leukemia. The mean patient age is 48 years, and most (85%) are solitary lesions. In the head and neck, osseous lesions have been reported in the skull, face, orbit, and paranasal sinuses, whereas extramedullary tumors have been reported in the nasal cavity, paranasal sinuses, nasopharynx, tonsil, mouth, lacrimal gland, salivary glands, and thyroid gland.[76]

An associated myeloproliferative disease is found in 48% of patients, and acute myeloid leukemia in 22% of the cases. However, 30% of patients with granulocytic sarcoma have no hematologic disease at the initial diagnosis. However, they develop acute myeloid leukemia within a few months after the diagnosis. The prognosis of patients with acute myeloid leukemia is not altered by the development of a chloroma; however, in patients with chronic myeloid leukemia and other myeloproliferative disorders, the granulocytic sarcoma is an ominous sign, since it is associated with the acute or blastic phase of the disease.[76] On CT scans chloromas are enhancing, homogeneous masses.[77] On MRI they have intermediate to high signal intensities on all imaging sequences.

PLASMA CELL DYSCRASIA

Multiple myeloma is the most common member of a group of diseases known collectively as plasma cell dyscrasias. These diseases (Waldenström's macroglobulinemia, heavy chain disease, and primary amyloidosis) all have a malignant proliferation of plasma cells or lymphocytoid plasma cells and the presence of monoclonal immunoglobulin or immunoglobulin fragments in the patient's urine. The proliferation of neoplastic cells is associated with bone destruction and involves the red marrow of the axial skeleton. However, the soft tissues can also be involved. Multiple myeloma usually affects patients over the age of 40 (mean age, 63) and has a roughly equal sex distribution. The most frequent complaints are bone pain (63%), weakness (23%), and weight loss (15%). An extraosseous plasmacytoma is the initial manifestation of the disease in only 5% of patients.[76]

In the head and neck, soft tissue masses occur primarily in the nose, paranasal sinuses, nasopharynx, and tonsils. Patients may have oronasal bleeding as a primary manifestation of hyperviscosity. Skeletal lytic lesions are found in 85% of patients, and a combination of lytic bone lesions, osteoporosis, and pathologic fractures is found in 63% of patients at disease onset.[76] An extraosseous tumor at the initial appearance of the disease is rare, but it is found in two thirds of patients at autopsy. Paraosseous tumor extension through destroyed cortical bone occurs in 50% of patients at autopsy. In 10% to 12% of patients with multiple myeloma, amyloidosis is present. Infection and renal failure are the primary causes of death. With the use of alkylating agents, steroids, and local irradiation, the median survival time is 20 months, with 66% of patients alive at 1 year, 32% at 3 years, and 18% at 5 years.[76]

EXTRAMEDULLARY PLASMACYTOMA

Extramedullary plasmacytoma is a rare soft tissue malignancy composed of plasma cells. Eighty percent of these tumors occur in the head and neck, mainly in the upper respiratory tract and oral cavity. They represent 3% to 4% of all sinonasal cavity tumors.[77-79] About 20% of the head and neck extramedullary plasmacytomas are initially associated with multiple myeloma, and of all of these tumors, 95% occur in patients over the age of 40 years (mean, 59 years).[76] The tumors have a 4:1 male predominance, and 90% of the patients are white.[76] The most common presenting symptoms are a soft tissue mass (80%), airway obstruction (35%), epistaxis (35%), local pain (20%), proptosis (15%), and nasal discharge (10%). The mean duration of symptoms is 4½ months. Of the head and neck lesions, 28% occur in the nasal cavity and 22% occur in the paranasal sinuses.[76]

The differential diagnosis includes not only anaplastic carcinomas, esthesioneuroblastomas, melanomas, histiocytic lymphomas, and embryonal rhabdomyosarcomas, but benign lesions such as plasma cell granulomas and pseudolymphomas.[76] Radiation therapy and surgery are the treatments of choice, with alkylating agents and steroids being helpful for painful bone lesions and in patients with systemic disease. Eventually, 35% to 50% of patients with primary extramedullary plasmacytomas develop disseminated disease and regional lymph node disease. Local bone destruction and persistent primary tumors after radiation are not necessarily poor prognostic indicators. Between 31% and 75% of patients are alive at 5 years; however, the median survival after the onset of dissemination is less than 2 years.[76]

On CT imaging extramedullary plasmacytomas of the sinonasal cavities are homogeneous, enhancing, polypoid masses that remodel the surrounding bone.[80] On MRI they have an intermediate signal intensity on all imaging sequences and because of their high vascularity, they may have vascular channel voids within the tumor substance (Figs. 2-279 and 2-280).

HISTIOCYTOSIS X

Hystiocytosis X comprises three diseases: eosinophilic granuloma, Letterer-Siwe disease, and Hand-Schüller-Christian disease. Although these diseases have manifestations in the skull and temporal bones, sinonasal disease is virtually unreported.[76]

RHABDOMYOSARCOMA

Rhabdomyosarcoma is a malignant tumor of striated muscle. It accounts for 84% percent of all soft tissue

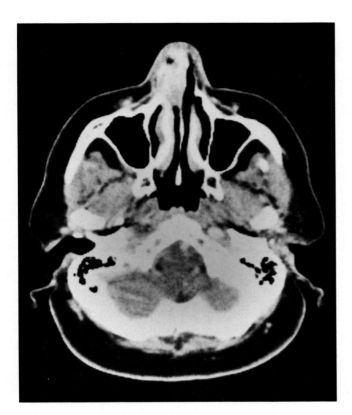

Fig. 2-279 Axial postcontrast CT scan shows enhancing right nasal mass that has caused little, if any, bone destruction. Extramedullary plasmacytoma.

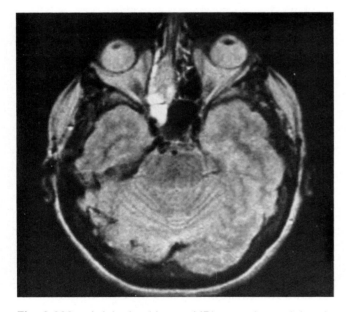

Fig. 2-280 Axial mixed image MRI scan shows right ethmoid and nasal mass *(arrow)*, which has a low-to-intermediate signal intensity. Surrounding the mass are chronically obstructed secretions with high signal intensity. Extramedullary plasmacytoma.

sarcomas and 35% to 45% of those occurring in the head and neck. It is primarily a pediatric disease, with 43% of patients being under 5 years old, and 78% being under 12 years old. About 7% occur in the second decade of life and 2% to 4% occur in each subsequent decade. Rhabdomyosarcoma is the seventh most common malignancy in children after leukemia, central nervous system tumors, lymphoma, neuroblastoma, Wilms' tumor, and bone cancer.[81] Of the fatal cases, 43.2% originate in the head and neck region, 28.6% in the genitourinary tract, 16% in the trunk, and 12.2% in the extremities.[68]

Embryonal rhabdomyosarcoma occurs primarily in the first decade of life, although 25% of the cases are in persons over the age of 20 years. Embryonal tumors 79% arise in the head and neck or genitourinary tract; with modern chemotherapy and radiation therapy, 5-year survival rates have risen from 8%-21% to 65%.[82] Between 10% and 38% of these cases metastasize to regional lymph nodes. Embryonal rhabdomyosarcoma can be histologically confused with anaplastic carcinoma, esthesioneuroblastoma, melanoma, histiocytic lymphoma, and extramedullary plasmacytoma.[35]

Alveolar rhabdomyosarcomas occur primarily in 15- to 25-year-olds. These tumors arise in the extremities in 54% of cases, the trunk in 28%, and the head and neck in 18%.[68] The median survival time is only 8¾ months, and the 5-year survival rate is only 2%.[83] Alveolar rhabdomyosarcomas have a great propensity for lymph node metastases, with 33% of cases having regional node involvement at initial tumor presentation and 75% to 85% involving regional or distant nodes during the course of the disease.[68]

The *pleomorphic rhabdomyosarcoma* occurs primarily between ages 40 and 60; only 6% of the tumors are found in patients under the age 15. Most of these tumors develop in the extremities, and only 7% develop in the head and neck. The 5-year survival rate is 25% to 35%. Most metastases result from hematogenous spread and only 9% involve regional lymph nodes.[68]

In the head and neck, the most common sites for all rhabdomyosarcomas are the orbit (36%), nasopharynx (15.4%), middle ear and mastoid (13.8%), sinonasal cavities (8.1%), face (4.5%), neck (4.1%), and larynx (4.1%). In the nasal cavity and paranasal sinuses, the most common presenting findings are nasal obstruction, rhinorrhea, epistaxis, sinusitis, local pain, otalgia, headache, toothache, proptosis, decreased visual acuity, and cranial nerve defects.[68] About 42% of patients have cervical lymph node metastases and 58% have distant metastases. After treatment, distant metastases may be a greater threat to survival than local recurrence.[84]

Although rhabdomyosarcomas can remodel bone or aggressively destroy it, on imaging most tumors show

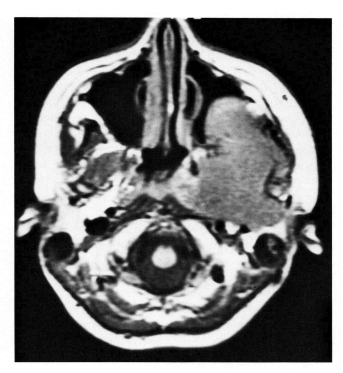

Fig. 2-281 Axial T_1W MRI scan shows homogeneous mass in the left infratemporal fossa extending into the left antrum and the skull base. The mass has an intermediate signal intensity. Rhabdomyosarcoma.

some elements of both. On postcontrast CT scans these tumors enhance little to moderately and are homogeneous in appearance. On MRI they also are remarkably homogeneous and have intermediate signal intensities on all imaging sequences (Fig. 2-281).

FIBROSARCOMA

Fibrosarcomas account for 12% to 19% of all soft tissue sarcomas and are found predominantly in the lower extremities and trunk; only 15% occur in the head and neck. Most of head and neck tumors involve the sinonasal cavities (18.3%), larynx (14.8%), neck (6.1%), and face (4.9%), and they usually arise in patients between 20 and 60 years of age.[68]

These tumors can be well differentiated, with well-developed collagen production and few mitoses (grades I and II), or they may be poorly differentiated, with little collagen production and frequent mitoses (grades III and IV). On the average, local recurrences develop within 18 months of initial treatment, and metastases occur within 2 years of local recurrences.[68]

The prognosis depends on the adequacy of the surgical resection, the degree of tumor differentiation, the number of mitoses, the size and location of the lesion, and the presence of pain or cranial nerve symptoms. Of these parameters, the resection margins are probably the

most important. Complete surgical excision with ample margins is the treatment of choice. Only 1% to 11% of patients develop positive regional lymph nodes; however, the 5-year survival rates are only 33% to 69%.[68]

Fibrosarcomas can occur in patients under 20 years old. Of all pediatric fibrosarcomas, 16% manifest in the head and neck. Most of these tumors are grades II or III, and, compared to the adult population, younger patients have a better prognosis. Although the local recurrence rate is similar to that for adults (17% to 47%), younger patients only have metastases in 10% to 14% of cases, and they have a higher 5-year survival rate of 85%. In addition, the younger the patient when the tumor appears, the better the prognosis.[68]

Less than 20% of all fibrosarcomas originate in the skeleton, where they account for 3% to 5% of all primary malignant bone tumors. Of these tumors, 15% occur in the head and neck, usually involving the jaw or maxilla. Medullary fibrosarcomas tend to spread more aggressively than their soft tissue counterparts. Most of these tumors arise in males between 35 to 40 years of age. Those occurring in the older population (30%) are usually the secondary type, arising in previously irradiated or diseased bone. Among the lesions so associated with the tumor are fibrous dysplasia, Paget's disease, giant cell tumors, bone infarcts, and osteomyelitis.[63] Most are grade II or III lesions, and the 5-year survival rate for all of these lesions varies from 27% to 40%. The higher the grade and the larger the tumor, the worse the prognosis. Metastases occur to the lungs and other bones; only 3% spread to regional lymph nodes.[53]

Fibrosarcomas have either a homogeneous or slightly nonhomogeneous, nonenhancing CT appearance. They remodel bone and on MRI have low to intermediate signal intensities on all imaging sequences.

FIBROUS HISTIOCYTOMA

The term fibrous histiocytoma refers to a variety of heterogeneous benign and malignant tumors that comprise an admixture of histiocytes and fibroblasts. Most fibrous histiocytomas of soft tissue or osseous origins are malignant. The vast majority occur in the extremities, retroperitoneum, and abdomen. Only about 3% occur in the head and neck, and most of these occur in the skin, orbit, or sinonasal cavities.[68] Most head and neck fibrous histiocytomas are malignant (71.6%), and they occur primarily in males (61%), with a median age of 46 years. Local recurrences develop in 27% of cases, and 75% of these appear within 2 years of diagnosis. Cervical nodal metastases occur in 12% and distant metastases in 42% of cases. The 2-year survival rate for all malignant fibrous histiocytomas is 60%. An accurate survival rate just for head and neck tumors cannot be obtained, since most of the reported tumors in this area have only recently appeared in the literature.[68]

Fibrous histiocytomas are histologically classified as benign or malignant, and those of uncertain histology are called *atypical*. The clinical outcome is not always predicted by this classification, although in general, patients with malignant lesions have a worse prognosis.

Fibrous histiocytomas may be confused histologically with pleomorphic rhabdomyosarcomas, pleomorphic liposarcomas, and anaplastic carcinomas. Electron microscopy and histochemical testing may be necessary for a definitive diagnosis.

The current treatment of choice is wide surgical excision; the role of radiation therapy remains difficult to assess.[68]

On postcontrast CT scans, these tumors usually enhance moderately or not at all. Aggressive bone destruction dominates the CT appearance and makes this lesion similar in its imaging characteristics to squamous cell carcinoma.[85] Similarly, on MRI fibrous histiocytomas have intermediate signal intensities on all imaging sequences.

LIPOSARCOMA

Liposarcomas comprise 15% to 18% of all malignant soft tissue sarcomas, and in some centers they are either the most commonly encountered sarcoma or the second most common type after malignant fibrous histiocytoma. Most occur in men, with an average age of 43 years; however, only about 3% occur in the head and neck. Of these, only isolated cases have been reported in the sinonasal cavities.[68] They can be well differentiated, myxoid, round cell, pleomorphic, or mixed in histologic appearance. The 5-year survival rate for well-differentiated tumors is 85% to 100%; for myxoid, 71% to 95%; round cell, 12.5% to 55%; pleomorphic, 0% to 45%; and mixed, 31% to 33%. The overall incidence of metastases is 25% to 45% with most of these tumors being of the round cell or pleomorphic types. The treatment of choice is wide surgical excision. The role of postoperative radiation remains controversial.

Based on the general experience with liposarcomas elsewhere in the body, these lesions have an overall low (fatty) attenuation value (−65 to −110 HUs) on CT scans, and irregular areas of soft tissue density are seen inside the lesion. The tumor margins may infiltrate adjacent soft tissues. MRI reveals a nonhomogeneous, high T_1-weighted signal of lower intensity than normal fat and a nonhomogeneous intermediate signal intensity on T_2 WIs.[86]

LEIOMYOSARCOMA

Leiomyosarcomas represent only 5% to 6% of all soft tissue sarcomas and occur primarily in the uterus, gastrointestinal tract, and retroperitoneum. Only 3% to 10% of these tumors arise in the head and neck; of these, 19% arise in the sinonasal cavities. Three types appear histologically: conventional, vascular, and epithelioid tumors. However, unpredictable clinical behavior is associated with these tumors, and pathologists often have difficulty in determining accurate criteria for distinguishing benign from malignant lesions. In general, the degree of mitotic activity and tumor size are the most important criteria.[68] In the nose and paranasal sinuses, these tumors have an equal sex distribution, with an average age incidence of 50 years.[87] The symptoms are nonspecific. On biopsy the malignant potential is often underestimated and the lesions may be confused with other soft tissue tumors. Treatment involves radical extirpation. Little response has been found with either radiation therapy or chemotherapy. About 75% of patients have a local recurrence and 35% develop metastases. At least 50% of these patients die of the disease, usually within 2 years of diagnosis.[87]

Leiomyosarcomas are bulky, lesions that remodel bone and enhance little; they may have multiple areas of necrotic and cystic liquefaction within.[88]

HEMANGIOPERICYTOMA

Hemangiopericytomas are uncommon vascular lesions that arise primarily in the lower extremities, retroperitoneum, and pelvis. However, 15% occur in the head and neck, and of these 55% arise in the nose.[89] The median age of onset is 45 years, and 40% to 60% of sinonasal hemangiopericytomas recur locally. Metastases, usually to the lungs and rarely to regional lymph nodes, are reported in 10% of the cases.[68] The 10-year survival rate is 77% for tumors with zero to three mitoses per 10 high-power fields and 29% for tumors with four or more mitoses per 10 high-power fields. One or more local recurrences typically precede metastases. The median interval to local recurrence is 17 months, whereas from diagnosis to metastases it is 4½ years.[88] Surgery remains the treatment of choice; the lesion is relatively radioresistant. The role of chemotherapy is still evolving, but initial reports show promise.[68]

Children account for 10% of all hemangiopericytomas, but no children's cases have been reported in the sinonasal cavities. In general, 20% to 35% of the tumors in pediatric patients are malignant, and most of these occur in older children.[90]

On CT scans hemangiopericytomas are expansile, bone-remodeling lesions with a variably enhancing, fairly homogeneous appearance (Fig. 2-282).

SOFT TISSUE ANGIOSARCOMA

Angiosarcomas account for only 2% to 3% of all soft tissue sarcomas. They have been reported in virtually every site of the body, but most arise in the skin, liver, and breast. Sinonasal tumors are uncommon, and the

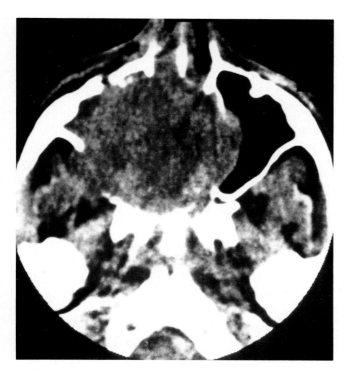

Fig. 2-282 Axial CT scan shows slightly nonhomogeneous expansile nasal cavity mass that extends into the right antrum, right infratemporal fossa, and central skull base and bulges into the left antrum. Hemangiopericytoma.

presenting symptoms include epistaxis, nasal obstruction, headaches, and proptosis. The average age of onset is 42 years, and the male-to-female ratio is 3:2. From the limited number of reported cases, the 5-year survival rate runs 60%. Sinonasal tumors appear to have a better prognosis than skin and soft tissue lesions. If head and neck soft tissue lesions behave similarly to other angiosarcomas, 30% spread to regional lymph nodes and 20% metastasize to distant sites within 2 to 3 years of initial treatment.[68] Surgery with or without radiation therapy is the treatment of choice, and therapy must take into account that angiosarcomas often extend several centimeters beyond their apparent limits.

On CT scans these tumors are aggressive, bone destroying lesions that enhance well.

OSSEOUS ANGIOSARCOMA

The term angiosarcoma describes malignant tumors that arise from endothelial cells of blood or lymphatic vessels. More specific terms, such as hemangioendothelioma, hemangioendothelial sarcoma, and hemangiosarcoma, describe tumors that arise in bone. Most of these tumors arise de novo, although they have been reported at sites of chronic osteomyelitis. They represent less than 1% of all primary malignant tumors of bone and can occur as solitary lesions (77%) or as multifocal tumors involving several bones (23%). Most oc-

cur in the bones of the extremities, pelvis, and spine. The solitary tumors are twice as common in males, and 60% of patients are between 20 and 49 years of age.[63]

Head and neck tumors make up 15% of solitary intraosseous angiosarcomas. Most arise in the mandible and skull. The symptoms vary with the specific bone involved; however, most patients complain of dull local pain and swelling of the affected region. Complete surgical excision is the treatment of choice, with radiotherapy being reserved for inaccessible lesions, incompletely excised tumors, or palliative treatment. Grade I lesions recur locally, but do not metastasize, as do grade II and III lesions. For patients with solitary lesions, the 5-year survival statistics are 20%, and for patients with multifocal lesions, the rate is 36%, reflecting the predominance of grade I tumors in these latter patients. Most metastases are to the lungs, rarely to other viscera, regional lymph nodes, and bones.[63]

MESENCHYMAL CHONDROSARCOMA

The mesenchymal chondrosarcoma is a rare neoplasm of bone (60% to 70% of cases) or soft tissues (30% to 40% of cases). The mandible is one of the preferred osseous sites, and the craniospinal meninges and orbital soft tissues are the most common extraskeletal sites. These tumors also have been reported in the ethmoid sinuses. Over half of the patients are 10 to 30 years of age, and radical excision appears to offer the best chance of cure. Few patients have responded to radiation therapy, and survival is highly variable. Most patients die within months, whereas others survive for many years. The 5-year survival figures do not always correspond with clinical cures. Metastases are hematogenous and are preceded by one or more local recurrences. The osseous and extraosseous lesions do not differ significantly in their clinical behavior.[68]

CHONDROMA AND CHONDROSARCOMA

Chondrogenic tumors of the sinonasal cavities are rare and, in contrast to those which occur in the larynx, are most often malignant. The average patient is 44 years old, and males predominate by a 3:2 ratio. About 60% of the tumors arise in the anterior alveolar region of the maxilla, and patients usually consult their physician with complaints of nasal obstruction, epistaxis, chronic nasal discharge, loose teeth, poorly fitting dentures, an expansile painless mass, proptosis, or headache.[63] Most tumors are either grade I or II chondrosarcomas, with grade III lesions being uncommon. The incidence for metastases for grades I, II, and III are 0%, 10%, and 71%, respectively.[91] Early, wide excision is the only modality that results in a cure, since these lesions are not radiosensitive and chemotherapy results have been unrewarding. The 5-year survival rate is 40% to 60%, and at least 60% of patients have a local recurrence within 5 years. However, some recurrences have been reported 10 to 20 years after initial treatment. Overall, only 7% of sinonasal chondrosarcomas develop metastases, which predominantly go to the lungs and bones. Uncontrolled local disease is the most common cause of death.[63]

True chondromas of the sinonasal cavities have been reported in the nose, ethmoid, sinuses, maxilla, sphenoid sinuses, and nasopharynx. They are equally divided between males and females, and about 60% occur in patients less than 50 years old. Since 20% of head and neck chondrosarcomas may be misdiagnosed initially as benign, wide surgical excision is the treatment of choice.[91,92]

Radiographically, calcifications within the tumor matrix are not often seen either on plain films or CT scans. These lesions tend to be expansile lesions that remodel bone and have an attenuation value less than muscle, but greater than fat.[93,94] They do not provoke sclerotic bone at their margins.

MALIGNANT MESENCHYMOMA

Malignant mesenchymomas are rare tumors composed of two or more sarcomatous elements that ordinarily are not found together. As diagnostic criteria have become more refined, the frequency of malignant mesenchymoma has declined from a peak incidence in the 1950s and 1960s. Most tumors that might have been diagnosed as malignant mesenchymomas in the past are currently being classified as malignant fibrous histiocytomas. Collectively, the death rate is 60% in adults and 43% in children.[68]

Two cases of malignant mesenchymoma studied with CT scans appeared as aggressive lesions that were indistinguishable from squamous cell carcinomas.

HEMANGIOMA

Experts disagree as to whether hemangiomas are true neoplasms or malformations. In the nasal cavity, they usually occur on the septum (65%), followed in frequency by the lateral wall (18%) and vestibule (16%). Most arise in the anterior septum near Kisselbach's plexus, and most are of the capillary type. Lesions arising on the lateral wall usually are of the cavernous type. Epistaxis and nasal obstruction are the most common presenting complaints. Simple excision is generally curative for these lesions, which rarely exceed 2 cm in their greatest dimension. This small size at discovery is attributed to the frightening initial complaint of severe epistaxis. Rarely, intranasal hemangiomas may develop in the second trimester of pregnancy. Most of these lesions spontaneously regress within 4 to 8 weeks after delivery.[68]

Hemangiomas of the paranasal sinuses are very rare, with two being described in the maxillary sinuses and two in the sphenoid sinuses. On CT scans these are enhancing lesions. The sphenoid sinus cases showed destruction of the skull base.[68] Hemangiomas have an intermediate signal intensity on all MR imaging sequences, and vascular flow voids occasionally may be present.

Solitary Hemangioma of Bone

This lesion accounts for only 0.7% of all primary bone tumors. In the head and neck, the most common sites are the skull (53%), mandible (10.7%), nasal bones (9%), and cervical vertebrae (6%). Although many patients have a history of prior local trauma, a cause-and-effect relationship remains doubtful. The lesions most often occur in females by a 2:1 ratio, with the average age of onset at 31 years. Most commonly, patients experience a firm, nonpainful swelling that is associated with a pulsating sensation. Actual bruits are rarely heard.

When hemangiomas involve the facial bones and mandible, angiograms have revealed that the blood supply is from the facial artery or the internal maxillary artery. The inadvertent surgical violation of an intraosseous hemangioma can be associated with an exceptionally rapid blood loss, often as much as 3500 ml. Even so, surgery is the primary treatment of choice. Embolization may greatly reduce operative blood loss, provided that the operation is performed very shortly after embolization, before a collateral circulation can develop.[63]

Radiographically, these lesions have a "soap bubble" or "honeycomb" appearance and enhance on postcontrast CT scans.

LYMPHANGIOMA

Lymphangiomas virtually are unreported in the sinonasal cavities and are located primarily on the neck, face, floor of the mouth, and tongue.[68]

RHABDOMYOMA

Rhabdomyomas represent less than 2 percent of all primary skeletal muscle neoplasms. Although they occur in the head and neck, they have not been reported in the sinonasal cavities.

LEIOMYOMA

Leiomyomas are benign smooth muscle tumors, only eight of which have been reported in the nose and paranasal sinuses. Knifelike pain has been reported with this lesion, and it is believed that the pain is due to spasmodic contraction of the tumor with resultant ischemia. Of the head and neck tumors, 71% are conventional leiomyomas, 27% are angiomyomas, 1.2% are epithelioid leiomyomas, and 0.8% are mesectodermal leiomyomas.[68]

LIPOMA AND LIPOMA-LIKE LESIONS

These lesions, which include the ordinary lipoma, myxoid lipoma, angiolipoma, pleomorphic lipoma, spindle cell lipoma, myelolipoma, hibernoma, and lipoblastomatosis, are of various reported frequencies; however, they have not been reported to arise within the sinonasal cavities.

MYXOMA

A myxoma is a mesenchymal neoplasm comprising undifferentiated stellate cells in a myxoid stroma. Only about 130 cases have been reported, and their occurrence in descending order of frequency is in the heart, subcutaneous tissues, bone, genitourinary tract, and skin. Only 7 cases have been reported in the head and neck. Bone myxomas occur almost exclusively in the jaws and represent 40% to 50% of all head and neck myxomas. Next most commonly they occur in the palate. On CT scans they are cystic lesions that do not enhance.[95]

FASCIITIS AND FIBROMATOSIS

These lesions also represent a wide variety of pathologic entities that include nodular fasciitis, proliferative fasciitis, focal myositis, myositis ossificans, myositis ossificans circumscripta or progressiva, the fibromatoses, and desmoid fibromatoses. None of these entities have been described in the sinonasal cavities.[68]

FIBROOSSEOUS LESIONS

Of all the nonepithelial tumors that involve the sinonasal cavities, 25% are osseous or fibroosseous lesions.

Osteoma

Osteoma is a benign proliferation of bone that occurs almost exclusively in the skull and facial bones. Although 20% to 30% of patients with osteomas have a history of prior trauma and 15% to 30% have a history of sinusitis, no cause-and-effect relationship has been proven.[63] These tumors occur mainly in the frontal sinuses, followed in descending order by the ethmoid, maxillary, and sphenoid sinuses. The high prevalence of osteomas in the frontal and ethmoid sinuses may relate to the fact that this region is the junction of membranous and enchondral development of the frontal and ethmoid bones.

Several histologic types exist. The compact, or "ivory," type is composed of dense, hard, mature bone, with only small amounts of fibrous tissue. The cancellous, or "mature," type has sparse intertrabecular spaces that may be empty or filled with fat, fibrous tissue or hematopoietic elements.[63] Fibrous osteomas contain abundant mature lamellar bone, but have greater amounts of intertrabecular fibrous tissue. As a result, on plain films, bone density varies from a very dense, sclerotic lesion for the ivory-type osteoma to a progressively less dense and less ossified lesion for the fibrous osteoma. In fact, some fibrous osteomas may be confused on plain films with a retention cyst or polyp (Figs. 2-283 and 2-284).

Osteomas usually are small and incidental findings on plain films. However, they can obstruct the frontal sinus in 17% of cases, and this results in the need for immediate surgery.[96] Almost all osteomas remain confined to the sinuses, often conforming to the contour of the sinus. However, osteomas are the most common benign paranasal sinus tumors to be associated with spontaneous cerebrospinal fluid rhinorrhea.[97]

When multiple osteomas are seen, primarily in the skull and mandible, the diagnosis of Gardner's syndrome should be considered. The osteomas in this syndrome can arise in the teenage years and be diagnosed before the appearance of intestinal polyps, which often do not arise until the third decade of life (Fig. 2-285).

On CT scans osteomas arise from one of the sinus walls or the intersinus septum. The differences between the compact, cancellous, and fibrous types correlate with the degree of bone matrix density seen within the lesion. On MRI these lesions give a nonhomogeneous, low to intermediate signal intensity on all imaging sequences. Based purely on MRI findings, their osseous nature may go undetected (Figs. 2-286 and 2-287).

Osteochondroma

Osteochondromas represent 40% to 50% of benign osseous lesions and 10% to 15% of all osseous tumors. It is not clear whether they represent a true neoplasm or a developmental abnormality. They can arise from any bone that develops from enchondral ossification. Since most of the craniofacial bones develop by intramembranous ossification, osteochondromas in the sinonasal cavities are rare. Of the approximately 77 cases reported in this region, most arose in the mandible. They have been reported in the sphenoid bone, maxillary tuberosity, zygomatic arch, and nasal septum.[63] Most osteochondromas stop growing with maturation of the remaining skeleton. However, it is not unusual to find a lesion that either stops growing before or continues to grow after skeletal maturation. Surgery is the treatment of choice, and only 1% to 2% of lesions recur. Similarly, only 1% to 2% of solitary osteochondromas undergo malignant change, usually into chondrosarcomas.[63] Radiographically, these tumors tend to have a pedunculated mushroom shape. The cartilaginous cap is often not visible and when seen may be focally calcified. On MRI they have a nonhomogeneous low to intermediate signal intensity on all imaging sequences (Figs. 2-288 and 2-289).

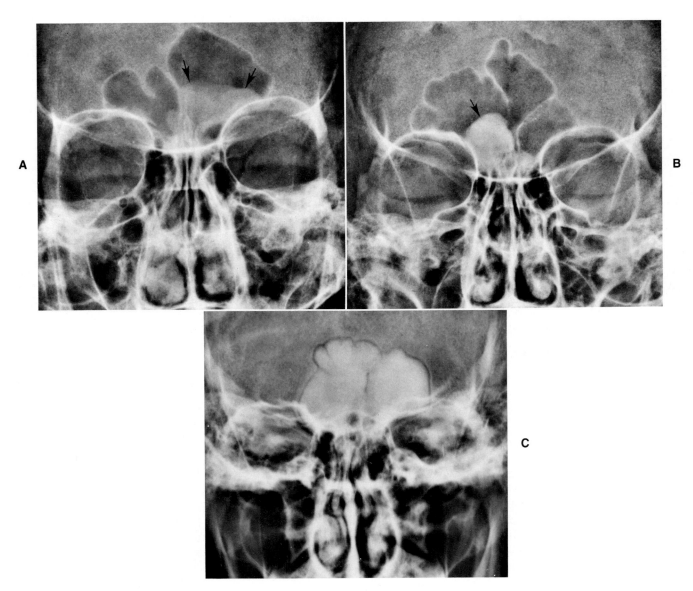

Fig. 2-283   A, Caldwell view shows polypoid mass *(arrows)* that is slightly denser than the adjacent frontal bone. Fibrous "soft" osteoma. **B,** Caldwell view shows ivory osteoma *(arrow)* in right frontal sinus. The sinus is not obstructed. **C,** PA view shows bilateral frontal osteomas. Note how osteomas have conformed to the sinus contour.

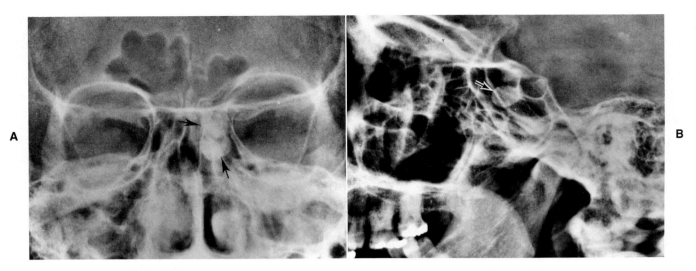

Fig. 2-284   **A,** Caldwell view shows osteoma in left ethmoid sinuses *(arrows)*. **B,** Lateral view shows osteoma *(arrow)* in sphenoid sinuses.

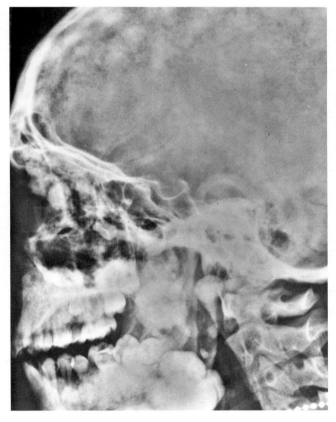

Fig. 2-285   Lateral view shows multiple osteomas of the facial bones, mandible, and calvarium. Gardner's syndrome.

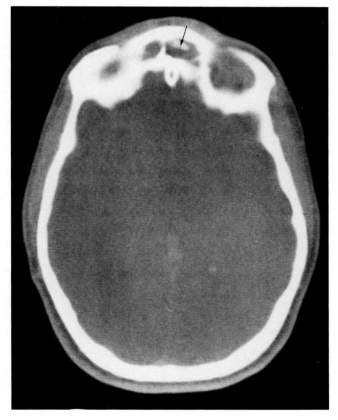

Fig. 2-286   Axial CT scan shows osteoma *(arrow)* obstructing the left frontal sinus.

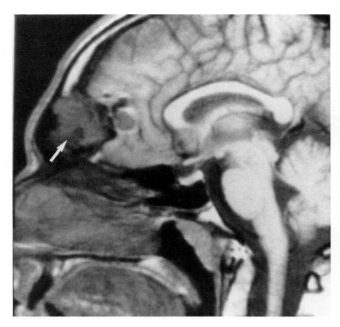

Fig. 2-287   Sagittal T$_1$W MRI scan shows low signal intensity mass in the frontal sinuses that has extended into the anterior cranial fossa causing pneumocephalus. Osteoma.

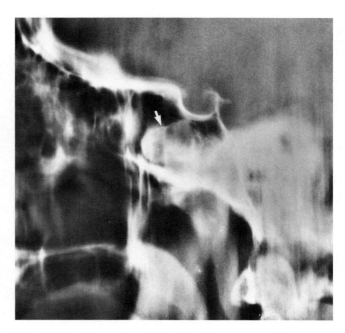

Fig. 2-288   Lateral multidirectional tomogram shows partially ossified pedunculated mass in the sphenoid sinus (arrow). Osteochondroma.

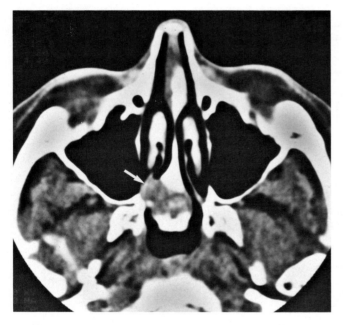

Fig. 2-289   Axial CT scan shows expansile, partially calcified mass in the posterior nasal septum (arrow). Osteochondroma.

Osteoid Osteoma

These lesions represent 11% of benign bone neoplasms. They occur twice as commonly in males, and 80% of the patients are between 5 and 25 years of age. Only 26 cases have been reported in the head and neck, mostly in the mandible and cervical vertebrae. Osteoid osteomas have been reported in the frontal, ethmoid, and maxillary bones. Patients describe a dull pain that usually worsens at night, is intensified by activity, and is relieved by rest. Radiographically, the classic lesion is a dense cortical ovoid mass with a 1- to 2-mm, low-density nidus. However, the nidus also may be dense and difficult to identify.[63] Surgery is the treatment of choice.

Osteoblastoma

Osteoblastomas represent only 3% of all benign bone tumors and possess histologic features that are virtually identical to osteoid osteoma. Those lesions greater than 2 cm in diameter usually are diagnosed as osteoblastomas. Most occur in the vertebrae (30% to 40%); however, at least 15 cases have been reported in the maxilla, ethmoid, and sphenoethmoid regions.[63] In contrast to osteoid osteomas, the pain of osteoblastomas usually is more severe, is not nocturnal, and is not relieved by aspirin. Osteoblastomas are divided into the classic benign type and the aggressive type.

Conservative surgery consisting of local excision or curettage cures 80% to 90% of the cases of benign osteoblastoma. The aggressive type recurs locally, but unlike osteogenic sarcoma (with which it may be confused histologically), it does not metastasize.[63]

Radiographically, these tumors have a variable appearance, with some lesions having large discrete areas of organized bone density and others having a mixed

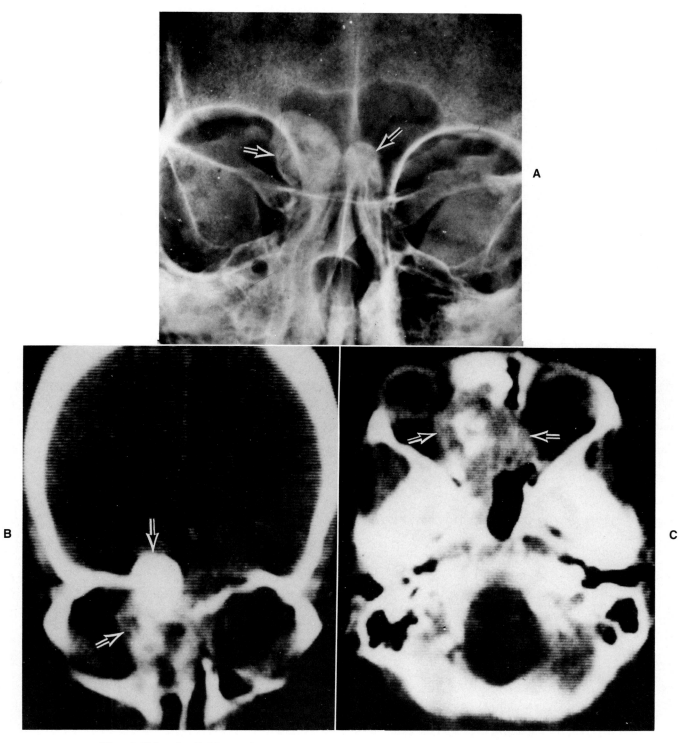

Fig. 2-290   **A,** Caldwell view shows bony masses *(arrows)* in the ethmoid sinuses, which are projected over the frontal sinuses. There is also disease in the ethmoid sinuses. **B,** Coronal CT scan and **C,** axial CT scan show the partially ossified ethmoid mass *(arrows)* that has extended into the right orbit and broken intracranially. Osteoblastoma.

osseous and fibrous appearance. The latter is more nodular and coarsely organized than that seen with most ossifying fibromas and some fibrous dysplasias. The lesions tend to be expansile and remodel the adjacent bone (Fig. 2-290).[98-100]

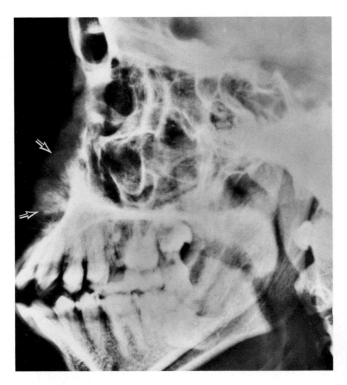

Fig. 2-291 Lateral view shows aggressive tumor of the maxilla that has caused a "sunburst" periosteal reaction. Osteogenic sarcoma.

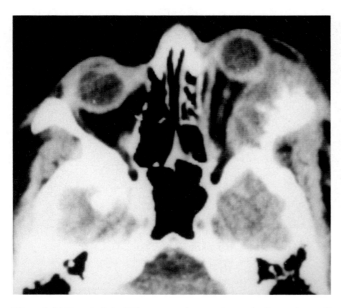

Fig. 2-292 Axial CT scan shows irregularly enlarged bony lesion in the left zygoma with surrounding soft tissue mass. Osteogenic sarcoma.

Osteogenic Sarcoma—Osteosarcoma

Osteosarcomas comprise 2% of all primarily malignant bone neoplasms. After multiple myelomas, they are the second most common malignant tumors of the skeleton. Osteosarcoma is twice as common as chondrosarcoma, three times more common than Ewing's sarcoma, and four to six times more common than medullary fibrosarcoma. It can arise as a primary lesion or be related to prior irradiation, exposure to Thorotrast, or a variety of benign conditions that include Paget's disease, fibrous dysplasia, giant cell tumor, osteoblastoma, bone infarct, and chronic osteomyelitis.[63,101] Osteosarcomas represent between 0.5% and 1% of all sinonasal tumors, and they can be classified as conventional, juxtacortical, and extraosseous.

Head and neck lesions account for 5% to 9% of conventional osteosarcomas, with the mandible and maxilla being the most common locations. In the maxilla, the most common sites are the alveolar ridge, the anterior midline, and the sinus. Pain occurs in half of the cases, and 25% have dental symptoms. Osteosarcomas occur primarily in males in their third or fourth decades of life and have a better prognosis than their extrafacial counterparts. The 5-year survival figures for tumors of

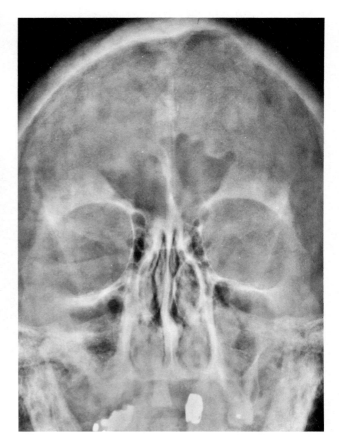

Fig. 2-293 Caldwell view shows scattered nodular densities in the calvarium and facial bones. Paget's disease.

the craniofacial bones range from 23% to 59% compared with 13% to 20% for all osteosarcomas. Of the head and neck tumors, 11% are grade I; 41%, grade II; 41%, grade III; and 7%, grade IV. This compares with 85% of the extrafacial tumors being grade III or IV. Of the osteosarcomas, about 53% are osteoblastic, 24% are chondroblastic, 24% are fibroblastic, and 2% to 11% are telangiectatic.[63]

The radiographic appearance depends on the degree of osteoblastic tumor present. As a result, these tumors vary from a purely lytic, aggressively destructive mass to a blastic zone within the facial bones. Classically, the rapid tumor growth can cause a "sunburst" periosteal reaction of the bone. Variable-sized areas of dense calcification or bone can be seen within some tumors (Fig. 2-291).

On CT scans these lesions appear as soft tissue, aggressively destructive masses. In about 25% of cases, regions of amorphous and irregular calcification occur both in the central and peripheral regions of the tumor. New tumor bone is present in only 25% of cases; however, purely blastic lesions can be seen, especially in the posterior maxillary alveolus.[101] On MRI these tumors have a nonhomogeneous appearance of low and intermediate signal intensity on all imaging sequences (Fig. 2-292).

Paget's Disease

Paget's disease is a bone disorder of unknown etiology. Increased osteoclastic and osteoblastic activity results in the disorderly production of abnormal, but highly characteristic bone.[76] The disease usually occurs in patients over the age of 50 years, and it primarily involves the vertebrae (76%), calvaria (65%), pelvis (43%), femur (35%), and tibia (3%). Its incidence increases with longevity, with between 3% and 3.7% of people older than 40 years of age affected.[102] In 80% of patients, the degree of skeletal involvement is limited and found fortuitously on radiographic studies or at autopsy. The facial bones are rarely involved; however, whenever the maxilla and mandible are affected, the calvarium is involved (Fig. 2-293).[103]

The initial radiographic and CT appearance of Paget's disease of the calvarium often reveals a lytic phase that produces osteoporosis circumscripta, usually involving the frontal region to the greatest degree. A "mixed" phase may follow. This phase shows foci of sclerotic, woven bone within areas of lower density, which repre-

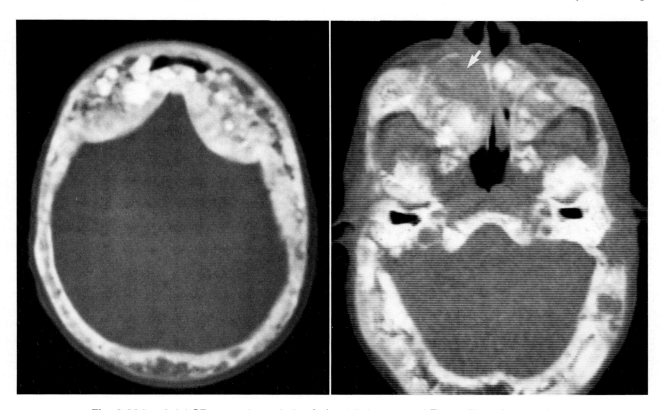

Fig. 2-294 Axial CT scans through the **A,** frontal sinuses and **B,** maxillary sinuses show marked thickening of the calvarium with localized areas of dense "woven" bone. The expanded bone is encroaching on the frontal sinuses. The facial bones are slightly thickened and dense and they have obliterated the maxillary sinuses and most of the nasal fossa. A localized area of nonossified tissue is seen in the right maxilla *(arrow)*, which was an osteogenic sarcoma. Paget's disease with osteogenic sarcoma.

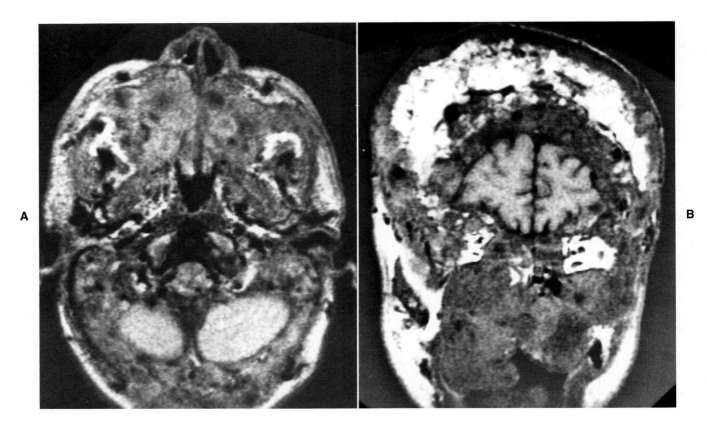

Fig. 2-295 **A,** Axial mixed image and **B,** coronal T₁W image MRI scans show diffusely thickened bone in the facial region and the calvarium. The areas of high signal intensity in the calvarium on **B** correspond to marrow. The thickened calvarium has reduced the size of the intracranial compartment. The majority of the abnormal bone has a nonhomogeneous low-to-intermediate signal intensity. Paget's disease.

sent sites of fibrous myeloid production. The remaining bone often gives a moderately diffuse radiopacity. The calvaria are thickened, usually with the greatest degree of thickening being anteriorly. One side of the skull tends to be more affected than the other. Any irregularity of the inner table is usually more extensive than that of the outer surface. When the facial bones are involved, it is by the sclerotic form of Paget's disease. This form results in a thickened, dense bone with slightly irregular cortical surfaces (Fig. 2-294).[103]

On MRI the dense foci of bone give rounded foci of signal void on all imaging sequences. The marrow tissues give high T₁-weighted and proton density–weighted signals and fairly high T₂-weighted signals. This reflects the fat and blood protein in these regions. The background matrix gives an intermediate signal on all imaging sequences. The facial area demonstrates a mixed low to intermediate signal intensity on all imaging sequences (Fig. 2-295).[103]

The reduced size of the cranial cavity secondary to bony ingrowth of the calvaria and skull base has led to an altered patient mentality, dementia, and other neurologic abnormalities. Basilar invagination is associated with cranial nerve deficits. Encroachment into the orbits, neurovascular canals, and sinonasal cavities has lead to proptosis, visual loss, neurologic deficits, facial deformity, and nasal congestion.

Sarcomas may develop in 5% to 10% of patients who have extensive Paget's disease and in less than 2% of patients with limited bone involvement. The prognosis is grave, with most patients dying within 2 years after the diagnosis is established. The development of multiple lesions is frequent; autopsy studies suggest a multicentric rather than a metastatic origin for these tumors. Most of these sarcomas are osteogenic sarcomas (50% to 60%) or fibrosarcomas (20% to 25%). In the facial area, giant cell tumors can also occur. On plain films and CT scans these tumors usually appear sharply localized. Because the bone seen in Paget's disease, as well as the sarcomas, tends to give intermediate signals on all imaging sequences, it is more difficult to diagnose and map these bone tumors on MRI than on CT scans.[103]

Fibrous Dysplasia

Fibrous dysplasia is an idiopathic skeletal disorder in which medullary bone is replaced and distorted by poorly organized, structurally unsound, fibroosseous tissue that is composed of woven-type bone with few osteoclasts. The disease can occur in a monostotic form, a polyostotic form, and as Albright's syndrome. The monostotic type accounts for 75% to 80% of all cases and most often involves the ribs and femurs. Bones of the head and neck comprise 20% to 25% of the cases of monostotic fibrous dysplasia, with the maxilla and mandible being the most common sites.[104]

Polyostotic disease accounts for 20% to 25% of all cases. Usually only the bones on one side of the body are involved, except in severe cases, where bilateral disease can occur. Of these patients 40% to 60% have involvement of the skull and facial bones.[102,104]

Almost exclusively a disease affecting females, Albright's syndrome consists of polyostotic fibrous dysplasia, cutaneous pigmentation, and sexual precocity. The ratio of monostotic fibrous dysplasia to Albright's syndrome is 40:1. The skin pigmentations have irregular margins (coast of Maine) as opposed to the smoother bordered pigmentations (coast of California) of neurofibromatosis. For all types of fibrous dysplasia, most patients are under 30 years of age when the disease is discovered.[102]

Bone expansion can encroach on the paranasal sinuses, nasal fossae, orbits, and neurovascular canals. With extensive involvement of the facial bones, the resulting distortion of the face has been referred to as the *lion face*, or *leontiasis ossea*.

Fibrous dysplasia undergoes malignant transformation in about 0.5% of cases. This occurs more often with the polyostotic form. About 50% of the sarcomas that complicate the monostatic disease occur in the skull and facial bones, whereas 62% of the sarcomas associated with polyostotic disease occur in the femur.[105] The tumors develop in bone affected by fibrous dysplasia; there may be a relationship to irradiation of the bone. The average time from the diagnosis of fibrous dysplasia to the appearance of the sarcoma is 13½ years. Of the sarcomas, 65% are osteogenic sarcomas, 18% are fibrosarcomas, 10% are chondrosarcomas, and 7% are "giant cell" sarcomas.[102]

It is generally accepted that fibrous dysplasia and the appearance of new lesions decrease or stop after skeletal growth ceases. It is also believed that the radiographic appearance of the lesion becomes more sclerotic with aging. However, some lesions continue to grow after skeletal maturation and after they become sclerotic. In addition, serial biopsies of lesions reveal no conversion of woven bone into lamellar bone.[102]

Surgery is used only to correct deformities, relieve pain, correct functional problems, or resect sarcomatous disease. Fibrous dysplasia recurs in 20% to 30% of cases, and recurrences usually appear within 2 to 3 years of initial therapy.[102]

The radiologic appearance varies according to the degree of fibrous tissue present. Thus the bone texture

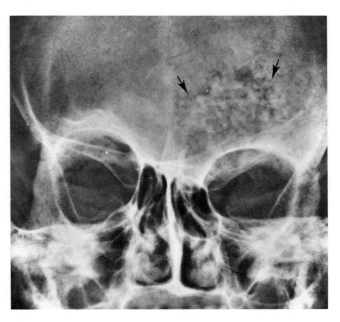

Fig. 2-296 Caldwell view shows mixed "lytic" and "blastic" expansile lesion of the left frontal bone *(arrows)* that has depressed the superior orbital margin. Fibrous dysplasia.

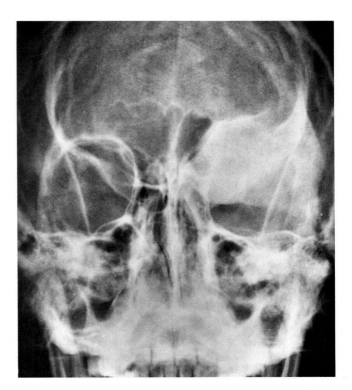

Fig. 2-297 Caldwell view shows very dense expansile lesion of the left frontal and zygomatic bones that has encroached on the left orbit. Fibrous dysplasia.

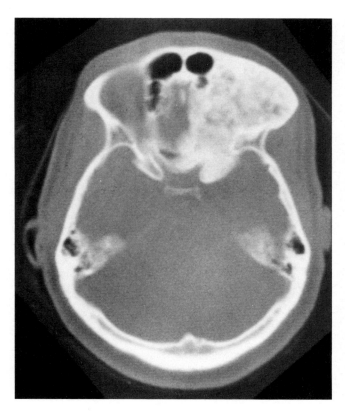

Fig. 2-298 Axial CT scan shows expansile dense lesion of the left frontal, zygomatic, and sphenoid bones. Small nonossified areas (fibrosis) are present within the lesion. Fibrous dysplasia.

can range from a nonhomogeneous mixture of bone and fibrous tissues to a predominantly fine bony (ground-glass) appearance. The disease expands the diploic or medullary space and widens the bone. A thin intact rim of cortical bone is often seen over the outer margins of the involved bone (Figs. 2-296 to 2-299).

MRI shows a low-to-intermediate intensity signal on all imaging sequences, and often the cortical bone overlying the medullary disease can be identified as a zone of low signal intensity (Fig. 2-300).

Ossifying Fibroma

This lesion has more highly cellular fibrous tissue and less mature and less organized osseous tissue than is found in the fibrous osteoma. Unlike fibrous dysplasia, the ossifying fibroma contains lamellar rather than woven bone and has lining osteoblasts. On CT scans the lesion is expansile and usually has larger, nonossified areas of fibrous tissue density than those in fibrous dysplasia.[102] The internal organization of the lesion shows discrete ovoid zones of either osseous or fibrous tissue. However, in some cases, the appearance is indistinguishable from fibrous dysplasia, and the pathologist also may have difficulty in differentiating these lesions. Compared to fibrous dysplasia, ossifying fibroma has a

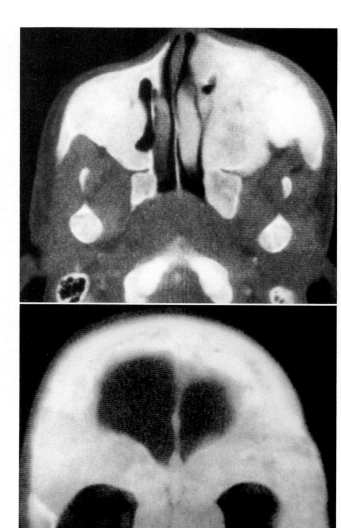

Fig. 2-299 A, Axial and **B,** coronal CT scans show ground glass density expansile bony process that has encroached on the orbits and obliterated the maxillary sinuses. Fibrous dysplasia (Leontiasis ossea).

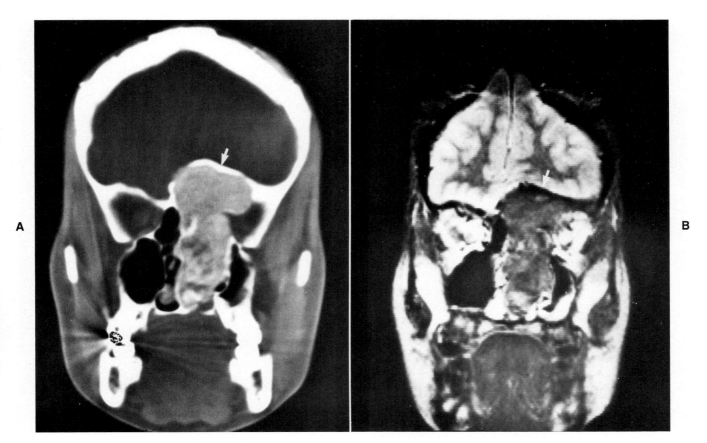

Fig. 2-300   A, Coronal CT scan and **B,** T₁W MRI scan show an expansile mass in the left nasal cavity, ethmoid and frontal region. There is marked encroachment on the left orbit. A thin rim of cortical bone is seen over the lesion *(arrow)*. In **A** the lesion has a "ground glass" appearance, while in **B** it has a nonhomogeneous low signal intensity. Fibrous dysplasia.

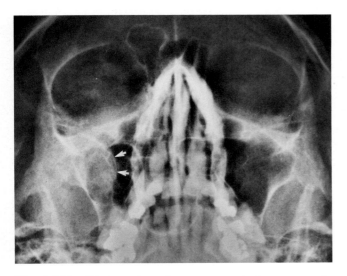

Fig. 2-301   Waters view shows expansile bony mass in the lateral wall of the right maxillary sinus. The mass has displaced the lateral sinus wall toward the midline *(arrow)*. Ossifying fibroma.

greater tendency to behave aggressively (grow faster and recur more quickly after surgery) and to expand internally toward the orbits, nasal fossae, and sinus cavities rather than to deform the outer surface bones (Figs. 2-301 and 2-302).

Cherubism

Cherubism is an autosomal dominant disease with variable expressivity often referred to as *congenital fibrous dysplasia.* However, some of the cases may arise as a result of a spontaneous mutation, which results in a non–sex linked dominant gene.[102] Usually a 50% to 75% penetrance exists in females and 100% in males. The disease appears between the ages of 6 months to 7 years and is characterized by bilateral fullness of the jaws and an upward-looking appearance caused by more exposed sclera in the lower portion of the eye. The disease often develops rapidly until age 7 years and then gradually regresses. First the mandible is involved and then, in about two thirds of the cases, the maxilla. Most of the radiographic changes occur in the mandible, where expansile cystic masses are seen in the an-

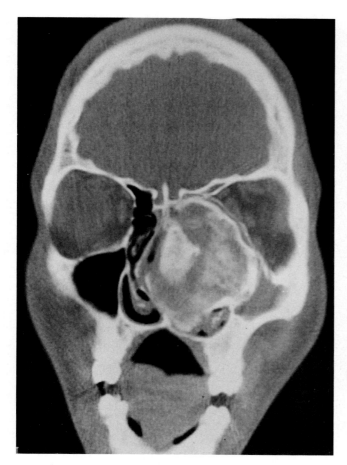

Fig. 2-302 Coronal CT scan shows expansile left nasal cavity mass that has extended into the left ethmoid sinuses, the maxillary sinus, and the orbit. The surrounding bone is intact and the central portion of the lesion has both ossified and nonossified segments. Ossifying fibroma.

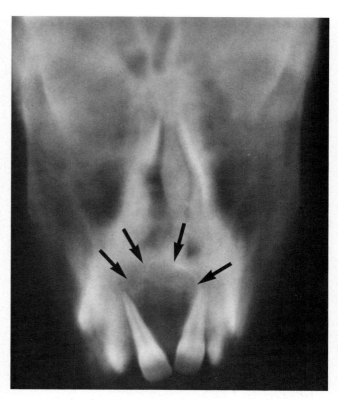

Fig. 2-303 Coronal multidirectional tomogram shows expansile erosion of the maxillary alveolus and hard palate (arrows). Central type giant cell granuloma.

gles and ramus. As the disease progresses to the maxilla, the sinus opacifies, and the orbital floor may be bulged upward. This latter finding is one of the causes of the upward-looking eye of cherubism.[102]

GIANT CELL TUMOR

True giant cell tumors (osteoclastomas) make up 4% to 5% of all primary bone neoplasms. Their biologic spectrum ranges from benign to malignant. More than 75% are located in the epiphyseal region of long bones, with half of the cases occurring about the knee. About 2% of all giant cell tumors occur in the head and neck, with most located in the sphenoid, temporal, and ethmoid bones. Symptoms depend on the tumor site and include headache (93%), diplopia (71%), decreased vision (43%), infraorbital hypesthesia (14%), proptosis (14%), and endocrinopathy (7%).[102,106,107]

On small biopsy specimens it may be impossible to distinguish these tumors confidently from giant cell (re-parative) granulomas and brown tumors of primary and secondary hyperparathyroidism.[106]

Approximately 10% to 15% of giant cell tumors show clinical or histologic evidence of malignancy. These malignant lesions can be primary or arise secondarily as a malignant transformation in a benign tumor. Almost all of the secondary type have been irradiated previously.

The recommended treatment of choice is complete surgical excision; since most tumors are not radiosensitive and this treatment may induce malignant transformation, radiation therapy should be reserved only for surgically inaccessible tumors. Based on all giant cell tumors occurring in the body, 30% to 50% recur with curettage, and most local failures recur within 2 years of initial therapy.[68]

Radiographically, the head and neck tumors are lytic lesions with no distinguishing features. Adjacent bone may be destroyed or remodeled, and the tumors enhance moderately on postcontrast CT scans.[106,107]

GIANT CELL GRANULOMA

Giant cell granuloma is the current name of choice because the older term reparative granuloma suggests a posttraumatic etiology, which usually is not the case.

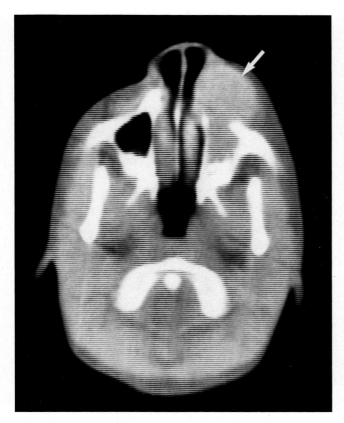

Fig. 2-304 Axial CT scan shows bulky lesion of the left antrum, which has destroyed the anterior maxillary wall and extended into the cheek *(arrow)*. Giant cell granuloma.

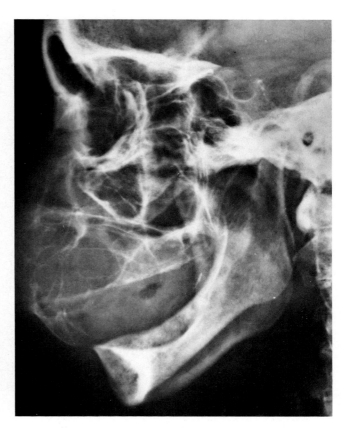

Fig. 2-305 Lateral view shows expansile, loculated, and destructive lesion of the maxilla. Aneurysmal bone cyst.

Most giant cell granulomas affect the mandible or the maxillary alveolus, and the tumor can be classified as peripheral or central. The peripheral (soft tissue) type is four times more common than the central type, and involves the gingiva and alveolar mucosa. Underlying bone is rarely involved. The tumor usually develops in women over 20 years of age and is related to a prior tooth extraction or ill-fitting denture. The central (bone) type can have extensive bone destruction and most often manifests in patients 10 to 20 years of age. Typically it has a multiloculated plain film appearance (Fig. 2-303).[68,106-109] The central type of giant cell granuloma is unrelated to preceding trauma.

These lesions may be histologically indistinguishable from the osteoclastoma or brown tumor of hyperparathyroidism, and curettage or surgery are the treatments of choice.

On CT scans these lesions enhance, are bulky, and can aggressively erode the maxillary sinus walls or have an expansile, remodeling appearance (Fig. 2-304).

ANEURYSMAL BONE CYST

An aneurysmal bone cyst is neither an aneurysm nor a true cyst. Rather, it is a benign, nonneoplastic os-

seous lesion characterized by the presence of numerous blood-filled, usually nonendothelialized, cavities. This lesion occurs mainly in females over the age of 20 years and represents only 1% to 2% of all primary bone "tumors." Between 3% and 12% of aneurysmal bone cysts occur in the head and neck, and they have been reported in the maxilla, orbit, ethmoid, and frontal bones.[63] They can be slowly or rapidly enlarging masses, and nonthrobbing pain is usually present. Surgical excision or curettage are the treatments of choice; in the jaws this treatment approach has resulted in a 26% recurrence rate. Recent use of cryosurgery and curettage has produced better results, with a recurrence rate of only 8%.[63] Radiographically, this lesion may be unilocular or demonstrate a multilocular "soap bubble" or "honeycomb" radiolucency. The peripheral bone margins demonstrate bone remodeling and destruction (Fig. 2-305).

THALASSEMIA

Thalassemia can reduce either the α-chains of globulin (α-thalassemia) or the beta-chains (β-thalassemia). The β-form has major osseous abnormalities.

Beta-thalassemia is an autosomal recessive disorder

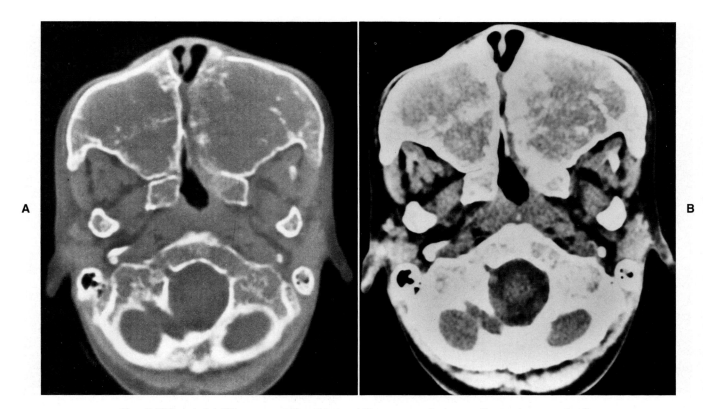

Fig. 2-306 Axial CT scans at **A,** wide and **B,** narrow window settings show markedly expanded maxilla with no development of the maxillary sinuses. The surrounding cortical bone is intact. The central portions of each maxilla are filled with expanded marrow. Thalessemia.

that occurs primarily in patients of Mediterranean origin. Patients who have thalassemia major have the most severe form of the disease, are homozygous for the trait, and have symptoms related to active marrow hyperplasia. Patients with thalassemia intermedia are also homozygous, but have a milder form of the disease. Patients with the mildest form, thalassemia minor, are heterozygous for the trait and are usually asymptomatic.

The classic radiographic changes of thalassemia in the skull include a thickened calvarium and a hair-on-end appearance. In the facial area, secondary to marrow expansion, sinus pneumatization is delayed and the maxilla expanded, which can result in both malocclusion and a cosmetic deformity. On CT scans a soft tissue–density material (marrow) is seen filling and expanding the maxilla, and this process may extend into the central skull base and mandible (Fig. 2-306).[110]

EWING'S SARCOMA

Ewing's sarcoma is a highly malignant, small, round cell tumor that accounts for 5% to 10% of all primary osseous malignancies. About 60% of cases occur in the lower extremities and pelvis. At the time of diagnosis,

almost 90% of patients are between 5 and 30 years of age. Only 1% to 4% of all Ewing's sarcomas occur in the head and neck. Most commonly, the mandible is involved, followed in frequency by the maxilla, calvarium, and cervical vertebrae.[63]

Patients typically have pain and localized swelling; radiographically a destructive lesion shows periosteal "onion skinning" or a "sunburst" appearance. The present treatment of choice is local excision with radiation therapy for the incompletely excised lesions. Micrometastases, which are present in 15% to 30% of patients, are treated with chemotherapy. The 5-year survival rates have risen from less than 10% in the prechemotherapy era to the current 60% to 79%. Ewing's sarcoma recurs locally in 13% to 20% of patients (65% at postmortem), usually coinciding with the completion of chemotherapy. The tumors metastasize to the lungs (86%), skeleton (69%), pleural cavity (46%), lymph nodes (46%), dura and meninges (27%), and central nervous system (12%).[63] Because of its rarity in the facial area, Ewing's sarcoma of the sinonasal cavities probably should be considered as a metastasis from an infraclavicular primary tumor until proven otherwise.

KAPOSI'S SARCOMA

Kaposi's sarcoma is a neoplastic vascular disorder that until recently was rare in the United States, but represented 12.8% of all cancers in the black population of central and south Africa. The incidence of this tumor has risen in recent years with the human immunodeficiency virus epidemic. It occurs in both mucosal and cutaneous sites; a few cases have been reported in the nasal mucosa. Fundamentally, Kaposi's sarcoma is not a sinonasal lesion; most of the head and neck tumors have been reported in the conjunctiva, oral cavity, and tonsils.[111]

ODONTOGENIC CYSTS

Odontogenic cysts arise from the various components of the dental apparatus. As a group, they are uncommon, and only those which grow sufficiently large to extend into the maxillary sinuses and palate will be discussed. Odontogenic cysts can be classified as follicular cysts, periodontal cysts, odontogenic keratocysts, and calcifying odontogenic cysts.

Follicular Cyst

These cysts can be subclassified as primordial or dentigerous. The *primordial cyst* represents only 5% of the follicular cysts and 1.75% to 6.9% of all odontogenic cysts. It results from degeneration of the enamel, and, since this occurs before any calcified dental structures have been formed and before the tooth germ has erupted, the cyst fills a place normally occupied by a tooth. Only if a primordial cyst arises from a supernumerary tooth germ will the patient have a normal complement of teeth.[111,112]

The cyst usually is an incidental finding on radiographs, since most are asymptomatic. The lesions are unilocular and well circumscribed. They are differentiated from residual cysts by the patient's history (with this latter cyst) of a prior tooth extraction in the area of the missing tooth. Treatment involves thorough curettage.

The *dentigerous cyst* represents 95% of follicular cysts and nearly 34% of all odontogenic cysts. Most occur in the second and third decades of life. The cyst arises in an unerupted tooth after the crown of the tooth has developed. Radiographically it appears as a cystic lesion into which the crown of the tooth projects. As the cyst grows, it pulls the unerupted tooth with it. When the cyst is large, the involved tooth may be displaced from its normally expected location. When small, dentigerous cysts are unilocular; however, when large, they may be multilocular and resorption of the roots of neighboring teeth is common.[112]

Radiographically, the dentigerous cyst must be distinguished from a normal dental follicle. If a dental fol-

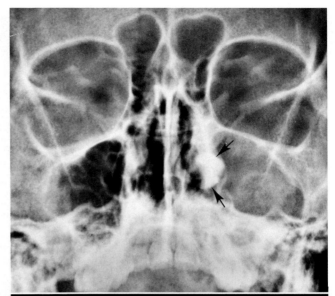

A

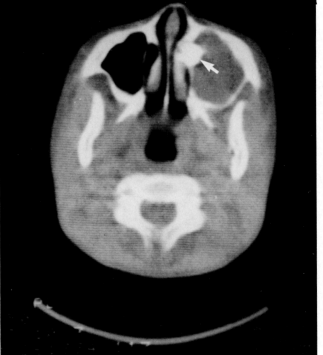

B

Fig. 2-307 **A,** Caldwell view and **B,** axial CT scan show expansile process in the left maxillary sinus with a tooth in the medial antral wall *(arrows).* Dentigerous cyst.

licle measures 2 cm or greater in width, it is highly likely that the unerupted tooth will become a dentigerous cyst. Similarly, a pericoronal space of 2.5 mm or more in width signals an 80% chance that the unerupted tooth will become a dentigerous cyst.[113] If the cyst breaks through into the maxillary sinus, it may grow rapidly, remodeling the antral walls. Often the in-

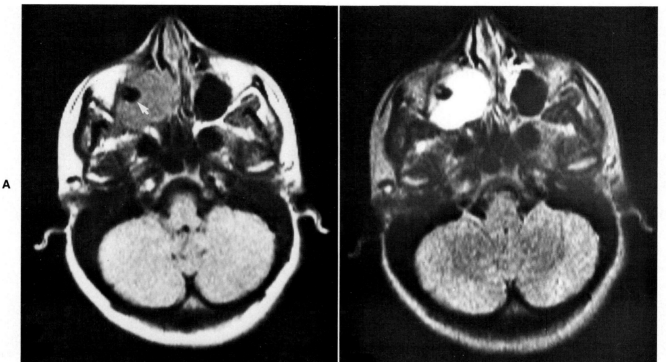

Fig. 2-308 **A,** Axial mixed image and **B,** T$_2$W MRI scans show expansile mass in the right maxillary sinus. The mass has a low-to-intermediate signal intensity in **A** and a high signal intensity in **B**. Within the mass is an area of low signal intensity (tooth) on all images *(arrow)*. Dentigerous cyst.

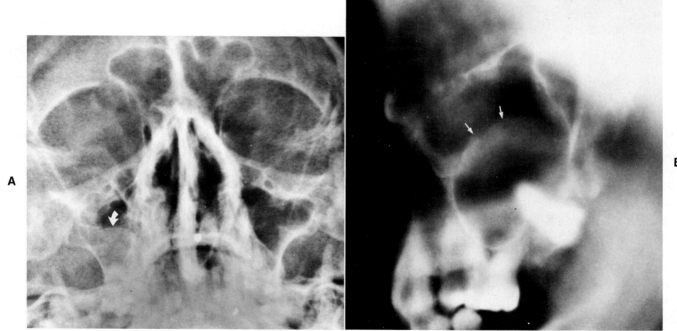

Fig. 2-309 **A,** Waters view shows mass in the lower right antrum that has elevated the inferior mucoperiosteal white line *(arrow)*. This indicates that the mass arose below the sinus in the alveolus. **B,** A lateral multidirectional tomogram shows cystic mass extending from a partially unerupted tooth and extending into the maxillary sinus. Radicular cyst.

ferior maxillary sinus cortex is elevated over portions of the cyst. In the axial view, this can be detected by noting what appears to be two posterior recess walls of the sinus. In these instances, the posterior bone is the true sinus wall, whereas the more anterior bone is the elevated sinus floor.

If multiple dentigerous cysts are present, the patient should be examined for the basal cell nevus syndrome.

An ameloblastoma may arise within the wall of the dentigerous cyst. This mural ameloblastoma is often diagnosed only by the pathologist; the radiographic findings in such cases are those of a simple dentigerous cyst.[112,113] On MRI the cyst fluid has intermediate signal intensities on T_1-weighted images and a high signal intensity on T_2-weighted images. The displaced tooth gives no signal on any imaging sequence. In this regard, the MRI appearance is similar to that of an antral aspergilloma (Figs. 2-307 and 2-308).

Periodontal Cyst

The apical periodontal, periapical, radicular, or dental cyst is the most common cyst of the jaws. It arises in erupted, infected teeth and usually is the sequela of a preexisting periapical granuloma. The cyst most commonly involves the maxillary teeth, and, if it breaks through into the maxillary sinus, it can grow rapidly, remodeling the antral walls and elevating portions of the inferior sinus cortex (Fig. 2-309).[112,113]

The residual periodontal cyst generally results from a retained periapical cyst after the involved tooth has been extracted. The residual cyst also occurs most often in the maxilla and is differentiated from a primordial cyst by the history of a tooth extraction. Treatment of these cysts consists of simple enucleation.[112]

Odontogenic Keratocyst

Most odontogenic keratocysts are of the parakeratotic type. These aggressively growing lesions tend to recur (12% to 62.5%) after removal. These cysts are associated with Marfan's syndrome and the basal cell nevus syndrome, and they may have a neoplastic potential.[112]

The parakeratotic odontogenic keratocyst represents 3.3% to 16.5% of all jaw cysts, and most occur in patients in their second and third decades of life. The mandible is affected two to four times more often than the maxilla, and most lesions occur in the posterior aspect of the jaws. In about half the patients, the lesion is asymptomatic, and in the other half pain is the most frequent complaint. The symptoms last an average 22 months. In the maxilla, parakeratotic odontogenic keratocysts can cause nasal obstruction and extend into the maxillary sinus.[112]

These cysts may be destructive and invade the adjacent bone or have a thin reactive sclerotic bony rim, and they can have smooth or scalloped margins. The re-

currence rate does not correlate with standard treatments (marsupialization or enucleation). However, no recurrences have been reported of cysts removed in one piece.

In 13% of cases the keratocyst is of the orthokeratotic type. These cysts are less aggressive, recur infrequently, and virtually all are unilocular.[112]

Calcifying Odontogenic Cyst

This cyst has a variety of names, including keratinizing ameloblastoma, keratinizing and calcifying ameloblastoma, and melanotic ameloblastic odontoma. The lesion probably occupies an anomalous pathologic position between that of a cyst and that of a neoplasm.[112] The calcifying odontogenic cyst is an uncommon lesion, affecting the maxilla and mandible equally. About 78% are intraosseous and 22% are confined to the soft tissues. They are either unilocular or multilocular radiolucent cysts that frequently contain radiopaque material ranging from small flecks to large masses. The lesion can be well circumscribed or poorly demarcated, and it radiographically resembles a calcifying epithelial odontogenic tumor, an odontoma, an ossifying fibroma, and fibrous dysplasia.[112]

Treatment can be by curettage, enucleation, or conservative surgical excision; unlike the keratocyst, recurrences are unlikely.

FISSURAL CYSTS

In general, fissural cysts are believed to be derived from entrapped epithelium in the fusion lines of the frontonasal and maxillary processes during facial development. As a group, fissural cysts are uncommon. They are lined by stratified squamous epithelium, respiratory epithelium, or a combination of the two. The capsule is composed of fibrous connective tissue. Because of their histologic similarities, fissural cysts are distinguished from one another by anatomic location.[112]

Fissural cysts are classified as midline or lateral cysts (Fig. 2-310). Those occurring along the midline fusion line of the maxillary processes (nasopalatine cysts [incisive canal cysts, cysts of the palatine papilla] and median palatal cysts) do not extend into the paranasal sinuses. Radiographically, they appear as well-delineated cystic lesions within the hard palate (Fig. 2-311).

Of the lateral cysts (nasolabial or nasoalveolar cysts and globulomaxillary cysts), only the latter involve the maxillary sinuses. The nasoalveolar cyst is entirely a soft tissue lesion and thus is not strictly a true fissural cyst. It appears as a small cystic mass in the upper lip and lateral aspect of the nose. The globulomaxillary cyst is found between the maxillary lateral incisor and canine teeth and is believed to be either a true fissural cyst or possibly of odontogenic origin. These cysts represent less than 3% of all cysts of the jaws and 20% of

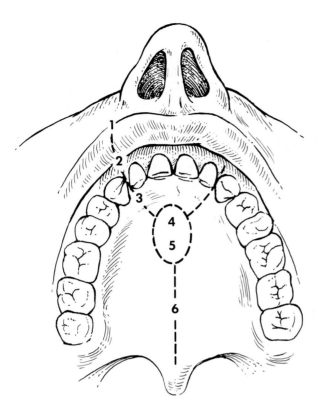

Fig. 2-310 Diagram of distribution of fissural cyst. *1,* Nasolabial cyst, *2,* nasoalveolar cyst, *3,* globulomaxillary cyst, *4,* nasopalatine cyst, *5,* cyst of palatine papilla, and *6,* median palatal cyst.

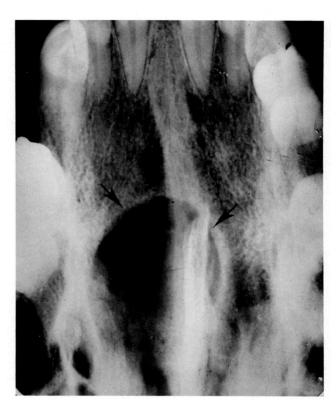

Fig. 2-311 Intraoral occlusal film shows well demarcated cyst *(arrows)* of the palate. Fissural cyst.

the maxillary fissural cysts. Most occur in patients under 30 years of age, and the lesions are usually painless unless secondary infection develops.[112,114]

Radiographically, the globulomaxillary cyst appears as an inverted pear-shaped radiolucency in the maxillary alveolus. The cyst often pushes apart the roots of the lateral incisor and canine teeth and, when large, can distort the lower anterior aspect of the maxillary sinus.

ODONTOGENIC TUMORS

Odontogenic tumors, like odontogenic cysts, arise from the dental apparatus; unlike the cysts, these tumors also mimic various stages of odontogenesis. A whole host of tumors of various histologic types exists; this section describes only the ameloblastoma, cementoma, odontoma, and fibromyxoma, since these are the most common odontogenic tumors to involve the paranasal sinuses.

Ameloblastoma

This tumor is derived from the odontogenic apparatus, but does not undergo differentiation to the point that a hard structure is formed. The prior terminology for this lesion, adamantinoma, suggests a hard tumor

and thus its use has been abandoned.

Although the ameloblastoma is the most common tumor that arises from the epithelial components of the embryonic tooth, this tumor comprises only 1% of all jaw cysts and tumors. Most occur in patients in the third and fourth decades of life, and 90% of the maxillary lesions involve the premolar-molar area. Few, if any, early clinical symptoms appear. As the tumor enlarges, a painless swelling forms, and in the maxilla large lesions have caused nasal obstruction. Other signs and symptoms include pain, bleeding, unhealed extraction sites, trismus, and neural involvement.[115,116]

Ameloblastomas represent 17% of dentigerous cysts; however, the percentage drops notably in patients older than 30 years of age. This drop suggests that the potential for ameloblastoma formation is lost as the cyst's odontogenic epithelium changes to squamous epithelium as the patient ages.[116] Primordial and residual cysts rarely convert to ameloblastomas.

Radiographically, the ameloblastoma appears as a multiloculated, lytic lesion with no mineralized components. If the tumor extends into the antrum, the sinus is clouded and the sinus walls are remodeled and destroyed. On CT scans these tumors tend to have a nonenhancing, nonhomogeneous appearance, and on MRI

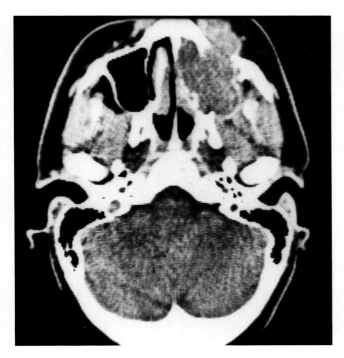

Fig. 2-312 Axial CT scan shows partially expansile and partially destructive mass in the lower left maxillary sinus. Ameloblastoma.

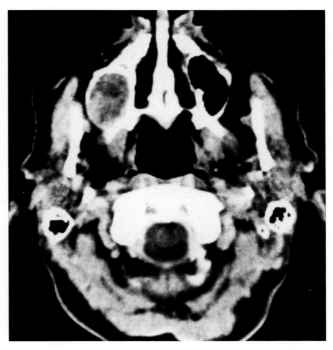

Fig. 2-313 Axial CT scan shows expansile nonhomogeneous mass in the right maxillary alveolus and lower antrum. Ameloblastoma.

they have nonhomogeneous mixed signal intensities. On T_1- and proton density-weighted images, these tumors demonstrate intermediate-intensity signals, whereas on T_2-weighted studies ameloblastomas have variable intermediate and high signal intensities (Figs. 2-312 and 2-313).

Ameloblastomas occur in two forms, the more common follicular and the plexiform. Although histologically benign, slow-growing, and nonmetastasizing, these tumors tend to recur and can even cause death secondary to skull base invasion with extension to the brain. In rare instances, two malignant variants may be found, the malignant ameloblastoma and the ameloblastic carcinoma.

The malignant ameloblastoma histologically resembles benign ameloblastoma, except that the former metastasizes. These metastases are also histologically benign and occur after a long history of multiple unsuccessful attempts at surgical cure or after radiation therapy. Most metastases go to the lungs, pleura, and regional lymph nodes.[116]

The ameloblastic carcinoma is an obviously histologic malignancy, and the metastases are less well differentiated than the primary tumor.

Complete surgical resection is the treatment of choice for all ameloblastomas. Chemotherapy appears to be relatively ineffective against both the primary lesion and the metastases, and most lesions are not radiosensitive.[116]

Cementoma

These tumors are believed to arise from the mesodermal periodontal ligament. This ligament surrounds and attaches the roots of the teeth to the adjacent alveolar bone. Its cells can form cementum, bone, and fibrous tissue. The four distinct tumor types include the cementifying fibroma, benign cementoblastoma, periapical cemental dysplasia, and gigantiform cementoma.

The *cementifying fibroma (ossifying fibroma)* is initially an asymptomatic lesion that is found on routine dental radiographs. When large, these lesions can produce a firm, painless swelling and facial asymmetry. Most lesions occur in the mandibular-premolar-molar region; however, the maxilla can be affected. Because cementifying fibromas contain varying amounts of calcified material, their radiographic appearance varies from a radiolucent process to a radiopaque lesion.[116] In all cases the lesion is well demarcated from the adjacent bone, and in most instances it is unilocular and ovoid. The presence of distinct margins differentiates this lesion from fibrous dysplasia, which is histologically similar, but has indistinct borders. Conservative excision is the treatment of choice and recurrences are rare (Figs. 2-314 and 2-315).

These lesions have been reported not only in the maxillary sinuses, but also in the ethmoid sinuses. Whether this latter occurrence results from differentiation of primitive mesenchymal cells or an ectopic periodontal ligament is an unresolved point; however, this

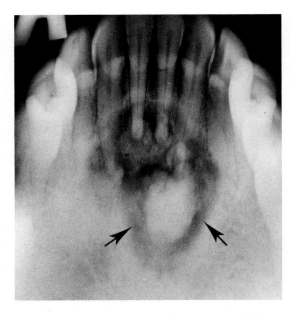

Fig. 2-314 Intraoral occlusal film shows calcified mass with a surrounding lucent zone in the palate *(arrows).* Note the small radiopague densities surrounding the tooth roots (hypercementosis). Cementoma.

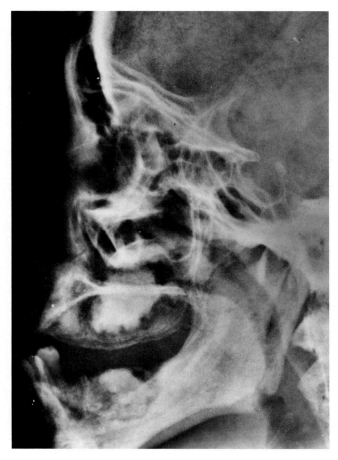

Fig. 2-315 Lateral view shows calcified mass with a surrounding lucent zone in the maxillary alveolus. Cementoma.

lesion is included in the differential diagnosis of fibrous dysplasia and meningioma.

The *benign cementoblastoma (true cementoma)* is an uncommon cementum-producing lesion that is fused to the root(s) of a tooth. Most of the teeth affected are in the premolar-molar region of the jaws and the lesion may disrupt the tooth innervation by surrounding the root apex. As a result, many of the involved teeth are not viable.[116]

Radiographically, these lesions appear as well-defined radiopaque mass(es) that are continuous with the root apices of affected teeth. A zone of lucency, or "halo," surrounds each lesion. The radiographic differential diagnosis is primarily with the condition known as *hypercementosis*. In this process, excessive amounts of cementum accumulate along the surface of the involved tooth root(s). Hypercementosis is associated with Paget's disease, periapical inflammation, and elongation of a tooth as a result of the loss of its antagonistic opposing tooth.[116]

Periapical cemental dysplasia (cementoma, periapical fibrous dysplasia) is more a reactive lesion than a true neoplasm. It is the most frequently encountered cementoid lesion and occurs almost exclusively in females. Initially the lesion appears radiolucent, similar to a periapical cyst or granuloma, but then it calcifies. The involved tooth is always vital to testing and the radiopaque mass is separated from the tooth root by a narrow radiolucent zone, rather than being on the root surface as in hypercementosis. The cementoma is a benign self-limiting process and surgical excision is not necessary.

The *gigantiform cementoma (familial multiple cementoma)* is a rare tumor that may be neoplastic or dysplastic. It is characterized by nodular, irregularly shaped radiopacities in several portions of one or both jaws. Asymptomatic expansion of the cortical plates is frequent, with concomitant, simple bone cysts. The term *florid osseous dysplasia* has been proposed as a better name for this entity, which is self-limiting, affects only the alveolar process, and seems to be independent of teeth. Paget's disease can be ruled out on the basis of a normal serum alkaline phosphatase level in patients with gigantiform cementoma. Treatment depends on the clinical course. The most common complication is the development of low-grade osteomyelitis in the edentulous areas.

Odontoma

Odontomas contain epithelial and mesenchymal components of the dental apparatus that have complete differentiation, resulting in the presence of enamel, dentin, cementum, and pulp. The complex odontoma has a haphazard arrangement of the elements. In compound odontomas the elements have a normal relationship to

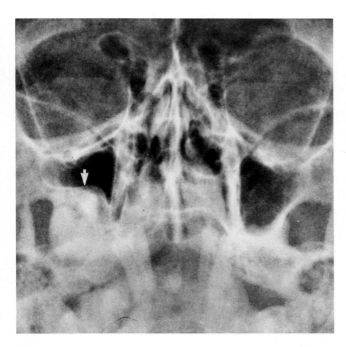

Fig. 2-316 Caldwell view shows mass in the maxillary alveolus that has pushed up the inferior mucoperiosteal white line *(arrow).* The mass itself has several very dense areas. Complex odontoma.

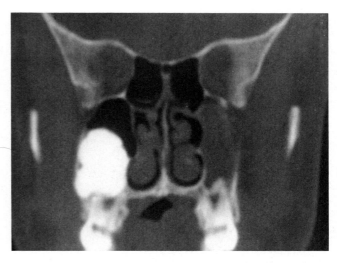

Fig. 2-317 Coronal CT scan shows very dense mass arising from the right maxillary alveolus and extending into the right antrum. Complex odontoma.

one another.[116] Complex and compound lesions occur equally, and 95% are detected in the second decade of life. Most lesions are asymptomatic, and 75% occur in the maxilla. Radiographically, the complex odontoma appears as an amorphous radiopacity. The compound odontoma has anywhere from 3 to 2000 miniature teeth (or denticles) with only single roots or no roots. All odontomas are surrounded by a thin radiolucent halo that represents the fibrous capsule. Treatment involves complete surgical excision; recurrences are rare (Figs. 2-316 to 2-318).

Fibromyxoma

This term applies to several lesions, which, as a group, are fibrous variants of a myxoma. These tumors include the nonossifying fibroma, the desmoplastic fibroma, and the odontogenic fibroma.[117] Possibly the odontogenic myxoma also should be included in this group. Fibromyxomas tend to occur in the second and third decades of life. When they appear in the maxilla and paranasal sinuses, these tumors can be locally aggressive and have a high recurrence rate.

Radiographically, fibromyxomas are primarily expansile when they involve the sinuses, although focal areas of aggressive bone destruction may be present. These lesions usually have flecks or thin strands of calcification dispersed within the tumor substance. Complete surgical excision is the treatment of choice (Fig. 2-319).

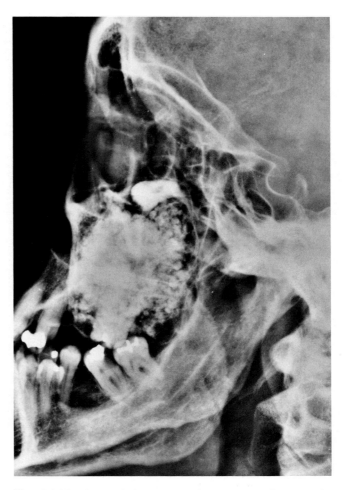

Fig. 2-318 Lateral view shows large expansile mass in the left maxillary alveolus and antrum. There are innumerable discrete toothlike densities (denticles). Compound odontoma.

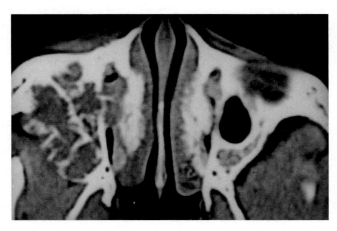

Fig. 2-319 Axial CT scan shows partially destructive and partially expansile mass in the right maxillary sinus with lacelike areas of calcification. Fibromyxoma.

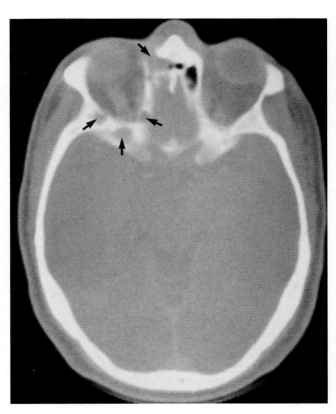

Fig. 2-321 Axial CT scan shows multiple discrete areas of lytic bone destruction *(arrows)*. Metastatic lung carcinoma.

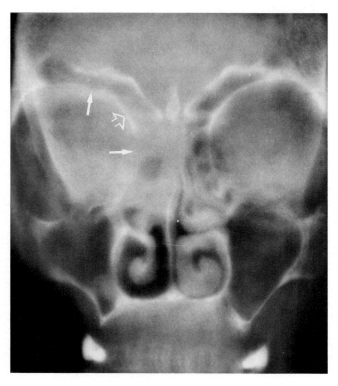

Fig. 2-320 Coronal multidirectional tomogram shows two discrete areas of bone destruction *(arrows)* in the medial and superior orbital walls. A portion of intact bone *(open arrow)* remains between the destructive areas. Metastatic lung carcinoma.

METASTASES TO THE SINONASAL CAVITIES

Metastasis from primary tumors below the clavicles to the sinonasal cavities is infrequent. The reported cases number only about 100. The most common primary tumor with signs and symptoms referable to the sinonasal cavities is the renal cell carcinoma. Tumors found in the sinonasal cavities precede the diagnosis of the primary tumor in 8% of patients.[118] Next in frequency are tumors of the lung and breast; these are followed considerably less frequently by tumors of the testis, prostate, and gastrointestinal tract.[2,119] The average age of patients with metastases from renal cell tumors to the sinonasal cavities is near the end of the sixth decade of life, similar to that of patients with breast carcinoma metastases. Bronchogenic and gastrointestinal tract metastases generally appear in the fifth decade of life. Symptoms of metastases are nonspecific, except for the renal cell lesions, which commonly cause epistaxis.[119]

The presence of metastases in the sinonasal cavities does not appear to alter the prognosis in patients with generalized carcinomatosis. However, if a sinonasal metastasis is the only one from a primary renal cell carcinoma, the surgical removal of the metastasis and the primary tumor may result in a good survival time.[120]

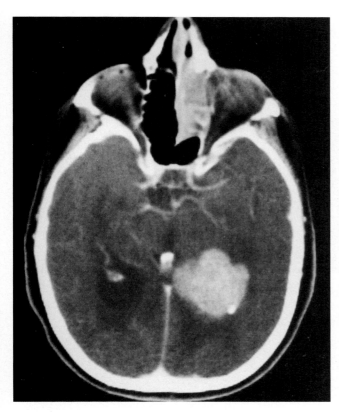

Fig. 2-322 Axial contrast enhanced CT scan shows enhancing mass in the left ethmoid sinuses and nasal cavity and a second mass in the occipital horn. Metastatic melanoma.

Squamous and basal cell carcinomas of facial and scalp skin may metastasize to the central skull base, usually along neurogenic pathways. These metastases can occur despite clean specimen margins of the resected primary skin tumor. In these cases, the most accurate prognostic finding is perineural tumor invasion in the primary lesion.[121-123]

Skin melanomas in rare instances metastasize to the sinonasal cavities. Along with the metastases from renal cell carcinomas, these lesions are the most vascular metastases and often manifest with epistaxis.

On CT metastases from lung, breast, distal genitourinary tract, and gastrointestinal tract tumors are aggressive, bone-destroying soft tissue masses that enhance minimally, if at all. The metastases are usually indistinguishable from a primary sinonasal squamous cell carcinoma. By comparison, metastases from primary renal cell carcinomas and melanomas are enhancing masses that may remodel the sinonasal walls, as well as destroy them.

Prostate carcinoma is one of the few primary tumors that may give a purely blastic metastasis to the facial bones and skull. Although a soft tissue mass may occur, often only a sclerotic, slightly thickened bone with an

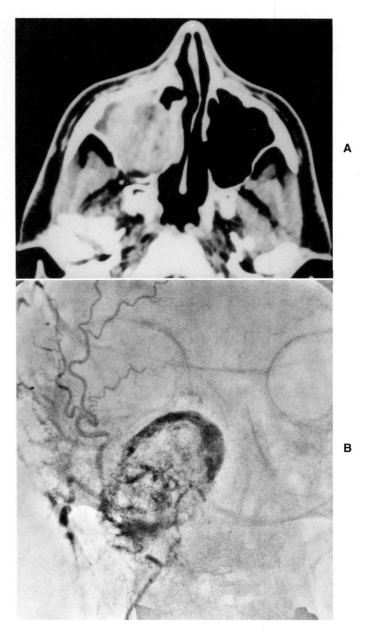

A

B

Fig. 2-323 **A,** Axial post contrast CT scan and **B,** coronal subtraction angiogram show expansile enhancing and vascular mass in the right maxillary sinus. Metastatic hypernephroma.

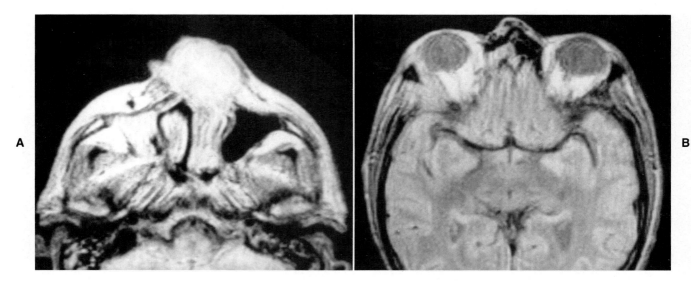

Fig. 2-324 Axial mixed image MRI scans through the level of **A,** the lower nasal fossa and **B,** the orbits show two distinct masses *(arrows);* one in the nose and one in the right lateral orbital wall. Both masses are homogeneous and of an intermediate-to-high signal intensity. Metastatic lung carcinoma.

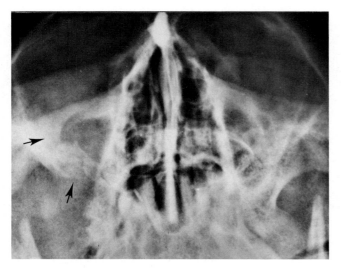

Fig. 2-325 Waters view shows destructive lesion of the lateral wall of the right antrum *(arrows).* This could be a squamous cell carcinoma but is instead metastatic ovarian carcinoma.

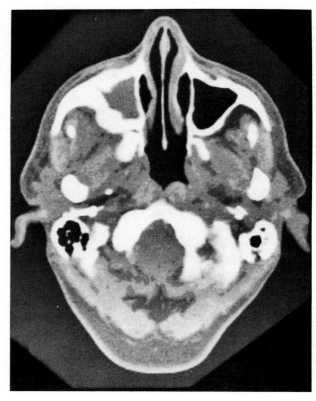

Fig. 2-326 Axial CT scan shows thickened, sclerotic bone in the right maxilla, zygoma, and lateral pterygoid plate. The right antrum is obstructed. Metastatic prostate carcinoma.

abnormal, irregular trabecular pattern is seen. On CT scans this pure bone disease can be overlooked unless wide windows are used to evaluate the bone.

The most important radiographic indication of metastasis is the presence of more than one lesion, particularly because sinonasal tumors usually do not erode multiple areas of bone. Rather, contiguous sites of bone erosion spread from an area of initial involvement. Thus two areas of bone erosion with intervening normal bone suggests metastatic disease (Figs. 2-320 to 2-326).

REFERENCES

1. Batsakis JG: Tumors of the head and neck: clinical and pathological considerations, ed 2, Baltimore, 1979, The Williams & Wilkins Co, pp 177-187.
2. Barnes L, Verbin RS, and Gnepp DR: Diseases of the nose, paranasal sinuses, and nasopharynx. In Barnes L, editor: Surgical pathology of the head and neck, vol 1, New York, 1985, Marcel Dekker, Inc, pp 403-451.
3. Harrison DFN: The management of malignant tumors of the nasal sinuses, Otolaryngol Clin North Am 4:159, 1971.
4. Harrison DFN: Problems in surgical management of neoplasms arising in the paranasal sinus, J Laryngol 90:69, 1976.
5. Jeans WD, Gilani S, and Bullimore J: The effect of CT scanning on staging of tumours of the paranasal sinuses, Clin Radiol 33:173, 1982.
6. Curtin HD, Williams R, and Johnson J: CT of perineural tumor extension: pterygopalatine fossa, AJNR 5:731, 1984.
7. Lloyd GAS et al: Magnetic resonance imaging in the evaluation of nose and paranasal sinus disease, Br J Radiol 60:957, 1987.
8. Som PM et al: Sinonasal tumors and inflammatory tissues: differentiation with MR, Radiology 167:803, 1988.
9. Dubois PJ et al: Tomography in expansile lesions of the nasal and paranasal sinuses, Radiology 125:149, 1977.
10. Som PM and Shugar JMA: When to question the diagnosis of anaplastic carcinoma, Mt Sinai J Med 48:230, 1981.
11. Som PM and Shugar JMA: The significance of bone expansion associated with the diagnosis of malignant tumors of the paranasal sinuses, Radiology 136:97, 1980.
12. Hyams VJ: Papillomas of the nasal cavity and paranasal sinuses: a clinicopathologic study of 315 cases, Ann Otol Rhinol Laryngol 80:192, 1971.
13. Lasser A, Rothfeld PR, and Shapiro RS: Epithelial papilloma and squamous cell carcinoma of the nasal cavity and paranasal sinuses: a clinicopathologic study, Cancer 1976 38:2503, 1976.
14. Vrabec DP: The inverted schneiderian papilloma: a clinical and pathological study, Laryngoscope 85:186, 1975.
15. Norris HJ: Papillary lesions of the nasal cavity and paranasal sinuses. I. Exophytic (squamous) papillomas: a study of 28 cases, Laryngoscope 72:1784, 1962.
16. Momose KJ et al: Radiological aspects of inverted papilloma, Radiology 134:73, 1980.
17. Lund VJ and Lloyd GAS: Radiological changes associated with inverted papillomas of the nose and paranasal sinuses, Br J Radiol 57:455, 1984.
18. Apostol JV and Frazell EL: Juvenile nasopharyngeal angiofibroma, Cancer 18:869, 1965.
19. Som PM et al: The angiomatous polyp and the angiofibroma: two different lesions, Radiology 144:329, 1982.
20. Som PM et al: The nonspecificity of the antral bowing sign in maxillary sinus pathology, JCAT 5:350, 1981.
21. Bryan RN, Sessions RB, and Horowitz BL: Radiographic management of juvenile angiofibromas, AJNR 2:157, 1981.
22. Som PM et al: Extracranial tumor vascularity: determination by dynamic CT scanning. II. The unit approach, Radiology 154:407, 1985.
23. Lufkin R et al: Magnetic resonance imaging of vascular tumors of the head and neck, Clear Imaging 1:14, 1987.
24. Fitzpatrick PJ, Briant DR, and Berman JM: The nasopharyngeal angiofibroma, Arch Otolaryngol 106:234, 1980.
25. See reference 1, pp 139-143.
26. Barton RT: Nickel carcinogenesis of the respiratory tract, J Otolaryngol 6:412, 1977.
27. Penzin KH, Lefkowitch JH, and Hui RM: Bilateral nasal squamous carcinoma arising in papillomatosis: report of a case developing after chemotherapy for leukemia, Cancer 1981 48:2375, 1981.
28. Weimert TA, Batsakis JG, and Rice DH: Carcinoma of the nasal septum, J Laryngol Otol 92:209, 1978.
29. Baredes S, Cho HT, and Som ML: Total maxillectomy. In Blitzer A, Lawson W, and Friedman WH, editors: Surgery of the paranasal sinuses, Philadelphia, 1985, WB Saunders Co, pp 204-216.
30. Harrison DFN: Critical look at the classification of maxillary sinus carcinoma, Ann Otol 87:3, 1978.
31. Chaudhry AP, Gorlin RJ, and Mosser DG: Carcinoma of the antrum: a clinical and histopathologic study, Oral Surg 13:269, 1960.
32. Larsson LG and Martensson G: Maxillary antral cancers, JAMA 219:342, 1972.
33. St Pierre S and Baker SR: Squamous cell carcinoma of the maxillary sinus: analysis of 66 cases, Head Neck Surg 5:508, 1983.
34. Som ML: Surgical management of carcinomas of the maxilla, Arch Otolaryngol 99:270, 1974.
35. Ogura JH and Schenck NL: Unusual nasal tumors: problems in diagnosis and treatment, Otolaryngol Clin North Am 6:813, 1973.
36. Conley J: Concepts in head and neck surgery, Stuttgart, Germany, 1970, Georg Thieme Verlag.
37. Spiro RH et al: Tumors of minor salivary origin: a clinicopathologic study of 492 cases, Cancer 31:117, 1973.
38. Conley J and Dingman DL: Adenoid cystic carcinoma in the head and neck (cylindroma), Arch Otolaryngol 100:81, 1974.
39. Acheson ED, Gowdell RH, and Jolles B: Nasal cancer in the Northamptonshire boot and shoe industry, Br Med J 1:385, 1970.
40. Hadfield EH: A study of adenocarcinoma of the paranasal sinuses in woodworkers in the furniture industry, Ann R Coll Surg Engl 46:301, 1970.
41. See reference 1, pp 76-99.
42. Klintenberg C et al: Adenocarcinoma of the ethmoid sinuses: a review of 38 cases with special reference to wood dust exposure, Cancer 54:482, 1984.
43. Compagno J and Wong RT: Intranasal mixed tumors (pleomorphic adenomas): a clinicopathologic study of 40 cases, Am J Clin Pathol 68:213, 1977.
44. Freedman HM et al: Malignant melanoma of the nasal cavity and paranasal sinuses, Arch Otolaryngol 97:322, 1973.
45. Batsakis JG and Sciubba J: Pathology. In Blitzer A, Lawson W, and Friedman WH, editors: Surgery of the paranasal sinuses, Philadelphia, 1985, WB Saunders Co, pp 74-113.
46. Holdcraft JH and Gallagher JC: Malignant melanomas of the nasal and paranasal sinus mucosa, Ann Otol Rhinol Laryngol 78:1, 1969.
47. Gallagher JC: Upper respiratory melanoma pathology and growth rate, Ann Otol 70:551, 1970.
48. See reference 2, pp 408-451, 659-724.
49. Som PM et al: Parapharyngeal space masses: an updated protocol based upon 104 cases, Radiology 153:149, 1984.
50. Oberman HA and Sullenger G: Neurogenous tumors of the head and neck, Cancer 20:1992, 1967.
51. D'Agostino AN, Soule EH, and Miller RH: Sarcomas of the peripheral nerves and somatic soft tissues associated with multiple neurofibromatosis (von Recklinghausen's disease), Cancer 16:1015, 1963.
52. Hunt JC and Pugh DG: Skeletal lesions in neurofibromatosis, Radiology 76:1, 1961.
53. Guccion JG and Enzinger FM: Malignant schwannoma associated with von Recklinghausen's neurofibromatosis, Virchows Arch 383:43, 1979.
54. Cadotte M: Malignant granular cell myoblastoma, Cancer 33:1417, 1974.
55. Elkon D et al: Esthesioneuroblastoma, Cancer 44:1087, 1979.

56. Kadish S, Goodman M, and Wine CC: Olfactory neuroblastoma: a clinical analysis of 17 cases, Cancer 37:1571, 1976.

57. Som PM et al: Ethmoid sinus disease: CT evaluation in 400 cases. III. Craniofacial resection, Radiology 159:605, 1986.

58. Regenbogen VS et al: Hyperostotic esthesioneuroblastoma: CT and MR findings, JCAT 12:52, 1988.

59. Stowens D and Lin TH: Melanotic progonoma of the brain, Hum Pathol 5:105, 1974.

60. Farr HW et al: Extracranial meningioma, J Surg Oncol 5:411, 1973.

61. Lopez DA, Silvers DN, and Helwig EB: Cutaneous meningioma: a clinicopathologic study, Cancer 34:728, 1974.

62. Som PM et al: "Benign" metastasizing meningioma, AJNR 8:129, 1987.

63. See Reference 2, pp 912-1044.

64. Shugar JMA et al: Primary chordoma of the maxillary sinus, Laryngoscope 90:1825, 1980.

65. Wright D: Nasopharyngeal and cervical chordoma: some aspects of their development and treatment, J Laryngol 81:1337, 1967.

66. Yuh WTC et al: MR imaging of unusual chordomas, JCAT 12:30, 1988.

67. Enziger FM and Weiss SW: Soft tissue tumors, ed 2, St Louis, 1988, The CV Mosby Co.

68. See reference 2, pp 725-880.

69. Rosenberg SA et al: Sarcomas of the soft tissue and bone. In De Vita VT, Hellman S, and Rosenberg SA, editors: Cancer: principles and practice of oncology, Philadelphia, 1982, JB Lippincott Co, pp 1036-1093.

70. Bortnick E: Neoplasms of the nasal cavity, Otolaryngol Clin North Am 6:801, 1973.

71. Lee Y-Y et al: Lymphomas of the head and neck: CT findings at initial presentation, AJNR 8:665, 1987.

72. Wilder WH, Harner SG, and Banks PM: Lymphoma of the nose and paranasal sinuses, Arch Otolaryngol 109:310, 1983.

73. Harnsberger HR et al: Non-Hodgkin's lymphoma of the head and neck: CT evaluation of nodal and extranodal sites, AJNR 8:673, 1987.

74. Kondo M et al: Computed tomography of sinonasal non-Hodgkin's lymphoma, JCAT 8:216, 1984.

75. Duncavage JA, Campbell BH, and Hanson GH: Diagnosis of malignant lymphomas of the nasal cavity, paranasal sinuses and nasopharynx, Laryngoscope 93:1276, 1983.

76. See reference 2, pp 1045-1209.

77. Pomeranz SJ et al: Granulocytic sarcoma (chloroma): CT manifestations, Radiology 155:167, 1985.

78. Castro EB, Lewis JS, and Strong EW: Plasmacytoma of paranasal sinuses and nasal cavity, Arch Otolaryngol 97:326, 1973.

79. Fu Y-S and Perzin KH: Nonepithelial tumors of the nasal cavity, paranasal sinuses and nasopharynx: a clinicopathologic study—IX plasmacytomas, Cancer 42:2399, 1978.

80. Kondo M et al: Extramedullary plasmacytoma of the sinonasal cavities: CT evaluation, JCAT 10:841, 1986.

81. Young JL Jr and Miller RW: Incidence of malignant tumors in US children, J Pediatr 86:254, 1975.

82. Hajdu SI: Soft tissue sarcomas: classification and natural history, Cancer 31:271, 1981.

83. Enzinger FM and Shiraki M: Alveolar rhabdomyosarcoma: an analysis of 110 cases, Cancer 24:18-31, 1969.

84. Makishima K, Iwasaki H, and Horie A: Alveolar rhabdomyosarcoma of the ethmoid sinus, Laryngoscope 85:400, 1975.

85. Merrick RE, Rhone DP, and Chilis TJ: Malignant fibrous histiocytoma of the maxillary sinus, Arch Otolaryngol 106:365, 1980.

86. Dooms GC et al: Lipomatous tumors and tumors with fatty component: MR imaging potential and comparison of MR and CT results, Radiology 157:479, 1985.

87. Dropkin LR, Tang CK, and Williams JR: Leiomyosarcoma of the nasal cavity and paranasal sinuses, Ann Otol Rhinol Laryngol 85:399, 1976.

88. McLeod AJ, Zornoza J, and Shirkhoda A: Leiomyosarcoma: computed tomographic findings, Radiology 152:133, 1984.

89. Enzinger FM and Smith BH: Hemangiopericytoma: an analysis of 106 cases, Hum Pathol 7:61, 1976.

90. Kauffman SL and Stout AP: Hemangiopericytoma in children, Cancer 13:695, 1960.

91. Evans HL, Ayala AG, and Romsdahl MM: Prognostic factors in chondrosarcoma of bone: a clinicopathologic analysis with emphasis on histologic grading, Cancer 40:818, 1977.

92. Chaudhry AP et al: Chondrogenic tumors of the jaws, Am J Surg 102:403, 1961.

93. McCoy JM and McConnel FMS: Otolaryngol 107:125, 1981.

94. Gay I, Elidan J, and Kopolovic J: Chondrosarcoma of the skull base, Ann Otol Rhinol Laryngol 90:53, 1981.

95. Shugar JMA et al: Intramuscular head and neck myxoma: report of a case and review of the literature, Laryngoscope 97:105, 1987.

96. Fu Y-S and Perzin KH: Nonepthelial tumors of the nasal cavity, paranasal sinuses and nasopharynx: a clinicopathologic study, Cancer 33:1289, 1974.

97. Shugar JMA et al: Nontraumatic cerebrospinal fluid rhinorrhea, Laryngoscope 41:114, 1981.

98. Osguthorpe JD and Hungerford GD: Benign osteoblastoma of the maxillary sinus, Head Neck Surg 6:605, 1983.

99. Som PM et al: Osteoblastoma of the ethmoid sinus: the fourth reported case, Arch Otolaryngol 105:623, 1979.

100. Coscina WF and Lee BCP: Concurrent osteoblastoma and aneurysmal bone cyst of the ethmoid sinus: case report, CT J Comput Tomogr 9:347, 1985.

101. Oot RF, Parizel PM, and Weber AL: Computed tomography of osteogenic sarcoma of nasal cavity and paranasal sinuses, JCAT 10:409, 1986.

102. See reference 2, pp 883-1044.

103. Som PM et al: Paget disease of the calvaria and facial bones with an osteosarcoma of the maxilla: CT and MR findings, JCAT 11:887, 1987.

104. Dehner LP: Fibro-osseous lesions of bone. In Ackerman LU, Spjut HJ, and Abell MR, editors: Bones and joints, International Academy of Pathology, Monograph No 17, Baltimore, 1976, The Williams & Wilkins Co, pp 209-235.

105. Schwartz DT and Alpert M: The malignant transformation of fibrous dysplasia, Am J Med Sci 274:35, 1964.

106. Som PM, Lawson W, and Cohen BA: Giant cell lesions of the facial bones, Radiology 147:129, 1983.

107. Rhea JT and Weber AL: Giant cell granuloma of the sinuses, Radiology 147:135, 1983.

108. Friedman WH, Pervez N, and Schwartz AE: Brown tumor of the maxilla in secondary hyperparathyroidism, Arch Otolaryngol 100:157, 1974.

109. Smith GA and Ward PH: Giant cell lesions of the facial skeleton, Arch Otolaryngol 104:186, 1978.

110. Smithson LV, Lipper MH, and Hall JA Jr: Paranasal sinus involvement in thalassemia major: CT demonstration, AJNR 8:564, 1987.

111. See reference 2, pp 1834-1836.

112. Ibid 2, 1233-1329.

113. Stafne EC and Gibilisco JA: Oral roentgenographic diagnosis, ed 4, Philadelphia, 1975, WB Saunders Co, pp 147-168.

114. See reference 1, pp 531-560.

115. Mehlisch DR, Dahlin DC, and Masson JK: Ameloblastoma: a clinicopathologic report, J Oral Surg 30:9, 1972.

116. See reference 2, pp 1331-1409.

117. See reference 2, pp 410.
118. Som PM et al: Metastatic hypernephroma to the head and neck, AJNR 8:1103, 1987.
119. Ibid Batsakis: pp 240-251.
120. Bernstein JM, Montgomery WW, and Balogh K: Metastatic tumors to the maxilla, nose and paranasal sinus, Laryngoscope 76:621, 1966.

121. Cottel WI: Perineural invasion by squamous cell carcinoma, J Dermatol Surg Oncol 8:589, 1982.
122. Goepfert H et al: Perineural invasion in squamous cell skin carcinoma of the head and neck, Am J Surg 148:542, 1984.
123. Hanke CW et al: Chemosurgical reports: perineural spread of basal cell carcinoma, J Dermatol Surg Oncol 9:742, 1983.

SECTION FIVE
FRACTURES

The paranasal sinuses develop within and are protected by the facial bones. These bones also serve as attachments for the facial muscles, support the maxillary dentition, and surround the orbits, nasal fossae, and mouth. The facial skeleton is a somewhat honeycombed structure of varying thicknesses and form that develops strength along stress zones by forming buttressed arches. In general, the most superficial portion of the facial skeleton is physically the strongest and serves the additional function of protecting the more delicate central part of the face.[1,2]

FACIAL BUTTRESSES

The supporting buttresses of the facial skeleton can be analyzed in several ways. One analysis identifies two sagittal buttresses on each side of the face. A medial strut extends from the maxillary alveolus up the lateral wall of the piriform aperture and into the medial orbital wall. This buttress comprises the lower maxilla, frontal process of the maxilla, lacrimal bone, and nasal process of the frontal bone. Together they form a medial structural pillar on each side of the facial midline. A lateral strut is formed on each side by the lateral wall of the maxilla, the body of the zygoma, and the orbital process of the frontal bone in the lateral orbital wall.[2]

Another analysis divides the facial bones into three groups of interconnecting osseous struts that are oriented in the horizontal and sagittal planes. In addition to the medial and lateral struts already described, this second analysis recognizes a median strut formed by the nasal septum. These three sagittal buttresses interconnect with three horizontal struts formed by the floor of the anterior cranial fossa, orbital floor and zygomatic arches, and hard palate. Together they form an interconnecting facial support system. Conceptually two coronal buttresses can exist: an anterior plane, formed by the frontal bone, orbital rims, anterior maxilla, and alveolus, and a posterior plane, formed by the posterior wall of the maxilla and pterygoid processes.[3]

These analyses help explain why certain fractures follow an overall predictable course. Le Fort studied the lines of weakness in the facial skeleton experimentally, and the results of his efforts are recognized today by the Le Fort types I, II, and III fractures.[4] Although the forces he used experimentally are small compared with those exerted in high-speed vehicular accidents today, the same fracture lines are still encountered, albeit in various combinations other than those Le Fort observed.

CLINICAL DIAGNOSIS AND TREATMENT

Fractures currently are described in terms of the bones they involve rather than what buttresses or struts are fractured. The actual diagnosis of facial fractures usually is accomplished by a combination of clinical and radiologic examinations. The clinician is primarily concerned with the detection of malocclusion, abnormal mobility, and crepitation as signs of fracture. Often deformity of the facial skeleton is initially concealed by overlying edema, hemorrhage, and soft tissue injury. Any evidence of a palpable step off at the orbital rim, diplopia, hypertelorism, midfacial elongation, cerebrospinal fluid (CSF) rhinorrhea, or flattening of the cheek further helps the clinician identify the type of fracture present. However, it is only after radiographic studies that the fractures can be completely identified and characterized. Radiographs are essential for proper treatment planning.

Some clinicians wait several days after the trauma before correcting the deformity. This delay allows some of the soft tissue injury to subside and may be necessary if the patient has other life-threatening injuries that require immediate attention before the less critical facial fractures are addressed. However, a delay of more than 7 days is to be avoided, if possible, since after this time fibrous fixation of the fracture occurs, and realignment of the fracture is more difficult, often requiring refracturing to attain normal positioning.

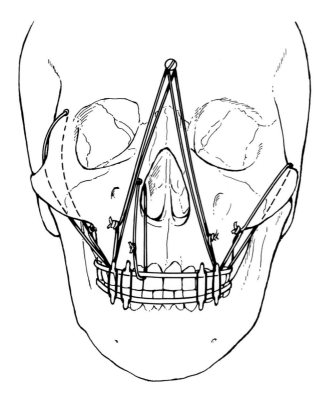

Fig. 2-327 Frontal diagram of different types of intraosseous wiring. The maxillary and mandibular teeth are fitted with arch bars, which are held together with rubber bands. With the patient in good occlusion, fixation can be achieved by frontomalar suspension, glabella (screw) suspension, pyriform aperture suspension, or circumzyomatic suspension.

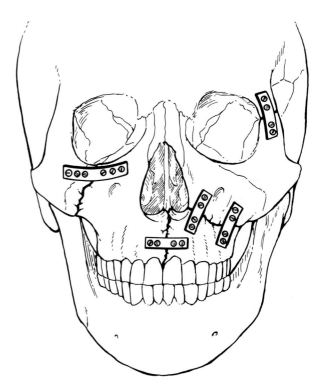

Fig. 2-328 Frontal diagram of use of miniplate osteosynthesis plates as they are used in the fixation of midfacial fractures at typical fracture sites.

In the treatment of simple maxillary fractures, some surgeons place a Foley catheter within the maxillary sinus through an antrostomy. The catheter is filled with radiopaque contrast material until its balloon fills the entire sinus cavity. This technique is useful when minimal to moderate fixation and support are required. A simple plain film allows a check on the balloon positioning.

The basic principles of treating midfacial fractures are the reduction and fixation of the fractured bones to one another and to the skull. Absolute immobilization of the fractures is the main prerequisite for rapid and undisturbed healing. The main interferences in fracture healing are local mechanical factors. In the early phase of fracture healing, mobility can disturb the normal course of bone regeneration and lead to faulty differentiation of the callus.[5,6]

Of primary clinical concern is the restoration of occlusion and facial form, since these provide a means of restoring the essential masticatory function. Midfacial restoration is accomplished by means of arch bars applied to the maxillary and mandibular teeth and then held in good occlusion, after manipulation, by fixing the

arch bars together with small rubber bands. Such fixation of the midface must be maintained either by internal or external skeletal fixation until bony union and consolidation are achieved (Fig. 2-327), about 6 to 8 weeks. Intermaxillary fixation alone requires 3 to 4 weeks to prevent further occlusal malalignment.[5] If the miniplate osteosynthesis technique is used for fixation, intermaxillary fixation is accomplished without a waiting interval. In addition, with the growing use of osteosynthesis fixation, external fixation is no longer necessary in many cases (Fig. 2-328).[5,7] Complex internal fixation also can be accomplished with wire sutures and wire suspensions. These suspension wires extend from the maxillary arch bars to the zygomatic processes of the frontal bones or the zygomatic arches, from a glabella screw, or the margins of the piriform aperture. External fixation is accomplished by use of a halo frame with fixation bars.

Infections of the fracture line are among the most serious complications of facial skeleton fractures. Any fracture must be considered as potentially infected if it traverses the alveolus, walls of the nasal skeleton or paranasal sinuses or if it communicates with a soft tissue wound. Such fractures are called *compound fractures.* Appropriate antibiotic therapy reduces the chances of infection in compound fractures.[6]

With good treatment, the risk of infection of a maxillary or midfacial fracture is only about 2%, and the risk of osteomyelitis is 0.5%. However, a treatment delay of 2 to 3 weeks raises the incidence of osteomyelitis to 1.3%.[6]

Similarly, posttraumatic sinusitis occurs in 7.25% to 9% of all the patients with midfacial fractures. A therapeutic consideration must be the proper maintenance of sinus drainage.[5]

IMAGING

A noncontrast CT scan is the modality of choice for the most complete evaluation of the facial skeleton, facial soft tissues, and brain and dural spaces, which so often are damaged in severe accidents that cause facial trauma.[8]

Axial and coronal CT scans currently provide the most diagnostic information to the clinician.[9] A single-plane study (i.e., axial or coronal) does not provide as much information as an orthogonal two-plane examination; specialized sagittal or oblique plane studies, although helpful in specific cases, are considered optional.[10] If direct coronal CT scans cannot be obtained because of the patient's clinical status, coronal multidirectional tomograms or coronal CT reconstructions from the axial study are acceptable, albeit less desirable, alternatives.

Magnetic resonance imaging (MRI) can be helpful in differentiating blood from inflammatory reactions and edema fluid. This is especially so if the imaging is performed at least 48 hours after the injury. By this time, intrasinus blood will have broken down into methemoglobin and can be distinguished by its high T_1-weighted signal intensity from edema and infection, which have intermediate to low T_1-weighted signal intensities.[11] However, because MRI does not visualize the bone directly, small, yet unstable, nondisplaced facial fractures may not be seen. As a result, CT scanning is the modality of choice in facial trauma patients.

Careful analysis of CT and MRI scans provides all of the information necessary for treatment planning. However, some clinicians find it difficult to conceptualize the information from the scans into a meaningful picture. These clinicians prefer three-dimensional reconstructions, which combine all the information from many scans into just a few images. However, a drawback of three-dimensional reconstruction is that it offers no means of finding fractures not visualized on the initial planar study (coronal or axial). In general, three-dimensional reconstructions are better if the CT study is performed as thin-section (1.5 to 3 mm), contiguous scans. The skull base also must be carefully examined because fractures of the anterior cranial fossa are found in 7.1% of central midfacial fractures, 14.7% of centrolateral midfacial fractures, and 1.1% of lateral midfacial fractures.[5]

The midfacial area is formed by the paired maxillae, palatal bones, inferior turbinates, lacrimal bones, nasal bones, zygomas, and solitary vomer and ethmoid bones. Central midfacial fractures include all forms of fractures that occur between the root of the nose and the alveolar processes of the maxillae, without involvement of the zygomas. These fractures include the alveolar process fracture of the maxilla with detachment of teeth, the transverse fracture just above the floor of the nasal cavity with separation of the palate and alveolus (Le Fort I, or Guérin's, fracture), the median or paramedian sagittal fracture of the hard palate, the pyramidal fracture with separation of the midface either with the nasal bones (Le Fort II and Wassmund II) or without the nasal bones (Wassmund I), and fractures of the nasal bones and nasoethmoidal region.[5]

NASAL FRACTURES

Nasal injuries are the most common fractures of the facial skeleton; about 50% of facial fractures are isolated fractures of the nasal pyramid.[7,12] Nasal fractures can occur as isolated fractures or with other facial injuries. A distinction should be made between fractures of the cartilaginous nasal structures and the nasal bones, since they represent completely different types of fractures.[13] The extent of disruption of the nasal structure relates to the direction and degree of force causing the injury (Fig. 2-329). Most nasal bone fractures involve the thinner distal third of the nasal bones, and the nasoethmoid margin remains intact.[7,13] A lateral blow to the nose usually causes a simple depression or fracture of one nasal bone (Fig. 2-330). However, an anteriorly placed nasal blow fractures both nasal bones at their lower ends, and the force is absorbed by the nasal septum, displacing and fracturing it. With a greater force, the entire nasal pyramid, including the frontal processes of the maxillae, may become detached (Fig. 2-331).[7] When the nasal bones and septum are displaced posteriorly, a saddle nose deformity and splaying of the nose result.[13] In more severe fractures, traumatic hypertelorism and telecanthus may occur, and hemorrhage caused by rupture of the anterior or posterior ethmoidal arteries may be severe.

In adults the internasal suture is solidly ossified so that the nasal bones function as a unit between the frontal processes of the maxilla. However, in children the internasal suture is not yet ossified, and the nasal bones are essentially hinged on each other while resting on the frontal processes of the maxillae. As a result, the frontal processes usually are not fractured in childhood nasal injuries.[13]

When the nose is struck from the side and near its base, the lateral cartilaginous walls may intrude. This type of trauma is not seen radiographically. Clinically, edema and hemorrhage fill in the resulting depression

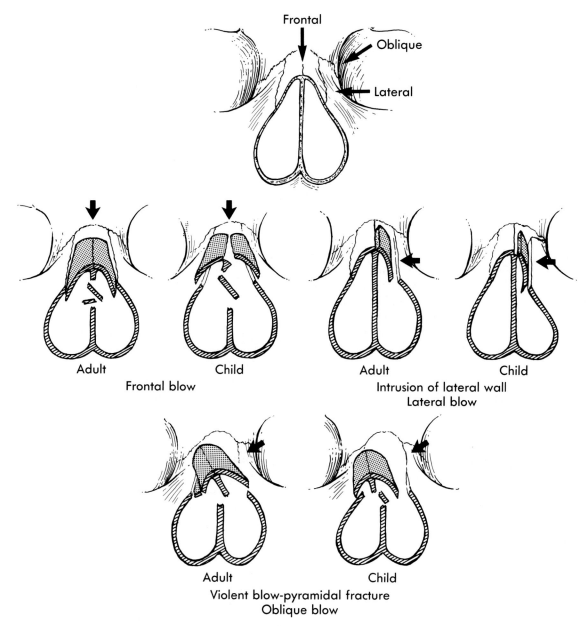

Fig. 2-329 Frontal diagram showing different common types of nasal fractures in children and adults that result from frontal, lateral, and oblique blows.

and obscure the deformity. If these injuries and simple nasal fractures are initially overlooked, especially if they are in conjunction with more serious injuries, the inadequately treated nasal fracture may result in cosmetic deformity and functional impairment.[13]

If the nasal trauma results in buckling of the nasal septal cartilage, the fractured fragments of cartilage can overlap one another, separating the perichondrium from the cartilage. This event in turn allows a hematoma to develop in the space between the perichondrium and the cartilage. A hematoma interferes with the vascular supply of the cartilage from the mucoperi-

osteum. Eventual cartilage necrosis occurs. If a septal hematoma is not initially identified and treated, it becomes an organized hematoma, which leads to an unyielding thickening of the septum and impaired breathing.

The septal hematoma that becomes infected after mucosal injury is called a septal abscess. A septal abscess may lead to the onset of fever, pain, septal swelling, and eventual cartilage necrosis with loss of the support for the nose, causing a saddle nose deformity.[13]

Careful clinical examination of the nasal septum and early evacuation of a septal hematoma are essential. If

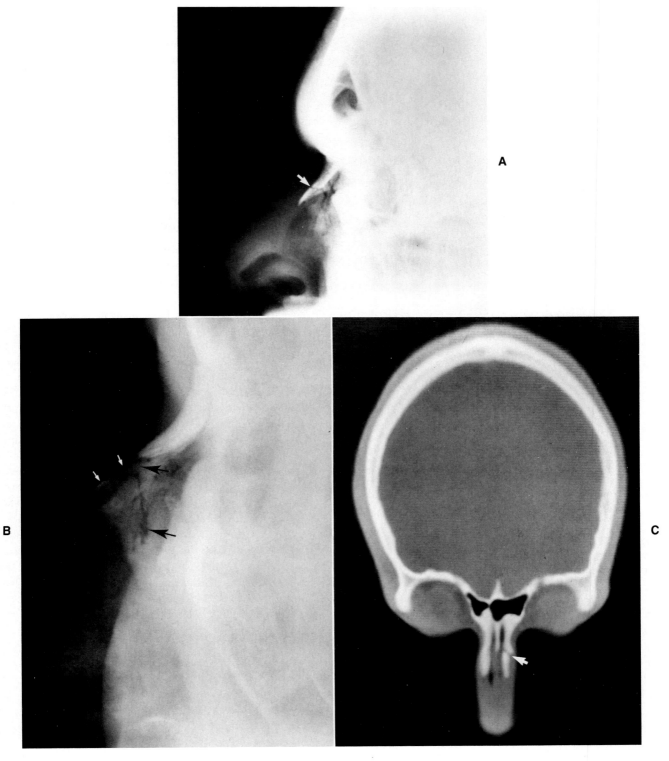

Fig. 2-330   Lateral view. **A,** Nondisplaced fracture *(arrow)* is seen extending from the midline nasal bones laterally. **B,** Lateral view shows communicated nasal bone fracture *(small arrows)* with extension of the fracture into the lateral nasal bones and frontal processes of the maxilla *(arrows)*. **C,** Coronal CT scan shows isolated minimally depressed left nasal fracture *(arrow)*.

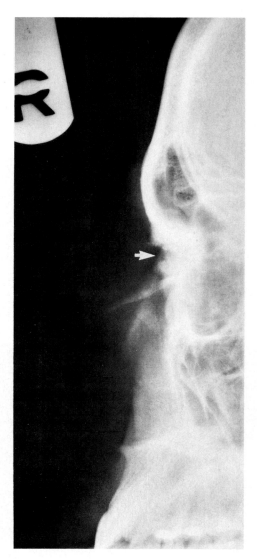

Fig. 2-331 Lateral view shows nasal fracture through the frontonasal suture *(arrow)* with posterior displacement of the nasal bones.

imaging studies of the nose and nasal fossae are also performed, the radiologist should direct attention to the septum to identify any localized septal swelling or deviation. If such a condition is seen, the radiologist should bring it to the clinician's attention.[13]

In the floor of the anterior cranial fossa, the dura is thin and firmly adherent to the bone. Thus the skull base and dura in the anterior cranial fossa function as a unit, and a fracture through this region invariably tears the dura. Dural tears provide a pathway for CSF rhinorrhea and the development of an intracranial pneumocele or infection.[13]

NASOORBITAL FRACTURES

The nasoorbital fracture most often results from a blow over the bridge of the nose. The force displaces the nasal pyramid posteriorly, fracturing the nasal bones, frontal processes of the maxillae, lacrimal bones, ethmoid sinuses, bones of the frontal sinuses, cribriform plate, and nasal septum. The ethmoid lamina fractures on itself in an accordion fashion, which is best visualized in the axial plane. Posttraumatic hypertelorism and telecanthus may result, as well as associated damage to the lacrimal apparatus (Fig. 2-332). On lateral films the nasion appears displaced posteriorly, and the degree of this displacement should be noted. Careful attention also should be given to the bones near the optic canal, since a surgical attempt at repositioning the displaced facial bones might move such an optic canal fracture and cause blindness.

MAXILLARY FRACTURES

Alveolar fractures are the most common isolated maxillary fractures. An upward blow to the mandible can thrust the mandible into the maxilla and push the maxillary teeth upward and outward. This movement in turn fractures the alveolus. Because of the strong soft tissue support over the alveolus, these isolated fractures rarely are displaced. The involved teeth often are displaced or devitalized and such alveolar fractures in children may damage the tooth germs.[5]

Partial fractures of the maxilla can result from a blow delivered by a narrow object directly over the anterior maxillary wall. The fractures involve the anterior and lateral antral walls and extend toward the piriform aperture and down into the maxillary alveolus (Fig. 2-333).

Sagittal fractures of the palate result from either an axial or an oblique blow to the chin or a direct blow to the upper jaw. The fracture passes through the weakest portion of the palatine process of the maxilla, which is sagittally oriented just off of the midline. The midline itself is reinforced by the vomer, whereas the lateral hard palate is supported by the alveolus. In more violent trauma, a sagittal midline fracture can occur; comminuted palatal fractures are associated with other central or centrolateral facial fractures.[5]

LE FORT I FRACTURES

The Le Fort I fracture results from a blow delivered over the upper lip region and is characterized by detachment of the upper jaw with the tooth-bearing segments (at a level just above the floor of the nasal cavity) and the caudal portions of the maxillary sinuses. The fracture extends through the lower nasal septum, the lower walls of the maxillary sinuses, and the lower pterygoid plates. Thus the fracture segment includes the entire palate, maxillary alveolus and teeth, and portions of the pterygoid plates. This "floating palate" is displaced posteriorly, resulting in malocclusion and hemorrhaging into the antra (Fig. 2-334).[5]

Text continued on p. 238.

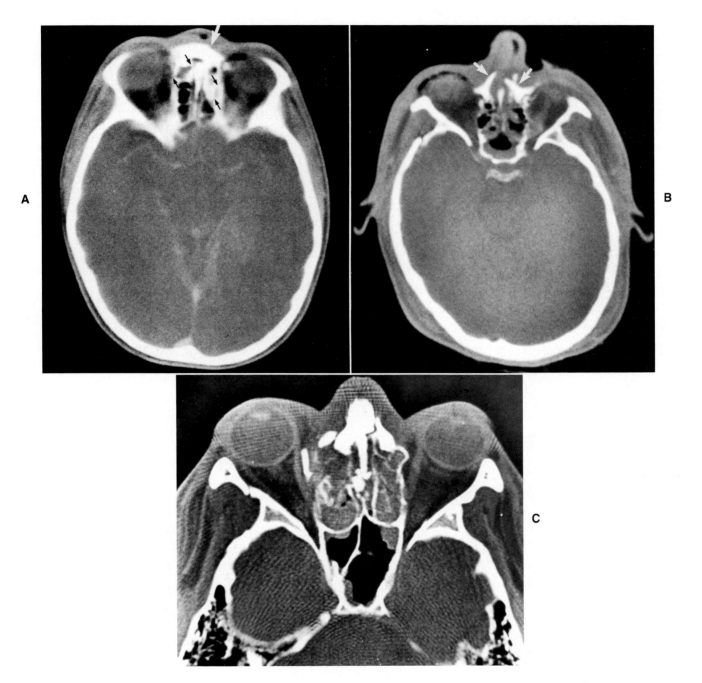

Fig. 2-332   A, Axial CT scan shows nasoorbital fracture with posterior displacement of the nasion *(arrow)* and fractures through the fovea ethmoidalis *(small arrows).* **B,** Axial CT scan shows nasoorbital fracture with posterior and medial displacement of the nasal bones and frontal processes of the maxilla *(arrows).* There are also fractures of the ethmoids with some hypertelorism of the ethmoids. **C,** Axial CT scan shows nasoorbital fracture with posterior displacement of the nasal bones and fractures and hypertelorism of the ethmoids.

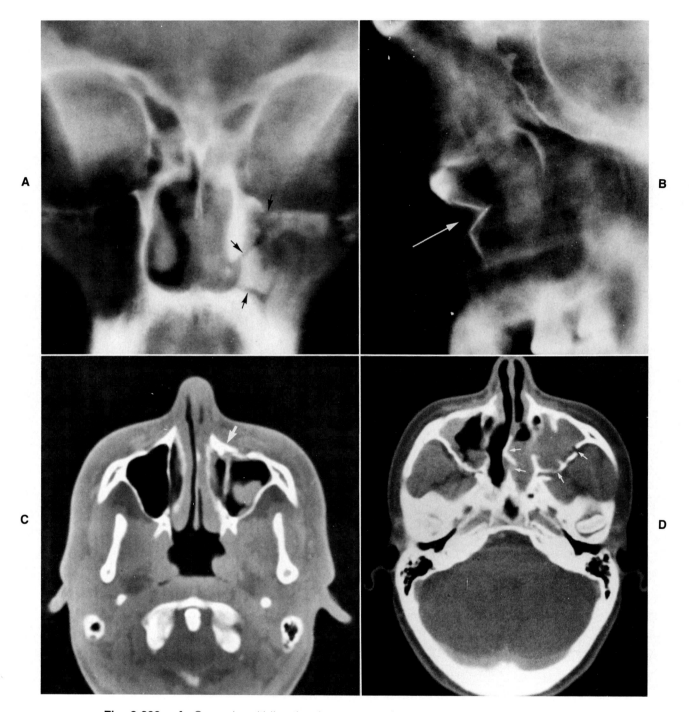

Fig. 2-333 A, Coronal multidirectional tomogram shows comminuted fractures of the left anterior and medial maxilla *(arrows)*. **B,** Lateral multidirectional tomogram shows isolated fracture of the anterior maxillary sinus wall *(arrow)*. This type of fracture usually results from a blow from a narrow object. **C,** Axial CT Scan shows isolated fracture of the anteromedial left maxilla *(arrow)*. Hemorrhage is present in the left antrum. **D,** Axial CT scan shows fractures of left maxillary sinus posterolateral and medial walls and a fracture of the nasal septum *(arrows)*.

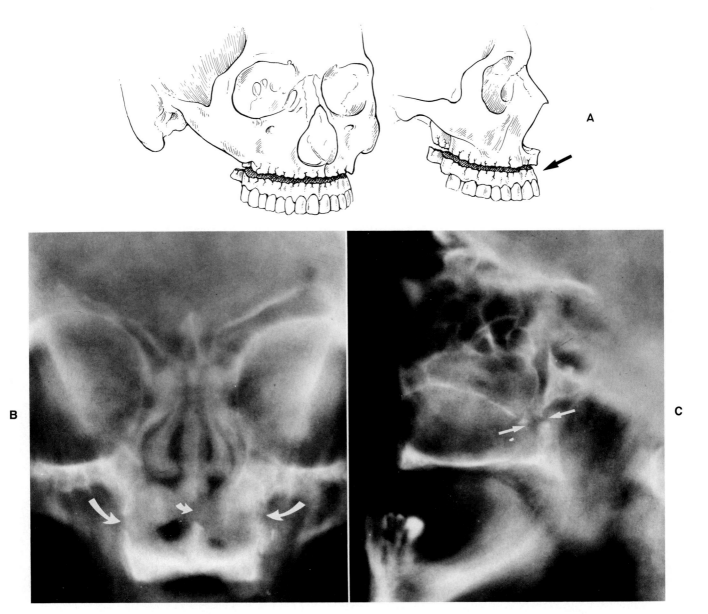

Fig. 2-334   A, Diagrams of Le Fort I fracture results in a "floating palate." **B,** Coronal multidirectional tomogram shows Le Fort I fracture *(arrows)*. **C,** Lateral multidirectional tomogram shows Le Fort I fracture. The extension of the fracture through the pterygoid plates is seen *(arrows)*.

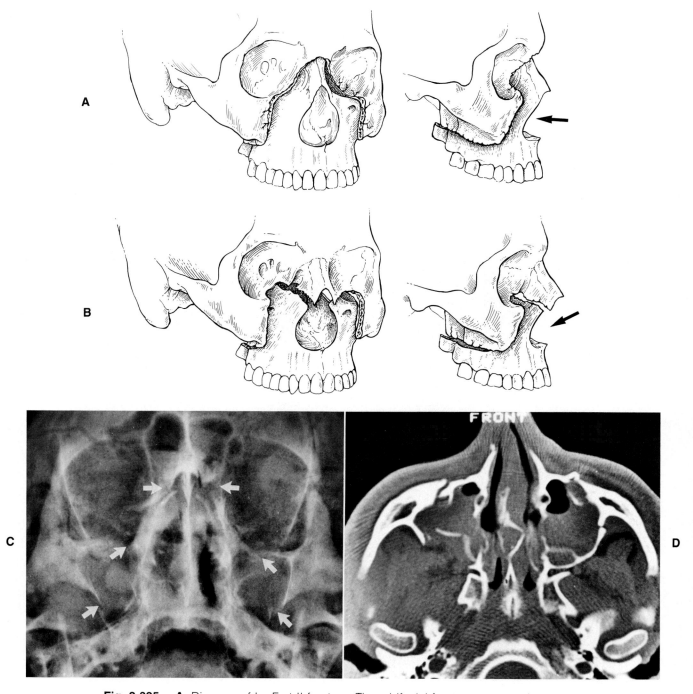

Fig. 2-335 **A,** Diagram of Le Fort II fracture. The midfacial fracture segment is pyramidal in shape and these fractures are often called pyramidal fractures. **B,** Diagram of Wassmund I fracture. This is the same type of fracture as Le Fort II except that the nasal bones are spared. **C,** Waters view shows Le Fort II fracture *(arrows)* that creates a pyramidal shaped fracture segment. **D,** Axial CT scan shows Le Fort II fracture. On more caudal scans the pterygoid plates were fractured, while on more cranial scans the ethmoid sinuses and orbital floors were fractured.

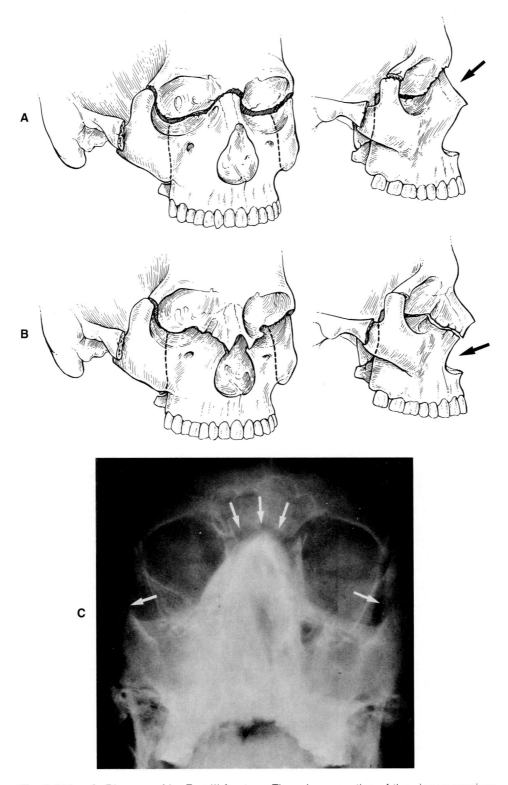

Fig. 2-336   A, Diagram of Le Fort III fracture. There is separation of the viscerocranium and the facial bones. The dotted fracture lines extend down the posterior maxillary sinus walls. **B,** Diagram of Wassmund III fracture. This is a similar fracture to the Le Fort III except the nasal bones are not involved. The dotted fracture lines extend down the posterior maxillary sinus walls. **C,** Waters view shows Le Fort III fracture *(arrows)*. Hemorrhage is present in both antra.

LE FORT II FRACTURES

A strong, broad blow over the central facial region causes a pyramidal fracture, one of the most severe midfacial fractures. The high central midface fracture (Le Fort II) is characterized by a fracture line that extends through the root of the nose, lacrimal bones, and medial orbital walls, and then turns anteriorly along the floor of the orbits near the infraorbital canals, down the zygomaticomaxillary sutures and anterior walls of the maxillae, posteriorly and down across the infratemporal surface of the maxillae, and finally to the lower pterygoid plates. The deep central midface (Wassmund I) fracture spares the nasal bones and extends from the lateral edges of the piriform aperture back across the lacrimal bones into the medial orbital walls. From this point, the fracture is the same as the Le Fort II (Fig. 2-335).[5]

In the Le Fort II fractures the zygomatic bones remain attached to the cranium. The pyramidal-shaped fracture segment—the central midface—is posteriorly displaced, resulting in a "dishface" deformity, malocclusion, and hemorrhage. Anesthesia or paresthesia of one or both of the infraorbital nerves occurs in 78.9% of the cases.[7]

LE FORT III FRACTURES

Centrolateral midfacial fractures are characterized by separation of the entire facial skeleton from the skull base. Such a craniofacial dysjunction usually has a fracture line extending through the root of the nose, across the lacrimal bones and medial orbital walls, and then posterolaterally across the floor of the orbits to the inferior orbital fissure. At this point, one portion of the fracture line extends laterally and upward across the lateral orbital walls to end near the zygomaticofrontal sutures. A second fracture line extends from the orbital floor down across the back of the maxillae to the lower

ends of the pterygoid plates. The zygomatic arches also are fractured, thereby completing the separation of the viscerocranium. Such a fracture is called a Le Fort III, or Wassmund IV, fracture (Fig. 2-336). The same fracture without inclusion of the nasal bones is called a Wassmund III fracture (Fig. 2-336). Wassmund III fractures extend from the piriform apertures up to the lacrimal bones and then continue as in a Le Fort III fracture. Thus, the distinguishing feature of Le Fort III fractures from the central pyramidal fractures is the inclusion in the fractured segment of the zygomas and lateral orbital walls. These patients have a dishface deformity, CSF rhinorrhea, hemorrhage, damage to the lacrimal apparatus, and malocclusion. The infraorbital nerves are involved in 69.3% of cases.[7]

Lateral midfacial fractures include the zygomatic fractures (trimalar, or tripod), zygomatic arch fractures, zygomaticomaxillary fractures, zygomaticomandibular fractures, and fractures of the floor of the orbit (blowout fractures).[14]

TRIMALAR (ZYGOMATIC) FRACTURES

Zygomatic (trimalar) fractures extend along the zygomaticofrontal suture (the lateral orbital wall, including the zygomaticosphenoid suture), the inferior orbital fissure to the orbital floor near the infraorbital canal, then down the anterior maxilla near the zygomaticomaxillary suture, up the posterior maxillary wall back to the inferior orbital fissure, and the zygomaticotemporal suture (zygomatic arch). The infraorbital nerve is impaired in 94.2% of the cases.[7]

Several classifications of lateral midface fractures have been proposed.[14-16] Each considers the displacement of the zygoma as it relates to the clinical severity of the fracture and how malar position may be used to plan the treatment.

Zygomatic fractures account for 49% to 53% of the

Table 2-1 Type, frequency, and postreduction stability of zygomatic fractures

Fracture type	Frequency (%)	Postreduction stability (%)
Nondisplaced	11	100
Isolated arch	16	93
Rotation around vertical axis	12	
Medial	3.5	57
Lateral	8.5	88
Rotation around horizontal axis	6	
Medial	1	0
Lateral	5	50
Displacement without rotation	31	
Medial	11.5	39
Lateral	1	0
Posterior	12	92
Inferior	6.5	0
Isolated rim	9.5	47
Complex	14.5	0

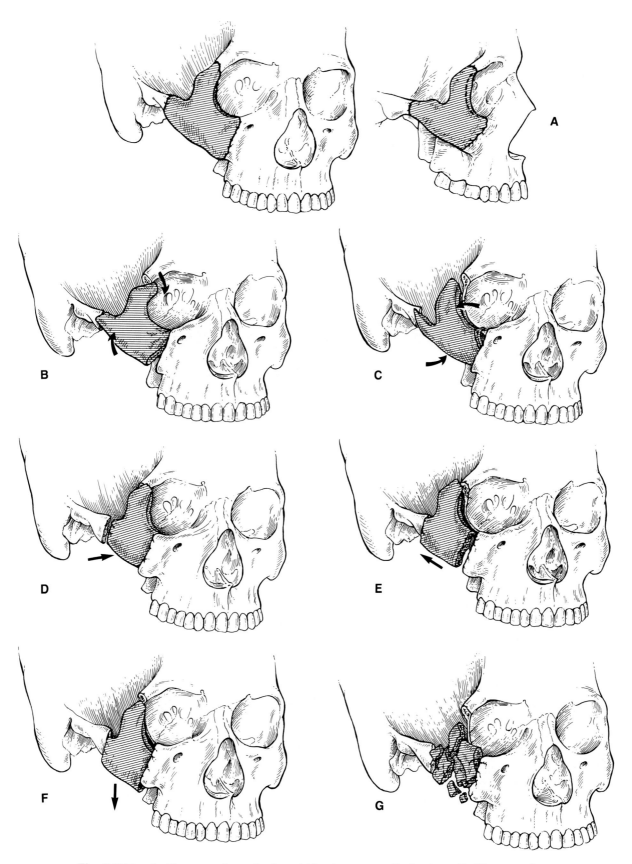

Fig. 2-337   **A,** Diagram of nondisplaced trimalar zygomatic fracture. **B,** Diagram of zygomatic fracture with clockwise (medial) rotation around a horizontal axis (anterior-to-posterior) through the zygoma. **C,** Diagram of zygomatic fracture with counterclockwise (lateral) rotation around a horizontal axis (anterior-to-posterior) through the zygoma. **D,** Diagram of zygomatic fracture with pure medial displacement. **E,** Diagram of zygomatic fracture with pure posterior displacement. **F,** Diagram of zygomatic fracture with pure inferior displacement. **G,** Diagram of zygomatic comminuted (complex) fracture.

midface fractures, and in one study, 69% of midfacial fractures involved the zygomatic complex either alone or in combination with other midface fractures.[5,15] The reports vary considerably as to the frequency of the different malar fracture positions. One of the more complete classifications, including the fracture type, frequency, and postreduction stability, is shown in Table 2-1.[15]

If the radiologist uses the type of classification shown in Table 2-1 the clinician is better able to predict which cases will require internal fixation, osteosynthesis fixation, or external fixation (Figs. 2-337 to 2-340).

Isolated fractures of the zygomatic arch usually involve at least three discrete fracture lines, which create two fracture segments. These pieces are displaced me-

dially and downward, reflecting the impact from the blow that caused them. The fracture pieces may impinge on the coronoid process of the mandible and interfere with movement of the lower jaw (Fig. 2-341).

Zygomaticomaxillary fractures differ from zygomatic fractures in that they include a maxillary segment. In distinction to the trimalar fracture line, zygomaticomaxillary fractures involve the orbital floor, extend down the anterior maxilla near the infraorbital foramen, run to the premolar region, and then extend across the palate to the maxillary tuberosity and lower pterygoid plates.

Zygomaticomandibular fractures differ from zygomatic fractures only by the additional fracture of the mandibular condyle, coronoid process or both.[14]

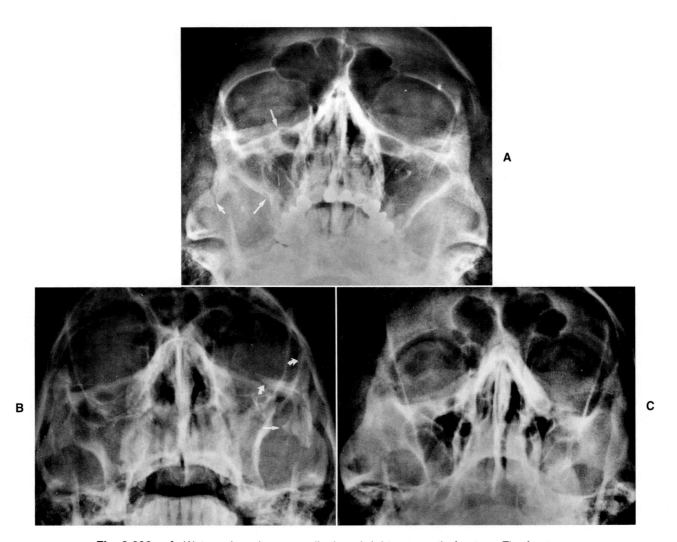

Fig. 2-338   A, Waters view shows nondisplaced right zygomatic fracture. The fractures through the maxilla and the zygomatic arch are seen *(arrows)*. However, the zygomaticofrontal fracture is not visualized because there was only a slight diastasis at this point. **B,** Waters view shows left zygomatic fracture that is laterally displaced *(arrow)* and slightly clockwise (laterally) rotated *(curved arrows)*. **C,** Waters view shows left zygomatic fracture that is inferiorly and medially displaced.

Fractures of the orbit floor may occur as either simple or comminuted fractures, in conjunction with midfacial fractures, with atypical periorbital fractures (orbital roof), or as isolated blow-out fractures.

BLOW-OUT AND BLOW-IN FRACTURES

The term orbital blow-out fracture describes the injury from a blow to the orbit by an object that is too large to enter the orbit (fist, baseball, etc.). The force of the blow is absorbed by the orbital rim and is transmitted to the thinner orbital floor, which shatters, usually in the middle third near the infraorbital canal. As the eye is pushed back into the conic orbital apex, it increases infraorbital pressure; this "blows out" the fractured floor into the maxillary sinus. Usually the orbital rim is not fractured (pure blow-out fracture) and the globe remains undamaged. Less commonly, the inferior orbital rim also is fractured; this is referred to as an impure blow-out fracture. Blow-out fractures represent only 3% to 5% of all midface fractures (Figs. 2-342 to 2-345).[14,17]

Herniation of orbital fat, inferior rectus muscle, and inferior oblique muscle can occur with occasional muscle entrapment in the fracture line, resulting in diplopia on upward gaze. However, diplopia is the most frequent complaint in all patients with blow-out fractures and may occur solely because of periorbital edema and hemorrhage, which exert pressure on the globe. This type of diplopia resolves in several days, whereas entrapment diplopia remains. If the cause of diplopia is in doubt, a traction test can be performed on the inferior

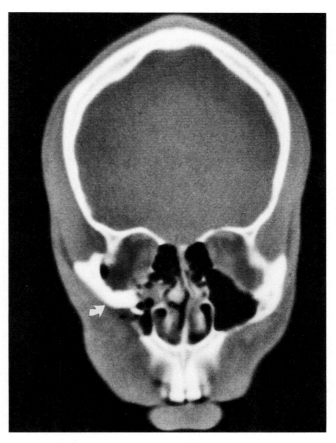

Fig. 2-339 Coronal CT scan shows right zygomatic fracture, which is superiorly displaced and considerably counterclockwise (laterally) rotated *(arrow)*. There is also subcutaneous emphysema.

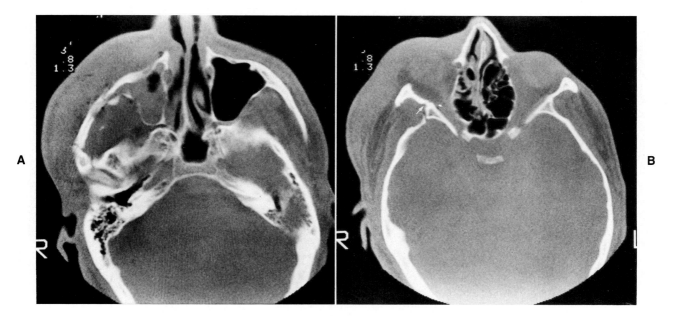

Fig. 2-340 **A,** Axial CT scan shows right zygomatic fracture with posterior displacement and clockwise (medial) rotation of the zygoma. **B,** Axial CT scan more cranial than **A** shows zygomatic frontosphenoid fracture *(arrow)*.

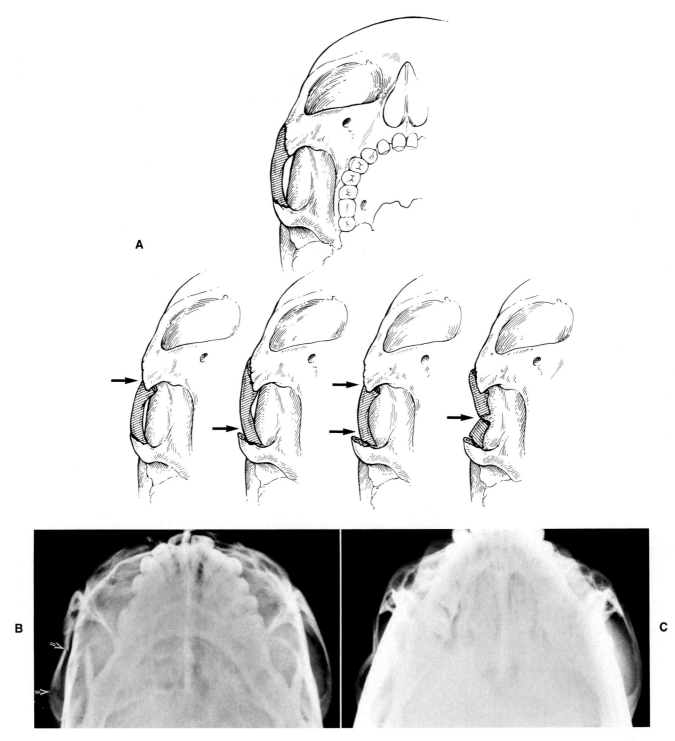

Fig. 2-341 **A,** Diagram of different types of isolated zygomatic arch fractures. The last type may impinge medially on the coronoid process of the mandible. **B,** Underpenetrated base view shows slightly depressed right zygomatic arch fractures *(arrows).* **C,** Underpenetrated base view shows markedly depressed right zygomatic arch fractures.

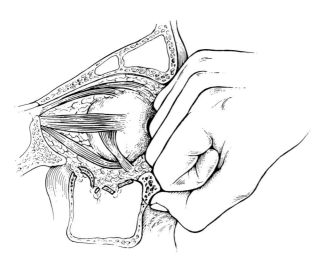

Fig. 2-342 Diagram of blowout fracture. The impacting object is larger than the orbital rim diameter. The blow fractures the orbital floor and pushes the eye back. The eye then displaces the fractured floor into the antrum.

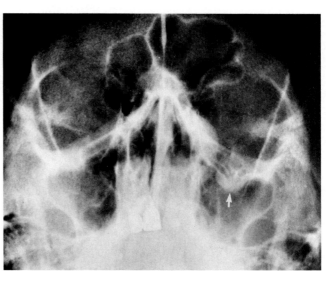

Fig. 2-343 Waters view shows polypoid soft tissue mass in roof of left antrum *(arrow)*. Blowout fracture.

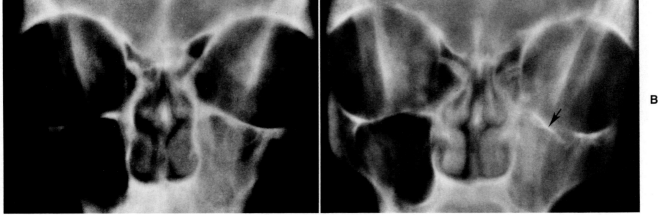

Fig. 2-344 Coronal multidirectional tomograms show **A,** an intact orbital rim anteriorly and **B,** a "trap-door" type of orbital floor fracture *(arrow)* posteriorly behind the rim. Pure blowout fracture.

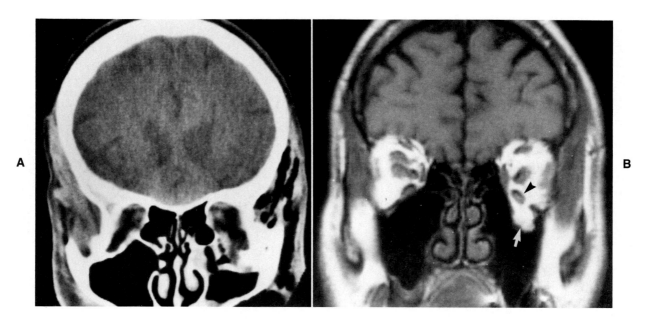

Fig. 2-345 **A,** Coronal CT scan shows blowout fracture of the left orbit with herniation of the orbital fat down into the antrum. **B,** Coronal mixed image MRI scan shows a left blow-out fracture. Fat has herniated into the left antrum *(arrow)*, and there is minimal depression of the inferior rectus muscle *(arrowhead)*.

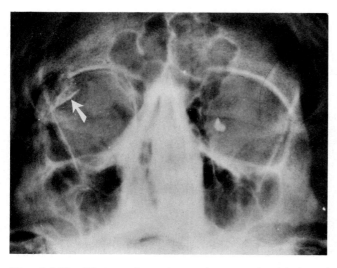

Fig. 2-346 Waters view shows depressed orbital roof fracture *(arrow)* that impinged on the globe and clinically mimicked a blowout fracture of the orbital floor with entrapment. A foreign body is also seen in the left eye.

muscles. Rarely, a depression fracture of the orbital roof or superior orbital rim can impinge on the globe, prohibiting upward gaze, and clinically can mimic inferior muscle entrapment (Fig. 2-346). Radiographic studies clarify this situation.[18] In these latter cases, communication with the base of the anterior cranial fossa can lead to CSF leakage into the orbit or herniation of meninges or brain through the fracture line.

Rarely, the orbital floor fracture segments can herniate upward into the orbit. This unusual occurrence has been called a *blow-in fracture* and must be clearly identified so that the fractured bone can be repositioned and does not impair vision.[7]

On plain films, soft tissue swelling over the inferior orbital rim and antral opacification or mucosal thickening are often the only indirect signs of a blow-out fracture. An actual depressed or displaced orbital floor bone fragment may not be seen. Occasionally, a soft tissue polypoid density can be visualized in the antral roof. This may represent the site of the blow-out fracture filled with orbital contents and hemorrhage, or it may represent an unrelated antral cyst or polyp. Only on coronal CT scans or coronal tomograms can the actual fracture be seen clearly. A completely displaced piece of bone or a trap-door or hinged fracture can then be identified, as can the typical "teardrop" herniation of orbital contents. On CT scans the orbital fat may be of a higher than expected attenuation because of hemorrhage; in rare cases an antral air-blood level may be present.[12]

Fracture of the medial orbital wall can occur in conjunction with orbital floor fractures. They may be present in as many as 50% of orbital floor fracture cases. Often the fracture is poorly visualized on plain films, with only some clouding of the ethmoid cells being evident. Even on CT scans these fractures may not be identified if there is no bone displacement. However, fat that has herniated into the ethmoid complex is

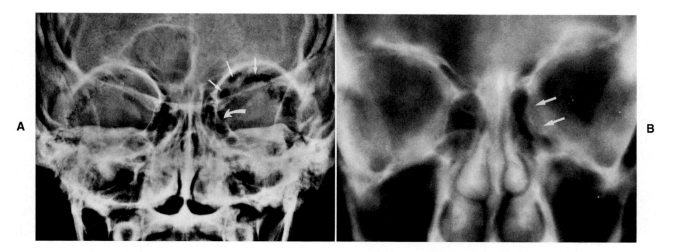

Fig. 2-347 **A,** Caldwell view and **B,** coronal multidirectional tomogram show orbital emphysema *(three arrows)* and a defect in the left lamina papyracea *(curved arrow).* The tomogram better shows the medial wall depressed fracture *(two arrows).*

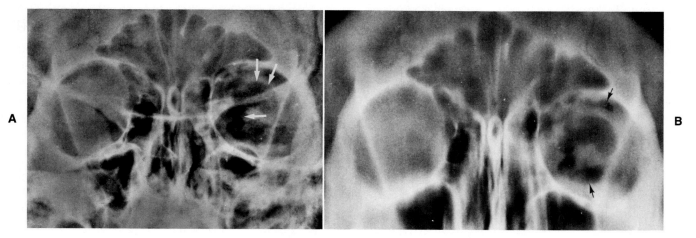

Fig. 2-348 **A,** Caldwell view and **B,** coronal multidirectional tomogram show orbital emphysema *(arrows).* Some opacification is present in the left ethmoid sinuses. These findings are better seen on the tomogram, however, the fracture is not identified. This is not uncommon with medial wall orbital fractures.

well visualized on CT scans. Muscle entrapment in these fractures is rare.[19] Herniated fat can also be clearly identified on MRI scan, although the small fracture segments may not be identified.

Medial wall fractures can be inferred by the presence of orbital emphysema. Such orbital air most commonly comes from an ethmoid sinus fracture and only rarely results from an antral fracture (Figs. 2-347 to 2-349). The infrequent occurrence of emphysema with orbital floor blow-out fractures is attributed to the rapid sealing of the fracture by edema, hemorrhage, and periorbital herniation of orbital fat and muscle. Orbital emphysema develops after the trauma when nose blowing by the patient increases intranasal pressure, which in

turn raises the intrasinus pressure and forces air into the orbit. In most patients, refraining from nose blowing allows the fracture line to seal and the orbital air to resorb.[7,14]

Rarely, air can enter the orbit from a complex fracture involving the frontal or sphenoid sinuses. However, these cases are associated with severe facial trauma, and the source of the air becomes evident on imaging studies.

The two clinical indications for immediate surgery on an orbital blow-out fracture are definite muscle entrapment and acute enophthalmos. In the most dramatic case, the globe is almost completely displaced into the maxillary sinus.[20] However, milder and more common

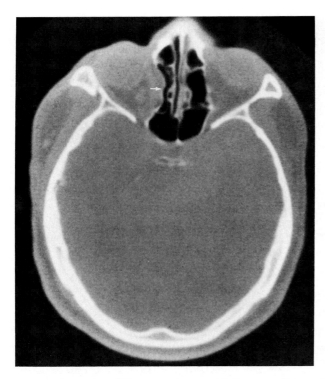

Fig. 2-349 Axial CT scan shows old right medial wall blowout fracture *(arrow)*.

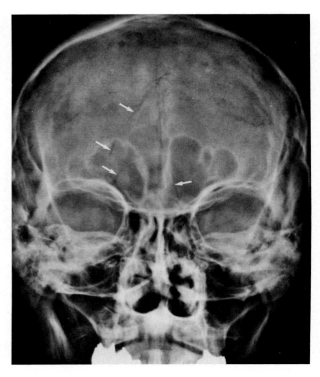

Fig. 2-350 Caldwell view shows comminuted fracture of the frontal bone *(arrows)* that extend into the right frontal sinus.

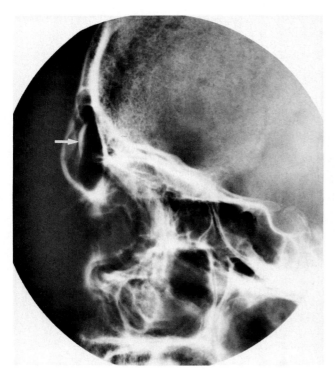

Fig. 2-351 Lateral view shows depressed anterior frontal sinus wall fracture *(arrow)*.

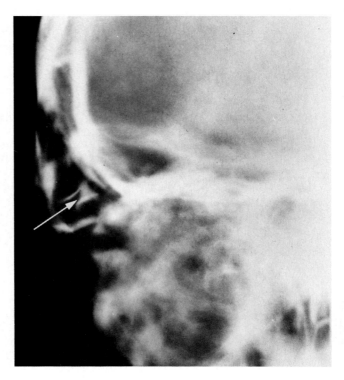

Fig. 2-352 Lateral view shows depressed fracture *(arrow)* of the anterior wall and floor of the frontal sinus.

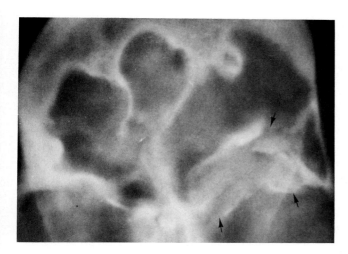

Fig. 2-353 Coronal multidirectional tomogram shows comminuted fracture of the anterior wall and floor of the left frontal sinus that involves the superior orbital rim *(arrows)*.

degrees of acute enophthalmos may take several days to clinically confirm because of the presence of periorbital edema and hemorrhage.[17]

The development of chronic enophthalmos is also to be avoided because it leads to cosmetic deformity and in some cases diplopia. Enophthalmos becomes chronic when too much orbital fat has herniated from the orbit. Subsequent scarring and lipogranulation of the herniated tissue causes sufficient volume loss that the eyeball recedes. The patients at greatest risk are those who have sizable herniations of fat into one sinus or moderate herniations into both medial wall and orbital floor fractures. The radiologist should draw the clinician's attention to such cases even in the absence of acute enophthalmos or muscle entrapment.[17]

FRONTAL SINUS FRACTURES

Frontal sinus fractures are either the result of direct trauma or an extension of a calvarial fracture into the sinus. Of all fractures involving the frontal sinuses, 67% are limited to the anterior table, 28% involve both the anterior and posterior sinus walls, and only 5% are lim-

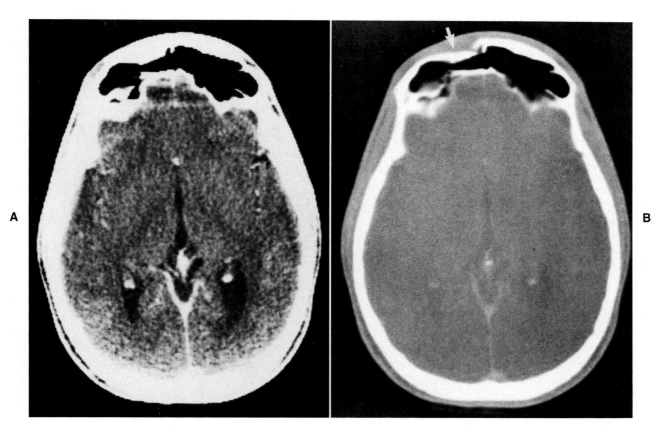

Fig. 2-354 Axial CT scans at **A,** narrow window and **B,** wide window settings. The fracture of the anterior right frontal sinus wall *(arrow)* can be missed on the "soft tissue" narrow window scan because hemorrhage fills in the soft tissue depression in the forehead.

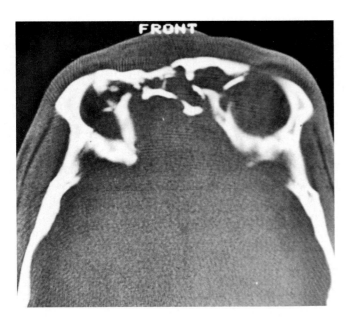

Fig. 2-355 Axial CT scan shows comminuted midfacial fracture that involves the frontal bone and frontal sinuses.

ited to the posterior sinus table.[21] Most commonly, a linear fracture occurs in the anterior sinus wall.[22] This tears the mucosa and produces hemorrhage, edema, and sinus opacification. The fracture line may extend downward, often involving the superomedial orbital rim (Figs. 2-350 to 2-355).

Comminuted fractures also occur and frequently reflect the size and shape of the object causing the fracture. Only a vague density may appear in the frontal sinus on plain film Caldwell and Waters views. However, the lateral view identifies bone fragments in the sinus. Axial CT scans most clearly confirm the presence of such depression fractures, which often are unobserved clinically, since the forehead depression is hidden by edema and hemorrhage.

Complex fractures of both the anterior and posterior frontal sinus tables usually are associated with other midfacial fractures.

Isolated fractures of the posterior sinus wall are rare. They occur from a fracture of the skull base or when a fracture of the calvarium extends into the posterior sinus wall.[23] Any fracture involving the posterior frontal sinus wall opens communication with the dural spaces. CSF leakage into the sinus and intracranial infection or pneumocele can develop. Rarely, orbital emphysema or CSF leakage can result from frontal sinus fractures.

SPHENOID SINUS FRACTURES

Fractures of the sphenoid sinus seldom occur, but when they do, they are associated with severe cranial trauma and basilar skull fractures. Rarely, milder trauma to the midfacial region may extend back into the sphenoid sinus. Sinus opacification or a sphenoid sinus air-fluid level may indicate the presence of CSF, hemorrhage, or simply poor sinus drainage. If the fracture injures the adjacent internal carotid arteries or cavernous sinuses, these events may be life threatening.

PEDIATRIC FACIAL FRACTURES

When compared with the adult skeleton, the pediatric facial bones behave differently with regard to fracture patterns, healing, and treatment. The inherent elasticity of the facial bones in the young patient is advantageous in trauma, because the bone yields more easily and does not fracture as readily as it does in an adult.[24] When a fracture occurs, the thick, elastic periosteum prevents displacement of the fragments and results in a green-stick fracture.

Fractures heal faster in children than in adults, so the period of immobilization is shorter. However, if treatment is delayed, the fragments may become fixed, making fracture reduction more difficult. Malocclusions in the primary dentition that are not completely corrected may be spontaneously compensated for by the secondary dentition or may be treated by orthodontic therapy.[24]

Although children have many advantages in terms of healing, they are at a disadvantage with regard to dentition. In 30% to 50% of pediatric facial fractures, the tooth germs lie in the fracture. These teeth fall out during healing or have delayed development and deformities that do not manifest clinically until the permanent teeth erupt.

Facial fractures also can damage the bony growth centers and result in osseous hypoplasia, functional abnormalities, and cosmetic deformities. Some clinicians believe that the child's parents should be informed of these potential problems at the time of the initial injury.

Children generally have too few teeth for fixation splints. Treatment plans must be modified from those used in adult patients. No wire ligatures can be placed in children under 2 years old. After this age, it may be possible to fix interdental wires and arch bars if the primary teeth have not been damaged by caries or their crowns have an adequately retentive form. However, with the appearance of interdental spaces caused by eruption of the secondary teeth, the possibility of fixing dental splints becomes less likely. Similarly, erupted permanent teeth can only accept such ligatures after their greatest convexity has passed the gingival margin. This period lasts from about the fifth to eighth years of life.[24]

REFERENCES

1. Smith HW and Yanagisawa E: Paranasal sinus trauma. In Blitzer A, Lawson W, and Friedman WH, editors: Surgery of the paranasal sinuses, Philadelphia, 1985, WB Saunders Co, pp 299-315.

2. Mancuso AA and Hanafee WN: Computed tomography and magnetic resonance imaging of the head and neck, ed 2, Baltimore, 1985, Williams & Wilkins, pp 42-60.

3. Gentry LR et al: High-resolution CT analysis of facial struts in trauma. I. Normal anatomy, AJR 140:523, 1983.

4. Le Fort R: Etude experimentale sur les fractures de la machoire superieure, Rev Chir 23:208, 360, 479, 1901.

5. Schwenzer N and Kruger E: Midface fracture. In Kruger E, Schilli W, and Worthington P, editors: Oral and maxillofacial traumatology, vol 2, Chicago, 1986, Quintessence Publishing Co, Inc, pp 107-136.

6. Kreipke DL et al: Computed tomography and thin-section tomography in facial trauma, AJNR 5:423, 1984.

7. Rowe NL and Williams JL, editors: Maxillofacial injuries, vol 1, Edinburgh, 1985, Churchill Livingstone, pp 363-558.

8. Brant-Zawadzki MN et al: High-resolution CT with image reformation in maxillofacial pathology, AJR 138:477, 1982.

9. Zilkha A: Computed tomography in facial trauma, Radiology 144:545, 1982.

10. See reference 6, pp 185-189.

11. Zimmerman RA et al: Paranasal sinus hemorrhage: evaluation with MR imaging, Radiology 162:499, 1987.

12. Dodd GD and Jing B-S: Radiology of the nose, paranasal sinuses, and nasopharynx, Baltimore, 1977, The Williams & Wilkins Co, pp 146-170.

13. See reference 6, pp 223-235.

14. See reference 6, pp 158-222.

15. Yanagisawa E: Symposium on maxillofacial trauma. III. Pitfalls in the management of zygomatic fractures, Laryngoscope 83:527, 1973.

16. Knight JS, North JF, and Chir B: The classification of malar fractures: an analysis of displacement as a guide to treatment, Br J Plast Surg 13:325, 1961.

17. Smith B, Grove A, and Guibor P: Fractures of the orbit. In Jones IS and Jakobiec FA, editors: Diseases of the orbit, Hagerstown, Md, 1979, Harper & Row, Publishers, Inc, pp 571-580.

18. McClury FL and Swanson PJ: An orbital roof fracture causing diplopia, Arch Otolaryngol 102:497, 1976.

19. Coker NJ, Brooks BS, and Gammel TE: Computed tomography of orbital medial wall fractures, Head Neck Surg 5:383, 1983.

20. Berkowitz RA, Putterman AN, and Patel DB: Prolapse of the globe into the maxillary sinus after orbital fracture, Am J Ophthalmol 91:253, 1981.

21. Shockley WW et al: Frontal sinus fractures: some problems and some solutions, Laryngoscope 98:18, 1988.

22. Valvassori GE and Hord GE: Traumatic sinus disease, Semin Roentgenol 3:160, 1968.

23. Bergeron RT and Rumbaugh CL: Skull trauma. In Newton TH and Potts DG, editors: Radiology of the skull and brain, St Louis, 1971, The CV Mosby Co, pp 763-818.

24. See reference 6, pp 259-296.

SECTION SIX
POSTOPERATIVE SINONASAL CAVITIES

RADIOGRAPHIC EVALUATIONS

To properly evaluate the postoperative patient, the radiologist must be knowledgeable about a number of facts, some of which are often obscure at the time of radiologic examination or film interpretation. Ideally, the radiologist should know the answers to the following questions: What operative procedure was done? How long ago was it performed? What disease prompted the surgery?

Familiarity with various otolaryngologic surgical procedures enables the radiologist to determine which bone, if any, was removed; what soft tissue defects were created, and what soft tissue or foreign material was placed to repair the surgical defect. This knowledge is essential for proper film interpretation and should help prevent the erroneous diagnosis of a surgical defect as a site of bone erosion or a muscle-fascia graft as a tumor recurrence.

The interval between the operation and the time of radiographic examination helps the radiologist determine the type of soft tissue reaction present. For recent surgery, the primary healing reaction is an active inflammation with some edema and possible hemorrhage. However, if the surgery was performed months to years ago, the primary expected healing reaction is a mature granulation tissue with varying degrees of fibrosis. In addition, reactive bone sclerosis that may occur after some procedures will have had time to develop and produce bone thickening or a reduction in sinus cavity size.

Finally, knowledge of the disease process that initially prompted the surgery allows the radiologist to anticipate the types of radiologic changes to be expected. Thus if the initial disease was chronic infection, one may commonly expect recurrent sinus mucosal thickening, reactive bone sclerosis and thickening, and possible nasal polyposis. If the initial disease was a granulomatous process, one may expect sinus mucosal thickening, nasal mucosal changes, septal erosions, and bone erosions intermixed with areas of reactive bony changes. If the initial disease was a tumor, the concern will be with characterizing nodular or localized soft tissue disease, differentiating recurrent tumor from infection, and observing the presence of progressive bone erosion or soft tissue extension to areas not normally involved by the surgery.

The best and most efficacious way to interpret an imaging study postoperatively is to compare the present examination to a prior one or a baseline study. The concept of a baseline study is an important one when monitoring a patient after surgery. The baseline examination provides an anatomic reference to which all future examinations can be compared. The question arises as to the best time to obtain such a baseline study. The closer to the time of surgery, the less chance there is for recurrence of the disease that prompted surgery. However, in the immediate postoperative period the scans can be dominated by the soft tissue changes of hemorrhage and edema and give a false image of what the eventual stable postoperative appearance will be. The best compromise appears to be a postoperative waiting period of 6 to 8 weeks. This time allows most of the hemorrhage and edema to resolve, whereas few, if any, tumors will recur within this period. The baseline study is less important in patients with inflammatory disease, but still provides a reference standard.

On subsequent follow-up scans, any progressive soft tissue resolution can be interpreted as a further reduction in the amount of postoperative hemorrhage and edema or resolution of inflammatory disease. However, the appearance of any new soft tissue changes or sites of bone erosion must be considered recurrent disease until proven otherwise. Patients who have been operated on for inflammatory disease usually do not need periodic follow-up scans and are only reimaged if symptoms reappear.

By comparison, those patients who have been operated on for tumors should have scheduled, periodic follow-up scans if early tumor recurrences are to be diagnosed. The time interval between these examinations varies from 4 to 6 months for the first 3 years postoperatively and then at 6- to 12-month intervals thereafter for 2 to 3 more years.

Plain film examinations do not allow detailed evaluation of the postoperative patient. This reflects the overall survey nature of the routine film examination and the unique anatomy of the paranasal sinuses, where focal soft tissue disease is assessed by its relationship to the adjacent bone (which now may be resected) and sinus cavity air (which may be obscured by fibrosis or disease).

Thus computer-generated sectional imaging is the examination of choice in monitoring the course of postoperative patients. Computed tomography (CT) allows the detailed evaluation of both bone and soft tissues. When studies include axial and coronal scans, the radiologist has a thorough examination with which to follow up the patient. Postcontrast scans are most desirable, since they allow distinction between inflammatory tissue, tumor, and scar tissue. However, such differentiation is not always easily accomplished on these examinations.

Magnetic resonance imaging (MRI) offers the further possibility of differentiating recurrent tumors from sites of active infection. This distinction can be made more accurately with MRI than with contrast-enhanced CT scans and without the attendant morbidity of iodinated contrast material. However, scars and tumors may not be easily distinguished with MRI, and early bone changes will be undetected.

Ultimately, the examination of choice depends on the surgical procedure done, if bone erosion is an important consideration, and if the major diagnostic problem is differentiating tumor from active infection or scar from active infection.

On noncontrast CT scans, inflammatory secretions and reactions tend to have a lower attenuation value than most sinonasal tumors, whereas on contrast-enhanced CT scans, active inflammatory changes tend to have a higher attenuation value than most tumors. However, variations in this pattern commonly exist, and scar tissues cannot be confidently differentiated from either inflammatory tissue or tumor.

On MRI inflammatory tissues have a low to intermediate signal intensity on T_1-weighted and proton density images, and a high signal intensity on T_2-weighted images. By comparison, about 95% of sinonasal tumors

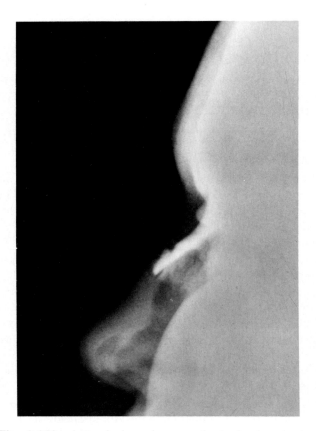

Fig. 2-356 Lateral view shows patient who has had a prior rhinoplasty. The irregularity of the nasal bone contour is postsurgical in etiology.

have an intermediate signal intensity on all imaging sequences. Only some minor salivary gland tumors and a rare cystic neuroma appear to have high T_2-weighted signal intensities. Unfortunately, mature granulation tissue with its combination of fibrosis and vascular, watery tissue also has an intermediate signal intensity on all image sequences.

OPERATIVE PROCEDURES
Nasal Surgery

Surgery on the nose is primarily cosmetic, and only those procedures which remodel the nasal bone have any noticeable radiographic manifestations. The saw, chisel, and file removal of bone during rhinoplasty may leave some slight irregularity of the midline nasal bones; this may give a nodular, somewhat unusual nasal bone profile on lateral plain films (Fig. 2-356). Nasal bones are also purposely fractured in cases of nasal bone hump removal. Once this bony mound has been removed, the broad nasal base would clinically appear too wide. Because of this, the lateral nasal walls are fractured and turned inward, recreating a thin, nasal contour. Such iatrogenic fractures may mimic a recent traumatic fracture, and only the patient's history may resolve any confusion. After 6 to 12 months, the sharp edges of all nasal fractures become smooth, and the fracture lines are less sharply seen on plain films. Old fractures also can prove confusing when there has been recent nasal trauma.[1,2]

In more severe nasal injuries, in which the nasal bones have been crushed, cartilage or rib implants may be used to reconstruct a normal nasal contour. These implants give a unique radiographic appearance that, once identified, always indicates reconstructive surgery was performed (Fig. 2-357).

Frontal Sinus Surgery

Statistically, most frontal sinus disease stems from infection and can be classified as acute or chronic. In acute infections, especially if an air-fluid level is found, factors such as the time to diagnosis and the immediate patient response to treatment determine whether or not a trephination (essentially an incision and drainage) procedure should be performed. The operation consists of the drilling of a small hole 0.5 to 1 cm to the side of the midline, usually near the upper edge of the eyebrow. After the sinus is entered and drained (the sinus mucosa is not stripped), a drainage tube or cannula is placed in the sinus for 8 to 14 days, after which it is removed to prevent a foreign reaction in the sinus mu-

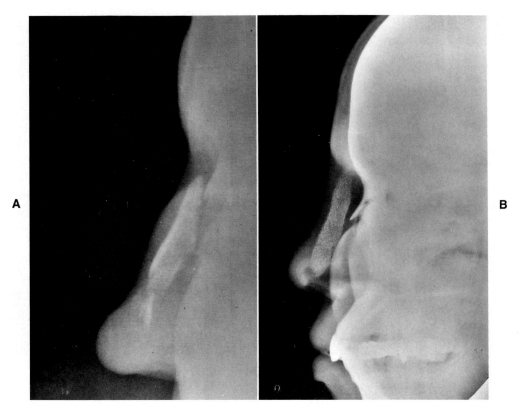

Fig. 2-357 **A,** Lateral view shows patient with a rib nasal graft replacing the badly fractured nasal bones. **B,** Lateral views shows patient with partially calcified cartilage nasal graft replacing the badly fractured nasal bones.

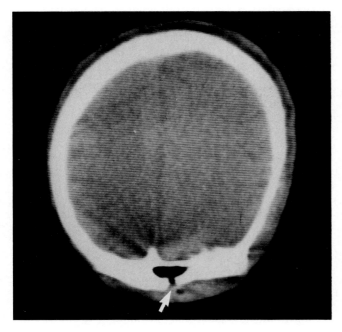

Fig. 2-358 Coronal CT scan shows posttrephination frontal sinus. The site of the trephination is seen as a hole in the anterior sinus wall *(arrow).*

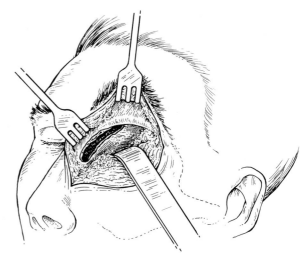

Fig. 2-359 Diagram of Lynch procedure. The ethmoid sinus, supraorbital ethmoid cells, and small frontal sinuses can be approached by this procedure. The incision is buried in the creases of the lateral nose and superomedial orbital rim.

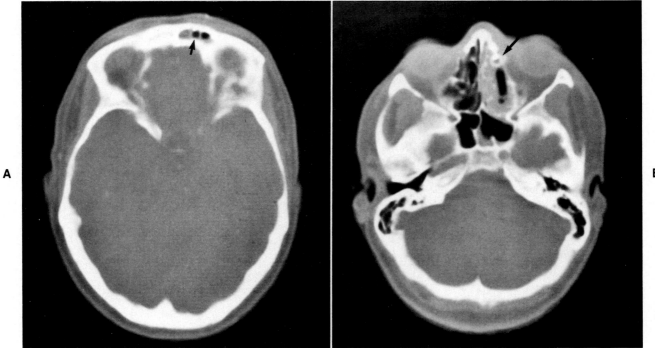

Fig. 2-360 **A,** Axial CT scan shows tube *(arrow)* in the left frontal sinus. The sinus is partially filled with secretions. **B,** Axial CT scan through the ethmoid sinuses of same patient shows the drainage tube *(arrow)* extending down into the nose. The anterior lamina papyracea has been removed as have most of the ethmoid septa because the patient has had an external ethmoidectomy. The ethmoid cavity and the left sphenoid sinus have inflammatory changes.

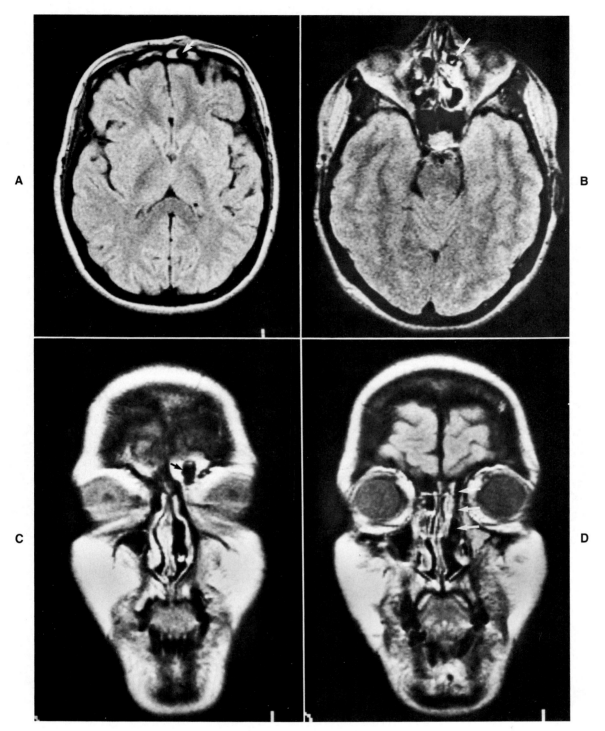

Fig. 2-361   **A,** Axial mixed image MRI scan shows drainage tube in the left frontal sinus *(arrow).* Inflammatory secretions are present in the sinus. **B,** Axial mixed image MRI scan shows drainage tube in the ethmoid sinuses *(arrow)* and inflammatory changes in the ethmoid sinuses. It is almost impossible to appreciate that an external ethmoidectomy has been performed (see Fig. 2-360, *B*). **C,** Coronal mixed image MRI scan shows frontal sinus tube *(arrow)* and frontal sinus secretions. **D,** Coronal mixed image MRI scan posterior to **C** shows the drainage tube extending through the ethmoid sinuses into the nasal fossa *(arrows).*

cosa.[1] The surgeon should ascertain by means of a Caldwell view the sinus size and its possible loculation. Care must be taken that the drill does not enter the orbit below or the anterior cranial fossa through the posterior sinus wall. The surgical defect is poorly visualized on coronal and axial CT scans unless the scans happen to pass directly through the bony hole (Fig. 2-358). If the scan is performed while the drain is in place, the drain can be followed to its exit point from the sinus.

In patients with chronic inflammatory disease, two types of procedures can be performed: those which do not obliterate the sinus cavity and the more commonly performed procedures that obliterate the sinus cavity.

The nonobliterative procedures include the Lynch, Killian, and Riedel approaches.

The *Lynch procedure* primarily is directed to the ethmoid sinuses and supraorbital ethmoid cells more than to the frontal sinus. However, it provides good entrance into a small- to moderate-size frontal sinus. The Lynch incision is buried in the creases and concavity of the lateral nose and superomedial orbital margin. The sinus is entered below and behind the orbital rim, and the nasofrontal duct is exposed as a lateral ethmoidectomy is performed. The diseased mucosa is removed and a tube placed in the nasofrontal duct to promote sinus drainage by attempting to reconstruct this duct. This tube remains in place for 6 to 8 weeks and then is removed intranasally (Figs. 2-359 to 2-361).[1,2]

If the frontal sinus is too large for all of its mucosa to be effectively reached and removed by the standard Lynch procedure, an extended Lynch incision can be used, running the incision more laterally over the orbit, or a larger bony defect can be made in the anterior

frontal sinus wall, using the Killian or Riedel procedures.

In the *Killian procedure*, a larger entrance into the frontal sinus is accomplished through two bony defects. The first is above the orbital rim in the anterior frontal sinus wall, and the second is below and behind the orbital rim in the sinus floor (the Lynch incision). The remaining superior orbital rim stops the overlying soft tissues from collapsing into the sinus and thereby minimizes the resulting cosmetic deformity (Fig. 2-362). However, the soft tissue of the forehead region partially prolapses into the sinus cavity through the surgical defect in the anterior sinus wall. This prolapsed forehead tissue creates a noticeable cosmetic deformity on axial scans. As in the Lynch procedure, the nasofrontal duct is reconstructed.

For reliable removal of the sinus mucosa in a larger frontal sinus, the *Riedel procedure* can be used. In this approach, the two surgical defects created in the Killian procedure are joined into one large defect, which includes the superior orbital rim (Fig. 2-363). At the completion of the procedure, the soft tissues of the forehead are laid on the posterior frontal sinus wall, which has been denuded of its mucosa. This effectively obliterates the upper sinus cavity, but creates an unpleasant soft tissue defect in the forehead. The nasofrontal duct is reconstructed as in the Lynch procedure.[1,2]

Because of the cosmetic deformities associated with these procedures, particularly the latter two techniques, and because the nasofrontal duct becomes obstructed postoperatively in about 50% of patients, the cosmetically less deforming, obliterative osteoplastic flap procedure has gained great recent popularity, es-

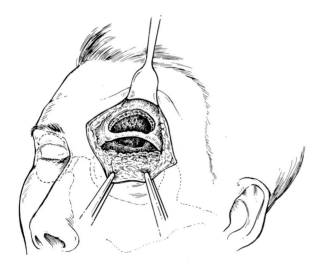

Fig. 2-362   Diagram of Killian procedure. Because of the forehead deformity, this procedure has for the most part been abandoned.

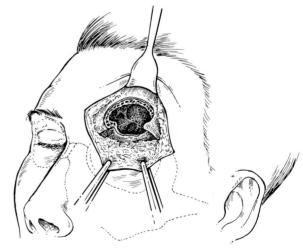

Fig. 2-363   Diagram of Riedel's procedure. Because this operation causes a large deformity of the forehead, it has been almost entirely abandoned.

pecially in the moderate to large sinuses in which mucosa cannot be removed by a Lynch approach.

The osteoplastic flap is approached through a curved coronal incision that is hidden in the scalp hair or through an incision that extends from one eyebrow to the other, crossing the intervening skin crease near the root of the nose. Once the periosteum over the frontal bone is exposed, a template made from a Caldwell view is used to trace the frontal sinus contour on the bone and periosteum. The template should come from a film taken on a dedicated head unit such as the Franklin Head Unit. On such a machine the magnification factor is only 3.4% compared with 10.3% on a standard 40-inch posteroanterior Caldwell film.[3] The outline of the sinus should be traced just inside of this line. The periosteum is incised on all except its inferior margin, and the frontal sinus contour is drilled into the anterior frontal sinus table. The drill line is beveled medially and downward to ensure that the frontal sinus and not the anterior cranial fossa is entered. The inferior margin of this anterior wall is not drilled, but is fractured from side to side and turned downward off of the sinus with its overlying periosteum intact. This technique yields a viable bone flap. The sinus mucosa is then drilled out, and the sinus cavity is obliterated with fat or muscle, usually taken from the abdominal wall. The anterior sinus wall is then replaced, the periosteum sutured, and the skin closed, leaving literally no cosmetic deformity (Fig. 2-364).

The fat gradually undergoes fibrosis until the fibrosis represents one third to one half the volume of the obliterating material. Throughout this process no volume loss occurs, so the sinus remains obliterated. Infection

of the bone flap or the operative margins with or without associated osteomyelitis and infection of the obliterating fat are the two most significant complications of the osteoplastic flap procedure and usually necessitate a second operation to remove the infection. This procedure often results in removal of the anterior sinus wall bone flap with obliteration of the remaining sinus cavity by the forehead tissues. A plastic reconstruction can then be performed at a later date, once the infection has healed.

If the osteoplastic flap procedure was performed for a mucocele and if the mucocele thinned or destroyed a portion of the posterior sinus table, then the posterior table defect and the surgically related anterior wall defect are visualized on subsequent radiographic studies.

On plain films the osteoplastic bone flap can be identified by a variably thin zone of lower density at its margins, which represents the surgically drilled-out anterior table. Because this portion of the bone is no longer present, the bone flap, by comparison, is easily identified (Figs. 2-365 and 2-366). In a few cases, the flap fit may be so good as to make visualization of the surgical margin almost impossible on Caldwell or Waters views. However, a lateral view clearly shows the surgical defect. In fact, if a surgical history is not obtained, the defect may be misinterpreted as an anterior frontal table fracture (Fig. 2-367). If the sinus margin was altered before surgery, it will remain so after surgery. Thus the mucoperiosteal white line may be absent or replaced by a thick zone of sclerosis, and the sinus contour may be remodeled. Although this appearance can be confusing and suggests that whatever caused these changes is still present in the sinus, these sinus alterations merely re-

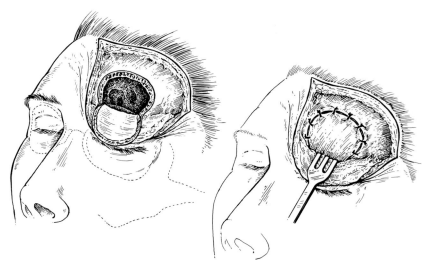

Fig. 2-364   Diagram of osteoplastic flap procedure. The anterior sinus wall is flipped down with the inferior periosteum left intact. After the sinus mucosa and disease are removed, the sinus is obliterated with fat and then the flap is replaced. This procedure leaves almost no cosmetic deformity.

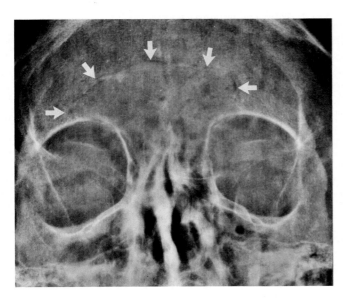

Fig. 2-365 Waters view shows patient to be status post a bilateral osteoplastic flap. The flap margins can barely be identified *(arrows)*.

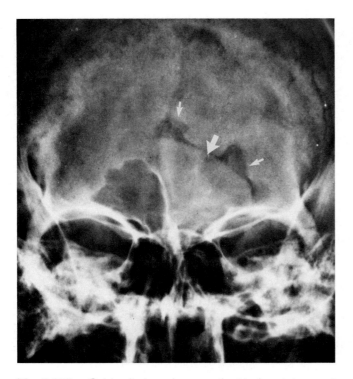

Fig. 2-366 Caldwell view shows patient to be status post a left osteoplastic flap. The margins of the flap are well seen *(arrows)*. The space between the flap and the sinus margin is a normal postoperative finding that results from the bone removed during the drilling to open the sinus and eliminate the inflammatory disease.

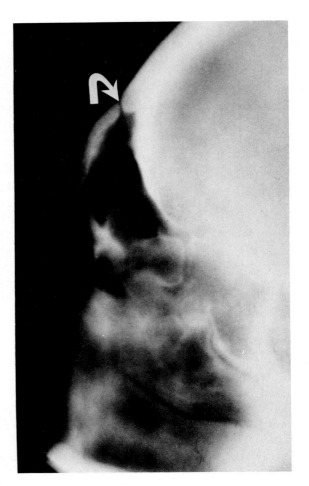

Fig. 2-367 Lateral multidirectional tomogram shows patient to be status post an osteoplastic flap procedure. The surgical margin of the flap *(arrow)* is seen and may simulate a fracture.

flect whatever process originally caused the surgery. If the sinus was obliterated, a hazy soft tissue density may appear in the sinus, suggesting sinusitis. The surgical bony margins should be sharp and of a normal texture even though the bone flap does not fit precisely against the adjacent frontal bone. An air-fluid level indicates reinfection of the sinus, a serious complication.

On CT scans the bone flap may go unnoticed if only narrow windows are used. At wide window settings, the bone has a normal texture (Fig. 2-368). The flap edges and adjacent frontal bone occasionally have a ragged, unsharp appearance that reflects the beveling surgical procedure and drill defects. Without any associated clinical or soft tissue changes, this bony appearance should not elicit a diagnosis of osteomyelitis. Frank osteomyelitis appears as areas of bone demineralization, erosion, or sequestration accompanied by swelling and cellulitis of the overlying forehead soft tissues and evidence of infection in the underlying fat (Fig. 2-369).

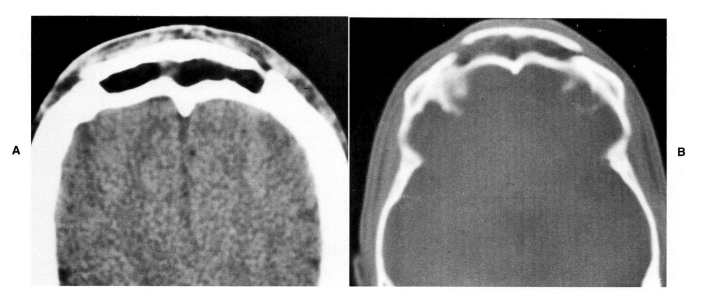

Fig. 2-368   Axial CT scan at **A,** narrow and **B,** wide window settings. The sinus is filled with fat, and the flap is sharply seen in good position.

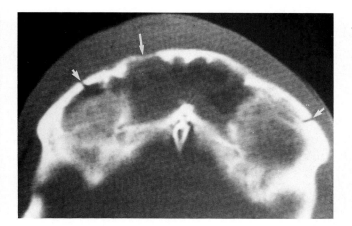

Fig. 2-369   Axial CT scan shows margins of the osteoplastic flap *(small arrows)*. There is a focal area of bone demineralization *(arrow)* in the flap with swelling of the overlying soft tissues. Osteomyelitis and cellulitis.

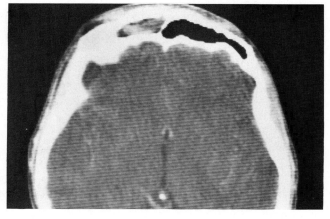

Fig. 2-370   Axial postcontrast CT scan shows patient to be status post a right osteoplastic flap. The obliterating fat is dense. Early postoperative infection of the fat.

The obliterated sinus is best examined at both narrow and wide windows. The entire sinus cavity should be filled with fatty material with randomly scattered strands of soft tissue density and fibrous tissue. No sinus air should be present. Whenever a focal mass of soft tissue density is seen within the fat or whenever more than half the fat content is of fibrous density, the radiologist should suspect infection of the obliterating material (Fig. 2-370). This type of infection is usually associated with elevation of the flap secondary to swelling of the fibrous fatty material (Fig. 2-371). In these cases, the intracranial compartment should also be examined for spread of the infection.

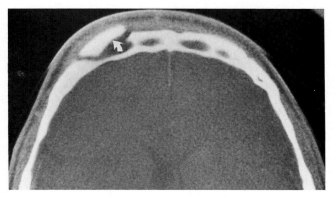

Fig. 2-371   Axial CT scan shows elevation of the top of a right osteoplastic flap *(arrow)*. This usually indicates swelling and infection of the obliterating fat.

Occasionally, the osteoplastic flap fractures during surgery; however, as long as the overlying periosteum remains intact, the fracture pieces remain viable. The radiologist should verify that the bony pieces have a normal texture and are not sites of osteomyelitis and that such bone pieces are not elevated, suggesting an underlying infection (Fig. 2-372).

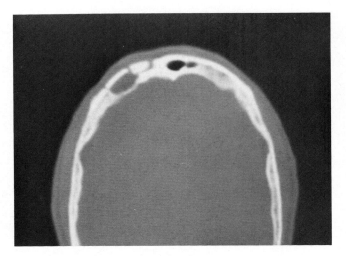

Fig. 2-372 Axial CT scan shows fracture of the osteoplastic flap on the right side. This occurred at surgery and is a normal postoperative finding.

In rare instances, after many years, some calcification can occur in the obliterating fat; this in and of itself should only be considered a normal postoperative variant.

On MRI the T_1-weighted and proton density images have a fairly high signal intensity, whereas the T_2-weighted studies reveal an intermediate signal intensity (Fig. 2-373). Infection gives a high T_2-weighted signal within the fat and possibly in the surrounding forehead tissues.

Ethmoid Sinus Surgery

The ethmoid complex can be partially resected or a biopsy specimen obtained by three major approaches: the external, the internal (intranasal), and the transmaxillary (transantral) (Fig. 2-374). In inflammatory disease, the aim of these procedures is to progressively remove the disease from each cell until all of the pathologic material is removed. The primary areas of complication are entrance into the floor of the anterior cranial fossa and damage to the orbital contents.[1,2,4]

The external approach provides the best access and overall visualization. The lamina papyracea is viewed on its surface so that prior fractures are more easily identified, and surgically related fractures are more easily prevented. If the anterior and posterior ethmoidal canals are exposed, a line connecting them lies just be-

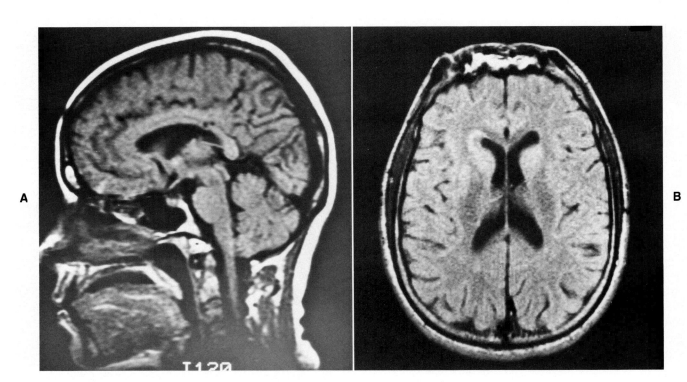

Fig. 2-373 **A,** Sagittal T_1W and **B,** axial mixed image MRI scans show (fat) high signal intensity material within the obliterated sinus. The flap is often hard to identify on MRI scans.

low the floor of the anterior cranial fossa. If the surgeon stays caudal to this level, intracranial entrance should not occur. The surgical field can be enlarged to the base of the skull, frontal sinus, supraorbital cells, or orbit; the nasofrontal duct is best opened with this approach. However, a Lynch incision must be made, despite its associated cosmetic defect. In this approach

the anterior cells are first entered through the lamina papyracea, and then the posterior cells are progressively opened as needed.

The internal ethmoidectomy is performed intranasally and includes resection of the middle turbinate to provide better access to the cells. The ethmoid complex is entered by way of the bulla ethmoidalis region, the more posterior cells are then opened, and then the anterior cells are resected. In experienced hands, the lamina papyracea is not violated in this procedure. This approach is used for isolated ethmoid sinus disease, for biopsies, in patients who do not have coexistent antral disease, and in patients who do not wish to have an external incision.

The transantral approach is used when the antral cavity has coexistent sinusitis or the intranasal approach is not possible because of anatomic or technical reasons. The antrum is entered using a Caldwell-Luc approach, and the medial, upper maxillary sinus wall (ethmoidomaxillary plate) is taken down so that the ethmoid cells can be entered.

In virtually all of these procedures, the surgeon is forced to blindly cut through the most inaccessible ethmoid septa located at the cranial and posterior margins of the ethmoid complex. Even when it appears that the surgeon went so far posteriorly that the sphenoid sinus was opened, scans often reveal the contrary. Typically

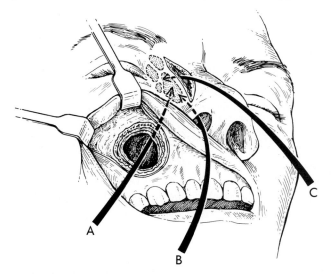

Fig. 2-374 Diagram of the three major surgical approaches to the ethmoid sinuses: *A,* transmaxillary or transantral, *B,* internal or intranasal, and *C,* external (Lynch).

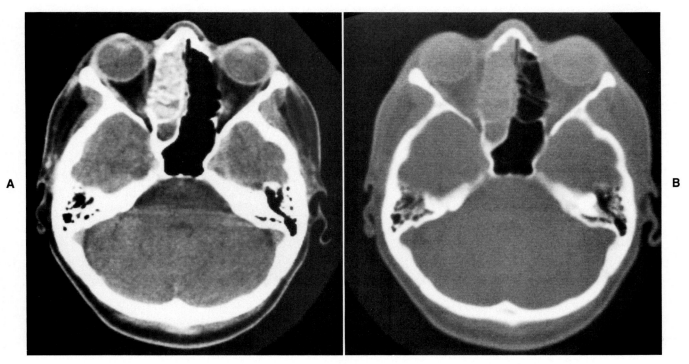

Fig. 2-375 Axial CT scans at **A,** narrow and **B,** wide window settings show inflammatory disease in the right ethmoid and sphenoid sinuses and, in **A,** an apparent prior left sphenoethmoidectomy. However, in **B,** the left ethmoid septa are present indicating that no surgery was performed.

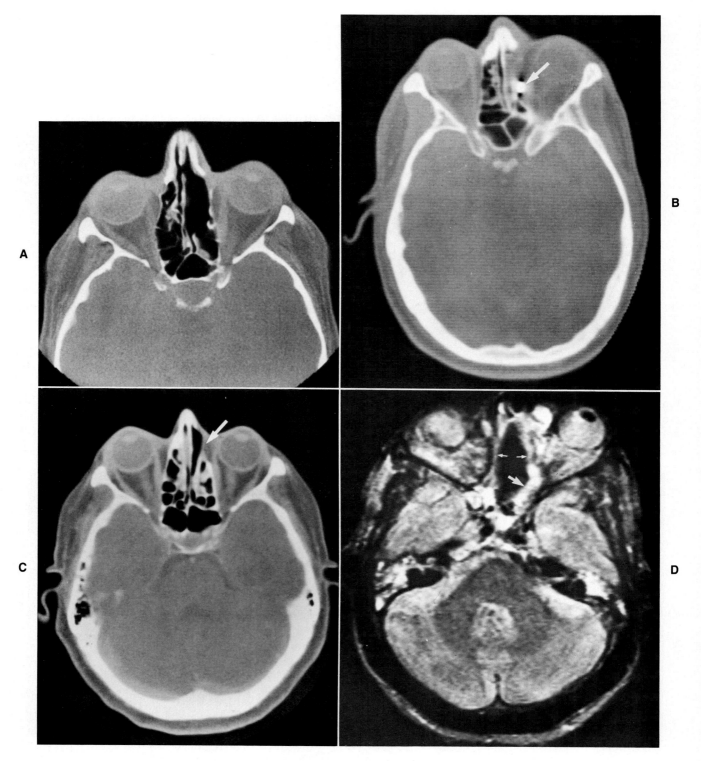

Fig. 2-376 **A,** Axial CT scan shows postoperative appearance of a complete left internal ethmoidectomy. **B,** Axial CT scan shows patient to be status post left external ethmoidectomy. The surgical clip *(arrow)* is used to control bleeding from ethmoidal vessels. The soft tissue in the anterior ethmoid cavity is fibrosis and granulation tissue. **C,** Axial CT scan shows postoperative appearance of left external ethmoidectomy. The anterior lamina papyracea has been surgically removed and is replaced by fibrosis (arrow). **D,** Axial T_2W MRI scan shows the appearance of prior complete bilateral internal ethmoidectomies. Part of the postoperative cavity is lined with fibrotic tissue *(small arrows)*, while other areas have inflammatory tissue with a high T_2W signal intensity *(arrow)*.

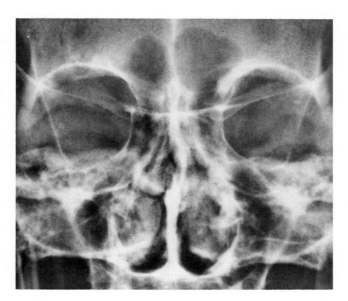

Fig. 2-377 Caldwell view shows clouding of the left ethmoid sinuses. This appearance suggests infection. However, in this patient, this was due to fibrosis after an ethmoidectomy.

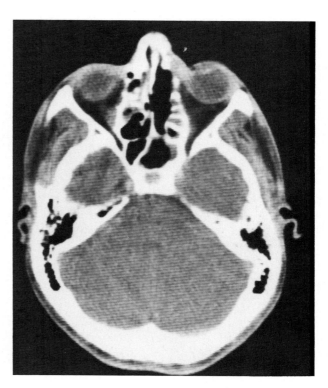

Fig. 2-378 Axial CT scan shows appearance of left ethmoidectomy. Several of the posterior and more cranial ethmoid septa are still seen. This is a common finding, and these areas may be sites of residual disease.

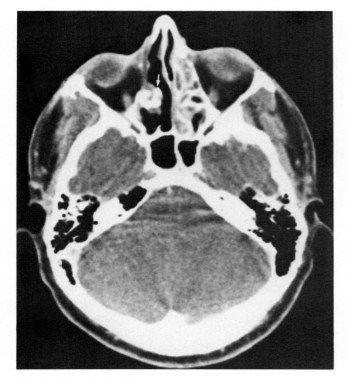

Fig. 2-379 Axial CT scan shows patient who has had a right ethmoidectomy. There is a focal area of bone production within the postoperative cavity *(arrow)*. This represents reactive bone response to surgery and has no pathologic significance.

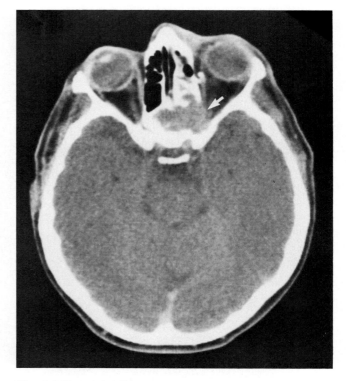

Fig. 2-380 Axial CT scan shows destructive mass in the left posterior sphenoethmoid region *(arrow)*. This patient had a limited left ethmoidectomy for suspected infectious disease. No preoperative scan was obtained. It was only when left eye signs developed that a scan was obtained. Infection and carcinoma.

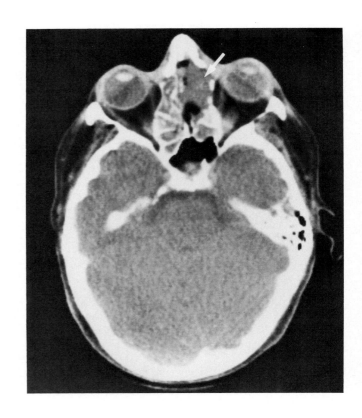

Fig. 2-381 Axial CT scan shows appearance of left ethmoidectomy and accumulation of mucoid material within the postoperative cavity *(arrow)*. Postoperative mucocele.

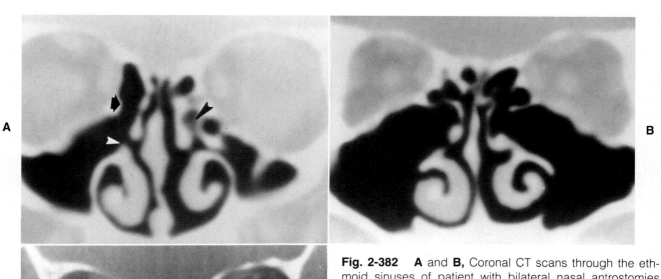

Fig. 2-382 **A** and **B,** Coronal CT scans through the ethmoid sinuses of patient with bilateral nasal antrostomies who subsequently had endoscopic removal of the right uncinate process *(white arrowhead)* and ethmoid bulla *(arrow)*. Minimal mucoperiosteal thickening is present in the contralateral middle meatus *(black arrowhead)*. **C,** Coronal CT scan through the anterior ethmoid sinus of patient with endoscopic removal of the right ethmoid bulla and partial resection of the uncinate process. Mucoperiosteal thickening persists along the lamina papyracea *(white arrowhead)* and remaining uncinate process *(white arrow)*. The right middle turbinate *(black arrow)* is fused to the nasal septum. (Courtesy of SJ Zinreich, MD.)

the most posterior ethmoid cells and the sphenoid sinus remain untouched by the procedure. This discrepancy points out the difficulty of clinically estimating the anatomy of the area, and it is precisely because of these limitations that postoperative scans should be obtained if the patient's symptoms persist or recur (Figs. 2-375 to 2-380).[4]

Because of the small, boxlike anatomy of the ethmoid cells, postoperative hemorrhaging can fill some cells and, on occasion, rather than resorb, the blood becomes fibrosed. Such en bloc fibrosis does not often occur after surgery in the other paranasal sinuses, but is fairly common in the ethmoid complex. Differentiating recurrent disease from fibrosis can be difficult. The recurrent inflammation enhances on postcontrast CT scans, and the fibrosis does not. However, the differences in attenuation values frequently are not sufficient to establish a definitive diagnosis. If enough time has passed after surgery so that a significant fibrotic component is present in the granulation tissue, this scar can be distinguished from active infection with T_2-weighted MRI.

In addition to removal of the ethmoid septa, the main bony defects the radiologist should key in on are (1) an absent anterior third to half of the lamina papyracea from an external approach, (2) an absent medial ethmoid wall and possible absent middle turbinate from an internal approach, and (3) a Caldwell-Luc defect in the lower anterior antral wall with absent bone in the upper medial antral wall from a transantral approach. Any residual soft tissue disease in the remaining ethmoid cells should be clearly noted by the radiologist for future reference.

If a postoperative ethmoid cavity becomes obstructed after mucosal reepithelialization, a mucocele develops (Fig. 2-381). This mucocele may not behave like a typical ethmoid mucocele, which usually expands laterally into the orbit. Rather, this postoperative mucocele takes the course of least resistance and expands within the enlarged postoperative ethmoid cavity. It is only after the entire ethmoid cavity is filled that the mucocele bulges into the orbit. On imaging this noninfected mucocele may be confused with infected tissue on both CT scans and with MRI.[5]

Maxillary Sinus Surgery

Today the most common diagnostic and therapeutic procedures performed on the antrum and its drainage area (the ostiomeatal complex) are endoscopic techniques, an intranasal antrostomy, and a Caldwell-Luc operation. The endoscopic techniques can vary from limited procedures, such as an uncinectomy and resection of the bulla ethmoidalis region, to more extensive procedures that resect most of the ethmoid cells. Any soft tissue disease in the ostiomeatal complex that is ob-

served on thin-section coronal CT scans should be reported to the surgeons (Fig. 2-382).

In an intranasal antrostomy, the membranous and bony lateral nasal wall of the inferior meatus is partially resected in an attempt to create better gravity drainage of the sinus. This defect is easily seen on axial and coronal CT scans (Fig. 2-383).

In the Caldwell-Luc procedure, in addition to the intranasal antrostomy, the maxillary sinus is entered by way of the canine fossa region of the lower anterior antral wall. An under–the–upper lip approach prevents facial scarring. Once the sinus is entered, the mucosa is removed. Thus, in addition to the antrostomy defect, the patient has a bony defect in the lower anterior sinus wall. Initially the bony defect is closed by a hematoma, which eventually undergoes fibrosis. The hematoma can become infected, however, and in rare instances an oroantral fistula may be created. If this unusual complication occurs, it is usually within the first or second postoperative week. With the Caldwell-Luc approach, the bone of the posterior sinus wall can be removed to provide access for internal maxillary artery ligation or to expose the pterygopalatine fossa, vidian nerve, and pterygopalatine ganglion.[1] In such cases, a bony defect in the upper, medial, and posterior antral wall also can be seen on scanning.

In some patients synechiae develop between the lateral margin of the canine fossa/Caldwell-Luc defect in the anterior sinus wall and the posterior sinus wall. Persistent synechiae may form the basis for a membrane that extends across the sinus between the anterior and posterior walls. Once formed, this membrane obstructs the drainage of the lateral portion of the maxillary sinus and leads to the appearance of a postoperative antral mucocele (Figs. 2-202, 2-203, and 2-384).

Another postoperative complication arises once the mucosa has been stripped from the sinus wall. This process may elicit a bony reaction that results in reactive bone formation, thickening of the sinus wall, and reduction or obliteration of the sinus cavity. Such a reaction is an expected consequence of the procedure and should not signify to the radiologist that active infection is present (Figs. 2-383 and 2-385).[6]

In patients with thyroid ophthalmopathy who have decreasing vision secondary to optic nerve compression, surgical orbital decompression procedures can be performed in an attempt to save vision. These procedures most commonly use a lateral orbitotomy (Krönlein's operation), an antral decompression performed using a Caldwell-Luc approach, an ethmoid decompression using an external ethmoidectomy, and an orbital roof decompression using a craniotomy. Of these procedures, the greatest degree of decompression is accomplished when the orbital floors are removed surgically. This procedure must be performed bilaterally so

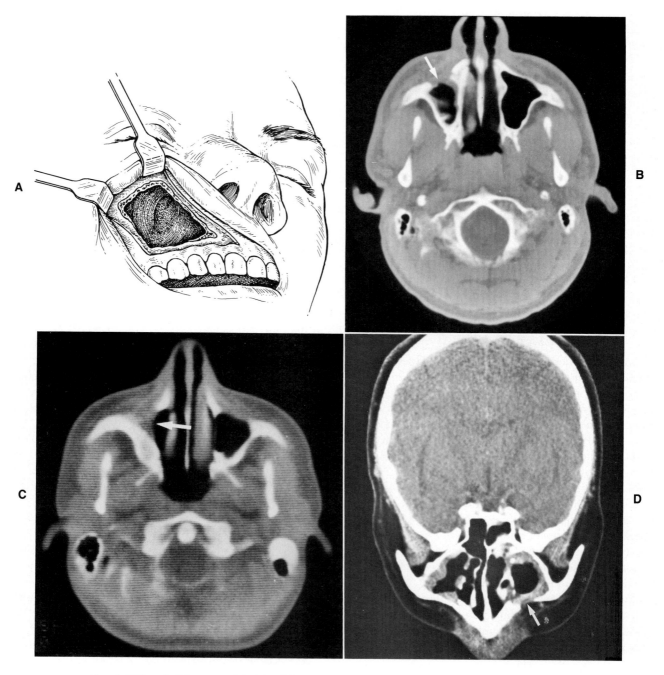

Fig. 2-383   A, Diagram of Caldwell-Luc approach. The maxillary sinus is entered ante-riorly from the canine fossa. The hole in the sinus can be of a variable size. **B,** Axial CT scan shows anterior sinus wall Caldwell-Luc defect *(arrow).* The soft tissues in the sinus were senechia. **C,** Axial CT scan shows anterior Caldwell-Luc defect, the antrostomy de-fect *(arrow),* and thickening of the remaining sinus wall. The soft tissue in the sinus is fibrosis. **D,** Coronal CT scan shows Caldwell-Luc defect in the anterior sinus wall *(arrow)* and inflammatory mucosal thickening in both antra.

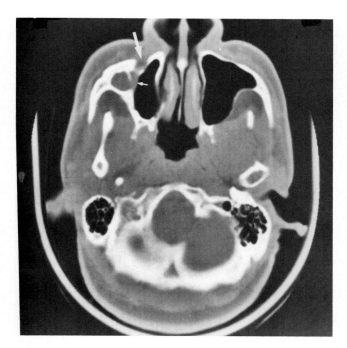

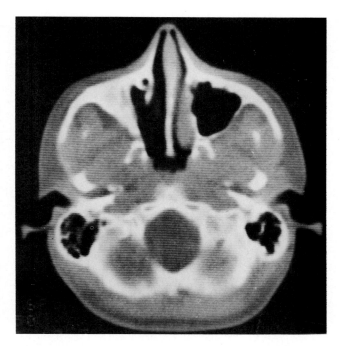

Fig. 2-384 Axial CT scan shows anterior Caldwell-Luc defect in the right maxillary sinus wall *(large arrow)*. There is an expansile mass in the lateral portion of the right antrum *(small arrow)*. Postoperative antral mucocele.

Fig. 2-385 Axial CT scan shows post Caldwell-Luc right maxillary sinus in which the remaining antral wall bone has thickened to almost obliterate the sinus cavity.

that the visual axes are not asymmetric, resulting in diplopia and cosmetic deformity. The lateral and ethmoid decompressions can be combined with antral decompressions to achieve maximal relief of exophthalmos and a decrease in intraorbital pressure. The orbital roof approach provides relatively little decompression, and, because it is a more dangerous surgical approach, it is reserved for only the most severe cases.

On sectional imaging the absence of the lateral portion of the orbital wall may at first elude detection, the radiologist's attention being drawn by pronounced proptosis with muscle enlargement. However, careful evaluation of the bony orbital margins reveals that Krönlein procedure was performed (Fig. 2-386). The ethmoid decompression has the same appearance as an external ethmoidectomy, and it is the orbital muscle findings of thyroid ophthalmopathy that suggests the diagnosis (Fig. 2-387). The antral decompression reveals prolapse of the orbital fat and inferior muscles into the upper maxillary sinuses. On axial scans this operation may present a confusing picture; however, coronal scans reveal that the orbital floor bone is missing, a finding that differentiates this postoperative appearance from the rare event of bilateral orbital blow-out fractures (Fig. 2-388).

Sphenoid Sinus Surgery

The sphenoid sinuses can be approached through the anterior sinus wall for biopsy, to improve sinus drain-

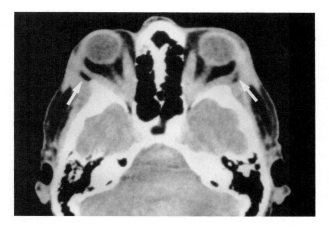

Fig. 2-386 Axial CT scan shows patient with the changes of thyroid ophthalmopathy. All of the extraocular muscle bellies are enlarged, and there is bilateral proptosis. The lateral orbital walls *(arrows)* have been surgically removed. Patient status post bilateral lateral orbitotomies (Kronlein approaches).

age, or to remove inflammatory tissue. The sphenoid sinusotomy opens the anterior wall of the sinus and creates a wide, open cavity that leads into the nasopharynx (Fig. 2-389). The sinus can be reached by intranasal, transseptal, transmaxillary, or transethmoidal approaches.

In the transnasal approach, portions of the posterior middle turbinate, the superior turbinate, and some of the posterior ethmoid cells are removed to gain exposure. In the transseptal approach, portions of the cartilaginous and bony nasal septum (vomer) are removed. The transmaxillary approach is an extension of a Caldwell-Luc procedure in which a transmaxillary ethmoidectomy is carried up to include the anterior sphenoid sinus wall. The transethmoidal approach is simply a posterior extension of an external ethmoidectomy pro-

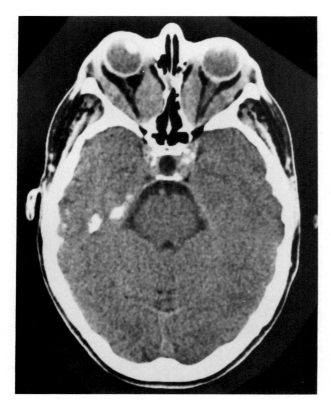

Fig. 2-387 Axial CT scan shows large muscle bellies in the extraocular muscles with tapering at the anterior tendon insertions. The ethmoid complexes have been collapsed for decompression. Thyroid ophthalmopathy.

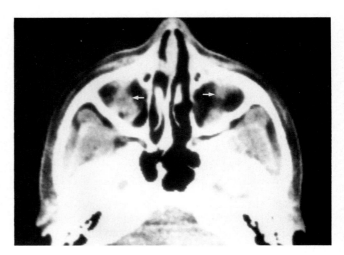

Fig. 2-388 Axial CT scan through the maxillary sinuses shows inferior rectus muscles *(arrows)* to lie in the upper antra. The orbital floors have been surgically removed. Thyroid ophthalmopathy in patient status post bilateral orbital floor decompressions.

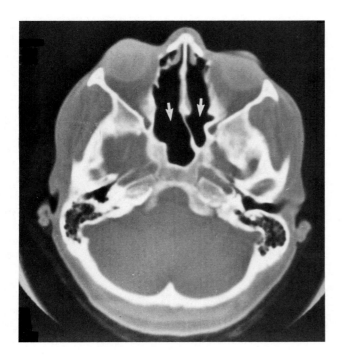

Fig. 2-389 Axial CT scan shows patient with bilateral ethmoidectomies and sphenoid sinusotomies. The anterior sphenoid sinus walls have been removed *(arrows)*.

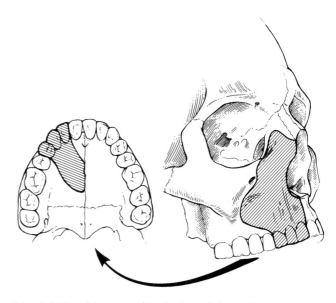

Fig. 2-390 Diagram of typical medial maxillectomy resection. A portion of the palate is removed if needed to obtain a tumor free margin. The medial antral wall and inferior turbinate are also included in the resection.

cedure. Thus, depending on the approach used, in addition to an absence of one or both anterior sphenoid sinus walls, the respective surgical defects just described should be observed on scans.[1,2]

When a sphenoid sinusotomy is performed, care must be taken to avoid trauma to the carotid artery. In 17% of patients, the bony wall separating the sinus and artery is so thin that it provides little if any protection from trauma. Carotid artery damage may lead to a post-traumatic aneurysm or a carotid-cavernous fistula.[7,8]

A transsphenoidal hypophysectomy can be performed as an extension of the sphenoid sinusotomy. Once the sphenoid sinus cavity is exposed surgically, portions of the sellar anterior wall and floor can be removed and the pituitary fossa entered from below. Muscle, fat, cartilage, or bone may be used to help seal the surgical defect. On sectional imaging, in addition to the site of surgical bone removal, sclerotic thickening of the remaining portions of the anterior sellar wall and floor may be observed. Some prolapse of sellar contents can occur, and, without benefit of the surgical history, the imaging picture can simulate that of a large pituitary tumor with extension down into the sphenoid sinus.

In the preoperative evaluation of patients for a transsphenoidal hypophysectomy, the radiologist must direct special attention to the thickness of the bone between the posterior sphenoid sinus margin and the anterior sellar cortical surface. In nearly 99% of patients the sphenoid sinus development is sufficient to extend up to or posterior to this lamina dura. However, in the 1% of patients in whom a thick margin of bone remains between the sinus and sella, the transsphenoidal approach is not desirable, and instead an intracranial approach is used.[9]

Endoscopic Nasal Surgery

The concept that ostiomeatal complex obstruction can perpetuate maxillary, ethmoid, and frontal sinusitis is not new. However, with recent technical developments, the otolaryngologist can now perform an endoscopic antrostomy and ethmoidectomy with restoration of mucociliary clearance. The inability to restore this mucociliary clearance when the more conventional Caldwell-Luc or ethmoidectomy approaches are used has been blamed for some of the failures of these procedures. Generally, these failures occur secondary to undiagnosed focal disease in the ostiomeatal complex.

The major advantages of the endoscopic middle meatal antrostomy are the ability to restore ostial patency and to remove associated anterior ethmoid sinus disease under direct visualization with minimal morbidity. The best preoperative visualization of the ostiomeatal complex is obtained on thin-section coronal CT scans (Fig. 2-382). The radiologist should direct attention to the infundibulum, uncinate process, ethmoid bulla, and middle meatus. Any focal soft tissue disease in these areas that partially or completely obstructs the normal airways should be localized for the surgeon.[10]

Surgery for Sinus Malignancy

Depending on the primary location of the tumor, one of several operations can be performed that involve the maxillary sinus. For localized nasal tumors that involve the lower portion of the lateral nasal vault, a partial maxillectomy (medial maxillectomy) can be performed. Rarely, portions of the hard palate and maxillary alveolus are included in the resection to obtain a tumor-free margin on all aspects of the lesion (Fig. 2-390). In a partial maxillectomy, the medial antral wall, the inferior turbinate, often the middle turbinate, the lower ethmoid cells, and, if appropriate, portions of the hard palate and alveolus are absent on the scans. The lateral portion of the antrum and its mucosa remain intact.

For more extensive tumors, a total maxillectomy can be performed (Fig. 2-391). Such surgery includes the maxilla, the body of the zygoma, the ipsilateral hard palate and alveolus, the inferior turbinate, and often the pterygoid plates and portions of the ethmoid sinuses.[1,2,11] Modifications are made to fit the specific tumor location. Thus the orbital floor may be left in place, or it may be included along with an orbital exenteration. The latter is performed for gross tumor extension into the orbit or for a tumor in the periosteum of the bones of the orbit, when such tumor is observed at surgery. The created surgical cavity is then lined with a split-thickness skin graft so that an epithelial surface immediately lines the defect. If the orbital floor was re-

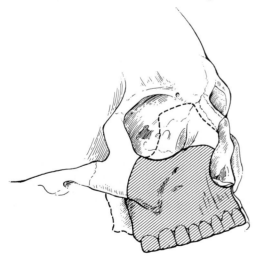

Fig. 2-391 Diagram of typical total maxillectomy resection. Variable portions of zygoma and pterygoid plates may be included in the resection. Similarly, the orbital floor may be taken in its entirety and an ethmoid resection *(dotted line)* may also be included in order to obtain a tumor-free margin.

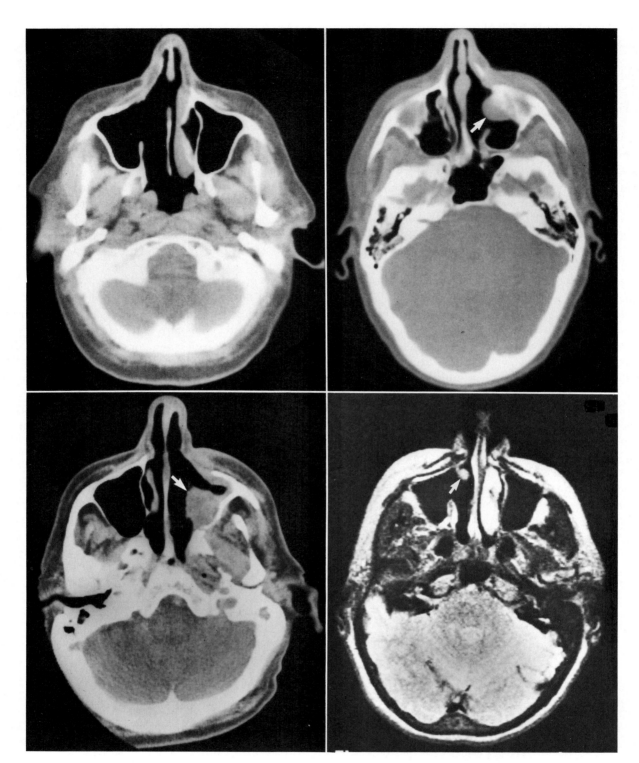

Fig. 2-392 **A,** Axial CT scan shows postpartial right maxillectomy appearance. The soft tissues in and around the antrum should be smooth. **B,** Axial CT scan shows postpartial left maxillectomy appearance with a nodular mass *(arrow)* in the antrum. Although this could be an inflammatory mass, the suspicion of tumor should be raised until proven otherwise. Tumor Recurrence. **C,** Axial CT scan shows postpartial left maxillectomy appearance with an irregularly nodular tumor recurrence *(arrow)* in the antrum. The smooth soft tissues lining the anterior left antrum represented scar tissue. **D,** Axial T$_2$W MRI scan shows postpartial right maxillectomy appearance. There is a small nodule *(arrow)* with intermediate signal intensity along the anterior resection margin that was a tumor recurrence.

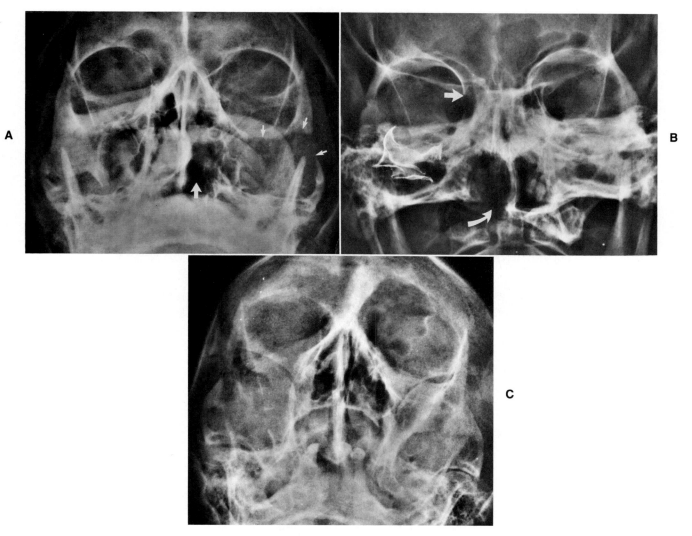

Fig. 2-393   A, Waters view shows post total left maxillectomy appearance. The orbital floor and zygoma have been removed *(arrows),* and a portion of the palate *(large arrow)* has been resected. **B,** Caldwell view shows post total right maxillectomy and ethmoidectomy. A graft to support the right orbital floor is seen. The margin of the ethmoid resection *(arrow)* and palatal resection *(curved arrow)* are also visualized. **C,** Waters view shows post total right maxillectomy appearance without palatal resection.

moved, various synthetic grafts can be placed to help support the orbital contents. Similarly, prostheses are placed to fill the surgical defects created in the hard palate and alveolus. These foreign substances can cause imaging problems either because they may degrade the image quality or because, in the case of some plastics and musculofascial grafts, on MRI they may simulate normal bone. Eye prostheses also may cause degradation artifacts on scans.

With a partial maxillectomy, normal mucosa lines the postoperative defect, whereas with a total maxillectomy, a split-thickness skin graft lines the cavity. In both cases, after the 6- to 8-week postoperative inter-

val, nearly all of the edema and hemorrhage have subsided, and a baseline scan should be performed. This scan not only maps the patient's new anatomy, but establishes the contour and thickness of the postoperative mucosal areas. The normal postoperative mucosal surfaces are smooth and moderately thin. Any localized areas of soft tissue nodularity or mucosal-submucosal thickening must be suspected of representing recurrent tumor until proven otherwise. If such areas develop where they were not noted on the baseline scan, the radiologist should direct the clinician to these sites (Figs. 2-392 to 2-394). This approach has led to more positive biopsy specimens than those obtained with the multiple

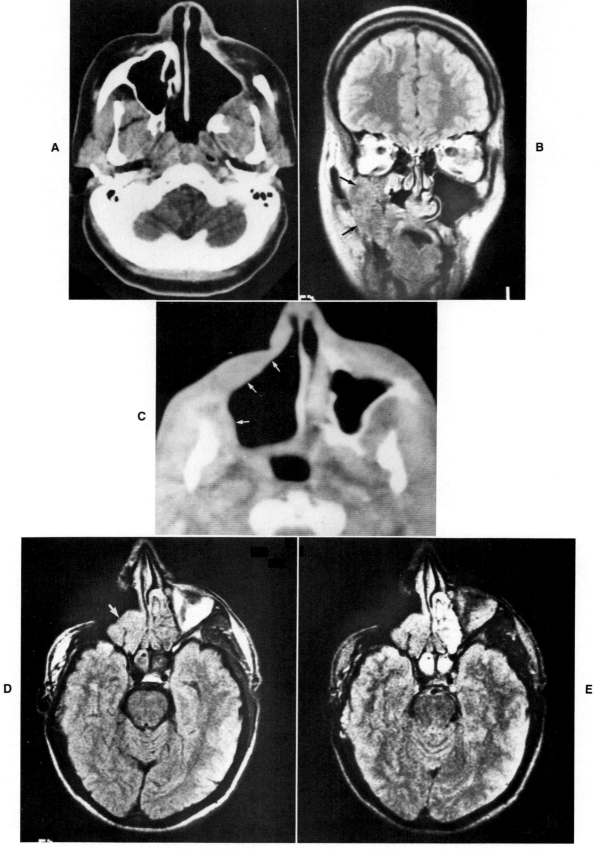

Fig. 2-394 For legend see opposite page.

Fig. 2-394   **A,** Axial CT scan shows total left maxillectomy appearance. The postoperative cavity is smooth. The pterygoid plates were not resected. **B,** Axial CT scan shows total right maxillectomy appearance. The pterygoid plates were resected. The cavity is smoothly lined *(arrows)*. **C,** Coronal mixed image MRI scan shows a large right tumor recurrence with an intermediate signal intensity *(arrows)* in a patient who had a total right maxillectomy. **D,** Axial mixed image MRI scan shows patient who has had a total right orbital extenteration and a total maxillectomy. Tumor recurrence is seen in the right orbital apex *(arrow)*. However, it is impossible to tell if the left ethmoid sinuses and the sphenoid sinuses are also involved. **E,** Axial T_2W MRI scan on same patient shows high signal intensity in the left ethmoid sinuses and both sphenoid sinuses, indicating the presence of entrapped inflammatory secretions and not tumor. The actual tumor is seen as an intermediate signal intensity mass.

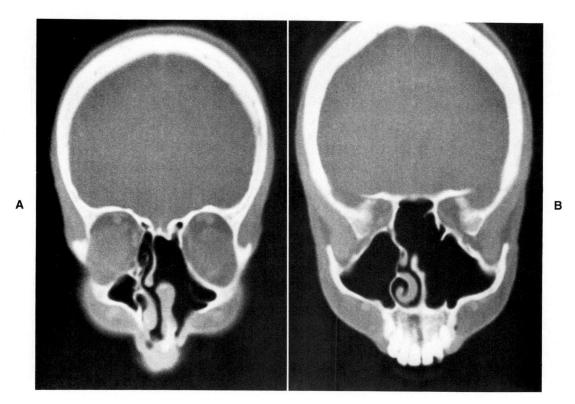

Fig. 2-395   Coronal CT scan through the **A,** anterior antrum and **B,** posterior antrum and sphenoid sinus in patient who has had a left lateral rhinotomy.

blind biopsy technique and has identified small early recurrences that were overlooked on clinical follow-up.[12]

Extensive Nasoethmoid Surgery

The lateral rhinotomy provides access to the entire nasal cavity and the maxillary, ethmoid, and sphenoid sinuses. Modifications and extensions of this approach can be used to include access to the frontal sinuses. The typical incision extends from just below the medial end of one eyebrow, caudally between the nasal dorsum and medial canthus of the eye, down the nasofacial crease, and along the nasal alar rim. The incision can be extended down the upper lip if necessary.[13] The nose is turned to the side, thereby exposing the piriform aperture. This procedure gives access, through a relatively short skin incision, to the entire lateral nasal wall and nasal septum for extirpation of both benign and malignant nasal disease. The medial antral wall, ethmoid cells, and inferior and middle turbinates usually are removed. The anterior sphenoid wall can be included in the procedure, and the operation can be extended to

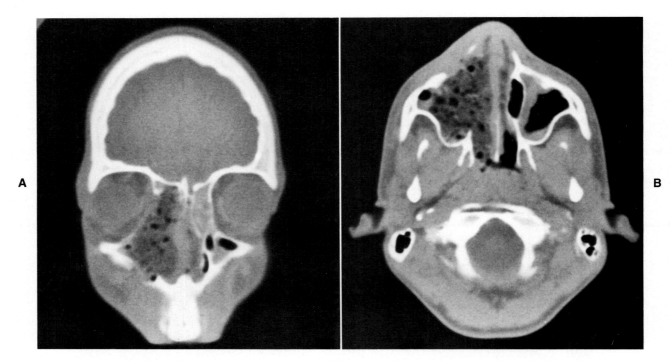

Fig. 2-396 **A,** Coronal and **B,** axial CT scans show patient who has had a right lateral rhinotomy. The postoperative cavity is filled with postoperative packing.

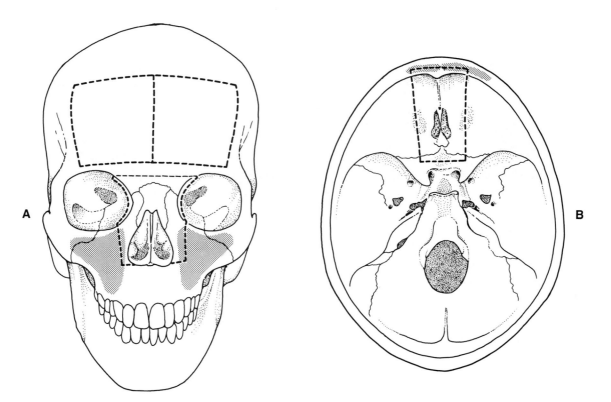

Fig. 2-397 Diagrams of the skull in the **A,** frontal view and **B,** axial view as seen from above with the calvarium removed. The osteotomies typically performed in the craniofacial procedure *(dashed lines)* are outlined.

include the entire nasal septum for a total rhinotomy. In general, the operation of choice for a unilateral nasal tumor is a medial maxillectomy with a lateral rhinotomy and ethmoidectomy. Despite the extent of the resection, the cosmetic and functional results are excellent. Regarding patient follow-up, the same general imaging rules of suspecting tumor at sites of soft tissue nodularity and mucosal thickening apply as in the post maxillectomy patents (Figs. 2-395 and 2-396).

Craniofacial Resection

This large operation is reserved for patients with tumors of the superior nasal cavity, ethmoid sinuses, frontal sinuses, and orbits. The operation essentially combines a frontal craniotomy and resection of the middle portion of the floor of the anterior cranial fossa with an extended lateral rhinotomy.

The operation is often performed first by a neurosurgical team and then by an otolaryngologic team. Initially, one of several types of frontal or bifrontal craniotomies are performed, the frontal lobes are elevated, and any tumor extension into the brain is resected. The bone and dura are then incised with a typical incision, including the posterior walls of the frontal sinuses, the cribriform plates, both foveae ethmoidalis, and as much of the medial orbital roof as is necessary to obtain a margin around the tumor. The posterior incision runs along the posterior roof of the sphenoidal sinus. An ex-

tended lateral rhinotomy, which includes the ethmoidal sinuses, nasal septum, and, if necessary, a portion of the medial orbital roof or the medial maxilla, is then performed. Once all of the specimen margins are freed, the surgeon proceeds with en bloc extirpation. An anterior dural flap and a temporalis free musculofascial graft are used to close and support the cranial floor defect, while the lateral rhinotomy is closed separately (Fig. 2-397).[14,15]

Postoperative CT scans reveal several areas that may cause diagnostic difficulties. First, the anterior dura adjacent to the frontal osteotomy becomes thickened and enhances on contrast studies. This appearance may persist indefinitely and relates to a low-grade granulomatous process that obliterates the dural spaces (Fig. 2-398). Second, the musculofascial flap that supports the central region of the floor of the anterior cranial fossa can bulge slightly downward into the upper postoperative nasoethmoid cavity (Fig. 2-399). This can simulate a tumor mass on axial CT scans and MRI, but usually can be resolved as representing the graft region on coronal studies. This is especially true during the period before the free flap becomes completely fibrosed, anywhere from 2 to 8 months.

Although the CT appearance is not effectively altered once the flap is completely fibrosed, the MRI findings are changed. The initial intermediate T_1-weighted and proton density–weighted signals and the higher (in-

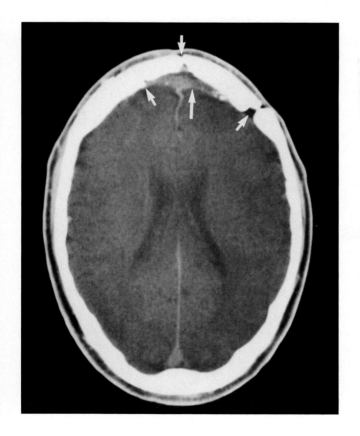

Fig. 2-398 Axial postcontrast CT scan shows dural thickening and enhancement *(large arrow)* that normally is seen as a postoperative finding in patient who has had craniofacial resection. The osteotomy sites in the frontal bones are also seen *(arrows)*.

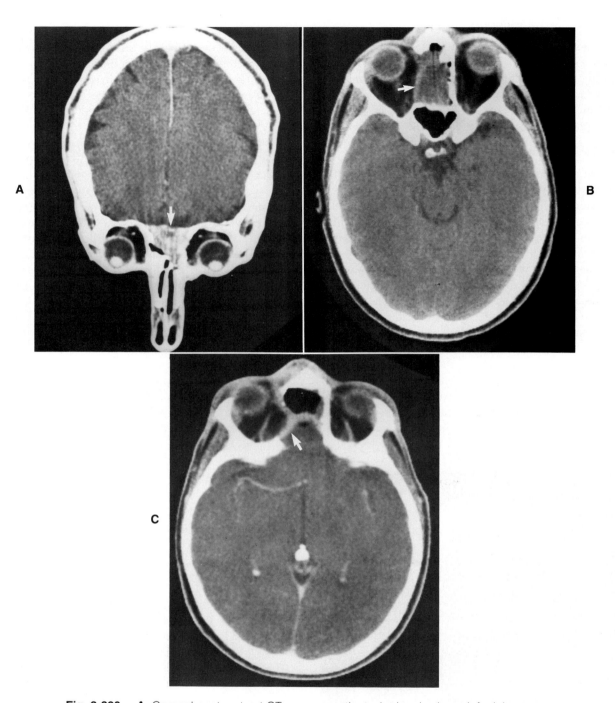

Fig. 2-399 **A,** Coronal postcontrast CT scan on patient who has had craniofacial resection. The fascial and muscle graft and the dural enhancement are seen *(arrow)* filling the surgical defect in the floor of the anterior cranial fossa. The graft hangs down into the postoperative nasoethmoidal cavity. **B,** Axial CT scan shows soft tissue mass *(arrow)* in the postoperative upper nasoethmoid cavity. This is the fascial-muscle graft of an osteoplastic flap procedure as it prolapses slightly below the level of the anterior skull base. **C,** Axial postcontrast CT scan shows dural and granulation tissue enhancement *(arrow)* just below the level of the fascial-muscle graft in patient who has had craniofacial resection. The air anteriorly is actually in the upper postoperative nasoethmoid cavity.

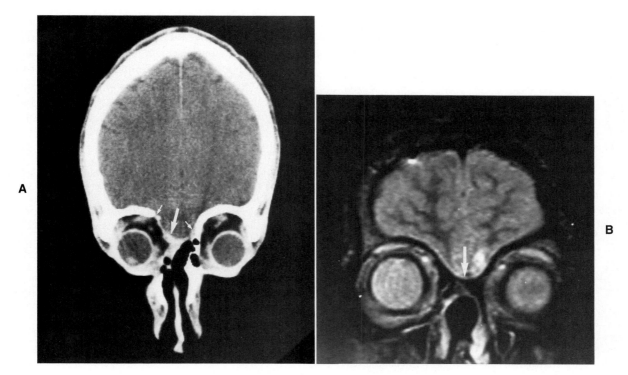

Fig. 2-400   **A,** Coronal postcontrast CT scan shows fascial-muscle-dural enhancement *(large arrow)* and margins of the bony resection *(small arrows)* in this patient who has had craniofacial resection. **B,** Coronal T$_2$W MRI scan shows same region as in **A.** The fibrosed graft *(arrow)* cannot be clearly delineated from the adjacent intact bone.

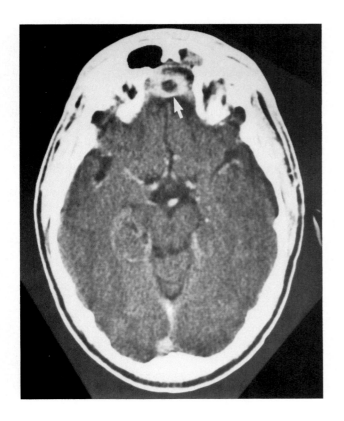

Fig. 2-401   Axial postcontrast CT scan shows ring enhancing mass *(arrow)* just cranial to the fascial-muscle graft in patient who has had craniofacial resection. Postoperative abscess.

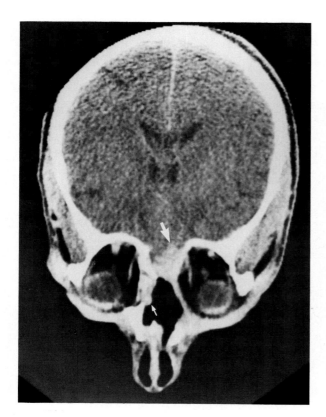

Fig. 2-402 Coronal postcontrast CT scan on patient who has had craniofacial resection. The fascial-muscle graft is nodular in appearance *(arrow)*. This should raise the possibility of an early tumor recurrence (compare to Figs. 2-399, *A,* and 2-400, *A*). Recurrent tumor.

flammatory) T_2-weighted signals are gradually replaced by low to no signal intensities on all imaging sequences as scar replaces the graft. On coronal images the thickness of this sheet of fibrosis may be sufficiently similar to that of the remaining bony floor of the adjacent anterior cranial fossa that the imager may not detect the absent bone (Fig. 2-400). Only the altered contour of the bony floor of the anterior cranial fossa may signify that the surgery included the bone in this re-

gion. Such bone defects are seen easily on coronal CT scans. In the more radical surgical cases, it is especially helpful to compare studies to a baseline examination, a fact that should be kept in mind at the time of the surgery. Any alteration from these expected CT and MRI appearances should raise the possibility of a postoperative infection or tumor recurrence (Figs. 2-401 and 2-402).

REFERENCES

1. Naumann HH and Buckingham RA: Head and neck surgery: indications, techniques, pitfalls, vol 1, Face and facial skull, Philadelphia, 1980, WB Saunders Co, pp 173-462.
2. Ballantyne JC and Harrison DFN, editors: Operative surgery: nose and throat, London, 1986, Butterworth, pp 1-177.
3. Urken ML et al: The abnormally large frontal sinus. I. A practical method for its determination based upon an analysis of 100 normal patients, Laryngoscope 97:602, 1987.
4. Som PM, et al: Ethmoid sinus disease: CT evaluation in 400 cases. II. Postoperative findings, Radiology 159:599, 1986.
5. Som PM and Shugar JMA: The CT classification of ethmoid mucoceles, JCAT 4:199, 1980.
6. Unger JM et al: The radiological appearance of the post Caldwell-Luc maxillary sinus, Clin Radiol 37:77, 1986.
7. Johnson DM et al: The unprotected parasphenoidal carotid artery studied by high-resolution computed tomography, Radiology 155:137, 1985.
8. Pedersen RA, Troost BT, and Schramm VL: Carotid-cavernous sinus fistula after external ethmoid-sphenoid surgery, Arch Otolaryngol 107:307, 1981.
9. Yanagisawa E and Smith AW: Normal radiographic anatomy of the paranasal sinuses, Otolaryngol Clin North Am 6:429, 1973.
10. Kennedy DW et al: Endoscopic middle meatal antrostomy: theory, technique, and patency, Laryngoscope 97(suppl 43):1, 1987.
11. Baredes S, Cho HT, and Som ML: Total maxillectomy, Arch Otolaryngol 107:204, 1981.
12. Som PM, Shugar JMA, and Biller HF: The early detection of antral malignancy in the postmaxillectomy patient, Radiology 143:509, 1982.
13. Lawson W and Biller HF: Lateral rhinotomy. In Blitzer A, Lawson W, and Friedman WH, editors: Surgery of the paranasal sinuses, Philadelphia, 1985, WB Saunders Co, pp 197-203.
14. Lund VJ, Howard DJ, and Lloyd GAS: CT evaluation of paranasal sinus tumors for craniofacial resection, Br J Radiol 56:439, 1983.
15. Som PM et al: Ethmoid sinus disease: CT evaluation in 400 cases. III. Craniofacial resection, Radiology 159:605, 1986.

3 Salivary Glands

PETER M. SOM

In the larger sense, lesions of the salivary glands are not common; nonetheless, they have as great a diversity of pathology as that found in any other organ system in the body. Some lesions are obviously inflammatory, some have an uncertain pathogenesis, some are reactive but can be mistaken for a malignancy, and fi-

277

nally there is a wide spectrum of both benign and malignant neoplasms.[1]

Most enlargements of the salivary glands are caused by inflammatory or nonneoplastic conditions, and neoplasms of the salivary glands make up less than 3% of all tumors in the head and neck. As to the relative incidence of salivary gland involvement, it is estimated that for every 100 parotid tumors, there are 10 submandibular tumors, 10 minor salivary tumors, and 1 sublingual tumor.[2]

It is generally accepted that the basal cells of the excretory duct and the intercalated duct cells act as the reserve cells for the more differentiated cells of the salivary gland unit, and all of the epithelial tumors appear to arise from these reserve cells rather than from the acini.[1,3] The basal cells of the excretory duct give rise to the columnar and squamous cells, while the intercalated duct cells give rise to the acinar cells, striated duct cells, other intercalated duct cells, and probably the myoepithelial cells.

SECTION ONE

INTRODUCTION TO THE SALIVARY GLANDS

EMBRYOLOGY

All of the salivary glands share a common embryogenesis in that they all develop from the ingrowth of local proliferations of surface epithelium and they have a similar overall structure. The parotid anlagen are the first to develop, are of an ectodermal origin, and appear between the fourth to sixth weeks (10 mm stage) of embryonic life. The submandibular gland anlagen appear later in the sixth week (18 mm stage) of embryonic life and probably are of endodermal origin. The sublingual gland anlagen arise in the seventh to eighth weeks (22 mm stage) of embryonic life; the minor salivary glands do not start to develop until late in the twelfth week (62 mm stage) of embryonic life (Fig. 3-1).[3-6]

The epithelial buds of each gland enlarge, elongate, and branch, the last process being induced by the mes-

enchyme surrounding the epithelium. Initially these buds are solid structures, but they eventually hollow out, creating lumina. The distal ends of the buds have bulbous terminals that develop into the acini; the secretory cells do not assume function during fetal development.[2]

Although the parotid anlagen are the first to emerge, they become encapsulated only after the submandibular and sublingual glands have done so. This delayed encapsulation is critical to the parotid gland's adult anatomy because although all of the glands are developing within a loose condensation of mesenchymal tissue, the emergence of the lymphatic system occurs after encapsulation of the submandibular and sublingual glands, but before that of the parotid glands. Thus, at the completion of embryogenesis, the parotid glands have lymph nodes and lymphatic channels within the gland's capsule, while the submandibular and sublingual glands do not. In addition, salivary epithelial cells can be included within the intraparotid and periparotid lymph nodes during the process of their encapsulation. This unusual situation of including salivary tissue within lymph nodes is unique to the parotid and periparotid nodes and is not found in any other lymph nodes in the body.

NORMAL ANATOMY

The bilaterally paired parotid, submandibular, and sublingual glands are referred to as the *major salivary glands*. Each has unique characteristics.

Parotid Gland

The parotid gland is the largest of the salivary glands and lies beneath the skin and over the ramus of the mandible. The gland is surrounded by a fascia of varying thickness, being thickest over the lateral and infe-

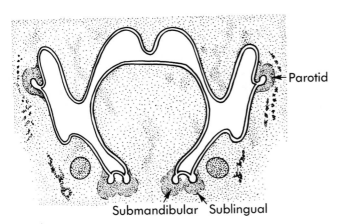

Fig. 3-1 Diagram of coronal section of human embryo at approximately 7 weeks. Anlagen of major salivary glands can be seen extending into adjacent mesenchyme. (From Mason DK and Chisholm DM: Salivary glands in health and disease, Philadelphia, 1975, WB Saunders Co.)

rior aspects of the gland. Deep extensions of this fascia divide the gland into lobules. The gland weighs between 14 and 28 g, and most of the gland (80%) lies on the outer surface of the masseter muscle and the ascending ramus and angle of the mandible. About 20% of the gland is situated between the posterior edge of the mandibular ramus and the anterior borders of the sternocleidomastoid muscle and the posterior belly of the digastric muscle. This smaller deep portion of the gland is referred to as its retromandibular portion; it lies in the stylomandibular tunnel and forms part of the lateral margin of the parapharyngeal space. The parotid gland lies below and anterior to the external auditory canal and mastoid tip, inferior to the zygomatic arch, and extends inferiorly to about the level of the angle of the mandible (Fig. 3-2).[3,4] Despite common belief, the parotid glandis not divided anatomically into superficial and deep lobes. Rather, this convention uses the facial nerve as a reference plane, within the gland, terming anything deep to this plane in the deep "lobe" of the gland and that lying external to the nerve as within its "superficial lobe."

The main trunk of the facial nerve exits the skull base via the stylomastoid foramen and immediately gives off three small branches, the posterior auricular, the posterior digastric, and the stylohyoid nerves. The facial nerve then courses laterally around the styloid process to rest upon the lateral surface of the posterior belly of the digastric muscle and then pierces the posterior capsule of the parotid gland and runs lateral to the posterior facial vein and external carotid artery. It then usually divides in one of several anatomic patterns into the temporal, zygomatic, buccal, mandibular, and cervical branches (Fig. 3-3).[7]

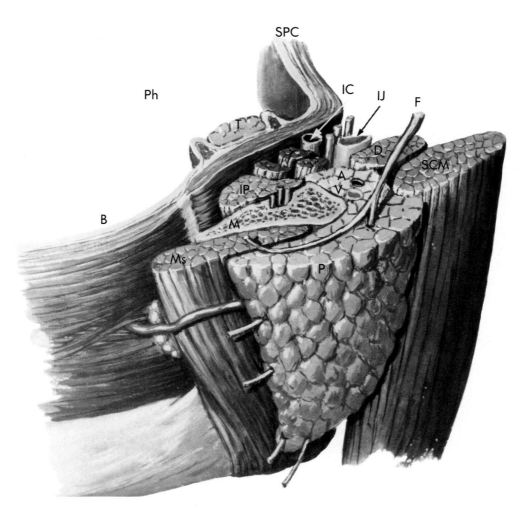

Fig. 3-2   Normal anatomy of left parotid gland and parapharyngeal space viewed obliquely and from above: Pharynx *(Ph)*, superior pharyngeal constrictor muscle *(SPC)*, tonsil *(T)*, buccinator muscle *(B)*, masseter muscle *(Ms)*, sternocleidomastoid muscle *(SCM)*, posterior belly of the digastric muscle *(D)*, internal pterygoid muscle *(IP)*, mandible *(M)*, internal carotid artery *(IC)*, internal jugular vein *(IJ)*, parotid gland *(P)*, facial nerve *(F)*, external carotid artery *(A)*, posterior facial vein *(V)*. (From Som PM and Biller HF: Radiology 135:387-390, 1980.)

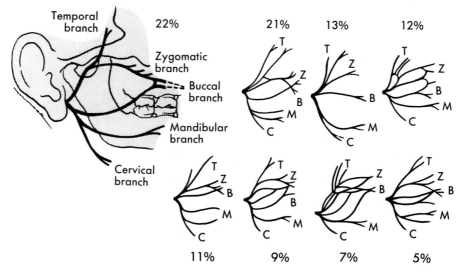

Fig. 3-3   Variations of facial nerve branching in parotid gland. (From Davis PA et al: Surg Gyn Obstet 102:384, 1956.)

The ductal organization within the salivary glands has an overall treelike branching pattern. As one moves proximally from the main duct toward the gland's acini, the ducts become progressively smaller and the number of side branches increases. This arborization pattern progresses from the largest main duct to the excretory ducts, the striated ducts, the intercalated ducts,

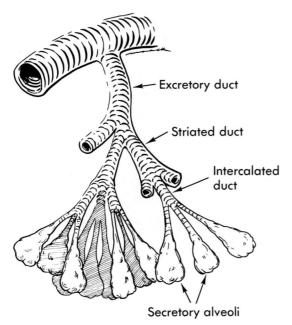

Fig. 3-4   Diagram of major salivary gland ductal system. (From Batsakis JG: Tumors of the head and neck: Clinical and pathological considerations, ed 2, Baltimore, 1979, Williams & Wilkins.)

and finally the acini. The latter are either serous or mucous producing (Fig. 3-4).

Some general differences exist between the duct appearances in the major salivary glands. In the parotid gland the intercalated ducts are long and thin, but in the submandibular gland they are shorter and wider. The sublingual gland has the shortest and widest intercalated ducts of the major salivary glands.

The main parotid duct (Stensen's duct) emerges from the anterior parotid gland, courses over the masseter muscle and buccal fat pad, and then turns medially to pierce the buccinator muscle and buccal mucosa to open intraorally opposite the second upper molar tooth (see Fig. 3-2).

Accessory parotid gland tissue is found in about 20% of people and lies along the course of Stensen's duct, usually about 6 mm anterior to the main parotid gland and most often on or above the duct. Usually these accessory glands have only one major excretory duct and that enters Stensen's duct. In the adult the parotid gland is a pure serous gland; only in the neonatal period are some mucous cells found.[3,4]

The lymph nodes within and immediately adjacent to the parotid gland drain into the superior deep cervical nodes.

Submandibular Gland

The submandibular gland is the second largest salivary gland, weighing between 10 and 15 g, or about one half the size of the parotid gland. By convention (not anatomy) it is divided into a superficial and deep lobe. The superficial lobe lies in the digastric triangle and is bounded anteriorly and inferiorly by the anterior

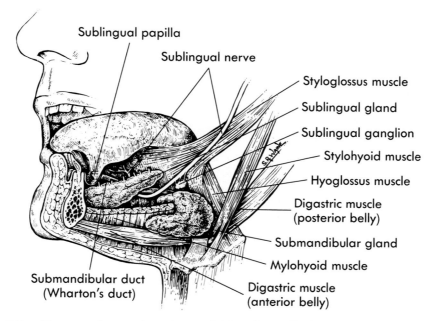

Fig. 3-5 Diagram of normal anatomy of left submandibular and sublingual glands viewed obliquely from the left side.

belly of the digastric muscle, posteriorly by the posterior belly of the digastric and stylohyoid muscles, and laterally by the lower border of the mandible and medial pterygoid muscle (Fig. 3-5). Posteriorly, the stylomandibular ligament separates it from the parotid gland. The floor of the triangle is formed by the mylohyoid muscle in front and the hyoglossus muscle behind. This portion of the submandibular gland is covered by the platysma muscle and is traversed by the anterior facial vein and marginal mandibular nerve. The facial artery runs upward on its posterior aspect, then turns downward and forward between the submandibular gland and the mandible.

The so-called deep portion of the submandibular gland lies deep to the posterior edge of the mylohyoid muscle. The lingual nerve lies above it and the hypoglossal nerve below it. The main salivary excretory duct is Wharton's duct, which exits the gland anteriorly, often making a sharp turn around the posterior edge of the mylohyoid muscle, and then runs forward and upward, lying medial to the sublingual gland and lateral to the genioglossus muscle. The duct makes an approximately 45-degree angle with both the sagittal and horizontal planes, and it opens into the anterior floor of the mouth on the sublingual papilla. As the duct courses upward, the lingual nerve winds around it, being first lateral, then inferior, and finally medial to it. The submandibular gland is a mixed serous and mucous gland, and its lymph drains into the submandibular nodes.

Sublingual Gland

The sublingual gland is the smallest of the major salivary glands, weighing only about 2 g. It lies just under the sublingual mucosa in the floor of the mouth and rests on the mylohyoid muscle. The gland is the shape of a flattened almond and usually measures about 2.5 cm in length. It is about half the size of the submandibular gland (see Fig. 3-5). The capsule is not well defined, and the gland is a mixed serous and mucous gland; however, the mucous elements predominate. About 20 individual minor ducts (ducts of Rivinus) open independently into the floor of the mouth along the sublingual papilla and fold. Occasionally some of these minor ducts fuse to form Bartholin's duct, which in turn opens into Wharton's duct.[4] The gland's lymph drains into the submental and submandibular lymph nodes.

Minor Salivary Glands

The minor salivary glands lie beneath the mucosa of the oral cavity, palate, pharynx, larynx, trachea, and paranasal sinuses. They are particularly concentrated in the buccal, labial, palatal, and lingual regions. Only the gingivae and the anterior hard palate are devoid or have only a few of these glands. The minor salivary glands are predominantly mucous glands.

The total daily production of saliva is between 1000 ml and 1500 ml. Of this total the parotid glands contribute about 45% (450 to 675 ml), the submandibular glands about 45% (450 to 675 ml), the sublingual glands 5% (50 to 75 ml), and the minor salivary glands 5% (50 to 75 ml).[8]

The formation of fluid occurs in the acini, where the secretory process is an isotonic water transport in which the major active process is a sodium transport from the intracellular to the intercellular space. Sodium enters along the basal cell membrane following an electrochemical gradient, which is the result of acetylcholine-induced enhanced permeability of the basal cell membrane to potassium and sodium. The result of this process is the formation of an isotonic, high-sodium, low-potassium fluid that becomes further modified primarily by the striated ducts, where reabsorption of sodium chloride occurs in excess of water. In some glands there is secretion of potassium and bicarbonate. These transport processes are mediated by the autonomic nervous system, as are the acinar functions.

It is most probable that the layer of salivary mucus that lines the mucosa of the mouth protects this underlying mucosa from the harmful effects of microbial toxins, noxious stimuli, and minor trauma. The salivary mucins are basically glycoproteins, which display some properties associated with polysaccharides. It is the characteristics of this group of glycoproteins that give the saliva its lubricating properties. The mucus in direct contact with the superficial epithelial cells of the oral mucosa is most likely derived from the secretions of the minor salivary glands, whose ducts open directly onto the mucosal surface. It may be this factor that primarily relates the clinical presence of xerostomia to minor salivary gland disease, despite the fact that the minor salivary glands produce only 5% of the total volume of saliva.[9]

The antibacterial activity of saliva is caused by the presence of lysozyme, thiocyanate-dependent factors, lactoferrin, its hydrogen ion concentration, and its buffering capacity. The normal range of salivary pH is 5.6 to 7.0, with an average value of 6.7.[9]

Developmental Anomalies

Developmental defects of the salivary glands are rare and are usually associated with other facial abnormalities. Anomalies of the salivary glands are associated with xerostomia and, thus, sialadenitis and dental caries. Aplasia and agenesis of a major salivary gland are uncommon and can occur unilaterally or bilaterally. Parotid gland agenesis has been reported with hemifacial microstomia, mandibulofacial dysostosis, cleft palate, and anophthalmia. Agenesis of the parotid duct has also been reported. Atresia of one or more major salivary gland ducts is very rare and is associated with xerostomia and possibly the development of a retention cyst. This condition usually occurs in the sublingual and submandibular ducts.[4]

Hypoplasia of the parotid gland has been reported in the Melkersson-Rosenthal syndrome, and congenital fistula formation of the ductal system has been associated with branchial cleft abnormalities, accessory parotid ducts, and diverticula.[4]

Aberrancy or salivary gland ectopia refers to the presence of salivary tissue at an abnormal site. Such heterotopic salivary tissue (choristoma) has been reported in an amazing variety of locales: middle ear cleft associated with ossicular abnormalities, external auditory canal, lower neck near the sternoclavicular joints, upper neck, inner-posterior mandible (Stafne cyst), anterior mandible, pituitary (pars nervosa), and cerebellopontine angle.[1,4] Congenital intraglandular cysts occur in a variety of forms and are discussed in Section Three, pp. 311-319.

REFERENCES

1. Peel RZ and Gnepp DR: Diseases of the salivary glands. In Barnes L, editor: Surgical pathology of the head and neck, vol 1, New York, 1985, Marcel Dekker, Inc, pp 533-645.
2. Thackray AC: Salivary gland tumors, Proc P Soc Med 61:1089, 1968.
3. Batsakis JG: Tumors of the head and neck, clinical and pathological considerations, ed 2, Baltimore, 1979, Williams & Wilkins, pp 1-120.
4. Mason DK and Chisholm DM: Salivary glands in health and disease, London, 1975, WB Saunders Co, Ltd, pp 3-18.
5. Johns ME: The salivary glands: anatomy and embryology, Otolaryngol Clin North Am 10:261, 1977.
6. Moss-Salentijn L and Moss ML: Development and functional anatomy. In Rankow RM and Polayes IM, editors: Diseases of the salivary glands, Philadelphia, 1976, WB Saunders Co, pp 17-31.
7. Davis RA et al: Surgical anatomy of the facial nerve and parotid gland based upon a study of 350 cervico-facial halves, Surg Gynecol Obstet 102:385, 1956.
8. Wotson S and Mandel ID: The salivary secretions in health and disease. In Rankow RM and Polayes IM, editors: Diseases of the salivary glands, Philadelphia, 1976, WB Saunders Co, pp 32-53.
9. See reference 4, pp 37-69.

SECTION TWO
IMAGING

RADIOLOGIC APPROACH

The radiographic and imaging modalities of choice for investigating a patient with salivary gland disease depends greatly on the clinical presentation of the patient. If the history is one of an acute, painful, diffuse swelling of the parotid or submandibular glands, an inflammatory process should be suspected. Similarly a history of recurrent subacute episodes of mildly painful and tender parotid or submandibular swelling indicates an inflammatory related process, and such inflammatory disease is best studied by plain films, ultrasound, sialograms (when clinically possible) and computed sectional imaging (CT or MRI) in limited cases. By comparison the clinical findings of a mass, whether slightly

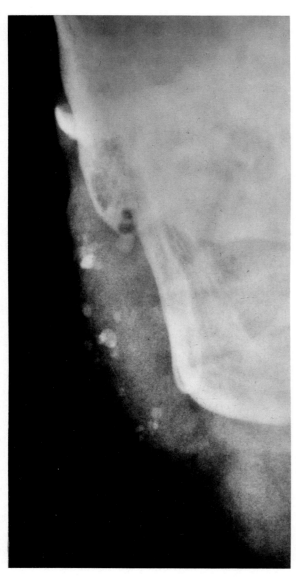

Fig. 3-6 Frontal plain film of parotid region shows multiple glandular calculi. These could easily be obscured by the contrast material of a sialogram in this patient with chronic recurrent sialadenitis.

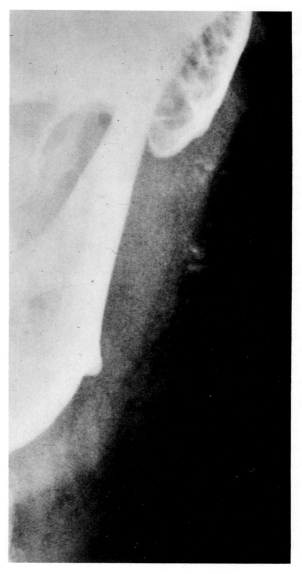

Fig. 3-7 Frontal plain film of parotid region shows faint dystrophic calcification within a pleomorphic adenoma.

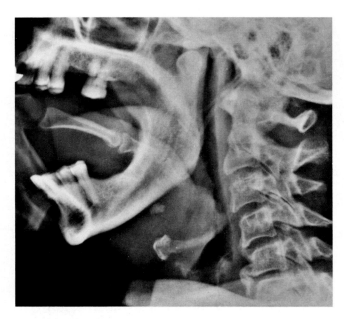

Fig. 3-8 Lateral plain film with patient's index finger depressing the tongue demonstrates a submandibular gland calculus that was hidden by the mandible on routine lateral films.

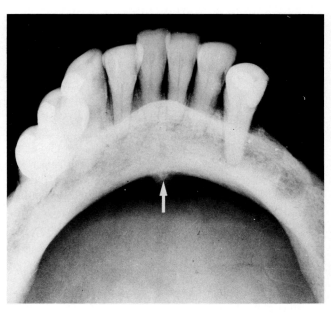

Fig. 3-9 Normal intraoral occlusal film. The arrow indicates the normal mental spines that act as the origin for the genioglossus and geniohyoid muscles.

tender or nontender, indicate a focal lesion, and this is best studied initially by cross-sectional imaging (CT or MRI).

Plain Films

The primary use of plain films is to detect radiopaque sialolithiasis, dystrophic calcifications, or adjacent mandibular bone disease (local, systemic, or metastatic disease). This procedure can be accomplished quickly and with little radiation exposure. However, such plain films will detect only gross calcifications, and often if such studies are normal, a noncontrast CT scan may identify the calculus. This reflects the fact that CT has about a ten to one increased sensitivity over plain films in detecting such calcifications.

For the parotid gland, an extended chin, open-mouth lateral film, posteroanterior views (with or without the cheeks blown out for detection of Stensen's duct stones), and oblique views provide a survey examination (Figs. 3-6 and 3-7). For the submandibular gland an extended chin, open-mouth lateral view with the patient's finger depressing the tongue, an intraoral occlusal film, and oblique views comprise the routine examinations (Figs. 3-8 to 3-10). Fluoroscopy may help detect a small calculus by allowing the radiologist to visualize its motion and/or by optimizing patient positioning to demonstrate the calculus.[1]

Sialography

Sialography employs positive contrast media in the radiographic demonstration of the ductal anatomy of the parotid or submandibular glands. The sublingual and minor salivary glands cannot be studied by this technique because of their small and numerous openings into the oral cavity, which cannot be routinely cannulated.

Sialography remains the only modality for examining the fine anatomy of the salivary ductal system. On CT and MRI only the most gross ductal detail (i.e., dilatation) can be imaged, and small to moderate degrees of functional and anatomic alteration cannot be identified. Thus sialography, and not computed sectional imaging, is the examination of choice for those diseases (subacute and chronic sialadenitis, autoimmune related disease, and sialosis) in which the ductal sialographic findings are distinctive. Their sectional imaging characteristics are similar and often the clinical presentations are inseparable.[2,3]

Sialography is an invasive retrograde procedure in which radiopaque contrast material is injected into the gland via the intraoral opening of either Wharton's or Stensen's duct. If the patient has an active infection, the procedure is contraindicated because it tends to propagate the infection back into the gland. In addition, because of pain the patient will not tolerate such

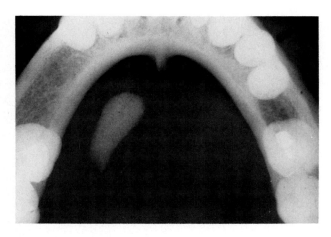

Fig. 3-10 Intraoral occlusal film shows large calculus in Wharton's duct in the floor of the mouth. This calculus was poorly visualized on other routine films. Smaller such calculi may be seen only on plain films using intraoral occlusal view.

an injection. Similarly if the patient has had a recent acute sialodenitis, although the gland may be clinically normal at the time of examination, the sialographic procedure can precipitate a recurrence of a clinically quiescent infection. In such cases if the procedure is clinically necessary, the patient may be given antibiotics to attempt to abort such a reinfection. The other major deterrent to performing a sialogram is a patient history of allergic sensitivity to iodine compounds (contrast materials).

The primary reasons a sialogram is performed include: (1) detection or confirmation of small parotid or submandibular gland sialoliths or foreign bodies; (2) evaluation of the extent of irreversible ductal damage present as a result of infection; (3) differentiation of diseases such as chronic sialadenitis, Sjögren's syndrome, and sialosis; (4) evaluation of fistulae, strictures, diverticula, communicating cysts, and ductal trauma; and (5), rarely, as a dilating procedure for mild ductal stenosis.[4]

Classically the contrast material once used to perform a sialogram was a fat-soluble agent. This reflected the fact that the fat-soluble contrast agents were more viscid, had higher iodine concentrations, and produced sharper boundaries with the salivary secretions than did the water-soluble agents. These desirable factors were, in part, negated by the moderate frequency of eliciting a foreign body reaction in the salivary parenchyma should perforation occur during the procedure with agents such as Lipiodol or Pantopaque. This possibility led later to the use of Ethiodol, which is a fat-soluble contrast material with a much lower clinical incidence of such foreign body reactions. In addition, most such

reported cases involving Ethiodol reflect the pathologic finding of a clinically silent granulomatous reaction in an autopsy specimen.[5]

The water-soluble agents in general are less viscid and are more miscible with saliva than the fat-soluble agents. Water-soluble Sinografin has a similar iodine content (38%) to Ethiodol (37%) and a workable viscosity that makes injection easy, while not being so watery that it will not stay within the main ductal system. In addition, there is no reported incidence of any foreign body reaction subsequent to perforation. Thus if the sialogram radiographs are taken quickly, before admixture of the Sinografin and saliva occurs, the study demonstrates clear and sharp ductal anatomy, equivalent to that seen on an Ethiodol study. Because of this, water-soluble agents such as Sinografin have literally replaced the fat-soluble agents as the contrast material of choice for a sialogram.

The equipment used to perform a sialogram may vary according to the examiner's particular preferences. However, a general list includes the following:

1. Sialographic cannulas. The most commonly employed are the Rabinov cannulas with tips ranging from 0.012 to 0.033 inches (Fig. 3-11).[6] Variations such as the Manashil modification of the Rabinov cannula and cannulas designed by Lowman and Belleza are also commercially available. Modifications of butterfly needles also can be used for parotid cannulizations.[7] In general, the larger diameter cannulas are used for the parotid gland, the smaller ones for the submandibular gland. Although cannulas without a polyethylene connecting tube can be used, the examiner has greater mobility during the procedure if such a flexible connecting tube is employed.
2. A set of lacrimal dilators ranging from 0000 through 0 caliber.
3. A 5 ml or 10 ml syringe.
4. 4 × 4 inch gauze sponge pads.
5. Sinografin.
6. Secretogogue such as fresh lemon, lemon extract, or lemon concentrate.
7. Adequately focused lighting, usually a head-light unit.
8. High-powered magnifying glasses.

Once the salivary duct is cannulated, the injection is usually made with hand pressure.[5] The patient may complain of local pressure or mild pain during the injection; however, a slow constant injection technique usually can accomplish complete ductal filling without much patient discomfort. The patient's sensation of glandular fullness and pressure usually abates within a few minutes of the end of the study. The patient should be alerted that there should be no residual discomfort

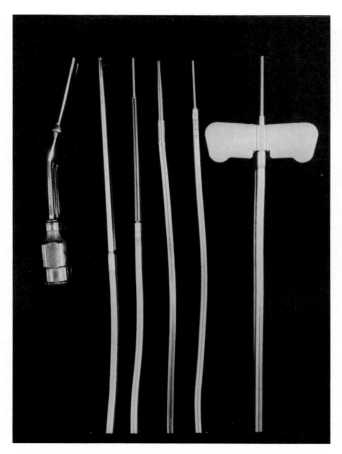

Fig. 3-11 Sampling of some of the sialography catheters and needles commonly used. They are available with end-holes, side-holes, or both.

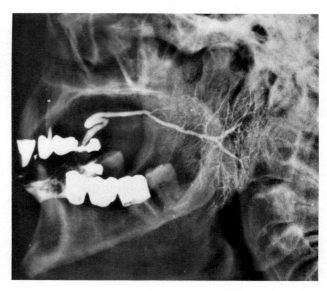

Fig. 3-12 Lateral view of normal parotid sialogram. Anteriorly Stensen's duct bends around the buccinator fat and then passes over the outer surface of the masseter muscle. There is a diffuse ductal "arborization" pattern and no portion of the gland parenchyma is "ductless."

by 24 hours after the examination. If, instead, local pain increases and becomes more intense 24 to 36 hours after the examination, a postsialogram infection is probably present and antibiotic therapy should be started immediately. In this manner the chances of a severe acute sialadenitis and/or an abscess can be diminished.

Parotid Gland Study. The intraoral opening of Stensen's duct is opposite the second upper molar tooth. In some patients this opening is easily seen; however, in others it may be very difficult to identify, especially in individuals who have a dry, obstructed gland or a mucosal bite ridge across the region. After drying the mucosa with gauze, milking of the gland and Stensen's duct may produce a drop of saliva that allows identification of the duct opening. In this regard the use of a secretogogue (lemon) may also be helpful. Once the opening is identified, the dilators can be used to widen the opening for easier cannula placement. Slight abduction of the cheek with the thumb and index finger often provides a better exposure and angle for cannula insertion. The cannula is then gently inserted and 0.5 to 1.5

ml of contrast material is slowly injected. The injection is best made under fluoroscopic control so that optimal ductal filling and gland positioning can be achieved, and spot-filling is used to document the examination.

Stensen's duct is approximately 6 cm long and has a small C-shaped curve anteriorly as it bends around the buccal fat pad and pierces the buccinator muscle to open opposite the second upper molar tooth. The duct's normal luminal caliber is only 1 to 2 mm, and on a direct PA film, the duct should lie within 15 to 18 mm of the lateral mandibular cortex. If the duct is more laterally placed, an anterior mass is present either in or near the masseter muscle (Figs. 3-12 and 3-13).

There is no specific parotid ductal branching pattern, and variation is noted from side-to-side within the same person as well as among different people.[8] Usually there is a main upper and lower duct; from these the arborization pattern takes form. The overall appearance is that of a leafless tree, and no area of the gland should be without some peripheral ducts. As the ducts arch behind the ramus of the mandible, they may appear slightly stretched on frontal films. This appearance should not be confused with a mass lesion; on lateral films, no mass effect will be seen (Figs. 3-12 and 3-13). No areas of the gland should have ducts positioned parallel. If present, this appearance indicates a mass displacing some of the ducts, since in the normal arborization pattern, no parallel ducts occur.

Acinar filling can be accomplished in most patients

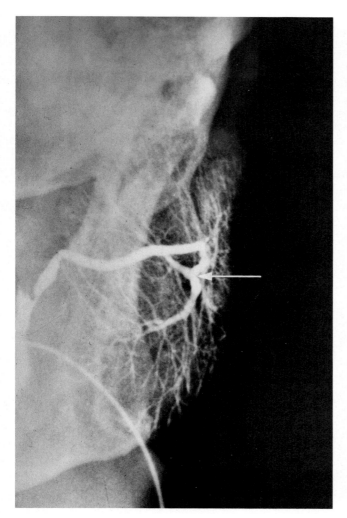

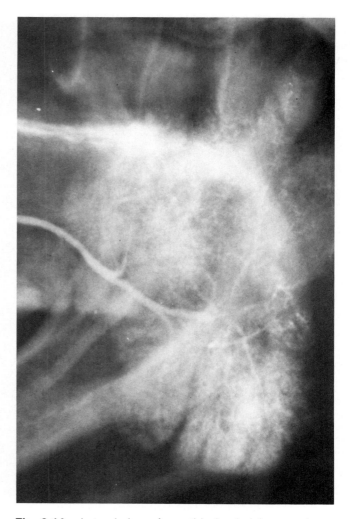

Fig. 3-13   Frontal view of normal parotid gland sialogram. The hilum of the gland *(arrow)* is within 15 to 18 mm of the lateral cortex of the mandible on a standard 40 inch TSD film. The posterior "deep lobe" ducts often appear stretched or splayed as they arch behind the mandible. The lateral view in the normal case, however, will show no splaying; and thus demonstrates that no mass is present.

Fig. 3-14   Lateral view of parotid gland sialogram showing acinar filling throughout the gland with most of the main ducts still being clearly identified.

and is a normal effect of slight overfilling of the ductal system.[9] It can be a useful technique to help identify small masses; however, the acinar filling should be carefully limited so that it does not obscure the ductal anatomy (Fig. 3-14).

The evacuation film should reveal complete and rapid ductal emptying. In some patients a more complete evacuation can be achieved if a secretogogue is given. On the other hand, any acinar filling will remain until the water-soluble contrast material is absorbed. Any delayed ductal emptying or trapping of the contrast material indicates the presence of a functional obstruction.[10]

Multiple or solitary accessory parotid glands may be present and are usually situated above Stensen's duct, anterior to the main parotid gland.[10] These accessory glands are routinely filled in a retrograde manner as the contrast material courses through Stensen's duct. These glands have a normal branching ductal pattern.

Submandibular Gland Study. The orifice of Wharton's duct lies in the floor of the mouth on or near the sublingual papilla. The opening is smaller than that of Stensen's duct and, to visualize it, the area should be dried with gauze and the tongue pushed upward and backward to put some tension on the papilla. Milking of the gland or a secretogogue can aid in identifying the orifice by producing a drop of saliva.[9] Once the duct is cannulated, only 0.2 to 0.5 ml of contrast material should be injected. Wharton's duct is seen to run downward and laterally at about a 45-degree angle to both the sagittal and horizontal planes.[10,11]

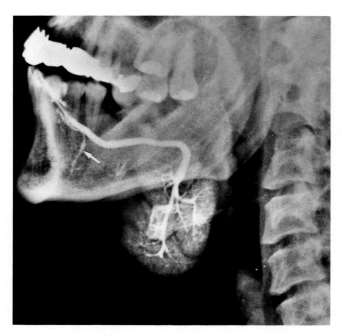

Fig. 3-15   Lateral view of normal submandibular gland sialogram demonstrates some acinar filling with shorter, more tapered ducts than those that are seen in the parotid gland. The posterior bend that Wharton's duct makes around the posterior edge of the mylohyoid muscle is clearly seen. There is partial filling of a Bartholin's duct *(arrow)*.

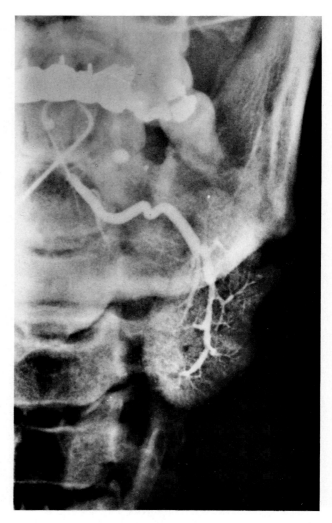

Fig. 3-16   Frontal view of normal submandibular gland sialogram shows the usual 45 degree downward and lateral angulation of Wharton's duct. The ducts are well seen, and, in this example, there is some acinarization, which demonstrates the gland parenchyma.

Wharton's duct is about 5 cm long and has a luminal caliber of 1 to 3 mm. Just before the duct enters the submandibular gland, it curves caudally over the back edge of the mylohyoid muscle. The intraglandular ducts are shorter and taper more abruptly than those in the parotid gland. The duct walls are also thinner so that perforation occurs easily (Figs. 3-15 and 3-16). If not monitored by fluoroscopy, such perforation and acinarization can routinely obscure the ductal system and ruin the examination.

Occasionally, Bartholin's duct will be filled, extending from Wharton's duct (Fig. 3-15). In some cases the sublingual gland may be visualized; it resembles an accessory gland with a normal branching ductal pattern.

The most common causes of sialogram failure or a poor sialogram are (1) failure to locate and cannulate the salivary duct, (2) perforation of the duct either into the cheek or the floor of the mouth, (3) suboptimal filling of the ductal system so that areas of the gland are not visualized, and (4) complete acinarization of the gland so that all ductal detail is obscured. The latter problem is especially prone to occur in the submandibular gland and can best be avoided by fluoroscopically monitoring the injection volume.

If there has been previous surgery in the floor of the

mouth, the scarring and altered anatomy probably account for more failures to cannulate Wharton's duct than any other single reason. A "dry" duct may be caused from prior surgery, scarring, irradiation, or obstruction by either a stone or a tumor. The absence of this saliva is the overall major cause of failure to identify the openings of either Stensen's or Wharton's ducts.[10]

Computed Sectional Imaging

CT and MRI are the examinations of choice for evaluating mass lesions. They can identify: the presence of a mass; its location within the gland and its position relative to the facial nerve; whether the mass is smoothly marginated or infiltrating; whether the mass is confined to the gland or has extended outside the gland capsule into the upper neck and skull base; whether the mass is necrotic, cystic, or solid; and whether there is more than one mass or bilateral disease that is clinically occult.

Because the parotid gland has a normally fatty interstitial structure and produces serous secretions, the CT attenuation of the gland (-25 to 15 Hounsfield units [HU]) is lower than that of muscle, but more than that of fat.[12] The intraglandular ducts are not normally visualized, and Stensen's duct is seen consistently only if abnormally dilated. There is usually a faint nonhomogeneity to the gland that represents the fibrous-vascular-epithelial elements seen as scattered strands of higher attenuation material arching and bending throughout the fatty-serous background matrix. The external carotid artery and posterior facial vein are usually seen positioned posterior to the ramus of the mandible (Figs. 3-17 and 3-18). The more cranial the level in the gland, the more laterally these vessels course. Some normal lobulation of the gland can be seen primarily along the upper margin of the gland; and normal areas of higher attenuation occur near the root or attachment of the pinna of the ear, which may mimic a small mass in the

upper pole of the parotid gland. In children and some adults the parotid gland may be uniformly dense, approaching the attenuation of muscle (20-45 HU). The reason this occurs in patients with no history of clinical disease is not known. Subclinical inflammation or a wide normal variation in glandular fat content may exist. In either case it is in these denser glands that small mass lesions will be more difficult to identify, and it is in these patients that MRI is a more sensitive examination.

In addition to not being able to visualize fine ductal anatomy, the facial nerve cannot be seen on CT scans. The course of the nerve, however, can be traced on the scans. The nerve runs from the skull base stylomastoid foramen, lateral to the styloid process, down along the lateral surface of the posterior belly of the digastric muscle, pierces the gland, and runs lateral to the posterior facial vein and external carotid artery. With these landmarks, an accurate estimate can be made in almost all cases as to whether a mass is medial or lateral to the facial nerve.

Because of artifacts from metallic dental restorations, several of the axial CT scans through the parotid gland are often badly degraded. In these cases exaggerated

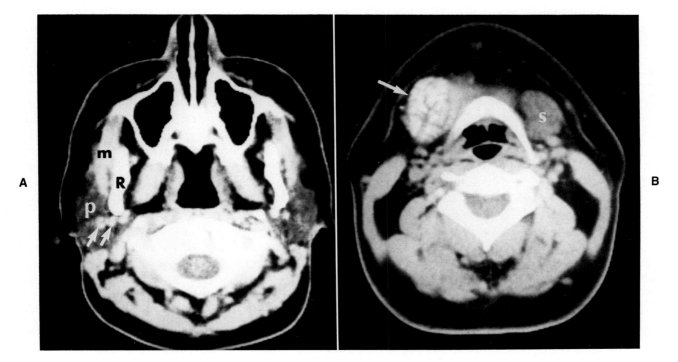

Fig. 3-17 **A,** Axial post contrast CT scan reveals the normal parotid gland *(P)* to be of a lower attenuation than muscle *(M* = masseter muscle), but higher than that of fat. The posterior facial vein and the external carotid arteries *(arrows)* are seen just behind the ramus of the mandible *(R).* **B,** Axial noncontrast CT scan taken after a right submandibular sialogram. Contrast material is seen filling the gland *(arrow).* The left submandibular gland *(S)* is well seen and is of a lower attenuation than muscle, but a higher attenuation than the surrounding fat.

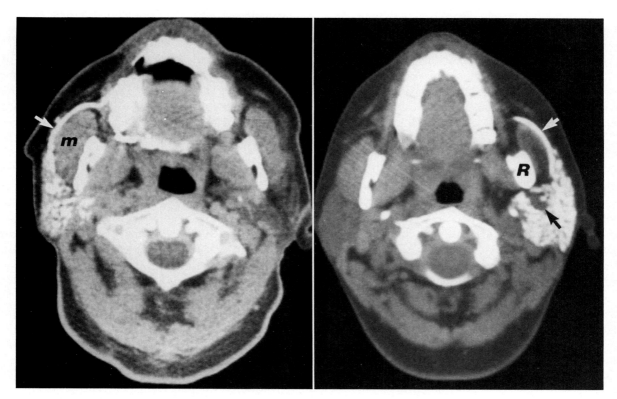

Fig. 3-18 Normal axial CT-sialograms of the parotid gland. Contrast material is seen in the parotid gland and in Stensen's duct *(white arrow)* as it bends around the masseter muscle *(m)*. The location of the vascular bundle in these nonintravenous contrast scans can be identified *(black arrow)*. Ramus of mandible, *(R)*, is also shown.

inferior orbitomeatal (IOM) angled scans or modified coronal scans should be obtained that cover the region of the parotid gland, which is poorly seen on the routine axial study.

On MRI, the fat content of the parotid gland primarily accounts for an intermediate-to-bright intensity T_1-weighted signal.[13,14] This signal is nonhomogeneous, with multiple irregular areas of lower signal intensity that represent the remaining interstitial tissue, epithelium, and serous secretions of the gland. The major vessels are identified by the absent (flow void) signal, and the facial nerve may be imaged in some cases. On T_2 WIs the parotid gland has a nonhomogeneous intermediate intensity signal that predominantly reflects the serous secretion and water content of the gland (Fig. 3-19).

Many similarities and some differences exist between the type of information that can be obtained from CT and MRI. CT has the ability to detect calcium deposits with a sensitivity approximately 10 times that of plain films. Thus in elusive clinical cases in which the plain film examinations are normal and a sialogram cannot be performed either because the gland is obstructed and

"dry" or there is active inflammation, a noncontrast CT scan may localize the calculus and resolve the problem. Gross calcifications are uncommon in salivary gland tumors and most often occur in pleomorphic adenomas. Therefore if a mass with focal calcifications is identified on CT, it is most likely to be a benign mixed tumor. The lack of ability to detect such calcifications is one of the limitations of MRI.

A cystic salivary gland lesion has a differential diagnosis distinct from that of a solid mass. Additionally, the character of the cyst wall (i.e., thickness, nodularity, and smoothness) will refine the differential diagnosis. CT provides an excellent means of evaluating these findings. Because the fluid that fills such cysts or cystic areas within a mass is primarily composed of water and because most major salivary gland tumors have a high water content, both a mass and a cyst (or cystic areas) may be indistinguishable on MRI. Certainly the ease with which these areas are identified is greater on CT than it is on MRI. For example, a small intraparotid branchial cleft cyst may look similar to a small benign mixed tumor on MRI, but these appear as distinctly different lesions on CT.

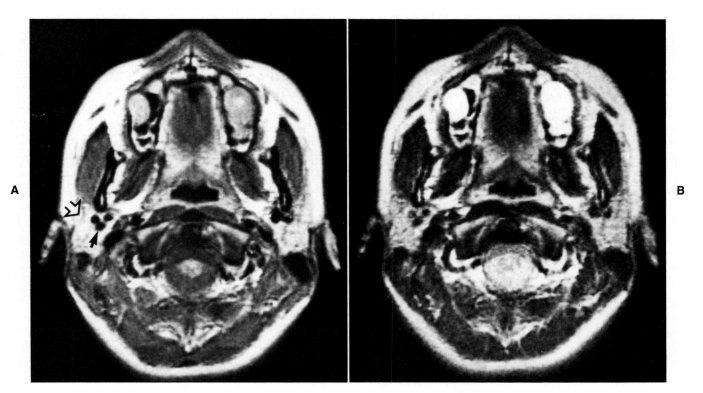

Fig. 3-19 **A,** Axial mixed image MRI scan (TR 1800 msec, TE = 30 msec) shows an intermediate-to-high signal intensity in the parotid glands *(open arrow)*. The posterior facial veins and external carotid arteries are identified as sites of flow voids *(arrow)* just posterior to the ramus of the mandible. **B,** Axial T$_2$-weighted MR scan (TR 1800 msec, TE = 80 msec) shows an intermediate, slightly nonhomogeneous signal intensity within the normal parotid glands.

On the other hand, MRI usually outlines the margins of a salivary gland mass more sharply than CT. What may appear as a vague fullness of the parotid gland on CT will usually be seen as a discrete mass on MRI. What appears to be probably several different masses on CT can be seen as either a highly lobulated solitary mass or several discrete masses on MRI. Evaluation of tumor extension outside the gland can be well achieved by either CT or MRI, and gross erosion of the mandible or skull base can be equally well seen on either modality. However, focal bone erosions or subtle bone sclerosis must be evaluated with CT. Thus each modality offers some benefits over the other. The final choice of whether to use CT or MRI may depend on the clinical presentation of the case and what the expected differential diagnosis is. More than occasionally the preferred examination is recognized only in retrospect.

CT is highly sensitive in *detecting* salivary gland masses with a reported overall sensitivity that may approach 100%.[12] Since MRI is as sensitive for detection, if not moreso than CT, it is evident that either modality could localize and map a clinically evident (and often clinically occult) mass. These nearly perfect figures should be compared to the sensitivity of sialography for detecting a mass of 85%. In addition, this figure is achieved only by very experienced sialographers.[15-17]

The distinction between a benign and a malignant mass frequently cannot be made purely on the basis of morphology as demonstrated by sectional imaging. However, by combining the radiologic and clinical findings, such a distinction can be made in almost 90% of the cases.[12] The sectional imaging problem arises because most benign salivary lesions (i.e., cysts, tumors, and nodes) have a capsule and are smoothly contoured and sharply delineated from the adjacent salivary tissues. However, low-grade malignancies (i.e., low-grade mucoepidermoid carcinomas, some acinic cell carcinomas, and adenoidcystic carcinomas) develop pseudocapsules and on sectional imaging are also smoothly outlined and "benign" in appearance.

Alternatively high-grade malignancies (i.e., high-grade mucoepidermoid carcinomas, adenocarcinomas, and squamous cell carcinomas) have irregular, infiltrating, indistinct margins as compared to the adjacent salivary tissue. However, a benign mass with some surrounding low-grade inflammation and/or hemorrhage (possibly from vigorous palpation) can present the same aggressive sectional imaging appearance.

In a similar manner a confident distinction between benign and malignant solid salivary gland tumors cannot be made based on their sectional imaging internal architecture. However, on MRI highly cellular tumors (usually high-grade malignancies) tend to have low to intermediate signal intensities on all imaging sequences, while the less cellular masses (benign, low grade malignancies) tend to have bright T_2-weighted signal intensities.

Clinically, benign tumors are slow growing, painless, nontender, mobile, firm masses that do not cause facial paralysis. Benign cysts usually develop quickly over several days, are tender and/or painful if infected, are moderately firm to palpation, and often have a history of prior recurrent episodes. Malignant tumors tend to enlarge rapidly over several weeks, may be slightly painful and minimally tender, are hard on palpation and fixed, and often have associated facial nerve paralysis.

CT Sialography. The CT sialogram was performed to provide better definition of major salivary gland masses than was attainable on the lower resolution, early CT scanners.[18-21] The study was a combination of the sialographic injection of contrast material (usually of the parotid gland) and the simultaneous CT scanning of the gland. Acinarization of the gland provided a background density that would silhouette any mass (see Fig. 3-18). However, with the development of higher resolution CT scanners and MRI, this more cumbersome double examination is, for the most part, no longer necessary.

Noncomputed Tomographic Sialography. In a manner similar to CT sialography, conventional multidirectional (or complex-motion) tomography of the parotid gland can be performed immediately after the gland is injected (with acinarization) as part of a sialogram. A mass is silhouetted by the contrast material and can be more easily identified than on the routine sialogram. In the present era of high resolution CT and MRI, this technique is no longer employed.

Ultrasound

The primary application of ultrasound to salivary gland disease has been the differentiation of solid and cystic masses. More recently it has been used to identify calculi. Although some differentiation of an intraparotid from an extraparotid mass can also be achieved by ultrasound, this technique is not used frequently, reflecting the superior visualization of the deep spaces of the upper neck and skull base attainable by CT and MRI.[22,23]

Radionuclide Salivary Studies

The salivary glands normally concentrate technetium Tc99m pertechnetate. However, a radionuclide sialogram cannot localize a mass as accurately as either CT or MRI and even then only identifies those masses that excessively accumulate the radionuclide. These lesions are primarily Warthin's tumors and oncocytomas.[10,24] Salivary gland function can also be assessed and hyperfunction can be demonstrated in acute sialadenitis, granulomatous disease, lymphoma, and sialosis. A cold area within a gland that has an overall increased activity may represent an abscess in a patient with an acute purulent sialadenitis. Decreased glandular activity is seen in Sjögren's syndrome and most primary and metastatic tumors. A viral sialadenitis and normal aging give a generalized decreased uptake, and ductal obstruction can be estimated by the degree of prolongation of the secretory phase of the radionuclide study. Patchy decreased uptake may indicate chronic and atrophic salivary disease.[10,25-27]

Angiography

Interventional vascular studies play little role in the diagnosis and treatment of most salivary gland disease and, with the exception of the embolization of some hemangiomas, angiographic studies are practically not used.

SKINNY NEEDLE BIOPSY

Skinny needle biopsy of salivary masses is being used increasingly. The biopsy is performed with a 22-gauge needle and can be done with or without CT or MRI guidance.[28-30] As more pathologists and cytologists gain expertise with this technique, the concurrence between the cytologic and histologic findings can be expected to rise above the present 91%.[10]

REFERENCES

1. Kushner DC and Weber AL: Sialography of salivary gland tumors with fluoroscopy and tomography, AJR 130:941, 1978.
2. Som PM et al: Manifestations of parotid gland enlargement: radiologic, pathologic and clinical correlations, part I: the autoimmune pseudosialectasias, Radiology 141:415, 1981.
3. Som PM et al: Manifestations of parotid gland enlargement: radiologic, pathologic and clinical correlations, II. The diseases of Mikulicz's syndrome, Radiology 141:421, 1981.
4. Osmer JC and Pleasants JE: Distension sialography, Radiology 87:116, 1966.
5. Lowman RM and Cheng GK: Diagnostic radiology. In Rankow RM and Polayer IM, editors: Diseases of the salivary glands, Philadelphia, 1976, WB Saunders Co, pp 54-98.
6. Rabinov KR and Jaffe N: A blunt-tip side injecting cannula for sialography, Radiology 92:1438, 1969.
7. Som PM and Khilnani MT: Technical note: a modification of a butterfly infusion set for sialography, Radiology 143:791, 1982.
8. Yoel J: Pathology and surgery of the salivary glands, Springfield, Ill, 1975, Charles C Thomas Publisher, pp 31-87.
9. Ollerenshaw R and Ross SS: Radiological diagnosis of salivary gland disease, Br J Radiol 24:538, 1951.

10. Rabinov K and Weber AL: Radiology of the salivary glands, Boston, 1985, GK Hall & Co, pp 1-221.
11. Manashil GB: Clinical sialography, Springfield, Ill, 1978,: Charles C Thomas Publisher, pp 19-28.
12. Bryan RN et al: Computed tomography of the major salivary glands, AJR 139:547, 1982.
13. Mandelblatt SM: Parotid masses: MR imaging, Radiology 163:411, 1987.
14. Teresi LM et al: Parotid masses: MR imaging, Radiology 163:405, 1987.
15. Calcaterra TC et al: The value of sialography in the diagnosis of parotid tumors, Arch Otolaryngol 103:727, 1977.
16. Potter GD: Sialography and the salivary glands, Otolaryngol Clin North Am 6:509, 1973.
17. Work WP and Johns ME: Symposium on salivary gland diseases, Otolaryngol Clin North Am 10:261, 1977.
18. Som PM and Biller HF: The combined CT-sialogram: a technique to differentiate deep lobe parotid tumors from extraparotid pharynomaxillary space tumors, Ann Otolaryngol 88:590, 1979.
19. Som PM and Biller HF: The combined CT-sialogram, Radiology 135:387, 1980.
20. Carter BL and Karmody CS: Computed tomography of the face and neck, Sem Roentgenol 13:257, 1978.
21. Mancuso A, Rice D, and Hanafee W: Computed tomography of the parotid gland during contrast sialography, Radiology 132:211, 1979.
22. Neiman HL et al: Ultrasound of the parotid gland, J Clin Ultrasound 4:11, 1976.
23. Gooding GA: Gray scale ultrasound of the parotid gland, AJR 134:469, 1980.
24. Cogan MI and Gill PS: Value of sialography and scintigraphy in diagnosis of salivary gland disorders, Int J Oral Surg (suppl 1) 10:216, 1981.
25. Schall GL: The role of radionuclide scanning in the evaluation of neoplasms in the salivary glands: a review, J Surg Oncol 3:701, 1971.
26. Schall GI, Smith RR, and Barsocchini LM: Radionuclide salivary imaging usefulness in a private otolaryngology practice, Arch Otolaryngol 107:40, 1981.
27. Pretorius D and Taylor A: The role of nuclear scanning in head and neck surgery, Head Neck Surg 4:427, 1982.
28. Gatenby RA, Mulbern CB, and Strawitz J: CT-guided percutaneous biopsies of head and neck masses, Radiology 146:717, 1983.
29. Lufkin R, Teresi L, and Hanafee W: New needle for MR-guided aspiration cytology of the head and neck, AJR 149:380, 1987.
30. Abemayor E et al: CT-directed aspiration biopsies of masses in the head and neck, Laryngoscope 95:1382, 1985.

SECTION THREE
NONNEOPLASTIC DISORDERS

INFLAMMATORY CONDITIONS

The major salivary glands have a limited ability to respond to an inflammatory insult; because of this, a great variety of processes may have a similar clinical presentation. In the case of solitary episodes of acute inflammation this fact does not present a clinical problem. However, in patients with chronic inflammatory disease, the signs and symptoms of the chronic infections may merge with those of the granulomatous diseases, the autoimmune diseases, sialosis, and certain neoplasms. Thus although the patient may clearly have a sialadenitis on sialography, the clinical presentation may not be as definitive, and the radiologist can play a major role in resolving this diagnostic dilemma.

Acute Inflammatory Diseases

As a group the viral and bacterial inflammatory diseases are the most common salivary gland abnormalities. Most of the bacterial infections ascend from the oral cavity and are related to a decrease in the salivary flow. It is the maintenance of a normal salivary flow that is the single best deterrent to such infections, and a variety of entities can decrease the production of saliva. These include prior infections, radiation, dehydration, trauma, surgery, and some medications.[1] The ascending infections are more common in the parotid gland than in the submandibular gland because the orifice of Stensen's duct is larger than that of Wharton's duct and the parotid duct orifice is more easily injured by cheek biting, dental prostheses, and other mechanical trauma. In addition, the overall smaller caliber of Stensen's duct may allow for an easier interruption of salivary flow by epithelial tears and thickened secretions.[2,3]

Viral Infections. By far the most common cause of viral parotitis is mumps. Mumps, in fact, is probably the most common of all salivary gland diseases.[4] It primarily involves the parotid glands but can occur in the submandibular glands. The disease is most reliably diagnosed during epidemics, and the diagnosis can be confirmed by measuring serum antibody titers.[3] The incubation period is between 2 and 3 weeks, and the parotid involvement is unilateral in about one third of the cases and bilateral in two thirds of the patients. The disease is characterized by an acute, painful swelling of the involved gland. Mumps can be subclinical, and this type of infection may account for some misdiagnosed or apparently idiopathic cases of parotid gland enlargement. One attack of the disease provides immunity. Other viral agents can cause parotitis, including coxsackieviruses, parainfluenza viruses (types I and III), influenza virus type A, herpes virus, echo virus, and choriomeningitis virus.[1,3]

Bacterial Infections. Acute suppurative sialadenitis is an acute, painful, diffuse disease primarily of the parotid gland. The gland is swollen and tender, and purulent exudate can be seen in the buccal orifice of Stensen's duct. About two thirds of the cases are associated with the postoperative period (from surgery unrelated to the oral cavity) and occur in debilitated, dehydrated patients, usually with poor oral hygiene.[5]

The incidence varies between 0.004% and 0.74% of patients who have had a major surgical procedure.[1] Good hygiene and hydration have markedly reduced the incidence of the entity. The most common offending agents are *Staphlyococcus aureus*, *Streptococcus viridans*, and *Streptococcus pneumoniae*. Treatment is with antibiotic therapy; intraparotid and periparotid lymph nodes may be involved in the inflammatory reaction.

Suppurative parotitis can also occur in neonates, usually affecting premature infants (35% to 40% of cases), and dehydration is the main predisposing factor.[6] The onset is usually between 7 and 14 days after delivery, and there is erythema of the skin overlying the parotid glands. The offending agents are staphylococci, *Pseudomonas aeruginosa*, streptococci, pneumococci,

and *Escherichia coli*.[1] Hydration and antibiotic therapy usually cure the infection.

An undiagnosed or incompletely treated acute suppurative sialadenitis can develop an intraglandular abscess (Fig. 3-20) irrespective of the patient's age. Small abscesses may form (Figs. 3-21 and 3-22) and coalesce to form a larger abscess, or a solitary abscess may develop. Patients with such an abscess have fever and malaise, and the abscess may extend into the parapharyngeal space or upper neck. Surgical drainage with adequate antibiotic therapy is the treatment of choice.

Acute suppurative sialadenitis can also involve the submandibular glands, in the absence of parotid disease. The lower incidence in these glands is related not only to the protective anatomy of Wharton's duct but also to the fact that submandibular secretions may be more bacteriostatic than the parotid secretions. They also have a faster rest salivary flow rate.[7] The presence of sialolithiasis is a major factor in the development of

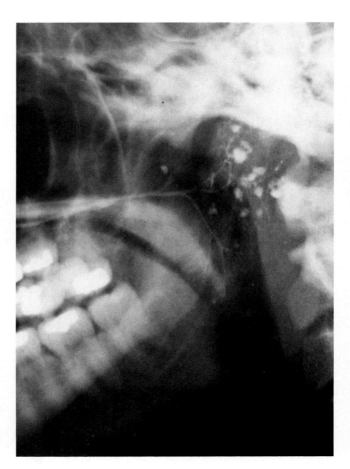

Fig. 3-21 Lateral view of parotid sialogram shows multiple collections of contrast material that are of varying size and are primarily located in the posterior portion of the gland: Small intraglandular abscesses in patient who had no clinical evidence of active disease at the time of this examination.

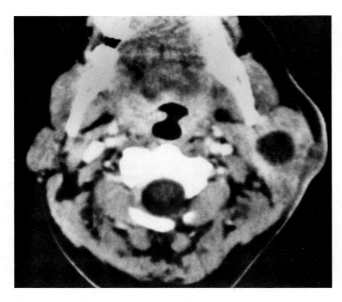

Fig. 3-20 Axial post contrast CT scan shows solitary low attenuation area within left parotid gland. There is a thick, indistinct, partially enhancing surrounding rim, and the remaining parotid tissue is denser than normal. There is also some thickening of the overlying skin and increased attenuation in the subcutaneous fat: Parotid abscess with cellulitis.

submandibular sialadenitis. Such a calculus is found initially in most cases of acute submandibular sialadenitis (Fig. 3-23).[1] The periglandular submandibular nodes are often enlarged, and painful swelling of the gland and these nodes is the characteristic clinical presentation.

Sialodochitis refers to inflammation of the *main* salivary duct. Usually the duct is dilated secondary to a distal obstruction. The enlarged duct can have a fusiform shape or appear as a "string of sausages" resulting from multiple areas of ductal stenosis (Figs. 3-24 and 3-25).

Because of the acute, painful nature of these inflammatory diseases and their usually short duration, sialography is rarely performed. In fact, radiography is contraindicated in these patients since the retrograde injection of contrast may drive the infection back into the gland and cause a recurrence of the process. If a sialogram is performed on a patient with *acute sialadenitis,*

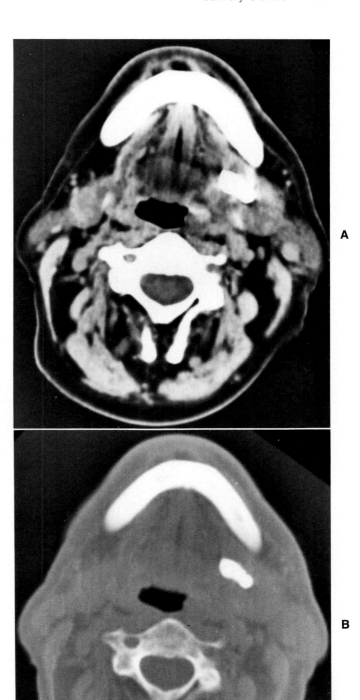

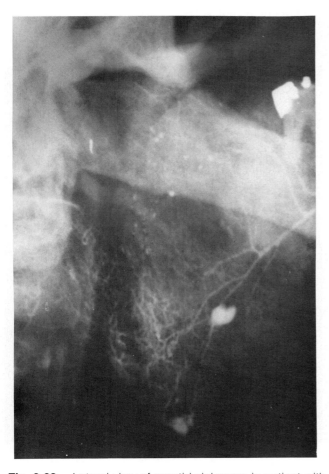

Fig. 3-22   Lateral view of parotid sialogram in patient with a vaguely palpable mass (superiorly, just below the mandible, where there is an absence of ducts). There are also scattered collections of contrast material in upper and lower poles of the gland: Tuberculosis.

Fig. 3-23   **A,** Axial noncontrast CT scan with enlargement of left submandibular gland and a calculus in the hilum of the gland. The structures of the floor of the mouth are otherwise normal. **B,** The same image seen at wide window settings shows the densely calcified nature of this left submandibular sialolith.

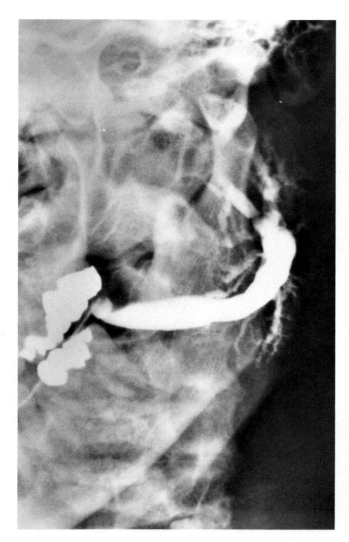

Fig. 3-24 Frontal oblique view of left parotid sialogram. The entire Stensen's duct is dilated, commencing at its buccal opening and continuing posteriorly into the gland. Central parotid ducts are also dilated; peripheral ducts are not visualized: Sialodochitis secondary to obstruction at the buccal orifice. This gland had to be surgically removed because it did not produce sufficient salivary flow to prevent recurrent infections.

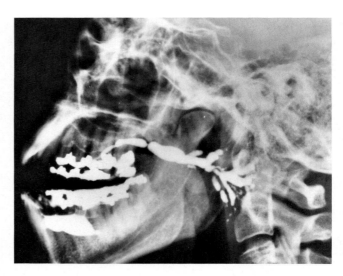

Fig. 3-25 Lateral view of parotid sialogram shows dilatation of Stensen's duct and central parotid ducts. Peripheral ducts are not visualized. Strictures along Stensen's duct create a "string of sausages" appearance: Sialodochitis in a gland that required a parotidectomy because of damage of the acini.

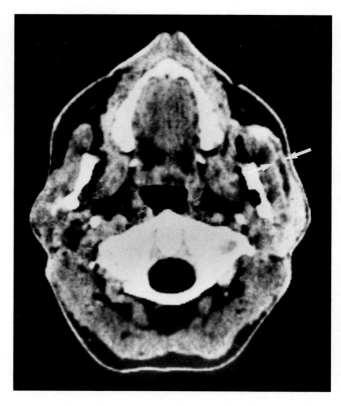

Fig. 3-26 Axial postcontrast CT scan demonstrates increased attenuation in the left parotid gland. There is also thickening and enhancement of the walls of Stensen's duct *(arrows)* and two lower attenuation areas are present within the dilated duct: Noncalcified sialolithiasis with sialodochitis and sialadenitis.

there is peripheral tapering of the ducts, causing a pruned appearance. This picture results from the periductal cellular infiltration of this acute process, which is confined by the gland capsule. Focal areas of dilatation and narrowing may also be seen in the major ducts, especially at the ductal junctions, and these most probably reflect areas of ectasia and functional spasm.[6]

On CT the gland is enlarged and has an increased attenuation reflecting its cellular infiltration.[8] Some diffuse enhancement usually exists on postcontrast studies, most probably reflecting the associated increased

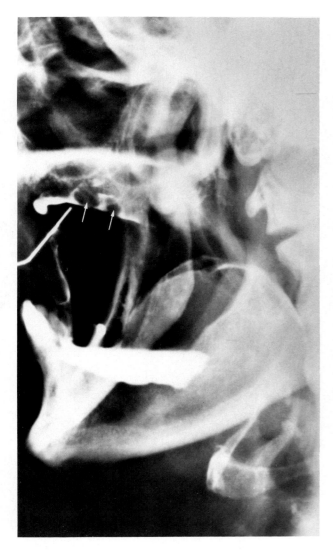

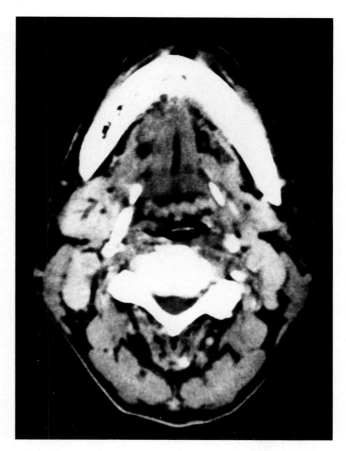

Fig. 3-28   Axial postcontrast CT scan showing enlargement and increased attenuation of right parotid gland. Dilatated mucus filled ducts are seen within the gland secondary to an obstruction in the floor of mouth: Sialadenitis.

Fig. 3-27   Lateral view of left parotid sialogram on same patient as in Fig. 3-26. Two noncalcified stones are seen in Stensen's duct *(arrows).*

vascularity of the gland. *Sialolithiasis* can be seen clearly if calcified and often is identified as a mass in Stensen's duct even if not calcified (Figs. 3-26 and 3-27). *Sialodochitis* is seen as a thickening and enhancing of the walls of Stensen's duct, and mucoid density secretions (10 to 18 HUs) can often be identified within the enlarged duct.

On MRI the gland can have either higher or lower signal intensity than normal on T_2 WIs, depending on whether edema or cellular infiltration is the predominant pathologic change.

The submandibular glands tend to be more cellular than the parotid glands. As a result they appear denser and more homogeneous on CT scans and of a lower signal intensity and more homogeneous on MRI se-

quences. On CT mucoid secretions can often be identified in the major collecting ducts (Fig. 3-28).

Sialolithiasis.   Between 80% and 90% of salivary gland stones occur in the submandibular gland, 10% to 20% occur in the parotid glands, and only 1% to 7% occur in the sublingual glands.[1,3] Most stones are solitary; however, about 25% of patients have multiple stones, with 32% of parotid calculi and 22% of submandibular stones being multiple. The incidence of bilateral salivary stones is 2.2%.[1,9] In patients with chronic sialadenitis, at least one calculus is present in two thirds of the cases, and 80% of submandibular and 60% of parotid stones are radiopaque on plain films.[4]

Some of the reasons given for the increased incidence of sialolithiasis in the submandibular gland as compared to the parotid gland include: the thicker, more mucous nature of the submandibular gland secretions, the more alkaline pH of submandibular saliva which helps precipitate salts, the higher submandibular concentration of hydroxyl-apatite and phosphatase, the

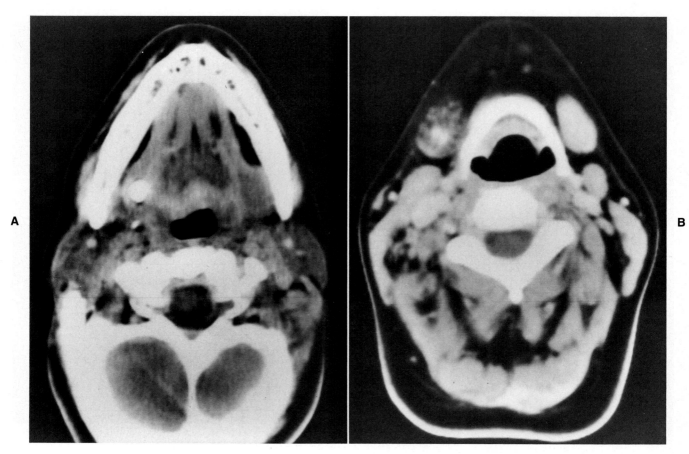

Fig. 3-29   **A,** Axial post contrast CT scan demonstrates a calculus near the hilum of the right submandibular gland. There is also some inflammatory thickening of the right mylohyoid muscle. **B,** More caudal axial CT scan shows the lower margin of the calculus in a somewhat fatty, partially atrophic gland.

narrower orifice of Wharton's duct when compared to the caliber of the duct itself, and the uphill grade in the erect position of Wharton's duct.[1,3,4]

About 85% of submandibular gland stones occur in Wharton's duct. The distribution of submandibular stones is such that 30% are located near the duct ostium, 20% are in the middle portion of the duct, 35% are at the bend in the duct as it goes around the back of the mylohyoid muscle, and only 15% occur in the hilum and gland proper (see Figs. 3-8, 3-10, 3-23, and 3-29).[1]

Symptomatic parotid gland stones occur primarily in Stensen's duct; however, incidental asymptomatic small intraparotid ductal calculi are not uncommonly seen on CT scans.

Because Wharton's duct is larger than Stensen's duct and because many stones can occur in pseudodiverticula of Wharton's duct that do not result in obstruction to the flow of saliva, the time between diagnosis and

the onset of symptoms for sialolithiasis is estimated to be 1 to 2 months in the parotid gland and 1 to 1½ years in the submandibular gland.

The initial radiographic investigation of sialolithiasis starts with the plain film examination. The larger, well-calcified stones can be well seen with this technique (Fig. 3-30). However, small or partially calcified stones may elude detection on plain films. Because CT has a 10 to 1 advantage over plain films for detecting focal calcium deposits, noncontrast CT scans can identify some of the stones that are unobserved on the plain film examinations (Figs. 3-31 to 3-35). Such small, faintly calcified stones may also be obscured on a sialogram and pass undiagnosed unless a plain scout film was obtained before the sialographic contrast medium was introduced. Noncalcified stones are best seen on a sialogram; however, some of the larger ones can also be identified on postcontrast CT scans (see Figs. 3-26 and 3-27).

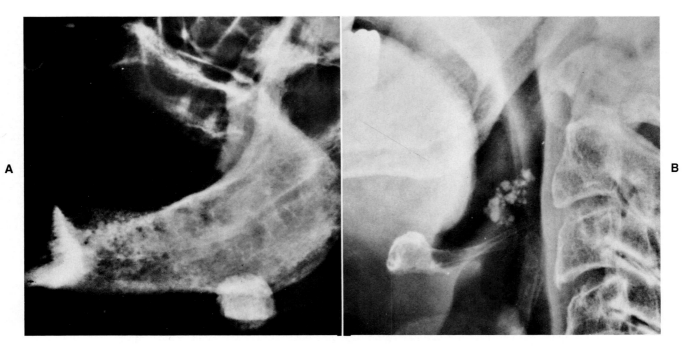

Fig. 3-30 **A,** Lateral plain film showing a large calculus in the submandibular gland. **B,** Lateral plain film showing multiple small calculi within the periphery of the parotid gland.

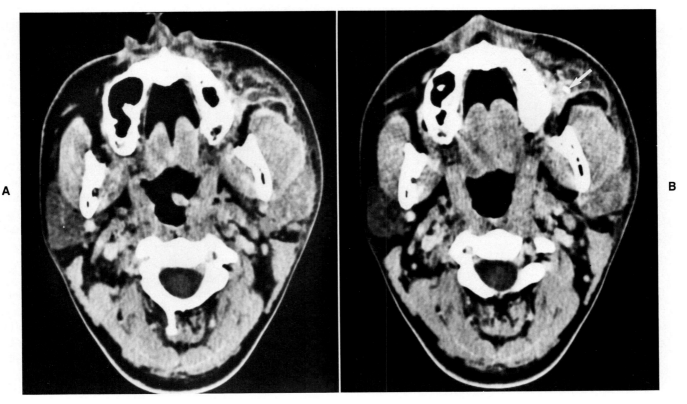

Fig. 3-31 **A,** Axial noncontrast CT scan showing increased attenuation of left parotid gland, thickening of left masseter muscle, and increased attenuation around buccal fat pad in the region of the anterior Stensen's duct. Areas of linear increased density are the inflammed walls of Stensen's duct. There is also increased attenuation in the subcutaneous soft tissues in this patient with normal plain films of this region. **B,** More caudal CT scan demonstrates a small calculus *(arrow)* in Stensen's duct that was not seen on the plain films: Sialodochitis, sialadenitis, sialolithiasis, myositis, and celluitis.

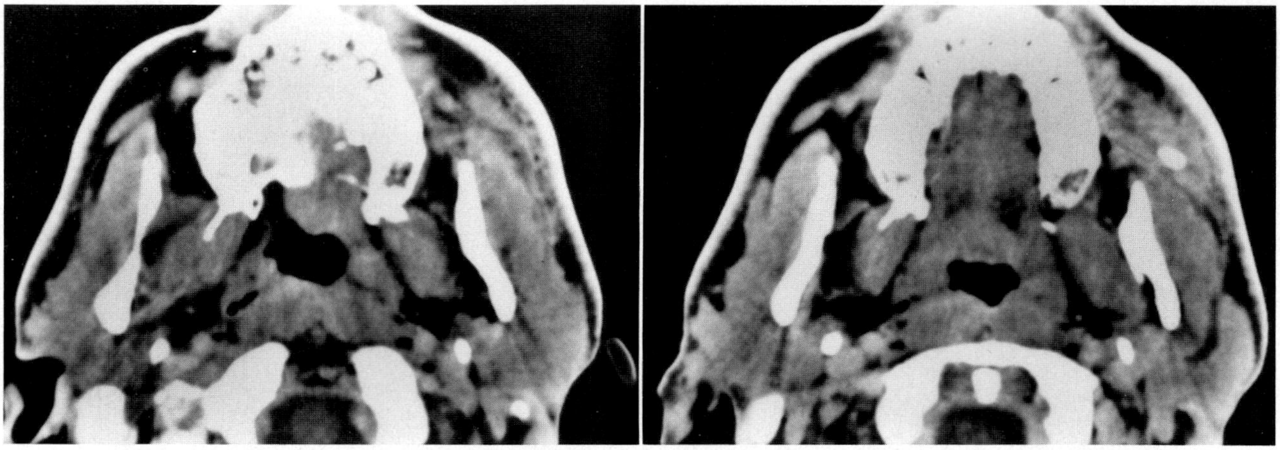

Fig. 3-32 **A,** Axial postcontrast CT scan showing increased attenuation in subcutaneous soft tissues overlying the region of Stensen's duct. There may be thickening of the left masseter muscle as well. **B,** More caudal axial CT scan shows a small calculus in Stensen's duct with surrounding inflammatory changes. The routine plain films on this patient were normal: Sialodochitis, sialolithiasis, and cellulitis.

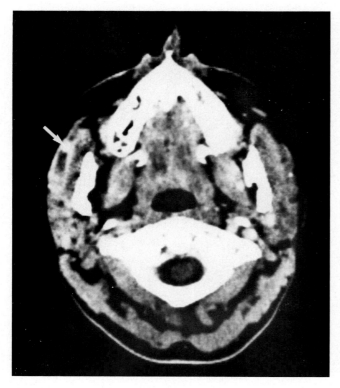

Fig. 3-33 Axial postcontrast CT scan showing increased attenuation in right parotid gland, enhancement and thickening of the walls of Stensen's duct, a small calculus *(arrow)* not seen on plain films and mucoid secretions in Stensen's duct behind the calculus. A small calculus is also present in the anterior superficial portion of the left parotid gland: Sialodochitis, sialadenitis, sialolithiasis.

Chronic Inflammatory Diseases

The chronic inflammatory diseases of the salivary glands can either have specific etiologies, such as a granulomatous process or prior irradiation, or obscure etiologies. The clinical presentation of these chronic conditions varies among three general types. The first presentation is that of repeated episodes of acute sialadenitis with painful swelling of the involved gland. The intervals between these episodes are characterized by the gland's return to normal size and the patient being asymptomatic. The second presentation is that of a slowly progressive enlargement of the gland that has periodic episodes of acute sialadenitis. The third clinical presentation is that of a slowly progressive painless enlargement of the salivary glands. It is this group of patients that may be confused clinically with those having neoplasms.

An attempt should be made to differentiate the obstructive and nonobstructive diseases, since the treatment and prognosis often vary considerably. The chronic nonobstructive diseases involve the parotid glands with a greater frequency than they do the submandibular glands. Conversely the obstructive disorders are more common in the submandibular glands.

Chronic Recurrent Sialadenitis

Chronic recurrent sialadenitis is characterized by recurrent diffuse or localized painful swelling of the salivary gland. It usually is associated with an incomplete obstruction of the ductal system.[5] A sialogram performed during a clinically quiescent period usually shows a focal narrowing of the main duct and central

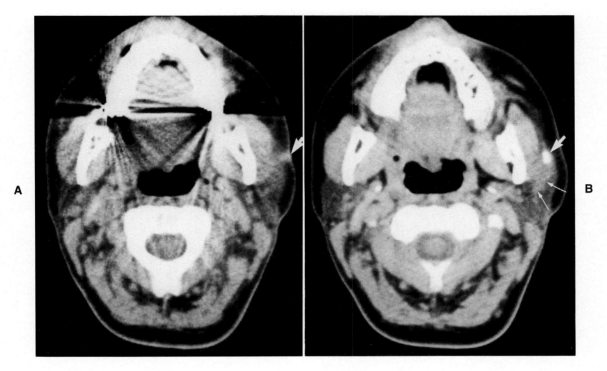

Fig. 3-34 **A,** Axial CT scan showing a small sinus tract *(arrow)* opening to the skin of the cheek. Clear fluid was draining from this site. **B,** More caudal axial CT scan shows a small calculus *(short arrow)* which caused obstruction of the saliva and which was not seen on routine plain films. There is increased attenuation in the obstructed parotid ducts just behind the calculus *(arrows):* Sialodochitis, sialadenitis, sialolithiasis, and sinus tract.

ductal dilatation (sialectasia); these dilated ducts often taper down rather dramatically to normal peripheral ducts (and acini). In these patients if the obstruction (stricture) in the main salivary duct can be relieved, the gland may function normally and not require a parotidectomy (Figs. 3-36 to 3-39). Alternately the peripheral ducts and acini may not be visualized on the sialogram. In these cases the acini are not visible because they are compressed by a cellular infiltrate and destroyed. As a result, saliva production decreases (see Figs. 3-24, 3-25, and 3-40). In turn, this decrease eventually results in the development of further sialadenitis. Thus if the peripheral ducts and acini are not visualized on a technically adequate sialogram, it is unlikely that this gland will function normally; eventually, a parotidectomy (partial) will probably have to be performed.

Areas of ductal branch point narrowing may in part represent focal inflammatory changes. In addition, scattered localized globular collections of contrast material may be encountered. These represent focal abscesses. When multiple, they usually are nonuniform in size and distribution throughout the gland, a factor that distinguishes most cases from the autoimmune diseases (Fig. 3-41).

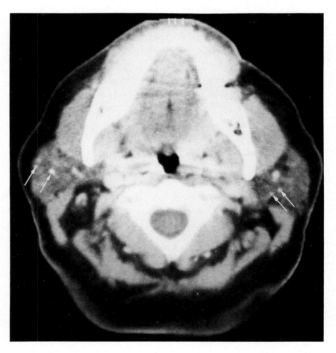

Fig. 3-35 Axial postcontrast CT scan demonstrates several minute calcifications *(arrows)* in both parotid glands. These were not seen on routine plain films: Chronic sialadenitis.

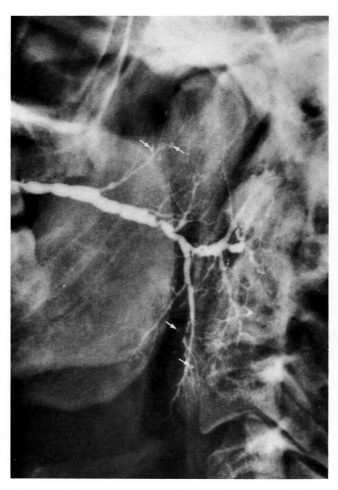

Fig. 3-36 Lateral view of parotid sialogram showing dilatation of Stensen's duct and some of the central parotid ducts. The peripheral ducts are not dilatated. There are scattered small collections of contrast material (arrows), which probably represent small abscesses. Areas of stricture and functional spasm are seen in the central ducts: Sialadenitis.

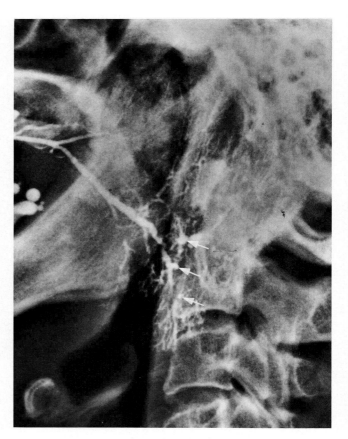

Fig. 3-37 Lateral view of parotid sialogram showing mild dilatation of Stensen's duct and central parotid ducts. Areas of narrowing are present primarily at branch points and small abscesses are seen in the gland (arrows). The majority of the peripheral ducts are visualized: Chronic sialadenitis.

Sialodochitis Fibrinosa (Kussmaul's Disease)

Sialodochitis fibrinosa is an unusual disease characterized by recurrent, acute, painless attacks of parotid or submandibular gland swelling secondary to a mucous or fibrinous ductal plug. The clinical appearance of this plug in either Stensen's or Wharton's duct orifice is diagnostic. This disease occurs primarily in dehydrated and debilitated patients, and the treatment is glandular massage and the use of secretogogues to release the plug.[10]

AUTOIMMUNE DISEASES

The autoimmune diseases form a clinically heterogeneous group of disorders that all share a common histology, the benign lymphoepithelial lesion (BLL) (of Godwin).[11] Microscopically the diffuse process initiates as a collection of small lymphocytes centered around the intralobular ducts. As the lymphoid infiltration increases, acinar atrophy occurs; eventually a replacement of the acinar tissue by the lymphocytes follows. Lymphoid follicles with germinal centers may develop; and plasma cells, eosinophils, and polymorphonuclear leukocytes are present in small numbers. An associated proliferation of ductal epithelium results in the obliteration of ductal lumina and the production of epithelial (epimyoepithelial) islands, which may undergo complete hyalinization. Although these islands may be few in number, their identification is necessary for a pathologic diagnosis of BLL to be made.[12]

Clinically the autoimmune diseases are a diffuse exocrinopathy with the lacrimal (keratoconjunctivitis sicca) and salivary glands being primarily affected. However, atrophic vaginitis, tracheobronchitis, and dry skin are not uncommonly associated findings, while involvement of the glands of the gastrointestinal tract occurs less frequently.[12,13]

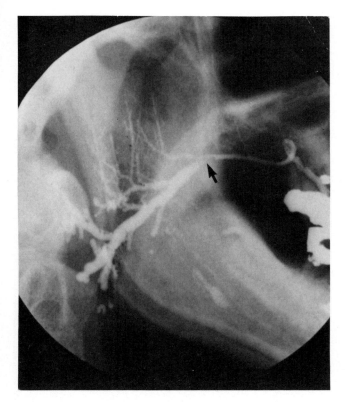

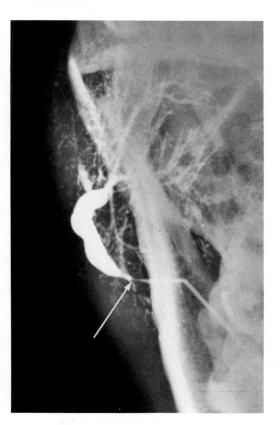

Fig. 3-38 Lateral view of parotid sialogram showing dilatation of Stensen's duct and central parotid ducts behind a noncalcified stone *(arrow)*. Most of the peripheral ducts are not visualized, and the patient eventually required a parotidectomy because of recurrent infections after initial surgery for removal of the stone: Sialadenitis, sialolithiasis, and stricture.

Fig. 3-39 Frontal view of parotid sialogram showing a stricture *(arrow)* in anterior portion of Stensen's duct. There is marked dilatation of Stensen's duct and the central parotid ducts behind the stricture. The peripheral ducts are almost normal. The patient did well after dilatation of the stricture site: Sialodochitis, sialadenitis, and stricture.

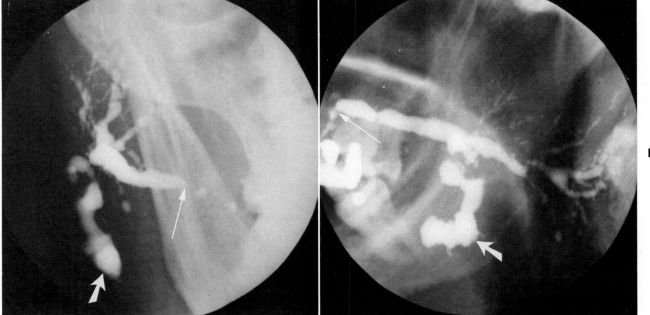

Fig. 3-40 **A,** Frontal and, **B,** lateral views of right parotid sialogram showing a stricture *(arrow)* of the anterior portion of Stensen's duct. There is dilatation of Stensen's duct and the central and peripheral parotid ducts with a fistulous tract *(short arrow):* Sialodochitis, sialadenitis, stricture, and fistula.

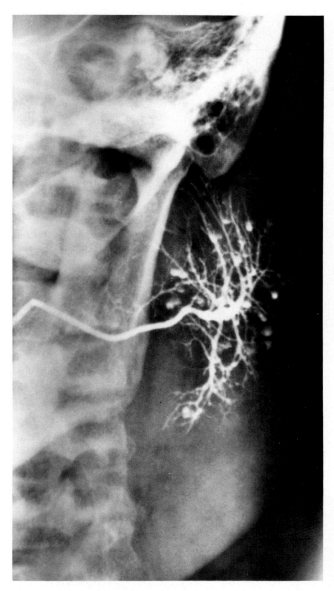

Fig. 3-41 Frontal view of left parotid sialogram showing a fairly normal Stensen's duct and parotid ducts with the exception of multiple scattered collections of contrast material in small abscesses: Chronic sialadenitis.

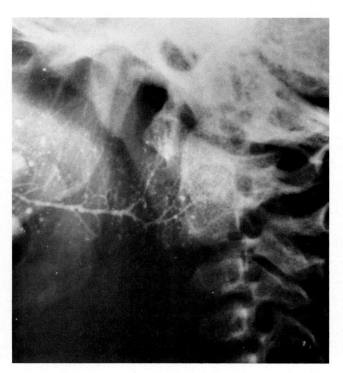

Fig. 3-42 Lateral view of parotid sialogram showing normal central ductal system with multiple uniform in size punctate collections of contrast material evenly distributed throughout the gland: Autoimmune disease. (From Som et al, Radiology 141:415, 1981.)

The BLL can be seen in several different clinical settings. Mikulicz's disease was the name used to describe the disease when it was limited clinically to the salivary and/or lacrimal glands. However, today these patients are described as having either (a) recurrent parotitis (in children) or (b) the sicca syndrome (primary Sjögren's syndrome).[12,14] When a systemic connective tissue disease (usually rheumatoid arthritis, but rarely scleroderma or lupus) is associated with the sicca syndrome, the patient is said to have secondary Sjögren's syndrome.

Recurrent parotitis in children occurs over an age range of 8 months to 15 years, with most cases being evident in the 3- to 6-year age group. The childhood form of the disease is one tenth as common as the adult form, with children having a lower incidence of developing the advanced form of parotid disease.[14] Males are affected slightly more often than females. Since most cases resolve spontaneously at puberty, the diagnosis must be established so that surgery can be delayed, if possible, until the attainment of puberty. In a few cases of recurrent parotitis in children the disease has progressed into adult life.[12]

The parotid gland enlargement is slightly more common in the primary form of Sjörgen's syndrome than it is in the secondary type of the disease. The incidence of parotid enlargement has varied from 25% to 55% of cases, and either parotid or submandibular gland enlargement occurs in 80% of all patients with Sjögren's syndrome.[15] About 90% to 95% of all affected adults are women.[1]

The clinical presentations vary from recurrent acute episodes to chronic glandular enlargement with superimposed acute attacks, to nontender, nonpainful, glandular enlargement.[11] Although the gland is usually diffusely affected, in some patients a localized area may be more involved, clinically simulating a mass. If accessory

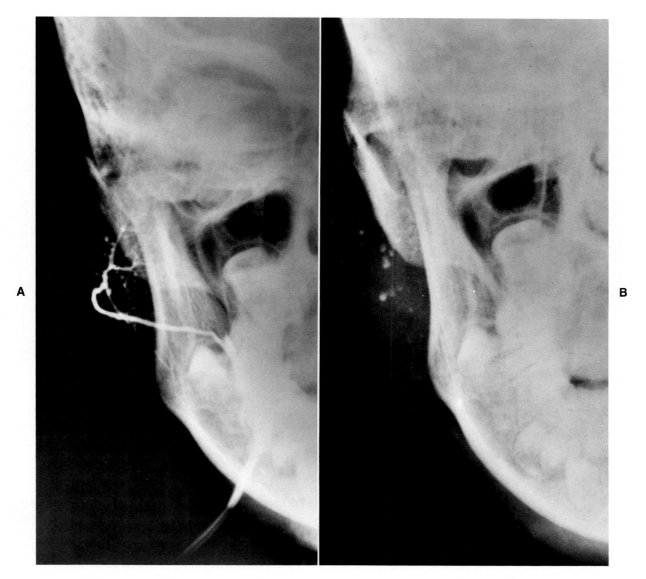

Fig. 3-43 **A,** Frontal view of right parotid sialogram showing normal Stensen's duct and central parotid ducts. Punctate collections of contrast material are uniformly scattered throughout the gland. **B,** Frontal post evacuation film on same patient as in **A** showing residual contrast within the punctate collections and good drainage of the ducts: Autoimmune disease.

parotid glands are present, they also are affected by Sjögren's syndrome, often being manifest as a mass in the cheek.

Submandibular gland enlargement is less common than that of the parotid gland, with a clinical incidence varying between 2.5% and 16% of cases with parotid gland disease.

Patients with Sjögren's syndrome have an increased risk of developing a lymphoma, which often has an aggressive biologic course.[14,16]

Because the autoimmune disease initially involves the most peripheral ducts and acini, the central ducts are normal in the initial stages of the disease. The sialogram reveals a normal central system and numerous punctate (1 mm or less in diameter) collections of contrast material uniformly scattered throughout the gland. These punctate changes are the earliest diagnostic sialographic findings of Sjögren's syndrome (Figs. 3-42 and 3-43). If the collections of contrast material are larger or globular in size (1 to 2 mm in diameter), the globular form of the disease is present and probably represents a progression of the punctate form (Figs. 3-44 and 3-45).

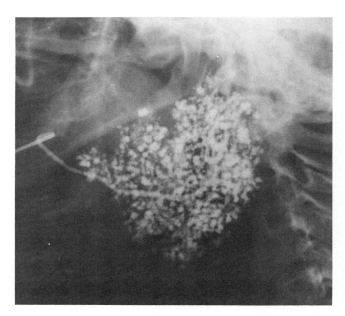

Fig. 3-44 Lateral oblique view of parotid sialogram showing larger punctate (globular) collections of contrast material that are fairly uniform in size and distribution throughout the gland. The central ductal system is normal: Autoimmune disease.

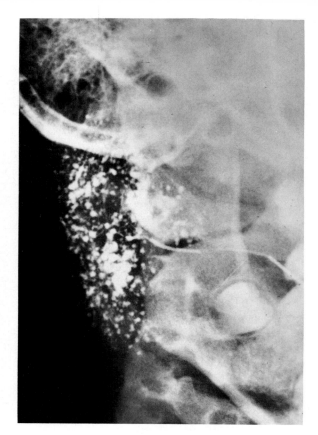

Fig. 3-45 Frontal oblique view of parotid sialogram showing diffuse globular collections of contrast material uniformly distributed throughout the gland. The central ducts are normal: Autoimmune disease.

Once sufficient acinar destruction has occurred, ascending infection can develop and its sialographic changes can be superimposed on those of the autoimmune disease. Thus the cavitary and destructive forms of the disease represent progressive changes in the gland that involve larger peripheral collections of contrast material combined with the central changes of sialodochitis and sialadenitis. This action eventually leads to an abscess formation that may involve the entire gland (Figs. 3-46 to 3-49).

If a secretogogue is given at the end of the sialographic examination, the contrast material will drain from the main ducts but remain within the punctate and globular collections.

The sialographic changes of the autoimmune disease are sufficiently specific; they allow the sialographer to differentiate such cases from patients with sialosis and most cases of chronic sialadenitis.

On CT the involved gland(s) is usually enlarged and denser than normal. The appearance is similar to that seen in patients with either chronic sialadenitis or sialosis (Figs. 3-50, 3-51, and 3-54). If a prior sialogram has been performed with fat-soluble contrast material, the agent's droplets that formed the punctate and globular collection seen on the sialogram can be identified on the CT scan many years after it was performed (Fig. 3-52). A honey-combed appearance in the paratid gland can be seen on CT or MRI, however, the sialographic findings remain the most characteristic method to establish the diagnosis.

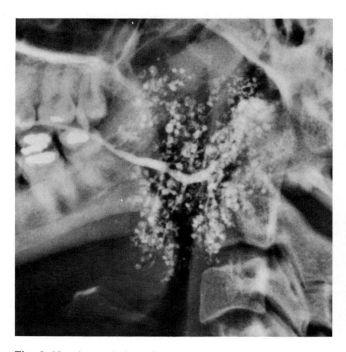

Fig. 3-46 Lateral view of parotid sialogram showing globular collections of contrast material uniformly distributed throughout the gland with some dilatation of Stensen's duct: Early sialodochitis and autoimmune disease. (From Som et al, Radiology 141:415, 1981.)

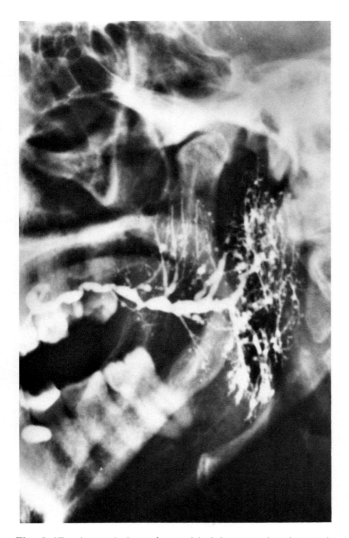

Fig. 3-47 Lateral view of parotid sialogram showing multiple punctate collections of contrast material uniformly scattered throughout the gland. Several collections in the inferior pole of the gland are larger, and there are changes of sialodochitis and central ductal sialadenitis: Early cavitary autoimmune disease.

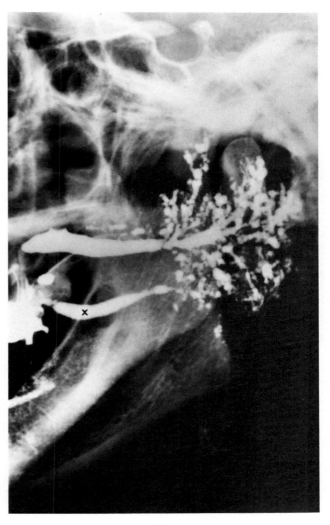

Fig. 3-48 Lateral view of parotid sialogram showing changes of sialodochitis and sialadenitis superimposed on those of autoimmune disease. Several focal areas appear to be coalescing to form larger collections. Some contrast material is seen layering-out in the floor of the mouth *(x):* Early destructive autoimmune disease.

SIALOSIS OR SIALADENOSIS

Sialosis refers to a nonneoplastic, noninflammatory, nontender, chronic or recurrent enlargement of the parotid glands.[17,52] Far less commonly the submandibular, sublingual, and minor salivary glands can be affected.[2]

The parotid disease is usually bilateral and symmetrical but can be unilateral and/or asymmetrical. The onset is usually insidious, with no symptoms of inflammation. The disease may worsen or improve depending on whether the underlying condition is treated, and resolution of the sialosis can occur in only a few days if fatty replacement of the gland has not taken place. A decreased salivary flow and/or xerostomia may or may not occur; however, these findings usually reflect the underlying disease and are not specific findings of sialosis.[18]

Sialosis is associated with a variety of endocrine diseases, nutritional and metastatic states, and certain medications. Sialosis is found in patients with diabetes, and the parotid gland enlargement may be the first clinical evidence of the underlying disease. Sialosis has also been reported with abnormalities of the ovaries and thyroid glands, and it has been associated with acromegaly.[17,18]

Sialosis is found in 26% to 86% of patients with chronic alcoholism, alcoholic cirrhosis, and with other chronic malnutrition states. Hypertension, hyperlipidema, obesity, prolonged starch ingestion, pregnancy,

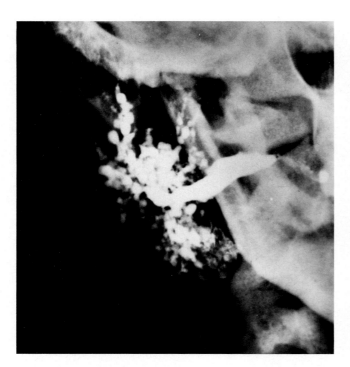

Fig. 3-49 Frontal oblique view of right parotid sialogram demonstrates coalescent abscesses and changes of sialodochitis and sialadenitis superimposed on those of autoimmune disease: Destructive autoimmune disease.

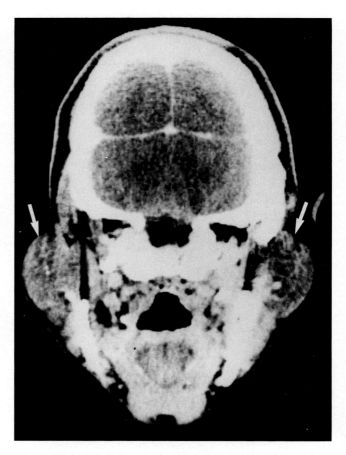

Fig. 3-50 Coronal postcontrast CT scan showing both parotid glands (arrows) to be larger and slightly denser than normal: Chronic sialadenitis. Note similarity to Figs. 3-51 and 3-54.

pellagra, kwashiorkor, brucellosis, and celiac disease are also associated with sialosis.

Sialosis has also been associated with a variety of medications, including phenylbutazone, oxyphenbutazone, sulfisoxazole, iodide, isoproterenol, atropine, imipramine, phenothiazides, benzodiazepines, monoamine oxidase (MAO) inhibitors, reserpine, guanethidine, heavy metals, methimazole, thiocyanates, and thiourea drugs such as thiouracil and propylthiouracil. With these pharmacologic sialoses both the submandibular and parotid glands may be involved, and the glandular swelling may be painful.[17,18]

Pathologically enlargement and degranulation of the parenchymal cells and/or fatty replacement of the parenchyma can occur. Usually acinar hypertrophy with increased zymogen granulation is the predominant early finding, while fibrosis and fatty atrophy dominate the later stages of the process. The fibrosis is confined to the interlobular septa, and there is no pathologic evidence of inflammatory changes.

On sialography the parotid gland is enlarged and the ducts are fairly normal in appearance, but splayed by the increased gland volume. There may be some compression of the smaller peripheral ductal branches by the increased interstitial fibrosis and/or fat. Because these sialographic changes are sufficiently different from those of chronic sialadenitis or the autoimmune

diseases sialosis can be sialographically distinguished from them (Fig. 3-53).

On computed sectional imaging the parotid glands are enlarged but may appear dense or fatty depending on the dominant pathologic change. As such the CT and MRI appearances are similar to those seen in the autoimmune diseases and chronic sialadenitis (Fig. 3-54).

POSTIRRADIATION SIALADENITIS

Postirradiation sialadenitis can occur in an acute or chronic form. The acute type is rare today and is characterized by a tender, painful swelling of the gland within 24 hours after it has been irradiated, usually by a single dose of 1000 rads or more. These manifestations usually subside within 3 to 4 days, and there may be an associated transient xerostomia. The chronic form occurs in glands irradiated as part of a curative treatment plan, usually for oral cavity or pharyngeal tumors. Clinically the gland atrophies; there is xerostomia that may in part be secondary to the decreased saliva production

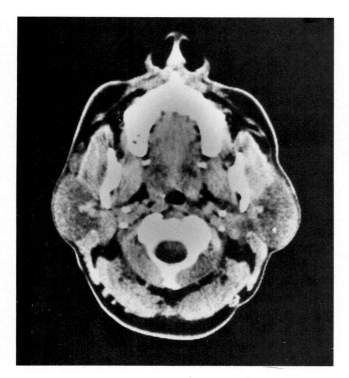

Fig. 3-51 Axial postcontrast CT scan showing larger, slightly denser parotid glands than normal: Autoimmune disease. Note the similarity to Figs. 3-50 and 3-54.

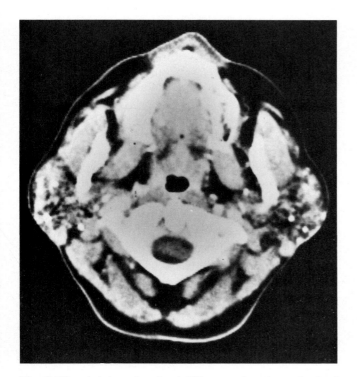

Fig. 3-52 Axial postcontrast CT scan of patient who had a bilateral parotid sialogram 15 years earlier. The glands are enlarged and globular collections of contrast material can be seen scattered throughout both salivary glands: Autoimmune disease.

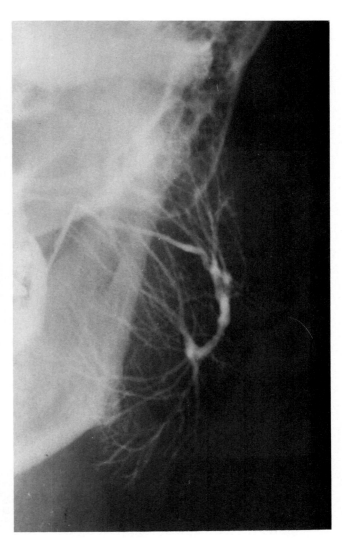

Fig. 3-53 Frontal view of left parotid sialogram showing normal Stensen's duct. The intraparotid ducts are normal with the exception of being widely separated as they fill the enlarged gland: Sialosis. (From Som et al, Radiology 141:421, 1981.)

of the major salivary gland but probably is produced primarily by the radiation effect on the minor salivary glands of the oral cavity. A sialogram reveals patchy areas of lack of acinar filling and focal areas of ductal pruning.

NECROTIZING SIALOMETAPLASIA

Necrotizing sialometaplasia is a benign, self-limiting disorder that can be mistaken for a malignancy. This entity is found three times more commonly in males than in females, and most patients are over the age of 40 years. It usually involves the mucoserous glands of the hard palate, although it can arise in any salivary gland tissue. Most often there is a painless, round, deep ulcer in the palate. Less commonly, the ulcers

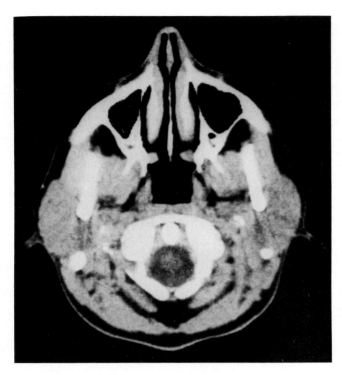

Fig. 3-54 Axial noncontrast CT scan demonstrating enlarged and dense parotid glands: Sialosis. Note the similarity to Figs. 3-50 and 3-51.

can be linear and multiple. The lesion(s) undergoes a slow but spontaneous healing over a 6- to 10-week period. It most often is misdiagnosed as either squamous cell carcinoma or mucoepidermoid carcinoma. The process probably is reparative in nature secondary to ischemic necrosis of the minor salivary gland tissue.[2] On imaging, a nonspecific soft tissue mass is seen in the palate without any associated bone erosion.

HYPERPLASIA OF MUCOUS SALIVARY GLANDS

Hyperplasia of mucous salivary glands is a rare entity that arises as a nonulcerated, asymptomatic, tumorlike sessile mass in the hard or soft palate. It is usually mistaken for a salivary gland neoplasm or fibroma, and the histology is that of hypertrophied lobules of normal mucinous acini. The etiology is unknown and local excision is curative.[2] Such masses are usually biopsied and excised without any imaging procedures.

GRANULOMATOUS DISEASES

Of the granulomatous diseases that affect the salivary glands, most arise within juxtaglandular lymph nodes, or in the case of the parotid gland, the intraparotid nodes. The gland parenchyma can also be directly involved. In the majority of these diseases the major salivary glands are secondarily involved by either an adjacent or systemic process.

In most cases a nontender, nonpainful, chronic en-

largement of the gland occurs. The gland is often multinodular and clinically may mimic a malignancy. The diseases that produce these findings include sarcoidosis, tuberculosis, atypical mycobacterial infection, syphilis, cat-scratch fever, toxoplasmosis, and actinomycosis.[1]

Sarcoidosis is a systemic disease of undetermined etiology characterized by noncaseating granulomas involving multiple organ systems. The parotid glands are affected in 10% to 30% of patients, and in some cases the parotid disease may be the initial and only manifestation of the disease. In 83% of these patients bilateral parotid gland enlargement is present and there is a decreased salivary flow. In some patients involvement of the minor salivary glands can cause xerostomia.[1,19]

The parotid glands can also be enlarged in patients with sarcoidosis who have uveitis and facial nerve paralysis. This triad of findings is called Heerfordt's syndrome. It is important to be aware of this syndrome so that the combination of a parotid fullness and an ipsilateral facial nerve paralysis is not erroneously interpreted as being indicative of a malignancy. Most cases of such salivary gland sarcoidosis usually resolve as the underlying disease is treated.

On CT or MRI, usually the parotid granulomas are multiple, benign-appearing masses that are not cavitated. This appearance can be present in association with cervical adenopathy (Figs. 3-55 to 3-58). In this circumstance the diagnosis can be suggested on the basis of the radiologic findings. However, if the sarcoid granuloma is a solitary parotid mass, it cannot be differentiated from the other benign parotid lesions such as a pleomorphic adenoma, a Warthin's tumor, or a hyperplastic lymph node.

Primary tuberculous involvement of the salivary glands is rare. Seventy percent of the cases involve the parotid glands, 27% involve the submandibular glands, and only 3% involve the sublingual glands.[1] Most often the salivary disease arises from a focus in the tonsils or teeth and spreads to the gland via the regional lymph nodes. Secondary salivary tuberculous involvement occurs in cases of generalized tuberculosis and tends to affect the submandibular glands.[3]

The sialographic findings are primarily those of bacterial sialadenitis, and focal abscesses tend to develop within the gland. Adjacent tuberculous cervical adenitis may either have an appearance similar to that of benign hyperplastic adenopathy or have more extensive findings, which are described in Chapter 8.

Atypical myobacterial infections of the salivary glands similarly tend to represent extensions from cervical adenopathy and are radiographically indistinguishable from tuberculous disease.[3]

Syphilis is extremely rare in the parotid glands. When it does occur, it is reported to have a similar distribution and appearance to that of tuberculosis, and its

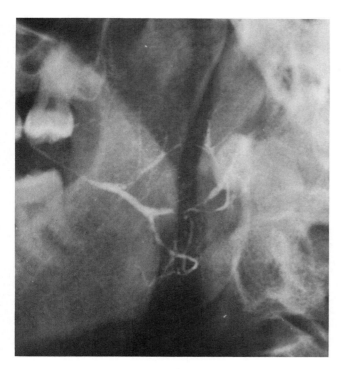

Fig. 3-55   Lateral view of parotid sialogram showing the ductal system to be "pruned" and displaced around several masses: Sarcoid. (From Som et al, Radiology 141:421, 1981.)

imaging findings are similar to those of sarcoidosis.[3]

Cat-scratch (animal) fever and toxoplasmosis are granulomatous diseases that may involve the parotid lymph nodes and mimic primary salivary gland disease.[1,3] Their radiographic findings can resemble either those of sarcoidosis or tuberculosis and as such, they are indistinguishable from these diseases.

Actinomycosis is an indolent, chronic fungal inflammatory disease that invades the salivary glands from a focus usually in the mandible. Sinus tracts are common, and nodal disease can occur in and around the parotid gland and in the submandibular lymph nodes.[1] An inflammatory infiltration of the soft tissues usually occurs in association with the nodal disease.

CYSTS

Cystic lesions account for up to 5% of all salivary gland masses; however, many of these happen to be cystic neoplasms rather than true cysts.[3] The majority of the true cysts occur in the parotid gland and may be classified as either congenital or acquired.

Congenital Cysts

Congenital cysts include branchial cleft cysts, lymphoepithelial cysts, or, rarely, dermoid cysts. Although these cysts are present at birth, they do not become ev-

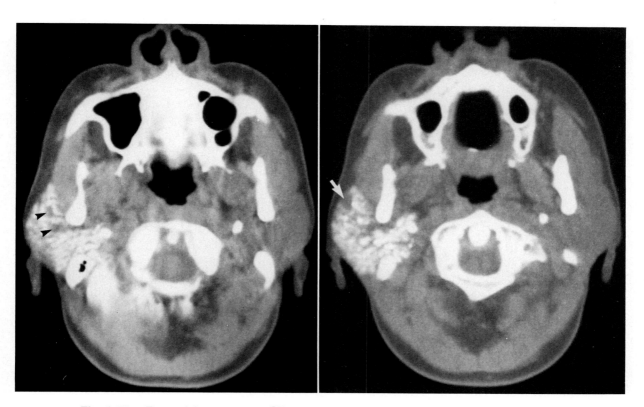

Fig. 3-56   Two axial noncontrast CT scans on a patient who had a right parotid sialogram immediately prior to the CT study. Arrows point to focal filling defects, which were granulomas that were no longer present on a follow-up study after the patient was treated with steroids: Sarcoid.

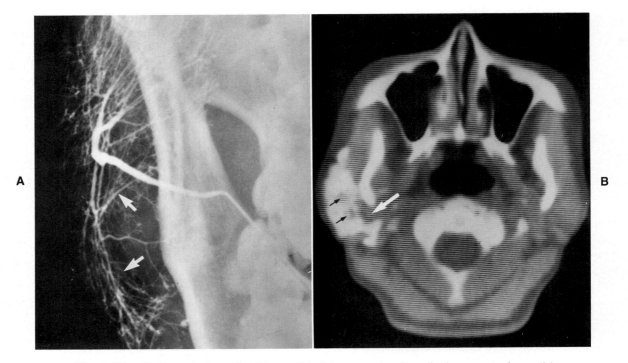

Fig. 3-57 A, Frontal view of right parotid sialogram showing displacement of parotid ducts around a solitary benign appearing mass: Sarcoid. **B,** Axial CT-sialogram showing the larger mass *(white arrow)* seen on the sialogram and two smaller masses *(black arrows),* which were not detected on the sialogram: Sarcoid.

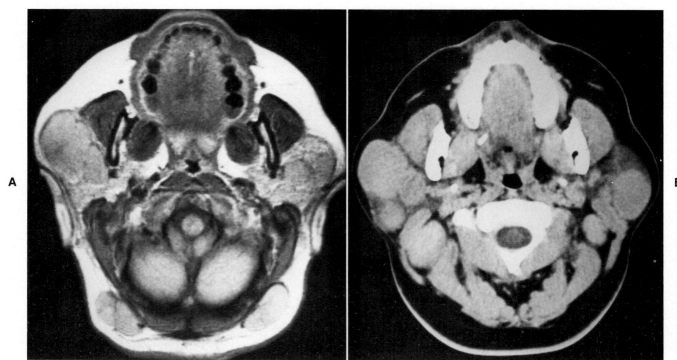

Fig. 3-58 A, Transverse mixed image MRI scan (0.5T, TR 1800 msec, TE 80 msec) showing multiple masses within both parotid glands and enlarged occipital and posterior triangle lymph nodes: Sarcoid. **B,** Axial CT scan shows multiple bilateral enlarged, homogeneous parotid lymph nodes: Sarcoid.

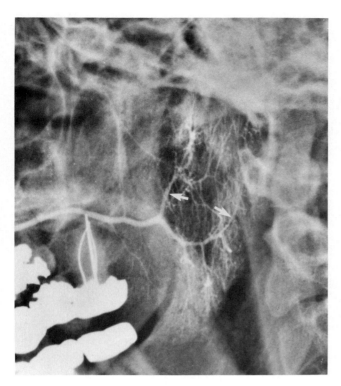

Fig. 3-59 Lateral view of parotid sialogram showing smooth displacement of the parotid ducts around a benign-appearing mass *(arrows):* Mucous cyst.

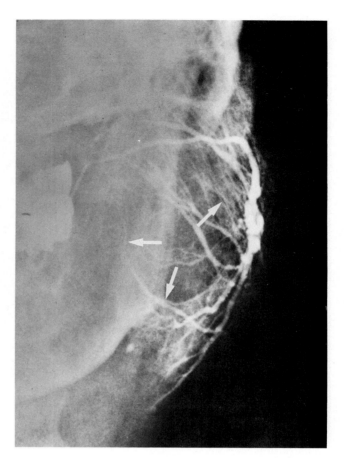

Fig. 3-60 Frontal view of parotid sialogram showing a benign-appearing mass *(arrows)* that displaces the parotid ducts: Mucous cyst.

ident clinically until adulthood. Their usual presentation is that of a painless unilateral parotid swelling. Pain may be present if the cyst becomes infected; sinus tracts and fistulas to the skin and external auditory canal may coexist (Figs. 3-59 to 3-64).[2]

Most of the branchial cleft cysts are classified as type II, which are believed to represent duplication defects of the membraneous external auditory canal and pinna. The cysts can vary from 1 to 7 cm in diameter, and histologically they have a lining of squamous epithelium, ciliated columnar epithelium, or a mixture of both. The cyst wall often has lymphoid tissue with germinal centers. Most of these cysts contain both skin appendages and cartilage.[2,20]

Some of the lymphoepithelial cysts arise within intraparotid and periparotid lymph nodes, most likely representing intranodal parotid inclusions. Branchial pouch cysts have also been reported to occur in the deep portion of the parotid gland, near the eustachian tube; and fibrocystic and polycystic disease can rarely affect the parotid glands.[10]

Complete surgical excision of all such congenital cysts and any sinus or fistulous tracts is curative.

Acquired Cysts

Acquired cysts of the major salivary glands develop secondarily to an obstruction that may be caused by a postinflammatory stricture, a calculus, trauma, a postsurgical complication (from stenosis or ligature of a duct), a benign lymphoepithelial lesion, or a neoplasm. Usually the obstruction is incomplete or intermittent, since an initial complete obstruction, such as a ligation of a duct, most often results in acinar atrophy rather than cyst formation (Figs. 3-65 to 3-67).[2,21]

These cysts are often referred to as retention cysts or mucoceles; and when they arise in the sublinqual gland, they are called *ranulas* (Fig. 3-68). Histologically, these acquired cysts have a layer of cuboidal, columnar, or squamous epithelium, and the lymphoid tissue present in the walls of the congenital cysts is usually not present in these acquired cysts.[2]

If a duct ruptures with escape of mucus into the surrounding tissues, a salivary mucocele results (Fig. 3-69). This is in reality a pseudocyst; no epithelial lining exists. These pseudocysts most often develop after trauma. However, such mucoceles can also result from any of the other causes of intermittent or partial obstruction with rupture. Surgery is the treatment of choice.

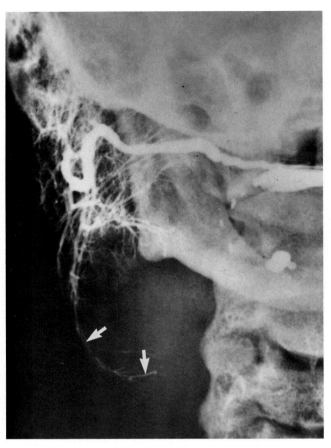

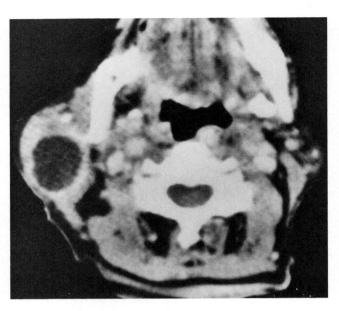

Fig. 3-62   Axial postcontrast CT scan showing low attenuation (10-18 HUs) cystic mass in right parotid gland. The cyst wall enhances and is farily smooth and uniform in appearance: Intraparotid branchial cleft cyst. Note similarity to Fig. 3-20.

Fig. 3-61   Frontal view of right parotid sialogram showing a large benign-appearing mass in the lower pole of the parotid gland *(arrows):* Intraparotid branchial cleft cyst.

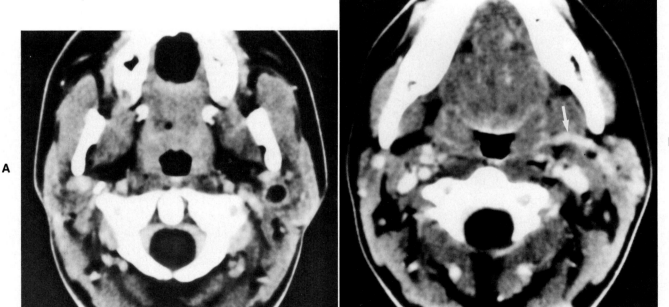

Fig. 3-63   Axial postcontrast CT scan through **A,** the parotid glands and **B,** a more caudal scan in the neck. There is a solitary smooth walled cyst in the retromandibular portion of the left parotid gland. Extending from it is an enhancing sinus tract *(arrow)* that leads to the left palatine tonsil: Intraparotid second branchial cleft cyst with infected tract.

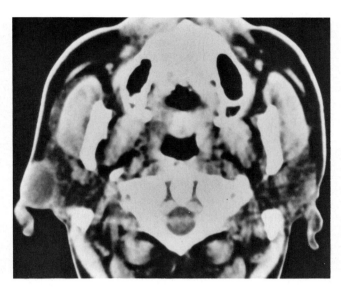

Fig. 3-64 Axial noncontrast CT scan demonstrating a smooth walled cyst in the superficial portion of the right parotid gland: Intraparotid branchial cleft cyst.

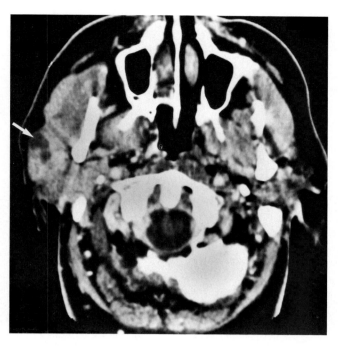

Fig. 3-65 Axial postcontrast CT scan showing several small cysts in the anterior superficial portion of the right parotid gland *(arrow)*. The right parotid gland is denser than normal: Post traumatic acquired cysts.

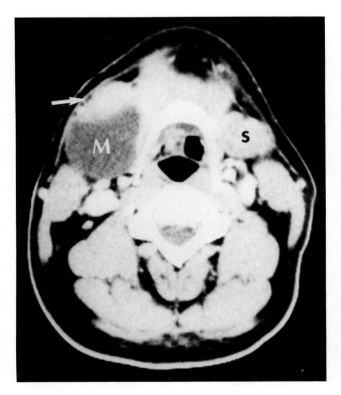

Fig. 3-66 Axial postcontrast CT scan showing a large, low attenuation mass in the posterior margin of the right submandibular gland *(M)*. The mass has no soft tissue plane separating it from the gland, but it is separated from the adjacent neck structures. *S* = normal left submandibular gland: Mucocele of a portion of the submandibular gland.

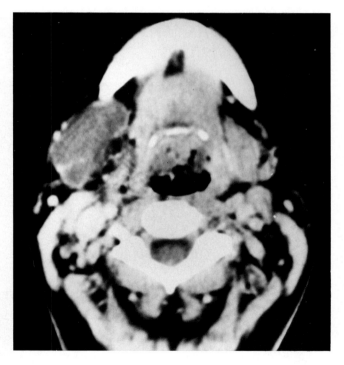

Fig. 3-67 Axial postcontrast CT scan showing right submandibular gland entirely replaced by a mucoid attenuation (10-18 HU) mass: Mucocele of the submandibular gland.

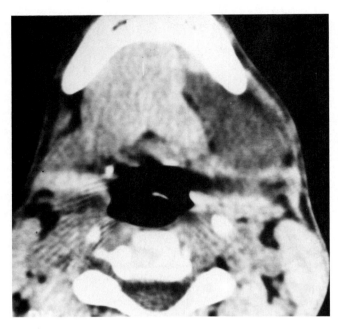

Fig. 3-68   Axial postcontrast CT scan demonstrating low attenuation (mucoid) mass in the left submandibular triangle of the neck. The mass is just anterior to the left submandibular gland and extends from the floor of the mouth: Ranula.

The salivary injury may occur secondary to either blunt nonpenetrating trauma or a penetrating injury. The main salivary duct is injured in about half of the cases, and ductal laceration may result in the development of a fistula that can communicate either with the overlying skin or the oral cavity.[22] The gland parenchyma can also be injured either separately or in conjunction with ductal trauma.

Stensen's duct orifice stenosis can occur from repeated cheek biting or ill-fitting dentures while ductal stenosis results secondary to epithelial injury from stones or surgical manipulation. Injury to the gland parenchyma can result in either a parenchymal laceration or an intracapsular hematoma. Calcification of such intraparenchymal hemorrhage can occur.[1]

A sialogram performed on a patient with a cyst reveals smooth displacement of the glandular ducts around the mass (see Figs. 3-59 to 3-61). In general, no direct communication with the ductal system is demonstrated (Fig. 3-70). In patients with main ductal stenosis the site and degree of this stenosis can be accurately assessed by a sialogram, provided the stenosis is not at the main ductal orifice. Similarly, lacerations of the ducts can be identified by sialography, and in some cases any fistulas or sinus tracts can be identified. In cases of parenchymal laceration or intracapsular hematoma, the sialogram reveals an area(s) of absent parenchymal filling with splaying of the ducts around the area(s).

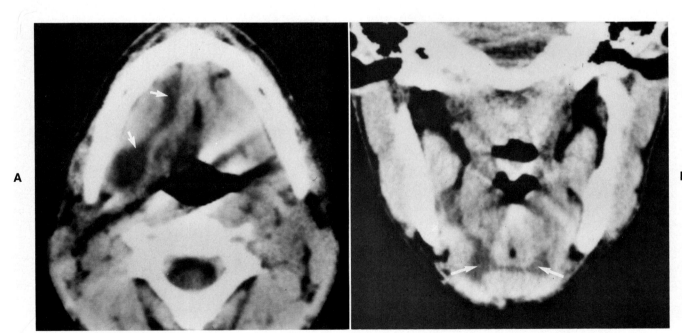

Fig. 3-69   **A,** Axial and **B,** coronal noncontrast CT scans reveal a low attenuation (mucoid) collection *(arrows)* in the right floor of the mouth that has tracked down and across the midline: Plunging ranula.

A sialocele arises when saliva accumulates within a cystic area developed from a complete or incomplete traumatic interruption of the excretory ducts draining the region. If some communication persists with the main ductal system, a sialogram will reveal a communicating cystic mass within the gland (Fig. 3-71). If no such communication exists, the sialocele will appear as a benign mass that displaces the adjacent ducts. These sialoceles develop rapidly after trauma, and needle aspiration of the cyst confirms the diagnosis.[23]

On CT scans, a cyst is identified as a smooth, well-delineated, ovoid mass that usually has a homogeneous, low central attenuation of 10 to 20 HU. The cyst wall in these cases is easily identified and usually thin and uniform in appearance. If the cyst contents are very proteinacious (usually after repeated episodes of infection), the attenuation of the cyst contents and the cyst wall may be the same, in which case the cyst will appear on CT as a homogeneous, benign-appearing solid mass. If the cyst has become infected, the cyst wall enhances and becomes thicker and less well delineated from the adjacent glandular parenchyma. The central portion is of lower attenuation. This CT appearance is indistinguishable from that of an abscess. The adjacent parenchyma in such cases usually has an increased attenuation (compared to the normal gland appearance), reflecting the cellular infiltration associated with the inflammation. In some cases fistulas or sinus tracts can be demonstrated on CT scans (see Fig. 3-63); however, these are usually better identified by sialography.

On MRI the cysts have low signal intensity on T_1-weighted images, intermediate signal intensity on proton density–weighted images, and high signal intensity on T_2-weighted images (see Fig. 3-75). These signal intensities reflect the predominant water content of the secretions within these masses. Definition of the wall thickness, smoothness, or uniformity may occasionally be made on T_1-weighted images, but this is usually better accomplished on postcontrast CT scans.

Multiple parotid cysts can be found unilaterally or bilaterally in association with benign hyperplastic cervical lymphadenopathy. The cysts have a lymphoepithelial origin. They arise secondary to an incomplete ductal obstruction from periductal lymphocytic infiltration and/or as intralymph node cysts by some process analogous to that believed to play a role in the development of Warthin's tumors. The association of such pa-

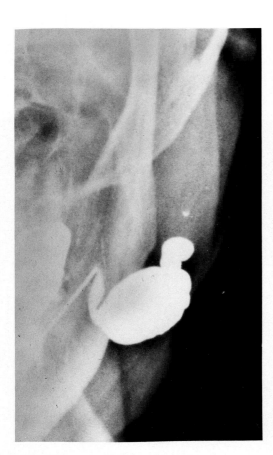

Fig. 3-70 Frontal view of left parotid sialogram demonstrating a cystic dilatation of Stensen's duct with no evidence of communication with the main parotid ductal system: Post traumatic stricture of Stensen's duct near the hilum of the gland.

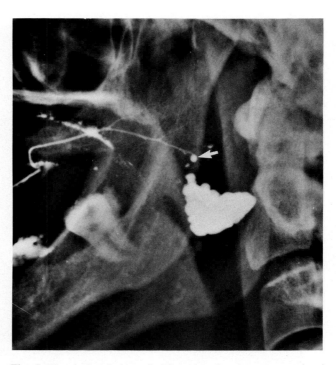

Fig. 3-71 Lateral view of sialogram showing a normal caliber Stensen's duct from which droplets of contrast material (arrow) fill a large cyst within the parotid gland: Posttraumatic communicating cyst-sialocele.

rotid cysts and benign cervical adenopathy (and occasionally hyperplastic adenoids) is most suggestive that the patient is HIV positive, and this may be the first manifestation of this disease. Overt clinical AIDS need not be present. On CT the cysts are homogeneous and have thin, smooth walls, while on MRI the cysts have high T_2-weighted signal intensities (Figs. 3-72 to 3-75).[24-26]

Ranulas. The ranula is a mucous retention cyst phenomenon that occurs in the sublingual gland. It occurs in two forms. The first, or simple type, is the most common, with the retention cyst remaining in the floor of the mouth above the level of the mylohyoid muscle. The second type is the deep or plunging ranula, which is a mucocele that develops from the rupture of the wall of a simple ranula. As such, it usually extends below the level of the mylohyoid muscle and, in reality, is a pseudocyst.

The simple ranula occurs as a mass in the floor of the mouth, off the midline in the area of the sublingual gland. The elevated mucosa of the floor of the mouth often has a characteristic bluish color; because of the simple ranula's location, the differential diagnosis includes a lateral dermoid or epidermoid cyst, a lipoma, or a salivary gland tumor. The plunging ranula appears clinically as a painless mass in the submandibular or submental triangles of the neck, with or without evidence of a mass in the floor of the mouth; and the differential diagnosis includes dermoid and epidermoid cysts, thyroglossal duct cysts, cystic hygromas, and adenopathy.[22]

On CT the simple ranula is cystic in appearance with a homogeneous central attenuation region of 10 to 20 HU. The cyst wall is either very thin or not seen, and the lesion is lateral to the genioglossal muscles and medial and above the mylohyoid muscle (see Fig. 3-68). The plunging ranula often infiltrates the tissue planes, extends to the submandibular gland, and may cross the midline to the contralateral floor of the mouth (see Fig. 3-69). The CT differential diagnosis includes dermoid, epidermoid, cystic lymphangioma, lipoma, lateral thyroglossal duct cyst, and a lymph node.[23]

On MRI the ranula's characteristics are dominated by its high water content, and thus it has a low T_1-weighted signal intensity, an intermediate proton density–weighted signal intensity, and a high T_2-weighted signal intensity. This appearance is similar to that of a lymphangioma and thyroglossal duct cyst and possibly an inflamed lymph node; however, the dermoid, epidermoid and lipoma usually are fat dominated on MRI with intermediate to high T_1-weighted signal intensities and intermediate T_2-weighted signal intensities.

Incomplete obstruction of intraglandular ducts may result in the development of a cystic mass that on CT

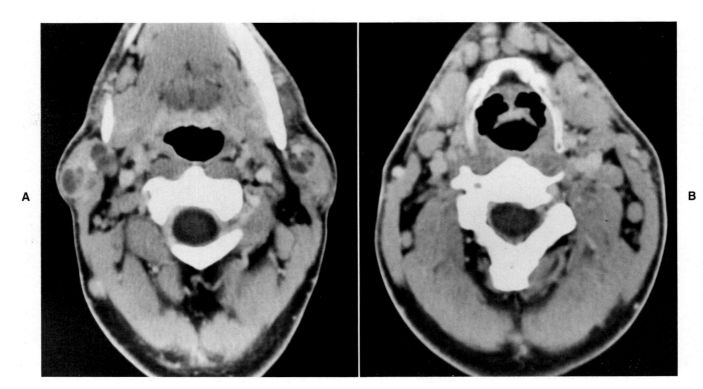

Fig. 3-72 Axial postcontrast CT scan showing **A,** multiple cystic masses in both parotid glands and **B,** diffuse cervical adenopathy. HIV positive patient with parotid lymphoepithelial cysts.

has an appearance of a very thin walled cyst with a central homogeneous collection of material with an attenuation of 10 to 20 HU. Such a condition has also been called a mucocele of the major salivary glands, and it occurs most often in the submandibular gland. Other names for this process include a retention cyst or an extravasation cyst reflecting the various interpretations of its pathogenesis (see Figs. 3-66 and 3-67).

A pneumocele of the salivary gland is a recurrent soft tissue mass produced by the retention of air in the gland parenchyma. This occurs after an increase in intrabuccal pressure that is often associated with occupations such as glass blowing, with trumpet playing, and with retrograde insufflation of the gland via Stensen's or Wharton's duct. The clinical presentation establishes the diagnosis.[23]

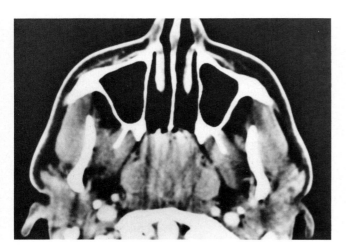

Fig. 3-73   Axial postcontrast CT scan reveals typical adenoidal prominence that may be present in HIV positive patients.

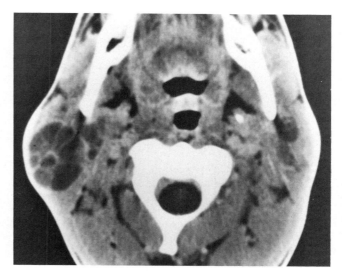

Fig. 3-74   Axial postcontrast CT scan demonstrating multiple bilateral parotid cysts with cervical adenopathy. HIV positive patient with parotid lymphoepithelial cysts. (From Shugar et al, Laryngoscope 98:772, 1988.)

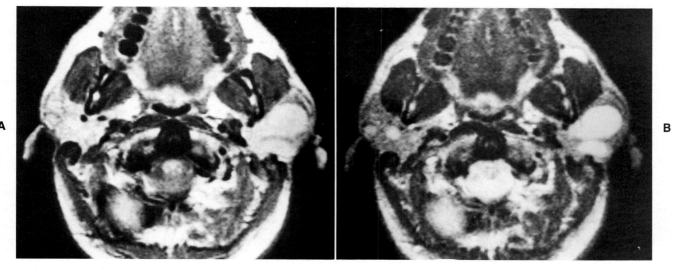

Fig. 3-75   **A,** Transverse mixed image and **B,** T_2-weighted MRI scans (0.5T, TR 1800 msec, TE 30, 90 msecs) demonstrating multiple cysts in both parotid glands. They are more easily identified on the T_2-weighted scans because their high water content gives them a high signal intensity: Lymphoepithelial cysts in a HIV positive patient. (**B** from Shugar et al, Laryngoscope 98:772, 1988.)

REFERENCES

1. Rabinov K and Weber AL: Radiology of the salivary glands, Boston, 1985, GK Hall & Co, pp 1-221.
2. Peel RZ and Gnepp DR: Diseases of the salivary glands. In Barnes L, editor: Surgical pathology of the head and neck, vol 1, New York, 1985, Marcel Dekker, Inc, pp 533-645.
3. Batsakis JG: Tumors of the head and neck, clinical and pathological considerations, ed 2, Baltimore, 1979, Williams & Wilkins, pp 1-120.
4. Moss-Salentijn L and Moss ML: Development and functional anatomy. In Rankow RM and Polayes IM, editors: Diseases of the salivary glands, Philadelphia, 1976, WB Saunders Co, pp 17-31.
5. Travis LW and Hecht DW: Acute and chronic inflammatory diseases of the salivary glands: diagnosis and management, Otolaryngol Clin North Am 10:329, 1977.
6. Leake D and Leake P: Neonatal suppurative parotitis, Pediatrics 46:203, 1970.
7. Spratt J: Etiology and therapy of acute pyogenic parotitis, Surg Gynecol Obstet 112:391, 1961.
8. Bryan RN et al: Computed tomography of the major salivary glands, AJR 139:547, 1982.
9. Levy DM, ReMine WH, and Devine KD: Salivary gland calculi, JAMA 181:1115, 1962.
10. Work WP and Hecht DW: Inflammatory diseases of the major salivary Glands. In Paparella MM and Shumrick DA, editors: Otolaryngology, vol 3, Philadelphia, 1973, WB Saunders Co, pp 258-265.
11. Godwin J: Benign lymphoepithelial lesion of the parotid gland (adenolymphoma, chronic inflammation, lymphoepithelioma, lymphocytic tumor, Mikulicz disease), report of eleven cases, Cancer 5:1089, 1952.
12. See reference 1, pp 222-264.
13. Bloch KJ: Sjögren's syndrome. In Stein JH, editor: Internal medicine, Boston, 1983, Little Brown & Co, pp 1034-1036.
14. Mason DK and Chisholm DM: Salivary glands in health and disease, London, 1975, WB Saunders Co, Ltd, pp 167-206.
15. Moutsopoulos HM et al: Sjögren's syndrome (sicca syndrome): current issues, Ann Intern Med 92:212, 1980.
16. Som PM et al: Manifestations of parotid gland enlargement: radiographic, pathologic, and clinical correlations. I. The autoimmune pseudosialectasias, Radiology 141:415, 1981.
17. See reference 14, pp 167-206.
18. See reference 1, pp 265-291.
19. Som PM, Shugar JMA, and Biller HF: Parotid gland sarcoidosis and the CT-sialogram, JCAT 5:674, 1981.
20. Mihalyka EE: Congenital bilateral polycystic parotid glands, JAMA 181:634, 1982.
21. Work WP: Cysts and congenital lesions of the parotid gland, Otolaryngol Clin North Am 10:339, 1977.
22. Manashil GB: Clinical sialography, Springfield, Ill, 1978, Charles C Thomas Publisher, pp 74-81.
23. Som PM: Cystic lesions of the neck, Postgrad Radiol 7:211, 1987.
24. Shugar JMA et al: Multicentric parotid cysts and cervical adenopathy in AIDS patients; a newly recognized entity: CT and MR manifestations, Laryngoscope 98:772, 1988.
25. Morris MR, Moore DW, and Shearer GL: Bilateral multiple benign lymphoepithelial cysts of the parotid gland, Otolaryngol Head Neck Surg 97:87, 1987.
26. Olsen WL et al: Lesions of the head and neck in patients with AIDS: CT and MR findings, AJNR 9:693, 1988.

SECTION FOUR
TUMORS AND TUMORLIKE CONDITIONS

In the general population salivary gland neoplasms represent less than 3% of all tumors.[1] However, a higher incidence of such salivary lesions has been reported in Eskimos and survivors of the atomic bomb blasts.[2,3]

Between 75% to 80% of parotid gland tumors, 40% to 50% of submandibular gland tumors, 15% of sublingual gland tumors, and 20% to 40% of minor salivary gland tumors are benign. Since very few sublingual gland tumors are encountered in absolute numbers, these figures indicate that the smaller the salivary gland involved, the greater the likelihood that a tumor is malignant. In addition, a given tumor histology tends to behave more aggressively as the gland of origin diminishes in size.[2,3]

The TNM staging of salivary gland tumors according to the American Joint Committee on Cancer is weighted heavily on the size of the primary lesion (i.e.,

T_0 = no evidence of primary tumor, T_1 = tumor ≤ 2.0 cm in diameter, T_2 = tumor >2.0 cm but ≤ 4.0 cm in diameter, T_3 = >4.0 cm but ≤ 6.0 cm in diameter, T_4 = 6.0 cm in diameter). All categories are subdivided into (a) no local extension or (b) local extension, which is defined as clinical or macroscopic evidence of tumor invasion of the skin, soft tissues, bone, or lingual or facial nerves.[4]

By using this staging system it is evident that the higher the stage, the greater the recurrence rate, the greater the incidence of metastases and the lower the survival rate. Although the overall cure rates traditionally are calculated on the basis of no evidence of disease for 5 years, several of the major salivary gland tumors may have late recurrences, some appearing 10 to 25 years after the initial treatment. Because of this, statistics citing 5 years of curability must be viewed with circumspection.[2,5]

There have been many classifications of salivary gland tumors proposed.[6-8] The one used here is based on a combined clinical and pathologic grouping and is useful as a basis to organize a discussion of these tumors:

I. Epithelial tumors
   A. Adenomas—related tumors
      1. Pleomorphic adenoma
         a. Benign mixed tumor
         b. Carcinoma ex pleomorphic
         c. Malignant mixed tumor
      2. Monomorphic adenoma
         a. Adenolymphoma—Warthin's tumor
         b. Oncocytoma (oxyphilic adenoma)
         c. Oncocytic papillary cystadenoma
         d. Basal cell adenoma
         e. Clear cell adenoma
            (1) Clear cell tumor
         f. Sebaceous lymphadenoma
   B. Mucoepidermoid carcinoma
   C. Adenoid cystic carcinoma
   D. Acinic cell carcinoma
   E. Undifferentiated carcinoma
   F. Primary squamous cell carcinoma
   G. Adenocarcinoma
      1. Low-grade papillary adenocarcinoma
      2. High-grade adenocarcinoma
   H. Malignant tumors of large salivary duct origin
   I. Adenosquamous carcinoma
   J. Sebaceous neoplasms of salivary gland origin
   K. Carcinoma metastatic to salivary glands
II. Nonepithelial tumors
   A. Hemangioma
   B. Lymphangioma
   C. Lymphoma
   D. Intraparotid lymphadenopathy
   E. Lipoma
   F. Neurogenic tumors
      1. Neuroma (schwannoma)
      2. Neurofibroma
III. Miscellaneous lesions
   A. Masseteric hypertrophy
   B. Temporomandibular joint and mandibular lesions
   C. Other miscellaneous conditions

EPITHELIAL TUMORS
Pleomorphic Adenoma—Mixed Tumors

The pleomorphic adenoma is the most common salivary gland tumor and represents 70% to 80% of all benign tumors of the major salivary glands. Eighty-four percent of all pleomorphic adenomas occur in the parotid gland, 8% in the submandibular gland, 6.5% in the minor salivary glands, and 0.5% in the sublingual glands. Of the parotid tumors 90% arise lateral to the plane of the facial nerve.[2,9]

Typically these tumors occur as a slow-growing painless mass that has an average interval between the onset of signs and symptoms and initial work-up of almost 6 years. The tumors vary greatly in size from a few millimeters to several centimeters, and they occur most often in women over the age of 40 years.

The lesions are usually solitary, ovoid, well-demarcated masses despite their having a capsule of variable thickness and completeness. The larger tumors may have pedunculated outgrowths from the main lesion that grossly simulate multiple masses. The larger lesions can have sites of necrosis, hemorrhage, and focal calcification.[10]

The recurrence rate varies between 1% and 50% and is directly related to the initial surgical procedure. The higher reported recurrence rates are in studies that included patients who were treated by enucleation rather than a parotidectomy, as well as patients who had capsular rupture at surgery. Conversely some studies have very low reported recurrence rates because their follow-up period was of insufficient duration, since some recurrences take many years to become obvious. When recurrences happen, they are often multiple and clustered about the region of the original tumor. True multiple pleomorphic adenomas are rare with only isolated reports, and a primary multicentric origin is estimated to occur in 0.5% of parotid mixed tumors. The less common Warthin's tumors and acinous cell carcinomas are far more often multicentric than are pleomorphic adenomas.[9,10]

Three types of malignancies are associated with pleomorphic adenomas: the malignant mixed tumor, the carcinoma ex pleomorphic adenoma, and the metastasizing benign mixed tumor.[7]

The true malignant mixed tumor is very rare and contains both epithelial and stromal malignant elements. It is thus a true carcinosarcoma and has a grave prognosis.

The carcinoma ex pleomorphic adenoma is a carcinoma that arises in a benign mixed tumor in which elements of the benign lesion can still be identified. Usually the malignancy is an adenocarcinoma, but any epithelial subtype can occur and does in approximately 2% to 5% of all mixed tumors.[7,9,10] The usual clinical presentation is in a patient with a long history (average 10 to 15 years) of a benign mixed tumor that suddenly demonstrates a period of rapid growth (average 3 to 6 months). Pain and facial nerve paralysis are often present; these patients most commonly are about 60 years of age.[7]

The carcinoma ex pleomorphic adenomas also have an accelerated recurrence rate and a high metastatic rate, which varies from 25% to 75%.[10] The main sites of metastases are the regional lymph nodes, lungs, bones, and brain.[3] Death usually occurs within 1 year of the

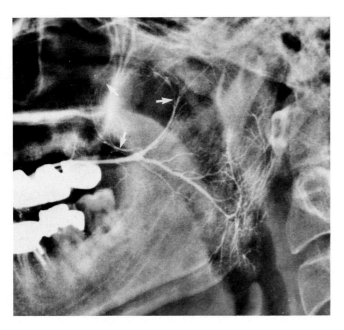

Fig. 3-76   Lateral view of parotid sialogram showing a mass *(arrows)* that smoothly displaces adjacent parotid ducts around it: Benign mixed tumor.

discovery of metastases. The malignant change may be a function of time, and it has been estimated that left untreated, nearly 25% of all pleomorphic adenomas may undergo malignant change.[10]

The metastasizing benign mixed tumor is the rarest form of malignancy associated with pleomorphic adenomas. These tumors metastasize and there is no histologic evidence of malignant elements in either the primary tumor or the metastases. It is generally considered only as a rare curiosity.[9,10]

On sialography pleomorphic adenomas displace the parotid ducts smoothly around the tumor mass (Figs. 3-76 and 3-77). On CT most benign mixed tumors are smoothly marginated, spherical tumors that have a higher attenuation than the surrounding parotid parenchyma, and they do not enhance significantly on postcontrast studies (Figs. 3-78 to 3-84). The smaller lesions are usually fairly homogeneous in appearance; however, the larger masses have a nonhomogeneous appearance with sites of lower attenuation representing areas of necrosis, old hemorrhage, and cystic change (Figs. 3-85 and 3-86). Localized areas of increased attenuation most often represent sites of recent hemorrhage and are associated with a sudden increase in tumor size and often with localized pain. The larger tumors tend to develop a lobulated appearance that may

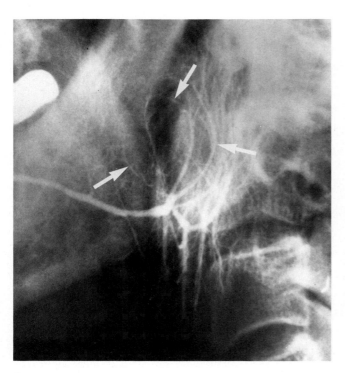

Fig. 3-77   Lateral view of parotid sialogram showing benign-appearing mass that displaces intraparotid ducts around it: Benign mixed tumor.

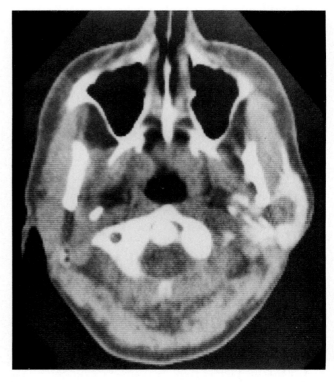

Fig. 3-78   Axial noncontrast CT-sialogram showing a smoothly marginated, benign-appearing mass in the left parotid gland: Benign mixed tumor.

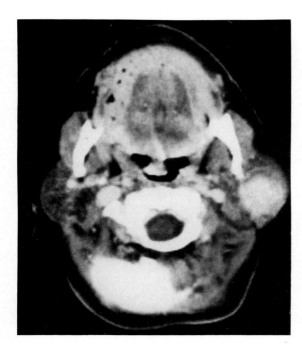

Fig. 3-79 Axial postcontrast CT scan showing slightly enhancing mass in superficial lobe of left parotid gland. The lesion has a smooth border along all of its margins except the lateral aspect, where hemorrhage and edema from vigorous palpation were present as demonstrated on pathological examination. This lesion enhances more than the usual pleomorphic adenoma and illustrates how, on occasion, a benign tumor may simulate a malignant lesion: Benign mixed tumor.

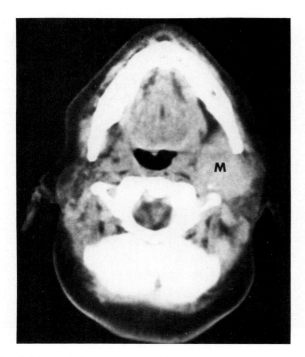

Fig. 3-80 Axial postcontrast CT scan showing benign-appearing deep lobe tumor *(M)* in the left parotid gland: Benign mixed tumor.

be confused with multiple masses rather than a solitary lesion that has a highly nodular surface (Fig. 3-87). Dystrophic calcification can be seen occasionally and is highly suggestive of this tumor (Figs. 3-88, 3-89, and 3-92).

On occasion the outer contour of a pleomorphic adenoma may be slightly indistinct. This is usually secondary to surrounding inflammation and/or hemorrhage. In these cases the CT appearance can simulate that of a more aggressive tumor.

On MRI these tumors have a nonhomogeneous appearance with intermediate signal intensities on T_1-weighted and proton density–weighted images (WIs). On T_2-weighted images there usually is a mixture of intermediate and high signal intensities. Areas of hemorrhage appear as regions of high signal intensity on T_1-weighted images; however, the regions of focal low attenuation seen on CT may not have directly corresponding sites of either high or low signal intensity on T_2-weighted images. The nonhomogeneous MRI appearance is not unique for this tumor and can be seen in other lesions, including malignancies. The dystro-

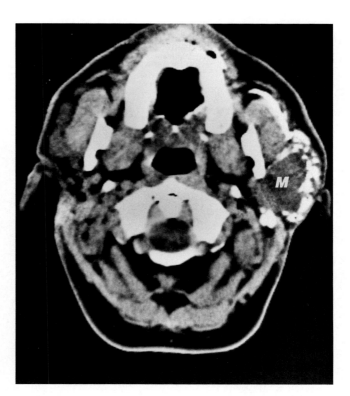

Fig. 3-81 Axial noncontrast CT-sialogram showing sialography contrast material in Stensen's duct and the superficial portion of the gland. This contrast outlines a benign appearing mass *(M)*. No normal deep lobe tissue is seen: Deep lobe benign mixed tumor that was superficially placed because it was prohibited from extending into the parapharyngeal space by the limiting size of the stylomandibular tunnel.

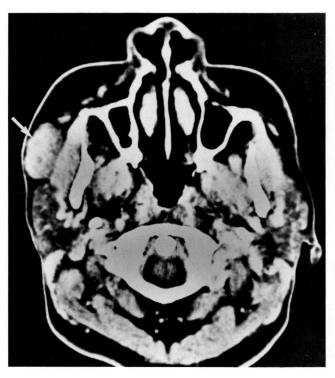

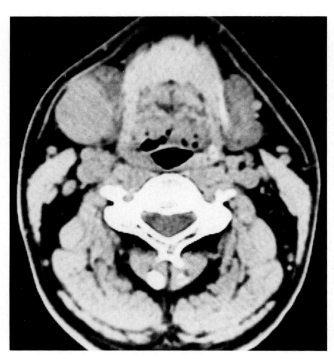

Fig. 3-82   Axial postcontrast CT scan showing a mass *(arrow)* in the right cheek overlying the masseter muscle. The parotid glands are normal: Benign mixed tumor of the right accessory parotid gland.

Fig. 3-83   Axial noncontrast CT scan showing benign-appearing mass in the posterolateral aspect of the right submandibular gland: Benign mixed tumor.

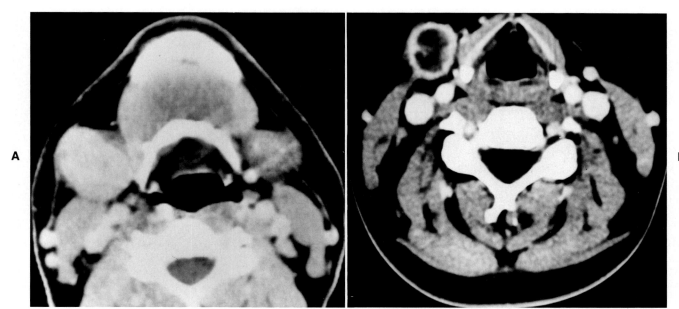

Fig. 3-84   **A,** Axial postcontrast CT scan showing minimally enhancing, benign-appearing right submandibular mass: Benign mixed tumor. **B,** Axial postcontrast CT scan showing well demarcated, cystic-appearing mass in the right submandibular gland. The walls of the cyst are irregular, suggesting a tumor: Degenerated cystic benign mixed tumor.

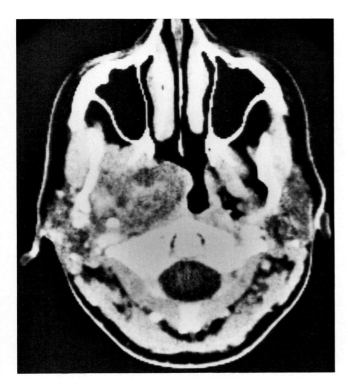

Fig. 3-85 Axial postcontrast CT scan showing large right deep lobe parotid tumor. The lesion is nonhomogeneous with cystic areas of lower attenuation (necrosis and mucoid degeneration) and areas of increased attenuation (hemorrhage). The mass is inseparable from the right parotid gland: Benign mixed tumor. (From Som et al, Radiology 153:149, 1984.)

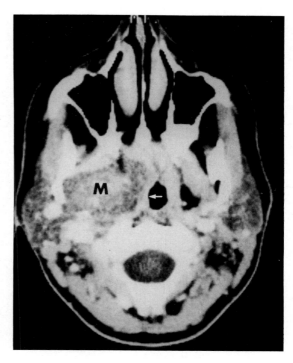

Fig. 3-86 Axial postcontrast CT scan showing large "deep lobe" tumor *(M)* of the right parotid gland. It has a slightly nonhomogeneous appearance, is inseparable from the parotid gland, and displaces the right pharyngeal wall *(arrow)* to the midline: Benign mixed tumor.

phic calcifications cannot be visualized or distinguished from focal areas of fibrosis (Figs. 3-90 to 3-92).[11-13]

If a carcinoma ex pleomorphic adenoma is present, it may have one of several CT appearances: (1) It may look like a large pleomorphic adenoma with no CT evidence of malignancy. (2) It may look like a benign mixed tumor that has an aggressive tumor appearance in a portion of the lesion. This aggressive area has a necrotic center, thick, irregular walls, and infiltrating margins. (3) Last, the tumor may be entirely aggressive in its CT appearance, with no remaining evidence of any benign pleomorphic adenoma. On MR a similar variation can be encountered; however, if a necrotic, thick-walled area is present, it may be poorly seen, if at all (see Fig. 3-92).

Monomorphic Adenoma

Monomorphic adenomas are benign neoplasms that presumably arise from ductal epithelium. They are distinguished from the pleomorphic adenomas by the absence of a chondromyxoid stroma and the presence of a uniform epithelial pattern. The primary tumors in this group are Warthin's tumors; oncocytomas; and a group of rare lesions that includes basal cell adenomas, clear cell adenomas, and sebaceous lymphadenomas.[9]

Warthin's Tumor. Warthin's tumor (adenolymphoma or papillary cystadenoma lymphomatosum) is the second most common benign lesion of the parotid gland, representing 2% to 10% of all parotid tumors. Only benign mixed tumors are more common benign parotid neoplasms.[7,9,14]

The lesion is unique among salivary gland tumors because of the presence of lymphoid tissue, a male predominance of 3-5:1 and multiplicity, including bilaterality. The tumor is benign, with only a very rare disputed malignant transformation being reported.[14] Similarly, facial nerve involvement is extremely rare. Eighty percent of the patients are in the fourth to seventh decade. This tumor is rarely found in nonwhites.

Grossly the tumor is ovoid, encapsulated, and either cystic or semisolid. This tumor has a greater tendency to undergo gross cystic change than any of the other parotid neoplasms.

The most likely pathogenesis of this tumor is heterotopic salivary gland ductal epithelial tissue that is trapped within intraparotid and periparotid lymph

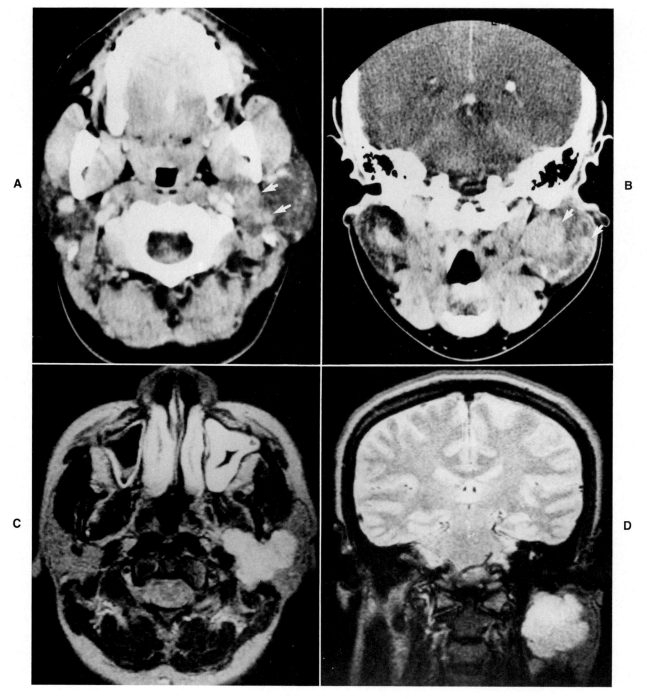

Fig. 3-87   **A,** Axial and **B,** coronal postcontrast CT scans showing what appear to be two adjacent masses in the left parotid gland *(arrows).* **C,** Transverse and **D,** coronal MRI scans (0.5T, TR 1800 msec, TE 80 msec) show a single, markedly lobulated mass in the left parotid gland. The mass has a fairly homogeneous high T₂-weighted signal intensity. This appearance is highly suggestive of the diagnosis. Incidentally noted are inflammatory changes in the maxillary sinuses: Benign mixed tumor. (From Som et al, JCAT 12:65, 1988.)

nodes; the histologic identification of such a normal nodal structure supports this hypothesis.[7,9] This subject is reviewed in the embryology section of this chapter (Section One, pp. 278-282).

Whatever the stimulus that leads to the development of this tumor, it can act on any such epithelial nodal inclusion, and therefore the possibility of multiple Warthin's tumors exists. Although the most common presentation of this tumor is that of a solitary mass in the tail of the superficial lobe of the parotid gland, this tumor presents bilaterally and as multiple masses within one or both parotid glands more frequently than any other salivary neoplasm. The commonly quoted figure

for bilateral occurrence is 6%; however, this is an erroneously low figure, and careful microscopic examination of pathology specimens has suggested that in almost 30% of the specimens, multiple lesions are present. Since these tumors may grow very slowly, they are often confused with postoperative recurrences. True recurrences appear to develop only if the capsule of the tumor is violated at the time of surgery.[7,9]

Microscopically, Warthin's tumors have a double layer of oncocytes that line the papillary projections that characteristically extend into the cystic spaces.[9] These oncocytes have a large number of mitochondria, and it is these cells that most probably accumulate Tc[99]m pertechnetate on salivary radionuclide scans in Warthin's tumors (Fig. 3-93). The only other tumor to so accumulate Tc[99]m pertechnetate is an oncocytoma.[14] Treatment is surgical excision.

On CT most Warthin's tumors appear as a small, ovoid, smoothly marginated mass in the posterior superficial lobe (tail) of the parotid gland. They are homogeneous soft tissue–density lesions that do not have dystrophic calcifications. Cavitation is common, and these tumors may have a cystic appearance on CT. The

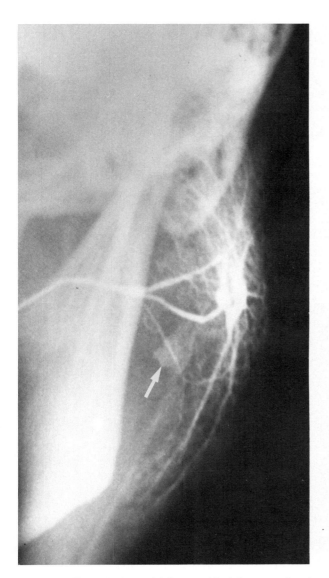

Fig. 3-88 Frontal view of left parotid sialogram showing vague mass effect on the medial aspect of the parotid gland that displaces the ducts around it (ball-in-glove appearance). Within the mass is a site of dystrophic calcification *(arrow):* Benign mixed tumor.

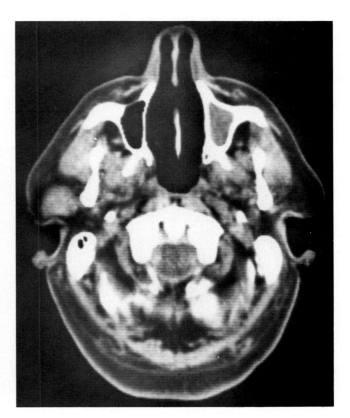

Fig. 3-89 Axial noncontrast CT scan showing solitary benign appearing mass in the right parotid gland. There are faint calcifications seen within the mass. Incidentally noted are inflammatory changes in the left antrum: Benign mixed tumor.

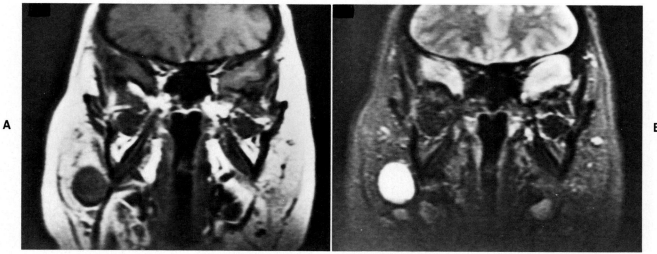

Fig. 3-90 **A,** Axial postcontrast CT scan showing moderately enhancing mass in superficial portion of the right parotid gland *(arrow)*. The mass is sharply delineated from adjacent parotid tissue. **B,** Transverse T$_2$-weighted MRI scan (1.5T, TR 500 msec, TE = 25 msec) shows the right parotid mass to have a high signal intensity and have almost the exact configuration as that seen in **A.** Incidentally noted is the very high signal intensity of the watery inflammatory tissue in the right maxillary sinus: Benign mixed tumor.

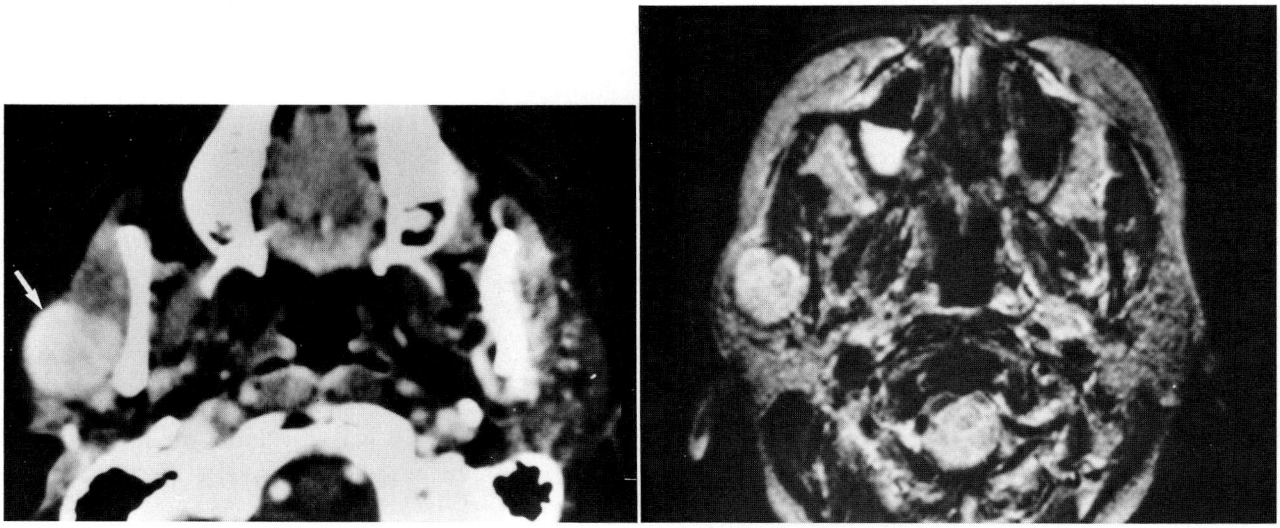

Fig. 3-91 **A,** Coronal T$_1$-weighted (1.5T, TR = 600 msec, TE 28 msec) and **B,** T$_2$-weighted (1.5T, TR = 2000 msec, TE 100 msec) MRI scans showing the right parotid mass to have a low intensity signal in **A** and a high signal intensity in **B.** These intensities are typical of tissues that are predominantly composed of water. The lesion is sharply defined: Benign mixed tumor.

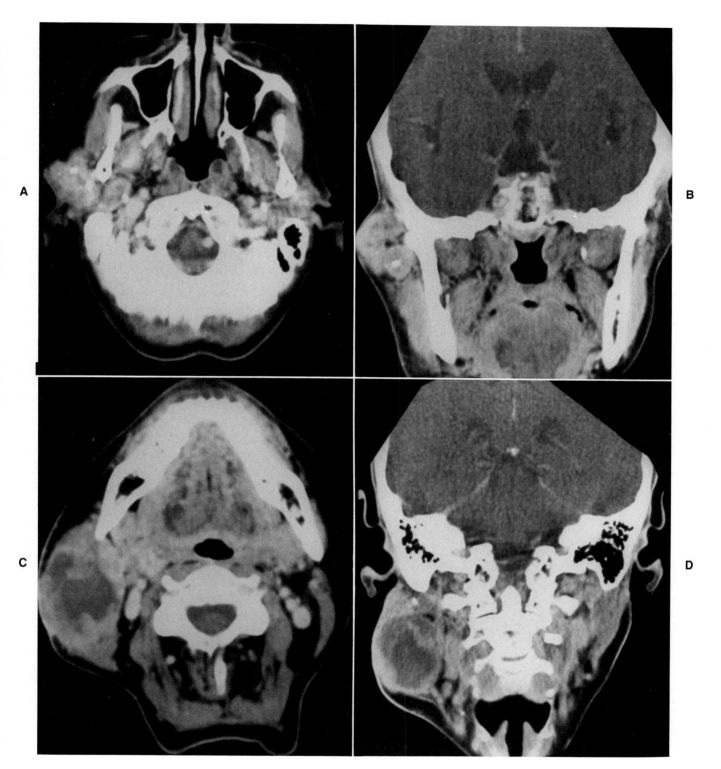

Fig. 3-92   **A,** Axial and **B,** coronal postcontrast CT scans showing multiple masses within the superior portion of the right parotid gland. Dystrophic calcifications are present within these lesions. **C,** Axial and **D,** coronal postcontrast CT scans through the more caudal aspect of the parotid gland show large, irregularly walled cystic mass in right parotid gland. The appearance is highly suggestive of a necrotic tumor. (**A** and **C** from Som et al, JCAT 12:65, 1988.)   *Continued.*

Fig. 3-92, cont'd   E, Coronal T$_1$-weighted, **F,** transverse mixed image, and **G,** T$_2$-weighted image MRI scans (0.5T, TR 500 msec, TE = 30 msec, TR 1800 msec, TE = 30, 80 msec) show a better definition of multiple distinct masses in the cranial portion of right parotid gland. The large necrotic portion of the tumor (**C** and **D**) has a very nonhomogeneous signal intensity (**F** and **G**) and the necrotic nature of the lesion is not well demonstrated. It has a similar appearance to that seen in benign mixed tumors: Multiple seeded recurrent benign mixed tumors with a large carcinoma ex pleomorphic adenoma.

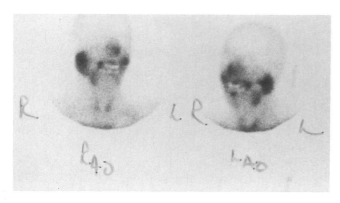

Fig. 3-93 Oblique frontal technetium sialograms showing intense bilateral uptake in parotid glands: Bilateral Warthin's tumors.

central cavity is filled with a homogeneous 10 to 18 HU material and the cyst wall is thin and fairly smooth. Usually there is a focal nodularity at some point in the tumor wall indicating that this lesion is a Warthin's tumor and not a branchial cleft cyst. When large and arising from the periphery of the parotid gland, most of the tumor may be outside the normal gland contour, and possible confusion with a branchial cleft cyst or necrotic node could exist (Figs. 3-94 to 3-101).

When multiple lesions are seen either in one parotid gland or bilaterally, the most likely diagnosis is Warthin's tumors. If the neoplasms are cystic, the differential diagnosis includes lymphoepithelial cysts of HIV positive patients (see Figs. 3-72 to 3-75) and possibly multiple cavitated metastatic nodes. If the multiple Warthin's tumors are not cavitated, the differential diagnosis is lymphoma, granulomatous disease, and benign adenopathy.

On MRI these tumors tend to be more homogeneous than pleomorphic adenomas and they have low to intermediate signal intensities on T_1-weighted images and proton density–weighted images and high signal intensities on T_2-weighted images. The cystic nature of some

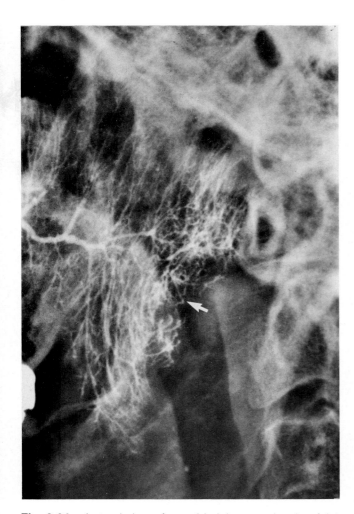

Fig. 3-94 Lateral view of parotid sialogram showing faint mass effect *(arrow)* at posterior margin of the parotid gland. Although not a specific finding, this is a typical location for a Warthin's tumor.

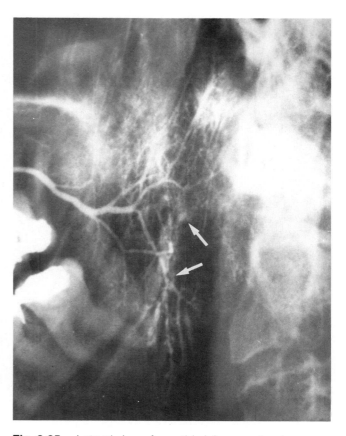

Fig. 3-95 Lateral view of parotid sialogram showing mass *(arrows)* in the "tail" of the parotid gland: Warthin's tumor.

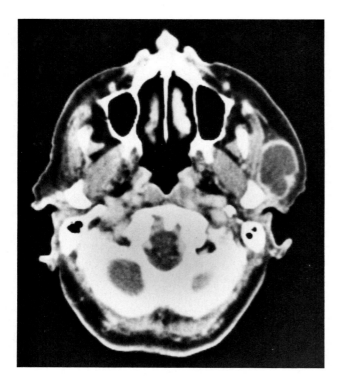

Fig. 3-96 Axial postcontrast CT scan showing cystic mass in left parotid gland. Most of the cyst wall is smooth, except for a small nodule at the posterior lateral side. This irregularity suggests that the lesion is a tumor rather than a cyst: Cystic Warthin's tumor.

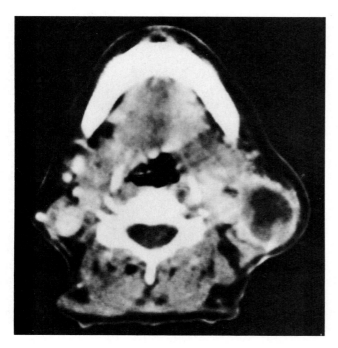

Fig. 3-97 Axial postcontrast CT scan showing cystic mass that projects caudally from the inferior pole of left parotid gland. The lesion has an irregular wall with several areas of nodularity: Cystic Warthin's tumor.

of these tumors is not as apparent with MRI as with CT.

Oncocytoma (Oxyphilic Adenoma). Oncocytes are large cells with granular eosinophilic cytoplasm that may be found individually or in groups in otherwise normal major and minor salivary glands. In the salivary glands they are rarely found in patients under the age of 50; they are seen with increasing frequency until age 70, after which they are nearly always present.[7,9] The granular eosinophilia results from mitochondrial hyperplasia. The term *oncocytoma* is used to describe a solid tumor that, unlike a Warthin's tumor, is composed entirely of oncocytes. The oncocytoma comprises less than 1% of all salivary gland tumors and most commonly occurs in the parotid gland. Most patients are between 55 and 70 years of age. These tumors are slow-growing masses that will accumulate $Tc^{99}m$ pertechnetate, similar to Warthin's tumors. Rarely, multiple tumors occur. Oncocytomas are well-encapsulated lesions when they

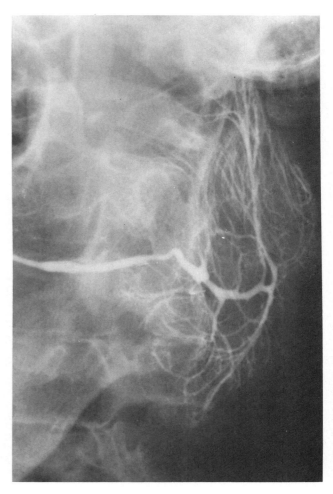

Fig. 3-98 Frontal oblique view of left parotid sialogram showing benign type ductal displacement around several masses throughout the gland: Multiple Warthin's tumors.

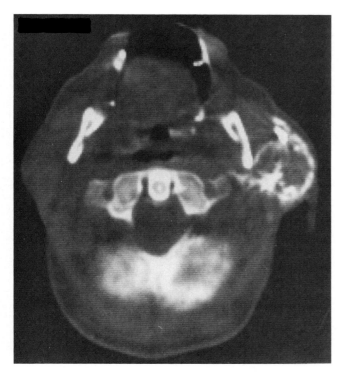

Fig. 3-99 Axial CT-sialogram study showing two distinct masses in left parotid gland. Other masses were also present at different scan levels: Multiple Warthin's tumors.

arise in the major salivary glands. Although most tumors are histologically benign, those lesions arising in the minor salivary glands often exhibit local invasion. Rarely, histologic evidence of malignancy is present and very rarely metastases have been reported. The treatment of choice is surgical excision; these tumors are radioresistant.[7,9] Their imaging characteristics are nonspecific and can be similar to those of a Warthin's tumor or a pleomorphic adenoma.

Oncocytic Papillary Cystadenoma. Oncocytic papillary cystadenoma is a rare lesion that can occur in the parotid gland, although it most often occurs in the larynx. It may represent an oncocytic metaplasia and hyperplasia of preexisting salivary gland ductal epithelial and not be a true neoplasm. This lesion is usually a rounded cyst and benign. Surgery is the treatment of choice.[9]

Basal Cell Adenoma. Although the basal cell adenoma is the most common of the other types of adenomas, it accounts for only 2% of all salivary gland tumors. There is no sex predilection; the mean age of patients is 60 years. Most occur in the superficial lobe of the parotid gland; nearly 80% of the minor salivary gland lesions arise near the upper lip. They are benign, slow-growing masses. Those in the parotid gland are encapsulated, while those arising from minor salivary glands may lack a capsule. They have been erroneously

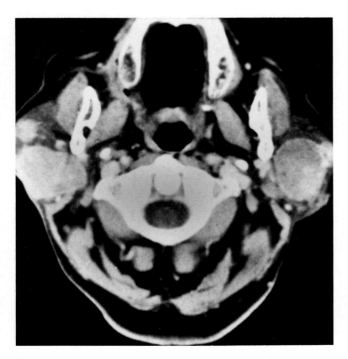

Fig. 3-100 Axial postcontrast CT scan showing multiple bilateral benign appearing masses. The largest mass on the left side is starting to undergo cystic change: Multiple Warthin's tumors.

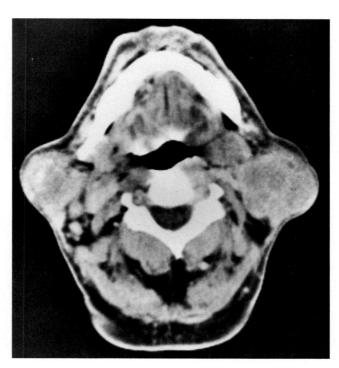

Fig. 3-101 Axial postcontrast CT scan showing multiple bilateral parotid masses. The lesions on the left form a large conglomerate mass. However, the cystic nature of the individual tumors can be identified as lower attenuation areas within the overall mass: Multiple Warthin's tumors.

diagnosed clinically as lymph nodes, cysts, lipomas, and mixed tumors. Surgical excision is curative.[7,9]

Clear Cell Adenoma (Clear Cell Tumor). Clear cell adenomas arise from the intercalated ducts of salivary glands and tend to occur in the parotid gland. They are well-circumscribed benign lesions. Histologically they may be confused with acinic cell carcinomas and mucoepidermoid carcinomas, both of which may contain clear cells. The adenoma has an orderly architecture and its clear cells are rich in glycogen. These are rare lesions reported to have infiltrative growth and occasional recurrences and metastases. There is a growing tendency pathologically to regard these tumors as low-grade carcinomas. Surgical excision is the treatment of choice.[7,9]

Sebaceous Lymphadenoma. Sebaceous lymphadenomas are rare and may arise from the blind ends of intralobular ducts. Most patients are 50 years or older. The lesions are slow growing and present as asymptomatic masses. They are composed of cysts that are lined by squamous epithelium and sebaceous cells arranged in a lymphoid stroma. They are benign, well-encapsulated tumors, and surgical excision is curative.[9]

Mucoepidermoid Carcinoma

Although mucoepidermoid carcinomas comprise less than 10% of all salivary gland tumors, they represent about 30% of the malignant salivary gland tumors. Nearly 60% of these lesions occur in the parotid gland, and about 30% arise in the minor salivary glands, primarily in the palate and buccal mucosa.[9] In adults mucoepidermoid carcinomas are the most common parotid gland malignancy, and the second most common malignancy in the submandibular gland, after adenoid cystic carcinoma. These tumors are also the most common malignant salivary gland tumors in children.[2,9] Most patients are in their third to fifth decades of life; and except for the intraosseous lesions (mandible, maxilla), which are more common in females, there is no sex predilection.

These tumors can be classified histologically as low grade, intermediate grade, or high grade tumors.[15] The low-grade lesions behave almost like benign lesions with the 5-year survival being nearly 90%. Although they are unencapsulated or incompletely encapsulated, they usually are well circumscribed. These tumors characteristically contain cysts filled with blood-tinged mucus. Hemorrhage and necrosis may be present. The tumors may recur locally after surgery; in cases with good surgical margins, the recurrence rate is only 6%.[9]

High-grade mucoepidermoid carcinomas are poorly circumscribed, with infiltrative borders. They tend to be solid neoplasms and behave as aggressive tumors with a 5-year survival of only 41.6%.[1] They metastasize primarily to the subcutaneous tissues, lymph nodes,

bone, and lung. They may be difficult tumors to separate from squamous cell carcinomas of the salivary glands. The presence of large numbers of clear cells may suggest the possibility of a metastatic renal cell carcinoma, and this must be excluded by a search for such a primary tumor.

Intermediate-grade carcinomas tend to behave more like the low-grade lesions. The recurrence rate is 20%, however, and there is a greater tendency to have positive margins at resection (35% versus 19%).[16]

Surgery is the treatment of choice, with wide local excision. Neck dissections are not indicated for low-grade lesions and are only performed for intermediate-grade lesions if positive nodes are suspected clinically. For high-grade lesions, radical neck dissection is combined with a wide block excision.[7,9]

The CT findings of mucoepidermoid lesions vary with the grade of the tumor. Low-grade lesions are benign in appearance, with apparently well-delineated, smooth margins. Cystic areas may be present with a low attenuation of 10 to 18 HU (Fig. 3-102). Rarely, focal calcification may be seen. The appearance is similar to that of a benign mixed tumor. On MRI, these low-

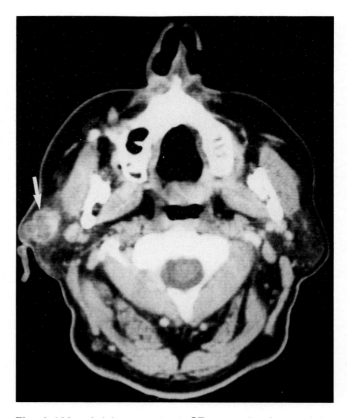

Fig. 3-102 Axial noncontrast CT scan showing nodular mass *(arrow)* in right parotid gland. The mass has cystic areas within it, and the medial wall of the lesion is nodular and slightly unsharp as it merges with the adjacent parotid gland: Low grade mucoepidermoid carcinoma.

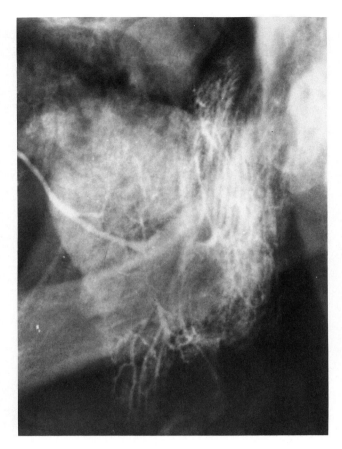

Fig. 3-103   Lateral view of parotid sialogram showing mass lesion that has caused ductal invasion and cutoff as well as a lack of parenchymal filling. This is the sialographic appearance of a malignant lesion: High grade mucoepidermoid carcinoma.

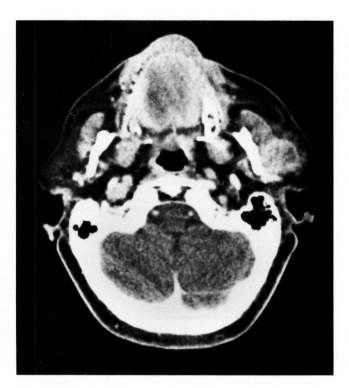

Fig. 3-104   Axial postcontrast CT scan showing partially necrotic mass with irregular walls in left parotid gland. The mass has an infiltrative margin with the adjacent parotid tissue: Mucoepidermoid carcinoma.

grade tumors also have signal intensities that are inseparable from pleomorphic adenomas. However, the high-grade lesions have indistinct infiltrating margins and on CT, have few cystic areas and usually are more homogeneous in appearance. On MRI these cellular tumors tend to have low-to-intermediate signal intensities on both T_1-weighted images and T_2-weighted images (Figs. 3-103 to 3-106).

Adenoid Cystic Carcinoma

Adenoid cystic carcinoma accounts for 2% to 6% of parotid gland tumors, 15% of submandibular gland tumors, 30% of minor salivary gland tumors, and 50% of lacrimal gland tumors.[9,17] Overall 4% to 8% of all salivary gland tumors are adenoid cystic carcinomas. Most arise in the minor salivary glands, primarily in the palate.

The tumor usually arises in patients between 20 to 80 years of age and is rare in patients who are under 20 years old. Most patients are in the fifth and sixth decades of life. The tumor may or may not involve pain;

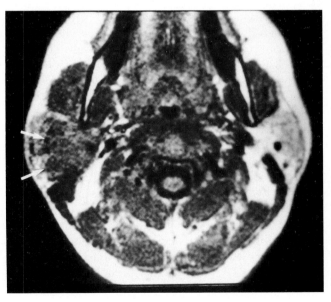

Fig. 3-105   Transverse T_1-weighted MRI scan (1.5T, TR 600 msec, TE = 28 msec) showing poorly defined mass occupying the medial three quarters of right parotid gland *(arrows)*. The mass had a low signal intensity on all imaging sequences: High-grade mucoepidermoid carcinoma.

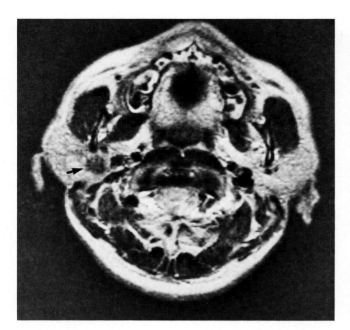

Fig. 3-106 Transverse mixed image MRI scan (0.5T, TR 1800 msec, TE = 30 msec) showing localized area of low signal intensity *(arrow)* in the "deep lobe" portion of the right parotid gland. This tumor had a low signal intensity on all imaging sequences: High grade mucoepidermoid carcinoma.

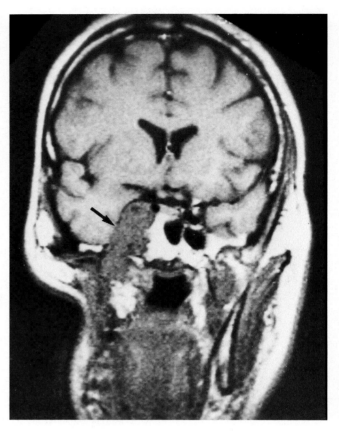

Fig. 3-107 Coronal T$_1$-weighted MRI scan (0.5T, TR 600 msec, TE = 30 msec). The patient had previously had a right parotidectomy. The recurrent tumor has grown from the parotid bed up along the third division of the trigeminal nerve via the foramen ovale to invade the right cavernous sinus *(arrow)*: Recurrent adenoidcystic carcinoma. (From Som et al, Radiology 164:823, 1987.)

and although a relentless tumor, it may often have a slow rate of growth, so that prolonged survivals are reported even after metastases are present. Because of this, the true survival must be evaluated by looking beyond the usual 5-year survival figures. Overall the 5-year survival is 69%; while the 15-year survival is 38%. When one considers the major salivary gland tumors alone, these figures are 76% and 57% respectively. When minor salivary gland lesions are considered alone, the survival figures are 64% and 23% respectively.[9,18] Thus the prognosis is worse when this tumor has a minor salivary gland origin.

The tumors are only partially encapsulated and have little tendency to have cyst formation and hemorrhage. Lymph node metastases are uncommon; however, hematogenous metastases go to the lungs and bones in 20% to 50% of cases.[2,9]

Perineural invasion is a pathologic hallmark of this tumor and accounts for the relatively frequent clinical presentation with pain. Perineural spread is also a common pathway for tumor extension, and such perineural disease can be present distally in a nerve that has a seemingly normal, uninvolved proximal segment. As a result, the clinical significance of "good" surgical margins plays less of a prognostic role in this tumor than in other malignancies that do not exhibit such perineural extension.

On imaging, these tumors may appear either as a be-

nign or malignant process, with the parotid lesions tending to appear as benign tumors, while the minor salivary gland neoplasms have infiltrative margins. Extension to the skull base via the facial nerve or mandibular nerve may be demonstrated by computed sectional scanning, especially when evaluating postoperative recurrences (Figs. 3-107 and 3-108).

Acinic Cell Carcinoma

Acinic cell carcinomas probably arise from reserve or stem cells in the terminal portion of the ductal system and represent only 2% to 4% of all major salivary gland tumors. They occur almost exclusively in the parotid gland and represent 15% to 17% of all malignant parotid tumors. Bilateral parotid gland tumors occur in 3% of cases, making these tumors second only to Warthin's tumor as being the most common parotid lesion to occur bilaterally.[2,9] Acinic cell carcinomas primarily occur in patients in their fifth and sixth decades of life. However, it should be noted that acinic cell carcinomas

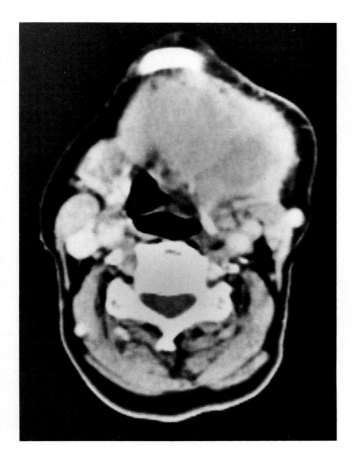

Fig. 3-108 Axial postcontrast CT scan showing large infiltrating mass of the left submandibular gland that has extended to invade the floor of the mouth: Adenoidcystic carcinoma.

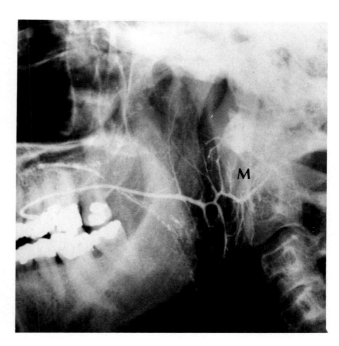

Fig. 3-109 Lateral view of parotid sialogram showing benign-appearing mass *(M)* in the posterior margin of the gland: Acinic cell carcinoma.

are the second most common parotid malignancy (after mucoepidermoid carcinoma) in childhood.[19] Usually the lesion is a painless, slow-growing mass. It may be solid or cystic and have (at best) a thin or incomplete capsule. The 5-year survival is 80% to 90%, but the 20-year survival is only 56%.[2,9] Metastases to regional lymph nodes occur in 10% of patients, and distant metastases (primarily to lung and bone) occur in nearly 15%.[15]

In general, if local excision is performed initially on the parotid lesion, 67% of cases recur and the death rate is 22%. However, if a total parotidectomy is performed initially, only 10% will ever recur and survival is nearly 100%.[9]

The imaging characteristics of these tumors are nonspecific, with most lesions having a generally benign appearance (Fig. 3-109).

Undifferentiated Carcinoma

Undifferentiated carcinomas are malignant epithelial salivary gland tumors that cannot be further subclassified. They comprise 1% to 3% of all parotid malignant tumors. They can occur in any age group, with most patients being near 60 years of age.[20] These tumors are painless, rapidly enlarging masses, and may develop along with squamous cell carcinoma or adenocarcinoma in a longstanding pleomorphic adenoma (carcinoma ex pleomorphic). These are highly aggressive, infiltrating tumors and the treatment of choice is radical excision, since most cases are radioresistant. The 5-year survival is 20% to 30%; about 50% of these patients die from distant metastases to lung, bone, and liver.[9] The imaging characteristics are those of a high-grade, infiltrating, cellular tumor (Figs. 3-110 and 3-111).

Primary Squamous Cell Carcinoma

Although squamous epithelium is not a normal component of the salivary glands, it can arise secondary to chronic inflammation (sialadenitis) as squamous metaplasia. The tumors apparently arise from these metaplastic cells and represent 0.1% to 0.5% of all parotid tumors and 3% to 10% of the malignant parotid neoplasms.[9,21] They comprise 3% of submandibular gland neoplasms and 4% of the carcinomas. These tumors usually arise in men in their sixth and seventh decades of life. These are firm, rapidly enlarging, high-grade tumors that often are fixed to the adjacent soft tissues and overlying skin. Facial paralysis is common. Metastases occur to regional lymph nodes, lungs, and liver; the five-year absolute cure rate is 30%.[9] Radical excision with a neck dissection is the treatment of choice. Their imaging characteristics are those of a high-grade infiltrating, cellular tumor.

Adenocarcinoma

Low-Grade Papillary Adenocarcinoma. Low-grade papillary adenocarcinomas can arise in major or minor salivary glands, but are most common in the latter, arising mainly in the palate. They are slow-growing, painless masses that can invade adjacent bone and metastasize to regional lymph nodes. Distant metastases are unreported. Wide local excision is the treatment of choice.[9]

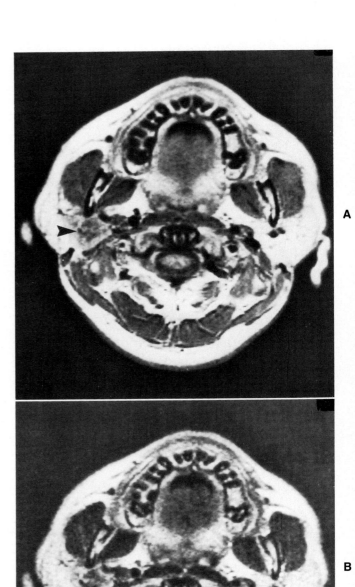

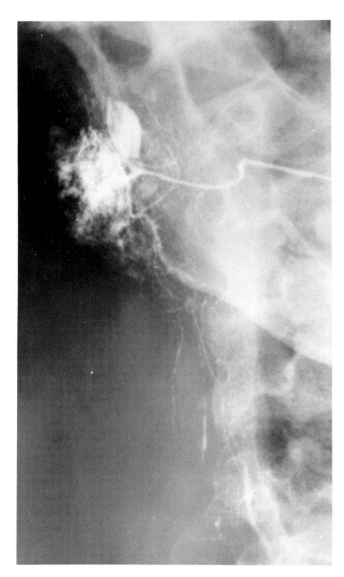

Fig. 3-110 Frontal view of right parotid sialogram showing amorphous pooling of contrast material within a necrotic high grade parotid tumor. Parotilymphatic backflow occurs to the lower cervical lymphatic ducts: Undifferentiated carcinoma. (From Som et al, Ann Otol Rhinol Laryngol 90:64, 1981.)

Fig. 3-111 **A,** Transverse mixed image and **B,** T_2-weighted MRI scans (0.5T, TR 1800 msec, TEs 3, 80 msec) showing poorly defined mass in the "deep lobe" of the right parotid gland *(arrowhead)*. The mass has low signal intensity on all imaging sequences: Undifferentiated carcinoma.

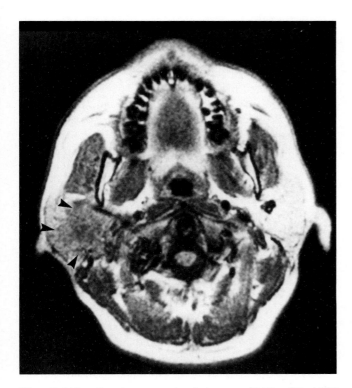

Fig. 3-112 Transverse mixed image (0.5T, TR 1800 msec, TE = 30 msec) MRI scan showing infiltrating mass in the deep portion of the right parotid gland *(arrowheads)*. The mass has low-to-intermediate signal intensity: High grade adenocarcinoma.

High-Grade Adenocarcinoma. High-grade adenocarcinomas cannot be placed into familiar histologic patterns. They often bear a close resemblance to adenocarcinomas of the colon. Most occur in males between 55 and 60 years of age. Actual metastasis from a colonic carcinoma must always be considered. These tumors represent about 2% of all parotid neoplasms; and while 46% of patients are alive at 5 years, only 15% are disease free. Radical surgery is the treatment of choice and the imaging characteristics are those of high-grade, cellular, infiltrating tumors (Fig. 3-112).[7]

Malignant Tumors of Large Salivary Duct Origin

Salivary duct carcinoma histologically resembles ductal carcinoma of the breast.[22] This salivary tumor may arise from either a major or minor salivary gland. Most arise in Stensen's duct, and they are rapidly enlarging masses that may be discrete or more commonly infiltrating. Central necrosis can occur, as well as metastases to the lung, bone, and brain. These are highly aggressive tumors that are capable of both hematogenous and lymphatic dissemination. Of the limited number of reported cases, 75% have died of their disease. Radical surgery with or without radiation is the treatment of choice.[9]

Squamous cell carcinoma of Stensen's duct is a rare tumor. Of the five reported cases, three patients are alive and free of their disease with a maximum follow-up period of 18 months. These are poorly differentiated squamous cell carcinomas, and treatment is surgical resection with or without radiation.[9]

Adenosquamous Carcinoma

Adenosquamous carcinoma is a rare malignant dimorphic salivary gland neoplasm occurring almost exclusively in minor salivary glands. These are aggressive lesions with 80% of patients developing regional and/or distant metastases. The 5-year survival is only 25%. Radical surgery with a neck dissection is the treatment of choice.[9]

Sebaceous Neoplasms of Salivary Gland Origin

Sebaceous neoplasms of salivary gland origin are extremely rare lesions.[23] Sebaceous differentiation probably occurs in most major salivary glands, with the parotid gland being the most common site. Despite this common differentiation, sebaceous neoplasms are very rare and are classified as adenomas, lymphadenomas, carcinomas, and lymphadenocarcinomas. The sebaceous carcinomas and lymphadenocarcinomas behave as low-grade malignant tumors, while the adenomas and lymphadenomas are benign in nature.[9]

Carcinoma Metastatic to the Salivary Glands

Of the major salivary glands the parotid gland is most frequently involved by metastatic disease. This fact reflects the presence of intraglandular lymph nodes. These nodes drain the face, external ear, and scalp. The most common primary tumor to metastasize to the parotid glands is melanoma of the temporal scalp, with such spread occurring in 80% of the cases. Metastatic squamous cell carcinoma of the mouth, pharynx, sinuses, and ear can also occur in the intraglandular parotid nodes. Less commonly, metastases from renal cell carcinoma, lung, breast carcinoma, and gastrointestinal carcinomas can occur both to the intraparotid and periparotid lymph nodes.[1,5,9]

NONEPITHELIAL TUMORS

Nonepithelial tumors of the salivary glands represent less than 5% of salivary gland neoplasms as a whole. In children alone, however, they may comprise over 50% of the lesions.[7,9] The only tumors of statistical consequence are the hemangiomas, lymphangiomas, and lymphomas. Rarely, neurogenic lesions, lipomas, and sarcomas are encountered.

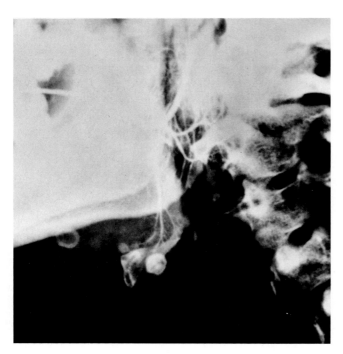

Fig. 3-113 Lateral view of parotid sialogram showing mass with multiple phleboliths in the lower pole region of the parotid gland: Hemangioma.

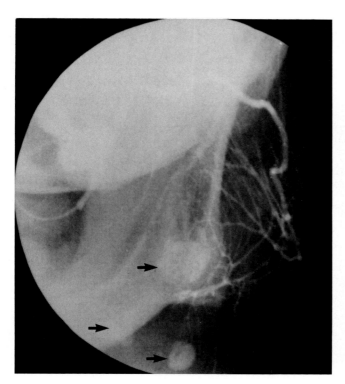

Fig. 3-114 Frontal view of left parotid sialogram showing benign mass displacing the parotid ducts laterally. Multiple phleboliths are present *(arrows):* Arteriovenous malformation which is radiographically indistinguishable from a hemangioma.

Hemangioma

Hemangiomas of the parotid gland are the most common salivary gland tumors in children.[7,9,24] Submandibular gland involvement is rare. The benign hemangioendothelioma or congenital capillary angioma is the predominant tumor in the first year of life, representing 90% of parotid gland tumors in this age group. This lesion is usually discovered shortly after birth, is unilateral, compressible, and soft. Rapid enlargement can occur and a bluish coloration can be seen in the overlying skin, especially when the infant is crying. There also may be an associated hemangioma in the overlying skin. These lesions are more common in girls and are nonencapsulated and lobulated. The differential diagnosis includes malignant hemangioendothelioma and cystic lymph angioma, both of which can be distinguished histologically. Surgery is to be avoided until adulthood if possible, since some tumors may spontaneously regress.[9]

Cavernous hemangiomas occur in older children and adults, with most patients older than 16 years of age. They tend to be well-circumscribed lesions, and surgery is the treatment of choice since spontaneous regression is unlikely.[9]

On CT these tumors enhance on postcontrast examinations, are often lobular in contour, may be seen to extend to the overlying skin, or have phleboliths within the tumor tissues (Figs. 3-113 to 3-115). On MRI the lesion can have sites of high signal intensity on T₁-

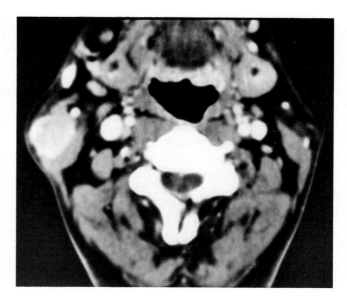

Fig. 3-115 Axial postcontrast CT scan showing enhancing benign-appearing mass in the right parotid gland: Hemangioma.

weighted images and T_2-weighted images, which are caused by blood protein and slow flow. The majority of the tumor has a low to intermediate, nonhomogeneous signal intensity (Fig. 3-116).

Lymphangioma

Lymphangiomas are benign tumors that are composed primarily of lymphatic vessels. These tumors are classified into three pathologic groups: the lymphangioma simplex, the cavernous lymphangioma, and the cystic lymphangioma or cystic hygroma. All three types may coexist within the same tumor. Most of the tumors found in the head and neck are cystic hygromas. Lymphangiomas represent 5% to 6% of all benign tumors of infancy and childhood. Between 50% to 60% are present at birth, and 80% to 90% are diagnosed by the age of 2 years. This corresponds to the period of greatest lymphatic growth. It is uncommon for cystic hygromas to be reported in adults.[25]

Most commonly these lesions arise in the posterior triangle of the neck. They can spread to invade the parotid and submandibular glands, muscles, and vessels. Most tumors are painless, soft or semifirm masses; some fluctuation in size is common. Sudden enlargement is associated with infection or hemorrhage. Facial nerve paralysis can occur secondary to nerve compression by the tumor with hemorrhage or secondary to an acute otitis media caused by eustachian tube obstruction by the tumor.[26]

Cystic hygromas can occur in adults and usually occur as a solitary cyst either in the submandibular triangle or the posterior triangle of the neck. Whether these lesions represent the congenital type or a posttraumatic type of lymphangioma is still unresolved.[27]

On CT these lesions are cystic masses usually with walls that are so thin, they cannot be identified on the images. Multiple cystic components are most common, and the cysts are filled with homogeneous low attenuation (10-18 HU) material. Areas of higher attenuation within the cysts usually correspond to sites of hemorrhage.[26] Septation can occur within the cysts even if they have not been previously aspirated. Infection is identified by an enhancing thickening of the cyst wall and adjacent soft tissues. In cases of multiple infections the attenuation of the cyst contents may approach that of muscle.

On MRI the dominant water content of the cysts is revealed in their signal intensities, which are low on T_1 WIs, intermediate on proton density-weighted images and high on T_2-weighted images.

Lymphoma

Primary lymphoma of the parotid gland is very rare. This diagnosis can be made only if there is histologic

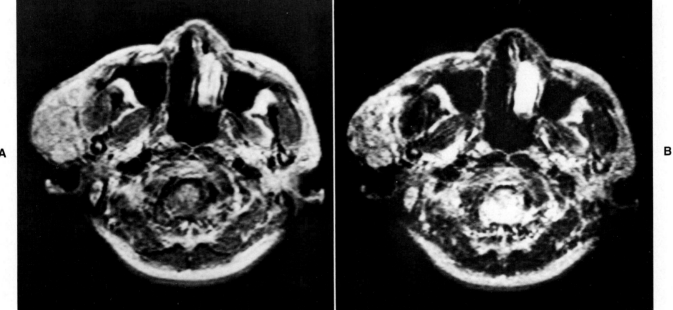

Fig. 3-116 **A,** Transverse mixed image and **B,** T_2-weighted MRI scans (0.5T, TR 2000 msec, TEs 30, 90 msec) showing poorly defined nonhomogeneous mass in right parotid gland. The gland is greatly enlarged, and the mass has an intermediate signal intensity background with areas of both low- and high-signal intensity scattered throughout it. One or two serpentine areas of low signal intensity may be flow voids from larger vessels: Hemangioma.

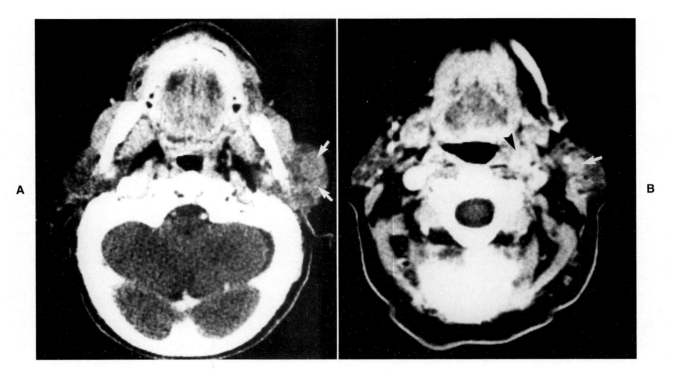

Fig. 3-117 **A,** Axial postcontrast CT scan showing two benign appearing masses in the left parotid gland. **B,** A more caudal scan reveals a third parotid mass *(arrow)* and a left internal jugular chain lymph node *(arrowhead):* Lymphoma.

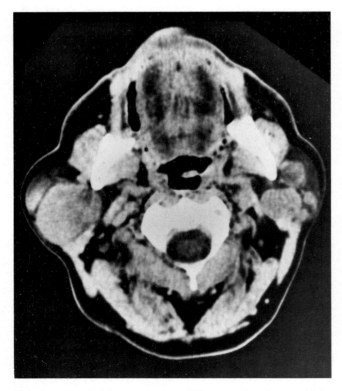

Fig. 3-118 Axial noncontrast CT scan showing multiple benign-appearing masses in both parotid glands: Lymphoma.

proof of lymphoma in the salivary parenchyma without any evidence of intra or extraparotid nodal involvement. Rarely the submandibular gland can be involved. These patients tend to do very well.[7]

Secondary involvement of the salivary glands is also rare, and the parotid gland is more commonly affected than is the submandibular gland. The incidence of such salivary gland lymphoma varies from 1% to 8% of the cases of lymphoma; 80% of these cases involve the parotid gland. Most commonly histiocytic lymphoma is the pathologic tumor type; however, all forms of non-Hodgkin's and Hodgkin's lymphomas have been reported.[2]

The CT appearance of secondary lymphoma of the parotid gland varies with the pathologic distribution of the disease. Most commonly, the lymphoma is confined to the intraparotid lymph nodes, and one or multiple benign appearing masses are identified within the gland. Each node is homogeneous and may enhance slightly on postcontrast CT scans (Figs. 3-117 and 3-118). If the parenchyma is involved, a diffuse infiltration will be seen either with poorly defined margins or involving the entire gland. Identification of extraparotid nodal disease can be helpful in suggesting the diagnosis. On MRI the lymphoma has a homogeneous intermediate signal intensity on all imaging sequences. In patients with Hodgkin's disease, on CT the nodes may be nonhomogeneous, with some sites of enhancement intermixed with scattered areas of low attenuation. This nonhomogeneity can also be seen on MRI.[28]

Intraparotid Lymphadenopathy

Enlargement of intraparotid lymph nodes can occur from a variety of causes. These include hyperplastic adenopathy, acute viral or bacterial adenopathy, lymphoma, and metastatic disease. The rapid, painful enlargement that may accompany the inflammatory adenopathy may simulate a parotid malignancy. In such cases the node(s) usually has a fairly bright T_2-weighted signal intensity, whereas the high-grade malignancies tend to have low-to-intermediate T_2-weighted signal intensities. This information can be helpful in distinguishing these entities, but in most cases needle aspiration or surgery will be necessary to establish the diagnosis. Such inflammatory nodes may enhance on postcontrast CT scans and have a slightly irregular margin, further simulating a malignancy (Fig. 3-119).

Lipoma

Lipomas comprise about 1% of parotid gland tumors. They also can arise in the immediate periparotid area and in these cases are often difficult or impossible to distinguish from an intraparotid lesion. Of the reported cases, 57% arose within the gland and 43% were of a periparotid origin. About 90% of the lipomas are ordinary lipomas, and the remaining lesions were examples of infiltrating lipomatosis or an infiltrating lipoma.[2,29]

The ordinary lipomas are discrete lesions that usually have a homogeneous low attenuation (−65 to −125 HU). They have no definable capsule, yet they are easily delineated from the adjacent soft tissues (Figs. 3-120 to 3-123). The infiltrating lipoma has poorly defined margins but is otherwise similar in appearance to the ordinary lipoma (Fig. 3-124). Hemorrhage and fibrotic changes can occur within the lipoma, and these cause increased attenuation within a lesion that may approach that of muscle. Usually these areas of increased attenuation are localized regions within the lipoma, but the entire lesion may be involved. It should be remembered, however, that a lipomatous mass with an overall heterogeneous, dense matrix may represent a liposarcoma.[29] On MRI lipomas have a high signal intensity on T_1-weighted images and an intermediate signal intensity on T_2-weighted images.

Neurogenic Tumors

Neurogenic tumors of the parotid gland can be either neuromas (schwannomas) or neurofibromas. Both lesions are usually ovoid, sharply delineated masses that

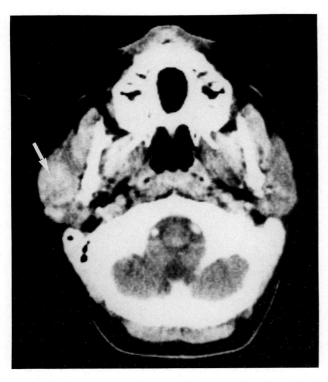

Fig. 3-119 Axial postcontrast CT scan showing slightly enhancing benign-appearing mass *(arrow)* in right parotid gland: Hyperplastic lymph node.

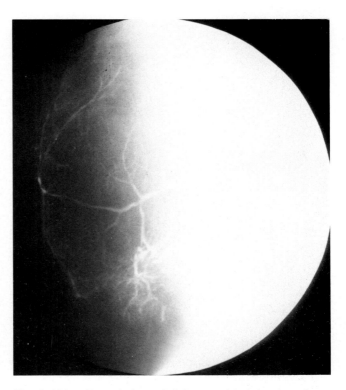

Fig. 3-120 Frontal view of right parotid sialogram showing large benign appearing mass that displaces the parotid ducts laterally. Note that this lipoma does not have a typical low fat density.

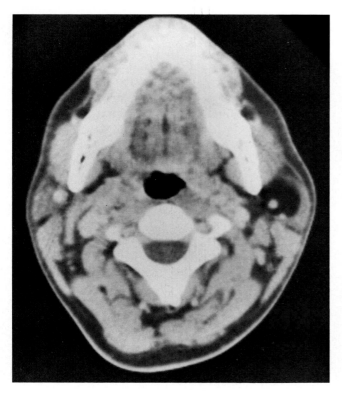

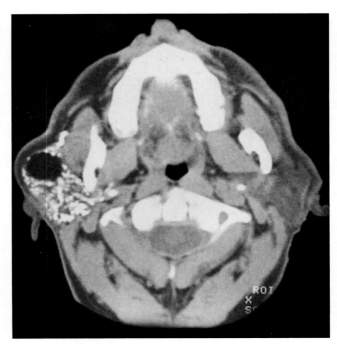

Fig. 3-121 Axial postcontrast CT scan shows fat attenuation well-defined mass in left parotid gland: Lipoma. (From Som et al, AJNR 7:657, 1986.)

Fig. 3-122 Axial CT-sialogram scan showing contrast material in right parotid gland and benign-appearing low attenuation mass in the anterior superficial lobe: Lipoma. (From Som et al, AJNR 7:657, 1986.)

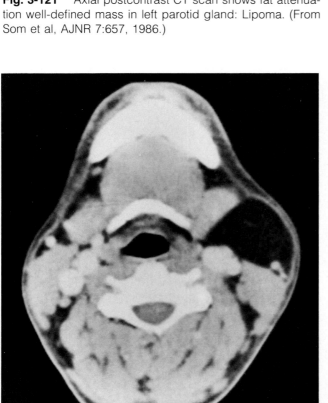

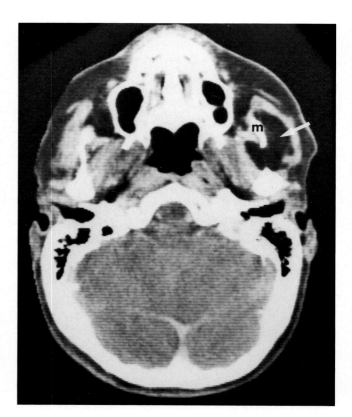

Fig. 3-123 Axial postcontrast CT scan showing large fat attenuation mass that simulated a left parotid mass clinically, but actually was in the soft tissues below the parotid gland: Lipoma. (From Som et al, AJNR 7:657, 1986.)

Fig. 3-124 Axial CT scan showing fat attenuation mass *(arrow)* that has extended from the superficial portion of the left parotid gland back around the mandible *(m)* into the deep portion of the gland: Infiltrating lipoma. (From Som et al, AJNR 7:657, 1986.)

arise primarily from the facial nerve trunk or its branches. The neuromas are solitary, whereas the neurofibromas may be multiple and associated with other manifestations of the von Recklinghausen's disease. On CT these tumors can enhance, be cystic, or be isodense with muscle. The cystic changes usually are small and multiple. The neurofibromas may have a low, almost fatty attenuation that may simulate a lipoma. On MRI these tumors in general have an intermediate background signal intensity on all imaging sequences. However, nonhomogeneous regions of higher signal intensities can occur that make these lesions indistinguishable from a pleomorphic adenoma.[30,31]

MISCELLANEOUS LESIONS
Masseteric Hypertrophy

Masseteric hypertrophy is an uncommon entity that usually is bilateral but may be unilateral. Muscle enlargement may be minimal or up to three times its normal size.[32] The temporalis muscle may also be enlarged on the involved side(s), and flaring of the mandibular angle(s) can occur. The process usually starts in adolescence or early adulthood; there is a history of slowly progressive muscle growth. The facial fullness is located anterior to the usual location of a parotid mass and enlarges when the patient's teeth are clenched. The mass feels like muscle on palpation.[33] Excessive gum chewing or teeth clenching has been suggested as playing an etiologic role, but many cases are of an unknown cause. Plain films may show an exostosis of the lateral aspect of the angle of the mandible at the line of attachment of the masseter muscle. A sialogram will demonstrate lateral bowing of Stensen's duct around the enlarged masseter muscle (Fig. 3-125). Computed sectional imaging will demonstrate the enlarged muscle mass(es), which otherwise appears as normal muscle tissue (Figs. 3-126 and 3-127).

Temporomandibular Joint and Mandibular Lesions

A variety of lesions can occur within the region of the temporomandibular joint (TMJ) that may clinically mimic parotid gland disease. Usually degenerative changes and internal joint derangements can be identified clinically as being of a primary TMJ origin. However, fibroosseous lesions of the temporal bone margin of the joint and/or the upper mandible can present as a parotid mass. Similarly, mandibular cysts, and odontogenic masses (i.e., dentigerous cysts and ameloblastomas) may be confused clinically with salivary lesions in some circumstances. Metastases to the mandibular ramus and TMJ region may also mimic salivary masses. In these patients computed sectional imaging will provide the most accurate assessment of the true anatomic

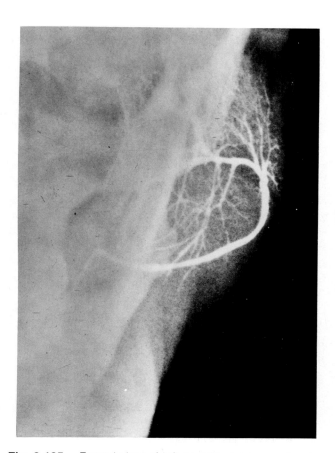

Fig. 3-125 Frontal view of left parotid sialogram showing benign-appearing lateral displacement of Stensen's duct and hilum of the gland: Masseteric hypertrophy.

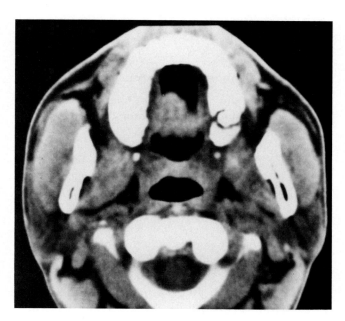

Fig. 3-126 Axial CT scan showing moderate enlargement of right masseter muscle: Unilateral masseteric hypertrophy.

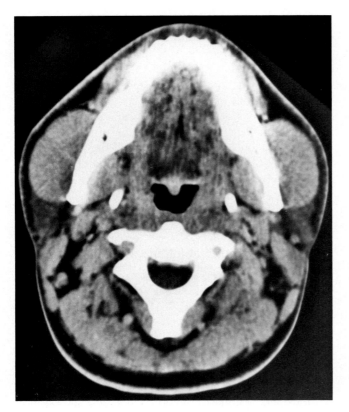

Fig. 3-127 Axial CT scan showing marked enlargement of both masseter muscles: Bilateral masseteric hypertrophy.

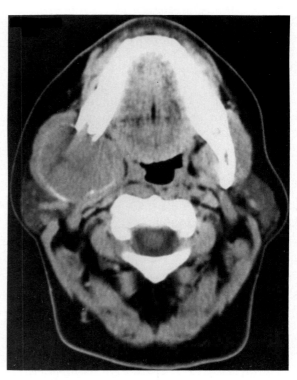

Fig. 3-128 Axial CT scan showing expansile mass of the right mandible, which simulated a parotid tumor clinically: Metastatic meningioma. (From Som et al, AJNR 8:127, 1987.)

origin of the process. Metastases often have a cystic, destructive appearance; the primary tumor usually arises in the lungs, breast, kidneys, or gastrointestinal tract (Figs. 3-128 to 3-131).

Other Miscellaneous Conditions

Rarely sebaceous cysts or dermoid cysts overlying the parotid gland may mimic a parotid tumor. Additionally, a prominent transverse process of the second cervical vertebra may be confused with a deep parotid mass on palpation. Tumors arising in the soft tissues around the parotid gland and masseter muscles may occur rarely and simulate a parotid mass. These include neuromas, Merkel cell tumors, and rare sarcomas.[2]

Frey's syndrome is an unusual entity that results from an injury to the auriculotemporal nerve. Clinically, sweating and flushing of the skin occurs in the area of this nerve's distribution when the patient has a stimulus to salivate. It most probably results from a communication between the postganglionic parasympathetic fibers from the otic ganglion and the sympathetic nerves from the superior cervical ganglion. Sialograms and computed sectional imaging studies are normal.[34]

SALIVARY TUMORS IN THE PEDIATRIC PATIENT

Salivary tumors in children are uncommon and represent less than 5% of tumors in all age groups. The most common tumor is a hemangioma, which represents over 50% of all lesions. Next in frequency are the pleomorphic adenoma, mucoepidermoid carcinoma, lymphangioma, and acinous cell carcinoma in declining order. Rarely, undifferentiated carcinoma, adenocarcinoma, and adenoid cystic carcinoma can occur. About 30% to 35% of the cases are malignant, a higher percentage than found in adults.[2,7]

Masses that result from autoimmune disease and chronic sialadenitis may on occasion simulate a parotid tumor, and intraparotid lymphadenopathy may also mimic a parotid neoplasm.

SUMMARY OF DISEASE PATTERNS

If the patient has a history of recurrent parotid swelling with or without associated pain, a sialogram is the modality of choice for initiating the radiographic workup. Dilatation of Stensen's duct and the central glandular ducts suggests a sialadenitis with or without obstruction. If the peripheral ducts and acini cannot be visual-

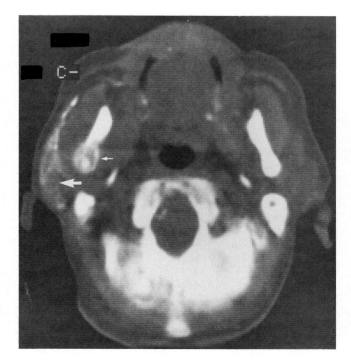

Fig. 3-129   Axial CT-sialogram scan showing invasive tumor of right parotid gland *(large arrow)* and a destructive lesion of posterior right mandible *(small arrow):* Metastatic lung carcinoma.

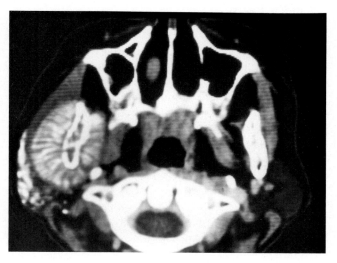

Fig. 3-130   Axial CT-sialogram scan showing normal contrast filled right parotid gland. The right mandible is expanded by an aggressive periosteal reaction causing a mass that clinically simulated a parotid tumor: Plasmacytoma.

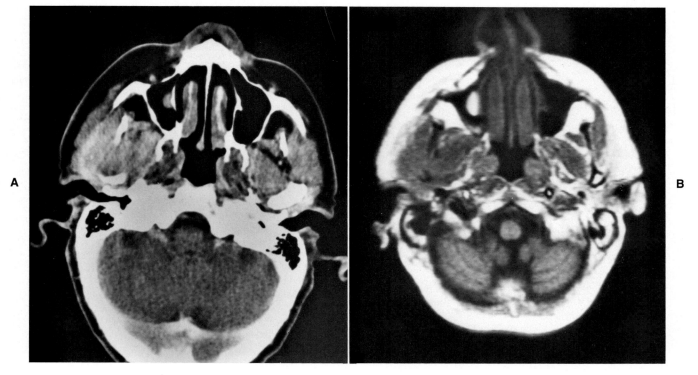

Fig. 3-131   **A,** Axial postcontrast CT scan showing infiltrating mass in the right infratemporal fossa and upper parapharyngeal space. The mass has eroded the head of the mandible and invaded the parotid gland. **B,** Transverse mixed image MRI scan (0.5T, TR 1800 msec, TE = 30 msec) shows the mass to have a low-to-intermediate signal intensity: Metastatic lung carcinoma.

ized, the gland most probably should be operated on since the production of saliva will be impaired. Scattered collections of contrast material usually indicate abscesses. Multiple collections of contrast material that are uniform in size and distribution throughout the gland suggest autoimmune disease. An enlarged gland with an otherwise normal sialogram makes sialosis most likely.

A solitary benign-appearing mass in a pediatric patient is most probably a lymph node, hemangioma, benign mixed tumor, low-grade mucoepidermoid carcinoma, or a lymphangioma.

A solitary benign-appearing mass in an adult patient is most probably a benign mixed tumor, Warthin's tumor, low-grade mucoepidermoid carcinoma, an adenoid cystic carcinoma, or an acinic cell carcinoma. A solitary malignant-appearing mass is most likely to be a high-grade mucoepidermoid carcinoma, an adenocarcinoma, or an undifferentiated carcinoma. Multiple masses suggest Warthin's tumors, acinic cell tumors, lymphoma, granulomatous disease, or metastases. Multiple cystic masses, especially in association with benign cervical adenopathy suggest that the patient is HIV positive. A solitary cystic mass could be a branchial cleft cyst, Warthin's tumor, or epithelial cyst.

Calcification within the mass suggests a benign mixed tumor or, less commonly, a mucoepidermoid carcinoma. Phleboliths indicate a hemangioma.

If the tumor accumulates $Tc^{99}m$ pertechnetate, a Warthin's tumor or oncocytoma is present.

If a tumor mass has low-to-intermediate signal intensity on all MRI imaging sequences, a high-grade malignancy should be suspected.

REFERENCES

1. Eneroth CM: Salivary gland tumors in the parotid gland, submandibular gland and the palate region, Cancer 27:1415, 1971.
2. Rabinov K and Weber AL: Radiology of the salivary glands, Boston, 1985, GK Hall & Co, pp 292-367.
3. Rankow RM and Polayes IM: Surgical treatment of salivary gland tumors. In Rankow RM and Polayes IM, editors: Diseases of the salivary glands, Philadelphia, 1976, WB Saunders Co, pp 239-283.
4. American Joint Committee on Cancer: Manual for staging of cancer, ed 3, Philadelphia, 1988, JB Lippincott Co, pp 51-56.
5. Johns ME: Parotid cancer: a rational basis for treatment, Head Neck Surg 3:132, 1980.
6. Thackray AC and Sobin LH: Histological typing of salivary gland tumors. In International histological classification of tumors, no. 7, Geneva, 1972, World Health Organization.
7. Batsakis JG: Tumors of the head and neck, clinical and pathological considerations, ed 2, Baltimore, 1979, Williams & Wilkins, pp 1-20.
8. Cornug JL and Gray SR: Surgical and clinical pathology of salivary gland tumors. In Rankow RM and Polayes IM, editors: Diseases of the salivary glands, Philadelphia, 1976, WB Saunders Co, pp 99-142.
9. Peel RZ and Gnepp DR: Diseases of the salivary glands. In Barnes L, editor: Surgical pathology of the head and neck, vol 1, New York, 1985, Marcel Dekker, Inc, pp 533-645.
10. Som PM et al: Benign and malignant parotid pleomorphic adenomas: CT and MR studies, JCAT 12:65, 1988.
11. Mandelblatt SM et al: Parotid masses: MR imaging, Radiology 163:411, 1987.
12. Mirich DR, McArdle CB, and Kulkarni MV: Benign pleomorphic adenomas of the salivary glands: surface coil MR imaging versus CT, JCAT 11:620, 1987.
13. Teresi LM et al: Parotid masses: MR imaging, Radiology 163:405, 1987.
14. Shugar JMA, Som PM, and Biller HF: Warthin's tumor, a multifocal disease, Ann Otol Rhinol Laryngol 91:246, 1982.
15. Batsakis JG et al: The pathology of head and neck tumors: salivary glands, part II, Head Neck Surg 1:167, 1978.
16. Healey WV, Perzin KH, and Smith L: Mucoepidermoid carcinoma of salivary gland origin, Cancer 26:368, 1970.
17. Batsakis JG and Regezi JA: The pathology of head and neck tumors: salivary glands, part IV, Head Neck Surg 1:340, 1979.
18. Conley J and Dingman DL: Adenoid cystic carcinoma in the head and neck (cylindroma), Arch Otolaryngol 100:81, 1974.
19. Batsakis JG et al: Acinic cell carcinoma: a clinico-pathologic study of 35 cases, J Laryngol Otol 93:325, 1979.
20. Evans RW and Cruickshank AH: Epithelial tumors of the salivary glands, Philadelphia, 1970, WB Saunders Co, pp 242-278.
21. Batsakis JG and Regezi JA: Selected controversial lesions of salivary tissues, Otolaryngol Clin North Am 10:309, 1977.
22. Chen KTK and Hafez GR: Infiltrating salivary ductal carcinoma; a clincopathologic study of five cases, Arch Otolaryngol 107:37, 1981.
23. Gnepp DR: Sebaceous neoplasms of salivary gland origin: a review, Pathol Ann 18:71, 1983.
24. Touloukian RJ: Salivary gland diseases in infancy and childhood. In Rankow RM and Polayes IM, editors: Diseases of the salivary glands, Philadelphia, 1976, WB Saunders Co, pp 284-303.
25. Barnes L: In Barnes L, editor: Surgical pathology of the head and neck, vol 1, New York, 1985, Marcel Dekker, Inc, pp 725-880.
26. Som PM, Zimmerman RA, and Biller HF: Cystic hygroma and facial nerve paralysis: a rare association, JCAT 8:110, 1984.
27. Som PM: Cystic lesions of the neck, Postgrad Radiol 7:211, 1987.
28. Johns ME: The salivary glands: anatomy and embryology, Otolaryngol Clin North Am 10:261, 1977.
29. Som PM et al: Rare presentations of ordinary lipomas of the head and neck: a review, AJNR 7:657, 1986.
30. Kuman AJ et al: Computed tomography of extracranial nerve sheath tumors with pathological correlation, JCAT 7:857, 1983.
31. Som PM et al: Parapharyngeal space masses: an updated protocol based upon 104 cases, Radiology 153:149, 1984.
32. See reference 7, pp 368-381.
33. Waldhart E and Lynch JB: Benign hypertrophy of the masseter muscles and mandibular angles, Arch Surg 102:115, 1971.
34. Mason DK and Chisholm DM: Salivary glands in health and disease, London, 1975, WB Saunders Co, pp 106-118.

4 Temporomandibular Joint Imaging

RICHARD WIER KATZBERG
PER-LENNART WESTESSON

The purpose of an imaging assessment of the temporomandibular joint (TMJ) is to depict clinically suspected disorders of the joint. For many years plain film radiography, mainly in a transcranial projection, was the most commonly used method of making this assessment. However, this modality has major limitations, since it is sensitive only to changes in the osseous com-ponents and depicts only the lateral aspect of the joint. With the evolution of newer imaging modalities such as arthrography, computed tomography, and magnetic resonance imaging, our ability to understand the anatomy and pathophysiology of internal derangement related to disc displacement has improved enormously.[1]

This chapter provides an overview of the various imaging modalities available for evaluating the TMJ, with the emphasis on the newer capabilities for direct soft tissue imaging. An algorithm for imaging of temporomandibular joint patients is suggested that is based on our own combined clinical experience.

ANATOMY OF THE TMJ

Interpreting each imaging modality and understanding the pathophysiology of the joint require a complete knowledge of both normal and pathologic anatomy of the joint and its surrounding structures. Therefore a description of joint anatomy, joint pathology, function and dysfunction is presented in some detail.

The osseous components of the TMJ consist of the mandibular condyle at the top of the condylar process of the mandible and the glenoid fossa and articular tubercle of the temporal bone (Fig. 4-1). The articulating surfaces in the joint are covered by a thin layer of dense fibrous tissue, unlike most other joints of the body, which have a cartilaginous covering.

The TMJ disc is a biconcave fibrous structure located between the mandibular condyle and the temporal component. The disc is round to oval and has a thick periphery and a thin central part. Thus, in a sagittal section, the normal disc appears biconcave. In a coronal plane the disc is crescent shaped (Fig. 4-2). The anterior and posterior parts of the disc as seen in the sagittal plane are called the anterior and posterior bands. In the normal joint, the posterior band is located over the condyle and the central thin zone is located between the condyle and the posterior part of the articular tubercle (Fig. 4-1). The anterior thick part (anterior band) is located under the articular tubercle. A joint capsule surrounds the joint. The capsule emerges from the temporal bone and extends like a funnel inferiorly to at-

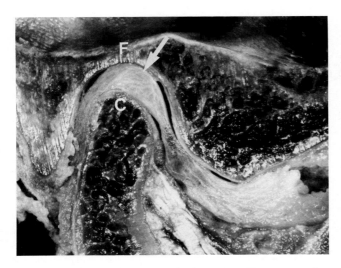

Fig. 4-1 Normal TMJ in sagittal section. Biconcave disc in normal superior position. The posterior band of disc *(arrow)* is lying over the condyle. The condyle *(C)* and glenoid fossa *(F)* are indicated.

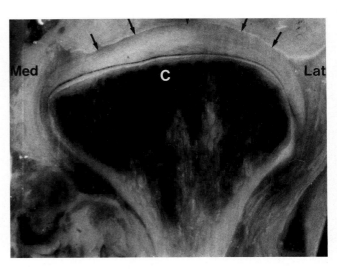

Fig. 4-2 Normal TMJ in coronal section. The disc (arrows) is crescent shaped and located over the condyle. Medially and laterally the disc is attached to the condyle and capsule. The condyle *(C)* is indicated.

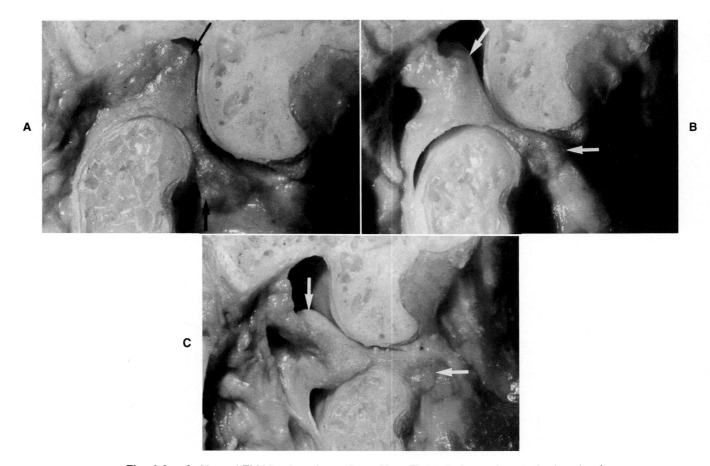

Fig. 4-3 **A,** Normal TMJ in closed mouth position. The anterior and posterior bands of the disc are indicated by arrows. **B,** Normal TMJ in half opened mouth position position. Anterior and posterior bands of the disc are indicated by arrows. **C,** Normal TMJ in open mouth position. Anterior and posterior bands of the disc are indicated by arrows.

tach to the neck of the condyle. Posteriorly, the disc is attached to the temporal bone and to the condyle by the posterior disc attachment synonymous with the bilaminar zone. The bilaminar zone consists of loose fibrous connective and elastic tissue components. The disc is also attached to the capsule and to the neck of the condyle both medially and laterally (Fig. 4-2). Anteriorly, the disc is attached to the joint capsule, and in the anteromedial portion of the joint, the disc sometimes also merges with the upper head of the lateral pterygoid muscle.

FUNCTION OF THE TMJ

The function of the temporomandibular joint is complex because the upper and lower joint compartments principally function as two small joints within this same joint capsule. This allows for proportionally great movements of the TMJ in relation to the actual size of the joint. Both rotation and translation occur in the upper and lower joint spaces. However, translation is predominantly seen in the upper space, and rotation is more prominent in the lower joint space. In the initial phase of jaw opening, the condyle rotates in the lower joint compartment. After this initial rotation, translation occurs in the upper and subsequently in the lower joint space. During translation the condyle and the disc translate together under the articular tubercle. During all mandibular movements the central thin part of the disc is located between the condyle and the articular tubercle. This suggests that the thick periphery of the disc and the thick posterior and anterior bands act as functional guides for the joint. The normal function of the joint is illustrated in Fig. 4-3.

INTERNAL DERANGEMENT RELATED TO DISPLACEMENT OF THE DISC

Internal derangement is a general orthopedic term implying a mechanical fault that interferes with the smooth action of a joint.[2] Internal derangement is thus a functional diagnosis, and for the TMJ the most common cause of internal derangement is displacement of the disc.[3-5] Most often the disc displaces in an anterior or anteromedial direction. Thus the posterior band of the disc prolapses anterior to the superior region of the condyle (Fig. 4-4) instead of being located between the condyle and glenoid fossa. As a consequence, the condyle functions under the inferior surface of the posterior disc attachment. The central thin part of the disc lies inferior to the articular tubercle.

Studies have shown that the disc frequently is also displaced in a medial direction.[6-9] A medially displaced disc is shown in Fig. 4-5. Lateral displacements of the disc also occur but not as commonly.[7-10] A general classification of the different types of disc displacement in the TMJ is shown in the box. The combina-

---

TERMINOLOGY FOR DESCRIBING THE POSITION OF THE DISC

Normal	Superior
Abnormal	Anterior
	Anteromedial rotational displacement
	Anterolateral rotational displacement
	Medial sideways displacement
	Lateral sideways displacement

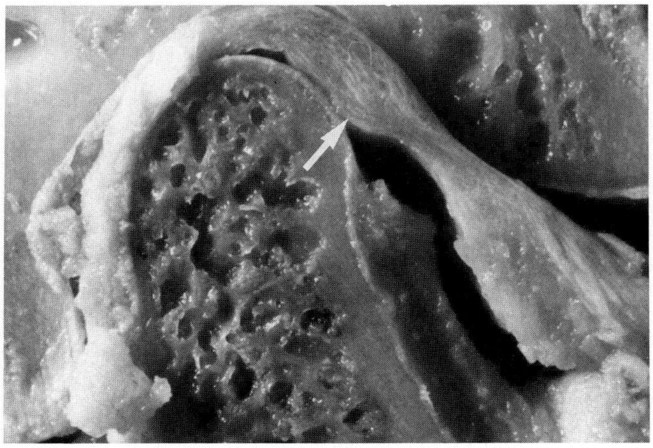

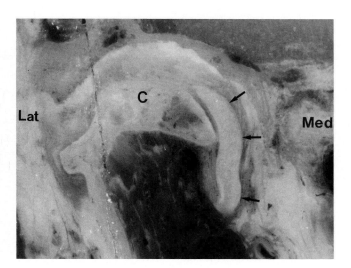

Fig. 4-4 Anterior disc displacement. The disc is anteriorly displaced with its posterior band *(arrow)* located slightly forward of the condyle.

Fig. 4-5 Coronal section of TMJ showing medial disc displacement. The disc is indicated by arrows. The condyle *(C)* is sclerotic.

tion of anterior and lateral or medial displacement is called *rotational displacement*,[7] whereas pure lateral or pure medial displacement is called *sideways displacement*.[7]

The functional aspects of disc displacement include displacement with or without reduction; this multiplies the possible combinations of TMJ abnormalities. The

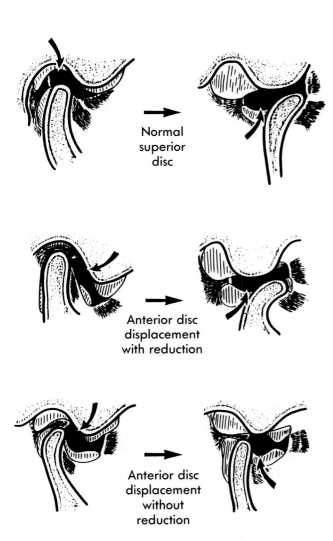

Fig. 4-6 Schematic drawing of normal TMJ and different categories of internal derangements. The disc is black and indicated by the curved arrows.

Normal superior disc

Anterior disc displacement with reduction

Anterior disc displacement without reduction

functional categories of internal derangement are illustrated in Fig. 4-6. In disc displacement with reduction (Fig. 4-6, *B*), the anteriorly displaced disc reverts to a normal superior position during opening. In disc displacement without reduction (Fig. 4-6, *C*), the disc lies anterior to the condyle during all mandibular movements and the normal condyle-disc relationship is not reestablished.

Disc Displacement with Reduction

When a displaced disc reduces to a normal position, a click is usually heard. When the jaw closes, the disc again displaces anteriorly, usually during the last phase of the closing movement of the jaw, and again a click is commonly heard. The closing click usually is less prominent than the opening one. The cyclic nature of disc displacement was described by Ireland[11] in 1951. The clicking sound has been shown to be caused by the impact of the condyle hitting against the temporal component of the articulation after the condyle has passed under the posterior band of the disc.[12,13]

Disc Displacement without Reduction

In disc displacement without reduction (Fig. 4-6, *C*), the disc remains displaced relative to the condylar head regardless of the jaw position. In the initial stages of this condition, jaw opening typically is limited and the jaw deviates to the side of the affected joint. However, this clinical characteristic is typical only during the initial (early) phase; with time the opening capacity of the TMJ increases and the jaw no longer deviates. This is probably the result of progressive elongation of the posterior disc attachment and deformation of the disc. Disc displacement without reduction is usually not associated with joint sounds in the early stage.

Disc Deformation

The normal disc is biconcave when viewed in the sagittal plane (Fig. 4-1). In the early stages of internal derangement, the disc remains normal in shape. However, the displaced disc begins to deform, as noted by a thickening of the posterior band and shortening of the entire anteroposterior length of the disc (Fig. 4-7).[6,14] Additionally, both the central thin part and the anterior band decrease in size. The end result is a biconvex disc configuration with a stretched, elongated, and thinned posterior disc attachment. The gross changes of the disc are also associated with histologic alterations within the disc that lead to metaplastic hyaline cartilage, hyalinization, and accumulation of foci of calcium deposits and abnormal collagen patterns.[15,16] Changes also occur in the posterior disc attachment itself, leading to fibrosis.[17,18]

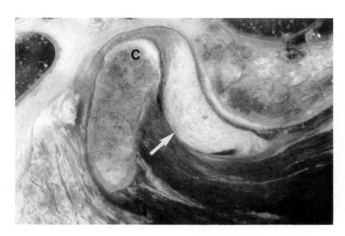

Fig. 4-7 Anterior displacement and deformation of disc. The disc *(arrow)* is biconvex. The condyle *(C)* articulates with the posterior disc attachment.

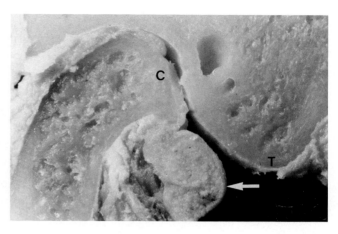

Fig. 4-8 Anterior displacement and extensive deformation of the disc *(arrow)* with perforation of the posterior disc attachment. The condyle *(C)* is flattened with an anterior osteophyte and surface irregularities.

Late-Stage Changes Following Disc Displacement

In the late or chronic stages of disc displacement without reduction, the disc is deformed and has a stretched, torn, or detached posterior attachment. Communications between the upper and lower joint spaces also are often seen in the late stages of disc displacement without reduction.[5,6,19] Most commonly the perforations are found in the posterior disc attachment at its junction with the disc itself (Fig. 4-8). Infrequently, perforations are found in the disc per se.[6] Osseous changes involving the condyle and temporal bone often occur as a sequela of disc displacement.[5,20,21] Osseous changes consist of flattening and osteophytosis of the mandibular condyle and flattening of the temporal component of the articulation. These changes are more commonly observed in the lateral part of the joint and can be detected by plain film imaging. It should be noted that osseous changes are relatively late findings in the disease process.

RELIABILITY OF CLINICAL EXAMINATIONS IN THE DIAGNOSIS OF TMJ DISC DISPLACEMENT

Internal derangement of the TMJ is an organic disease, and several attempts have been made to identify clinical symptoms indicative of TMJ disc displacement. The most extensive series of investigations[22-26] analyzed more than 200 patients with internal derangement. The aim of these studies was to identify clinical signs and symptoms that were predictive of the status of the joint. Signs and symptoms that showed a statistically significant relationship to the intraarticular status of the joint were related to abnormalities in the joint that led to functional alterations of jaw mechanics. Thus maximum jaw opening, forward translation of the condyle as assessed by fluoroscopy, deviation of the mandible from

Table 4-1 Comparison of clinical and arthrographic findings (N = 205 patients)[22-26]

Clinical finding	Arthrographic diagnosis		
	Normal disc position	Disc displacement	
		with reduction	without reduction
Pain in front of the ear	88%	82%	84%
Tender to palpation:			
Temporal tendon	61%	51%	54%
Medial pterygoid	24%	8%	16%
Superficial masseter	27%	27%	12%

the midline at maximal opening, and lateral movements of the jaw were associated with disc displacement. However, the overall clinical accuracy in predicting the various anatomic aspects of internal derangement was only about 70% (Table 4-1). As an example, the intensity and location of pain did not distinguish patients with internal derangement from those without internal derangement. No consistent relationship was found between the occlusion and the status of the joint.

The findings of these studies suggest that clinical examination per se is not reliable for determining the status of the joint.[22-26] The conclusion of these studies has been recently confirmed,[27] and it is reasonable to assume that there is a specific need for accurate imaging to be able to determine the status of the joint.

TRANSCRANIAL AND TRANSMAXILLARY PROJECTIONS

The commonest and most well-established technique for examining the TMJ radiographically is the transcranial projection (Fig. 4-9). The lateral aspect of the joint

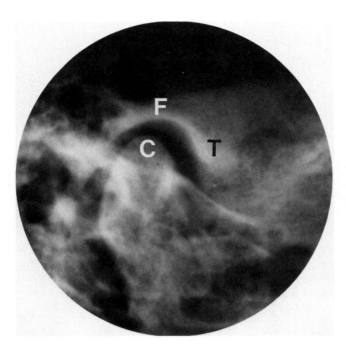

Fig. 4-9 Transcranial radiograph of TMJ. The condyle *(C)*, fossa *(F)*, and tubercle *(T)* are indicated.

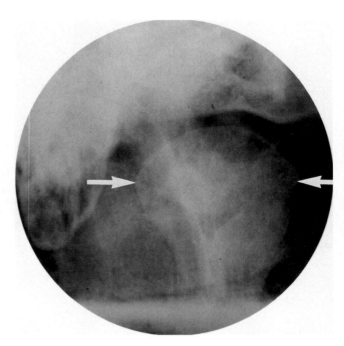

Fig. 4-10 Transmaxillary radiograph of TMJ. The lateral and medial poles of the condyles are indicated by arrows.

is well visualized on the transcranial radiograph. The central and medial parts of the joint are not clearly seen on the transcranial projection, since the x-ray beam is not tangent to these articular surfaces. This disadvantage is partly compensated for because most of the early osseous changes occur laterally in the joint.[28]

We recommend that in addition to the transcranial projection, an anteroposterior projection be obtained to depict the central and medial parts of the condyle. A transmaxillary projection[29] (Fig. 4-10) or a transorbital projection is acceptable.

TOMOGRAPHY

Complex motion tomography has been recommended for detection of early osseous changes (Fig. 4-11). Studies have demonstrated that a clearer depiction of the osseous anatomy can be gained from tomography than from transcranial radiography.[30] Tomography may also be performed in the coronal plane, providing information about the medial and lateral poles of the condyle, which are usually not adequately depicted on the sagittal tomograms. The disadvantage of tomography is the rather large radiation dose delivered to the lens of the eye. To a certain extent tomography has been replaced by computed tomography (CT) in the modern imaging department. CT probably represents the most effective modality to demonstrate osseous abnormalities.

ARTHROGRAPHY
Development of TMJ Arthrography

Early attempts with TMJ arthrography were undertaken by Nørgaard[31,32] in the 1940s. However, this procedure was not adopted by many clinicians because it was considered to be technically difficult and painful for the patient, and the information gathered was not considered of great value for treatment planning and evaluation of prognosis. Only a few descriptions of TMJ arthrography appeared in the literature over the ensuing quarter century.

Toward the end of the 1970s several articles appeared that described the clinical and arthrographic characteristics of internal derangement related to displacement of the disc.[33-36] These arthrographic studies were actually the first to depict displacement of the disc, a pathologic entity that had been suspected earlier.[11,37-41] During the following years considerable enthusiasm developed for TMJ arthrography, and a large number of publications describing the usefulness of the technique appeared in the literature. The changed attitude toward TMJ arthrography can be traced to several factors: (1) use of an image intensifier to facilitate the puncture of the joint[33-36]; (2) use of the technique to study and document the dynamics of the joint[42]; (3) identification of disc displacement as a common cause of TMJ pain and dysfunction[33,34]; and probably most importantly, (4) introduction of new, conservative

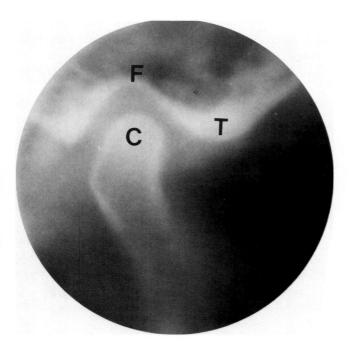

Fig. 4-11 Sagittal tomogram of TMJ. The condyle *(C)*, fossa *(F)*, and tubercle *(T)* are indicated.

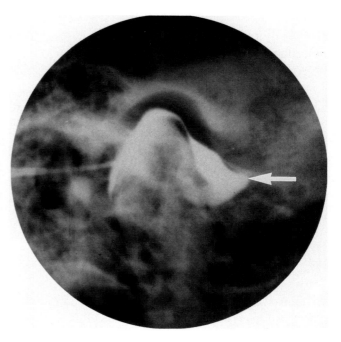

Fig. 4-12 Lower compartment arthrogram of TMJ showing anterior disc displacement. Prominent anterior recess *(arrow)* of the lower joint space is a sign of disc displacement.

methods[43-45] and surgical techniques[46,47] for treating disc displacement. These newer treatment methods required accurate information about the status and function of the joint. The use of nonionic contrast medium,[4,19] which made the examination less painful, and the combination of arthrography and tomography* also influenced the more frequent use of arthrography.

Single- and Double-Contrast Arthrography

Injection of contrast medium into the lower space only[3,36,43] is a simplification of the original arthrographic technique, in which contrast medium was injected into both upper and lower joint spaces (Fig. 4-12). This simplification further popularized the use of arthrography, and currently single-contrast lower compartment arthrography[3,43] is the most commonly used arthrographic technique.

Double-contrast arthrography is a variant of arthrography in which injection of iodine contrast medium is combined with an injection of air. Techniques for double-contrast arthrography of the TMJ have been described.[4,19,50-53] The double-contrast technique is superior to the single-contrast study in its demonstration of the configuration of the disc and the posterior disc attachment (Fig. 4-13). However, the double-contrast technique is technically more difficult to perform, since

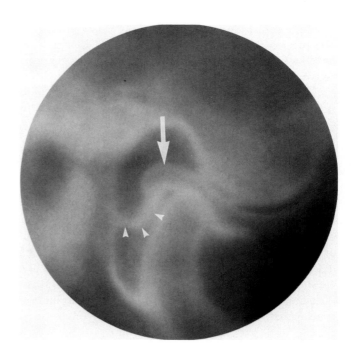

Fig. 4-13 Dual space double contrast arthrotomogram showing the disc *(arrow)* in a superior position. The mouth was halfway opened and the redundant posterior disc attachment *(arrow heads)* is seen between the disc and the posterior capsule. The upper and lower joint spaces are radiolucent due to the intraarticular injection of air.

*References 33, 34, 36, 48, 49.

Table 4-2 Indications and contraindications for arthrography

Indications	
Common	Assess position, function, and configuration of the disc
	Differential diagnosis in patients with diffuse facial and head pain
	Establish a jaw position for protrusive splint therapy
Infrequent	Diagnosis of loose bodies in the joint space
	Evaluation after trauma
	Aspiration of joint fluid
	Intraarticular injections
Contraindications	Infections in the preauricular area
	"Allergy" to contrast medium
	Bleeding disorder
	Anticoagulation medication

it requires cannulation of both upper and lower joint spaces and injection of both contrast medium and air.

Indications and Contraindications

The most common indication for arthrography is to assess the position and function of the disc in patients with pain and dysfunction that suggest internal derangement as the cause (Table 4-2). Arthrography can also be used in patients with TMJ disc displacement with reduction to determine the mandibular position that reestablishes a normal condyle-disc relationship.[54,55] The purpose of this would be to establish the optimum position for initiating protrusive splint therapy (conservative therapy).[54,55] Very infrequently, arthrography is performed to delineate loose bodies within the joint spaces, for one diagnostic aspiration of joint fluid, for one intraarticular injection of cortisone, or for evaluation of the TMJ after trauma.

An infrequent contraindication for TMJ arthrography is infection in the preauricular area, which could result in contamination of the joint during the arthrographic procedure. In patients with previous reactions to contrast medium, other modalities such as magnetic resonance imaging should be considered as alternative imaging techniques. However, arthrography has been performed on such patients without untoward reaction without any premedication. Bleeding disorders and anticoagulation medication also are relative contraindications to arthrography.

Radiologic Equipment

A fluoroscopic table or a C-arm unit with an x-ray tube and image intensifier is necessary equipment for this study. Because of the small dimensions of the TMJ, it is also useful to be able to magnify the image to about three times normal size. The capability for spot filming and videotape recording is valuable for docu-

mentation and the evaluation of dynamic joint movements. For double-contrast arthrography, tomography is also needed.

The methodology of the examination is explained to the patient. The patient is placed on the tabletop in a laterally recumbent position, and the head is oriented so that the side to be injected is located superiorly. The head is slightly tilted, and the transcranial projection is optimized with fluoroscopy. Opening and closing movements of the jaw, with attention to the condyle and fossa, are recorded on videotape before contrast medium is injected.

Technique for Single-Contrast Arthrography

The superoposterior aspect of the condyle is clinically and fluoroscopically identified and indicated on the skin by a metal marker. The area is marked with a pen, and local anesthesia (1% lidocaine) is injected. The joint is punctured with a 23 guage, ¾-inch scalp vein needle introduced perpendicular to the skin surface, and contrast medium (nonionic, 300 mg iodine/ml) is injected into the lower joint space (Fig. 4-14, A). Contrast medium is injected until optimum visualization of the joint space has been achieved. Usually between 0.2 and 0.5 ml of contrast medium is injected. The optimum amount of contrast material is determined by fluoroscopic observation of the joint space. The needle is then withdrawn, and the patient is asked to open and close the mouth several times while the image is recorded on videotape. The free flow of contrast medium around the top of the condyle onto the anterior aspect of the condylar head and into the anterior joint space indicates a successful injection. Simultaneous filling of the upper joint space indicates a perforation between these spaces. In joints with perforation, additional contrast medium usually needs to be injected for optimum image quality. Spot films are obtained in at least the closed and open mouth positions and at additional positions where abnormalities are clearly seen.

If the diagnosis is not clear from these images, it may be necessary to inject contrast medium into the upper joint space also (Fig. 4-14, B). This can be done either by withdrawing the needle slightly and then directing the needle superiorly into the upper joint space (if one needle was left in place after the initial injection) or by reinserting the needle while the patient is holding the mouth half open. This allows a clearer delineation of the disc, since both its under and upper surfaces are coated by contrast medium.

Technique for Double-Contrast Arthrography

If double-contrast arthrography is to be performed, additional local anesthesia must be used. Instead of puncturing the joint space with a needle, the joint spaces are punctured with catheters (Angiocath 0.8 mm

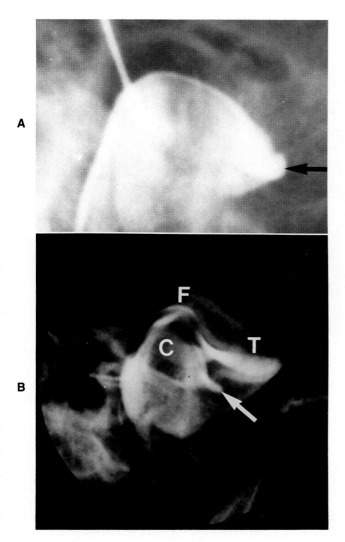

Fig. 4-14   A, Normal TMJ single contrast arthrogram with contrast injection into the lower joint compartment only. The small anterior recess of the lower joint compartment *(arrow)* suggests a normal superior disc position. **B,** Normal TMJ demonstrated by single contrast arthrogram with contrast injection into both upper and lower joint spaces. The condyle *(C)*, fossa *(F)*, and tubercle *(T)* are indicated. The arrow indicates the anterior recess of the lower joint space.

diameter and 25 mm length). The lower joint space may be entered in the same manner as for the single-contrast technique. The upper joint space is cannulated by guiding the cannula along and then into the fossa or along the posterior slope of the articular tubercle.

Correct placement of the catheter into the joint space can be felt when free movement of the catheter occurs without resistance. The inner metal needle is then removed, and the catheter is advanced into the joint space. Contrast medium is injected via the extension

tube that has already been filled with contrast medium. Usually about 0.2 to 0.5 ml is adequate for each joint space. Joint movements are recorded by videofluoroscopy in the same way as for single-contrast arthrography.

After recording the dynamic phase of the study, the outer parts of the catheters are taped to the skin so that they will stay in the proper position in the joint space during the next phase of the examination. After instructing the patient to open and close the jaw, contrast medium is aspirated from the joint spaces, new extension tubes filled with air are connected, and the patient is moved from the fluoroscopic unit to the tomographic unit. We have used a Phillips Polytome unit in which the patient can be placed in an upright position. A specially designed head holder that permits positioning of the patient in the same position for subsequent exposures is also helpful for the examination.

After the patient has been correctly positioned in the tomographic unit, about 1 ml of air is injected into both upper and lower joint spaces simultaneously. The correct amount of air is determined by the resistance to injection, and a different amount may be necessary for different jaw positions. Thus it is usually necessary to use more air at maximum jaw opening than for the closed mouth position. After the air is injected, a hemostat is placed on the extension tubes to prevent backflow of the air. After the examination has been completed, the air is aspirated from the jaw spaces and the catheters are removed.

We use a book cassette with five films, 3 mm apart for simultaneous tomography. In this way one exposure results in five different images representing five different layers of the joint. Use of a book cassette is advantageous because it guarantees that the condylar position is the same in all images, it saves time, and it also minimizes the total radiation dose.

Arthrographic Findings of the Normal TMJ

In a normal TMJ the posterior band of the disc is located superior to the condyle (Fig. 4-15). The lower joint space has a relatively small anterior recess, although studies of normal individuals without symptoms have shown a great variation in the size of this recess despite the disc's being located in the superior position.[56] At maximum opening the disc is located inferior to the articular tubercle, and the condyle articulates with the central thin zone and the posterior part of the disc, as seen in Fig. 4-15.

Abnormal Findings

Displacement of the disc with reduction (Figs. 4-16 and 4-17) and without reduction (Fig. 4-18) are the most frequent pathologic findings in TMJ arthrography. Principally, this means that the posterior thick part

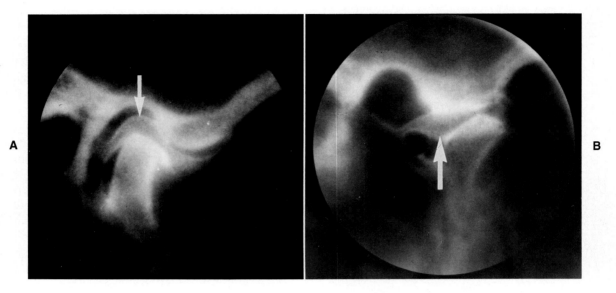

Fig. 4-15 **A,** Normal TMJ with dual space double-contrast arthrotomography in closed mouth position. The posterior band *(arrow)* of the disc is located over the condyle. **B,** Normal TMJ dual-space double-contrast arthrotomography in open mouth position. The posterior band *(arrow)* of the disc is located posterior to the condyle.

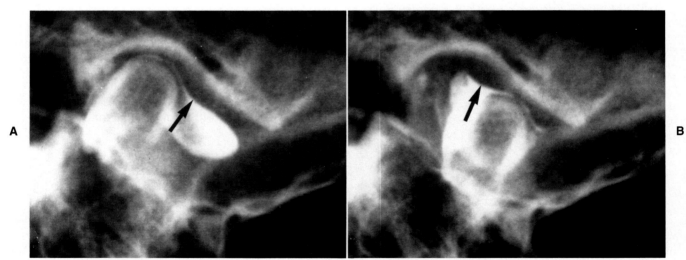

Fig. 4-16 **A,** Anterior disc displacement as demonstrated with single contrast lower compartment arthrography. The posterior band *(arrow)* of the disc is located anterior to the condyle. **B,** Same joint as in **A.** After reduction the disc is in a normal superior position. The posterior band *(arrow)* of the disc is located posterior to the condyle.

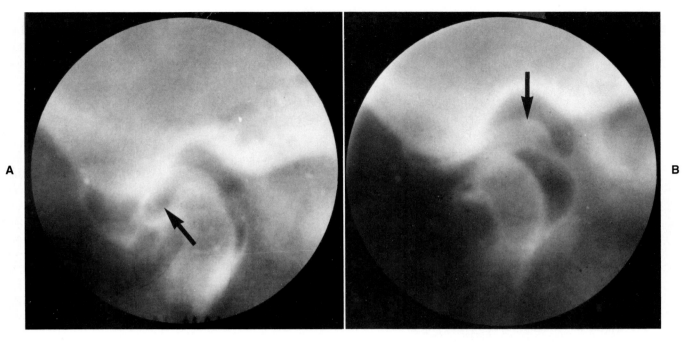

Fig. 4-17 Anterior disc displacement depicted with dual space double-contrast arthro-tomography. **A,** Before reduction the disc *(arrow)* is located anterior to the condyle. **B,** After reduction the disc is located superior to the condyle.

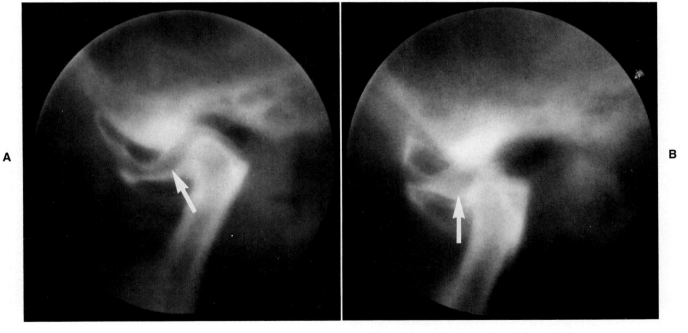

Fig. 4-18 Anterior disc displacement without reduction. In **A,** closed mouth and **B,** maximum mouth opening the disc is located anterior to the condyle. The position of the posterior band is indicated by arrows.

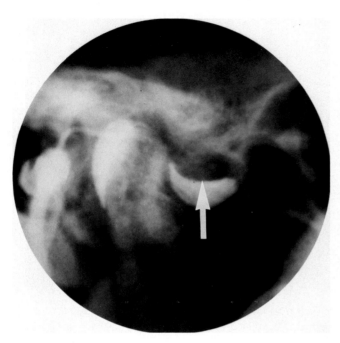

Fig. 4-19 Anterior disc displacement with associated enlargement of the posterior band of the disc *(arrow)*.

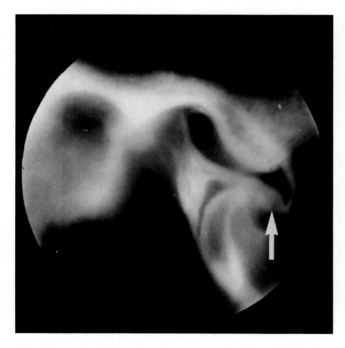

Fig. 4-20 Anterior disc displacement with extensive deformation of the disc. The disc is biconvex *(arrow)*.

(posterior band) of the disc is located anterior to the condyle in the closed mouth position. An arthrographic sign of disc displacement in single-contrast lower compartment arthrography is enlargement of the anterior recess of the lower joint space (Fig. 4-19).

In disc displacement with reduction, the disc is usually biconcave, although there may be some minor enlargement of the posterior band (Fig. 4-17). This corresponds to the early intermediate stage in the classification scheme described by Wilkes.[5] In disc displacement without reduction, a more extensive deformity of the disc is frequently encountered (Fig. 4-20), and this corresponds to the late stage in the same classification scheme.[5] This is consistent with the deformities observed in pathologic specimens, which include thickening and shortening of the anteroposterior dimension of the disc. Perforation of the posterior disc attachment is another sign of late-stage internal derangement. Perforation is indicated by overflow of contrast medium from the lower to the upper joint space. Occasionally, however, the perforation itself can also be demonstrated directly on double-contrast, double-space arthrotomograms.

In rare cases patients with symptoms such as clicking and locking may be suspected to have one or more loose bodies within the joint space.[57] Synovial chondromatosis, osteoarthrosis, or osteochondritis dessicans are the three principal causes of loose bodies in a joint.

Inflammatory arthritis, such as rheumatoid arthritis, is another pathologic entity that may affect the TMJ. However, this is usually diagnosed clinically, and patients with these diseases are rarely seen for TMJ imaging. However, osseous changes associated with rheumatoid arthritis can be clearly demonstrated with tomography.

Complications Following Arthrography

Serious complications after arthrography are rare; no cases of infection following arthrography have been reported. Transient facial nerve palsy may result from extensive injection of local anesthetic agent around the condyle and condylar neck, and the patient may have moderate discomfort for 1 to 2 days after the procedure. The use of nonionic or low-osmolality contrast media has been helpful in reducing the patient's discomfort. It is our experience that most of the major complications occur as a result of inexperience on the part of the physician in performing the examination.

COMPUTED TOMOGRAPHY (CT)

CT scanning of the TMJ can be performed either as direct sagittal scanning[58,59] (Fig. 4-21) or as axial scanning with sagittal reconstructions.[60] Both techniques have been reported to be successful in demonstrating internal derangement and osseous disease.[61-63] How-

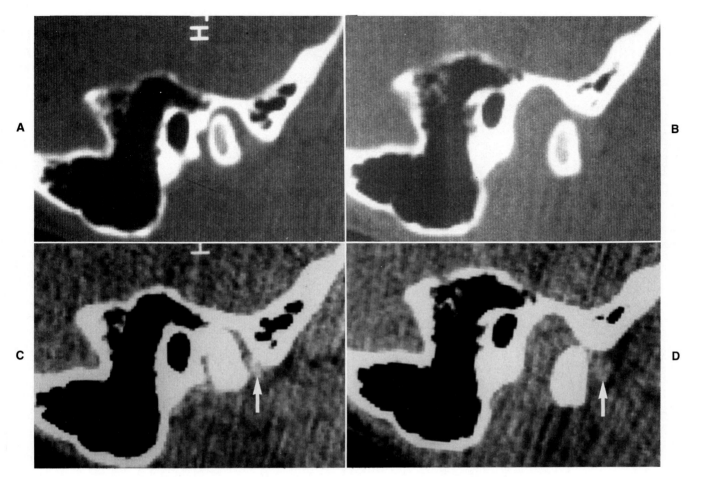

Fig. 4-21 **A,** Direct sagittal CT of TMJ showing posterior condylar position. **B,** Same joint as in **A** obtained at maximal mouth opening showing some limitation of anterior condylar translation. **C,** Same joint as in **A** and **B** with soft tissue setting showing disc *(arrow)* anterior to the condyle. **D,** Same joint as in **A, B,** and **C.** Soft tissue setting at maximal mouth opening showing the disc *(arrow)* anterior to the condyle, suggesting anterior disc displacement without reduction.

ever, the use of CT scanning for diagnosis of soft tissue changes in the TMJ has decreased rapidly during the past few years because of the superiority of magnetic resonance imaging with surface coils. The latter modality has been shown to be superior to CT scanning for imaging the soft tissues of the joint,[64] as illustrated in Fig. 4-22. However, CT scanning still represents the best means of examining the osseous structures of the joint.

The disadvantages common to computed tomography and magnetic resonance imaging are an inability to detect perforations and limitation to static images. Cine CT of the TMJ[65] has been reported but has not gained wide acceptance, partly because of the limited availability of cine CT scanners and the limited soft tissue detail.

Technique for CT Scanning

Direct sagittal CT scanning is preferred over axial acquisitions with sagittal reconstructions, based on our own experience. The design of most CT scanners requires an additional stretcher to position the patient in the direct sagittal CT imaging plane.[58,59] The stretcher is placed laterally at an angle with respect to the scanner table and the scanner gantry. Once the patient is in the correct position in the scanner, scans are performed at 1.5 to 2 mm intervals from the medial to the lateral poles of the condyle. Additional images are then obtained at maximum mouth opening. Coronal images can be obtained from reconstructions of the sagittal image. CT scans are filmed at settings for bone detail and soft tissues, and in this way the need for conventional radiography or tomography is eliminated.

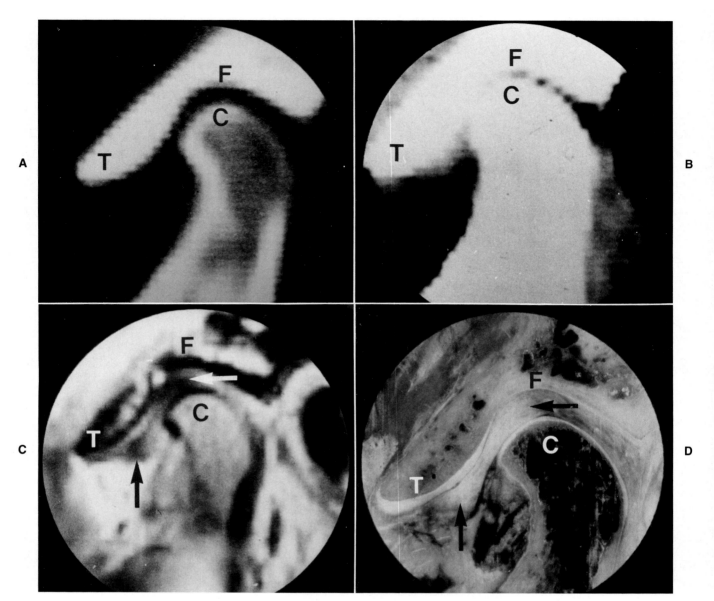

Fig. 4-22   CT in **A,** hard tissue and **B,** soft tissue setting, **C,** MRI, and **D,** corresponding cryosection of TMJ with normal superior disc position. The tubercle *(T),* fossa *(F),* and condyle *(C)* are indicated. The anterior and posterior bands of the disc are indicated by arrows.

CT Findings

When the disc is normal and thus positioned superior to the condyle, it is usually most difficult to visualize directly. Indeed, the inability to see the disc anterior to the condyle and inferior to the tubercle is interpreted as a diagnosis of normal disc position (Fig. 4-22). The lateral pterygoid fat pad is an important landmark used to determine disc displacement. CT scans that can be performed with wide mouth opening usually produce the optimum images of the disc (Fig. 4-23).

When the disc is anteriorly displaced, it appears as a high attenuation mass anterior to the condyle, inferior to the tubercle, and within the low attenuation lateral pterygoid fat pad (Figs. 4-22 and 4-23). The configuration of the disc typically cannot be determined by CT, since the anatomic resolution is not sufficient for this purpose. The depiction of the disc on CT depends on the disc's density and size. Thus if the disc is thin and small, it usually is not possible to demonstrate it on CT, leading to a higher incidence of false-negative diagnoses. On the other hand, if the disc is large, it can be readily demonstrated by CT.

MAGNETIC RESONANCE IMAGING (MRI)

MRI has been used to image the TMJ since 1984, and imaging quality has continuously improved since that time.[1,66-70] A major advantage of MRI over all other radiographic imaging techniques is the absence of radiation to the patient. MRI does not depend on the differences in electron density, but rather on the proton densities, the tissue magnetic relaxation characteristics, and the flow of blood. The physical principles of MRI have been described elsewhere[71-75] and thus are not reviewed here.

The objective of MRI of the TMJ is to document soft and hard tissue abnormalities of the joint and its surrounding structures. The ability of MRI to visualize the soft tissue structures around the joint is another advantage of this modality over arthrography. A comparison of arthrography and MRI of the same joint is shown in Fig. 4-24.

Magnetic Field Strength and Comparison with CT

The most significant characteristic of an MR scanner is probably its magnetic field strength. Scanners with magnetic field strengths from 0.05 up to 2 Tesla are currently in clinical use. Studies that have compared the image quality of scanners with different magnetic field strengths are scarce, and the results are somewhat contradictory. However, a recent study imaged a series of TMJs on two different scanners at 0.3 Tesla versus 1.5 Tesla[76] (Fig. 4-25). A comparison of the images obtained with the two scanners with equal acquisition times is shown in Fig. 4-25. The impression from this study was that the image quality was significantly better using the high-field system as compared to the midfield system when equivalent imaging times were used. The lower image quality of the 0.3 Tesla scanner could be compensated for to some degree by increasing the acquisition time (the number of excitations) by a factor of about 4.[76]

Some principal advantages and disadvantages of MRI as compared to CT are outlined in the box on p. 364. Contraindications for MRI scans are also outlined in the box on p. 364.

Surface Coil and Scanning Technique

The sagittal imaging plane is standard for MRI as for other imaging techniques of the TMJ. An imaging protocol that can be used for a high-field system is shown in Table 4-3. The use of the dual surface coil technique for imaging of left and right TMJs at the same time[77,78] (Fig. 4-26) has been of great value, since the time on the scanner can be significantly shortened for bilateral TMJ imaging. MRI is performed using the body coil as

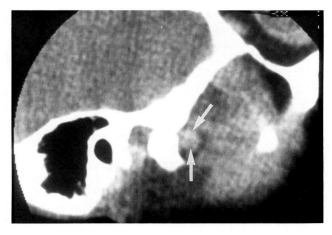

Fig. 4-23 CT scan with soft tissue setting depicting anterior disc displacement without reduction. The image of the disc is indicated by arrows and has a relatively high CT attenuation.

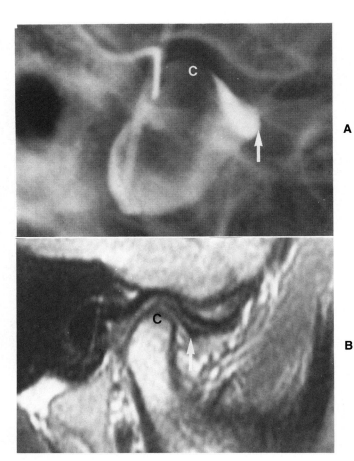

Fig. 4-24 **A,** Arthrogram and **B,** MRI scan on the same TMJ showing normal superior disc position. The anterior recess of the lower joint compartment is indicated by an arrow in the arthrogram and the anterior band of the disc is indicated by an arrow in the MRI scan. The condyle *(C)* is noted in both studies.

<table>
<tr><td colspan="2">

ADVANTAGES AND DISADVANTAGES OF MRI COMPARED TO CT

</td></tr>
<tr><td>Advantages</td><td>No ionizing radiation
Fewer artifacts from dense bone and metal clips
Imaging possible in several planes without moving the patient
Superior anatomic detail of soft tissues</td></tr>
<tr><td>Disadvantages</td><td>High initial cost of the scanner
Special site planning and shielding
Patient claustrophobia in magnet
Inferior image of hard tissues</td></tr>
</table>

<table>
<tr><td colspan="2">

CONTRAINDICATIONS FOR MRI

</td></tr>
<tr><td>Absolute</td><td>Patients with cerebral aneurysm clips
Patients with cardiac pacemakers</td></tr>
<tr><td>Relative</td><td>Claustrophobic or uncooperative patients
Pregnant patients
Metallic prosthetic heart valves
Ferromagnetic foreign bodies in critical locations (e.g., eye)
Implanted stimulator wires for pain control</td></tr>
<tr><td>No contraindications</td><td>Metallic prostheses
Orthodontic fixed appliances</td></tr>
</table>

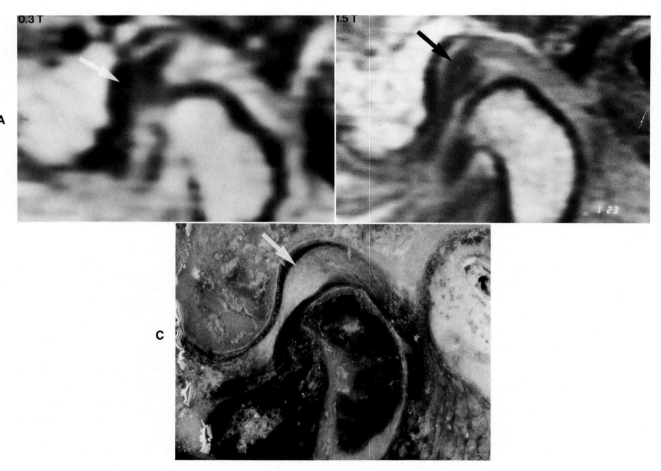

Fig. 4-25 MRI scan in **A,** 0.3 Tesla, **B,** 1.5 Tesla, and **C,** corresponding cryosection showing normal superior disc position *(arrow)*. Image quality of 1.5 Tesla scanner is superior to that of 0.3 Tesla scanner when comparable imaging times are used.

Table 4-3 Scanning parameters for MRI

Image*	Scanning time
Axial localizer	52 sec
TR = 400	
NEX = 1	
256 × 128 matrix	
Corrected sagittal	
(closed jaw)	4 min, 19 sec
(open jaw)	2 min, 21 sec
TR = 1,000	
NEX = 2 (closed jaw)	
NEX = 1 (open jaw)	
256 × 128 matrix	
Corrected coronal	
(closed jaw)	2 min, 21 sec
(open jaw)	2 min, 21 sec
TR = 1,000	
NEX = 1	
256 × 128 matrix	

If a splint is provided by the clinician, additional corrected sagittal scans may be performed with the splint in place. In this case the open coronal scans are replaced by corrected coronal scans with the splint in place.
Total scanning time for complete bilateral TMJ examination is 14 to 17 minutes. Table time is approximately 40 minutes.

*TE for all pulse sequences = 20 msec. Slice thickness = 3 mm, 0.5 mm between slices.

the transmitter and the two 6.5 cm circular surface coils as the receivers. The patient is placed supine in the magnet, and the surface coils are located lateral to the TMJs (Fig. 4-26). Closed and open mouth images in the sagittal and coronal planes are obtained. For acquisition of imaging in the closed mouth position, two excitations are usually needed to get excellent anatomic detail of the disc per se. For all other images one excitation is usually sufficient to determine disc position (Table 4-3). If the patient's oral splint is to be assessed, additional sagittal images are obtained with the splint in place. In this case the open jaw coronal scans are replaced by coronal scans with the splint in place. Syringes of variable sizes or commercially available bite block devices are used to stabilize the patient's jaw in the open mouth positions (Fig. 4-26).

The coronal images are helpful in identifying medial and lateral displacements of the disc. Additionally, the osseous anatomy of the condyle can sometimes be better visualized in the coronal plane.

The relative value of T_1- versus T_2-weighted images is not well established. The disc has a low signal intensity at all pulse sequences, and the lateral pterygoid fat pad has high signal intensity on T_1- and proton-weighted sequences. The need to document edema in the tissues behind the disc or fluid in the joint spaces may require T_2-weighted images[5,67,79,80] (Fig. 4-27).

MRI Findings of the Normal TMJ

The normal TMJ as demonstrated by MRI in the sagittal and coronal planes is shown in Fig. 4-28. In the sagittal plane the disc is biconcave with the posterior

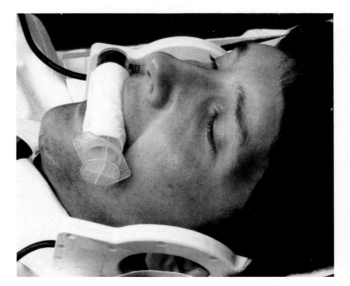

Fig. 4-26 Clinical positioning with dual surface coils and syringe between upper and lower teeth used as bite block.

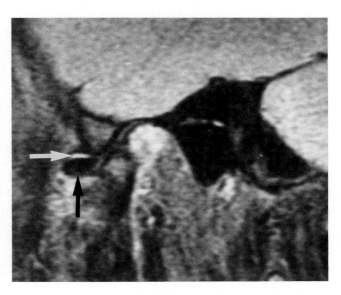

Fig. 4-27 T_2-weighted MRI showing joint effusion in the anterior part of the upper joint space *(white arrow)*. The position of the anteriorly displaced disc *(black arrow)* is also indicated.

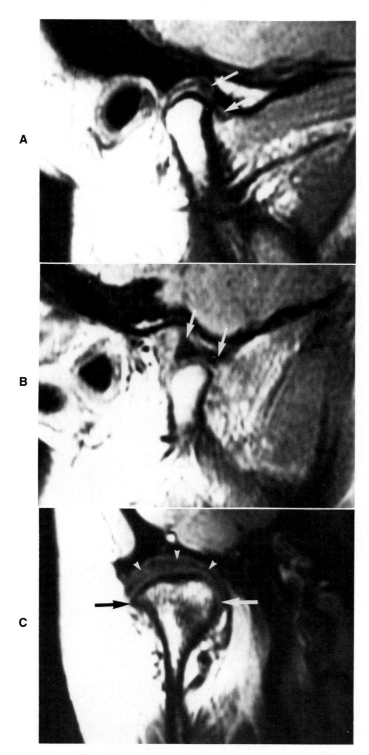

Fig. 4-28   **A,** MRI scan of normal TMJ with jaw closed. The posterior and anterior bands of the disc are indicated by arrows. **B,** Normal TMJ at three quarter open mouth. The disc is indicated by arrows. **C,** Normal TMJ in coronal MRI scan. The medial and lateral poles of the condyle are indicated by large arrows. The crescent shaped disc is indicated by arrowheads.

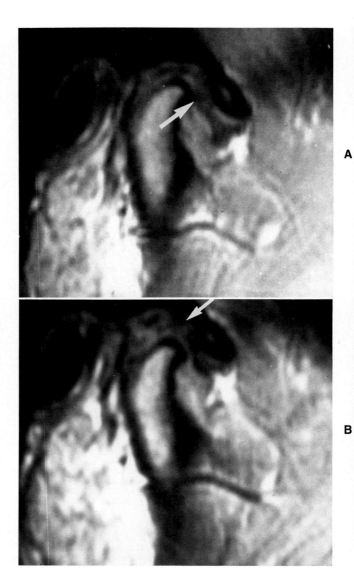

Fig. 4-29   **A,** The posterior band of the displaced disc is indicated by an arrow. **B,** Same joint as in **A** after reduction of the disc *(arrow)* to normal superior position with jaw opening.

thick part (posterior band) lying over the condyle. Because the fibrous connective tissue of the disc has a low signal intensity, the disc usually can be distinguished from the surrounding tissues, which have a higher signal intensity. The cortices of both the condylar and temporal components of the joint have a low signal intensity, but the articular coverings of the joint have a higher signal intensity. This makes the outline of the osseous components easily visible. The posterior disc attachment has a relatively high signal intensity compared to the posterior portion of the disc itself because of the fatty tissue in the posterior disc attachment. MRI is the only modality that can actually allow the disc to be distinguished from its posterior attachment.

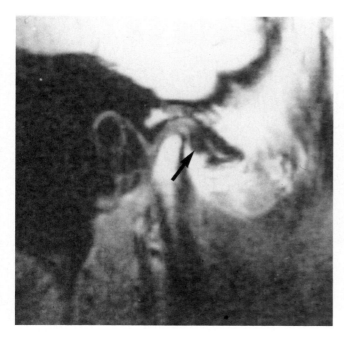

Fig. 4-30   MRI scan of TMJ depicting anterior disc displacement. The posterior band *(arrow)* is slightly enlarged and located anterior to the condyle.

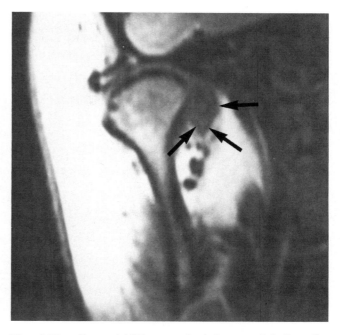

Fig. 4-31   Coronal MRI scan depicting medial disc displacement. The position of the displaced disc is indicated by arrows.

In the MRI scans obtained at maximum mouth opening, the central thin zone of the disc is visualized between the condyle and the tubercle (Fig. 4-28, *B*). The posterior band of the disc articulates against the posterior surface of the condyle, as has been demonstrated in anatomic specimens (Fig. 4-3).

In the coronal plane (Fig. 4-28, *C*) the disc has a crescent appearance. The medial aspect of the disc is attached to the medial pole of the condyle and to the medial capsule. The lateral part of the disc is attached to the lateral pole of the condyle and to the lateral capsule (Fig. 4-28, *C*).

Abnormal Findings

Displacements of the disc in the anterior (Fig. 4-29), anteromedial, or anterolateral directions are the most common findings observed when interpreting MR images from patients with clinical signs and symptoms of internal derangement. In the sagittal plane the disc is noted to be displaced when its posterior band is anterior to the condyle (Fig. 4-30). Most commonly, however, the disc is also displaced slightly medially. This is noted in the coronal images as a medial location of the disc off the top of the condyle (Fig. 4-31). When the disc is displaced medially or laterally in combination with an anterior displacement, this is called a rotational displacement.[7] A pure lateral displacement (Fig. 4-32) or a pure medial displacement is called sideways displacement[7] (see box on p. 352).

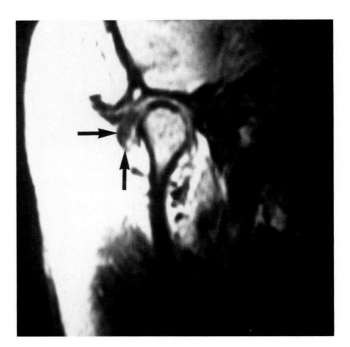

Fig. 4-32   Coronal MRI scan depicting lateral disc displacement *(arrows)*.

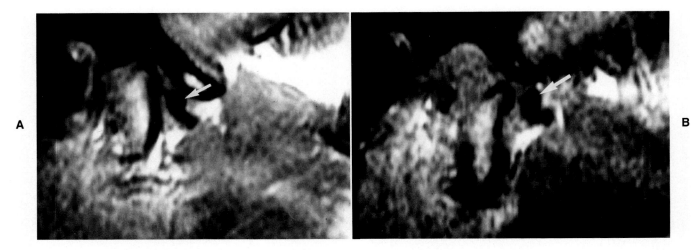

Fig. 4-33   Sagittal MRI scans showing anterior disc displacement without reduction. The disc *(arrow)* is located anterior to the condyle in **A,** the closed mouth position as well as in **B,** maximal mouth opening. At maximal mouth opening the disc is folding.

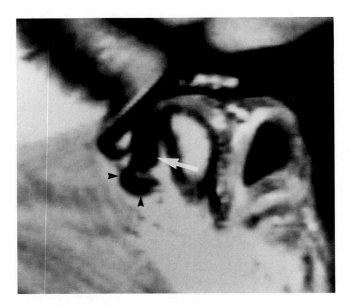

Fig. 4-34   MRI scan showing anterior displacement and deformation of disc. The posterior band *(arrow)* of the disc is enlarged and the anterior part is folded downwards *(arrow heads).*

MRI scans obtained at maximum mouth opening determine whether the disc displacement occurs with or without reduction. In displacement with reduction (Fig. 4-29), the position of the disc normalizes during jaw opening. In displacement without reduction (Fig. 4-33), the disc remains anterior to the condyle in all mandibular positions. Coronal imaging acquired at the open mouth position may demonstrate whether the medially or laterally displaced disc also reduces to a normal superior position in this anatomic plane.

Deformity of the disc resulting from chronic displacement can usually be demonstrated by MRI scans (Fig. 4-34). MRI clearly shows the characteristic signs of disc deformations such as enlargement of the posterior band (Fig. 4-34) and the biconvex shape. Late-stage degenerative joint disease with extensive hard and soft tissue changes can also be demonstrated exquisitely by MRI (Fig. 4-35). As previously mentioned, the inability to depict perforation and the limitation to static images are disadvantage of MRI (see box on p. 364). However, recent attempts with gradient-recalled acquisition in the steady state (GRASS) show promise in depicting the sequential positioning of the disc during incremental opening and closing movements.

A series of recent reports[79,80] has suggested that MRI of the TMJ may have the potential to provide information about the status of the bone marrow of the mandibular condyle. If the central marrow-containing area of the condyle (Fig. 4-36) has low signal (rather than the normal high signal of marrow fat on T_1-weighted images), it has been thought to be a sign of avascular necrosis of the condyle.[79] More research is needed, however, to clarify the pathophysiology of the alterations of the signal intensity of the mandibular condyle with correlation to histology before it is known what the reduced signal intensity of the bone marrow actually represents. It is clear that MRI is an exciting modality that allows further insights into the biology of the bone marrow of the mandibular condyle. This type of information currently is not possible with other imaging modalities.

A paper on MRI of the muscles of mastication[81] reported that abnormalities of the masticatory

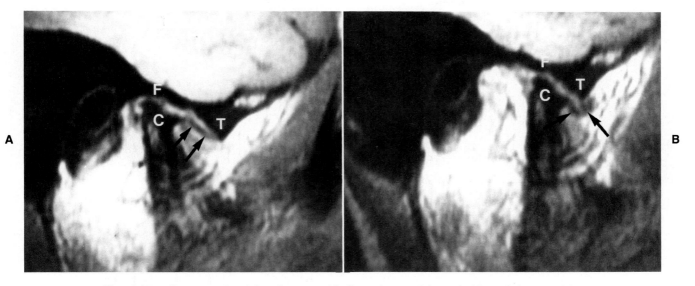

Fig. 4-35   Degenerative joint disease with flattening and irregularities of the condyle and temporal component in **A,** closed and **B,** open mouth position. The condyle *(C),* fossa *(F),* and tubercle *(T)* are indicated. The remaining part of the disc *(arrows)* is anterior to the condyle and folding at maximal mouth opening.

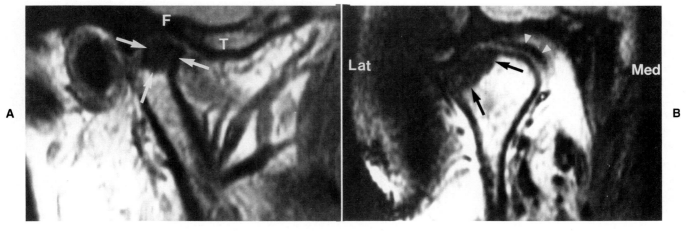

Fig. 4-36   **A,** Sagittal MRI scan showing decreased signal from the bone marrow in the upper part of the mandibular condyle *(arrows).* The fossa *(F)* and tubercle *(T)* are indicated. **B,** Coronal MRI scan of the same joint as in **A** showing the low signal intensity area *(arrows)* in the lateral part of the joint. In the medial part of the condyle the disc is seen superior to the condyle *(arrow heads)* and laterally the disc is absent, suggesting perforation.

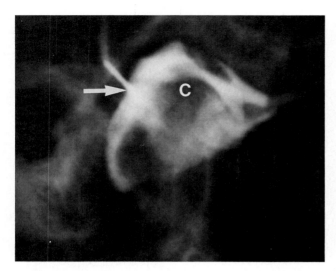

Fig. 4-37 Postsurgical arthrogram. Contrast medium was injected into the lower joint space *(arrow)* and there is a perforation to the upper joint space. Peripheral adhesions make the joint space smaller than normal. A disc plication had been performed two years before this arthrogram.

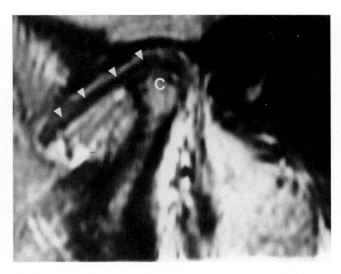

Fig. 4-38 MRI scan of TMJ with proplast teflon implant *(arrowheads)* in good position without extensive granulation tissue surrounding the implant. The condyle *(C)* is indicated.

muscles such as fatty replacement, fibrosis, and muscle contracture may accompany internal derangements. These alterations are relatively infrequent, but the possibility of depicting them, as well as alterations in related structures, represents another exciting potential for MRI.

IMAGING AFTER TREATMENT

Imaging after surgical treatment is indicated in patients who continue to have symptoms that might be related to intraarticular pathology such as recurrence of disc displacement, intraarticular adhesions, or inflammatory changes.

Before the availability of MRI as an imaging modality, plain films, tomography, and arthrography were used for this purpose. However, arthrography can be difficult to perform in surgically treated patients, since the anatomy is altered and the joint spaces are narrowed as a result of peripheral or intraarticular adhesions (Fig. 4-37). For this reason MRI is a preferable method of examination for postoperative complications.[1,82,83]

Postoperative MRI is helpful in confirming whether surgical treatment corrected the displaced disc and in understanding the nature of postoperative surgical failures. MRI is also a modality for imaging patients with surgical alloplastic disc implants. An example of a postsurgical MR image of a proplast Teflon implant in good position without extensive soft tissue granulation is seen in Fig. 4-38. MRI is valuable for distinguishing intraarticular pain from extraarticular pain after surgery in patients with implants. An example of a patient with

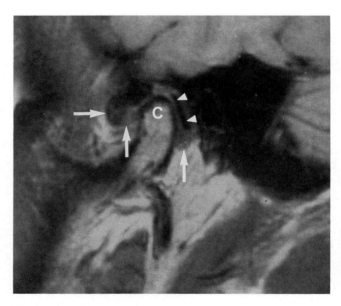

Fig. 4-39 Sagittal MRI scan of TMJ with displaced implant *(arrowheads)*. The implant is located posterior to the condyle and surrounded by granulation tissue *(arrow)*. There is also granulation tissue anterior to the condyle *(arrows)*.

an implant and granulation tissue around the implant is shown in Fig. 4-39. The Teflon proplast implant is correctly located within the mandibular fossa but is associated with a considerable amount of granulation tissue and osseous deformities.

For the patient with an alloplastic implant, CT scan-

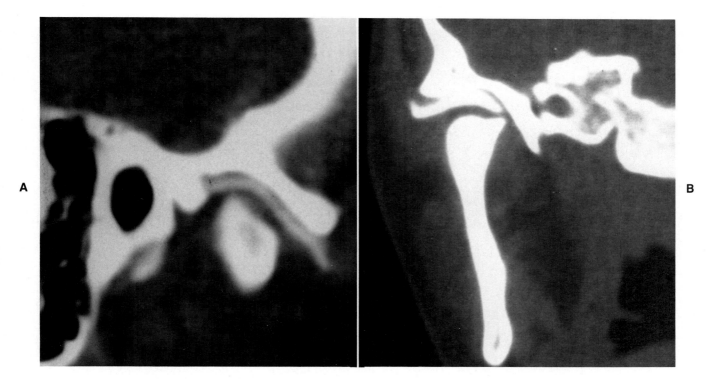

Fig. 4-40 CT scan in **A,** sagittal and **B,** coronal planes showing implant in good position.

ning represents an alternative postoperative imaging modality as long as a nonmetallic implant is used (Fig. 4-40). When erosions and osteolytic changes are suspected, CT scanning is well suited to demonstrate these changes. It should be mentioned, however, that the erosions of the bone usually are the result of granulation and inflammation in the soft tissues, changes that might be detected earlier by MRI. MRI with intravenous paramagnetic contrast medium might be a way to improve the differentiation between postoperative inflammation, granulation tissue, and fibrous scar tissue.

Arthrography after discectomy has been a valuable tool in the understanding of postdiscectomy remodeling of the joint. It has been reported that radiographically a distance is maintained between the condyle and the glenoid fossa even though the disc has been removed.[84] Arthrography has demonstrated that this distance between the mandibular condyle and the glenoid fossa is filled with thickened soft tissues that cover both the temporal component and the mandibular condyle.[84] However, arthrography is limited to the detection of intraarticular alterations or remodeling. If the changes occur outside the joint capsule, arthrography will not demonstrate them. Thus MRI is preferred in most patients after surgery or treatment. An example of fibrosis occuring in the lateral capsular wall after surgery as seen with MRI is shown in Fig. 4-41.

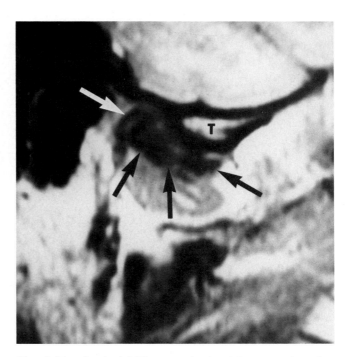

Fig. 4-41 Sagittal MRI scan obtained 2 years after disc plication surgery showing scar tissue formation *(arrows)* in the lateral capsule wall. The tubercle is shown by *(T).*

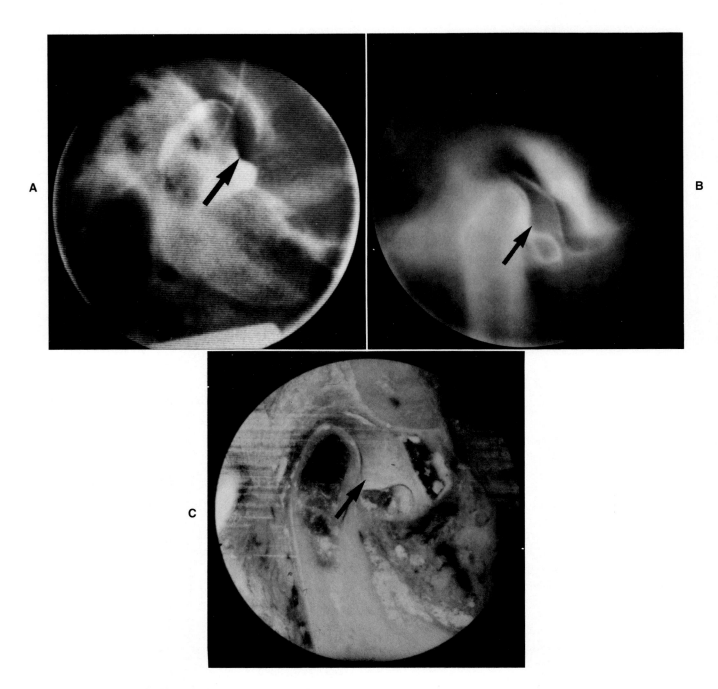

Fig. 4-42 **A,** Single space and **B,** dual space double-contrast arthrotomography, and **C,** corresponding cryosection of TMJ with anterior disc displacement. The location of the posterior band is indicated by arrows.

Table 4-4 Accuracy of different forms of imaging based on several anatomic studies[10, 64, 76, 86, 87]

Study number	Imaging modality	Number joints	Disc position	Disc configuration	Perforation
1	Single-contrast arthrography	58	84%	N/A	97%
2	Dual space, double-contrast arthrotomography	48	92%	92%	100%
	Computed tomography	15	67%	N/A	N/A
3	Magnetic resonance imaging	15	73%	60%	N/A
4	Magnetic resonance imaging	39	85%	N/A	N/A

Arthrography has been used as a research tool to gather information about the postsurgical status of joints operated on for disc repositioning.[85] The arthrograms obtained after disc repositioning surgery are difficult to interpret,[85] and Bronstein's study[85] was not able to state conclusively whether this type of surgery was successful in repositioning the displaced disc.

ACCURACY OF ARTHROGRAPHY, CT, AND MRI

Knowing the diagnostic accuracy of an imaging modality is essential for the clinical users of each method. The accuracy of arthrography, CT, and MRI has been investigated in several studies on fresh autopsy material.[10,64,86-88] All techniques have demonstrated a relatively high accuracy in determining disc position (Table 4-4). A comparison between single- and double-contrast arthrography obtained in the same joint is shown in Fig. 4-42. It is clear that dual space, double-contrast arthrotomography demonstrates the configuration of the disc better than the single-contrast lower joint space technique. However, the accuracy of determining displacement of the disc is similar (Table 4-4).

The accuracies noted in Table 4-4 are from investigations performed without the biases of clinical work. However, the figures are relevant for the comparison between the different techniques, since the studies were performed under the same conditions. In a clinical situation, however, additional information about the patient is available that might help in improving the capability of interpreting the images. Therefore it is reasonable to say that these figures represent a good estimate of the accuracy of these techniques. The multiplanar imaging capability of MRI may provide even greater accuracy rates, however. This can be obtained by avoiding false negative diagnosis of medially or laterally displaced discs.

RADIONUCLIDE IMAGING

Studies[89,90] have suggested that radionuclide imaging of the TMJ (Fig. 4-43) using conventional skeletal imag-

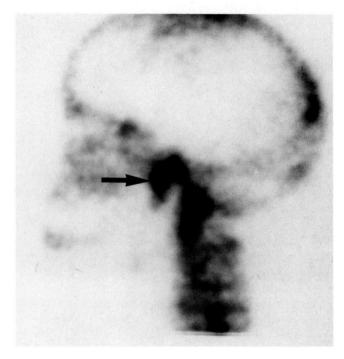

Fig. 4-43 Radionuclide imaging of patient with condylar hyperplasia of left TMJ *(arrow)*.

ing techniques may be a valuable screening test for osseous disease. The technique can be performed easily, and the radiation dose to the patient is low.[1] An advantage of the technique is that conditions outside the joint may also be easily detected.

MISCELLANEOUS CONDITIONS AND DIFFERENTIAL DIAGNOSIS

The main purpose of imaging is to help the clinician determine whether or not there is an intraarticular source for the clinical symptoms. In this context it is important to distinguish patients with intraarticular disorders from those who have other causes of their symptoms. In this chapter we have concentrated our presentation on the radiographic diagnosis of internal derange-

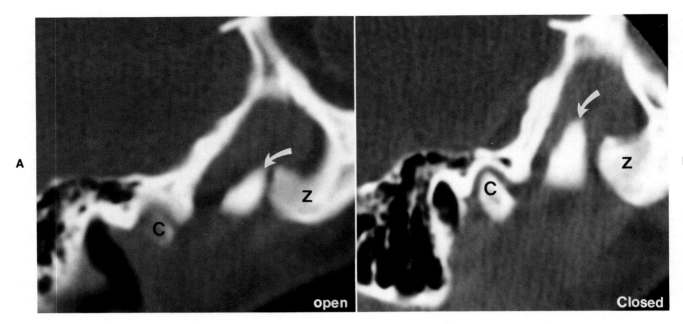

Fig. 4-44 Coronoid hyperplasia restricting mouth opening. Direct sagittal CT scan at **A** and **B,** opened and closed mouth positions showing the elongated coronoid process *(arrows)* to interfere with the zygomatic process *(z)* of the maxilla at the open mouth position. The condyle *(C)* is in the glenoid fossa.

ment and related conditions. This is our primary focus since the most common radiographic findings in patients presenting with symptoms of TMJ disorders are different manifestations of internal derangement and the related arthrosis. Occasionally, however, there are other causes of TMJ pain and limitation of jaw opening, and it is important that imaging clearly depicts the components of these changes.

Hyperplasia or elongation of the coronoid process of the mandible can mimic TMJ internal derangement. This condition has been extensively described[91-93] and a recent study indicates that elongation of the coronoid process may occur in up to 5% of patients with TMJ symptoms.[92] If the coronoid process is significantly elongated, it can impact physically on the zygomatic process of the maxilla, thus causing limitation of jaw opening. CT scanning in the axial and plane acquired at closed and open mouthed positions is a valuable imaging strategy for patients with clinical suspicion of coronoid hyperplasia. The mechanical limitation of jaw opening can be demonstrated in conjunction with coronoid impression on the maxilla (Fig. 4-44).

Another uncommon diagnosis in patients presenting with symptoms of TMJ disorders is enlargement of the condyle and condylar neck due to idiopathic hyperplasia or tumor of the mandibular condyle (Fig. 4-45). An example of a patient with osteochondroma of the mandibular condyle is seen in Fig. 4-45. The imaging modality of choice for this condition is MRI in sagittal and coronal planes. CT scans may be supplementary in these cases to more precisely delineate the extension of the tumor and its relation to anatomic structures medial to the TMJ region. The specific diagnosis between condylar hyperplasia and osteochondroma is difficult and the final assessment is often by histologic examination.

Other, more remote differential diagnostic considerations in patients with symptoms mimicking TMJ disorders should include tumors in the head and neck region that may affect the innervation of the muscles of mastication, resulting in facial pain and limitation of opening.

IMAGING STRATEGY AND CLINICAL CONSIDERATIONS

An imaging strategy for patients with symptoms of temporomandibular joint disorders is presented in the accompanying box.

IMAGING STRATEGY

I. Initial imaging of osseous structures: Plain film or panoramic radiography
II. Soft tissue imaging:
  1. MRI is the first choice
  2. Arthrography is the second choice if MRI is not available or if joint dynamic is of primary concern
  3. CT is the third choice if MRI or arthrography is not available or if the osseous components of the joint are of primary concern

---

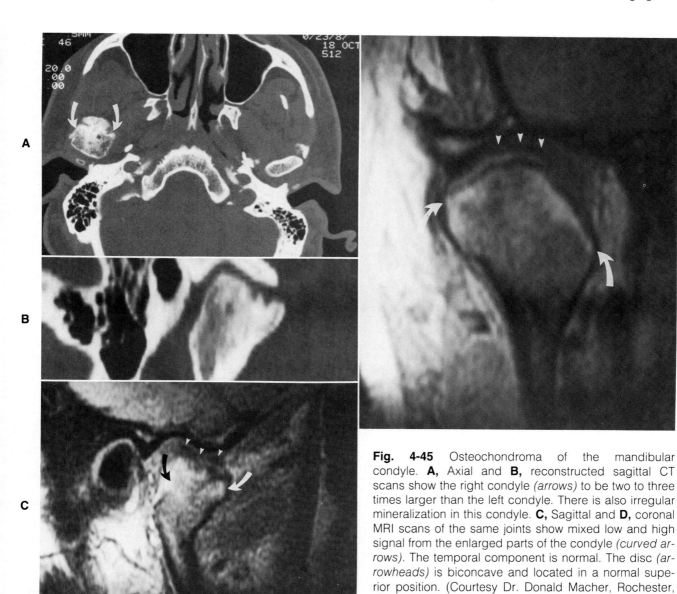

Fig. 4-45 Osteochondroma of the mandibular condyle. **A,** Axial and **B,** reconstructed sagittal CT scans show the right condyle *(arrows)* to be two to three times larger than the left condyle. There is also irregular mineralization in this condyle. **C,** Sagittal and **D,** coronal MRI scans of the same joints show mixed low and high signal from the enlarged parts of the condyle *(curved arrows)*. The temporal component is normal. The disc *(arrowheads)* is biconcave and located in a normal superior position. (Courtesy Dr. Donald Macher, Rochester, N.Y.)

1. The first step in imaging a patient with TMJ pain and dysfunction might be a plain film or a panoramic radiograph. If greater detail is necessary, tomography should be performed. However, these images are not diagnostic for internal derangement, and a negative study does not rule out the possibility of some pathologic change in the joint.

2. The most important radiographic objective should be soft tissue imaging. Studies have shown that CT is inferior to MRI in the detection of soft tissue abnormalities, and therefore CT does not represent a competitive modality. The capability of multiplanar imaging, the relatively high frequency of medial and lateral disc displacements, the absence of radiation, and the ease of imaging are all factors that should direct the radiologist's decision toward MRI instead of arthrography. For postsurgical or posttreatment imaging, MRI is definitely the modality of choice.

3. If altered dynamics are of primary concern, with regard to the patient's symptoms, arthrography is the procedure of choice. Arthrography can clearly depict the dynamics of the joint, and the correct mandibular position can be established for the initiation of protrusive splint therapy.

4. If MRI is not available, arthrography is the best alternative imaging technique.

5. CT scanning should be considered when MRI or arthrography are not available or when the osseous components of the joint are of primary concern.

REFERENCES

1. Katzberg RW: Temporomandibular joint imaging, Radiology 170:297, 1989.
2. Adams JC: Outline of orthopedics, ed 9, London, 1981, Churchill Livingstone, p 61.
3. Katzberg RW et al: Arthrotomography of the temporomandibular joint, AJR 134:995, 1980.
4. Westesson P-L: Double-contrast arthrography and internal derangement of the temporomandibular joint, Swed Dent J Suppl 13:1, 1982.
5. Wilkes CH: Internal derangements of the temporomandibular joint, Arch Otolaryngol 115:469, 1989.
6. Westesson P-L, Bronstein SL, and Liedberg J: Internal derangement of the temporomandibular joint: morphologic description with correlation to function, Oral Surg Oral Med Oral Pathol 59:323, 1985.
7. Katzberg RW et al: Temporomandibular joint: magnetic resonance assessment of rotational and sideways disc displacements, Radiology 169:741, 1988.
8. Liedberg J and Westesson P-L: Sideways position of the temporomandibular joint disk: coronal cryosectioning of fresh autopsy specimens, Oral Surg Oral Med Oral Pathol 66:644, 1988.
9. Liedberg J, Westesson P-L, and Kurita K: Sideways and rotational displacement of the temporomandibular joint disk: diagnosis by arthrography and correlation to cryosectional morphology, Oral Surg Oral Med Oral Pathol (in press).
10. Westesson P-L et al: Temporomandibular joint: comparison of MR images with cryosectional anatomy, Radiology 164:59, 1987.
11. Ireland VE: The problem of the "clicking jaw," Proc R Soc Med 44:363, 1951.
12. Isberg-Holm AM and Westesson P-L: Movement of disc and condyle in temporomandibular joints with clicking: an arthrographic and cineradiographic study on autopsy specimens, Acta Odontol Scand 40:153, 1982.
13. Isberg-Holm AM and Westesson P-L: Movement of disc and condyle in temporomandibular joints with and without clicking: a high speed cinematographic and dissection study on autopsy specimens, Acta Odontol Scand 40:167, 1982.
14. Eriksson L and Westesson P-L: Clinical and radiological study of patients with anterior disc displacement of the temporomandibular joint, Swed Dent J 7:55, 1983.
15. Bessette RW et al: Diagnosis and reconstruction of the human temporomandibular joint after trauma or internal derangement, Plast Reconstr Surg 75:192, 1985.
16. Kurita K et al: Histologic features of the temporomandibular joint disk and posterior disk attachment: comparison of symptom-free persons with normally positioned disks and patients with internal derangement, Oral Surg Oral Med Oral Pathol 67:635, 1989.
17. Blaustein DI and Scapino RP: Remodelling of the temporomandibular joint disk and posterior attachment in disk displacement specimens in relation to glycosaminoglycan content, Oral Surg Oral Med Oral Pathol 78:756, 1986.
18. Isberg AM and Isacsson G: Tissue reactions associated with internal derangement of the temporomandibular joint: a radiographic, cryomorphologic, and histologic study, Acta Odontol Scand 44:159, 1986.
19. Westesson P-L: Double-contrast arthrotomography of the temporomandibular joint: introduction of an arthrographic technique for visualization of the disc and articular surfaces, J Oral Maxillofac Surg 41:163, 1983.
20. Westesson P-L and Rohlin M: Internal derangement related to osteoarthrosis in temporomandibular joint autopsy specimens, Oral Surg Oral Med Oral Pathol 57:17, 1984.
21. Westesson P-L: Structural hard-tissue changes in temporomandibular joints with internal derangement, Oral Surg Oral Med Oral Pathol 59:435, 1985.
22. Roberts CA et al: Mandibular range of motion versus arthrographic diagnosis of the temporomandibular joint, Oral Surg Oral Med Oral Pathol 60:244, 1985.
23. Roberts CA et al: Chemical and arthrographic evaluation of temporomandibular joint sounds, Oral Surg Oral Med Oral Pathol 62:373, 1986.
24. Roberts CA et al: Comparison of internal derangements of the TMJ to occlusal findings, Oral Surg Oral Med Oral Pathol 63:645, 1987.
25. Roberts CA et al: Clinical and arthrographic evaluation of the location of TMJ pain, Oral Surg Oral Med Oral Pathol 64:1, 6, 1987.
26. Roberts CA et al: Comparison of arthrographic findings of the temporomandibular joint with palpitation of the muscles of mastication, Oral Surg Oral Med Oral Pathol 64:3, 275, 1987.
27. Anderson GC et al: Clinical vs. arthrographic diagnosis of TMJ internal derangement, J Dent Res 68:826, 1989.
28. Oberg T, Carlsson GE, and Fajers CM: The temporomandibular joint: a morphologic study of human autopsy material, Acta Odontal Scand 29:349, 1971.
29. McCabe JB, Keller SE, and Moffet BC: A new radiographic technique for diagnosing temporomandibular joint disorders, J Dent Res 38:663, 1959.
30. Omnell K-A and Peterson A: Radiography of the temporomandibular joint utilizing oblique lateral transcranial projections: comparison of information obtained with standardized technique and individualized technique, Odontol Rev 26:77, 1976.
31. Nørgaard F: Artografi av kaebeleddet. Preliminary report, Acta Radiol 25:679, 1944.
32. Nørgaard F: Temporomandibular arthrography. Thesis. Copenhagen Munksgaard, 1947.
33. Wilkes CH: Arthrography of the temporomandibular joint in patients with the TMJ pain-dysfunction syndrome, Minn Med 61:645, 1978.
34. Wilkes CH: Structural and functional alterations of the temporomandibular joint, Northwest Dent 57:287, 1978.
35. Farrar WB and McCarthy WL: Inferior joint space arthrography and characteristics of condylar paths in internal derangements of the TMJ, J Prosthet Dent 41:548, 1979.
36. Katzberg RW et al: Arthrotomography of the temporomandibular joint: new technique and preliminary observations, AJR 132:949, 1979.
37. Annadale T: Displacement of the inter-articular cartilage of the lower jaw, and its treatment by operation, Lancet 1:411, 1987.
38. Pringle JH: Displacement of the mandibular meniscus and its treatment, Br J Surg 6:385, 1918.
39. Burman M and Sinberg SE: Condylar movement in the study of internal derangement of the temporomandibular joint, J Bone Joint Surg (Br) 28:351, 1946.
40. Silver CM, Simon SD, and Savastano AA: Meniscus injuries of the temporomandibular joint, J Bone Joint Surg (Am) 38A:541, 1956.
41. Farrar WB: Diagnosis and treatment of anterior dislocation of the articular disc, NY J Dent 41:348, 1971.

42. Bell KA and Walters PJ: Videofluoroscopy during arthrography of the temporomandibular joint, Radiology 147:879, 1983.

43. Farrar WB and McCarty WL Jr: Inferior joint space arthrography and characteristics of condylar paths in internal derangements of the TMJ, J Prosthet Dent 41:458, 1979.

44. Dolwick MF and Riggs RR: Diagnosis and treatment of internal derangements of the temporomandibular joint, Dent Clin North Am 27:561, 1983.

45. Lundh H et al: Anterior repositioning splint in the treatment of temporomandibular joints with reciprocal clicking: comparison with a flat occlusal splint and an untreated control group, Oral Surg Oral Med Oral Pathol 60:131, 1985.

46. McCarty WL and Farrar WB: Surgery for internal derangements of the temporomandibular joint, J Prosthet Dent 42:191, 1979.

47. McCarty WL: Surgery. In Farrar WB and McCarthy WL, editors: A clinical outline of temporomandibular joint diagnosis and treatment, ed 7, Montgomery, Ala, 1982, Normandie Publications.

48. Campbell W: Clinical radiological investigations of the mandibular joints, Br J Radiol 38:401, 1965.

49. Frenkel G: Untersuchungen mit der Kombination Arthrographie und Tomographie zur darstellung des Discus articulares des Menschen: Dtsch Zahnarztl Z 20:1261, 1965.

50. Arnaudow M, Haage H, and Pflaum I: Die Doppelkontrastarthrographie des Kiefergelenkes, Dtsch Zahnarztl Z 23:390, 1968.

51. Arnaudow M and Pflaum I: Neue Erkenntnisse in der beurteilung bei der Kiefergelenktomographie, Dtsch Zahnarztl Z 29:554, 1974.

52. Westesson P-L, Omnell K-A, and Rohlin M: Double-contrast tomography of the temporomandibular joint: a new technique based on autopsy specimen examinations, Acta Radiol (Diagn Stock) 21:777, 1980.

53. Westesson P-L: Arthrography of the temporomandibular joint, J Prosthet Dent 51:163, 1984.

54. Manzione JV et al: Internal derangement of the temporomandibular joint: diagnosis by direct sagittal computed tomography, Radiology 150:111, 1984.

55. Tallents RH et al: Arthrographically assisted splint therapy, J Prosthet Dent 53:235, 1985.

56. Westesson P-L, Eriksson L, and Kurita K: Temporomandibular joint: variation of normal arthrographic anatomy, Oral Surg Oral Med Oral Pathol (in press).

57. Anderson QN and Katzberg RW: Loose bodies of the temporomandibular joint: arthrographic diagnosis, Skeletal Radiol 11:42, 1984.

58. Manzione JV et al: Direct sagittal computed tomography of the temporomandibular joint, AJNR 3:677, 1982.

59. Manzione JV et al: Internal derangement of the temporomandibular joint: diagnosis by direct sagittal computed tomography, Radiology 150:111, 1984.

60. Helms CA et al: Computed tomography of the meniscus of the temporomandibular joint: preliminary observations, Radiology 145:719, 1982.

61. Sartoris DJ, Neumann CH, and Riley RW: The temporomandibular joint: true sagittal computed tomography with meniscus visualization, Radiology 150:250, 1984.

62. Thompson JR et al: The temporomandibular joint: high resolution computed tomographic evaluation, Radiology 150:105, 1984.

63. Manco LG et al: Internal derangements of the temporomandibular joint evaluated with direct sagittal CT: a prospective study, Radiology 157:407, 1985.

64. Westesson P-L et al: CT and MRI of the temporomandibular joint: comparison with autopsy specimens, AJR 148:1165, 1987.

65. Helms CA et al: Cine-CT of the temporomandibular joint, J Craniomandibular Practice 4:247, 1986.

66. Katzberg RW et al: Magnetic resonance imaging of the temporomandibular joint meniscus, Oral Surg Oral Med Oral Pathol 59:332, 1985.

67. Harms SE et al: The temporomandibular joint: magnetic resonance imaging using surface coils, Radiology 157:133, 1985.

68. Katzberg RW et al: Normal and abnormal temporomandibular joint: MR imaging with surface coil, Radiology 158:183, 1986.

69. Manzione JV et al: Magnetic resonance imaging of the temporomandibular joint, J Am Dent Assoc 113:398, 1986.

70. Roberts D et al: Temporomandibular joint: magnetic resonance imaging, Radiology 155:829, 1985.

71. Lauterbur PC: Image formation by induced local interactions: examples employing nuclear magnetic resonance, Nature 242:190, 1973.

72. Bradley WC, Newton TH, and Crooks LE: Physical principles of nuclear magnetic resonance. In Newton TH and Potts DG, editors: Advanced imaging techniques, San Francisco, 1983, Clavadell Press, pp 15-61.

73. Bottomley PA et al. NMR imaging/spectroscopy system to study both anatomy and metabolism, Lancet 2:273, 1983.

74. Edelstein WA et al: Signal noise and contrast in nuclear magnetic resonance (NMR) imaging, J Comput Assist Tomogr 7:391, 1983.

75. Alfidi RJ and Haaga JR: Magnetic resonance imaging, Radiol Clin North Am 22:763, 1971.

76. Hansson LG et al: Comparison of MR imaging of the temporomandibular joint: images of autopsy specimens made at 0.3 T and 1.5 T with anatomic cryosections, AJR 152:1241, 1989.

77. Hardy CJ et al: Switched surface coil system for bilateral MR imaging, Radiology 167:835, 1988.

78. Shellock FG and Pressman BD: Dual-surface-coil MR imaging of bilateral temporomandibular joints: improvements in imaging protocol, AJNR 10:595, 1989.

79. Schellhas KP et al: MR of osteochondritis dissecans and avascular necrosis of the mandibular condyle, AJNR 10:3, 1989.

80. Schellhas KP and Wilkes CH: Temporomandibular joint inflammation: comparison of MR fast scanning with T_1- and T_2-weighted imaging techniques, AJNR 10:589, 1989.

81. Campbell W: Clinical radiological investigations of the mandibular joints, Br J Radiol 38:401, 1965.

82. Kneeland JD et al: Failed temporomandibular joint prosthesis: MR imaging, Radiology 165:179, 1987.

83. Schellhas KP et al: Permanent proplast temporomandibular joint implants: MR imaging of destructive complications, AJR 151:731, 1988.

84. Westesson P-L and Eriksson L: Diskectomy of the temporomandibular joint: a double-contrast arthrotomographic follow-up study, Oral Surg Oral Med Oral Pathol 59:435, 1985.

85. Bronstein SL: Postsurgical TMJ arthrography, J Craniomandibular Practice 2:165, 1984.

86. Westesson P-L and Rohlin M: Diagnostic accuracy of double-contrast arthrotomography of the temporomandibular joint: correlation with postmortem morphology, AJNR 5:463, and AJR 143:655, 1984.

87. Westesson P-L, Bronstein SL, and Liedberg J: Temporomandibular joint: correlation between single-contrast videoarthrography and postmortem morphology, Radiology 160:767, 1986.

88. Westesson P-L and Bronstein SL: Temporomandibular joint: comparison of single- and double-contrast arthrography, Radiology 164:65, 1987.

89. Collier DB et al: Internal derangement of the temporomandibular joint: detection by single-photon emission computed tomography, Radiology 149:557, 1983.

90. Katzberg RW et al: Radionuclide skeletal imaging and single photon emission computed tomography in suspected internal derangements of the temporomandibular joint, J Oral Maxillofac Surg 42:782, 1984.

91. Isberg A, Isacsson G, and Nah KS: Mandibular coronoid process locking: A prospective study of frequency and association with internal derangement of the temporomandibular joint, Oral Surg Oral Med Oral Pathol 63:275-279, 1987.

92. Langenbeck B: Angeborene Kleinheit des Unterkiefers; Kiefersperre verbunden, geheilt durch Resection der Processus coronoidei, Archiv für Klin Chir 1:30, 1860.

93. Munk PL and Helms CA: Coronoid process hyperplasia: CT studies, Radiology 171:783-784, 1989.

94. Hovell JH: Condylar hyperplasia, Br J Oral Surg 1:105-111, 1963.

95. Stanson AW and Baker HL: Routine tomography of the temporomandibular joint, Radiol Clin North Am 14:105-127, 1976.

5 The Mandible

ALFRED L. WEBER

SECTION ONE
NORMAL ANATOMY[1-6]

The mandible is a tubular structure formed by dense cortical bone that is filled with trabecular bone and marrow. The mandible is bilaterally symmetric and has a horseshoe configuration. When viewed from the side, it is L-shaped, with a horizontal body and a vertical ascending ramus. The body is capped by the alveolar process, which contains the tooth sockets. The body and ascending ramus joint at the angle of the mandible. The ascending ramus ends posteriorly and superiorly in the condyle and anteriorly in the coronoid process. The condyle and coronoid process are separated by the mandibular or sigmoid notch. The condyle consists of the head and neck; anteriorly on the neck is the insertion of the lateral pterygoid muscle. The insertion of the temporal muscle is on the coronoid process anteriorly. On the outer cortex anteriorly, a mental foramen is located on each side of the body near the level of the first premolar tooth; these foramina contain the mental nerves and vessels. The mental protuberance and mental tubercle are situated along the caudal anterior border of the mandible. The portion of the mandible between the mental foramina occasionally is referred to as the mandibular symphysis.

On the inner surface of the middle third of the ascending ramus is the mandibular foramen, which is the origin of the mandibular canal. The canal contains the inferior alveolar nerves and vessels. The mylohyoid groove, which contains the mylohyoid nerve and vessels, extends obliquely downward and forward from the mandibular foramen.

From the inner cortex in the midline, extending laterally, are the genial tubercle, the digastric fossae on either side, and the mylohyoid ridges on the inner surface of each side of the body of the mandible; these structures form the origins of the musculature of the tongue (genioglossus, geniohyoid, digastric muscles, and the mylohyoid muscle).

The angle and ascending ramus of the mandible serve as the main insertion of the muscles of mastication. (On the outer cortex is the masseter; on the inner cortex is the medial pterygoid; and bridging the inner and outer cortices of the coronoid process and anterior body are the temporalis muscles.) The mandible has several weak, bony areas that predispose toward fractures, including the mental foramina, tooth sockets, crypts of impacted teeth, and condylar neck.

Each tooth is contained in a socket (alveolus) within the alveolar process that is surrounded by cancellous bone. The alveolus is lined by dense cortical bone, called the cribriform plate. This is seen radiographically as a radiopaque line, referred to as the lamina dura. The space between the lamina dura and the tooth represents the periodontal ligament, which is seen radiographically as a lucent zone. The periodontal ligament attaches the tooth to the cribriform plate.

The center of the tooth is composed of dentin, which contains a hollow core, the pulp cavity. The pulp cavity is filled with connective tissue, vessels, and nerves. At the tooth root foramen the pulp is continuous with the periodontal ligament. The dentin is covered with enamel, which projects above the gingiva and is about 1.5 mm thick at the chewing surface. The cementum serves as an intermediate tissue between the dentin and the periodontal ligament.

Two sets of teeth (dentition) develop during life. The first 20 deciduous teeth erupt between 6 and 36 months of age and are composed of two incisors, one canine, and two molars in each quadrant of the mouth. The permanent dentitions develop with additional teeth that have no deciduous predecessors. The permanent teeth appear between 6 and 21 years of age and consist of two incisors (medial and lateral), one canine, two premolars, and three molars in each quadrant of the mouth, making a total of 32 teeth.

REFERENCES

1. Mustoe TM and Thaller SR: General concepts: overview of anatomy and basics of history and physical examination. In Thaller SE and Montgomery WW, editors: Guide to dental problems for physicians and surgeons, Baltimore, 1988, Williams & Wilkins.
2. Kerr D, Marsh M, and Millard HD: Oral diagnosis, St Louis, 1974, The CV Mosby Co.
3. Montgomery WW: Surgery of the upper respiratory system, vol 2, ed 2, Philadelphia, 1989, Lea & Febiger, pp. 1-31.
4. Scott JH, Barrington N, and Symons B: Introduction to dental anatomy, ed 7, London, 1974, Churchill Livingstone, Inc.
5. Sicher H and DuBrul EL: Oral anatomy, St Louis, 1975, The CV Mosby Co.
6. Reed GM and Sheppard VF: Basic structures of the head and neck: a programmed instruction in clinical anatomy for dental professionals, Philadelphia, 1976, WB Saunders Co.

SECTION TWO
IMAGING

RADIOLOGIC EXAMINATION[1-8]

Radiologic examination of the mandible can be performed on a head unit or on a horizontal radiography table. Intensifying screens are used to achieve detail of the anatomic structures. The film cassette is placed on the tabletop or in the head holder of the head unit. The standard routine views in radiologic evaluation of the mandible include the posteroanterior (PA) view, the left and right lateral oblique views, and the lateral view. When indicated, these radiographic techniques can be supplemented by views of the temporomandibular joints and by panoramic radiographs and intraoral dental views.

PA View (Fig. 5-1)

The PA view provides a look at the ascending ramus and the angle and body of the mandible as seen from the front. Because of the superimposition of the cervical spine, the symphysis of the mandible is poorly delineated. This can be partially circumvented by turning the head slightly to the left or right, depending on the area of interest. This view is obtained by having the patient's forehead and nose on the cassette. The sagittal plane of the head is perpendicular to the plane of the cassette. The central ray is perpendicular to the cassette.

Lateral Oblique View (Fig. 5-2)

The lateral oblique view is the most common and useful of the conventional projections. It is obtained by placing a 5- by 7-inch film cassette at the side of the lower jaw. The roentgen ray tube is angled 30 degrees cranially with the central beam at the angle of the mandible. This view depicts the body of the mandible, including the alveolus, angle, and ascending ramus, as well as the sigmoid notch, mandibular condyle, and coronoid process of the mandible. Portions of the mandibular canal in which run the nerves and vessels of the teeth are also well seen.

Lateral View (Fig. 5-3)

The lateral view provides limited information because of superimportion of both halves of the mandible. The film cassette is placed on the side of the face, including the jaw. The roentgen ray tube points toward the face from a straight lateral position, and the central beam is focused on the angle of the mandible.

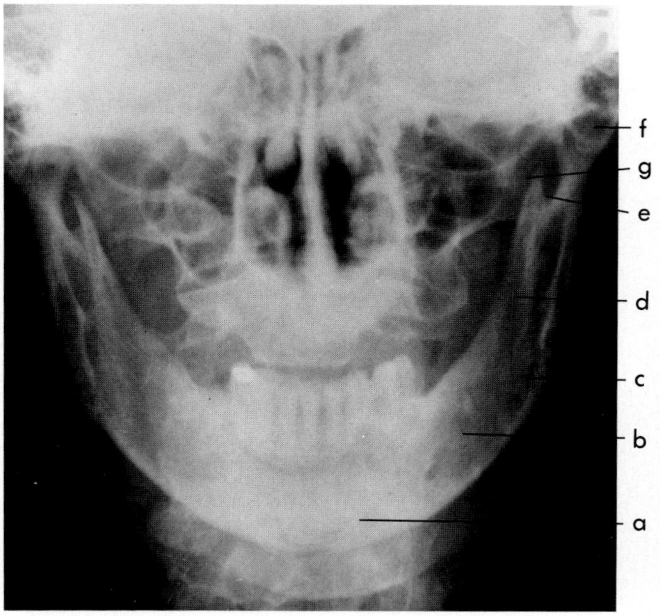

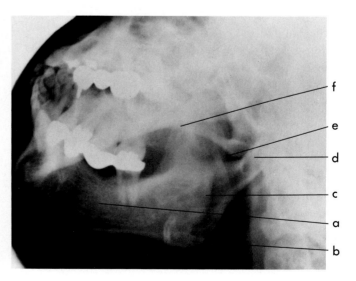

Fig. 5-1 PA view of mandible demonstrates normal anatomy: *a*, symphysis of mandible; *b*, body of mandible; *c*, angle of mandible; *d*, ascending ramus; *e*, sigmoid notch; *f*, mandibular condyle; and *g*, coronoid process.

Fig. 5-2 Oblique view of mandible demonstrates normal anatomy: *a*, body of mandible; *b*, angle of mandible; *c*, ascending ramus; *d*, mandibular condyle; *e*, sigmoid notch; and *f*, coronoid process.

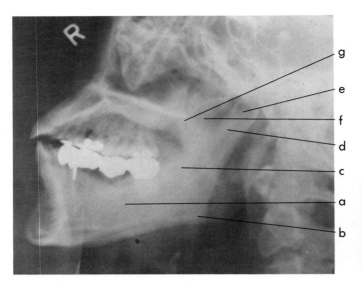

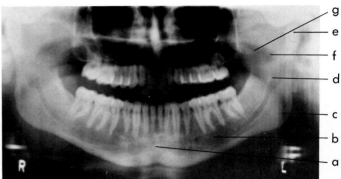

Fig. 5-3 Lateral view of mandible demonstrates normal anatomy: *a,* body of mandible; *b,* angle of mandible; *c,* ascending ramus; *d,* neck of mandibular condyle; *e,* mandibular condyle; *f,* sigmoid notch; and *g,* coronoid process.

Fig. 5-4 Panorex view of mandible demonstrates normal anatomy: *a,* symphysis of mandible; *b,* body of mandible; *c,* angle of mandible; *d,* ascending ramus; *e,* mandibular condyle; *f,* sigmoid notch; and *g,* coronoid process.

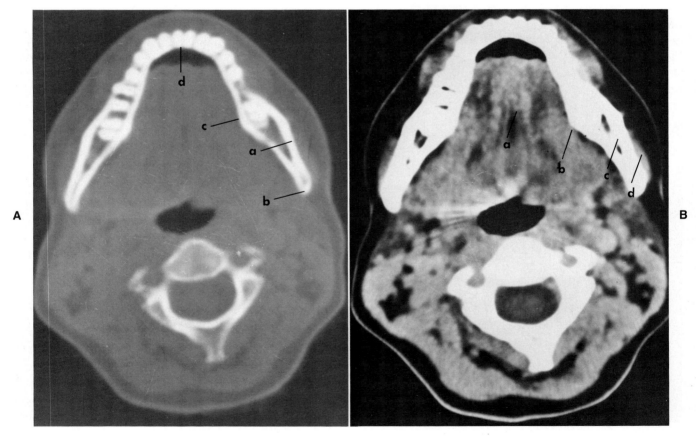

Fig. 5-5 **A,** Axial CT section through normal mandible (bone window setting). *a,* Ascending ramus; *b,* angle of mandible; *c,* body of mandible; and *d,* symphysis of mandible. **B,** Axial CT section of normal mandible (soft tissue window setting). *a,* Central floor of mouth; *b,* lateral floor of mouth; *c,* mandible; and *d,* masseter muscle.

Panoramic Radiograph (Fig. 5-4)

A panoramic radiography machine makes a curved planar tomogram of the upper and lower jaws, including the teeth. The image is obtained by a synchronous and reciprocal movement of the roentgen ray tube and the film cassette around the lower region of the patient's head. This single radiograph provides a survey examination of the entire mandible and the maxilla, including the lower portions of the nasal fossae and maxillary antra. The apices of the teeth, with the exception of the anterior teeth (because of the overlying cervical spine), are well depicted.

INTRAORAL RADIOGRAPHY

Intraoral dental radiography is performed with small dental film packets containing nonscreen high-speed radiographic film and a sheet of lead foil to reduce roentgen ray back scatter. The dental radiography machine consists of a small, lightweight, freely movable tube head with a tube current of 10 to 15 mA and a range of 60 to 100 kV(p). There are three basic intraoral projections: periapical, bite wing, and occlusal.

For a radiologist, the periapical view is important in evaluating the anatomy of the tooth apices and adjacent bone. The relationship of the tooth to pathologic conditions constitutes an important diagnostic parameter in many lesions. The intraoral view depicts the lingual and outer surface of the anterior mandible and can localize stones in the submandibular ducts. In addition, this view can be used to demonstrate the anterior hard palate.

COMPUTED TOMOGRAPHY (CT)[5-8]

CT has become an important diagnostic tool in the assessment of many mandibular lesions, especially malignant tumors within and adjacent to the mandible. A CT examination should include bone and soft tissue window settings; 4 to 5 mm axial contiguous sections, parallel to the inferior bony margin of the body of the mandible and extending from the level of the temporomandibular joint to the hyoid bone; and 4 mm coronal contiguous sections, extending from the external auditory canal to the anterior margin of the symphysis of the mandible and oriented perpendicular to the orbitomeatal plane (Fig. 5-5, *A* and *B*). CT delineates to best advantage bony expansion, especially of the lingual and outer surfaces of the mandible, bone destruction, and extraosseous extension of benign and malignant lesions. Lesions arising in the floor of the mouth and gingiva, with secondary invasion of the mandible, also are well seen.

MAGNETIC RESONANCE IMAGING (MRI)

MRI has limited application with most mandibular lesions. However, it can contribute to diagnostic assessment with some lesions by differentiating solid from cystic lesions, identifying invasion of the mandible by an adjacent malignant tumor, and by evaluating bone marrow abnormalities. On T_1-weighted images, a fluid-filled cyst has a low-intermediate signal intensity, whereas the T_2-weighted image discloses a high signal intensity. With a tumor, a T_1-weighted image most often shows a low to intermediate signal intensity, and a T_2-weighted image an intermediate to slightly higher intensity. Differentiating between a cyst and a tumor may be especially useful in a younger patient with a hemorrhagic bone cyst, a case in which surgical intervention is not indicated. Some tumors, including ameloblastomas, can exhibit an aggressive behavior with extraosseous extension. If the tumor is not completely extirpated, recurrence is likely. MRI is important in visualizing and delineating extraosseous extension before surgical removal.

The mandible frequently is eroded by carcinomas arising in the gingiva, floor of the mouth, and tongue. This bony erosion is characterized by loss of the normal signal void of the cortical bone of the mandible's lingual surface. The medullary portion of the mandible consists of fatty marrow, which has a high signal intensity on T_1-weighted images. Obliteration of this high signal intensity on the T_1-weighted images usually signifies tumor invasion. With tumors within the marrow (e.g., metastatic disease, leukemia, lymphoma, or multiple myeloma), the normal high signal intensity on T_1-weighted images is replaced by a low signal intensity.

REFERENCES

1. Stafne EC and Gibilisco JA: Oral roentgenographic diagnosis, ed 4, Philadelphia, 1975, WB Saunders Co.
2. Weber AL and Easter KM: Cysts and odontogenic tumors of the mandible and maxilla. I, Contemporary Diagnostic Radiology 5(25):1, 1982.
3. Weber AL and Easter KM: Cysts and odontogenic tumors of the mandible and maxilla. II, Contemporary Diagnostic Radiology 5(26):1, 1982.
4. Blaschke DP and Osborn AG: The mandible and teeth. In Bergeron RT, Osborn AG, and Som PM, editors: Head and neck imaging excluding the brain, St Louis, 1984, The CV Mosby Co.
5. Weber AL: Radiologic evaluation. In Thaller SR and Montgomery WW, editors: Guide to dental problems for physicians and surgeons, Baltimore, 1988, Williams & Wilkins.
6. Osborn AG, Hanafee WN, and Mancuso AA: Normal and pathologic CT anatomy of the mandible, AJR 139(3):555, 1982.
7. Hanafee WN and Mancuso AA: Pictorial essay: normal and pathologic CT anatomy of the mandible, AJR 139:555, 1982.
8. Seldin EB: Radiology of the mandible. In Taveras JM and Ferrucci JT, editors: Radiology: diagnosis, imaging, intervention, vol 3, Philadelphia, 1987, JB Lippincott Co.

SECTION THREE
PATHOLOGY

CYSTS[1]
Definition and Classification

A cyst is an epithelial lined cavity that usually contains fluid or semisolid material. Microscopic examination of the lining tissue, along with the clinical and radiographic findings, is necessary for diagnosis.

Cysts frequently occur in the jaw. They appear radiographically as unilocular or multilocular lucent areas of varying size and definition. A cyst's relationship to a tooth provides important features for the differential diagnosis. On the basis of development, cysts have been subdivided into *odontogenic* and *nonodontogenic* types.

Odontogenic cysts[2] arise from tooth derivatives. Histologic analysis of the epithelial layers, association with other clinical findings, the relationship to a tooth, and internal cyst calcification allow further subdivision. The term *residual cyst* is frequently used for any cyst (specifically a periodontal apical cyst) that remains or develops after surgical removal of a tooth.

Nonodontogenic cysts are developmental in origin. The fissural variety, as the name implies, arises along lines of fusion of various bones and embryonic processes. These cysts, like odontogenic cysts, are lined by epithelium and usually contain fluid or semisolid material. Fissural cysts are classified according to their anatomic location. Developmental cysts include other types derived from embyrologic structures (e.g., dermoid cysts) and cysts arising from other causes (e.g., solitary bone cysts, Stafne cysts, and aneurysmal bone cysts).

Odontogenic Cysts

Dentigerous (Follicular) Cyst.[3,4] After the radicular cyst (see following discussion on "Periodontal Cyst"), the dentigerous cyst is the most common type of odontogenic cyst. Most dentigerous cysts become evident during the third and fourth decades of life (20 to 40 years of age). Most of these cysts (75%) are located in the mandible, and they have been noted to occur in association with the crown of an unerupted tooth. In the usual case the crown of the tooth projects into the lumen of the cystic cavity, but with continued growth, only a limited portion of the tooth may be attached to the cyst's surface (Fig. 5-6). A number of dentigerous cysts may occur.

Dentigerous cysts vary greatly in size, ranging from less than 2 cm in diameter to cysts that cause massive

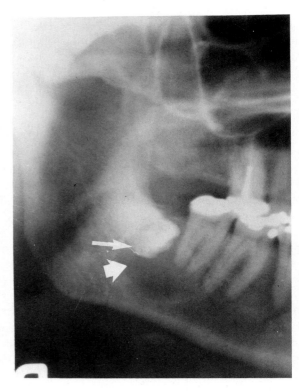

Fig. 5-6 Dentigerous cyst. Panorex view of mandible reveals sharply marginated, oval-shaped cyst in body of right mandible *(short arrow)*. Crown of impacted third molar tooth is incorporated into posterior portion of cyst *(long arrow)*.

expansion of the jaw. Dentigerous cysts do not demonstrate an extracystic soft tissue mass, as is seen in ameloblastomas. Dentigerous cysts may cause displacement of teeth, but apical resorption of tooth structures is uncommon. Fractures and superimposed infection may develop in the cyst. Ameloblastomas, mucoepidermoid tumors, and carcinomas may develop on the wall of a dentigerous cyst.

A dentigerous cyst in the mandible appears as a circumscribed, unilocular area of osteolysis that incorporates the crown of a tooth (Fig. 5-7, *A* and *B*). The adjacent teeth are displaced and may be partly eroded. Dentigerous cysts in the maxilla often extend into the antrum, with displacement and remodeling of the bony sinus wall. Large cysts may project into the nasal cavity and infratemporal fossa and may elevate the floor of the

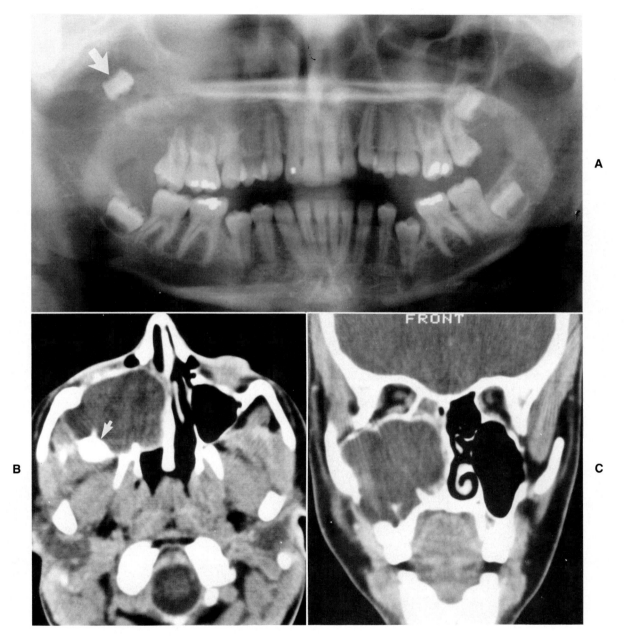

Fig. 5-7   Dentigerous cyst. **A,** Panorex view of mandible and maxilla reveals displaced tooth in upper lateral aspect of right maxilla *(arrow)*. Poorly defined expansile lesion is present in the same region, including maxillary antrum. **B,** Axial CT section demonstrates cystic lesion within right antral cavity with extension into right nasal cavity and pterygo-palatine and infratemporal fossae. Note localized density at posterior margin of cyst, rep-resenting tooth *(arrow)* that is incorporated into cyst. **C,** Coronal CT section also shows cyst arising from alveolar portion of right maxilla with extension into right antrum and right nasal cavity. Floor of right orbit is slightly elevated.

orbit. On MRI, the contents of the cyst show a high signal intensity on T_2-weighted images and low-to-intermediate signal intensity on T_1-weighted images.

Periodontal Cyst.[5] Periodontal cysts can be further classified as periapical (radicular) cysts or lateral cysts. Radicular cysts are by far the most common type of odontogenic cyst. They may form at any time during life, although the peak incidence occurs between 30 and 50 years of age; there is no sex predilection. This cyst is most often associated with teeth that reveal untreated caries, and it may originate asymptomatically in a per-

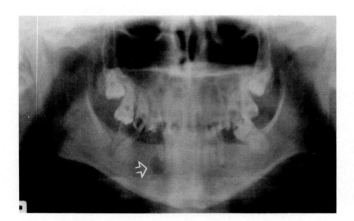

Fig. 5-8 Radicular cyst. Panorex view of mandible reveals cystic lesion around root of lower canine tooth *(arrow).* Note caries in crown of tooth. Second radicular cyst is present at apex of carious second lower right molar tooth.

sistent periapical granuloma. Swelling and pain may occur when the cyst enlarges. Most of these cysts are discovered incidentally on radiography, but expansion of the cyst may cause a clinically noticeable displacement of teeth.

Radiographically, a radicular cyst is a well-circumscribed radiolucency arising from the apex of the tooth and bounded by a thin rim of cortical bone (Fig. 5-8); large lesions may expand the cortical plates. A radicular cyst can displace tooth structures and may cause slight root resorption. Extension into the maxillary sinus may be observed if the cyst occurs in the maxilla (Fig. 5-9). Radiographically, radicular cysts cannot be differentiated from periapical granulomas, which usually are less than 1.6 cm in diameter.

Odontogenic Keratocyst.[6-8] Odontagenic keratocysts account for 3% to 11% of all jaw cysts, and they occur twice as often in the mandible as in the maxilla. These cysts are found in patients of all ages, but the peak incidence occurs in the second and third decades of life. This cyst has been classified as a separate type of bone cyst because of its differential clinical behavior and histologic structure. The recurrence rate following incomplete surgical excision has been reported as being between 20% and 60%.

An odontogenic keratocyst is lined by epithelial cells, with keratinization of the lining. The diagnosis depends on the cyst's microscopic features and is independent of its location and radiographic appearance. This cyst is a radiolucent lesion that often is multiloculated and has a

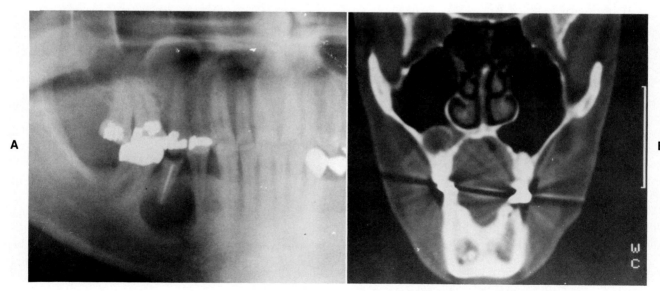

Fig. 5-9 Radicular cyst. **A,** Panorex view of mandible and maxilla reveals radicular cyst around apex of right second premolar tooth and first molar tooth within mandible and around apex of upper right first molar tooth. Upper radicular cyst bulges into right antral cavity. **B,** Coronal CT section of paranasal sinuses reveals maxillary radicular cyst projecting into floor of right antrum (see panorex view in **A**).

smooth or scalloped border; it characteristically is located in the body and ramus of the mandible. Odontogenic keratocysts often occur in conjunction with an impacted tooth (Fig. 5-10).

In many instances a keratocyst cannot be differentiated radiographically from an ameloblastoma. Several odontogenic keratocysts may occur, and they can be associated with the basal cell nevus syndrome.

Basal Cell Nevus Syndrome.[9,10] Basal cell nevus syndrome becomes apparent between 5 and 10 years of age; there is no sex predilection. The disorder is inherited as an autosomal dominant trait with variable penetrance and expressivity. Many patients with this syndrome have slight mental retardation.

The syndrome consists of a number of changes. Among the most common are multiple cysts of the jaw, multiple basal cell carcinomas, skeletal abnormalities, and ectopic calcifications. At least two of these findings must be present to make a diagnosis.

The multiple jaw cysts develop early in childhood. They may be either unilocular or multilocular and often prove to be keratocysts, varying in size from 1 mm to several centimeters. Nevoid basal cell carcinomas appear later than the cysts but before 30 years of age; they are found especially on the face, trunk, neck, and arms. The most common skeletal abnormalities are bi-

fid ribs, synostosis of ribs, kyphoscoliosis, vertebral fusion, mild ocular hypertelorism, prognathism, polydactyly, and frontal and temporoparietal bossing. The ectopic calcifications occur most frequently in the falx cerebri and other parts of the dura.

Nonodontogenic Cysts

Fissural Cyst. A *nasopalatine duct cyst (incisive canal cyst)*[11,12] is a nonodontogenic developmental cyst in the incisive canal near the anterior palatine papilla. These cysts probably arise from epithelial remnants in the incisive canal. The cysts can occur at any age but are most frequently found in patients in the fourth and sixth decades of life, with no sex predilection. These cysts are usually asymptomatic, but some patients note swelling in the palate, especially when the cyst is primarily in the incisive papilla. Occasionally patients notice a discharge of mucoid material and a salty taste.

Most of these cysts are small and are found on routine radiographic surveys. Radiographically, it may be difficult to differentiate between an enlarged incisive fossa and an incisive canal cyst. However, an incisive canal cyst is always located at or close to the midline and usually is round or ovoid, although it may be heart shaped (Fig. 5-11, *A* and *B*). A condensed rim of cortical bone is often seen along the periphery of the cyst, and the lesion may displace the roots of the central incisors.

A *globulomaxillary cyst*[13,14] is a cyst located between the lateral incisor and the canine tooth, at the site that corresponds to the incisive suture. Such a cyst usually extends toward the crest of the alveolar ridge and may cause the roots of these adjacent teeth to diverge. The cyst usually assumes a pear shape as it increases in size (Fig. 5-12). If a globulomaxillary cyst extends over the apex of the root of the incisor or canine tooth (or both), the vitality of the tooth must be determined to help differentiate a globulomaxillary cyst from a radicular cyst.

Solitary, Simple, or Hemorrhagic Bone Cyst.[15,16] Solitary, simple, or hemorrhagic bone cysts are seen more frequently in men than in women, and they usually occur in young people (70% occur in patients in the second decade of life). This type of cyst is believed to result from an injury unassociated with a fracture; the injury may cause an intramedullary hematoma that disintegrates and produces a cyst within the bone. A hemorrhagic bone cyst is a unilocular cavity that may be empty or partly filled with a clear or sanguineous fluid. The lining consists of a loose vascular connective tissue that may have areas of recent or old hemorrhage.

Since these cysts often are asymptomatic, most are discovered incidentally during examination of the teeth. It is believed that some of these solitary bone cysts regress spontaneously. These lesions are most commonly located in the mandibular marrow space that

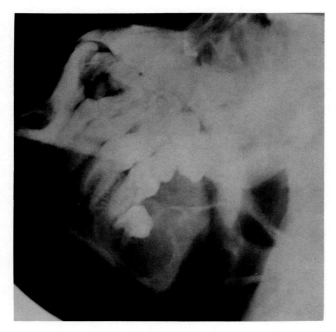

Fig. 5-10 Keratocyst. Oblique view of mandible reveals multiloculated cyst in posterior body of mandible, angle of mandible, and ascending ramus. Third molar tooth is incorporated into anterior part of cyst, and there is encroachment upon posterior aspect of second molar tooth. Note also expansion with thinning of anterior wall of ascending ramus.

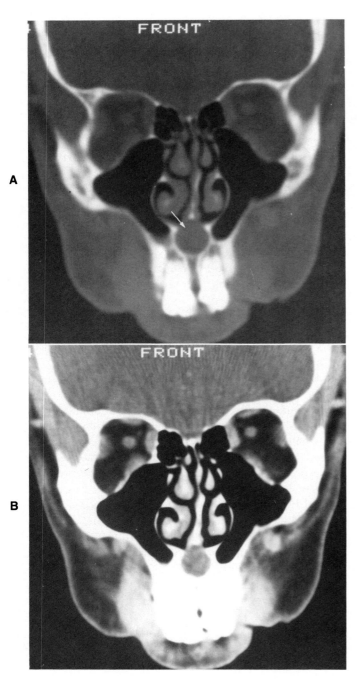

A

B

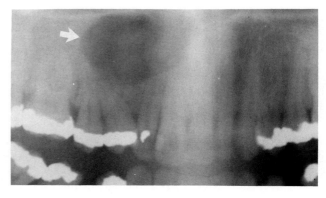

Fig. 5-12 Globulomaxillary cyst. Panorex view reveals cystic structure in right maxilla *(arrow),* causing roots of lateral incisor and canine tooth to diverge.

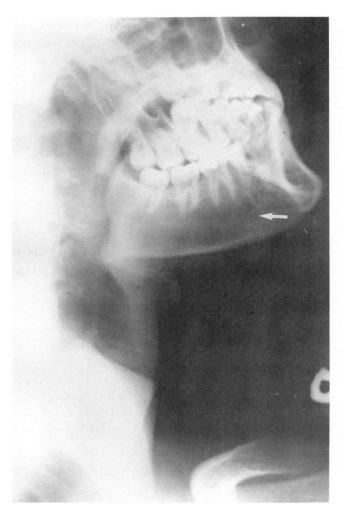

Fig. 5-11 Nasopalatine cyst. **A,** Coronal CT section (bone window setting) reveals cystic structure with bony expansion in nasopalatine duct between upper central incisor teeth *(arrow).* Slight bulge extends into adjacent nasal cavity. **B,** Coronal CT section (soft tissue window setting) reveals cystic structure that is isodense with muscle.

Fig. 5-13 Hemorrhagic bone cyst. Oblique view of mandible reveals large, oval-shaped cystic lesion within body of right mandible *(arrow).* Note interdigitations of this cyst between root parts of teeth.

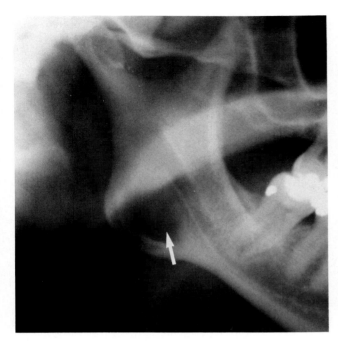

Fig. 5-14   Static bone cavity (Stafne cyst). Oblique view of mandible reveals oval-shaped cavity *(arrow)* in angle of mandible below mandibular canal.

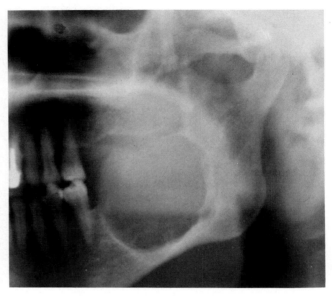

Fig. 5-15   Ameloblastoma. Oblique view of mandible reveals large cystic lesion in body and ascending ramus of mandible with attenuation and loss of bone superiorly. Lesion has broken through upper part of mandible.

extends posteriorly from the premolar region. They also may occur in the incisor area of the mandible, although this is a less likely site. Radiographically, these cysts are slightly irregular in shape and size and have poorly defined borders (Fig. 5-13). The outline of the cyst between the roots of the teeth has a scalloped appearance. Larger cysts may extend into the interdental space and the ramus, and the mandible may be slightly expanded. The radiographic features are not specific enough to be diagnostic.

Static Bone Cavity (Stafne Cyst).[17]   A Stafne cyst appears as an elliptical, ovoid, or round radiolucency usually located in the posterior mandible, often near the angle of the mandible below the mandibular canal (Fig. 5-14). Stafne cysts occur more frequently in men than in women and have been reported in patients from 20 to 70 years of age (most of these cysts are discovered by 50 years of age). These asymptomatic lesions are detected incidentally on routine radiographs of the mandible.

Radiographically, the radiolucency has a well-defined border, often showing slight sclerosis at the margin. The lesions vary in size from 1 to 2 cm in diameter and may be oval, round, or elliptic. Bilateral defects have been described. Submandibular salivary gland tissue has been demonstrated within the bone cavity of some Stafne cysts. The cyst is open on the lingual surface of the mandible, allowing salivary gland tissue to extend into its cavity.

BENIGN ODONTOGENIC TUMORS[18,19]

Odontogenic tumors result from an abnormal proliferation of the cells and tissues involved in odontogenesis. These tumors represent a diverse group of structures, and they are classified according to the origin of the various layers of tooth development. According to the histologic findings, these tumors have been divided into epithelial, mesodermal, and mixed tissue tumors of odontogenic origin. The radiographic appearance of odontogenic tumors varies, and many of them cannot be differentiated from the cysts previously described.

Ameloblastoma[20-22]

An ameloblastoma is a benign, epithelial odontogenic tumor thought to arise from ameloblasts. It is found with about equal frequency in men and women and has a peak incidence in the third and fourth decades (two thirds of the cases occur before 40 years of age). Ameloblastomas account for approximately 18% of odontogenic tumors. Eighty-one percent of ameloblastomas are located in the mandible, and the remaining 19% are found in the maxilla. Half of the mandibular lesions are located in the molar regions. An ameloblastoma is a slow-growing, painless mass that may reach a considerable size. Swelling is the only symptom.

Radiographically, an ameloblastoma is radiolucent and either multilocular or unilocular (Fig. 5-15). Unilocular lesions occur most often in the maxilla. In

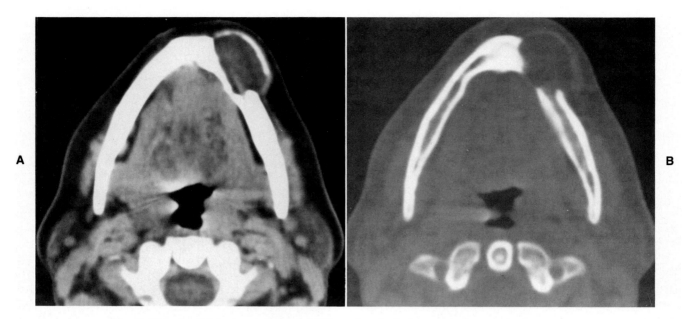

Fig. 5-16 Ameloblastoma. **A,** Axial CT section (soft tissue window setting) shows expansile lesion in body of left mandible and adjacent symphysis with marked lateral expansion. **B,** Axial CT section (bone window setting) defines boundary of this expansile lesion to better advantage. Also, note erosion of lingual surface of mandible with slight bulge.

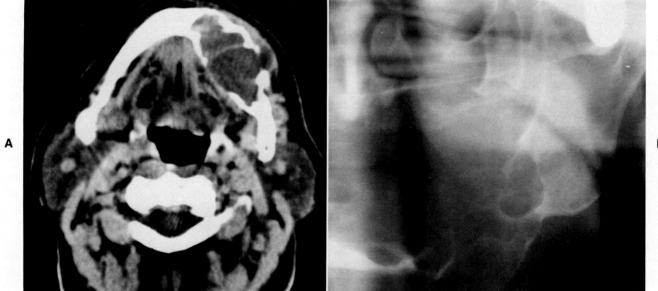

Fig. 5-17 Ameloblastoma. **A,** Panorex view of mandible reveals multiloculated, aggressive lesion in body and ascending ramus of mandible with considerable loss of bone. **B,** Axial CT section (soft tissue window setting) reveals expansile lesion in body and ascending ramus. Loss of bone has occurred medially and laterally. Low attenuation, slightly septated soft tissue densities are present in lesion. Small component of tumor has penetrated lateral cortex and extended into adjacent soft tissues.

the multilocular form, the lesion has a honeycomb or bubblelike appearance. These loculi may be oval or spherical and may vary in size. The size varies from a small cyst confined to the alveolar portion of the jaw to a cyst that causes extensive destruction of the mandible or maxilla. The tumor has a tendency to break through the cortex of the bone, with subsequent formation of a soft tissue mass (Fig. 5-16, *A* and *B*). Bony expansion of variable degrees, sometimes with a scalloped margin, also can be observed (Fig. 5-17, *A* and *B*). The lesion often has an oval configuration with distinct borders, slight marginal sclerosis, and no periosteal new bone formation. Loss of the lamina dura, erosion of the tooth apex, and displacement of the teeth are also encountered.

Calcifying Epithelial Odontogenic Tumor (Pindborg Tumor)[23-25]

A calcifying epithelial odontogenic tumor is composed of polyhedral epithelial cells in a fibrous stroma that contains acidophilic homogeneous structures that commonly calcify. The average age of the patient at first diagnosis is about 40 years (a range of 12 to 78 years of age), and there is no sex predilection. Most of these tumors are located in the premolar-molar area of the mandible, and they are associated with the crown of an impacted tooth in half of the cases.

Radiographically, the lesion is usually radiolucent. It may be unilocular but more often is multilocular (honeycombed) and has poorly defined, irregular borders, reflecting an aggressive behavior similar to that of an ameloblastoma (Fig. 5-18). In other manifestations of development, radiopaque densities of varying degrees are located close to the crown of an impacted tooth. Curettage is the preferred treatment, but recurrence or extensive tumor involvement should be treated by resection.

Odontoma[26-30]

An odontoma is a benign tumor made up of the various tissue components of teeth (e.g., enamel, dentin, cementum, and pulp). It is also designated as composite because of the admixture of several types of tissue. In its development an odontoma passes through the same stages as a developing tooth, but dentin and enamel are laid down in an abnormal pattern. In the initial stage of development a radiolucent area develops, caused by resorption of bone from the odontogenic tissues. In the intermediate and late stages, progressive calcification takes place, initially characterized by small, speckled calcific densities that eventually form radiopaque masses surrounded by a lucent ring. These tumors may be discovered in any location of the dental arches and are situated between the roots of teeth.

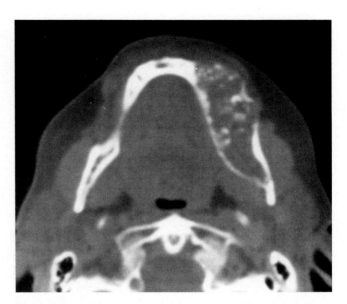

Fig. 5-18 Pindborg tumor. Axial CT section (bone window setting) reveals marked expansion of right mandible with loss of bone in lateral cortex. Several calcific densities are noted within lesion.

Both forms of odontoma (complex composite and compound composite) are frequently associated with unerupted teeth. It is noteworthy that compound composite odontomas occur most often in the anterior portion of the jaw, whereas complex composite odontomas occur in the posterior part. A developing odontoma without calcifications or with few calcifications presents difficulty in the radiologic diagnosis and cannot be differentiated from other similarly appearing lesions.

Complex Composite Odontoma.[27,28] Complex composite odontomas account for 24% of all odontomas. These lesions are composed of all dental tissues arranged in a disorderly pattern and bearing no morphologic similarity to normal or rudimentary teeth. Complex composite odontomas most commonly occur in patients 10 to 25 years of age, and males and females are affected equally. The lesion usually is asymptomatic and most frequently is located in the premolar and molar regions in the mandible, although it is sometimes found in the maxilla. Most lesions are small, measuring only a few millimeters, but some may reach a considerable size.

Radiographically, the lesion appears as a well-demarcated radiopaque mass, revealing radiating structures in some cases. Occasionally the tumor is surrounded by a narrow radiolucent zone. Usually an unerupted tooth is seen near the tumor. The preferred therapeutic treatment is enucleation. Cancellous bone grafting may be appropriate, depending on the size and location of the surgical defect.

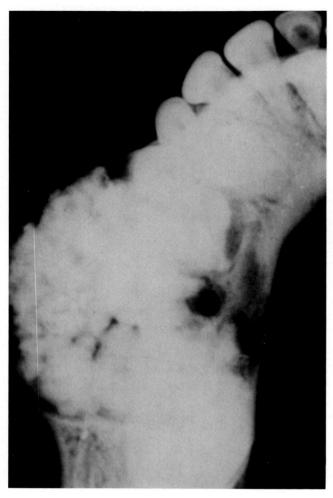

Fig. 5-19 Compound odontoma. Semiaxial view of mandible reveals calcified lesion arising from outer cortex of mandible. Lesion contains several malformed teeth. Note surrounding lucent zone between expanded cortex and malformed teeth.

Compound Composite Odontoma.[29,30] Compound composite odontomas consist of a malformation in which all dental tissues that have some similarity to a normal tooth are represented in a more orderly pattern than in the complex composite odontoma. The lesion is composed of many toothlike structures, with enamel, dentin, cementum, and pulp arranged as in a normal tooth. The differentiation of teeth varies from case to case, and the number of teeth involved may be surprisingly high.

Most compound composite odontomas (60%) occur in patients in the second and third decades of life, and there is no sex predilection. The tumor frequently is located in the incisor-canine region of the maxilla. It usually is small but occasionally may displace teeth or interfere with their eruption; the lesion is otherwise asymptomatic. Radiographically, several small, rather

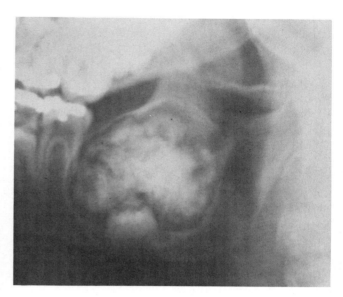

Fig. 5-20 Ameloblastic fibroodontoma. Oblique view of mandible reveals expansile lesion in posterior body and ascending ramus of mandible. Amorphous calcific densities are noted within lesion. Radiolucent zone is present between calcified mass and adjacent expanded cortex. Note impacted third molar tooth, which is incoporated into inferior part of lesion.

well-defined, malformed or rudimentary teeth are demonstrated, surrounded by a radiolucent zone that is caused by a fibrous capsule. The teeth contained in a compound composite odontoma are dwarfed and usually distorted, with simple roots (Fig. 5-19). Most of these lesions are well encapsulated and easily enucleated. Recurrences are not encountered after enucleation.

Ameloblastic Fibroodontoma. An ameloblastic fibroodontoma is a mixture of ameloblastic tissue and a composite odontoma. An ameloblastic odontoma is a rare lesion that can occur at any age but is more prevalent in children; it is rare after age 13. This type of tumor is more common in the mandible (premolar-molar region) than in the maxilla, and it always occurs in association with unerupted teeth. Painless swelling or absence or displacement of teeth are the most common signs leading to its diagnosis.

Radiographically, the tumor consists of a lucent, well-defined area with a solitary mass or several small radiopaque masses that may resemble miniature teeth (Fig. 5-20). Radiologic differentiation from other odontomas is not possible, and inadequate removal may be followed by a recurrence.

Odontogenic Myxoma[31-34]

An odontogenic myxoma appears to be a true odontogenic tumor, originating from the mesodermal portion

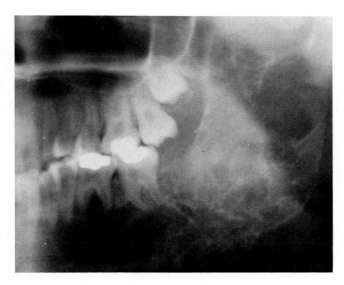

Fig. 5-21 Myxoma of mandible. Panorex view of mandible reveals several small, irregular, lucent areas in mandible bounded by thickened trabeculae. Lesion, more anteriorly, demonstrates ill-defined lucent area beneath molar teeth. Myxoma has extended through cortex of mandible, which is best illustrated inferiorly near angle of mandible.

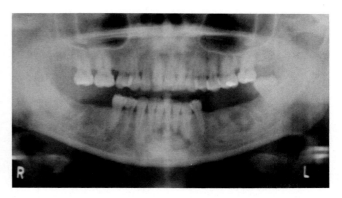

Fig. 5-22 Periapical cemental dysplasia. Panorex view of mandible reveals several sclerotic foci within mandible, especially at symphysis and body on left. Some of these sclerotic areas merge imperceptibly with mandible. Other densities are surrounded by lucent ring. Radiographic appearance shows evolution from lucent areas in early stages to mixed stage and, finally, sclerotic stage.

of the odontogenic apparatus. This tumor, which is not found in bones outside the jaw, accounts for about 3% to 6% of odontogenic tumors.

Odontogenic myxomas occur most often in the second and third decades of life, with no sex predilection. The tumor consists of rounded and angular cells lying in abundant mucoid stroma, and the lesion is painless, locally invasive, and slow growing. If untreated, odontogenic myxomas eventually may cause extensive destruction of bone and marked cortical expansion. Odontogenic myxomas involve the mandible and maxilla with about equal frequency. In the mandible, the body and ramus are most commonly affected.

Radiographically, several radiolucent areas of varying size are present, septated by straight or curved bony trabeculae that form triangular, quadrangular, or square-shaped compartments (Fig. 5-21). Unilocular cysts have also been described. The radiographic margins of the tumor may be well or poorly defined. An odontogenic myxoma may simulate an ameloblastoma, central giant cell granuloma, or hemangioma. When the tumor is very aggressive and rapid growing, it shows little encapsulation and often extends through bone into the adjacent soft tissues without any well-defined margin.

The treatment of choice is enucleation. A tumor-free margin must be resected because of the tumor's local invasiveness and resultant tendency to recur. A recurrence rate of 25% after curettage has been reported.

Cementoma[35-40]

Periapical Cemental Dysplasia.[36,37] A periapical cemental dysplasia is a rare lesion that occurs most often in the mandibular region, although in rare cases one may develop in the maxilla. It always occurs at the roots of teeth. This lesion is more common in women (average age at diagnosis is 40 years) and among blacks. In almost half of the patients, pain is the initial symptom; other patients develop only a hard swelling that may cause facial asymmetry.

The initial lesion, which is caused by proliferation of connective tissue from the periodontal membrane, appears as a well-defined radiolucency, but it subsequently may be transformed into a radiopaque calcified mass. These lesions can be divided radiographically into three stages: (1) a rather well-defined radiolucency at the apex of a tooth (osteolytic stage); (2) a lesion that is partly radiolucent and partly radiopaque (cementoblastic stage), with the hard tissue formation usually initiated centrally in the lesion; and (3) a lesion that is transformed into a mineralized radiopaque mass surrounded by a narrow radiolucent zone (mature incisive stage) (Fig. 5-22). The tooth is normal in color and responds normally to tests of vitality.

Periapical cemental dysplasia does not require treatment unless the lesion becomes infected or other disturbing symptoms occur. The treatment of choice is enucleation, with or without extraction of the involved tooth. No recurrences have been reported.

Cementifying Fibroma.[38] A cementifying fibroma is a slow-growing lesion of mesenchymal origin that is composed of cellular fibroblastic tissue that contains basophilic masses of cementum-like tissues. In some cases varying amounts of bony trabeculae are interspersed within the lesion, reflecting the name "cementoossifying fibroma." Cementifying fibromas occur most commonly in young and middle-aged adults, with predominant involvement in the mandible. The condition most often affects black women. The tumors usually are 1 to 2 cm in diameter, although larger lesions have been seen in rare cases.

The radiographic features depend on the tumor's stage of development. In the early stage, the tumor appears as a well-circumscribed, well-demarcated radiolucent lesion with no internal radiopacities. As with an osteoblastoma, the lesion in time becomes surrounded by a well-defined radiolucent zone, which appears as a unilateral or symmetrically bilateral mass of varying opacity. These tumors may be treated by enucleation.

Benign Cementoblastoma.[39,40] Also called a "true cementoma," a benign cementoblastoma is a rare neoplasm of functional cementoblasts, characterized by the formation of a cementum or cementum-like mass connected with a tooth root. The lesion occurs most frequently in individuals under 25 years of age and predominantly among men. The lesion is solitary and usually is located in the molar or premolar region, with the mandibular first molar being frequently involved. Benign cementoblastomas are most often associated with permanent teeth, but primary teeth may also be sites.

Radiographically, the tumor is well defined. The dense radiopaque central part is attached to the tooth root and commonly is surrounded by a radiolucent zone of uniform width, which represents the peripheral unmineralized tissues of the formative cellular layers. These tumors have a tendency to expand the cortical bone of the jaws. The lesion is easily enucleated, since it is benign and surrounded by a capsule.

BENIGN NONODONTOGENIC TUMORS

Benign nonodontogenic tumors are not unique to the jawbone; they are found in other parts of the skeleton. Their radiographic appearance in the jaw does not differ significantly from their appearance in other bones, taking into account any abnormalities a tumor may cause in adjacent tooth structures. The discussion of these lesions is based mainly on their tissue of origin.

Exostoses[41-43]

Exostoses are localized outgrowths of bone. They vary in size and appear as flat, nodular, or pedunculated protuberances on the surface of the mandible or maxilla. The cause of exostosis of the jaw is unknown. Three types, torus mandibularis, torus palatinus, and multiple exostoses, must be differentiated according to location.

Radiographically, exostoses are recognized as areas of increased bony density projecting from the mandible or

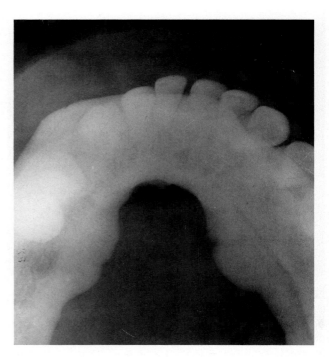

Fig. 5-23 Torus mandibularis. Dental view demonstrates bony exostoses along lingual surface of mandible bilaterally.

maxilla. The exostoses composed of compact bone are of uniform radiopacity, whereas others that contain a marrow space have trabeculations. Some exostoses are difficult to demonstrate radiographically, particularly small ones and those that are superimposed on the teeth. A counterpart of the exostosis is an enostosis, which originates from the inner cortex as an area of osteosclerosis.

Torus mandibularis[41] is an outgrowth of bone on the lingual surface of the mandible (Fig. 5-23). It usually is situated above the mylohyoid line, opposite the bicuspid teeth. The size, shape, and number of protuberances vary. The mandibular tori usually are bilateral, but this condition has been found to be unilateral in 20% of cases. The reported incidence in the United States ranges between 6% and 8%, with no sex predilection.

Torus palatinus[41,42] is a flat, spindle-shaped, nodular or lobular exostosis that arises in the middle of the hard palate (Fig. 5-24). The cause is unknown, but some theories suggest that it may be a hereditary condition. The incidence in the United States varies between 20% and 25% with women being the most often affected. The torus palatinus may occur at any age but reaches its peak incidence before 30 years of age. Radiographically, the torus palatinus is radiopaque with distinct borders, either of dense compact bone or of a shell of compact bone with a center of cancellous bone. Surgi-

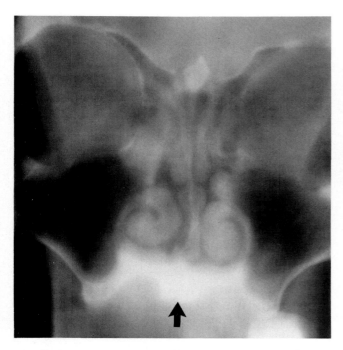

Fig. 5-24 Torus palatinus. Coronal tomographic section reveals bony exostosis of hard palate *(arrow)* projecting into upper oral cavity.

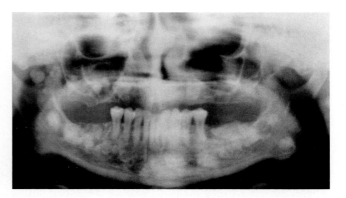

Fig. 5-25 Gardner's syndrome. Panorex view of mandible and maxilla demonstrates several osteomas within mandible and alveolar portion of maxilla. There is some conglomeration of some osteomas, especially in body of right mandible.

cal removal is indicated if the torus interferes with swallowing or if a denture must be constructed.

Multiple exostoses[43] of the jaw arise from the buccal surface of the maxilla in the molar region. They appear as small, nodular, bony masses.

Osteoma[44-50]

An osteoma is a benign neoplasm composed of compact or cancellous bone, usually in an endosteal or periosteal location. These tumors vary greatly in size, from small to large enough to cause disfiguration. The average age of patients with osteomas is 50 to 60 years of age, with twice as many women affected as men. These lesions occur most often in the paranasal sinuses, especially in the frontal sinus. The next most common site is the jaw. The mandible is more often affected than the maxilla.

Osteomas have a characteristic appearance. Radiographically, they are well circumscribed, sclerotic bony masses attached with a broad base or pedicle to the surface of the mandible. Root absorption may occur when the tumor is located in the vicinity of a tooth. The need for surgical removal is determined by the clinical indications, since the tumor has not been found to become malignant.

Gardner's syndrome,[47-50] which is inherited as an autosomal dominant trait, consists of multiple osteomas associated with multiple polyposis of the colon, epider-

moid and sebaceous cysts, desmoid tumors of the skin, and impacted supernumerary and permanent teeth (Fig. 5-25). The multiple osteomas often precede the onset of the colonic polyps, which eventually become malignant in virtually all cases. Osteomas have a predilection for the frontal bone, maxilla, and mandible, although they may be observed in any of the bones of the cranium or facial skeleton. With this syndrome, the osteomas of the jaw appear early in life (most often in the second decade).

Giant Cell Granuloma[51-53]

Giant cell granuloma occurs most frequently in the second and third decades of life, twice as often in women as in men. Painless swelling is the most common symptom, but some lesions may be noted as an incidental finding during routine roentgenographic screening. The mandible is affected in about two thirds of the reported cases, with most tumors located in the anterior part of the mandible from the second premolar to the second molar, often with extension across the midline.

Radiographically, the lesion most often has a radiolucent, multilocular, honeycombed appearance with tiny bony septae traversing the involved area (Fig. 5-26). The loculi are irregular in shape and vary in size. However, unilocular tumors without trabeculation do occur. Often there is a rather marked expansion with thinning of the cortical plates, and perforation may occur in large lesions. If the lesion is adjacent to the teeth, displacement and root resorption are encountered. Lesions in the maxilla produce "ground glass" radiopacities, especially in the antral region. Treatment consists of curettage and in rare cases en bloc resection. Recurrences (13% of cases) are managed in a similar fashion.

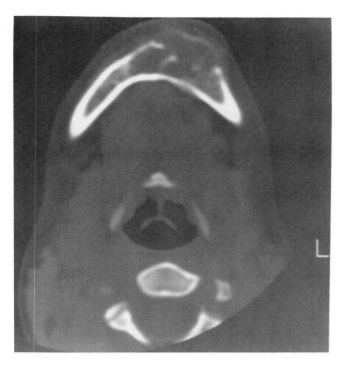

Fig. 5-26 Giant cell granuloma of mandible. Axial CT section (bone window setting) reveals loculated expansile lesion in symphysis and body of left mandible. Bony septae of varying thickness are present within the lesion. Note considerable bulge of anterior cortex of mandible.

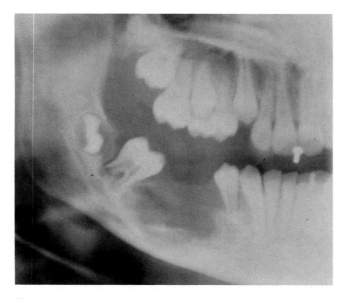

Fig. 5-27 Eosinophilic granuloma in right mandible. Panorex view of mandible reveals lucent, irregular area fairly well defined in body of mandible between second molar tooth and first premolar tooth. Some loss of lamina dura has occurred in lower second molar tooth.

Histiocytosis X[54-60]

Letterer-Siwe Disease.[58] Letterer-Siwe disease is the acute, widely disseminated form of histiocytosis X. It is generally fatal and usually occurs in infants under 1 year of age. Lesions usually are present in several bones and may appear as several small, rounded radiolucencies with well-defined borders. If teeth are present in the affected regions, they frequently are mobile and there is associated gingival bleeding.

Hand-Schüller-Christian Disease.[59] Hand-Schüller-Christian disease is a disseminated, chronic skeletal and extraskeletal form of histiocytosis X. It is the intermediary stage between eosinophilic granuloma and Letterer-Siwe disease. It occurs mostly in children (predominantly boys by a ratio of two to one) from the first to the tenth year of life.

The three classic signs of the disease (single or multiple sharply defined calvarial defects, unilateral or bilateral exophthalmos, and diabetes insipidus) are noted in about 10% of patients. Other organs such as the lymph nodes, liver, spleen, lungs, and skin also may be involved. The first indication of the disease appears in the oral structures, either in the form of red, spongy gingiva or premature loss of teeth. The typical radiographic appearance is one of irregular, lucent defects in the mandible and maxilla. The affected teeth appear to be "floating in space" as a result of marked destruction of alveolar bone. The disease is slowly progressive, and the mortality rate may be as high as 60%.

Eosinophilic Granuloma.[60] Eosinophilic granuloma is the mildest and most favorable form of histiocytosis X. There is a predilection for males, with a morbidity peak in the third decade. The average age of patients with eosinophilic granuloma of the jaw is higher than that of patients with the lesion in other parts of the body. The skull and the tooth-bearing areas of the jaw, predominantly the mandible, frequently are sites. The lesion may be found as an incidental radiographic finding or may manifest as local pain, swelling, tenderness, and occasionally fever and general malaise. Eosinophilic granuloma of the mandible causes well-demarcated areas of osteolysis that may appear "punched out." Maxillary lesions usually are not as well demarcated as those in the mandible.

The area of bone involvement is characterized by irregular lucent patches having no reactive sclerosis but often showing cortical destruction (Fig. 5-27). These patches may appear as single or multiple areas of rarefaction simulating jaw cysts, periapical granulomas, or periodontal disease (Fig. 5-28). Destruction of the crest of the alveolar bone and interdental septum may be an early radiographic finding, together with loss of the cortical outline of a tooth follicle or the lamina dura. The teeth in the involved regions become loose, float in space, and are exfoliated.

Unifocal lesions may be curetted and packed with

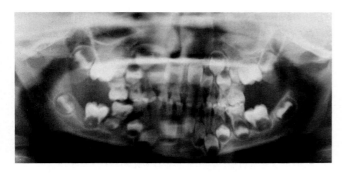

Fig. 5-28 Diffuse eosinophilic granuloma in mandible. Panorex view of mandible reveals loss of lamina dura of erupted and partially erupted tooth follicles. This is especially evident at second lower right molar tooth.

cancellous bone. With several recurrences or persistent residual granulomas, low-dose irradiation and cortisone treatment may be beneficial. Cytostatic agents (vinblastine, cyclophosphamide) also have been used successfully.

FIBROOSSEOUS LESIONS[61-69]
Fibrous Dysplasia[63-66]

Fibrous dysplasia of bone is a lesion of unknown cause, diverse histopathology, and an uncertain pathogenesis. It occurs more frequently in the maxilla than in the mandible, where it usually arises in the posterior regions of the bone. The lesion is most commonly seen in the first three decades of life. There are considerable microscopic variations in different lesions, as evidenced by fibrous tissue alternating with trabeculae of coarse, woven bone, and less well-organized lamellar bone. The three forms of fibrous dysplasia are *monostotic fibrous dysplasia*, *polystotic fibrous dysplasia* (in which multiple bony lesions, often unilateral, occur), and *Albright's syndrome.*

Monostotic[63] fibrous dysplasia occurs with equal predilection for males and females and is encountered frequently in children and young adults, with a mean age at diagnosis of 27 years. The clinical symptoms are painless swelling or bulging of the jaw (usually the labial or buccal plate), malalignment and displacement of teeth, and protuberance of the maxilla, as well as involvement of the maxillary sinus, zygomatic process, floor of the orbit, and sometimes extension to the base of the skull.

Polystotic fibrous dysplasia manifests itself early in life, often with an insidious onset. The disease is characterized by bone deformities such as bowing and thickening, and in some cases it is associated with bone pain. In this form of fibrous dysplasia, the skull and face, including the mandible and maxilla, frequently are involved, often with obvious asymmetry secondary to bony expansion.

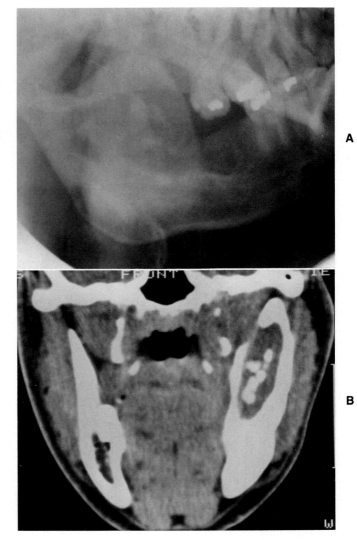

Fig. 5-29 Monostotic fibrous dysplasia of left mandible. **A,** Oblique view of left mandible reveals sclerotic expansile lesion in ascending ramus of mandible with extension into coronoid process. Some calcific densities are present in central anterior part of this lesion. **B,** Coronal CT section (soft tissue window setting) shows expansile nature of lesion in ascending ramus with some loss of cortex medially. Calcified densities are noted within lesion, which is isodense with muscle centrally.

Albright's syndrome is a developmental defect of unknown cause. It is represented by cutaneous pigmentation, precocious puberty, and multiple skeletal lesions. Young girls are most often affected.

The roentgenographic appearance of fibrous dysplasia varies considerably. In one form a unilocular or multilocular, radiolucent lesion with a well-defined border is seen. Interspersed bony trabeculae often are present in the lucent area, rendering the lesion radiopaque (Fig. 5-29, *A* and *B*). The degree of radiopacity depends on the amount of bone laid down within the lesion. An-

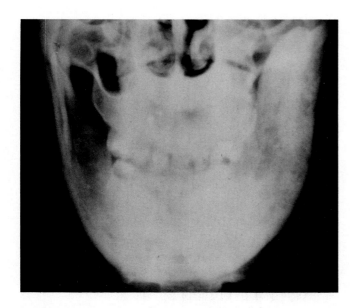

Fig. 5-30 Monostotic fibrous dysplasia. PA view of mandible reveals expansile sclerotic lesion involving ascending ramus of mandible with extension into angle and body of left mandible.

other pattern reveals a marked, homogeneous increase in bone density associated with bony expansion. In this lesion the predominant histologic finding is bony trabeculae with only a small amount of fibrous tissue (Fig. 5-30).

Cystic lesions of appreciable size cause thinning and expansion of the cortex but rarely perforate and produce new periosteal bone. The lesion may cause resorption of the roots of erupted teeth, but this is rarely seen.

Treatment may be limited to surgical contouring for correction of disfiguring asymmetries. Only small lesions can be removed by enucleation. Regular and careful follow-up should be maintained because of the danger of malignant transformation of this lesion.

Ossifying Fibroma (Fibroosteoma)[67-69]

An ossifying fibroma is an encapsulated, benign neoplasm consisting of fibrous tissue that contains various amounts of irregular bony trabeculae. As the lesion matures, the areas of ossification increase in number and coalesce. This transition accounts for the increased radiopaqueness on the roentgenogram. The disorder is most often found in females and may occur at any age, but most cases are reported in the third and fourth decades. The lesion develops predominantly in the mandible and is commonly situated at the roots of the teeth or in the periapical region. It generally is asymptomatic, but a progressive increase in size eventually may cause swelling of the jaw.

Radiographically, the lesion demonstrates a distinct boundary (unlike fibrous dysplasia) and in the early stages appears as a lucent area. As the tumor matures, bony densities are deposited, transforming the lesion into a radiopaque mass. One variety of ossifying fibroma is referred to as juvenile ossifying fibroma. This term is designated for a very actively growing destructive lesion that is histologically identical to the ossifying fibroma. This lesion affects individuals before age 15 and occurs exclusively in the maxilla.

VASCULAR TUMORS—HEMANGIOMA[70,71]

Hemangiomas are most often found in the skull and vertebrae; they are rarely located in the jaw. A hemangioma is a benign tumor composed of newly formed blood vessels of the capillary, cavernous, or mixed type. The tumor may be recognized incidentally on a roentgenographic study or may appear as a hard swelling of variable size. The clinical significance of a hemangioma is stressed by the occasional, severe bleeding that occurs spontaneously or after a tooth extraction. Most hemangiomas are seen in patients under 20 years of age, and they occur twice as frequently in females as in males. They are more often located in the mandible than the maxilla.

Roentgenographically, the lesion appears as a radiolucent area often traversed by delicate bony trabeculae, with formation of variably sized small cavities. In large hemangiomas the cortex is thinned and expanded and may be eroded. If the trabeculae are arranged in a radiating pattern, a sunburst appearance results. In some cases a single radiolucent lesion with a sclerotic or ill-defined border simulating a cyst may be encountered. Root absorption, loss of the lamina dura, and exfoliation of teeth have been reported.

NEUROGENIC TUMORS[72-75]

Benign neurogenic tumors, which include neurilemomas, neurofibromas, and traumatic neuromas, occasionally are found centrally within the jaw. They may occur at any age, and there is little or no sex predilection. Most of these slow-growing lesions arise in the mandible and cause pain or paresthesia.

A *neurilemoma or schwannoma*[73] is usually encapsulated and composed of two distinct histologic components: Antoni type A tissue and Antoni type B tissue. A *neurofibroma*[74,75] arises from the connective tissue sheath of nerve fibers and reveals neurites that traverse the unencapsulated tumor. Neurofibromas may occur as single nodules or as part of neurofibromatosis. Single neurofibromas may originate in the oral mucosa or may occur inside the jaws.

Radiographically, these lesions may appear as a solitary radiolucency associated with the inferior alveolar canal or as a multilocular radiolucency that has produced extensive bone damage, with cortical expansion and even perforation. On occasion the intraosseous tumor may perforate the cortex of the jawbone and extend into the overlying soft tissues. A neurilemoma, arising from the dental nerve within the inferior alveolar canal, may cause bulbous, elongated enlargement of the canal. A neurofibroma, adjacent to bone, may produce a saucer-shaped, erosive defect on the surface of the bone.

MALIGNANT TUMORS

Malignant tumors can be grouped into three categories: (1) lesions that invade the mandible and maxilla secondarily from adjacent soft tissue structures of the oral cavity and sinuses, (2) tumors that arise primarily within the mandible and maxilla, and (3) metastatic tumors from distant sites. The radiographic appearance of malignant lesions often allows them to be differentiated from benign tumors and cysts. However, in many instances a biopsy is indicated for the final diagnosis. It is important, nonetheless, to radiographically assess the extent of the malignant tumor before surgery or radiation therapy. CT has proved particularly valuable in assessing the extent of a tumor outside the mandible and maxilla.

Carcinoma[76-80]

Most carcinomas encountered in the jaw originate in the oral cavity (lip, tongue, buccal mucosa, gingiva, floor of mouth, and palate) and maxillary sinuses. They invade the mandible (and maxilla) secondarily. The mechanism of bone involvement occurs by extension through the nutrient channels or by direct erosion by the advancing tumor.

Radiographically, the osseous involvement manifests early at the alveolar ridge with a saucer-shaped erosive defect. Initially this defect may be shallow and well defined, but in time an irregular cavity is formed. Progressive invasion leads to considerable irregularity of the lytic area. Superficial erosion at the alveolar crest in the tooth-bearing regions may mimic periodontal disease. A pathologic fracture is a common complication in advanced cases. Usually there is no evidence of bony sclerotic reaction or periosteal reaction in carcinomatous involvement of the jaw.

A subgroup of carcinomas is referred to as *central epidermoid carcinoma of the jaw.* This tumor may develop from epithelial components that participated in the development of the teeth or from epithelial cells that became enclosed within the deeper structures of the jaw during embryonic development. About 90% of these lesions are found in the mandible, more frequently in men than in women. The lesions most often occur in patients in the sixth and seventh decades of life. This tumor is now recognized as a definite entity, although it is uncommon.

Radiographically, a carcinoma appears radiolucent with an irregular outline (Fig. 5-31, *A* and *B*). Several small areas of bone destruction may create a moth-eaten appearance. The radiographic findings are nonspecific, and the tumor cannot be differentiated from other malignant lesions.

Carcinomatous transformation of the epithelium in an odontogenic cyst is a rare event, although it has been reported in dentigerous cysts, radicular cysts, residual cysts, and keratocysts. None of the reported cases affected individuals over 40 years of age. On the roentgenogram, the lesion has a cystlike appearance, with a circumscribed margin. In the area of malignant degeneration, the margin becomes ill-defined and irregular or moth-eaten.

Mucoepidermoid Carcinoma[81,82]

Another carcinoma that may occur within the jaw is the mucoepidermoid carcinoma, which is derived from aberrant salivary gland tissue within the maxilla or mandible, almost always in the premolar-molar region. The tumor arises within the medullary portion of the mandible. Women are affected twice as often as men, and the average age at diagnosis is 46 years. The radiographic changes consist of ill-defined, lytic, or multilocular cystic areas (Fig. 5-32, *A, B,* and *C*).

Metastatic Jaw Tumor[83-88]

A metastatic tumor of the mandible or maxilla may be the first indication of malignancy from an undiscovered site or the first evidence of dissemination of a known primary tumor. Patients with metastatic lesions may be asymptomatic or may complain of pain, paresthesia, and anesthesia of the lip or chin. These symptoms are similar to those found with other primary malignant tumors. Soft tissue and bony swelling and loss of teeth are other occasional findings. Metastases to the mandible are four times more frequent than to the maxilla, an unexplained fact. The most common primary tumors are from the breast, lung, kidney (hypernephroma), thyroid, prostate, and stomach.

In most instances the bone destruction caused by a metastatic lesion is reflected radiographically by an irregular lucency with indistinct margins (Fig. 5-33, *A* and *B*). On occasion a mixed type of lesion (consisting of lytic and sclerotic areas) may be encountered, such as in a carcinoma of the breast. In rare cases metastasis from a carcinoma of the prostate causes diffuse osteoblastic changes. The area of destruction within the mandible may be localized, unilateral, bilateral, or diffuse through a large portion of the bone.

Sarcoma[89-95]

Osteogenic Sarcoma.[89-91] Osteogenic sarcoma is a malignant tumor of the bone in which neoplastic cells

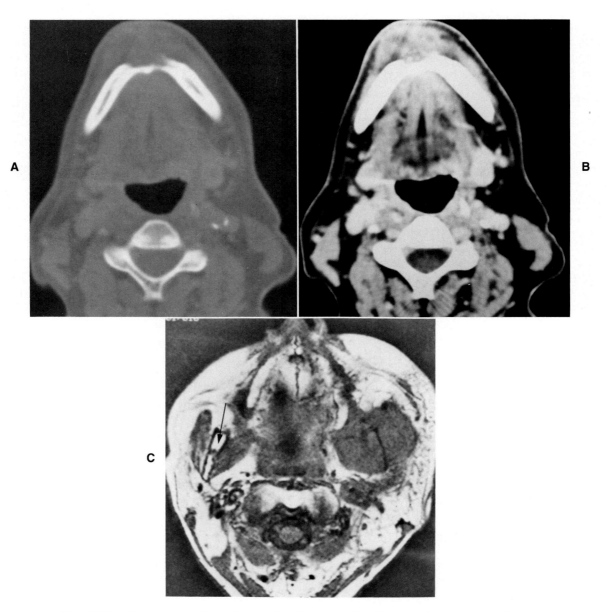

Fig. 5-31 Squamous cell carcinoma of anterior mouth with secondary invasion of mandible. **A,** Axial CT section of mandible (bone window setting) reveals erosion in central and anterior parts of mandible at symphysis. **B,** Axial CT section (soft tissue window setting) demonstrates lesion in anterior mouth with extension into mandible. Again, note erosion in anterior cortex and adjacent medullary portion of mandible. **C,** Axial T_1- weighted MRI scan shows a large squamous cell carcinoma in the left cheek and retromolar trigone, which has infiltrated the ramus of the mandible. The normal high signal intensity of the marrow *(arrow)* has been destroyed by the tumor.

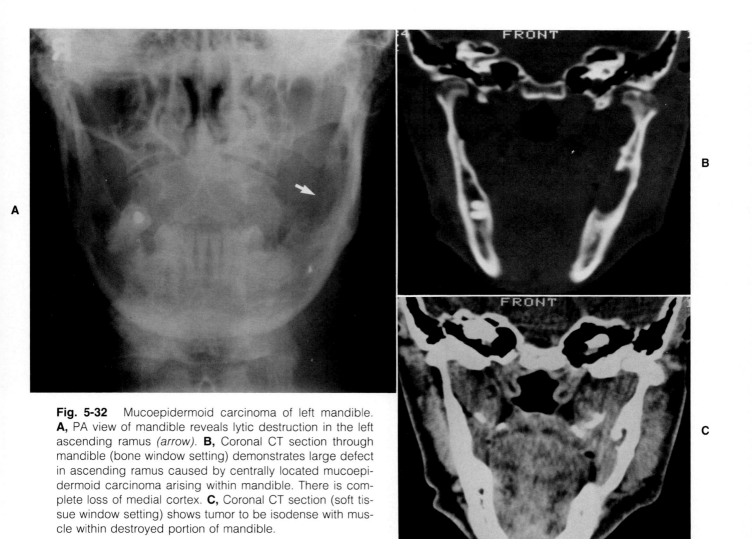

Fig. 5-32   Mucoepidermoid carcinoma of left mandible. **A,** PA view of mandible reveals lytic destruction in the left ascending ramus *(arrow).* **B,** Coronal CT section through mandible (bone window setting) demonstrates large defect in ascending ramus caused by centrally located mucoepidermoid carcinoma arising within mandible. There is complete loss of medial cortex. **C,** Coronal CT section (soft tissue window setting) shows tumor to be isodense with muscle within destroyed portion of mandible.

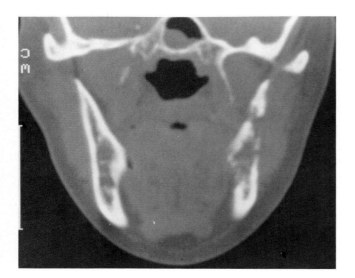

Fig. 5-33   Carcinoma of breast metastatic to right mandible. Coronal CT section through mandbile (bone window setting) shows lytic destructive lesion in ascending ramus of left mandible.

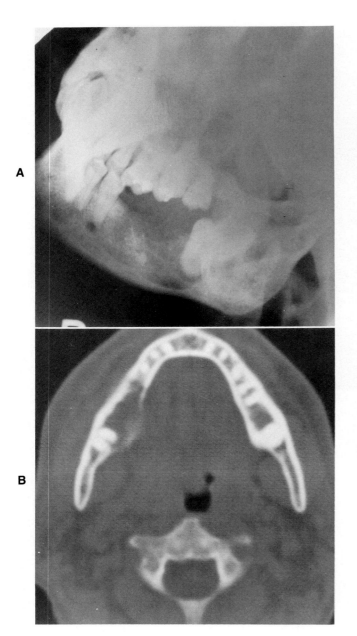

Fig. 5-34 Osteogenic sarcoma of mandible. **A,** Oblique view of mandible reveals ill-defined, lucent area in body of right mandible. Tumor has caused loss of lamina dura of remaining third molar tooth and has invaded mandibular canal. **B,** Axial CT section (bone window setting) shows ill-defined, lucent area in body of right mandible with expansion of cortex medially and loss of bone within cortex.

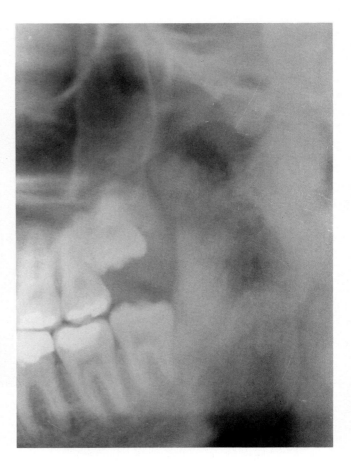

Fig. 5-35 Osteogenic sarcoma of left mandible. Panorex view of mandible reveals sclerotic lesion in ascending ramus with extension into mandible and coronoid process. Boundaries of mandible are poorly defined posteriorly. Tumor has extended into upper left mandibular canal.

produce a variable amount of osteoid. According to the predominant tissue observed microscopically, these lesions are classified as osteoblastic, chondroblastic, or fibroblastic. About 6.5% of osteogenic sarcomas arise in the jaw.

Primary osteogenic sarcoma affects children and young adults, with a peak incidence in the second decade; osteogenic sarcomas of the mandible and maxilla have their peak incidence a decade later. The mandible is more often affected than the maxilla, and there is no sex predominance. The main symptoms are swelling and pain, but paresthesias, loose teeth, and bleeding have been encountered.

Radiographically, osteogenic sarcoma causes lytic destruction of bone with indefinite margins (osteolytic type) (Fig. 5-34, A and B), sclerosis with increased radiopacity (osteoblastic type) (Fig. 5-35), or a mixed pattern. Some osteosarcomas show a sunray effect, caused by radiating mineralized tumor spicules. Cortical breakthrough with tumor outside the jaw is a common finding in advanced cases. Because a symmetrically widened periodontal membrane may be the earliest radiographic finding in osteogenic sarcoma, the disorder must be differentiated from other diseases such as scleroderma or acrosclerosis that also cause widening of the periodontal membrane.

Because lesions that contain calcium, osteoid, or both are easily identified by CT, the presence and extent of osteosarcoma can be easily assessed by that technique. Noncalcified or calcified osteoid within the tumor tissue is reflected by high attenuation values. The increase in density values is proportional to the amount of deposited calcium, ranging from 20 to 300 HU units. Destruction of the bony cortex, with variable attenuation densities that have no characteristic or specific features, is demonstrated by CT. The type and degree of bony permeation by tumor or subtle periosteal reaction in cortical bone may be better appreciated by conventional radiographic techniques.

Among the osteosarcomas of the jaw, most are the osteoblastic type. Patients with mandibular osteosarcomas have a better prognosis than those with maxillary osteosarcomas. Patients with mandibular or maxillary osteosarcomas are prone to developing a recurrence or distant metastases.

Fibrosarcoma.[92,93] Fibrosarcoma of the jaw is a rare lesion that occurs predominantly in the mandible. Onset can occur at any age but is most common before age 50, with a peak incidence between 20 and 40 years of age. Among these tumors, peripheral and central fibrosarcomas have been differentiated. The rare central form most frequently develops in the mandibular canal and causes bone destruction, located centrally, with gradual expansion leading to cortical erosion in larger lesions. The more prevalent peripheral type originates from the periosteum of the mandible or the periodontal membrane, frequently in the body and angle. Radiographically, erosive changes are encountered at the alveolar ridge or at the inferior border of the mandible. The depth of the erosive defect varies, depending on the stage of tumor development. Usually an extramandibular soft tissue mass of variable size is palpated.

Ewing's Sarcoma.[94,95] Ewing's sarcoma occurs predominantly in children and young adults between 5 and 25 years of age, and males are affected twice as frequently as females. In one series of studies, jaw involvement occurred in 13% of cases. This lesion has been found 10 times more frequently in the mandible than in the maxilla. Radiographically, the lesion has a mottled, irregular, lucent appearance, with sclerosis interspersed in a small percentage of tumors. Perpendicular bony spicules and extensive bone destruction may be found at the corticles. The characteristic onion-peel layering of new subperiosteal bone is often absent in the jaw.

Malignant Lymphoma[96]

Malignant lymphoma is derived from lymphocytes and reticulum (histiocytic) cells that are in different stages of development. The disease has a regional or systemic distribution. Lymphomas in the head and

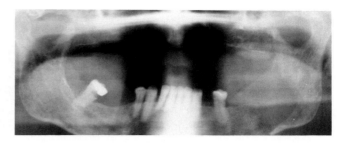

Fig. 5-36   Multiple myeloma of mandible. Panorex view of mandible reveals large destructive lesion in body and ascending ramus of mandible with extramandibular extension at alveolar margin. Pathologic fracture is suggested at anterior aspect of this lytic defect. Also, note several punched-out, lucent areas throughout mandible, especially at left ascending ramus, consistent with foci of multiple myeloma.

neck region occur predominantly in the neck nodes, oral cavity, and nasopharynx and occasionally in the sinuses. Primary lymphoma of bone may occur in the mandible and maxilla. Such bone lymphomas are predominantly reticulum cell sarcomas (histiocytic lymphoma) and less commonly Hodgkin's lymphomas. Reticulum cell sarcoma occurs more frequently in the mandible than in the maxilla, with a predominance in males. Radiographically, there are no pathognomonic findings. Most often seen are ill-defined, lytic destructive areas of variable size within the mandible.

Multiple Myeloma[97,98]

Multiple myeloma is characterized by multiple or diffuse bone involvement, although single lesions occasionally are seen. Myeloma occurs most frequently in people 40 to 70 years of age, with males being affected twice as frequently as females. In patients with multiple myeloma of the jaw, mandibular lesions are by far the most common; they have a predilection for the angle, ramus, and molar teeth regions. Punched-out, regular, circular, or ovoid radiolucencies with no circumferential bone reaction characterize the typical radiographic appearance, especially when the skull is involved (Fig. 5-36). The cortex of the mandible may be perforated, but expansion of bone is not demonstrated. If the lesion is extensive, the entire bone may be destroyed.

Leukemia[99,101]

Leukemia may involve the jawbones. In one series of patients with acute leukemia, 63% of patients showed alteration in the jaws. An early radiographic finding is loss of the lamina dura and loosening of the teeth. This is often followed by a varying degree of lytic bone destruction.

REFERENCES

1. Weber AL and Easter KM: Cysts and odontogenic tumors of the mandible and maxilla. I, Contemp Diagn Radiol 5(25):1, 1982.
2. Borg G, Persson G, and Thilander H: A study of odontogenic cysts with special reference to comparisons between keratinizing and non-keratinizing cysts, Swed Dent J 67:311, 1974.
3. Albright CR and Hannig GH: Large dentigerous cyst of the maxilla near the maxillary sinus, J Am Dent Assoc 83:1112, 1971.
4. Mourshed F: A roentgenographic study of dentigerous cysts, Oral Surg 18:47, 54, 1964.
5. Stafne EC and Milhorn JA: Periodontal cysts, J Oral Surg 3:102, 1945.
6. Donoff RB, Guralnick WC, and Clayman L: Keratocysts of the jaw, J Oral Surg 30:800, 1972.
7. Brannon RB: The odontogenic keratocyst: a clinicopathologic study of 312 cases. I. Clinical features, Oral Surg 42:54, 1976.
8. Brannon RB: The odontogenic keratocyst: a clinicopathologic study of 312 cases. II. Histologic features, Oral Surg 43:233, 1977.
9. Koutnik AW et al: Multiple nevoid basal cell epithelioma, cysts of the jaws, and bifid rib syndrome: report of case, J Oral Surg 33:686, 1975.
10. Gorlin RJ and Goltz RW: Multiple nevoid basal cell epithelioma, jaw cysts and bifid ribs, N Engl J Med 262:908, 1960.
11. Abrams A, Howell FV, and Bullock WK: Nasopalatine cysts, Oral Surg 16:306, 1963.
12. Campbell JJ, Baden E, and Williams AC: Nasopalatine cyst of unusual size: report of case, J Oral Surg 31:776, 1973.
13. Christ TF: The globulomaxillary cyst: an embryologic misconception, Oral Surg 30:515, 1970.
14. Little JW and Jakobsen J: Origin of the globulomaxillary cyst, J Oral Surg 31:188, 1973.
15. Huebner GR and Turlington EG: So-called traumatic (hemorrhagic) bone cysts of the jaw, Oral Surg 31:254, 1971.
16. Biewald HF: A variation in the management of hemorrhagic, traumatic, or simple bone cyst, J Oral Surg 25:627, 1967.
17. Stafne EC: Bone cavities situated near the angle of the jaw, J Am Dent Assoc 29:1969, 1942.
18. Regezi JA, Kerr DA, and Courtney RM: Odontogenic tumors: analysis of 706 cases, J Oral Surg 36:771, 1978.
19. Weber AL and Easter KM: Cysts and odontogenic tumors of the mandible and maxilla. II, Contemporary Diagnostic Radiology 5(26):1, 1982.
20. Small IA and Waldron CA: Ameloblastoma of the jaw, Oral Surg Oral Med Oral Pathol 8(3):281, 1955.
21. Hylton RP, McKean TW, and Albright JE: Simple ameloblastoma: report of case, J Oral Surg 30:59, 1972.
22. Mehlisch DR, Dahlin DC, and Masson JK: Ameloblastoma: a clinicopathologic report, J Oral Surg 30:9, 1972.
23. Franklin CD and Hindle MO: The calcifying epithelial odontogenic tumor—report of four cases: two with long term follow-up, Br J Oral Surg 13:230, 1976.
24. Franklin CD and Pindborg JJ: The calcifying epithelial odontogenic tumor, Oral Surg 42:753, 1976.
25. Pindborg JJ: A calcifying epithelial odontogenic tumor, Cancer 11:838, 1958.
26. Tratman EC: Classification of odontomas, Br Dent J 91:167, 1951.
27. Curreri RC, Messer JE, and Abramson AL: Complex odontoma of the maxillary sinus: report of case, J Oral Surg 33:45, 1975.
28. Caton RB, Marble HB Jr, and Topazian RG: Complex odontoma in the maxillary sinus, J Oral Surg 36(5):658, 1973.
29. Thompson RD, Hale ML, and McLeran JH: Multiple compound composite odontomas of maxilla and mandible: report of case, J Oral Surg 26:478, 1968.
30. Seth VK: Large compound composite odontoma: report of case, J Oral Surg 26:745, 1968.
31. Gundlach KK et al: Odontogenic myxoma—clinical concept and morphological studies, J Oral Pathol 6(6):343, 1977.
32. Hindler BH, Abaza NA, and Quinn P: Odontogenic myxoma: surgical management and an ultrastructural study, Oral Surg 47:203, 1979.
33. Davis RB, Baker RD, and Alling CC: Odontogenic myxoma: clinical pathologic conference. Case 24. I, Oral Surg 36:534, 1978.
34. Davis RB, Baker RD, and Alling CC. Odontogenic myxoma: clinical pathologic conference. Case 24. II, Oral Surg 36:610, 1978.
35. Zegarelli EV, Napoli N, and Hoffman P: The cementoma: a study of 235 patients with 435 cementomas, Oral Surg 17:219, 1964.
36. Vegh T: Multiple cementomas (periapical cemental dysplasia), Oral Sug 42:402, 1976.
37. Chaudhry AP, Spink JH, and Gorlin RJ: Periapical fibrous dysplasia (cementoma), J Oral Surg 16:483, 1958.
38. Hamner JE III, Scofield HH, and Cornyn J: Benign fibro-osseous jaw lesions of periodontal membrane origin: an analysis of 249 cases, Cancer 22:861, 1968.
39. Cherrick H et al: Benign cementoblastoma: a clinicopathologic evaluation, Oral Surg 37:54, 1974.
40. Eversole LR, Sabes WR, and Dauchess VG: Benign cementoblastoma, J Oral Surg 36:824, 1973.
41. Suzuki M and Sakai T: A familial study of torus palatinus and torus mandibularis, Am J Phys Anthropol 18:263, 1960.
42. King DR and Moore GE: An analysis of torus palatinus in a transatlantic study, J Oral Med 31:44-46, 1976.
43. Bhaskar SN and Cutright DE: Multiple exostoses: report of cases, J Oral Surg 26:321, 1968.
44. Weinberg S: Osteoma of the mandibular condyle: report of case, J Oral Surg 35:929, 1977.
45. Noren GD and Roche WC: Huge osteoma of the mandible: report of a case, J Oral Surg 36:375, 1978.
46. Alling CC et al: Clinical-pathological conference. Case 5. II, Osteoma cutis, J Oral Surg 32:195, 1974.
47. Halse A, Roed-Petersen B, and Lund K: Gardner's syndrome, J Oral Surg 33:673, 1975.
48. McFarland PH, Scheetz WL, and Kinisley RE: Gardner's syndrome: report of two families, J Oral Surg 26:632, 1968.
49. Neal CG: Multiple osteomas of the mandible associated with polyposis of the colon (Gardner's syndrome), Oral Surg 28:628, 1969.
50. Gorlin RJ, Pindborg JJ, and Cohen MM: Syndromes of the head and neck, ed 2, New York, 1976, McGraw-Hill, Inc, pp 324-328.
51. Waldron CA and Shafer WG: Central giant cell reparative granuloma of the jaws, Am J Clin Pathol 45:437, 1966.

52. Wesley RK et al: Central giant cell granuloma of the mandible: clinical-pathologic conference. Case 25. I, Oral Surg 36:713, 1978.

53. Smith GA and Ward PH: Giant-cell lesions of the facial skeleton, Arch Otolaryngol 104:186, 1978.

54. Rapidis AD et al: Histiocytosis X, Int J Oral Surg 7:776, 1978.

55. Scott J and Finch LD: Histiocytosis X with oral lesions: report of case, J Oral Surg 30:748, 1972.

56. Soskolne WA, Lustmann J, and Azaz B: Histiocytosis X: report of six cases initially in the jaws, J Oral Surg 35:30, 1977.

57. Sigala JL et al: Dental involvement of histiocytosis, Oral Surg 33:42, 1972.

58. Lieberman P et al: A reappraisal of eosinophilic granuloma of bone: Hand-Schüller-Christian syndrome and Letterer-Siwe syndrome, Medicine 48:375, 1969.

59. Maw RB and McKean TW: Hand-Schüller-Christian disease: report of case, J Am Dent Assoc 85:1353, 1972.

60. Ragab RR and Rake O: Eosinophilic granuloma with bilateral involvement of both jaws, Int J Oral Surg 4:73, 1975.

61. Waldron CA and Giansanti JS: Benign fibro-osseous lesions of the jaws: a clinical-radiologic-histologic review of sixty-five cases. II, Benign fibro-osseous lesions of periodontal ligament origin, Oral Surg 35:340, 1973.

62. Cangiano R, Stratigos GE, and Williams FA: Clinical and radiographic manifestations of fibro-osseous lesions of the jaws: report of five cases, J Oral Surg 29:872, 1971.

63. Hayward JR, Melarkey DW, and Megquier J: Monostotic fibrous dysplasia of the maxilla: report of cases, J Oral Surg 31:625, 1973.

64. Eversole LR, Sabes WR, and Rovin S: Fibrous dysplasia: a nosologic problem in the diagnosis of fibro-osseous lesions of the jaws, J Oral Pathol 1:189-220, 1972.

65. Waldron CA and Giansanti JS: Benign fibro-osseous lesions of the jaws: a clinical-radiologic-histologic review of sixty-five cases. I, Fibrous dysplasia of the jaws, Oral Surg 35:190, 1973.

66. Waldron CA and Giansanti JS: Benign fibro-osseous lesions of the jaws: a clinical-radiologic-histologic review of sixty-five cases. II, Benign fibro-osseous lesions of periodontal ligament origin, Oral Surg Oral Med Oral Pathol 35:340, 1973.

67. Schlumberger HG: Fibrous dysplasia (ossifying fibroma) of maxilla and mandible, Am J Orthod 32:579, 1946.

68. Sherman RS and Sternbergh WCA: Roentgen appearance of ossifying fibroma of bone, Radiology 50:595, 1948.

69. Waldron CA: Ossifying fibroma of mandible: report of two cases, Oral Surg Oral Med Oral Pathol 6:467, 1953.

70. Lund BA: Hemangioma of the mandible and maxilla, J Oral Surg 22:234, 1972.

71. Macansh JD and Owen MD: Central cavernous hemangioma of the mandible: report of cases, J Oral Surg 30:293, 1972.

72. Sdhklar G and Meyer I: Neurogenic tumors of the mouth and jaws, Oral Surg 16:1075, 1963.

73. Shimura K et al: Central neurilemoma of the mandible: report of case and review of the literature, J Oral Surg 31:363, 1973.

74. Prescott GH and White RF: Solitary, central neurofibroma of the mandible: report of case and review of the literature, J Oral Surg 28:305, 1978.

75. Singer CF, Gienger GL, and Kulborn TL: Solitary intraosseous neurofibroma involving the mandibular canal: report of case, J Oral Surg 31:127, 1973.

76. Nolan R and Wood NK: Central squamous cell carcinoma of the mandible: report of a case, J Oral Surg 34:260, 1976.

77. Coonar H: Primary intraosseous carcinoma of maxilla, Br Dent J 147:47, 1979.

78. Lapin R et al: Squamous cell carcinoma arising in a dentigerous cyst, J Oral Surg 31:354, 1973.

79. Shear M: Primary intra-alveolar epidermoid carcinoma of the jaw, J Pathol 97:645, 1969.

80. Sirsat MV, Sampat MB, and Shrikhande SE: Primary intra-alveolar squamous cell carcinoma of the mandible, Oral Surg 35:166, 1973.

81. Fredrickson C and Cherrick HM: Central mucoepidermoid carcinoma of the jaws, J Oral Med 30:80, 1978.

82. Schultz W and Whitten JB: Mucoepidermoid carcinoma in the mandible: report of case, J Oral Surg 27:337, 1969.

83. Adler CI, Sotereanos GC, and Valdivieso JG: Metastatic bronchogenic carcinoma of the maxilla: report of case, J Oral Surg 31:543, 1973.

84. Al-Ani S: Metastatic tumors to the mouth: report of two cases, J Oral Surg 31:120, 1973.

85. Appenzeller J, Weitzner S, and Long GW: Hepatocellular carcinoma metastatic to the mandible: report of case and review of literature, J Oral Surg 29:660, 1971.

86. Carter DG, Anderson EE, and Currie DP: Renal cell carcinoma metastatic to the mandible, J Oral Surg 35:992, 1977.

87. Cherrick HM and Demkee D: Metastatic carcinoma of the jaws, J Am Dent Assoc 87:180, 1973.

88. Moss M and Shapiro DN: Mandibular metastasis of breast cancer, J Am Dent Assoc 78:756, 1969.

89. Garrington GE et al: Osteosarcoma of the jaws, Cancer 20:377, 1967.

90. Caron AS: Osteogenic sarcoma of the facial and cranial bones: review of 43 cases, Am J Surg 122:719, 1971.

91. Wilcox JW et al: Osteogenic sarcoma of the mandible: review of the literature and report of case, J Oral Surg 31:49, 1973.

92. Taconis WK and Rigssel VA: Fibrosarcoma of the jaws, Skeletal Radiol 15:10, 1986.

93. Wright JA and Kuehn PG: Fibrosarcoma of the mandible, Oral Surg 36:16, 1973.

94. Borghelli RF, Barros RE, and Zampieri J: Ewing sarcoma of the mandible: report of case, J Oral Surg 36:473, 1978.

95. Carl W et al: Ewing's sarcoma, J Oral Surg 31:472, 1971.

96. Steg RF, Dahlin DC, and Gores RJ: Malignant lymphoma of the mandible and maxillary region, Oral Surg Oral Med Oral Pathol 12:128, 1959.

97. Miller CE, Goltry RR, and Shenasky JH: Multiple myeloma involving the mandible, Oral Surg 28:603, 1969.

98. Tabachnick TT and Levine B: Multiple myeloma involving the jaws and oral soft tissue, J Oral Surg 34:931, 1976.

99. Curtis AB: Childhood leukemias: osseous changes in jaws on panoramic dental radiographs, J Am Dent Assoc 88:844, 1971.

100. Michaud M et al: Oral manifestations of acute leukemia in children, J Am Dent Assoc 95:1145, 1977.

101. Sela MN and Pisanti S: Early diagnosis and treatment of patients with leukemia: a dental problem, J Oral Med 32:46, 1977.

6 The Pharynx and Oral Cavity

WILLIAM PATRICK DILLON

EMBRYOLOGY

During the first month of intrauterine life, the embryo undergoes rapid and complex differentiation. Progressive infolding at the cephalic and caudal end of the embryo produces an entoderm lined cavity that, at its cephalic end, is in direct contact with the ectoderm at the floor of the stomodeum. This entoderm-ectoderm membrane is known as the buccopharyngeal membrane. At the end of the third week, this membrane ruptures, establishing an open connection between the stomodeum and the foregut. This is the early pharynx and alimentary system. During the fourth and fifth weeks of development, four pharyngeal pouches form along the lateral wall of the pharynx, gradually penetrating the surrounding mesenchyme. Simultaneously, four lateral grooves become visible on the surface of the embryo. These are known as the pharyngeal clefts, which penetrate the underlying mesenchyme. The clefts on the lateral aspect of the embryo approach the pharyngeal pouches closely, although they rarely communicate with each other. The mesodermal tissue between the ectodermal pharyngeal clefts and the endodermal pouches is pushed aside, creating a number of mesodermal arches—the branchial or pharyngeal arches. The human embryo has five pharyngeal arches, the caudal one being poorly defined. The development of the pharyngeal arches is intimately associated with that of the pharyngeal pouches and clefts and will form many of the characteristic ectodermal orifices and pharyngeal parenchymal tissues (Table 6-1).[1-4]

Pharyngeal Arches

During the fourth to fifth weeks of gestation, the pharyngeal arches develop their own cartilage, muscle, arteries, and nerves. Some of the cartilaginous parts persist as adult bony or cartilaginous structures. The first pharyngeal arch, or mandibular arch, consists of a dorsal portion known as the maxillary process extending beneath the region of the eye and a much larger ventral portion called the mandibular process, or Meckel's cartilage. These retrogress except for two small portions at the dorsal end, which form portions of the ossicles of the middle ear—the incus and malleus. The mandible is formed secondarily by ossification of the mesodermal tissue surrounding Meckel's cartilage. The muscles of mastication, the anterior belly of the digastric muscle, and the tensor tympani muscle arise from the mandibular arch. These are innervated by the mandibular branch of the trigeminal nerve, which is the nerve of the first arch. This nerve also supplies sensation to the skin over the mandible and the anterior two-thirds of the mucosa of the tongue.

The second, or hyoid, arch contains Reichert's cartilage. This cartilage gives rise to the crura of the stapes, the styloid process of the temporal bone, the stylohyoid ligament, and the lesser horn and the upper part of the body of the hyoid bone. The muscles of the second arch include the stapedius, the stylohyoid, the posterior belly of the digastric, and the muscles of facial expression. These are supplied by the facial nerve, which is the nerve of the second arch.

Table 6-1 Embryologic origin of head and neck structures

Location	Pharyngeal cleft	Arch	Pouch
1st	External canal	Mandible Incus Malleus Stapedius muscle	Eustachian tube Tympanic cavity Mastoid
2nd	Cervical sinus of His	Muscles of facial expression Posterior belly of digastric Hyoid bone (part) Cranial nerve VII and VIII Stapes, styloid process	Palatine tonsil
3rd	Cervical sinus of His	Superior constrictor muscle Stylopharyngeus muscle Internal carotid artery Cranial nerve XI Hyoid bone (lower body and greater horn)	Inferior parathyroid Thymus gland Pyriform fossa
4th	Cervical sinus of His	Thyroid gland Cuneiform cartilage Superior laryngeal nerve Aortic arch and right subclavian artery	Superior parathyroid gland
5th & 6th		Laryngeal muscles Laryngeal cartilage Inferior pharyngeal constrictors Cranial nerve XI Recurrent laryngeal nerve	Thyroid cells

The third pharyngeal arch forms the lower part of the body and the greater horn of the hyoid bone. The musculature of this arch includes the stylopharyngeal muscle, which is innervated by the glossopharyngeal nerve. Part of the tongue is also derived from this arch.

The fourth and sixth pharyngeal arches fuse to form the thyroid, cricoid, and arytenoid cartilages of the larynx. The muscles of the fourth arch include the cricothyroid and constrictors of the pharynx and are innervated by the superior laryngeal branch of the vagus nerve. The intrinsic muscles of the larynx are supplied by the recurrent laryngeal branch of the vagus, which is the nerve of the sixth arch.

Pharyngeal Pouches

There are five pharyngeal pouches in the embryo. These pouches exist on the pharyngeal side of the developing embryo and thus are of entodermal origin. Each gives rise to a number of parenchymal organs (Table 6-1).

The first pharyngeal pouch forms a diverticulum referred to as the tubotympanic recess. This approaches the epithelial lining of the first pharyngeal cleft to contribute to the tympanic membrane. The distal portion of the pharyngeal pouch widens into the primitive middle ear cavity, whereas the proximal portion remains narrow, forming the eustachian tube.

The second pharyngeal pouch largely regresses during development. A small portion, however, remains to form the palatine tonsil. The tonsil is infiltrated with lymphatic tissue during the third to fifth months of gestation.

The third pharyngeal pouch consists of a dorsal and a ventral aspect. In the fifth week of development, the dorsal aspect gives rise to the inferior parathyroid gland, while the ventral portion forms the primordium of the thymus gland. At the sixth week of development, both the parathyroid and thymus glands lose their connection with the pharyngeal wall and migrate in a caudal and medial direction, eventually arriving at their "adult" location in the upper mediastinum and thyroid region. The parathyroid tissue of the third pouch comes to rest on the dorsal surface of the thyroid gland and in the adult forms the inferior parathyroid gland.

The fourth pharyngeal pouch gives rise to the superior parathyroid gland. During development, the parathyroid gland also loses its contact with the wall of the pharynx, attaching itself to the caudally migrating thyroid gland, and is found on the dorsal surface as the superior thyroid gland.

The fifth pharyngeal pouch is the last to develop and is often considered part of the fourth pouch. It gives rise to a structure called the ultimobranchial body, which is incorporated into the thyroid gland. Its function is unknown, but it can be seen histologically within the thyroid gland.

Pharyngeal Clefts

The four pharyngeal clefts separate the lateral aspect of the pharyngeal arches and give rise to ectodermal structures. The first pharyngeal cleft gives rise to the external auditory meatus. Its medial aspect contributes to formation of the tympanic membrane. The second pharyngeal arch grows rapidly during development and overlaps the third and fourth arches. As a result of this overgrowth, the second, third, and fourth pharyngeal clefts are buried and no longer open to the outside. Temporarily the clefts form a cavity lined with ectoderm referred to as the cervical sinus. With further development, this sinus usually disappears. However, persist growth of this sinus may give rise to branchial cleft anomalies.[3] A fistula may connect the cervical sinus to the outside. This fistula, referred to as the branchial fistula, is found in the lateral aspect of the neck, directly anterior to the sternocleidomastoid muscle. A cervical cyst may be found anywhere along the anterior border of the sternocleidomastoid muscle, although it usually is found at the angle of the jaw. Most often the cyst is located posterior to the submandibular gland and anterior to the sternocleidomastoid muscle. The lateral cervical cyst may not be visible at birth but will become evident as the result of enlargement later in life. Rarely, the cervical sinus may develop a fistula internally. The sinus is then connected to the lumen of the pharynx by a small canal that usually opens into the tonsillar region. Such a fistula indicates a rupture of the membrane between the second pharyngeal cleft and pouch at some time during embryologic development.

Table 6-1 summarizes the components of the pharyngeal arch and the organs formed by the pharyngeal cleft and pouches.

Floor of Pharynx

Tongue. The tongue appears at approximately four weeks of gestation. Two lateral lingual swellings and one medial swelling, called the tuberculum impar, result from proliferation of mesoderm in the ventral aspect of the mandibular arch. A second medial swelling, called the hypobranchial eminence, results from mesoderm of the second, third, and part of the fourth arch. A third medial swelling formed by the posterior part of the fourth arch marks the development of the epiglottis.

With proliferation and ingrowth of mesoderm, the lateral lingual swellings increase greatly in size and fuse with each other, forming the anterior two-thirds of the body of the tongue. Because the mucosa of the body of tongue originates from the first pharyngeal arch, it is innervated by a branch of the mandibular segment of the trigeminal nerve (lingual nerve). The posterior third of the tongue develops from the second, third, and part of the fourth pharyngeal arch. Its innervation is supplied by the glossopharyngeal nerve, which is associated with the third arch. The most posterior part of the tongue and the epiglottis are innervated by the superior laryngeal nerve, developing from the fourth arch. The anterior two-thirds and posterior one-third of the tongue are separated by a V-shaped sulcus called the terminal sulcus. At its apex, the foramen caecum marks the junction of the tuberculum impar and the hypobranchial eminence. It is from the foramen caecum that the thyroid gland develops and descends to its adult position in the neck. Bridging the foramen caecum and the thyroid gland is the thyroglossal duct, a primordial tract. Usually the duct becomes solid and disappears with development. However, the thyroglossal duct cyst, and infrequently thyroid carcinoma, may arise from remnants of this duct epithelium.[5] (See "Benign Lesions of the Oral Cavity and Oropharynx".)

NORMAL ANATOMY AND PHYSIOLOGY

Both CT and MRI are excellent modalities for imaging the upper aerodigestive tract.[6-27] The chief advantages of MRI include its capacity for high spatial and soft tissue contrast resolution, multiplanar imaging, its ability to clearly depict vessels without the use of intravenous contrast agents, and the dependence of tissue intensity on several operator-dependent imaging parameters. CT scan advantages include an ability to detail subtle bone erosion.

In this section, the various compartments of the nasopharynx are considered, detailing the normal and pathologic anatomy within each compartment as visualized by MRI sequences, emphasizing both T_1- and T_2-relaxation differences.

The Nasopharynx

The nasopharynx occupies the most superior extent of the aerodigestive tract, participating in both nasal respiration and deglutition.[28,29] Although the anatomy of the nasopharynx includes a small part of the extracranial head and neck soft tissues, its close proximity to the critical neurovascular anatomy of the skull base gives the nasopharynx special neuroradiologic importance. The jugular fossa (cranial nerves IX through XII), foramen ovale (cranial nerve V3), carotid canal, sella turcica, cavernous sinus (cranial nerves III through V1), and clivus all are within close proximity to the nasopharyngeal mucosa. Thus it is not surprising that invasive nasopharyngeal pathologic conditions frequently result in neurologic symptoms such as diplopia, trigeminal pain or anesthesia, and the jugular fossa syndrome.

The nasopharynx is an open airway lined by squamous epithelial mucosa. It measures approximately 4 cm in transverse diameter and height and 2 cm in its anterior-posterior dimension. Its roof slopes beneath the sphenoid sinus and upper clivus. The lower clivus and upper cervical spine form the posterior boundary of the nasopharynx. The posterior nasal margin represents the anterior limit of the nasopharynx. The medial

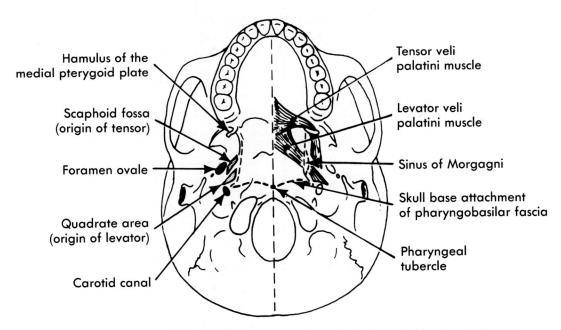

Fig. 6-1 Axial schematic of skull base demonstrates attachment of levator and tensor veli palatini muscles and pharyngobasilar fascia. (Courtesy of Wendy Smoker, MD, University of Utah.)

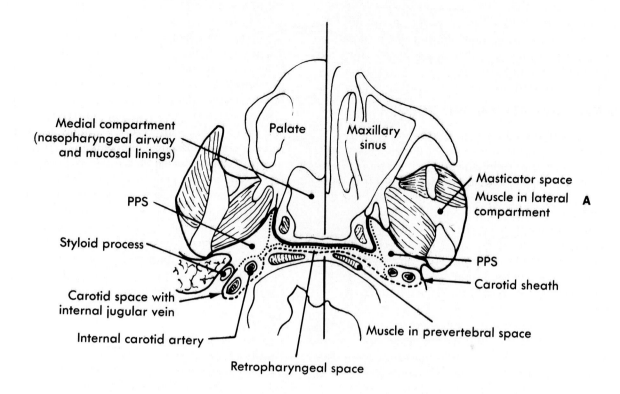

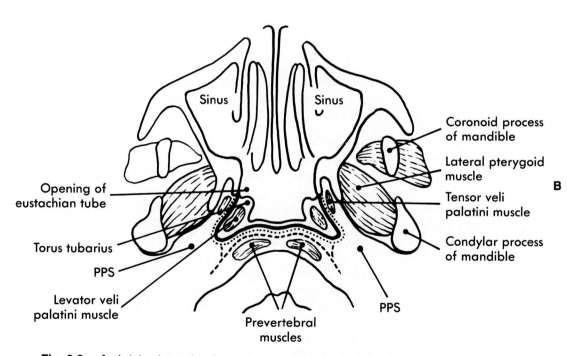

Fig. 6-2   A, Axial schematic of upper nasopharynx. Left side of image is at lower level than right side of image. Various deep spaces of head and neck include masticator space, parapharyngeal space (PPS), carotid space, and retropharyngeal and prevertebral spaces. Dense heavy line represents pharyngobasilar fascia; thin dotted line represents buccopharyngeal fascia. Note that carotid sheath is made up of components of all fascial layers. **B,** Axial schematic through mid/nasopharynx demonstrating relationship of levator and tensor palatini muscles to pharyngobasilar fascia and torus tubarius. (Courtesy Wendy Smoker, MD, University of Utah.)

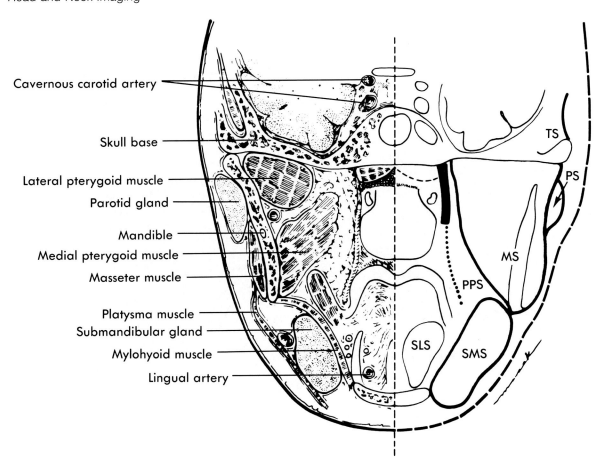

Fig. 6-3 Coronal schematic of nasopharynx and oropharynx demonstrates relationship of deep spaces of head and neck on right side of image to anatomic components on left side of image. *MS*, Masticator space; *SMS*, submandibular space; *PPS*, parapharyngeal space; *PS*, parotid space; *SLS*, sublingual space; *TS*, temporalis space. (Courtesy of H. Ric Harnsberger, MD, University of Utah.)

pterygoid plates form the bony margins of the anterior 5 mm of the lateral walls of the nasopharynx. More posteriorly, the lateral walls of the nasopharynx are formed by fascia, muscle, and deep tissue spaces surrounding the airway (Figs. 6-1 to 6-3).[28,29] Inferiorly, the nasopharynx is demarcated from the oropharynx by the soft palate. The soft palate hangs well into the oropharynx during quiet respiration. The levator and tensor veli palatini muscles arise from the skull base, inserting in the soft palate (Fig. 6-1). These muscles elevate and tense the palate, which opposes a ridge of pharyngeal musculature (Passavant's ridge) that forms the true inferior anatomic limit of the nasopharynx. This sphincteric function prevents nasopharyngeal reflux during speech and swallowing.

The airway is held patent by a firm fascial layer, the pharyngobasilar fascia, which surrounds the mucosa, the superior constrictor muscle, and the levator palatini muscle.[28,29] Some authors feel that the pharyngobasilar fascia may sometimes be detected on MRI as a thin band of low-signal intensity.[17] Others[30] believe this hy-

pointense line represents the cartilaginous portion of the eustachian tube. Nevertheless, the pharyngobasilar fascia effectively divides the superficial "mucosal" space of the nasopharynx from the deep fascial spaces (Figs. 6-2 and 6-3). Harnsberger has demonstrated that, through an understanding of the fascial spaces and their contents, pathologic conditions may be localized more effectively and a differential diagnosis tailored according to the space in which it originates (Table 6-2).[31]

Superficial (Mucosal) Space. The superficial or mucosal space of the nasopharynx contains the squamous mucosa, adenoidal (lymphoid) tissue, superior and middle constrictor muscles, torus tubarius, and levator palatini muscle (Figs. 6-1 to 6-3). These structures lie on the airway side of the pharyngobasilar fascia, which provides an initial barrier to the spread of mucosal disease into the deeper compartments.[6,15]

The mucosa of the nasopharynx comprises both stratified squamous and ciliated columnar epithelium. Columnar epithelium predominates during the first 10 years of life. Stratified squamous epithelium is more

Table 6-2   Deep compartments of the nasopharynx

Compartment	Contents	Pathologic conditions
Mucosal space	Adenoids Mucosa	Carcinoma, lymphoma Plasmacytoma, melanoma Pediatric rhabdomyosarcoma Juvenile angiofibroma Non-Hodgkin's lymphoma Minor salivary gland tumors
Parapharyngeal space	Fat Ascending pharyngeal artery 3rd division of trigeminal cranial nerve V3 Internal maxillary artery	Lipoma, cellulitis Abscess (tonsillar) 2nd brachial cleft cyst Schwannoma Salivary rest tumors
Carotid space	Carotid artery Jugular vein Cranial nerves IX-XII Sympathetic chain Lateral retropharyngeal lymph nodes	Paragangliomas, Schwannomas, Extracranial meningiomas Adenopathy, lymphoma Cellulitis, Abscess

Masticator space	Mandible
	Medial pterygoid muscle
	Lateral pterygoid muscle
	Temporalis muscle
	Masseter muscle
	Inferior alveolar nerve
		Abscess and cellulitis—odontogenic
		Benign masseteric hypertrophy
		Tumor
		   Benign:
		     Lipoma, hemangioma
		     Neurogenic tumors
		   Malignant:
		     Minor salivary gland
		     Metastatic to mandible
		     Sarcoma of muscle or mandible
		     Direct spread of squamous cell
		       carcinoma
		     Lymphoma

Retropharyngeal space	Fat Medial retropharyngeal lymph nodes	Lymphoma, lipomas Metastatic adenopathy Abscesses or cellulitis
Prevertebral space	Notochord elements Prevertebral muscles	Chordomas Metastatic disease to the spine Osteomyelitis with abscess, cellulitis

common with advancing age, especially in the lateral pharyngeal recesses of Rosenmüller. Normally about 60% of the nasopharyngeal mucosa in the adult is composed of squamous epithelium.[32] Mucous-secreting glandular elements are located in the submucosal lamina propria of the posterior pharyngeal wall. These structures probably give rise to the infrequent adenocarcinomas of the nasopharynx. Likewise, minor salivary glands abound within the oropharynx and nasopharynx. These are the origin of both benign and malignant tumors.

The adenoids are residual lymphatic tissue and occupy the superior recesses of the nasopharynx. They decrease in volume with age but may persist as small tags of tissue well into adulthood. Residual adenoidal tissue may be mistaken for a superficial malignancy both on clinical examination and on CT scans, but these

entities are usually easily differentiated by MR imaging (Figs. 6-4 and 6-5).

The mucosa and adenoidal tissue of the nasopharynx have a relatively prolonged T_1 and T_2 relaxation time, resulting in intermediate-signal intensity on T_1-weighted images and high-signal intensity on T_2-weighted images (Figs. 6-4 to 6-6). Children and young adults may have prominent adenoidal tissue that fills the superior recesses of the nasopharynx (Fig. 6-5). Degenerative or cystic changes can often be identified within the adenoidal tissue only on T_2-weighted MR images. These subtleties are not resolved by CT scans. Gradual involution of the adenoidal tissue begins at puberty, and although large amounts of lymphoid tissue may be seen into the sixth or seventh decade, most adults have lost this tissue by 30 years of age (Fig. 6-7). Benign adenoidal tissue is enclosed by the pharyn-

Fig. 6-4 **A,** Sagittal T₁-weighted MRI scan through the mid/oropharynx and nasopharynx. Note in this young individual, hypertrophied adenoidal tissue *(a)* occupying superior and lateral recesses of nasopharynx. Its signal intensity is slightly higher than that of surrounding muscle but much higher than that of fat. Also seen are elements of fatty marrow within crista galli *(closed white arrow)* and vomer bone *(open white arrow)*. Occipital sphenoid suture is hypointense line dividing midclivus *(black arrows)*. **B,** Parasagittal T₁-weighted MR images through lateral nasopharynx. Demonstrated here are longus colli muscles extending to skull base *(lc)* and lateral aspect of adenoidal tissue *(A)*. Fat and glandular elements within hard and soft palate *(white arrows)* exhibit high-signal intensity. *T,* tongue; *C,* clivus; *S,* sphenoid sinus; *es,* ethmoid sinus; *mt,* middle turbinate; *it,* inferior turbinate; *C2,* Second cervical vertebrae.

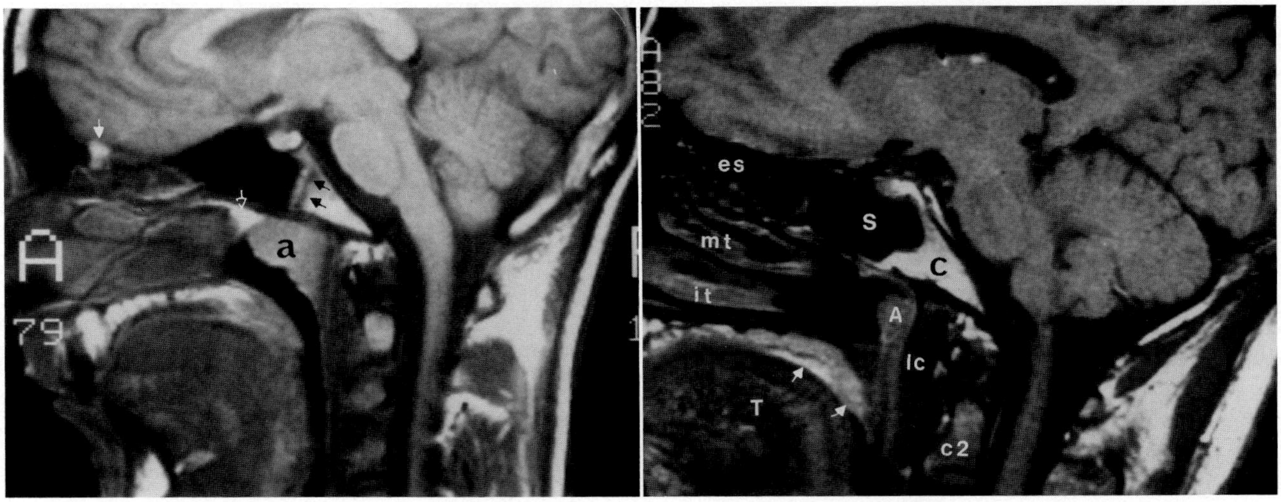

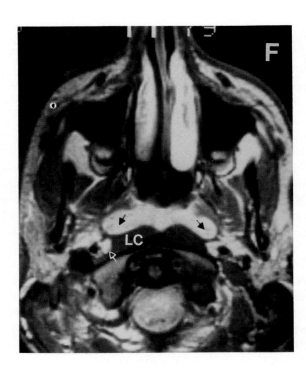

Fig. 6-5 Proton density axial view through nasopharynx demonstrates adenoidal tissue filling recesses of nasopharynx *(arrows)*. Notice sharp contrast between hyperintense adenoidal tissue and longus capitis-colli muscle *(LC)*. Also note reactive lateral retropharyngeal node *(open white arrow)* interposed between longus capitis muscle and internal carotid artery.

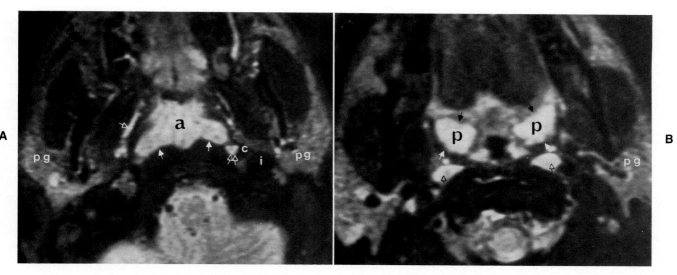

Fig. 6-6   A, Axial T$_2$-weighted MRI sequence through midnasopharynx demonstrates increased signal intensity within adenoidal tissue *(a)*. Lateral retropharyngeal node is again identified *(double open white arrows)*, adjacent to carotid artery *(c)* and internal jugular vein *(i)*. Parotid glands are noted to be of slightly increased signal intensity with respect to muscle *(pg)*. Veins within pterygoid plexus are identified adjacent to mucosal airway *(single open white arrow)*. These can demonstrate hyperintense signal on T$_2$-weighted images caused by echo rephasing. **B,** Axial T$_2$-weighted MRI view through oropharynx. Most prominent features of midoropharynx in young adults and children are palatine tonsils *(P)*. Lateral retropharyngeal nodes are also identified *(open black arrows)*. Surrounding palatine tonsils is area of hypointense signal posteriorly representing superior constrictor muscle *(white arrows)* and palatoglossus muscle *(black arrows)* anteriorly. *PG,* Parotid gland.

gobasilar fascia and lateral recesses of the nasopharynx. It never infiltrates structures deep to the pharyngobasilar fascia (Figs. 6-5 and 6-6, *A*). Obliteration of fascial planes deep to the pharyngobasilar fascia indicates an invasive pathologic condition.

The eustachian tubes connect the nasopharyngeal airway and the middle ear. Each tube terminates within the lumen of the nasopharynx in a lateral cartilaginous enlargement, called the torus tubarius (Figs. 6-2, *B*, 6-5, and 6-7). The nasopharyngeal end of the cartilaginous portion of the eustachian tube is C shaped in cross-sectional appearance. The tensor palatini, the levator palatini, and the salpingopharyngeal muscles arise on opposing margins of this cartilage in such a manner that during swallowing their contractions maximally open the eustachian tube to ensure pressure equilibration between the pharynx and the middle ear. Eustachian tube dysfunction rapidly produces negative pressures in the middle ear, often resulting in serous effusions within the middle ear and mastoid air cavities.

The lateral pharyngeal recess of Rosenmüller is formed on each side of the nasopharynx by the mucosal reflection over the lateral aspects of the prevertebral

longus colli and capitis muscles (the flexor muscles of the cervical spine) (Figs. 6-5 and 6-7). In elderly patients, the lateral pharyngeal recess may be quite shallow because of loss of muscle bulk. In such patients, the nasopharynx may assume a distended hypotonic configuration. In younger individuals, the lateral pharyngeal recesses may be obliterated by adenoidal tissue (Fig. 6-5).

The lateral pharyngeal recesses must be carefully evaluated, because they are the site of origin for approximately 50% of squamous carcinomas of the nasopharynx.[33] Close scrutiny of the superficial landmarks of the nasopharynx for asymmetry may lead to the discovery of infiltration of the deep musculofascial planes, which is the hallmark of malignancy or aggressive inflammatory disease.

The levator palatini muscle is identified on axial MRI scans as a muscular band located just lateral to the torus tubarius (Figs. 6-1, 6-2, and 6-7). The levator palatini muscle is surrounded by fat, which separates it from the longus colli and capitis muscles. Infiltration of this fat plane, which is adjacent to the lateral pharyngeal recess, is an early sign of nasopharyngeal carcinoma.[15] A

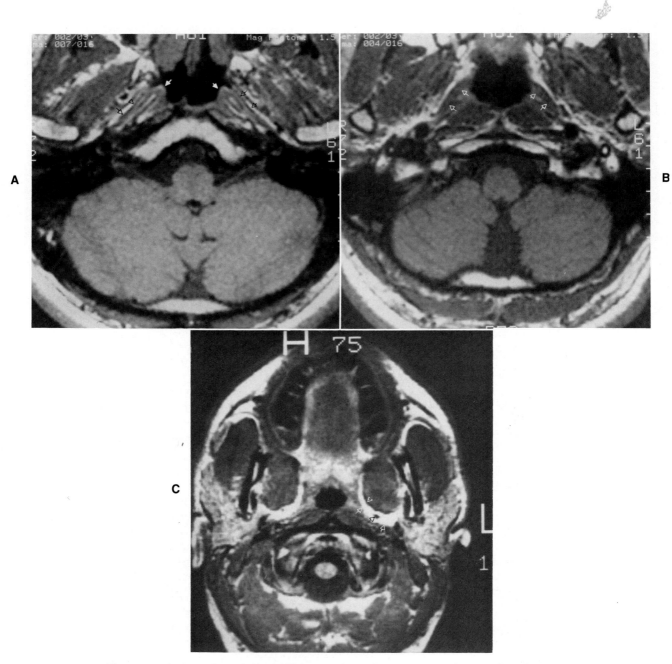

Fig. 6-7 **A,** Axial T₁-weighted MR image through upper nasopharynx. Prominent torus tubari extend into oronasal airway *(white arrow)*. Levator palatini muscle is located just lateral to these structures *(open black arrows)*. Further lateral, parapharyngeal space is seen. **B,** Axial T₁-weighted MR image through midnasopharynx. Tensor palatini muscle *(arrows)* extends from skull base down to palate. **C,** Axial T₁-weighted MR image through midoropharynx to lower oropharynx. Parapharyngeal space is medial to masticator space and contains high-signal intensity fat *(white arrows)*. In middle of parapharyngeal space, hypointense signals can sometimes be identified from either pharyngeal veins *(black arrow)*, branches of trigeminal nerve, or ascending pharyngeal arteries.

second palatal muscle, the tensor palatini muscle, courses laterally to the pharyngobasilar fascia and the levator muscle (Figs. 6-1, 6-2, *B*, and 6-7). Its contraction places lateral tension on the soft palate, elevating it to appose the pharyngeal musculature during swallowing (Fig. 6-2, *B*). The tensor palatini muscle can usually be identified on axial and coronal images, embedded within fat lateral to the nasopharyngeal airway and medial to the parapharyngeal space.

With modern CT scanners the structures within the confined compartment surrounding the levator palatini muscles can be studied in detail. Following intravenous contrast administration, the cartilaginous ends of the eustachian tube appear lower in density than the surrounding, enhancing mucosa and musculature. This appearance most likely reflects the avascular nature of the cartilage. Fat is usually not abundant in this space; however, in some patients definite fat planes are visible around the levator palatini muscle.

The density of the superior constrictor muscle and pharyngobasilar fascia is similar so that the two are inseparable on CT scans. These two structures do not create a definable thickness until the level of the lower nasopharynx.

Deep Musculofascial Spaces of the Nasopharynx and

Oropharynx. The tissues of the nasopharynx and oropharynx deep to the mucosa are best considered as spaces demarcated by layers of the deep cervical fascia. With an understanding of the anatomic contents of these spaces and the pathologic processes that can occur within them, a differential diagnosis is facilitated for mass lesions occurring in these regions.[25,31]

Parapharyngeal Space. The parapharyngeal space is a symmetric triangular fat-filled space lying deep to the pharyngobasilar fascia (Figs. 6-2 and 6-3). The parapharyngeal space is in direct contact with the basisphenoid and inferior petrous apex, as well as with the submandibular and parotid glands. This relationship provides a direct pathway for pathologic conditions of the nasopharynx and oropharynx to the basilar foramina and the greater wing of the sphenoid. Therefore pathologic processes in the parapharyngeal space may spread superiorly to the base of the skull, as well as inferiorly to the submandibular and parotid glands.

The tensor palatini muscle, the superior constrictor muscle, branches of the pharyngeal neurovascular structures, and the third division of the trigeminal nerve all course within the parapharyngeal space. Following contrast administration, on axial CT scans, branches of the ascending pharyngeal artery and the

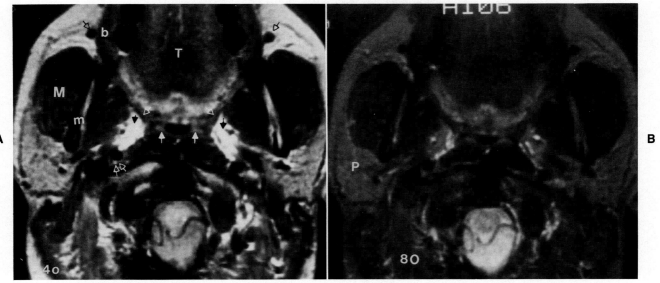

Fig. 6-8   A, Proton-density (TE-40) image through oropharynx demonstrates hyperintense parapharyngeal spaces located medial to masticator space *(closed black arrows).* Tensor and levator palatini muscles insert on palate *(open white arrows).* Mucosa of oropharynx has slightly hyperintense area surrounding airway *(closed white arrows).* Also identified are buccinator muscles *(b),* facial artery *(black arrows),* masseter muscles *(M),* mandible *(m),* and retropharyngeal nodes *(double open white arrows).* **B,** T$_2$-weighted MR image (TE 80 msec). Parapharyngeal space exhibits decreased signal intensity. Foci of increased signal intensity within this space represent pharyngeal veins. Note that parotid gland *(P)* decreases in signal, similar to fat.

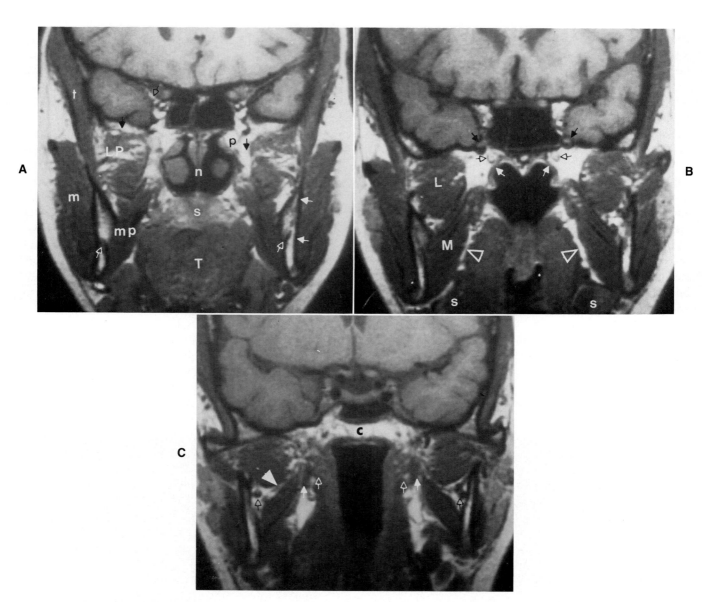

Fig. 6-9 A, Coronal view through anterior aspect of nasopharynx and oropharynx. At this region, masticator space muscles are seen in cross-section and include superior and inferior belly of lateral pterygoid *(LP)*, medial pterygoid *(mp)*, and masseter muscle *(m)*. Fatty marrow within pterygoid plate and skull base has high-signal intensity *(closed black arrows)*. Superior orbital fissure is seen as area of increased signal intensity near orbital apex *(open black arrows)*. Mandible consists of marrow that is high in signal and cortical bone that is low in signal *(closed white arrows)*. Neurovascular canal containing inferior alveolar artery and nerve exists within mandible *(open white arrows)*. *T,* Tongue; *s,* soft palate; *p,* pterygoid plate; *n,* nasal cavity; *t,* temporalis muscle. **B,** Coronal view at 1 cm posterior to **A** demonstrates parapharyngeal space *(arrowheads)* interposed between masticator space muscles and tonsillar tissue. Parapharyngeal space extends down to angle of mandible just above submandibular gland *(s)*. Also note in this view, superior lateral recesses of nasopharynx *(closed white arrows)*, pterygoid canal *(open black arrows)*, and foramen rotundum occupied by second division of trigeminal nerve *(closed black arrows)*. *L,* Lateral pterygoid muscle; *M,* medial pterygoid muscle. **C,** Coronal view at 1 cm posterior to **B.** High-signal intensity fatty marrow of clivus *(c)* is seen. Located within masticator space are branches of third division of trigeminal nerve *(white arrowhead)* and internal maxillary artery *(open black arrows)*. Levator *(open white arrows)* and tensor *(closed white arrows)* extend down toward palate from their skull base origin.

pharyngeal veins appear as multiple round high-density structures within the parapharyngeal space.

On MRI, the parapharyngeal space has a high-signal intensity on T_1-weighted images and an intermediate-to low-signal intensity on heavily T_2-weighted images (Figs. 6-8 and 6-9). This is due to the short T_1 and intermediate T_2 relaxation times of fat. Foci of low- and high-signal intensities represent branches of the ascending pharyngeal artery and slow flowing pharyngeal veins, respectively (Fig. 6-8).

The relationship of the parapharyngeal space to surrounding muscles is best demonstrated on coronal sections (Fig. 6-9). The deep lobe of the parotid gland abuts the parapharyngeal space posterolaterally. Alteration in the intimate relationship between the deep lobe of the parotid gland and the posterolateral aspect of the parapharyngeal space often indicates disease processes in the region (see Chapter 3). The CT density of the parotid gland in most adults approximates the attenuation of the fat in the parapharyngeal space.

Carotid Space. The so called carotid space spans the neck from the skull base to the aortic arch. It is enclosed in part by the carotid sheath, which receives contributions from all three layers of the deep cervical fascia (Fig. 6-2). This sheath is a well-defined structure below the carotid bifurcation, but it is often incomplete or absent in the area of the internal carotid artery. At the level of the nasopharynx, the carotid sheath contains the internal carotid artery, the internal jugular vein, cranial nerves IX through XII, and the cervical sympathetic plexus. On MR images, the cranial nerves, particularly the vagus nerve, may be recognized as intermediate-signal–intensity structures adjacent and posterior to the carotid artery (Fig. 6-8, *A*). They can be followed back through the cisterns of the posterior fossa to their origins in the brainstem. The retropharyngeal nodes of Rouvier lie medial to the internal carotid artery. This lymph node chain is divided into a medial and lateral group. The medial group may extend across the midline, whereas the lateral retropharyngeal nodes surround the neurovascular structures that are within the carotid sheath.[34] The retropharyngeal nodes are the first echelon nodes draining the pharynx and are almost always visualized on normal scans. They may number as many as two or three on either side and usually measure less than 3 to 5 mm in diameter.[34,35] Their signal intensity increases on T2-weighted scans; however, no signal differences are apparent between benign reactive nodes and small nodes harboring microscopic metastases (Fig. 6-6, *B*).

On axial MR scans, the internal carotid artery normally has an absent signal (flow void) caused by the wash-out of protons in high-velocity blood flow (Figs. 6-6 and 6-8). In most instances the internal jugular vein also has a low-signal intensity (Fig. 6-8, *A*). Slow blood flow within a small internal jugular vein sometimes has a high signal, which undergoes even-echo rephasing.[11] This may be due in part to impingement on the vein by the transverse processes of either or both of the first two cervical vertebrae. The carotid sheath may be difficult to distinguish from the aerated cortical bone of the petrous apex in the upper nasopharynx. It usually can be identified by its position posterior and lateral to the parapharyngeal space.

On contrast-enhanced CT studies, the carotid artery and internal jugular vein are normally enhanced.[22] Any other structures in the carotid sheath region that are enhanced should be considered abnormal. The small punctate low densities surrounding the carotid sheath represent cranial nerves IX through XII, as well as small retropharyngeal lymph nodes.

The internal jugular veins are often asymmetric, with the right being larger than the left in nearly 80% of people. This difference may be very dramatic and simulate a pathologic process. However, in the normal patient, the cortex of the jugular fossa, the jugular spur, and the bony septum, separating the carotid artery and jugular vein, are always intact.[36]

Masticator Space. The masticator space is defined by the superficial or investing layer of the deep cervical fascia (buccopharyngeal fascia), which splits at the angle of the mandible to enclose the muscles of mastication, the ramus and posterior body of the mandible, and the pterygoid venous plexus (Fig. 6-2) (Table 6-2). The muscles of mastication include the lateral and medial pterygoids, the temporalis, and the masseter muscles. All four muscles are supplied by the third division of the trigeminal nerve. Injury to this nerve may result in diminished volume (atrophy) of the masticator musculature.

The masticator space provides tumors and infections a route for spreading to the skull base (Fig. 6-3).[18,37] Because the temporalis muscle is within the masticator space, extension of tumor or infection along its fibers lateral to the skull is not uncommon. The most common masticator space masses are odontogenic infections. Postextraction infection or periodontal infection may lead to mandibular osteomyelitis and abscess. Masticator space neoplasms are rare (Table 6-2). Pathologic processes involving the masticator space often manifest clinically as trismus.

Anteriorly and inferiorly, the masticator space is in direct continuity with the buccinator space (Fig. 6-7, *B*). The fat-filled buccinator space lies just lateral and posterior to the lower aspect of the maxilla. The buccinator space separates the soft tissues of the cheek from the buccinator muscle, which is a thin muscle that inserts on the inferolateral surface of the maxilla and the pterygomandibular raphe.

Prevertebral Space. The prevertebral space lies be-

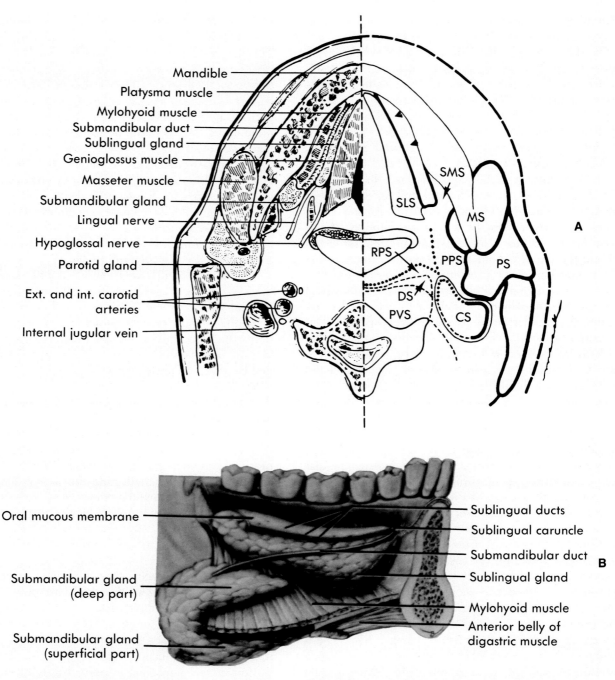

Fig. 6-10 **A,** Axial schematic view through floor of mouth demonstrates sublingual space *(SLS),* which contains sublingual salivary gland, and submandibular space *(SMS),* which contains submandibular salivary gland. Mylohyoid muscle separates these two spaces *(arrowheads). PVS,* Prevertebral space; *CS,* carotid space; *DS,* danger space; *PS,* parotid space; *PPS,* parapharyngeal space; *RPS,* retropharyngeal space; *MS,* masticator space. **B,** Sagittal schematic through floor of mouth demonstrating sublingual salivary gland, submandibular gland, and mylohyoid muscle. Note that submandibular gland has both superficial part and deep part that extends around posterior margin of mylohyoid muscle. Submandibular duct exits deep portion and travels within sublingual space, adjacent to sublingual salivary gland, to empty into sublingual caruncle. Sublingual salivary glands empty through numerous ducts that penetrate mucosa of oral cavity. Thus pathologic disorders within sublingual space may extend into submandibular space around posterior margin of mylohyoid muscle. (Courtesy of H. Ric Harnsberger, MD, University of Utah.)

tween the deep layer of the cervical fascia and the vertebral bodies, directly posterior to the retropharyngeal space (Figs. 6-1 and 6-2). It contains the vertebral column, the prevertebral muscles, the brachial plexus and phrenic nerves, and the vertebral arteries and veins (Figs. 6-1 and 6-2). It extends from the skull base to the coccyx. The most common prevertebral space lesions include infections or tumors of the cervical spine. In addition, extension to the prevertebral space may occur from retropharyngeal space tumors or infections (Table 6-2).[25]

Parotid Space. A full discussion of the pathologic processes of the parotid glands is given in Chapter 3. However, in summary, deep lobe masses may present clinically as submucosal tumors of the oropharynx or nasopharynx. Differentiation of such parotid masses from primary parapharyngeal or carotid space masses is easiest on MRI scans, which usually demonstrate contiguity between the parotid gland and the mass.

Retropharyngeal Space. The retropharyngeal space is a potential space that separates the prevertebral muscles and the pharyngeal constrictor muscles.[25] It is bound posteriorly by the posterior portion of the deep layer of the deep cervical fascia (prevertebral fascia) and anteriorly by the retrovisceral fascia. Laterally, the alar fascia (a portion of the deep layer of the deep cervical fascia) arises and crosses the retropharyngeal space from side to side, therefore dividing this space into an anterior and posterior portion. The retropharyngeal space extends from the skull base to the level of the third thoracic vertebral body and primarily contains fat and the medial retropharyngeal lymph nodes (Table 6-2). Inflammatory or postsurgical edema within the retropharyngeal space may enlarge the posterior retropharyngeal space and dissect it along its course into the posterior mediastinum.[38] In addition, reactive or metastatic adenopathy, cellulitis or abscess, and benign tumors such as lipoma and hemangioma may involve the structures within this space.

The Oral Cavity and Oropharynx

The oral portion of the upper aerodigestive tract is divided into two major components: the oral cavity and the oropharynx. The oral cavity contains the anterior two-thirds of the tongue, the buccal mucosa, the floor of the mouth (Fig. 6-10), and the supporting mandible and maxillary bones. The oropharynx is that region posterior to the circumvallate papilla of the tongue and includes the posterior one-third of the tongue (tongue base), the palatine tonsils, the soft palate, and the oropharyngeal mucosa and constrictor muscles from the level of the soft palate to the top of the epiglottis. Three major types of soft tissue are present in the oral cavity and oropharynx: muscle, lymphoid tissue, and fat.[39] They exhibit different MRI and CT signals, depending on the intrinsic properties mentioned above and the MR imaging parameters selected. On CT scans, muscle and lymphoid tissue are often difficult to discern from neoplastic tissues (Fig. 6-11). On MRI fat has a short T_1 relaxation time and has high-signal intensity on T_1-weighted images (Fig. 6-12). Most soft tissue structures such as the muscle of the tongue have an intermediate-signal intensity on both T_1- and T_2-weighted images (Fig. 6-8, *B*). Tumors generate increased amounts of water protons, which prolong relaxation times and result in higher signals on T_2-weighted images.

Lymphoid tissue, present in the palatine and lingual tonsils and on the inferior surface of the soft palate, has a signal intensity similar to muscle and most tumors on T_1-weighted images.[39-43] Lymphoid tissue has a relatively long T_2 relaxation time and therefore increases in signal intensity relative to muscle on a T_2-weighted image (Fig. 6-6). T_1-weighted MRI sequences afford the best contrast between fat and muscle, whereas T_2-weighted MRI sequences (long TR/TE) demonstrate the best contrast between muscle and lymphoid tissue (Figs. 6-5 and 6-6).

The oral tongue is supported by the floor of the mouth. The tongue consists of three intrinsic muscles that interdigitate on either side of midline. Fat separates the muscle fibers and can be visualized on both CT and T_1-weighted MRI scans (Figs. 6-11 and 6-12). On T_2-weighted MR images, the tongue decreases in signal intensity in a homogeneous fashion (Figs. 6-8, *B* and 6-12, *F*).

The floor of the mouth is a U-shaped area covered by squamous mucosa. It is bounded anteriorly by the gingiva of the mandible and posteriorly by the anterior faucial pillar. The sublingual and submandibular spaces are two important landmarks in the floor of the mouth. The sublingual space contains the sublingual salivary glands and the duct and hilum of the submandibular gland. The main body of the submandibular gland resides within the submandibular space. Thus the submandibular gland bridges these spaces by bending around the posterior free edge of the mylohyoid muscle (Figs. 6-3 and 6-10 to 6-12). The sling-shaped mylohyoid muscle and the anterior belly of the digastric muscle combine with the extrinsic tongue muscles to form the floor of the mouth (Figs. 6-10 to 6-12). On CT and MR scans, the fat planes between these muscles are important normal landmarks (Figs. 6-11 and 6-12). The extrinsic muscles of the tongue include the genioglossus, styloglossus, and hyoglossus muscles. Along with the geniohyoid, they form the majority of the muscles of the floor of the mouth and are innervated by the hypoglossal nerve (cranial nerve XII).

The lingual vessels, which are branches of the external carotid arteries, supply each half of the tongue and floor of mouth. They course within the fat plane be-

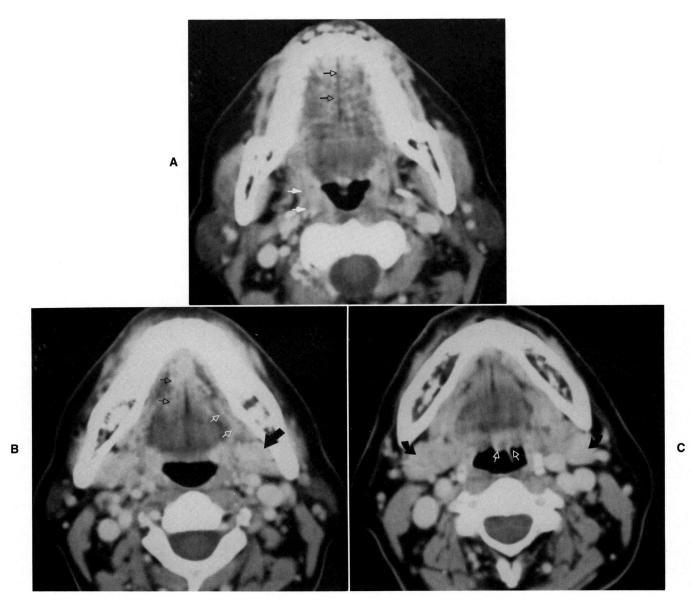

Fig. 6-11 **A,** Axial CT scan through midoropharynx. Muscular anatomy of oropharynx is demonstrated. Note similar density exhibited by palate, tonsillar tissue *(white arrows),* and surrounding musculature. A midline fat-filled septum divides tongue into halves *(black arrows).* This septum is hyperintense signal on T_1-weighted MRI scans. **B,** Axial CT scan of lower oropharynx and floor of mouth. Mandible encircles floor of mouth anteriorly. Midline low-density lingual septum divides two genioglossus muscles. Genioglossus muscles *(open black arrows)* extend from genu of mandible in midline to insert into intrinsic tongue muscles. Just lateral to genioglossus muscles is sublingual space. Interposed between sublingual space and mandible is mylohyoid muscle *(white arrows).* Mylohyoid muscle forms sling that supports floor of mouth. Its posterior margin demarcates sublingual space and submandibular space. Submandibular space contains submandibular gland, seen here as muscular density structure just below insertion of medial pterygoid muscle *(curved black arrow).* **C,** Axial CT scan through floor of mouth shown in **B.** Residual lymphoid tissue at base of tongue can be confused with superficial neoplasm *(white arrows).* Submandibular glands are located lateral to each aspect of airway adjacent to carotid arteries *(curved arrows).* Their density is similar to surrounding muscle.

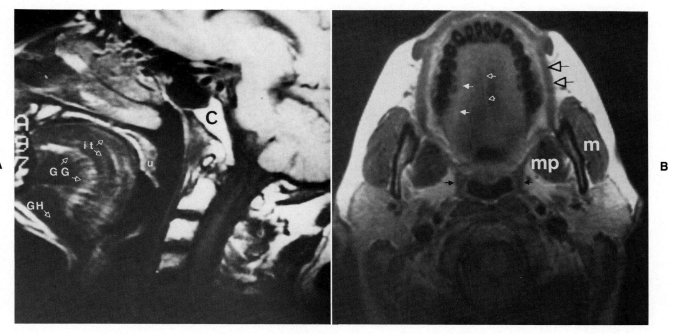

Fig. 6-12 **A,** Sagittal view of oropharynx. Muscles of tongue—geniohyoid *(GH)*, genio-glossus *(GG)*, and intrinsic muscles *(it)*—are characteristic features on sagittal image. Uvula *(u)* hangs into upper third of oropharynx. Hyperintense signal at superior aspect of nasopharynx is clivus *(C)*. **B** to **F,** Series of axial T_1-weighted MR images of oral cavity beginning at level of tongue and proceeding through floor of mouth. **B,** Section through oral tongue demonstrates intermediate-signal intensity of oral cavity musculature. Characteristic midline lingual septum is hyperintense *(open white arrows)*. This separates tongue into halves. Oral tongue itself consists of heterogeneous signal intensity containing both fat and muscle. Fat tends to be located just beneath surface of tongue and, in axial plane, can be seen best along lateral surfaces *(solid white arrows)*. Upper teeth outline anterior half of oral cavity. Buccinator muscle *(open black arrows)* is located just lateral to teeth. This muscle forms internal structure of cheek and attaches posteriorly to pterygomandibular raphe. At this level, muscles of mastication include masseter *(m)* and medial pterygoid muscle *(MP)*. Oropharyngeal airway is surrounded by superior and middle constrictor muscles *(closed black arrows)*.

Continued.

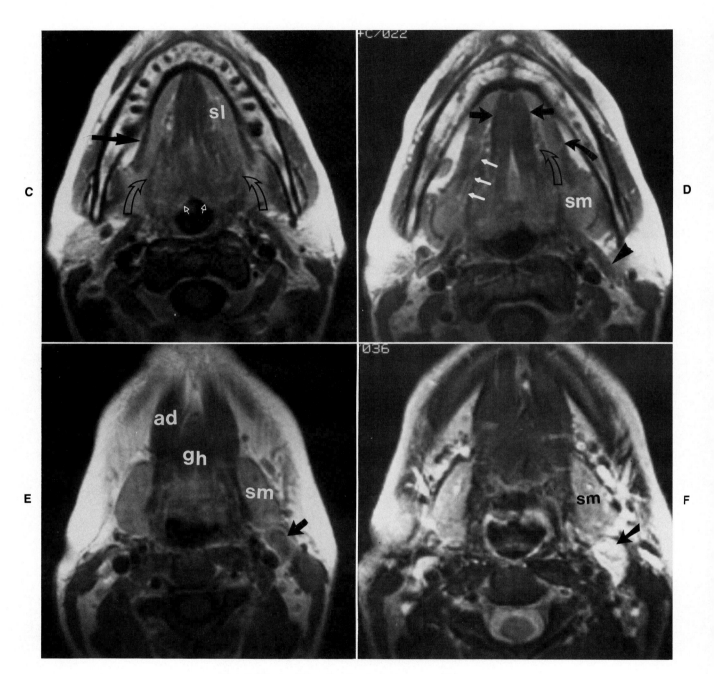

Fig. 6-12, cont'd For legend see opposite page.

Fig. 6-12, cont'd   C, T$_1$-weighted MR image through base of tongue *(open white arrows)* and floor of mouth. Mandible surrounds lower aspect of floor of mouth. Note its hypointense cortical surface and hyperintense marrow cavity. Genioglossus muscles emanate from inner surface of mandible and course posteriorly, and superiorly to insert in intrinsic tongue muscles. Genioglossus muscles are separated by fat-filled lingual septum in midline. Paired intermediate signal sublingual salivary glands *(sl)* lies lateral to genioglossus near anterior aspect of floor of mouth. Further posteriorly the hyoglossus muscles *(open curved arrows),* two curvilinear muscles on either side of genioglossus muscles emanate from hyoid bone and insert on intrinsic tongue muscles. Lateral to sublingual salivary gland and adjacent to mandible are mylohyoid muscles *(black arrow).* These originate from mylohyoid ridge of inner mandible; interdigitating with each other near hyoid bone, they provide sling support for floor of mouth. Free margin posteriorly exists, providing communication between sublingual salivary space and submandibular space. **D,** Axial section through inferior floor of mouth. Genioglossus muscles *(closed black arrows),* mylohyoid muscle *(curved black arrow),* sublingual space *(open curved arrow)* and the submandibular gland *(sm)* are located at posterior margin of mylohyoid muscle. Submandibular duct exits deep lobe of gland and travels in sublingual space between mylohyoid muscle and hyoglossus-genioglossus muscles *(open white arrows).* Also noted is the posterior belly of the digastric muscle *(arrowhead).* **E,** Axial T$_1$-weighted contrast-enhanced MRI scan beneath floor of mouth. At this level, supporting musculature of floor of mouth consists of anterior belly of digastric muscle *(ad)* and geniohyoid muscle *(gh).* Note submandibular glands *(sm)* behind which is necrotic, peripherally enhancing metastatic node *(arrow).* **F,** Axial T$_2$-weighted MRI sequence (TR 2800, TE 80 msec) through inferior floor of mouth and submandibular glands at same level as **E.** Submandibular glands *(sm)* retain intermediate-signal intensity between muscle and fat. Necrotic metastatic node has increased signal intensity *(arrow).*

---

tween genioglossus muscles and hypoglossus muscles, sending perforating branches to the tongue.

The lingual nerve, a branch of the trigeminal nerve, carries sensory fibers from the anterior tongue. It also travels within the floor of the mouth, adjacent to the hypoglossal nerves. Special sensory fibers for taste from the anterior two-thirds of the tongue merge with the lingual branch of the trigeminal nerve, but then separate from it to form the chorda tympani, which joins the facial nerve in the middle ear. The posterior one-third of the tongue is supplied with sensory taste fibers from the glossopharyngeal nerve (cranial nerve IX).

The extrinsic muscles in the floor of the mouth are separated by normal fat planes. Axial and coronal images clearly demonstrate this anatomy (Figs. 6-10 to 6-12). The most prominent landmark in the floor of the mouth is the midline fat-filled lingual septum separating the paramedian genioglossus muscles.[40,42,43] Deviation or obliteration of this septum is abnormal.

The submandibular gland, located primarily inferior to the mylohyoid muscle (Fig. 6-10, *B*) and beneath the mandible has an intermediate-signal intensity between muscle and fat on T$_2$-weighted MR images (Fig. 6-12, *D* and *E*). On CT scans, the submandibular gland is similar in density to muscle (Fig. 6-11, *C*). The proximal 3 to 4 mm of the submandibular duct may be normally seen on MR images as a tubular structure leaving the deep portion of the gland, just medial to the mylo-

hyoid muscle (Fig. 6-12, *D*). This anatomic structure is difficult to detect routinely on CT scans. The sublingual gland occupies the anterior one-third of the lateral floor of the mouth just deep to the mucosa over the floor of the mouth, in a position medial to the mylohyoid muscle (Fig. 6-10, *B*). It has a signal intensity that is similar to lymphoid tissue and the gland can be difficult to separate from tumor (Fig. 6-12, *C*).

The oropharynx consists of the oropharynx proper (pharyngeal constrictor muscles surrounding the mucosa, the palatine, and lymphoid tissue at the base of tongue) and the palatine arch complex (oral surface of the soft palate and anterior tonsillar pillars). As the dominant fat plane deep to the airway, the parapharyngeal space is best defined on T$_1$-weighted MRI sequences. Displacement of the parapharyngeal space fat often indicates deep invasion of neoplasms. Tumor and lymphoid tissue in the palatine fossa and lingual tongue base cannot be reliably differentiated from each other on the basis of signal intensity.

The tonsils and faucial pillars have a similar CT density[44,45]; they appear as bilateral symmetric soft tissue densities on either side of the airway (Fig. 6-11, *A*). These lymphoid structures are prominent features on MRI scans (Fig. 6-6, *B*). They have a slightly more intense signal than muscle on T$_1$-weighted images, and they increase in signal intensity on T$_2$-weighted images.[39] Tonsils are more prominent in children and young adults; they diminish in size with age and after radiation therapy. Dystrophic calcification from previous infections is commonly present on CT scans within the tonsillar beds.

The soft palate forms the roof of the oropharynx and the inferior boundary of the nasopharynx (Fig. 6-12, A). The CT density of the palate is similar to that of muscle.[44] The MRI appearance of the palate reflects the large number of glandular elements that are intermixed with fat.[39] This gives this structure a mixed appearance on T_1-weighted images (Fig. 6-12, A and B) and a high-signal intensity on T_2-weighted images.

Masses usually have lower-signal intensity on T_1-weighted images than does the surrounding normal glandular tissue. Differentiation from the parapharyngeal space fat is best obtained on T_1-weighted images (TR=600 msec, TE=20 msec). Masses that also have low-signal intensity on T_2-weighted images should be suspected of being highly malignant tumors, whereas benign soft tissue masses generally have high T_2-weighted signal intensities. MR images, however, can not be used to reliably differentiate between benign and malignant disease.

IMAGING TECHNIQUES
Specific Indications for CT and MRI Scans

Nasopharyngeal tumors are usually diagnosed late in the course of the disease. This delay reflects both the tendency for late development of signs and symptoms that might bring the patient to the physician and the clinician's difficulty in visualizing these tumors. Patients suspected of harboring nasopharyngeal pathologic conditions should have an MRI study, even if the endoscopic examination of the nasopharynx is normal.

Symptom complexes such as atypical facial pain or anesthesia, cervical adenopathy of uncertain etiologic factor(s), and epistaxis should initiate an investigation for a nasopharyngeal tumor. An MRI study of the neck and the entire upper aerodigestive tract is warranted before biopsy.[46-48] Most authors now agree that MRI is the imaging study of choice for evaluating the nasopharynx. Although late-generation CT scanners using 2 to 4 second exposures are capable of exquisite images of the head and neck, this technique is limited by the requirement for intravenous contrast, inferior soft tissue contrast resolution, and patient cooperation for orthogonal views. These disadvantages have been surmounted by MRI. However, CT scanning is still complementary to MRI in the assessment of the osseous structures of the face and skull base and is the modality preferred by many for the examination of the oral cavity.

Although the advantages of MRI over CT scanning in evaluation of the nasopharynx are clear cut, the optimal imaging modality for the evaluation of the oral cavity is controversial. This largely is a result of patient-induced-motion artifact, which degrades 5% to 15% of oral cavity MRI studies. In addition, benign cystic neck masses occasionally can be difficult to distinguish from solid masses on MR images, whereas this problem is unusual on CT scans. Clearly, in the cooperative patient, MRI has the same advantages in the oral cavity as in the nasopharynx and, in this author's experience, is preferred as the initial screening examination for tongue and floor of the mouth malignancies. Those individuals with severe obstructive lung disease or large tumors are imaged by CT, largely decreasing the number of inadequate MRI examinations.

Parapharyngeal space masses may present as neck masses, as asymptomatic bulges beneath the mucosa of the lateral pharyngeal wall, or as cranial nerve deficits. CT or MRI scans are often definitive for preoperative planning in such lesions.

The oropharynx is usually imaged because of the presence of a primary squamous cell carcinoma that shows evidence of deep infiltration. Nodal groups must also be studied carefully in such cases. Either CT or MRI scans can be utilized effectively. MRI optimally demonstrates the interface between a tumor and muscle; however, it lacks the specificity for nodal metastases enjoyed by CT scanning. Contrast-enhanced fat-saturated MRI sequences may alter this relative disadvantage of MRI in the near future.

CT Technique

Patient Positioning. The pharynx and oral cavity are best examined with the patient supine and the sections made parallel to the infraorbital-meatal line. The head should be carefully positioned so that it is not askew along the cephalocaudad axis, as this may result in an appearance that may simulate pathologic conditions. When positioning the patient for direct coronal examinations, the head must not be turned to one side, as the resulting anatomic distortion makes reliable diagnosis more difficult. A localizing lateral scout image is always obtained to avoid artifacts from dental hardware. A preliminary scan, performed about 1 cm inferior to the orbital-meatal line, will usually extend through the upper nasopharynx or skull base. The preliminary scan can also be used to choose an optimal field of view (usually 14 to 18 cm). If the study is limited to the nasopharynx, scans are then continued inferiorly to the maxillary alveolar ridge and superiorly to include the cavernous sinus. If the pathologic lesion extends beyond the nasopharynx or if cervical adenopathy is to be assessed, the scan is continued to encompass the full extent of disease. Direct coronal and axial scans should be performed in any patient suspected of having a nasopharyngeal or skull base mass.

The oropharynx and nasopharynx should be studied during suspended respiration. Proper gantry angulation is essential in the oropharynx to avoid dental-related artifacts. Sections that are parallel to the ramus of the mandible should be obtained from the top of the mandibular alveolar ridge to the hyoid bone. This plane of section is usually suitable for surveying the neck. If the larynx and hypopharynx are to be studied in detail, sections must be parallel to the true vocal cords in that portion of the study.

Scanning Parameters. Scans should be contiguous with a slice thickness of 3 to 4 mm or less, and the field of view should be kept as small as possible while still including all essential anatomic areas of interest. Algorithms optimizing bone detail are essential to evaluate pathologic bone conditions.

Significant mucosal masses usually alter the surrounding deep tissue planes. A clinical examination and biopsy, if necessary, can resolve the CT finding of a suspicious mucosal mass, although this is rarely a problem with MRI.

Intravenous Contrast. The aims of intravenous contrast infusion in the head and neck are to: (1) determine the margins of the lesion with greater clarity; (2) establish its vascularity; (3) distinguish normal vessels from pathologic processes (e.g., vessels versus lymph nodes); and (4) study the effects of pathologic conditions on regional vessels. MR images often achieve these goals without the use of contrast material. The goals are also met with CT scans in over 90% to 95% of cases by using a combined bolus-rapid drip-infusion method of contrast enhancement. Specific technique depends on whether a power injector is available:

Without a power injector, the following steps should be taken.

1. Start an IV infusion with 19 or 20 gauge intravenous catheter.
2. Plan the study; for instance, scout views, choose gantry angulation, and perform preliminary axial scan to set FOV.
3. Inject 40 to 60 cc bolus of 60% contrast medium over 1½ to 2 minutes (to avoid nausea and vomiting).
4. Open the IV to the maximum flow rate, giving up to 300 cc of 25% to 30% (low-viscosity) contrast and begin scanning.

With a power injector, the following steps should be taken:

1. Start an IV as without a power injector.
2. Plan study, as without a power injector.
3. Load injector with 60% contrast and infuse at 0.5 cc/sec; start scanning after an approximately 90-second delay.
4. *Optional:* With appropriate CT unit, if continuous monitoring of study is possible, multiple 35 cc boluses may be used, "titrating" the dose by the appearance of vessels in the images.

These techniques deliver about 42 to 50 grams of iodine to the patient. If more is used, poststudy hydration is encouraged.

Indications for CT contrast infusion include: (1) evaluation of primary malignancy; (2) evaluation of retropharyngeal and deep cervical lymph nodes; (3) definition of the extent of intracranial disease; (4) differential diagnosis of carotid sheath and parapharyngeal space masses; (5) elucidation of tumor invasion or obstruction of the paranasal sinuses; and (6) differentiation of an abscess and cellulitis. The first three indications mainly apply to the study of patients with known or suspected malignancies. The last three indications may apply to lesions of benign or malignant character. In none of these types of patients is a precontrast examination indicated.

MRI Technique

High-quality MRI of the head and neck is easy to obtain. First, patients are instructed that motion (swallowing, talking, snoring) will degrade images. Surprisingly, this bit of education probably has the greatest impact on image quality. Scans of the nasopharynx and oropharynx are accomplished with the routine head coil. The floor of mouth also can often be imaged with this coil, depending on the habitus of the patient. Scans of the neck must utilize an anterior or posterior neck coil (or a combination of the two) of sufficient size to cover the patient from the floor of the mouth to the supraclavicular region. Coil geometry plays a critical role in the coverage and depth of volume excitation. Permanent magnet systems may use solenoid type coils that encircle the neck. Coil position is critical, and coils should be centered on the region of greatest interest.

Selection of pulse sequences depends on the type and extent of the pathologic condition. For routine screening examinations, localize from a sagittal T_1-weighted spin-echo (TR=600 msec, TE=20 msec) sequence followed by an axial T_2-weighted spin-echo sequence (TR 2000, TE 35,80 msec) from the sella turcica to at least the midoropharynx. The second echo of this series usually results in scans with lower-signal intensity fat and muscle, and higher-signal intensity lymph nodes and areas of pathologic disorders. Finally a coronal T_1-weighted sequence provides an additional orthogonal image of the skull base and superior nasopharynx.

The use of intravenous paramagnetic contrast has yet to be defined in the upper aerodigestive tract. Initial reports[49,50] are encouraging, but there seem to be few instances in which contrast defines pathologic conditions that were inapparent on a combination of T_1- and T_2-weighted images. Such instances may include the detection of extradural disease, the definition of necrotic nodes, and perhaps the separation of an abscess

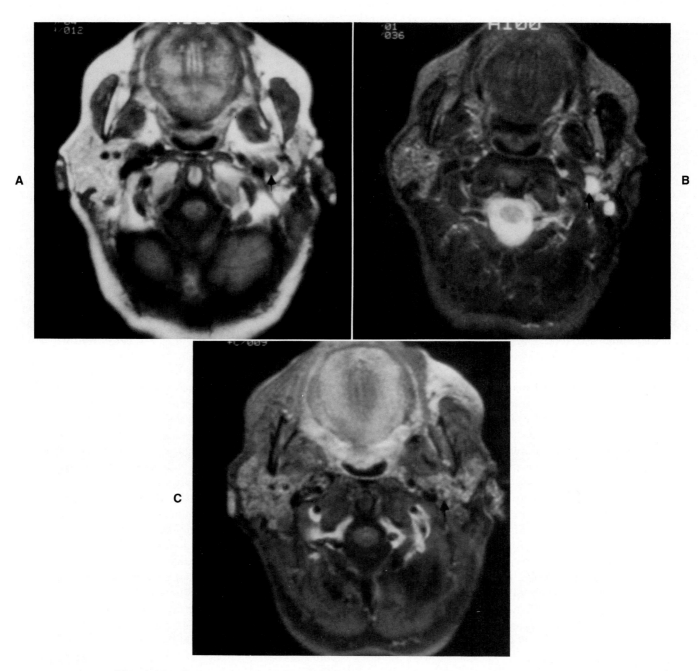

Fig. 6-13 Fat-saturation MRI with gadolinium-DTPA. Malignant mixed cell tumor with necrotic adenopathy. **A,** Noncontrast enhanced T_1-weighted MR image (600/20) through parotid gland demonstrates homogeneous low-signal intensity to mass deep to parotid gland. **B,** Noncontrast enhanced T_2-weighted MR image (2800/80). Note two foci of increased signal intensity *(arrows)* deep to left parotid gland. **C,** T_1-weighted MR image performed following gadolinium and with radiofrequency fat-suppression technique demonstrates peripheral enhancement surrounding necrotic parotid node *(arrow)*. Node was verified by surgical excision.

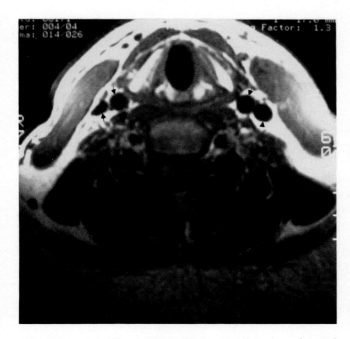

Fig. 6-14 Axial T_1-weighted MR image of neck performed with presaturation radiofrequency pulse inferior and superior to slice of interest. Note that lumen of carotid artery and jugular veins *(arrows)* have no internal signal. This is due to presaturation of entering blood by radiofrequency pulse and eliminates phase misregistration artifact and helps differentiate cervical nodal disease from blood vessels. In addition, this technique is useful in detecting intraluminal thrombosis.

from cellulitis. The use of contrast material in combination with fat-saturated T_1-weighted images appears to have great potential, as the saturation of the high-signal intensity fat allows better discrimination of any enhancing pathologic conditions. This seems certain to become routine in orbital imaging and may be of some use in the aerodigestive tract (Fig. 6-13).

When contemplating the use of an MRI contrast agent, it is helpful to acquire a noncontrast–T_1-weighted sequence in the same plane as the contrast sequence so as not to confuse either high-signal intensity fat or proteinaceous fluid with an area of enhancement.

MRI studies of the oropharynx and oral cavity are performed primarily in the axial plane. Coronal scans may be of use in assessing the anterior tongue or palate but have little role in assessing the tongue base or oropharynx. T_2-weighted axial sequences are performed following a T_1-sagittal localizing sequence. Scanning coverage should include at least the region between the palate and the hyoid bone. The cervical neck nodes must be examined with the neck coil. Sections 4 or 5 mm thick are mandatory to prevent volume averaging. Presaturation pulses designed to decrease an entry-slice signal within the lumen of blood vessels are extremely

useful in head and neck imaging. They have the effect of saturating the entry-slice signal (producing signal void) within the vessel lumen and secondarily reducing the phase-encoding flow artifact, which is so often troublesome in neck imaging (Fig. 6-14).

Additional technical features that are important for optimizing head and neck MR images include selection of the proper field of view and acquisition matrix (18-20 cm, 192-256 matrix), antialiasing techniques (no phase and no frequency wrap), offset field of view techniques, gradient moment nulling (flow compensation) and respiratory gating options, and interleave and concantenating features.

PATHOLOGY OF THE NASOPHARYNX
CT and MRI Localization of Pathology

The pharyngobasilar fascia divides the nasopharynx into superficial and deep anatomic spaces. Superficial "mucosal" lesions of the nasopharynx reside on the pharyngeal side of this tough fascia. Hypertrophied adenoids, Tornwaldt's cysts, and squamous carcinoma are examples of mucosal lesions of the nasopharynx.[51,52] Infiltrative nasopharyngeal lesions either penetrate the pharyngobasilar fascia or extend beneath its free inferior margin, spreading into the deep soft tissues. Masses arising within the deep spaces of the nasopharynx (the parapharyngeal, masticator, parotid, carotid, and retropharyngeal spaces) may all bulge the superficial mucosa medially. The differential diagnosis of nasopharyngeal pathologic conditions is facilitated by accurate localization of the origin of the lesion to a specific space. The vector of the pathologic disorder's spread may be inferred by its effect on the fat-filled parapharyngeal space. Lateral displacement of this space implies a lesion with a superficial or mucosal origin, such as a carcinoma of the nasopharynx (Fig. 6-15). Medial displacement of the parapharyngeal space is caused by masses within the deep lobe of the parotid gland or the masticator space (Fig. 6-16). Anterior displacement of the parapharyngeal space results from masses within the carotid space, such as vagus nerve schwannomas and carotid paragangliomas (Fig. 6-17).

As a general rule, T_1-weighted MR images (TR $\leq$ 600 msec, TE=25 msec) best outline musculofascial anatomy, whereas heavily T_2-weighted images (TR $\geq$ 2800 msec, TE $\geq$ 70 msec) best identify signal intensity differences between normal and pathologic anatomy (Fig. 6-17, *B*).

Benign Mucosal Lesions of the Nasopharynx

Benign primary mucosal masses of the nasopharynx are rarely symptomatic.[53] The most common lesions are hypertrophied adenoidal tissues and congenital Tornwaldt's cysts (Table 6-2). Other benign masses arising from tissues surrounding the nasopharynx are frontoeth-

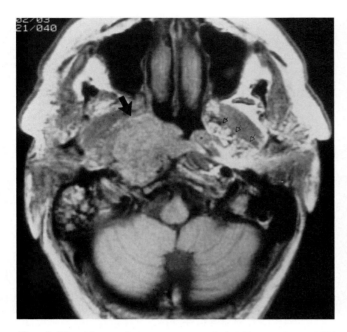

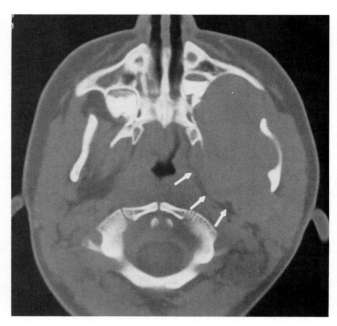

Fig. 6-15 Mucosal space mass. Axial T₁-weighted MRI scan through nasopharynx in patient with nasopharyngeal carcinoma. Mass arises from mucosal surface, displacing right parapharyngeal space laterally *(closed arrow)*. Normal parapharyngeal space is noted on right *(open arrows)*.

Fig. 6-16 Masticator space mass. 6-year-old patient with aggressive fibromatosis of masticator space with deviation of left mandible and left maxillary sinuses. This mass compresses parapharyngeal space posteriorly and medially *(arrows)*. This deviation is typical of masticator space masses.

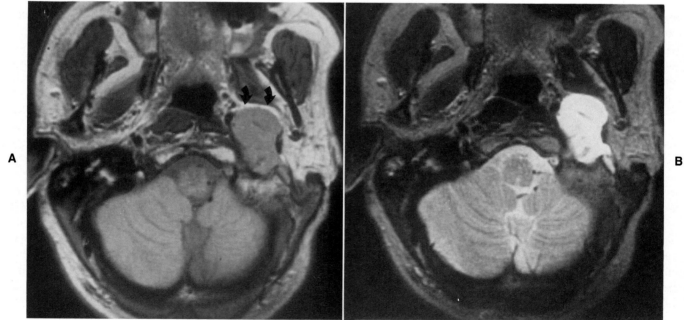

Fig. 6-17 Carotid space mass. Left jugular foramen chordoma. **A,** T₁-weighted MR image demonstrates homogeneous mass emanating from jugular fossa splaying and displacing carotid and jugular vein. Left parapharyngeal space is compressed and deviated anteriorly *(arrows)*. **B,** T₂-weighted MR images (TR 2800, TE 80 msec). Mass homogeneously increases in signal intensity. This feature allows distinction from paragangliono-mas.

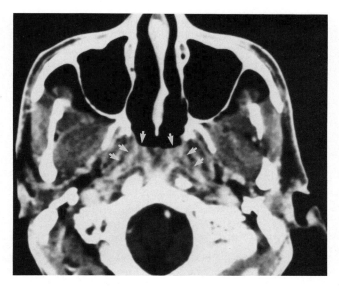

Fig. 6-18 Nasopharyngeal adenoidal tissue. Contrast-enhanced axial CT scan through nasopharynx demonstrates residual adenoidal tissue occupying mucosal side of nasopharynx *(arrows)*. This residual adenoidal tissue is commonly seen in young patients, including young adults. It does not invade deep planes and is usually isodense to surrounding musculature.

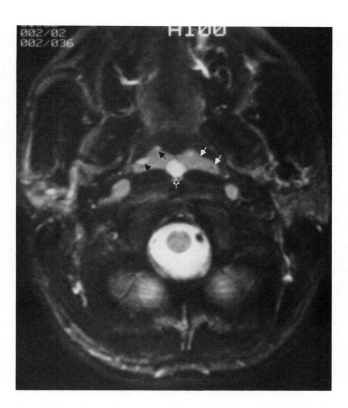

Fig. 6-19 Nasopharyngeal cysts. Axial T_2-weighted MRI sequence through upper nasopharynx demonstrates residual adenoidal tissues occupying mucosal side of nasopharynx *(closed white arrows)*. High-intensity Tornwaldt cyst is located in midline posteriorly *(open white arrow)*. Cyst has high-signal intensity on T1 weighted MR images (see Fig. 6-20). Also noted within adenoidal tissue are small retention cysts *(black arrows)*. These are commonly seen on MR images but rarely identified on CT scans.

moidal encephaloceles, teratomas, invasive pituitary neoplasms, nasal polyps, and malignant otitis externa, all of which may encroach on the mucosal space of the nasopharynx. Their origination is usually clear from their vector of growth.

Adenoidal Hypertrophy. Adenoidal tissue is prominent in children and young adults, appearing as a homogeneous, superficial mass of soft tissue, occupying the superior and lateral recesses of the nasopharynx. On CT scans, adenoidal tissue is often isodense with the surrounding musculature (Fig. 6-18). The intrinsic features of adenoidal hypertrophy are best appreciated on MR images. Adenoidal tissue has a high-spin density and a relatively long T_1 and T_2 relaxation time. These factors result in a signal intensity quite similar to muscle on T_1-weighted images, but a high-signal intensity on T_2-weighted images (Figs. 6-4, *A* and 6-6, *A*). Occasionally, small foci of higher-signal intensity may be detected within the adenoidal bed on T_2-weighted images (Fig. 6-19). These represent postinflammatory, degenerative, or obstructed glandular cysts. Benign adenoidal tissue never infiltrates the soft tissue planes deep to the mucosa or the pharyngobasilar fascia.[51] However, it may be quite difficult to differentiate residual adenoidal tissue from a small tumor on CT or MRI scans.[52] Endoscopy with biopsy is the only way to make this distinction. Reactive cervical adenopathy often accompanies prominent adenoidal tissue in children and in adults with the AIDS related complex syndrome.

Tornwaldt's Cyst. Tornwaldt's cyst is present in 4% of normal autopsy specimens and is related to the transient descent of the notochord into the nasopharynx. As the notochord ascends back into the developing skull base, it may pull a small tag of the developing nasopharyngeal mucosa with it, creating a midline pit or tract, usually located between the longus capitus muscles (Fig. 6-20). This tract may close over and result in a midline cyst that on occasion may become infected. Extension off of the midline is infrequently seen. The cyst varies from 1 to 5 mm in diameter and has a high-signal intensity on T_1- and T_2-weighted images, probably caused by its proteinaceous fluid contents (Fig. 6-20). Tornwaldt's cyst often has a CT density similar to that of the surrounding muscle and adenoidal tissue (Fig. 6-20, *A*). This appearance is probably also due to proteinaceous debris within the cyst. Infection may lead to a syndrome consisting of prevertebral muscular spasm and postnasal discharge. Tornwaldt's abscess must be surgically drained to prevent retropharyngeal abscess.

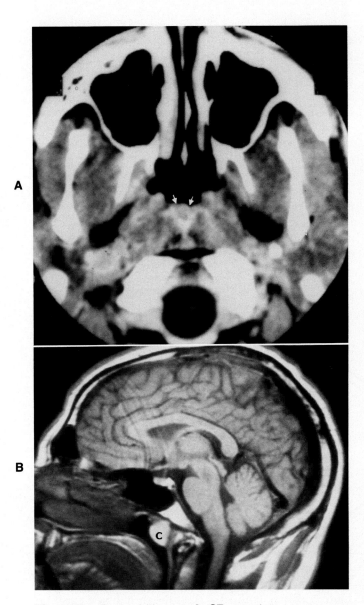

Fig. 6-20 Tornwaldt's cyst. **A,** CT scan through upper nasopharynx demonstrates midline Tornwaldt's cyst *(arrows)*. Note that its density is similar to surrounding muscle. High density of this cyst is probably related to high-protein concentration. **B,** Sagittal T₁-weighted MRI scan through upper nasopharynx demonstrates high-signal−intensity Tornwaldt's cyst *(c)*. High intensity is due to high-protein concentration within cyst. This shortens T1 relaxation time sufficiently to produce increase in intensity on T₁-weighted images.

Teratoma. Teratomas are true neoplasms that contain mixed elements representing all three germ layers, which are foreign to the part of the body in which they arise.[53-55] These congenital tumors occur predominantly in the midline or lateral wall of the nasopharynx and there is a female predominance.[53] The lesion contains elements including skin, hair, cartilage, muscle, and bone. Epignathus, a congenital lesion that consists of organs and limbs of a parasitic fetus, is quite unusual. Deformities of the skull may be present with complex teratomatous lesions. Surgery is the treatment of choice. CT scans may demonstrate a wide range of appearances; however, a midline mass containing calcification, fat, and soft tissue is diagnostic.

Heterotopic Pharyngeal Brain. Heterotopic brain within the nasopharynx is a rare condition, usually diagnosed in infancy or childhood. Respiratory distress is the most frequent presentation, and it may be life threatening. Associated congenital anomalies are noted in about 50% of the described cases and include pectus excavatum, cleft palate, unilateral choanal stenosis, and micrognathia. The embryogenesis of the lesion is poorly understood. Inferior displacement of neural tissue during the formation of Rathke's pouch or the presence of an isolated encephalocele have been suggested as possible causes. CT scans demonstrate a soft tissue or low-density mass occupying the nasopharynx, contiguous with the skull base.[56] MR images may demonstrate tissue contiguous with brain coursing through a defect in the base of skull. The differential diagnosis includes a transsphenoidal encephalocele in which the third ventricle and hypothalamic structures have herniated through the base of the skull into the nasopharynx.

Inflammatory Lesions of the Nasopharynx

Mucosal Infections. Primary inflammatory lesions of the nasopharynx are uncommon, and nasopharyngeal infections most often occur as extensions of infections from the immediate surrounding areas. Infection of adenoidal or tonsillar tissue in children is a common example. Infection of a Tornwaldt's cyst or extension of abscesses in the retropharyngeal and parapharyngeal spaces to the nasopharynx are less common causes of primary inflammatory lesions that involve the nasopharynx.

Masticator Space Infections. Most masticator space infections result from osteomyelitis of the mandible caused by uncontrolled dental infection. Other causes also include hematogenous osteomyelitis of the mandible (Fig. 6-21), fungal infections of the mandible such as actinomycosis, and rarely inferior extension of a malignant otitis externa. Masticator space infections may be differentiated from tumors by the surrounding soft tissue inflammatory cellulitis and the clinical history.[57]

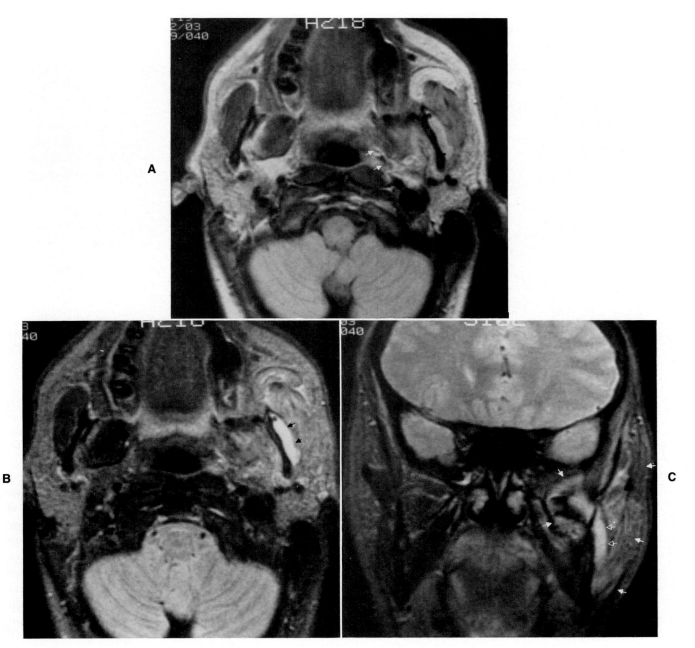

Fig. 6-21 Masticator space infection. **A,** T_1-weighted MR image through mid/na-soooropharynx demonstrates mass lesion surrounding left mandible. Note infiltration of parapharyngeal space *(arrows)*. **B,** Same level as in **A,** T_2-weighted MR image (TR 2800, TE 80) through mid/nasopharynx. Cellulitis surrounding masticator space is character-ized by diffuse high signal. Well-circumscribed focus of increased signal intensity adja-cent to mandible is consistent with pyogenic abscess in subperiosteal region found at surgery *(arrows)*. Patient's status was determined after dental extraction. **C,** Coronal T_2-weighted MRI view. Increased signal intensity within masticator space *(closed arrows)* is evident. Liquid abscess adjacent to mandible *(open arrows)* can be seen.

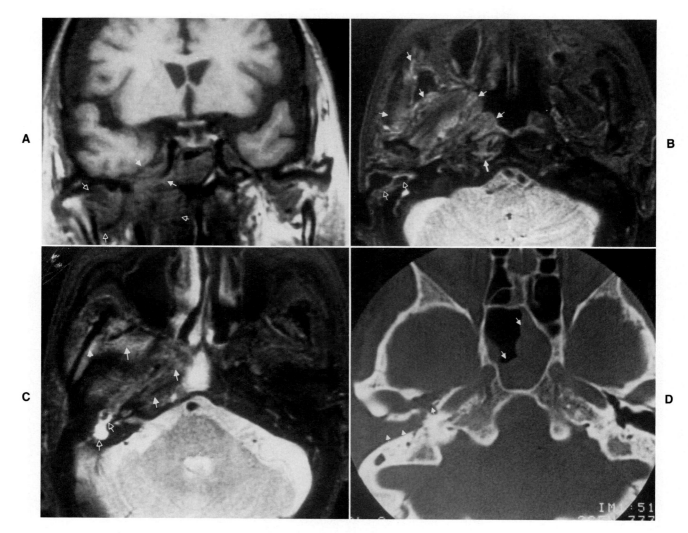

Fig. 6-22 Malignant external otitis involving upper masticator space in elderly diabetic male. **A,** Coronal T_1-weighted MRI view (600/20) of nasopharynx and skull base. Diffuse mass involves skull base and masticator space *(open arrows)*. Extension through foramen ovale is noted *(closed arrows)*. **B,** Axial T_2-weighted MR image demonstrates diffuse high-signal intensity—cellulitis involving masticator space *(closed arrows)*. In addition, evidence is present for involvement of external canal *(open arrows)*. This appearance is atypical for tumor and more typical of diffuse process, such as inflammatory disease. **C,** Axial T_2-weighted MR images and view through skull base demonstrate intense signal within upper masticator space and skull base *(closed arrows)*. In addition, there is fluid within tympanic cavity *(open arrows)*. Appearance is typical of malignant otitis externa. **D,** Axial CT scan with bone review through skull base. Extensive soft tissue fills external canal, middle ear structures, and sphenoid sinus *(arrows)*.

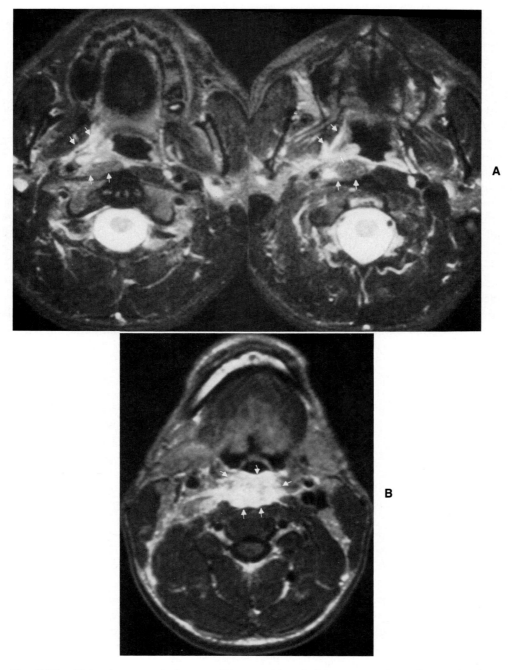

Fig. 6-23   Retropharyngeal abscess. 21-year-old male intravenous drug abuser developed inflammatory cellulitis of neck following internal jugular vein injection. **A,** Two contiguous T$_2$-weighted axial MRI views through nasopharynx and oropharynx. Mass with increased signal intensity occupies right nasopharynx, right prevertebral muscle, and right carotid vessel *(arrows)*. Appearance cannot be differentiated from nasopharyngeal carcinoma. **B,** Axial T$_1$-weighted postgadolinium MRI view through low oropharynx and upper neck. Retropharyngeal mass that increases in signal intensity following gadolinium is present *(arrows)*. *Staphylococcus aureus* was isolated from blood cultures. This retropharyngeal phlegmon consisted of small microabscesses that had not coalesced to form frank abscess. This mass improved following antibiotic therapy.

Malignant Otitis Externa. Malignant otitis externa is an opportunistic infection of the external auditory canal, seen primarily in elderly diabetic patients. The offending organism is usually a strain of *Pseudomonas aeruginosa*. The infection begins as an external otitis, and it can rapidly grow subperiosteally to involve the temporal bone and skull base, with a jugular foramen syndrome and facial palsy being ominous findings. The inflammatory process may extend anteriorly along the subperiosteal compartment of the skull base to involve the masticator space (Fig. 6-22). The presence of a nasopharyngeal mass, associated with skull-base osteomyelitis, obliteration of the external auditory canal by soft tissue, and the appropriate clinical history are the usual features. MR images demonstrate this condition as a diffuse increase in signal intensity on T_2-weighted images of the superior masticator space and skull base. Gadolinium-enhanced T_1-weighted sequences have been shown to result in intense subperiosteal and perimuscular enhancement.

Retropharyngeal Abscess. A retropharyngeal abscess most often arises secondary to an inflammatory extension from a tonsillar infection in children.[58] In adults, perforation of the posterior pharyngeal wall or retropharyngeal adenitis may result in inflammation of the retropharyngeal soft tissues. On CT scanning, a retropharyngeal abscess usually appears as an area of low density, located anterior to the prevertebral muscles and displacing the airway anteriorly. The retropharyngeal soft tissues are swollen. Necrotic neoplasms may have a similar appearance. Treatment consists of intraoral drainage and antibiotic therapy. The appearance on MR images often depends on whether the process is a frank abscess or in the phlegmonous stage. Both stages may appear as low intensity on T_1-weighted and high intensity on T_2-weighted sequences. However, the gadolinium T_1-weighted sequences can differentiate these stages, as cellulitis enhances, whereas frank abscess does not (Fig. 6-23).

Parapharyngeal Space Abscess. Abscesses in the parapharyngeal space may be the result of tonsillar infection or perforation of the pharynx, which may be iatrogenic or traumatic.[57] When the abscess gains access to the parapharyngeal space, it may extend from the skull base to the submandibular space. Infection of the submandibular gland may occasionally extend superiorly from the submandibular space into the parapharyngeal space.

On CT or MRI scans, a parapharyngeal space abscess deviates the nasopharyngeal airway medially and the medial pterygoid muscles laterally. The infection may be difficult to differentiate from neoplastic disease unless intense cellulitis, focal low density representing a fluid-filled cavity, or gas is seen within the abscess. Surgical drainage is required, because, among other

reasons, mycotic aneurysms of the carotid artery can occur within 10 days if the abscess is not drained.

Malignant Tumors of the Nasopharynx
Mucosal Space Masses

Squamous Cell Carcinoma. Squamous cell carcinoma represents 80% of all superficial epithelial carcinomas of the nasopharynx.[59,60] Of the remaining malignancies, most are adenocarcinomas, minor salivary gland tumors, or lymphomas.

Squamous cell carcinoma of the nasopharynx is rare in most countries of the world, with an incidence in the Caucasian population of less than 1 per 100,000 people per year.[60] This tumor is more prevalent in Asian countries, particularly in the southern provinces of China where an incidence as high as 18 to 20 cases per 100,000 people per year has been reported. Squamous cell carcinoma can develop in any age group; however, it favors middle-aged and older persons. Tobacco and alcohol abuse are not associated with the development of nasopharyngeal carcinoma; however, both environmental and genetic factors appear to play a role in Chinese patients. IGA antibodies to the Epstein-Barr virus have been associated with undifferentiated carcinoma of the nasopharynx and can be used as a marker for tumor in patients with this specific histology.

The clinical presentation varies depending on the size and location of the tumor. More than half of the patients present with asymptomatic enlargement of cervical lymph nodes in either the posterior triangle or the superior internal jugular chain. Other symptoms include serous otitis media secondary to dysfunction of the eustachian tube, nasal obstruction, epistaxis, trismus caused by involvement of the medial and lateral pterygoid muscles, and neurologic symptoms, which are noted in 25% of patients and include the cavernous sinus or the jugular fossa syndromes.

Patterns of Spread. The lateral pharyngeal recess or fossa of Rosenmüller is the most common site of origin for nasopharyngeal cancer (Fig. 6-24). The tumor tends to extend deep along musculofascial or neural pathways and to grow exophytically into the airway (Fig. 6-25). Superior extension medial to the pharyngobasilar fascia involves the foramen lacerum and sphenoid sinus. Extension to the skull base lateral to the pharyngobasilar fascia may involve the foramen ovale and the carotid canal or jugular fossa. The tumor may extend inferiorly along the musculature of the nasopharynx to involve the tonsillar pillars and soft palate. Anterior spread of nasopharyngeal carcinoma along the medial pterygoid muscle may result in destruction of the pterygoid plate or involvement of the nasal cavity and pterygomaxillary fissure. Posterior extension through the retropharyngeal space involves the clivus and prevertebral muscles (Fig. 6-26). Lateral extension is most common and is

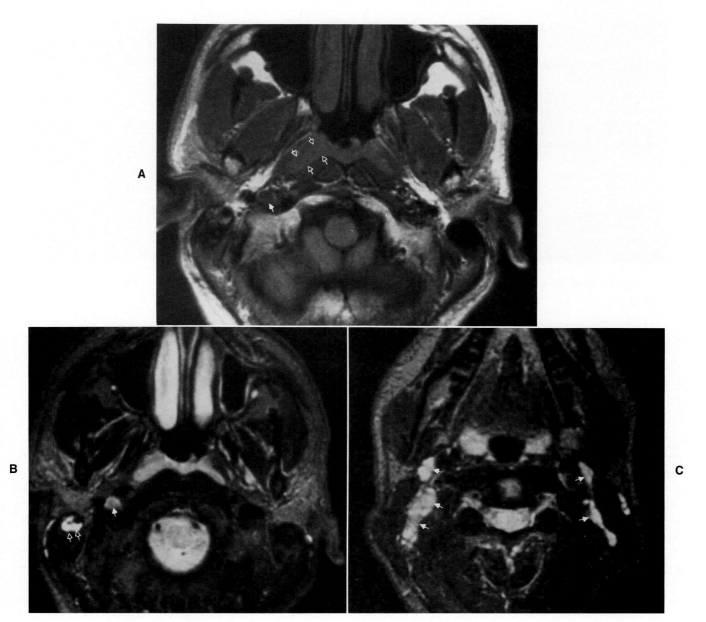

Fig. 6-24   Squamous cell carcinoma of right nasopharynx isolated to fossa of Rosen-müller. 28-year-old male presented with unilateral hearing loss. **A,** Axial T_1-weighted MR image (600/20) through upper nasopharynx demonstrates low-intensity mass occupying right nasopharynx and fossa of Rosenmüller *(open arrows)*. Also present is necrotic retropharyngeal node *(closed arrow)*. **B,** Axial T_2-weighted MRI view (2800/80) through same level as **A.** Mass has increased signal intensity similar to that surrounding adenoidal tissue. Note increased signal intensity of retropharyngeal node *(closed arrow)*. Fluid within mastoid *(open arrows)* is due to serous otitis media. **C,** Axial T_2-weighted MR image (2800/80) through lower neck demonstrates multiple bilateral posterior triangle and anterior cervical nodes *(arrows)*.

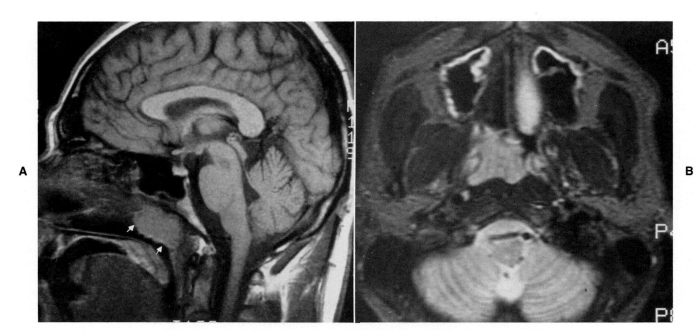

Fig. 6-25 Exophytic squamous carcinoma of nasopharynx. **A,** Sagittal T₁-weighted MRI view (660/20) of nasopharynx demonstrates soft tissue mass occupying superior aspect of nasopharynx *(arrows)*. This appearance is quite similar to residual adenoidal tissue seen in younger patients. **B,** Axial T₂-weighted MR image (2800/80) through nasopharynx. Mass is contained within right nasopharynx and has similar signal intensity to residual adenoidal tissue seen in previous images (Figs. 6-4, *A* and 6-6, *A*). Diagnosis cannot be certain based on image intensity; however, appearance of unilateral nasopharyngeal mass in middle-aged or elderly patient should require endoscopic examination and biopsy.

recognized by deviation or infiltration of the parapharyngeal space.

Retrograde spread of tumor along the trigeminal nerve may cause facial pain or anesthesia. In addition, atrophy of the muscles innervated by the motor division of the trigeminal nerve may be noted (Fig. 6-27). At the time of diagnosis 80% of patients have nodal disease, 50% being bilateral. The first nodes involved are the lateral retropharyngeal nodes. Subsequent involvement of the spinal accessory and internal jugular nodal chains is frequent (Fig. 6-28).

CT and MRI Appearance of Nasopharyngeal Carcinoma. Squamous cell carcinoma of the nasopharynx most often develops in the lateral pharyngeal recess of Rosenmüller (Fig. 6-24).[61-68] Superficial mucosal carcinomas usually are asymptomatic and may be difficult to differentiate both clinically and radiographically from superficial adenoidal tissue (Figs. 6-24 and 6-25). The earliest CT or MR imaging features of malignant disease are invasion of the deep musculofascial planes around the levator and tensor palatini muscles. Ipsilateral mastoid opacification and serous otitis media are common findings with nasopharyngeal carcinoma. MRI

is particularly sensitive to these early changes (Fig. 6-24). As the tumor invades laterally, it may initially displace and then invade the parapharyngeal space fat plane (Fig. 6-15). At this point, the tumor may grow in a caudal or cranial direction along the muscular planes deep to the nasopharyngeal mucosa.

Direct coronal MR images demonstrate skull-base erosion by replacement of the normal cortical and marrow bone by a signal similar to that of tumors (Figs. 6-26 and 6-27). These changes may be more subtle on MRI than CT scans; however, if particular attention is paid to the normal appearance of the skull base, early skull-base erosion may also be detected by MR imaging.

Metastatic nodal disease should be suspected in an adult with retropharyngeal nodes that are greater than 5 mm in diameter (in children these nodes are normally 5 to 10 mm in diameter) (Fig. 6-26).[69] On CT scans, the presence of a lucent or heterogeneous center within an enlarged retropharyngeal node, with surrounding peripheral enhancement in a patient with carcinoma of the nasopharynx, is highly suspicious for metastatic disease (Fig. 6-24).

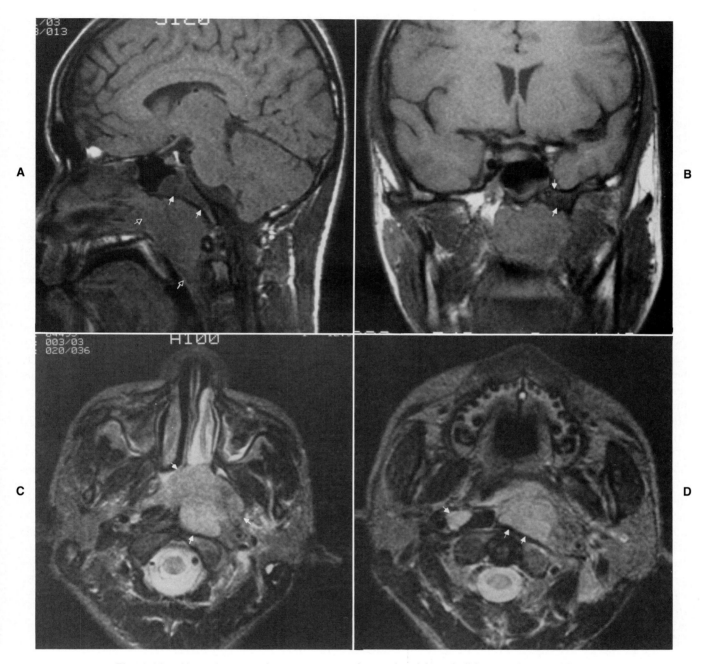

Fig. 6-26 Nasopharyngeal squamous carcinoma involving skull base. 42-year-old patient presented with anesthesia of third division of trigeminal nerve. **A,** T_1-weighted sagittal MRI view (600/20) of nasopharynx demonstrates soft tissue mass occupying upper nasopharynx *(open arrows).* Low-signal intensity has replaced normal high-signal intensity of clivus *(closed arrows).* **B,** Coronal T_1-weighted MRI views (600/20) demonstrates soft tissue mass adjacent to upper nasopharynx. Low intensity has replaced left sphenoid bone *(arrows).* This may either reflect early transosseous involvement by carcinoma or hyperostosis. **C,** Axial T_2-weighted MRI view of upper nasopharynx demonstrates large bulky nasopharyngeal carcinoma extending into upper nasopharynx, laterally into left parapharyngeal space, and posteriorly into prevertebral muscle *(arrows).* **D,** Axial T_2-weighted MR image of lower nasopharynx-oropharynx region. Large retropharyngeal nodes both lateral and medial *(arrows)* are present. These nodes are first echelon drainage nodes of nasopharynx.

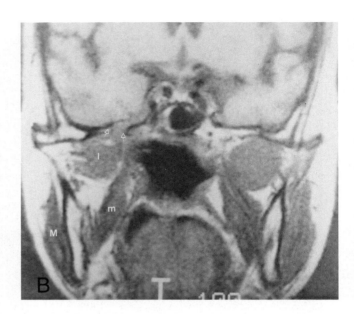

Fig. 6-27 Nasopharyngeal carcinoma and atrophy of masticator muscles. 67-year-old Chinese male with anesthesia of V3 division. Patient's status was determined after radiation therapy for nasopharyngeal carcinoma. T_1-weighted coronal MRI view (600/20) demonstrates residual carcinoma near foramen ovale *(arrows)*. Notice decreased bulk of right masticator muscles, which are supplied by third division of trigeminal nerve. This is common finding in patients with nasopharyngeal carcinoma involving skull base and extending into foramen ovale. *M,* masseter muscle, *m,* medial pterygoid muscle, *l,* lateral pterygoid muscle.

On MRI adenopathy usually has a homogeneous low-signal intensity on T_1-weighted images and a high-signal intensity on T_2-weighted images (Fig. 6-26). Node necrosis can best be identified on heavily T_2-weighted images as foci of heterogenous signal intensity. Gadolinium-enhanced T_1-weighted sequences may demonstrate a central low intensity surrounded by peripheral enhancement (Fig. 6-13).

Perineural spread of tumor may be detected on MR images or CT scans by either direct or indirect signs. Direct findings of perineural spread include enlargement of a cranial nerve near the skull base with occasional enlargement of basilar foramina and extension into the cavernous sinus. Indirect evidence of perineural tumor or neural compromise is indicated by muscular denervation atrophy (Fig. 6-27).[70] Intravascular spread of tumor is most unusual, occurring through invasion of the internal jugular vein. This may lead to thrombosis of the vessel.

Nasopharyngeal carcinoma is usually treated with radiation therapy. Neck dissection is reserved for bulky adenopathy. The prognosis depends on the tumor stage at the time of diagnosis. T_1-stage carcinomas are controlled in approximately 80% to 100% of patients. The overall control rate for all stages is 66% to 80%.[71,72] The presence of lower cervical adenopathy decreases the survival statistics by at least half.

Posttherapy CT evaluations of the nasopharynx have been recommended beginning 3 to 6 months following initial therapy and every 3 to 6 months within the initial 2 years to diagnose early recurrent disease.[73] However, CT scanning cannot differentiate between inflammatory tissue, tumor, or postradiation fibrosis. MRI is more capable of detecting the subtle changes of radia-

tion, and for this reason MR images are the preferred study for assessing posttherapy recurrences. Postradiation changes include mucosal fibrosis (low-signal intensity on T_1- and especially T_2-weighted sequences) and areas of high-signal intensity within the potential spaces separating muscles. These latter findings should be distinguished from the mass-like lesions, which are typical of recurrent tumor.

Lymphoma. Primary lymphoma of the nasopharynx is usually of the non-Hodgkin's type of lymphoma. Non-Hodgkin's lymphoma may involve any aspect of Waldeyer's ring, including residual lymphoid tissue in the nasopharynx. Lymphomas, which rarely involve only the nasopharynx, are essentially indistinguishable from squamous cell carcinoma by CT or MRI scans. However, a tumor with a rounded bulky appearance might suggest the diagnosis of lymphoma (Fig. 6-28). Radiation therapy and chemotherapy are the primary modes of treatment for lymphoma.

Rhabdomyosarcoma. Rhabdomyosarcomas are rare mesenchymal malignant tumors found throughout the body.[74,75] About 30% of rhabdomyosarcomas involve the head and neck. The orbit and nasopharynx are the most frequent sites of involvement, followed by the paranasal sinuses and middle ear. The tumor occurs primarily in young children of less than 6 years of age,[76] but may occur in adolescents. The tumor is thought to arise from rhabdomyoblasts within one of the muscles of the nasopharynx. The initial symptoms may be abrupt or insidious in onset depending on the location of the tumor. Nasopharyngeal rhabdomyosarcomas usually produce a rhinorrhea, sore throat, and serous otitis media. Invasion of the skull base is common and produces cavernous sinus syndrome (Fig. 6-29). Local re-

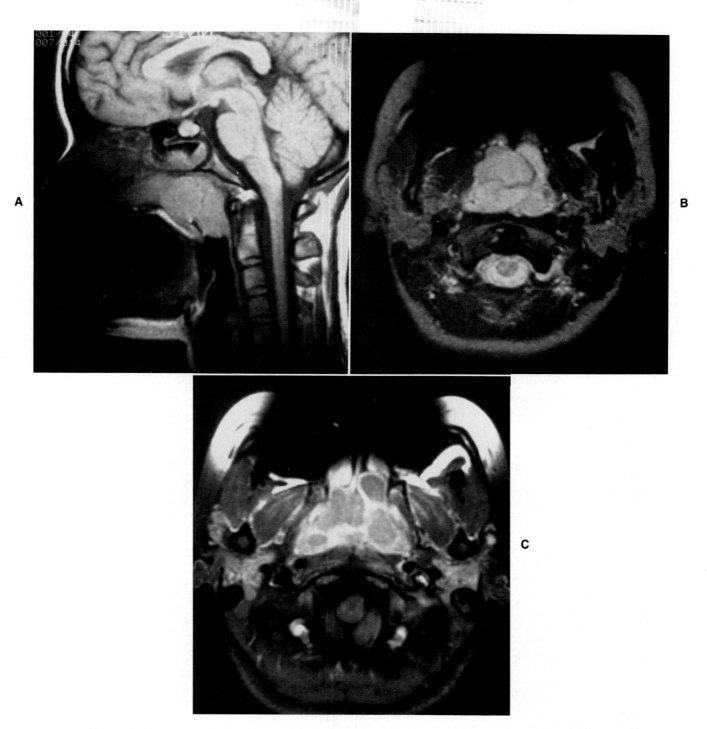

Fig. 6-28   Non-Hodgkin's lymphoma involving nasopharynx in 14-year-old female with nasal stuffiness and bilateral conductive hearing loss. **A,** Sagittal T_1-weighted MRI scan (660/20). Bulky soft tissue mass fills upper nasopharynx. **B,** Axial T_2-weighted MRI sequence (2800/80). Bulky mucosal spaced mass of increased signal intensity is seen filling nasopharyngeal lumen. Note that there is no deep invasion of soft tissue structures. **C,** T_1-weighted MRI sequence following gadolinium-DTPA. Peripheral enhancement is noted within mass. There is homogeneous appearance to mass without evidence of necrosis. Diagnosis is non-Hodgkin's lymphoma.

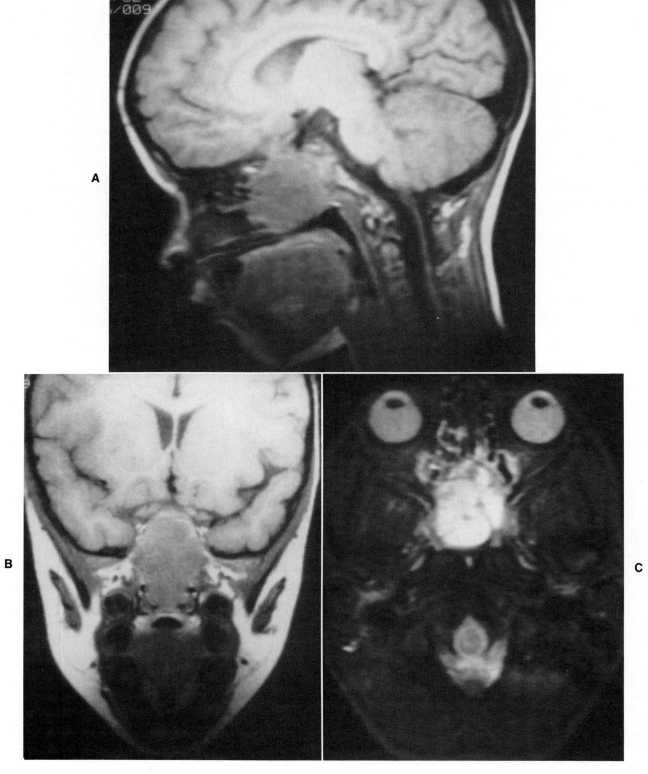

Fig. 6-29 For legend see opposite page.

Fig. 6-29 Six-year-old female with rhabdomyosarcoma of nasopharynx invading skull base and sphenoid sinus. **A,** Sagittal T_1-weighted MRI sequence demonstrates soft tissue mass of intermediate-signal intensity involving upper nasopharynx, sphenoid sinus, and skull base. Mass destroyed part of clivus and entered cranial cavity through planum sphenoidale. **B,** Coronal T_1-weighted MRI view demonstrates mass extending into sphenoid sinus and posterior ethmoid air cells. Mass extends upward to involve planum sphenoidale. **C,** T_2-weighted MRI sequence (2800/80) demonstrates diffuse homogeneous increased signal intensity. Intensity is nonspecific. Rhabdomyosarcoma must be included in differential diagnosis along with nasopharyngeal lymphoma and squamous carcinoma in young patient with nasopharyngeal mass.

---

currence and distant metastases are also common. Combined therapeutic regimens with chemotherapy, radiation therapy, and surgery have improved response rates to over 60% to 70%.[77] The 5-year survival rate after recurrence is less than 5%. On CT scans, nasopharyngeal rhabdomyosarcoma appears as an infiltrating soft tissue mass that produces destruction of the skull base and posterior maxillary sinus.[78] The MR image features of rhabdomyosarcoma are also similar to squamous cell carcinoma. However, rhabdomyosarcomas arise from muscle and may not involve the mucosal space. Prolonged T_1 and T_2 relaxation times are often noted along with frequent involvement of the skull base. Tumors may show a variable amount of enhancement following contrast administration.

Minor Salivary Gland Carcinoma. Carcinomas arising from minor salivary glands within the nasopharynx are rare. The appearance of this lesion is similar to that of squamous carcinoma; however, the tumor's response to therapy and its prognosis vary according to the histology. Perineural tumor extension is common, particularly with adenoid cystic carcinoma (see "Pathology of the oral cavity and oropharynx").

Deep Compartment Tumors. Tumors arising from structures adjacent to the nasopharyngeal mucosa—such as in the carotid space, masticator space, deep lobe of the parotid, and the oropharynx—may be difficult to differentiate on clinical examination. The site of origin of these malignancies, however, may be identified by CT and MRI scans and this in turn facilitates their diagnosis and treatment.

Carotid Space Masses

Masses within the carotid space are most commonly neoplastic. Tumors within the carotid space originate from vascular, neurogenic, or lymphatic elements. Inflammatory masses within the carotid space are infrequent. Benign tumors within the carotid space include paragangliomas and neurogenic tumors, such as neurofibromas and schwannomas. Malignant tumors within

the carotid space result from lymphatic involvement of the retropharyngeal nodes by lymphoma or carcinoma.

A mass in the carotid space can efface the fat planes surrounding the internal carotid artery and internal jugular vein, or it may displace these vessels. The mass may also cause characteristic deviation of the parapharyngeal space fat anteriorly (Fig. 6-17). The bony margins of the carotid canal or jugular foramen also may be eroded, and the styloid process may be deviated anteriorly.

Paraganglioma. Paragangliomas are usually benign and arise from paraganglion cells in the head and neck.[60] The paraganglion cells arise from amine precursor uptake and decarboxylation cells (APUD cells). These cells form bioactive amines such as norepinephrine, epinephrine, and serotonin. These substances are rarely secreted by paragangliomas in high enough concentrations to result in characteristic symptoms of hypertension, blushing, and tachycardia. The most common sites for paragangliomas include the common carotid bifurcation, jugular bulb, middle ear (tympanicum), and nodose ganglion of the vagus nerve. Paragangliomas may produce pulsatile tinnitus, a neck mass with bruits, isolated cranial neuropathy, jugular fossa syndrome, or hearing loss.

Paragangliomas are multiple in 3% to 5% of patients. This incidence rises to 20% to 30% in patients with a family history of the tumor. Therefore the other common sites of occurrence should be evaluated at the time of CT or MRI scanning, particularly when the patient has a family history of this lesion.

On CT scans, paragangliomas densely enhance. This finding is best shown by the use of a bolus infusion of iodinated contrast material.[79] Osseous erosion of the jugular bulb and inferior petrous bone may be noted with large lesions. The bone erosion is generally irregular and permeative in appearance, differentiating the paragangliomas from expansile benign neurogenic masses such as schwannomas (Fig. 6-30).

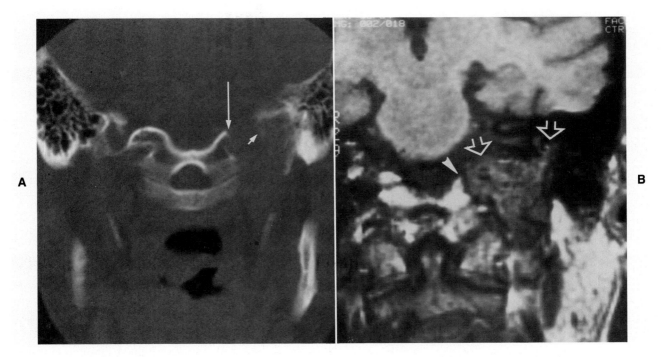

Fig. 6-30 Paraganglioma of left jugular foramen. **A,** Coronal CT scan through jugular foramen photographed with bone windows demonstrates irregular destructive mass involving jugular foramen. Jugular tubercle of clivus has been eroded *(long arrow)*. Tumor extends in invasive fashion into petrous apex *(short arrow)*. **B,** Coronal T_1-weighted MR image demonstrates paraganglioma involving left jugular foramen with inhomogeneous appearance caused by signal void from flowing vessels. Tumor can be seen eroding jugular spur *(arrowhead)* and extending into middle ear and skull base *(open arrows)*.

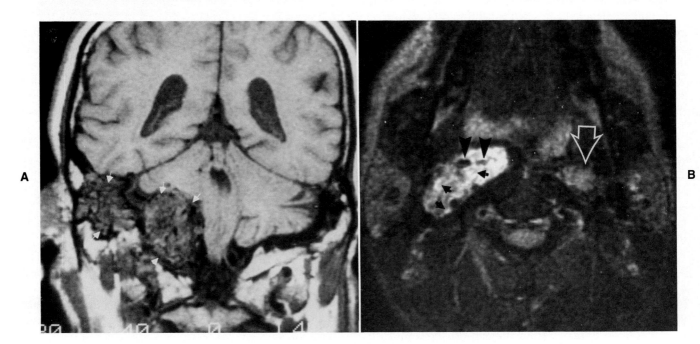

Fig. 6-31 Paraganglioma of right jugular fossa. **A,** Coronal T_1-weighted image (600/20). Large glomus jugulare invades CP angle *(arrows)*. Extension into mastoid is suggested. Numerous signal voids within mass are suggestive of hypervascular nature of this tumor. **B,** T_2-weighted MR image demonstrates hyperintense signal to mass with areas of signal void *(arrowheads)*. Hyperintense signal *(small arrows)* is probably caused by matrix of tumor. Small contralateral glomus jugulare can be seen on left *(large arrow)*.

On MR images, paragangliomas of 2 cm or greater in size have a relatively specific appearance, consisting of heterogeneous foci of high and low intensity on T_2-weighted sequences.[80] T_1-weighted sequences may demonstrate flow voids within vessels supplying the tumor (Figs. 6-30, A and 6-31, A). Prompt and intense enhancement occurs on both CT or MRI scans following contrast administration. Extension through the jugular foramen into the temporal bone and middle ear may be seen with larger lesions (Figs. 6-30 and 6-31). The heterogeneous appearance differentiates these lesions from other metastatic and neurogenic lesions of the carotid space; however, this same appearance has been seen with some vascular metastases such as thyroid and renal cell carcinoma.[81] Extension into the internal jugular vein may be detected in some patients (Fig. 6-30, B). The patient may be referred for angiography if surgical therapy or embolotherapy is planned.

Schwannoma (Neurilemmoma). Schwannomas are encapsulated benign tumors that arise from Schwann cells. Malignant change is rare. The tumor has two components: a cellular component (Antoni A) and a loose, myxoid component (Antoni B). These two pathologic features help differentiate schwannoma from neurofibroma.

Schwannomas most often develop in the third through the sixth decade of life. Although any peripheral nerve may be involved, the region of the head and neck, the cervical spinal rootlets, the vagus nerve, and the cervical sympathetics are most commonly affected. Although usually unifocal, multiple schwannomas may occur in patients with neurofibromatosis.[82]

Schwannomas tend to grow slowly, producing pain and focal neurologic symptoms only when they are large enough to compress surrounding structures. Pain and cranial neuropathy, related to compression of the nerves in the jugular foramen, are the most common symptoms of schwannomas of the head and neck. However, a painless parapharyngeal space or neck mass is an equally typical presentation.

On CT scans, schwannoma appears as a well-defined mass of soft tissue density. Splaying of the carotid vessels and anterior displacement of the parapharyngeal space is typical. Contrast enhancement of the tumor may be noted, especially in larger lesions that have undergone degenerative cystic or necrotic changes. Their slow expansile growth may cause a smooth scalloping of adjacent bone, a feature that differentiates them from the more invasive jugular paragangliomas. Treatment of schwannomas is by surgical excision.

On MR images, schwannomas usually have a homogeneous signal intensity on T_1-weighted images (Fig. 6-32), which increases with progressive T_2-weighting (Fig. 6-32, D). Internal necrosis or cystic degeneration is a feature of larger lesions and is best assessed on con-trast-enhanced T_1-weighted images. Smooth bony expansion and erosion may be detected. Intense enhancement occurs following gadolinium-DTPA administration.

Neurofibroma. Neurofibromas are benign, nonencapsulated, well-circumscribed tumors of the peripheral nerves. About 9% of patients with neurofibromas have von Recklinghausen's syndrome. Most patients with solitary neurofibromas are between 20 and 30 years of age. Clinical symptoms depend on the nerve involved. Most commonly, the neurofibroma presents as a solitary subcutaneous mass. However, if the tumor arises from a larger nerve, the tumor expands the nerve in a fusiform fashion. Degenerative cystic changes are rare.[83]

On CT scans, neurofibromas appear as well-circumscribed, solid, low-density masses that involve a peripheral nerve. The tumor may displace the parapharyngeal space. Unlike schwannomas, neurofibromas rarely have central degenerative cystic or necrotic changes. On T_2-weighted MR images, neurofibromas may have a characteristic central hypointense central fibrous core surrounded by areas of increased signal intensity (Fig. 6-33). These lesions may also enhance.

Meningioma. Meningioma may descend from the jugular fossa to involve the carotid space. True extracranial meningiomas are rare but do occur. On MR images, meningioma has a characteristic signal similar to gray matter on T_1-weighted images. Meningiomas can usually be differentiated from schwannomas on the basis of the latter's prolonged T_2 relaxation time. Both lesions enhance, but the meningioma intensely enhances and often will demonstrate a dural origin. On CT scans, meningiomas are usually either slightly hyperdense or frankly calcified on unenhanced scans and typically enhance after contrast administration. Angiography demonstrates a vascular tumor supplied primarily by branches of the external carotid arteries. Direct coronal scanning optimally shows the relationship of a meningioma to the intracranial compartment.[84]

Parapharyngeal Space Masses. Primary tumors within this space are unusual; they include lipoma, ectopic minor salivary gland tumor, atypical brachial cleft cyst (Fig. 6-34), neurogenic neoplasm, and sarcoma. Most so-called parapharyngeal space tumors actually arise from adjacent structures and secondarily displace or invade the fat-filled parapharyngeal space. True masses that arise in the parapharyngeal space are recognized on CT or MRI scans as being clearly surrounded by or arising from elements within this space (Fig. 6-34).

Lipomas. Lipomas of the parapharyngeal space may be benign or malignant. Most benign lipomas are characterized by the low attenuation of fat on CT (0 to −100 Hounsfield units) or high signal on T_1-weighted MR im-

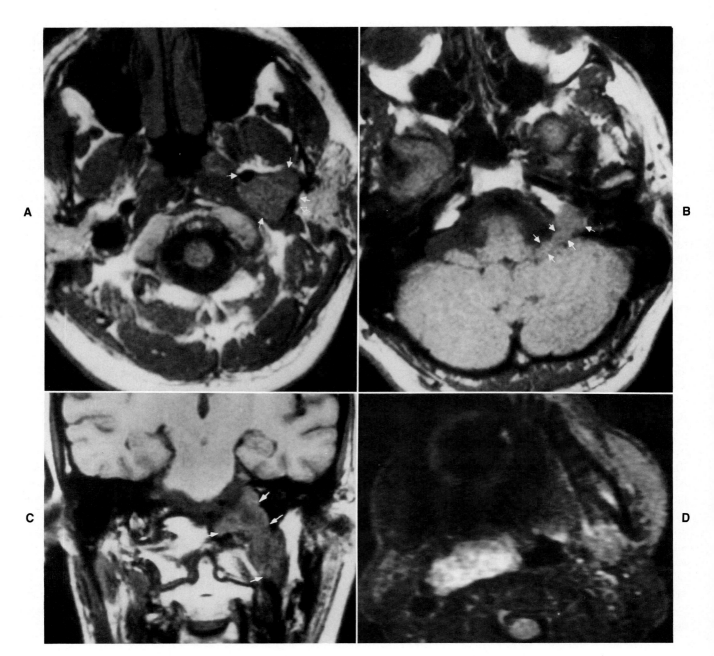

Fig. 6-32 Schwannoma of jugular foramen. 40-year-old patient presented with left vocal cord paralysis and fullness in left ear. (**A** to **D** courtesy W Kucharzyk, MD.) **A,** Axial T₁-weighted MRI sequence through upper nasopharynx demonstrates homogeneous mass in carotid space *(solid arrows)* that displaces carotid artery anteriorly and jugular vein laterally *(open arrow)*. Notice that parapharyngeal space is deviated anteriorly. **B,** Axial T₁-weighted MRI view superior to level A demonstrates extension of schwannoma along cranial nerves X and XI into cerebellopontine angle *(arrows)*. Perineural extension is typical of schwannoma. **C,** Coronal T₁-weighted MRI view demonstrates homogeneous feature to smoothly expansive schwannoma *(arrows)*. **D,** Axial T₂-weighted MRI sequence (different patient from **A** to **C**). 57-year-old female with right carotid schwannoma of cranial nerve X demonstrates diffuse increased signal intensity of carotid mass. Note that mass is somewhat heterogeneous, probably caused by small cystic degeneration.

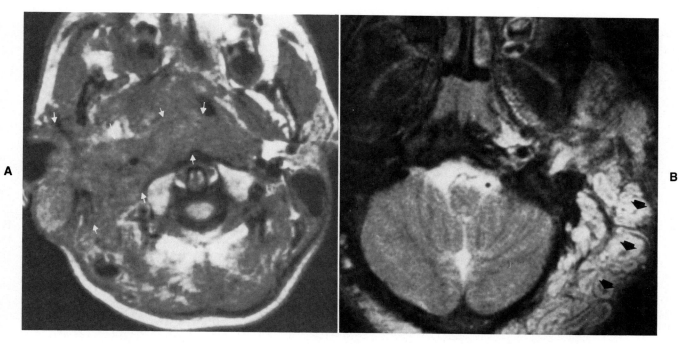

Fig. 6-33 Two different patients with neurofibromatosis involving nasopharynx. **A,** Axial T₁-weighted MR images through nasopharynx of 16-year-old demonstrates invasive mass that diffusely involves nasopharynx, retropharyngeal space, and carotid space. Mass is homogeneous and infiltrates throughout these spaces, as well as throughout subcutaneous tissue *(arrows).* **B,** Axial T₂-weighted MRI view of upper nasopharynx in another patient with neurofibromatosis. Plexiform neurofibroma involves subcutaneous tissues, as well as parotid and carotid spaces. Note punctate areas of focal hypointensity in centers of these neurofibromas characteristic of neurofibromatosis *(arrows).* Hypointensity relates to fibrosis at center of neurofibroma.

ages. The tumor may extend posteriorly into the retropharyngeal space or laterally into the carotid space. Lipomas are usually asymptomatic and discovered incidentally.

Minor Salivary Gland Tumors. Tumors of the minor salivary glands may arise from ectopic cell rests within the parapharyngeal space or deep infratemporal fossa (Fig. 6-34). Fifty percent of minor salivary gland tumors are benign mixed-cell tumors. Malignant varieties exist but can only be differentiated by histologic analysis. On CT scans, benign mixed-cell tumors of the parapharyngeal space are well-circumscribed heterogeneous masses with internal foci of low attentuation, representing islands of mucoid matrix (Fig. 6-34, A). This heterogeneous appearance is characteristic of both benign and malignant types of salivary gland tumors. On MRI minor salivary gland tumors often have a low signal on T₁-weighted images and a very high signal on T₂-weighted sequences (Fig. 6-34). These lesions cannot be histologically differentiated from other malignancies on the basis of signal intensities.

Masticator Space Neoplasms. A mass in the masticator space deviates the parapharyngeal space posteromedially and causes soft tissue infiltration of fat planes around the pterygoid and masseter muscles (Fig. 6-16). Infiltration of the marrow or frank osseous destruction of the mandible is common. Metastatic or primary tumors may occasionally involve the masticator space. Carcinoma of the lung, kidney, or breast are the most common sources of metastatic neoplasms to the masticator space. Chondrosarcoma, rhabdomyosarcoma, lymphoma, and neuroblastoma are other unusual tumors that may involve the masticator space. Primary dental lesions such as dentigerous cysts or ameloblastoma may also extend from the mandible to affect the masticator space. Retrograde perineural extension of tumor along the mandibular nerve (a branch of the third division of the trigeminal nerve) may occasionally result in extension of the tumor to the skull base and cavernous sinus (Fig. 6-35).[85]

A tumor in the masticator space can usually be differentiated from infection by virtue of the intense cellulitis, gas formation, and clinical symptomatology noted with infection (Fig. 6-16).

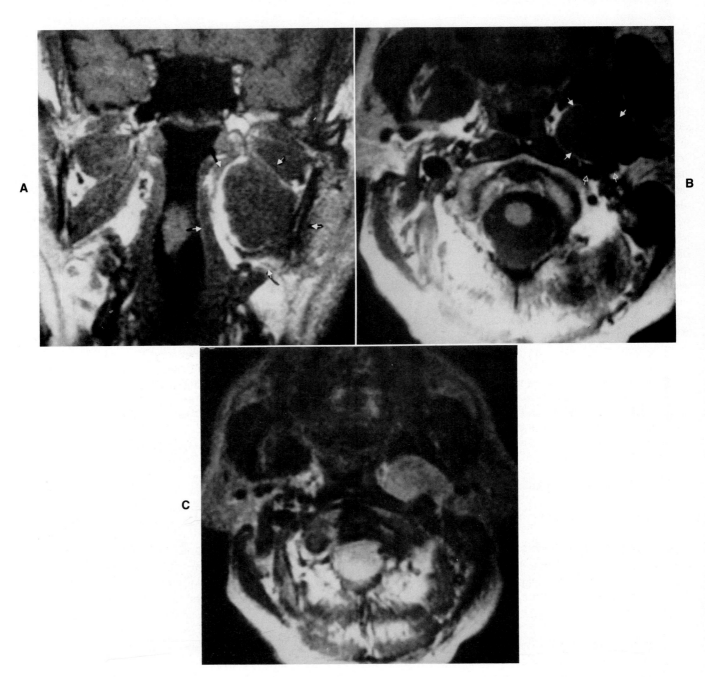

Fig. 6-34 Benign mixed cell tumor of left parapharyngeal space. 42-year-old female presents with left nasopharyngeal mass. **A,** Coronal T$_1$-weighted MR image demonstrates homogeneous mass located within left parapharyngeal space separate from masticator space and parotid gland *(arrows)*. **B,** Axial T$_1$-weighted MRI view (600/20) demonstrates left parapharyngeal space mass completely surrounded by parapharyngeal fat and separate from deep level of parotid gland *(closed arrows)*. Notice that carotid artery and jugular vein are displaced posteriorly *(open arrows)* as opposed to carotid space masses, which usually splay these vessels or displace them anteriorly. **C,** Axial T$_2$-weighted MR image demonstrates diffuse increased signal intensity to mass characteristic of benign mixed cell tumor. (Courtesy I Balcar, MD.)

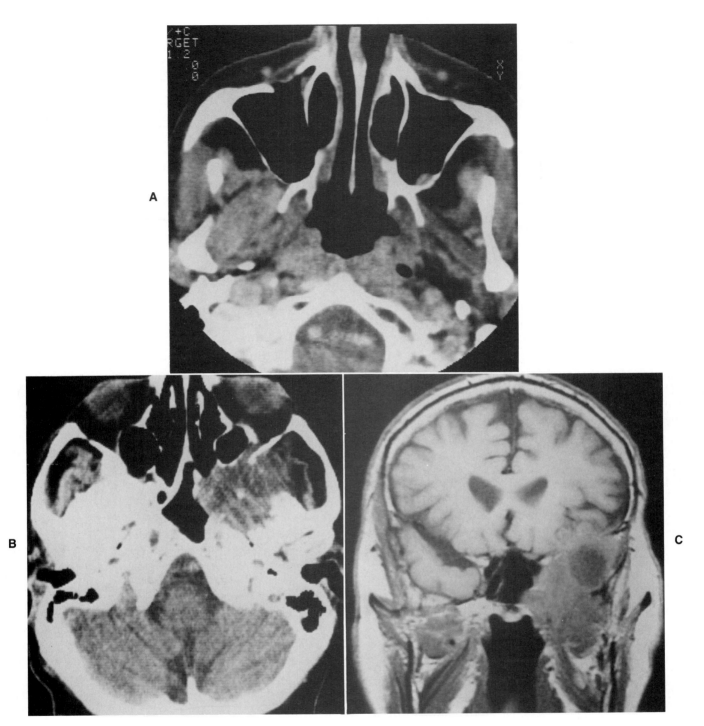

Fig. 6-35 Retrograde perineural extension of tumor along trigeminal nerve with atrophy. 60-year-old smoker presented with anesthesia involving third division of trigeminal nerve. **A,** Axial CT scan through nasopharynx demonstrates atrophy of masticator muscles on left without obvious tumor. **B,** Axial CT scan 6 months after initial scan **(A)** demonstrates mass involving left skull base and pterygopalatine fossa. In this individual, carcinoma was present at initial CT scan, but was obscured during physical examination and on CT scanning. Involvement of third division of cranial nerve V resulted in atrophy of muscles of mastication, which is indirect sign of perineural tumor extent. **C,** Coronal MRI scan 6 months after initial scan **(A)** demonstrates large mass involving left nasopharynx, skull base, and inferior temporal lobe.

PATHOLOGY OF THE ORAL CAVITY AND OROPHARYNX

Most lesions involving the oral cavity are dental in origin and usually do not require CT scans for diagnosis. Only 7% of all lesions in the oral cavity are malignant and 90% of these are squamous cell carcinomas.[86] Those benign and malignant processes of the oral cavity and oropharynx that may require CT evaluation are considered in the following discussion.

Malignant Tumors of the Oral Cavity

As stated, squamous cell carcinomas represent over 90% of malignant lesions in the oral cavity and oropharynx. A histologic gradient exists within the oral cavity and oropharynx from anterior to posterior. The more aggressive undifferentiated tumors tend to affect the posterior regions, whereas more benign lesions are found anteriorly. This gradient may be related to the fact that the squamous epithelium from the oral cavity anterior to the circumvallate papillae is derived from ectodermal elements, whereas the oropharyngeal mucosa posterior to the faucial pillars is derived from endodermal elements.[87,88]

Squamous cell carcinomas are often associated with a long history of alcohol and tobacco use. Other environmental agents associated with the development of squamous cell carcinoma include the exposure to betel nut and the HTLV-III virus, with the latter associated with the acquired immune deficiency syndrome (AIDS).[88-90] Although squamous cell carcinoma may arise from any mucosal surface, it has a predilection for the dependent portions of the mouth, including the floor of the mouth, gingival gutter, and retromolar trigone. Many squamous cell carcinomas infiltrate the deep musculofascial planes to some extent. Therefore the detection or evaluation of the full extent of tumor spread by clinical examination is difficult.[91,92] However, 5% of squamous cell carcinomas are exophytic in appearance, mimicking benign squamous papillomas.

Non-Hodgkin's lymphoma is the second most common malignancy of the oropharynx, comprising 5% of all malignancies in this region. Non-Hodgkin's lymphoma develops in the palatine and lingual lymphoid tissue and is indistinguishable from squamous cell carcinoma by CT scans.

Carcinomas other than the squamous cell variety are rare within the oral cavity and oropharynx. Most arise from the more than 1000 minor salivary glands scattered throughout the upper aerodigestive tract. The majority of minor salivary glands are located posterior to the plane of the second molar, an anatomic fact that is responsible for the higher frequency of minor salivary gland neoplasms in this region. Neoplasms of the minor salivary glands are identical to those of the major salivary glands. Malignant mixed cell, adenoid cystic carcinoma, mucoepidermoid carcinoma, and adenocarcinoma are the most common malignant tumors of the minor salivary glands.

Adenoid cystic carcinomas tend to invade and infiltrate along local nerves early in the natural history of the disease. In fact, 80% of tumors greater than 1 cm in size have invaded regional nerves at the time of surgery.[87] This factor is responsible for their high incidence of local recurrence after surgery, as tumor cells have often extended beyond the surgical resection. A wide radiation therapy port is often necessary to ensure inclusion of perineural tumor. When uncontrolled locally, this carcinoma almost always extends to either regional lymph nodes or to distant viscera with a tendency for pulmonary involvement. Early regional lymph node involvement is unusual. Regardless of the treatment, the disease tends to recur over a 10 to 15-year period.

Mucoepidermoid carcinoma arises from the mucous and basal cells of the salivary gland ducts. This histology represents 10% and 15% of all salivary gland tumors. Low-grade and high-grade forms exist but are often difficult to differentiate histologically; high-grade varieties are likely to recur locally and metastasize to regional nodes. Grossly, this tumor is often well circumscribed but usually is not encapsulated, and it often has numerous small cysts containing mucoid material.

Adenocarcinoma, a rare lesion in the oral cavity and oropharynx, may originate from the palate, buccal mucosa, tongue, floor of the mouth, or lips.[87] Local recurrences are common. Adenocarcinoma has the worst prognosis of any of the neoplasms of the minor salivary glands.

Melanomas and sarcomas are rare tumors of the oral cavity and oropharynx. Melanomas tend to grow rapidly, having multicentric, polypoid, or sessile appearances.[88] The histology of this lesion may be difficult to distinguish from undifferentiated carcinoma without the use of special melanin-specific stains. Sarcomas within the oral cavity and oropharynx include rhabdomyosarcomas, fibrosarcomas, angiosarcomas, liposarcomas, and myosarcomas.[89]

Clinical Presentation. Lesions within the oral cavity are most often detected by the patient or during routine dental examination. Early squamous cell carcinomas are often asymptomatic and grossly appear as erythematous mucosal lesions with ill-defined borders. Oral leukoplakia (white patches) may be present. These lesions are now believed to be related to cigarette use. However, only 10% of leukoplakic lesions eventually transform into carcinoma. Larger carcinomas may cause ill-fitting dentures or pain when drinking hot liquids.

Referred pain to the external auditory canal (referred otalgia) is a common symptom of carcinoma of the oral cavity and oropharynx. This occurs because both the external auditory canal and various sites in the upper aerodigestive tract are innervated by branches of the same cranial nerves. Otalgia is not a sign to be ignored, especially if the patient is at risk for head and neck carcinoma.

Carcinomas of the oropharynx and tongue base are usually advanced at the time of diagnosis because of their aggressive course and relatively mild symptomatology. Even rather large lesions involving the base of the tongue or pharyngeal wall may only cause a mild sore throat. The first sign of carcinoma of the posterior tongue or pharyngeal wall may be a palpable cervical lymph node metastasis. Dysphagia, nasal speech, foul breath, and ear pain may develop as the primary lesion enlarges.

Tonsillar lesions are frequently discovered during routine dental examination. Early symptoms of tonsillar malignancy also include sore throat and referred ear pain. Deep invasion with involvement of the medial pterygoid muscle may cause trismus in advanced lesions.

Clinical Staging (TNM Classification). The American Joint Committee on Cancer Staging (1988) has developed a clinical staging system for all primary malignancies of the oral cavity and oropharynx (see box).

Routes of Spread. Squamous cell carcinoma of the oropharynx tends to extend submucosally and along deep musculofascial planes in preference to exophytic mucosal growth.[91-93] CT scan and MR image assessment of submucosal growth is particularly important, as the mucosal surfaces may appear completely normal clinically.[91-96] CT scan assessment of the parapharyngeal space therefore is an important aspect of radiographic staging.

Tumors of the oropharynx may eventually invade the periosteum of the skull base or mandible. The tumor may grow along the periosteum and may invade the adjacent bone via a nutrient canal, neural canal, or muscular attachment. Once within bone, the marrow cavity is involved preferentially.

Tumor may spread in a retrograde manner along peripheral branches of the regional nerves to the central nervous system and base of the skull. The hypoglossal nerve (cranial nerve XII) and branches of the trigeminal nerve (cranial nerve V) are the nerves most often involved in this manner. Adenoid cystic carcinoma, recurrent squamous cell carcinoma, and sarcomas are the neoplasms that most commonly exhibit this pattern of spread. Non-Hodgkin's lymphoma may also occasionally extend along regional nerves. Perineural spread of squamous cell carcinoma at first presentation is unusual and, when present, probably indicates a very aggressive lesion.

Tumor extension to regional lymph nodes must be detected to offer the best therapy for carcinoma.

TNM CLASSIFICATION OF OROPHARYNGEAL MALIGNANCIES

Primary tumor (T)
TX, Primary tumor cannot be assessed
T0, No evidence of primary tumor
Tis, Carcinoma in situ

OROPHARYNX
T1, Tumor 2 cm or less in greatest dimension
T2, Tumor > 2 cm but not > 4 cm in greatest dimension
T3, Tumor > 4 cm in greatest dimension
T4, Tumor invades adjacent soft tissues or osseous structures

NASOPHARYNX
T1, Tumor limited to one subsite of nasopharynx
T2, Tumor invades more than one subsite of nasopharynx
T3, Tumor invades nasal cavity and/or oropharynx
T4, Tumor invades skull and/or cranial nerve(s)

HYPOPHARYNX
T1, Tumor limited to one subsite of hypopharynx
T2, Tumor invades more than one subsite of hypopharynx or an adjacent site, *without* fixation of hemilarynx
T3, Tumor invades more than one subsite of hypopharynx or an adjacent site, *with* fixation of hemilarynx
T4, Tumor invades adjacent structures (e.g., cartilage or soft tissues of neck)

Regional lymph nodes (N)
NX, Regional lymph nodes cannot be assessed
N0, No regional lymph node metastasis
N1, Single ipsilateral lymph node, 3 cm or less
N2, Single ipsilateral lymph node, > 3 cm but not > 6 cm in diameter; or multiple ipsilateral lymph nodes, none > 6 cm in diameter; or in bilateral or contralateral lymph nodes, none > 6 cm in diameter
N2a, Metastasis in single ipsilateral lymph node > 3 cm but not > 6 cm in greatest dimension
N2b, Metastasis in multiple ipsilateral lymph nodes, none > 6 cm in greatest dimension
N2c, Metastasis in bilateral or contralateral lymph nodes, none > 6 cm in greatest dimension
N3, Metastasis in a lymph node > 6 cm in greatest dimension

Distant metastasis (M)
MX, Presence of distant metastasis cannot be assessed
M0, No distant metastasis
M1, Distant metastasis

Lips and Gingival Buccal Region. Malignant tumors of the lip are usually squamous cell carcinomas. These tumors arise on the vermillion border and then invade the orbicularis oris muscle and adjacent skin.[97] Advanced lesions may involve the buccal mucosa, the mandible, and eventually the mental nerve. Involvement of the mental nerve, although rare, provides a route for centripetal extension of the tumor into the medullary cavity of the mandible and along the third division of the trigeminal nerve. Lymphatic spread to the submental, submandibular, and jugulodigastric nodes is noted in 10% to 20% of patients at the time of initial diagnosis. Cervical node metastases occur most frequently in patients with large lesions, with recurrent disease, and with undifferentiated cell types.

Gingival carcinomas tend to invade the tooth sockets and mandible, leading to local bone erosion and loose teeth. The larger retromolar trigone carcinomas may spread along the pterygomandibular raphe to the low infratemporal fossa. This spread is usually not evident clinically and may require an extended posterior maxillectomy for adequate surgical margins.

Carcinoma of the buccal mucosa may extend along the planes of the buccinator muscles, into the subcutaneous tissues of the cheek, and posteriorly to the retromolar trigone. Lymphatic drainage extends primarily to the submandibular nodes and eventually to the jugulodigastric and parotid nodes. Rarely, deep facial nodes in the buccinator space are enlarged by advanced buccal or retromolar trigone carcinoma.

Tongue. Tumors of the anterior two-thirds of the tongue are usually either squamous cell carcinomas or minor salivary gland tumors. CT or MRI scans have little to offer in the evaluation of superficial lesions without clinically palpable nodes. Larger lesions of the oral tongue (stage T2 to T4) invariable invade deeply into muscle. Tumors spread easily along the bundles of the intrinsic muscles of the tongue. Tumors may also spread along the extrinsic muscles of the tongue to their sites of attachment, such as the hyoid bone, symphysis menti of the mandible, styloid process, and soft palate. Submucosal spread may involve the floor of the mouth, tonsils, pharyngeal wall, and mandible.[92,98] The rich lymphatics of the tongue result in a high incidence of bilateral nodal disease. Thirty to forty percent of patients with T1- or T2-stage carcinomas have clinically palpable nodes. Lymphatic drainage occurs primarily to the submandibular and jugulodigastric nodes.

Surgical therapy of carcinoma of the tongue is usually limited to local laser resection or hemiglossectomy. Total glossectomy is poorly tolerated and often results in chronic aspiration. Therefore it is important to assess the spread of carcinoma across the midline of the tongue by CT or MRI scans for planning both surgery and radiation therapy ports.

Carcinoma of the tongue has density on CT scans that is similar to that of the surrounding normal tongue muscle. Tumors are recognized by infiltration and distortion of the normal fat planes within the tongue and by enhancing margins caused by a vascular response (Fig. 6-36). Occasionally on CT scans, the exact extent of muscular invasion may be difficult to assess. On MR images, tongue carcinomas have increased signal intensity on T_2-weighted images, and this is useful in assessing the depth of tumor invasion into the muscles. Tumors usually enhance with gadolinium (Fig. 6-37).

Floor of Mouth. Squamous cell carcinoma is the most common neoplasm to involve the floor of the mouth. Carcinomas arising from the sublingual salivary glands account for only 5% of tumors in this region. The anterior floor of the mouth is the most common site of origin. Penetration into the extrinsic tongue muscles is frequently shown on CT scans by obliteration of the fat planes surrounding these muscles. The carcinoma may also spread into the sublingual and submandibular spaces (Fig. 6-37).[99,100] Infiltration along the periosteum of the mandible occurs early in the course of the disease. Destruction of the mandible usually occurs later as tumor invades at an interruption of the periosteum, such as the mental or inferior alveolar foramina (Fig. 6-37). Encasement of the lingual artery by tumor is common; however, life-threatening arterial hemorrhage is infrequent. The submandibular duct may become obstructed by carcinomas of the floor of the mouth, resulting in inflammatory enlargement of the submandibular gland, which may be mistaken for a cervical lymph node (Fig. 6-37, C). Invasion of the hypoglossal and lingual nerves by carcinoma of the floor of the mouth may lead to motor and sensory changes such as denervation atrophy (Fig. 6-38).

Palpable submandibular and jugulodigastric adenopathy is present in 30% of all patients with carcinomas of the floor of the mouth of less than 2 cm diameter (stage T1). However, one-third of these nodes are enlarged by benign reactive changes.[87,101] Bilateral nodal metastases occur in approximately 50% of patients who receive no treatment to the nodal drainage sites in the neck. Therefore both the ipsilateral and contralateral neck nodes are routinely treated with radiation therapy or radical neck dissection. Carcinomas of the floor of the mouth do not usually spread to the submental lymph nodes.[97]

Surgical and radiation therapy are equally effective in treating carcinomas of the floor of the mouth of less than 4 cm diameter (stage T1 and T2). Stage-T3 and stage-T4 lesions (equal to or greater than 4 cm) are generally treated using a combined regimen of interstitial radiation implants and external beam radiation. The risk of osteoradionecrosis is increased if the tumor has invaded the mandible.[97] Partial mandibular resection

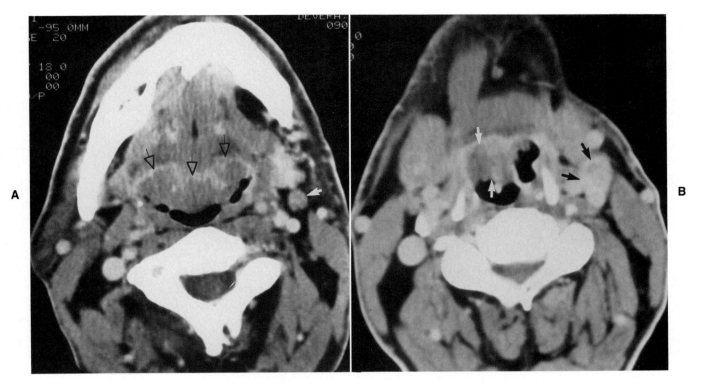

Fig. 6-36   Carcinoma of base of tongue. 57-year-old male with right ear pain and diffi-culty swallowing. **A,** Axial CT scan through base of tongue demonstrates homogeneous mass involving vallecula and base of tongue region. Mass is isointense to surrounding muscle. Minimal peripheral enhancement is noted *(open arrows)*. Also noted is small left subdigastric nerve *(solid arrow)*. **B,** Axial CT scan after contrast infusion through the val-lecula and lower base of tongue, demonstrates mass involving right vallecula *(white ar-rows)*. Note inhomogeneous necrotic metastatic subdigastric lymph node on left *(black arrows)*.

may be required for carcinomas that are immediately adjacent to the mandible, because occult microscopic invasion of the mandible often cannot be excluded. Carcinomas involving the lateral floor of the mouth are resected in continuity with an ipsilateral neck dissec-tion. The survival rates vary according to the stage of the lesion at the time of diagnosis and the treatment modality used. In general, overall 5-year survival rates of approximately 60% have been achieved, ranging from 100% survival for stage-T1 lesions to 20% or less for stage-T4 lesions.[97]

Malignant Tumors of the Oropharynx Proper

Palate. The majority of malignancies of the soft palate are squamous cell carcinomas; however, carcinomas of the minor salivary glands have their highest frequency in the posterior soft palate. Carcinomas of the palate usually affect the oral aspect of the palate. They tend to be well-differentiated lesions that have the best progno-sis of all the oropharyngeal carcinomas. The nasopha-ryngeal side of the soft palate is rarely involved, even

when the tumors are extensive. Extension of palatal carcinoma occurs in all directions, but the tonsillar pil-lars and hard palate are usually affected first (Fig. 6-39). Deep lateral invasion occurs along the levator or tensor palatini muscles and into the parapharyngeal space, the nasopharynx, and the base of the skull.

Lymphatic spread is present in 60% of all patients at the time of the diagnosis of carcinoma of the palate. The incidence of cervical node metastases depends on the size of the primary lesion. T1 carcinomas (less than 2 cm in diameter) are associated with an 8% incidence of cervical metastases. Larger (T4) tumors (greater than 4 cm in diameter with invasion) are associated with a 70% incidence of cervical metastases. Palatal carcino-mas drain first to the high internal jugular and subdi-gastric nodes with subsequent involvement of the lower internal jugular chain or retropharyngeal nodes. Exten-sion up the greater and lessor palatine nerve canals can occur, allowing spread of tumors into the pterygopala-tine fossa and cavernous sinus (Fig. 6-40). Treatment of palatal lesions depends on the stage of the disease pro-

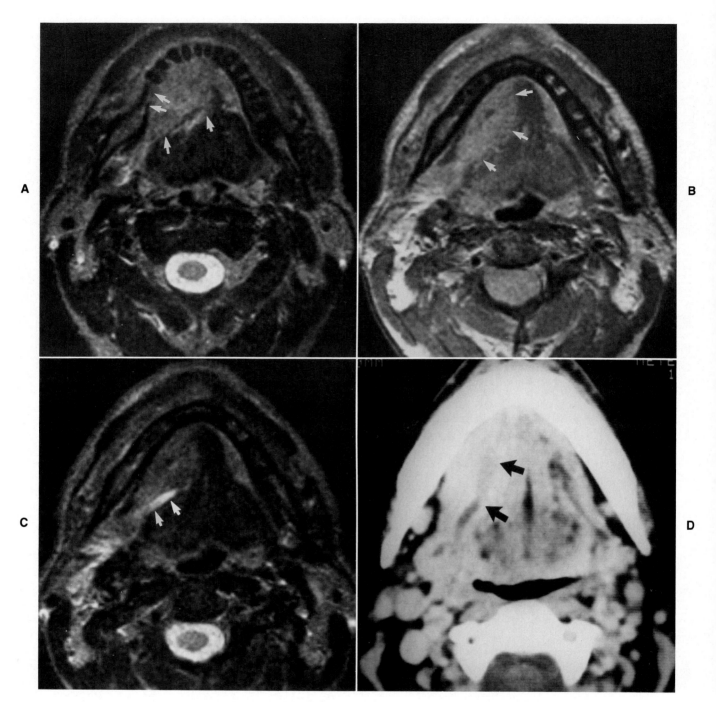

Fig. 6-37 Squamous cell carcinoma of right tongue and floor of mouth. **A,** T$_2$-weighted MRI sequence (2800/80) through midoropharynx. Large hyperintense mass is located in dorsal aspect of anterior tongue. It crosses midline and appears to erode part of internal cortex of mandible *(arrows)*. **B,** Proton density image (2800/30) through floor of mouth. Carcinoma extends down into right sublingual and submandibular space *(arrows)*. At this level cortex of mandible appears intact. **C,** Heavily T$_2$-weighted MRI sequence at same level as **B.** On this sequence obstructed submandibular duct *(arrows)* can be identified. This is common feature associated with carcinoma of floor of mouth. **D,** Axial CT scan in different patient with carcinoma in floor of mouth. Note obstruction of submandibular gland and duct with low-density tubular structure occupying right sublingual space *(arrows)*.

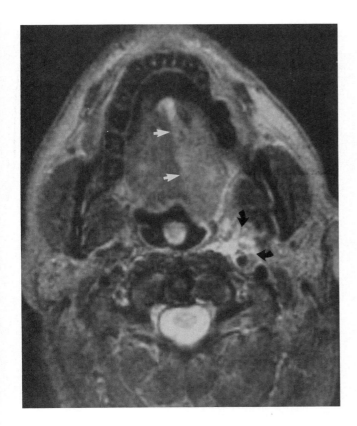

Fig. 6-38   Carcinoma of base of tongue with cranial nerve XII atrophy. T_2-weighted MRI sequence through midoropharynx demonstrates increased signal intensity to left half of tongue *(arrows)*. In addition, area of increased signal intensity with mass effect is noted in left posterior tongue base and carotid sheath region *(closed curved arrows)*. Hypointensity of left tongue is due to myositis, which occurs in patients with denervation atrophy. This will later evolve to fatty replaced, atrophic tongue evident as increased signal intensity on T_1-weighted MR images.

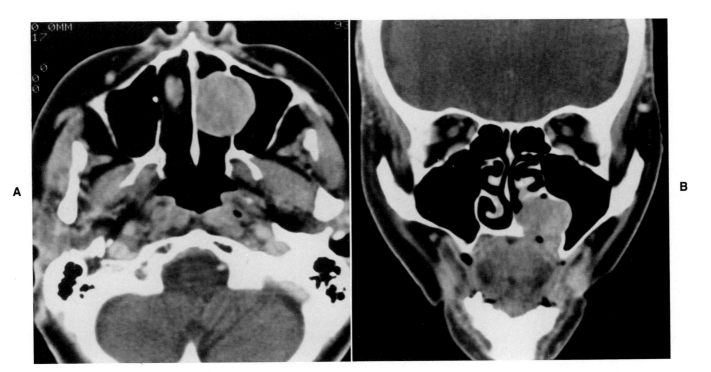

Fig. 6-39   Adenocarcinoma of palate in 57-year-old female with palpable mass in roof of mouth. **A,** Axial CT scan, after infusion of contrast through midnasal region, demonstrates well-circumscribed mass involving left nasal cavity and maxillary sinus. **B,** Coronal view through this same level demonstrates erosion of left hard palate and extension of carcinoma to left nares and maxillary sinus. Smooth margin of this tumor suggested benign lesion; however, adenocarcinoma was detected at biopsy.

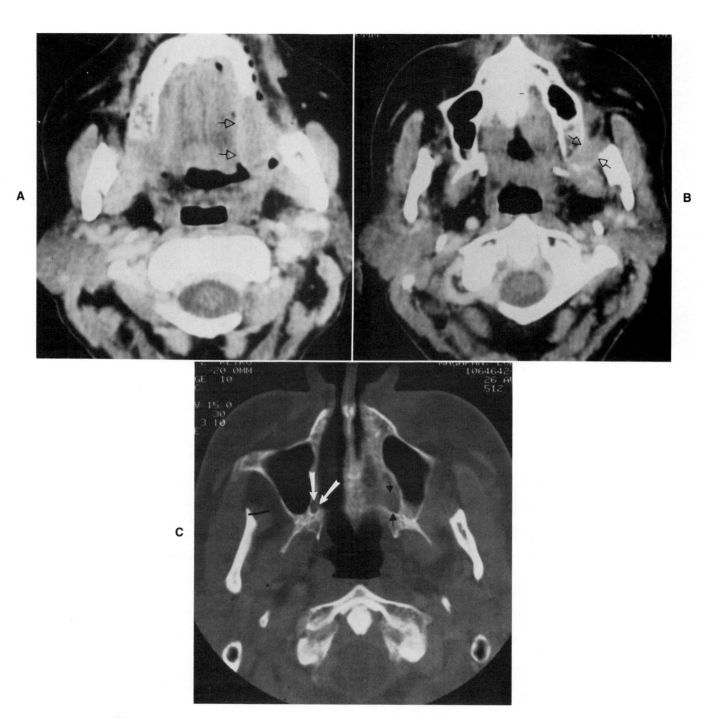

Fig. 6-40 Adenoid cystic carcinoma in left alveolar ridge with extension into greater palatine foramen. **A,** CT scan through upper oropharynx demonstrates subtle isointense mass involving left superior alveolar ridge *(arrows)*. **B,** Axial CT scan at higher level than **A** demonstrates extension of mass through buccinator space *(arrows)*, common finding in patients with lateral palate carcinoma. **C,** Bone window at level of hard palate demonstrates expansion of greater palatine foramen *(black arrows)*. Normal greater palatine foramen is seen on right *(white arrow)*. Extension up greater palatine foramen is common with palatal carcinomas. This may extend upward to pterygopalatine fossa and into cavernous sinus.

cess. Advanced lesions, such as T2 and T3 carcinomas, are usually treated with combined surgery and radiation to the primary mass and to the cervical lymph nodes at highest risk for metastases. Surgical excision of palatal carcinomas must encompass a wide area and may lead to significant problems with phonation and swallowing.[102]

The CT scan findings of carcinomas of the soft palate depend on the size and extent of the lesions. Subtle lesions along the oral surface of the soft palate may just increase the fullness of the soft palate on axial CT scans (Fig. 6-40, *A*). Large lesions may result in unilateral fullness in the region of the tonsil and soft palate and have invasion of the parapharyngeal space.[103] Direct coronal CT scans must be used to evaluate the soft and hard palate as these structures lie in the axial plane and therefore are poorly examined by axial CT scans. MRI is ideally suited to evaluate the palate in both the sagittal and coronal planes.[104] Generally, T_1-weighted images suffice, with T_2-serial images adding little information. The palate has intrinsically high signal, probably caused by the mucous glands and fat that are abundantly present. This gives a normally high signal on T_1-weighted images and allows tumors to be easily identified when they invade and replace this high signal with a lower T_1-weighted signal intensity. Extension up the greater and lesser palatine nerves is best assessed with thin section axial CT scans or enhanced MR images.

Tonsil. Tonsillar carcinoma is the most common malignancy of the oropharynx and oral cavity.[105] This lesion often develops in elderly men with a history of heavy cigarette and alcohol use. A mild sore throat may be the only clinical symptom. The tumor usually begins in the anterior tonsillar pillar or in the tonsil itself. Carcinoma of the posterior tonsillar pillar is less common. A tumor in this location may spread inferiorly along the palatopharyngeus muscle into the base of the tongue and thyroid cartilage. Small (less than 1 cm) tonsillar carcinomas are usually impossible to detect by CT or MRI scans because of the normal asymmetry of the palatine tonsils.[100] Larger lesions infiltrate surrounding tissue planes and extend into adjacent regions in a predictable manner. The high density of normal lingual tonsillar tissue near the base of the tongue is often indistinguishable from carcinoma. On MRI scans, tonsillar carcinoma has a low signal on T_1-weighted images and a high signal on T_2-weighted images (Fig. 6-41). Infiltration of surrounding muscles such as the tongue or pterygoids is easily seen.

The lymphatic spread of carcinomas of the tonsil to the internal jugular chain and submandibular nodes is similar to that of lesions of the soft palate. Carcinoma of the tonsil tends to be highly malignant with a propen-

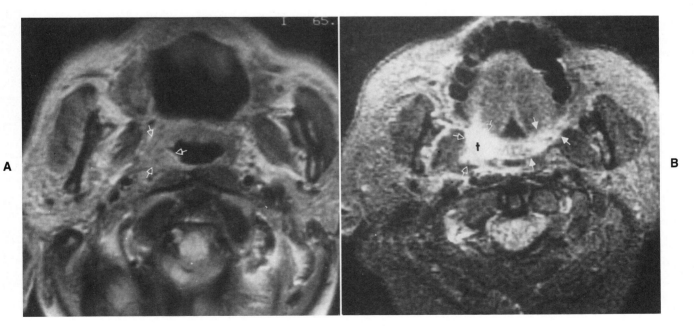

Fig. 6-41   Squamous cell carcinoma of right tonsil. **A,** Axial T_1-weighted MRI sequence through oropharynx demonstrates soft tissue mass involving right pharyngeal wall and tonsil *(arrows)*. **B,** Axial T_2-weighted MRI sequence (2800/80) demonstrates tumor *(t)* and its extension anteriorly into tongue, laterally into masticator space region, and posteriorly into carotid space region *(open arrows)*. Note, however, its interface with normal lymphoid tissue of palate *(closed arrows)* is difficult at best.

sity for early metastases. Tonsillar carcinoma has a 75% or greater chance of node involvement at presentation. Contralateral and bilateral cervical node metastases are frequent because of the rich lymphatic system in the oropharyngeal region.[87,105] Anterior pillar lesions have a 45% risk of clinical node metastases at presentation.[99]

Base of Tongue. The base of the tongue is that area posterior to the circumvallate papillae.[106] Of all carcinomas of the tongue, 25% involve this area; 90% are poorly differentiated squamous carcinomas, whereas the remaining 10% are either lymphoma or minor salivary gland carcinomas. The subtle initial symptoms of sore throat or referred ear pain are responsible for delay in diagnosis. Cervical node metastasis or bulky primary disease is usually the first clinically apparent sign. The delay in diagnosis and the more malignant nature of these tumors result in a poorer prognosis than that of the more anterior lesions.

Primary carcinoma of the tongue base tends to remain unilateral until it is quite extensive. The tumor often extends anteriorly into the substance of the tongue, inferiorly into the vallecula and hypopharynx or superiorly along the glossopalatini sulcus to the palatal arch complex (Figs. 6-36 and 6-38). Inferior extension into the preepiglottic space is common. Such extension is recognized by infiltration of the fat of this space, which separates the hyoid bone from the epiglottis (Fig. 6-36, B).

Cervical adenopathy frequently involves the internal jugular chain and submandibular triangle. Unilateral adenopathy is present in up to 75% of patients at the time of initial diagnosis. Bilateral cervical adenopathy occurs in 30% of patients (Fig. 6-36).[99] Accurate assessment of the primary lesion, as well as the extent of cervical adenopathy, is essential for treatment planning. Particular attention must be paid to the relationship of the carotid vessels to the surrounding nodes. The tumor may be unresectable if the carotid vessels are encased or compressed by adenopathy. The exact relationship between cervical adenopathy and the cervical vessels can be best determined by high-resolution ultrasound, dynamic bolus contrast-enhanced CT scans, or MRI.[107,108]

Lymphoma of the base of the tongue is usually of the non-Hodgkin's variety and occurs within the lymphatic tissues that are frequently present in the base of the tongue and vallecula. The CT scan findings are similar to those of squamous cell carcinoma (Fig. 6-42). A soft tissue mass or density similar to muscle may extend into the preepiglottic space or vallecula. MRI is also helpful in delineating the tumor margins from surrounding muscles.

All carcinomas of the tongue base appear similar to oral tongue lesions (*vide supra*). High-signal intensity on T$_2$-weighted sequences is typical. CT or MRI scan-

ning should be performed as part of the work-up for all tumors of the tongue base, particularly those that are greater than 1 to 2 cm in size. This evaluation is important in deciding whether partial glossectomy or radiation therapy is to be performed and the extent of therapy to be given. Extension of tumor into the preepiglottic space and hypopharynx requires partial laryngectomy and pharyngectomy as part of the curative surgical procedure.

The normal lymphatic tissue at the base of the tongue may occasionally simulate the appearance of carcinoma of the tongue on CT or MRI (Fig. 6-11, *C*). The lack of mass effect, the absence of cervical adenopathy, and the heterogeneous appearance of lymphatic tissue in this region are features that are used to help to exclude the presence of a tumor. However, occasionally normal lymphatic tissue simulates tumor on CT or MRI in both density (intensity) and location. In these instances, endoscopy with biopsy is required to exclude a tumor.

Pharyngeal Walls. The biologic behavior of neoplasms of the pharyngeal wall is similar to that of carcinomas of the hypopharyngeal wall. Both sites develop aggressive, less well-differentiated squamous cell carcinomas that have a high proclivity to bilateral cervical node metastases. Clinical symptoms are similar to those of carcinoma of the tonsil or soft palate. Palpable cervi-

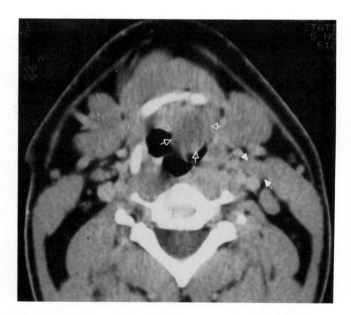

Fig. 6-42 Lymphoma at base of tongue. Axial CT scan through hyoid bone level demonstrates homogeneous mass involving left base of tongue and vallecula (*open arrows*). Mass is poorly distinguished from surrounding muscle but does have mass effect and could be easily differentiated from surrounding lymphoid tissue. Non-Hodgkin's lymphoma was detected at biopsy. Note also small subdigastric node adjacent to carotid sheath (*closed arrows*).

cal adenopathy is common at the time of diagnosis. Although retropharyngeal nodes are the first-order drainage nodes for lesions of the oropharyngeal wall, these nodes are not palpable at clinical examination.

On CT or MRI scans, carcinomas of the pharyngeal walls show a thickening of the pharyngeal wall over several contiguous centimeters (Fig. 6-41, *A*). Extension of tumor deep to the pharyngeal walls into the surrounding soft tissue planes is frequently detected. In older patients, the pharyngeal walls normally should not exceed 3 mm in thickness. An increase in thickness of the pharyngeal walls near the tongue base on the palatine tonsils must be differentiated from residual lymphoid tissue in younger patients. Recent biopsies or inflammatory lesions may thicken the pharyngeal walls and simulate carcinoma. For this reason, imaging studies should always be performed before or no less than 2 weeks following biopsy.

Large deeply invasive carcinoma of the pharyngeal wall may extend submucosally along the constrictor muscles into the nasopharynx and skull base.[91] The tumor may also extend into the base of the tongue, hypopharynx, carotid sheath, and parapharyngeal spaces. Spread along the constrictor muscles may result in recurrences at various points of their attachment. Invasion of the prevertebral fascia posterior to the pharyngeal wall allows access of the carcinoma to the cervical spine. Patients with pharyngeal wall cancers have a 15% to 25% incidence of a second primary cancer occurring in the cervical esophagus.

Benign Lesions of the Oral Cavity and Oropharynx

Thyroglossal Duct Anomalies. These are best considered in the chapter on the cervical neck. Nevertheless, some discussion is warranted. The thyroglossal duct cyst is located close to or in the midline of the neck along the tract of the primordial thyroid gland.[86] Fifty percent of these cysts are located close to or behind the hyoid bone; however, they may be found anywhere from the foramen caecum to the thyroid gland itself (Fig. 6-43).

Lingual Thyroid. Failure of thyroid tissue to completely descend from the foramen cecum of the tongue to the lower neck during embryologic development may result in a residual mass of thyroid tissue along this tract. The dorsal posterior third of the tongue is the most common site of such residual tissue. The ectopic thyroid tissue may enlarge to form a reddish mass; however, it is usually asymptomatic. Women are more frequently affected than men. If surgical excision is contemplated, a nuclear thyroid scan must be performed before resection of the ectopic thyroid mass to establish the presence of normal thyroid tissue in the neck. Car-

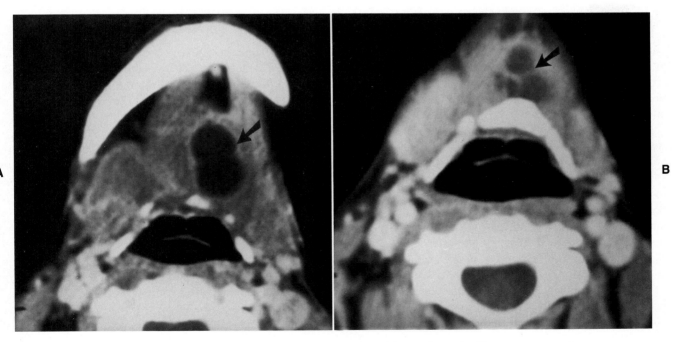

Fig. 6-43 Thyroglossal duct cyst involving midline of floor of mouth. (Case courtesy of Dr. Rob Lufkin, University of California, Los Angeles.) **A** and **B,** Contiguous transaxial sections demonstrate cystic mass involving midline structure of neck and floor of mouth. Cyst extends upward through anterior belly of digastric muscle and is associated with hyoid bone *(arrow)*.

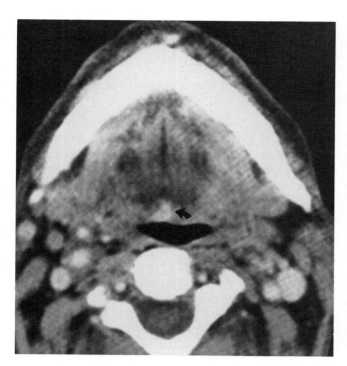

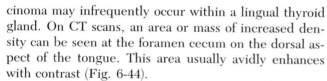

Fig. 6-44 Residual lingual thyroid tissue at foramen cecum. Contiguous transaxial CT section through tongue base demonstrates high-density focus near foramen cecum characteristic of residual lymphoid tissue *(arrow)*. This occurs as result of failure of descent of thyroid tissue from foramen cecum. Cysts may develop along this tract, or residual thyroid tissue may be present. Thyroid tissue may develop features of carcinoma.

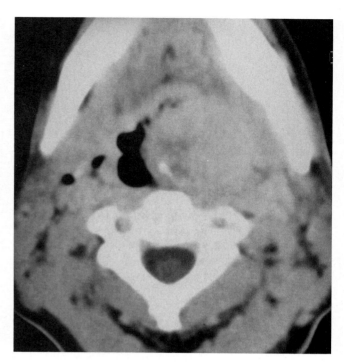

Fig. 6-45 Hemangioma of base of tongue. Transaxial CT scan following contrast administration in 6-year-old male demonstrates large base of tongue mass with focus of calcification. At resection this proved to be cavernous hemangioma.

cinoma may infrequently occur within a lingual thyroid gland. On CT scans, an area or mass of increased density can be seen at the foramen cecum on the dorsal aspect of the tongue. This area usually avidly enhances with contrast (Fig. 6-44).

Hemangioma. Hemangiomas are the most common tumor in the cervical region in children. They may involve the oropharynx or face (Fig. 6-45), usually as a sessile reddish submucosal mass near the base of the tongue. The cavernous type is most common. CT scans demonstrate a mass of muscle intensity that may or may not enhance. Phleboliths (venous calculi) are diagnostic, if present. MR images demonstrate an infiltrative mass of low-signal intensity on T_1-weighted images and high-signal intensity on T_2-weighted images (Fig. 6-46).[109] This reflects the pathologic processes of these lesions, which largely consist of stagnant nonclotted blood.

Fibrous Lesions

Fibromatosis. Fibrous lesions of the head and neck vary in their biologic activity and histologic appearance. Even though their histologic appearance is benign, some lesions are so locally aggressive that they are considered to be low-grade fibrosarcomas. The term *des-*

moid has also been applied to a subgroup of these lesions, which present as well-differentiated but locally infiltrating fibrous masses near the musculoaponeurotic junctions. Twelve percent of desmoids involve the region of the head and neck, most commonly the soft tissues of the supraclavicular region and face.[110] Involvement of the oral cavity or nasopharynx is rare in adults. The CT scan findings of the fibromatoses are nonspecific. Desmoids involving the head and neck usually encase and infiltrate the musculature of the supraclavicular region. They may infiltrate fat planes and cannot be differentiated from malignant lesions on the basis of their CT scan findings.

Skeletal Muscle Tumors. Benign tumors of muscles of the oral cavity and oropharynx include rhabdomyomas and benign masseteric hypertrophy.

Rhabdomyoma. Rhabdomyomas are rare benign skeletal tumors that have a predilection for the head and neck. Whereas cardiac rhabdomyomas affect patients with tuberous sclerosis, extracardiac rhabdomyomas have no relationship to this syndrome. Affected regions include the oropharynx, nasopharynx, larynx, and submandibular triangle. On CT and MRI scans, the tumors are well circumscribed with a density or intensity similar to muscle (Fig. 6-47).

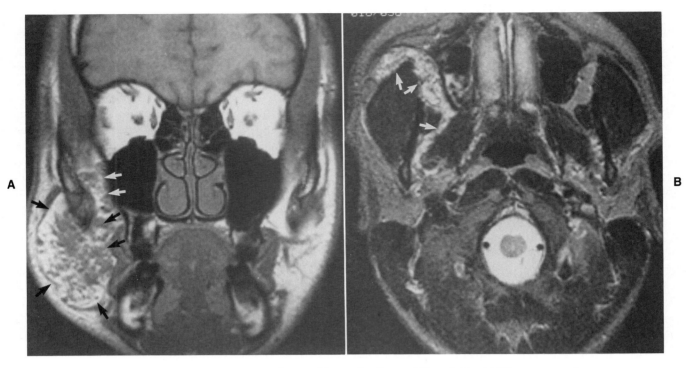

Fig. 6-46   Cavernous hemangioma of face. **A,** Coronal T_1-weighted MRI sequence in young patient with painless mass of cheek demonstrates inhomogeneous soft tissue mass with areas of both increased and decreased signal intensity *(white and black arrows)*. Decreased signal intensity presumably relates to residual areas of pooled blood within cavernous hemangioma. As hemangioma involutes, high-signal–intensity fatty deposition occurs. **B,** T_2-weighted MRI sequence. Hemangiomas characteristically have high-signal intensity reflecting areas of increased blood pooling. This is best seen on MRI scans on heavily T_2-weighted sequences *(arrows)*.

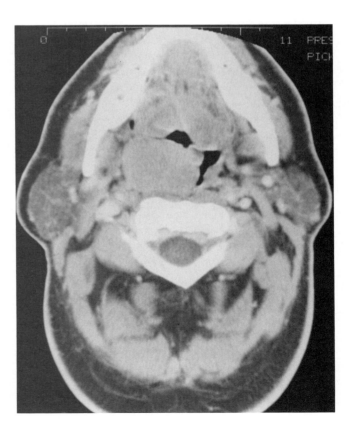

Fig. 6-47   Rhabdomyoma of posterior pharyngeal wall. Contrast-enhanced axial CT scan demonstrates well-circumscribed mass of muscular intensity involving posterior right lateral wall of pharynx. Note sharp interface with surrounding parapharyngeal space, tongue, and prevertebral muscle. Biopsy proved this to be benign rhabdomyoma.

A subgroup of rhabdomyomas occur in newborns and children below 3 years of age. These so-called fetal rhabdomyomas may actually be hamartomatous malformations rather than true neoplasms.[87]

Benign Masseteric Hypertrophy. Benign masseteric hypertrophy is an uncommon idiopathic enlargement of the masseter muscle. This condition must be included in the differential diagnosis of superficial masses in the parotid region. The lesion has a male predominance and approximately half the cases are bilateral. Enlargement of the masseter muscle may be congenital or acquired. The acquired form may result from dental malocclusion or from excessive tooth grinding habits.

On CT scans, benign masseteric hypertrophy appears as a focal enlargement of the masseter muscle.[111] MR images demonstrate an enlarged masseter that is isointense to surrounding muscles. A projection of cortical bone along the outer surface of the angle of the mandible may lie beneath the enlarged masseter muscle. The surrounding fatty and fascial planes are preserved—a finding that differentiates benign masseteric hypertrophy from aggressive tumors or inflammatory lesions.[87,110]

Neurogenic Neoplasms

Schwannoma and Neurofibroma. Twenty-five percent of schwannomas are located in the region of the head and neck. Most of these tumors involve cranial nerves in the jugular foramen or lateral neck. The tongue, palate, and floor of the mouth are the most frequent sites in the oral cavity. Most are diagnosed in the second and third decades of life as asymptomatic enlarging masses. They appear on CT scans as focal, well-encapsulated masses.[112] Small lesions are usually homogeneous on CT scans, whereas focal areas of central low density are often present in larger masses. On contrast-enhanced CT scans, these tumors are relatively hypovascular compared to the highly vascular paragangliomas.[112] On MR images, schwannomas have a low-signal intensity on T_1-weighted images and high-signal intensity on T_2-weighted images. Contrast enhancement is typical. Neurofibromas of the oral cavity are rare lesions, usually associated with von Recklinghausen's syndrome.[113] The tongue is the most frequent oral region affected. Unilateral macroglossia is a characteristic finding.

Granular Cell Tumors. Granular cell tumors are benign lesions that are considered neurogenic in origin, although they contain skeletal muscle and histiocytes, as well as fibrous and neurogenous elements. The tumor appears in two forms: a congenital infantile ("epulis") and an adult form, referred to as granular cell myoblastoma.

Granular cell myoblastoma usually occurs in young adults. Fifty percent of these lesions involve the tongue or floor of the mouth, and one-third are noted in subcutaneous tissues. Involvement of all anatomic sites throughout the body has been described. These lesions usually involve the lateral tip and dorsum of the tongue. Ten percent have multiple sites of involvement. Batsakis[87] believes that granular cell myoblastomas are always benign and do not metastasize. However, infiltration of surrounding soft tissues is common—a finding that accounts for the difficulty of complete surgical resection. Recurrences may occur if surgical resection is inadequate.

The CT scan findings of adult granular cell myoblastoma are nonspecific and may appear to be similar to carcinoma of the tongue. The findings are usually those of an infiltrative soft tissue mass in the dorsum and tip of the tongue, which may infiltrate deeper muscular fibers. The MR image features, however, may be a bit more specific. A low-signal intensity may be seen on both T_1-weighted and T_2-weighted images, perhaps reflecting the fibrous or skeletal components (Fig. 6-48).

Minor Salivary Gland Tumors. Over one-thousand microscopic salivary glands are present in the submucosal tissues of the upper aerodigestive tract. Fifty percent of these glands are located within the palate, upper lips, and buccal mucosa. Unlike neoplasms of the parotid glands (80% of which are benign mixed cell tumors), 50% of minor salivary gland tumors are malignant. Benign mixed cell neoplasms of the oral cavity are the most common benign variety (Fig. 6-49). Malignant minor salivary gland tumors take all of the forms found in their major salivary gland counterparts. The adenoid cystic carcinoma is the most common, representing approximately 30% to 50% (depending on the site of origin) of all minor salivary gland tumors in the oropharynx.[87]

Benign and malignant minor salivary gland tumors usually present clinically as a symptomatic swelling without pain or ulceration. Early invasion of the cranial nerves is a frequent feature of adenoid cystic carcinoma. Benign mixed cell tumors appear on CT scans as localized soft tissue masses, affecting the palate or mucosa surrounding the oral cavity or the parapharyngeal space. These tumors are well marginated, displacing rather than infiltrating the deep soft tissue planes. When large, they have a mixed internal CT density and MRI intensity on T_2-weighted images, reflecting islands of mucoid material interspersed among higher density (intensity) cellular nests (Fig. 6-49; see also Fig. 6-34).

Inflammatory Disease of the Oral Cavity and Oropharynx

Infections involving the mandible, teeth, salivary glands, and tonsils are responsible for most of the inflammatory processes in the oral cavity. Most dental infections are self-limited or localized processes that are cured by incision and drainage, extraction of the offend-

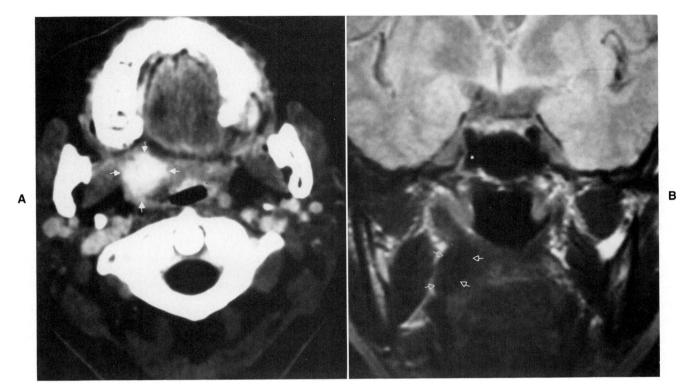

Fig. 6-48   Granular cell myoblastoma of right tonsillar pillar. **A,** Contrast-enhanced axial CT scan demonstrates enhancing mass, which involves right tonsil *(arrows)*. **B,** Coronal proton density MR (2000/30). Mass has decreased signal intensity *(arrows)*. This is typical for carcinoma. Low signal is reflection of fibrotic elements within granular cell myoblastoma. (**A** and **B** courtesy of H. Ric Harnsberger, MD, University of Utah.)

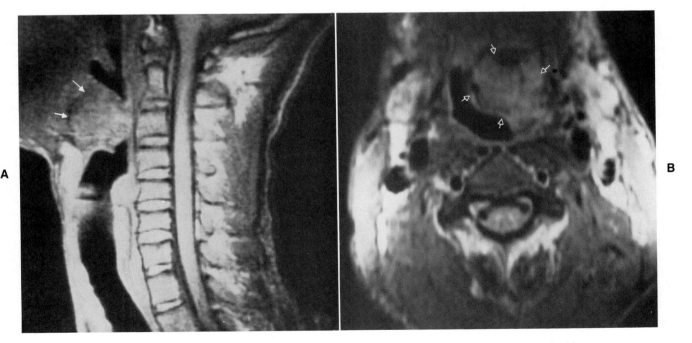

Fig. 6-49   Benign mixed cell tumor of tongue base. 38-year-old male presented with dysphasia. **A,** Sagittal T_1-weighted MR image. Homogeneous mass fills vallecula and indents base of tongue *(arrows)*. **B,** Proton density axial MRI through tongue base. Mass demonstrates intermediate-signal intensity *(arrows)*. Appearance is nonspecific. On biopsy this proved to be benign mixed cell tumor.

ing tooth, and antibiotics. Deep soft tissue infections, however, may extend from the alveolar ridge to involve the maxillary sinus, mandible, or masticator space. The resultant osteomyelitis may require long-term antibiotic therapy.

Inflammatory disease of the submandibular gland is usually caused by an obstructive calculus within the submandibular duct. Such obstruction causes acute dilatation of the submandibular duct and may result in an abscess within the gland if the obstruction is prolonged.

Ludwig's Angina. Ludwig's angina is the eponym applied to an extensive infection of the floor of the mouth, usually of dental or salivary gland origin.[114] Ludwig's angina is usually caused by streptococcal or staphylococcal bacteria. Before the advent of antibiotics, the infection often dissected inferiorly into the mediastinum within the fascial planes of the neck, resulting in substernal angina-like chest pain. The clinical syndrome consists of trismus, submandibular and intraoral cellulitis, and eventually, airway obstruction. Infections of the floor of the mouth disrupt the soft tissue planes separating the extrinsic tongue muscles. This appearance is similar to that caused by neoplasms; however, the presence of cellulitis of the subcutaneous soft tissues and platysma muscle may help to differentiate an infection from a tumor.

Tonsillar Abscess. Acute tonsillitis is usually a self-limited febrile disease of adolescents or young adults. The most common offending bacterial organisms include beta-hemolytic streptococcus, staphylococcus, pneumococcus, and hemophilus. Suppurative uncontrolled infection of the tonsils may result in a peritonsillar abscess (quinsy) or rarely in a tonsillar abscess. A peritonsillar abscess is an accumulation of pus around the palatine tonsils. If the peritonsillar abscess extends outside the tonsillar fossa, it may involve the lateral retropharyngeal or parapharyngeal spaces. Severe sore throat and pharyngeal edema that progresses despite antibiotic therapy are the usual clinical presentations. Trismus develops if the medial pterygoid muscle is involved.

On CT scans, the appearance of acute or chronic tonsillitis is nonspecific; focal homogeneous swelling of the palatine tonsil may simulate tumor. The inflammatory process may extend laterally into the parapharyngeal space, medial pterygoid muscle, and soft palate. If mature, the peritonsillar or tonsillar abscess has a low-density center surrounded by an enhanced margin. The abscess may extend from the tonsillar bed superiorly into the retropharyngeal space (Fig. 6-23) or inferiorly into the submandibular space.[114]

REFERENCES

1. Langman J: Medical embryology human development: normal and abnormal, ed 2, Baltimore, 1969, Williams & Wilkins Co.
2. Newton TH, Hasso A, and Dillon WP: Computed tomography of the head and neck, New York, 1989, Raven Press.
3. Wilson DB: Embryonic development of the head and neck. II. The branchial region, Head Neck Surg 2:59-66, 1979.
4. Wilson DB: Embryonic development of the head and neck. III. The face. Head Neck Surg 2:145-153, 1979.
5. Silverman PM et al: Papillary carcinoma in a thyroglossal duct cyst: CT findings, J Comput Assist Tomogr 9:806-808, 1985.
6. Mancuso AA et al: Computed tomography of the nasopharynx: normal and variants of normal, Radiology 137:113-121, 1980.
7. Mancuso AA and Hanafee WN: Elusive head and neck cancer beneath intact mucosa, Laryngoscope 93:133-139, 1983.
8. Nicholson RL and Kreeb L: CT anatomy of the nasopharynx, nasal cavity, paranasal sinuses and infratemporal fossa, J Comput Tomogr 3:13-23, 1979.
9. Kalovidoris A, Mancuso AA, and Dillon WP: A CT-clinical approach to patients with symptoms related to the V, VII, IX-XII cranial nerves and cervical sympathetics, Radiology 151:671-676, 1984.
10. Han JS et al: MR imaging of the skull base, J Comput Assist Tomogr 8:944-952, 1984.
11. Dillon WP et al: Magnetic resonance image of the nasopharynx, Radiology 152:731-735, 1984.
12. Dillon WP: Magnetic resonance of head and neck tumors, Cardiovasc Intervent Radiol 8:275-282, 1986.
13. Lufkin R, Larsson SG, and Hanafee WN: Work in progress: NMR anatomy of the larynx and tongue base, Radiology 148:173-175, 1983.
14. Lufkin RB et al: Tongue and oropharynx: findings on MR imaging, Radiology 161:69-75, 1986.
15. Mancuso AA and Hanafee WN: Computed tomography and magnetic resonance imaging of the head and neck, Baltimore, 1985, Williams & Wilkins Co.
16. Dooms GC et al: Characterization of lymphadenopathy by magnetic resonance relaxation times: preliminary results, Radiology 155:691-697, 1985.
17. Teresi LM et al: MR imaging of the nasopharynx and floor of the middle cranial fossa. I. Normal anatomy, Radiology 164:811-816, 1987.
18. Hardin CW et al: Infection and tumor of the masticator space: CT evaluation, Radiology 157:413-417, 1985.
19. Hardin CW et al: CT in the evaluation of normal and diseased oral cavity and oropharynx, Semin Ultrasound CT MR 7:133-153, 1986.
20. Harnsberger HR and Dillon WP: Major motor atrophic patterns in the face and neck: CT evaluation, Radiology 155:665-670, 1985.
21. Silver AJ et al: Computed tomography of the nasopharynx and related spaces, Radiology 147:725-731, 1983.
22. Silver AJ et al: Computed tomography of the carotid space and related cervical spaces. I. Anatomy, Radiology 150:723-728, 1984.
23. Som PM: The parapharyngeal space. In Bergeron RT, Osborn AG, and Som PM, editors: Head and neck imaging excluding the brain, St. Louis, 1984, The CV Mosby Co.
24. Som PM et al: Parapharyngeal space masses: an updated protocol based on 104 cases, Radiology 153:149-156, 1984.
25. Smoker WRK and Gentry LR: Computed tomography of the nasopharynx and related spaces, Semin Ultrasound CT MR 7:107-130, 1986.

26. Scotti G and Harwood-Nash DC: Computed tomography of rhabdomyosarcomas of the skull base in children, J Comput Assist Tomogr 6:33-39, 1982.

27. Teresi LM et al: MR imaging of the nasopharynx and floor of miccle cranial fossa. II. Malignant tumors, Radiology 164:817-21, 1987.

28. Last RJ: Anatomy: regional and applied, ed 5, Edinburgh, 1972, Churchill Livingston.

29. Hollingshead WH: Anatomy for surgeons: the head and neck, vol 1, ed 2, Hagerstown, Md, 1968, Harper & Row.

30. Naito Y et al: Magnetic resonance imaging of the eustachian tube, Arch Otolaryngol Head Neck Surg 113:1281-1284, 1987.

31. Harnsberger HR: CT and MRI of masses of the deep face, Curr Probl Diagn Radiol 16:141-173, 1987.

32. Batsakis JG: Tumors of the head and neck: clinical and pathologic considerations, ed 2, Baltimore, 1979, Williams & Wilkins Co.

33. Lederman M: Cancer of the nasopharynx: its natural history and treatment, Springfield, Ill, 1961, Charles C Thomas.

34. Rouvier H: Anatomy of the human lymphatic system, Ann Arbor, Mich, 1938, Edward Brothers.

35. Mancuso AA et al: Computed tomography of cervical and retropharyngeal lymph nodes: normal anatomy, variant of normal, and applications in staging head and neck cancer. I and II, Radiology 148:715-723, 1983.

36. Daniels DL, Williams AL, and Haughton VM: Jugular foramen: anatomic and computed tomographic study, AJR 142:153-158, 1984.

37. Braun IF and Hoffman JC: Computed tomography of the buccomasseteric region. I. Anatomy, AJNR 5:605-615, 1984.

37a. Braun IF and Hoffman JC: Computed tomography of the buccomasseteric region. II. Pathology, AJNR 5:611-616, 1984.

38. Everts EC and Ecatvarria J: Diseases of the pharynx and deep neck infections. In Paparella M and Shumrick D, editors: Otolaryngology, Philadelphia, 1980, WB Saunders Co.

39. Dillon WP et al: Magnetic resonance image of the nasopharynx, Radiology 152:731-735, 1984.

40. Unger JM: The oral cavity and tongue: magnetic resonance imaging, Radiology 155:151-153, 1986.

41. Lufkin RB, Larsson SG, and Hanafee WN: Work in progress: NMR anatomy of the larynx and tongue base, Radiology 148:173-175, 1983.

42. Lufkin R et al: Tongue and oropharynx: findings on MR imaging, Radiology 161:69-75, 1986.

43. Larsson SG, Mancuso AA, and Hanafee WN: Computed tomography of the tongue and floor of the mouth, Radiology 143:493-500, 1982.

44. Byrd SE et al: Computed tomography of palatine tonsillar carcinoma, J Comput Assist Tomogr 7:976-982, 1983.

45. Muraki AS, Mancuso AA, and Harnsberger HR: CT of the oropharynx, tongue base and floor of the mouth: normal anatomy and range of variations and applications in staging carcinoma, Radiology 148:725-731, 1983.

46. Mancuso AA and Hanafee WN: Elusive head and neck carcinomas beneath intact mucosa, Laryngoscope 93:133-139, 1983.

47. Mancuso AA and Hanafee WN: Computed tomography and magnetic resonance imaging of the head and neck, ed 2, Baltimore, 1985, Williams & Wilkins Co.

48. Muraki AS, Mancuso AA, and Harnsberger HR: Metastatic cervical adenopathy from tumors of unknown origin: the role of CT, Radiology 152:749-753, 1984.

49. Vogl T et al: Kernspintomographische untersuchungen non paraganglionen des glomus caroticum und glomus jugulare mit Gd-DTPA, Rofo 148:38-46, 1988.

50. Crawford SC et al: The role of gadolinium DTPA in the evaluation of extracranial head and neck mass lesions, Radiol Clin North Am 27:219-242, 1989.

51. Mancuso AA and Hanafee WN: Computed tomography and magnetic resonance imaging of the head and neck, Baltimore, 1985, Williams & Wilkins Co.

52. Dillon WP et al: Magnetic resonance image of the nasopharynx, Radiology 152:731-735, 1984.

53. Batsakis JG: Tumors of the head and neck, ed 2, Baltimore, 1979, Williams & Wilkins Co.

54. Heroman WH, Golden SM, and Yudt WM: Nasopharyngeal teratoma in the newborn, Ear Nose Throat J 59:203-207, 1980.

55. Howell CG, VanTassel P, and El Gamal T: High resolution computed tomography in neonatal nasopharyngeal teratoma, J Comput Assist Tomogr 8(6):1179-1181, 1984.

56. Faerber EN and Swartz JD: Heterotopic pharyngeal brain, AJNR 4:989-990, 1983.

57. Hardin CW et al: Infection and tumors of the masticator space: CT evaluation, Radiology 157:413-417, 1985.

58. Everts EC and Ecatvarria J: Diseases of the pharynx and deep neck infections. In Paparella M and Shumrick D, editors: Otolaryngology, Philadelphia, 1980, WB Saunders Co.

59. Cammoun M et al: Histologic types of nasopharyngeal carcinoma in an intermediate risk area. In de-The G and Ito Y, editors: Nasopharyngeal carcinoma: etiology and control, 20:13-26, 1978.

60. Batsakis JG: Tumors of the head and neck, ed 2, Baltimore, 1979, Williams & Wilkins Co.

61. Huang HN: Nasopharyngeal carcinoma in Peoples Republic of China: incidence, treatment and survival rates, Radiology 149:305-309, 1983.

62. Lederman M: Cancer of the pharynx: a study based on 2,417 cases with special reference to radiation treatment, J Laryngol Otol 81:151-172, 1967.

63. Mancuso AA and Hanafee WN: Computed tomography and magnetic resonance imaging of the head and neck, ed 2, Baltimore, 1985, Williams & Wilkins Co.

64. Million RR, Cassisi NJ, and Wittes RE: Cancer in the head and neck. In DeVita VT, Hellman S, and Rosenberg SA, editors: Cancer: principles and practice of oncology, Philadelphia, 1982, JB Lippincott Co.

65. Schaefer SD et al: Magnetic resonance imaging versus computed tomography: comparison in imaging oral cavity and pharyngeal carcinomas, Arch Otolaryngol Head Neck Surg 111:730-734, 1985.

66. Silver AJ et al: Computed tomography of the nasopharynx and related spaces. I and II, Radiology 147:723-738, 1983.

67. Schaefer SD et al: Computed tomographic assessment of squamous cell carcinomas of the oral and pharyngeal cavities, Arch Otolaryngol Head Neck Surg 108:688-692, 1982.

68. Smoker WRK and Gentry LR: Computed tomography of the nasopharynx and related spaces, Semin Ultrasound CT MR 7(2):107-130, 1986.

69. Mancuso AA et al: Computed tomography of cervical and retropharyngeal lymph nodes: normal anatomy, variant of normal, and applications in staging head and neck cancer. I and II, Radiology 148:715-723, 1983.

70. Harnsberger HR and Dillon WP: Major motor atrophic patterns in the face and neck: CT evaluation, Radiology 155:665-670, 1985.

71. Bedwinck JM, Perez CA, and Keys DJ: Analysis of failures after definitive irradiation for epidermoid carcinoma of the nasopharynx, Cancer 45(11):2725-2729, 1980.

72. Gefter JW: Carcinoma of the nasopharynx. Proceedings of the 10th Annual Radiation Therapy Clinical Research Seminar, Gainesville, University of Florida, 1981:229-235.

73. Harnsberger HR, Mancuso AA, and Muraki AS: The upper aerodigestive tract and neck: CT evaluation of recurrent tumors, Radiology 149:503-509, 1985.

74. Lee FA: Rhabdomyosarcoma. In Parker BR and Castellano RA, editors: Pediatric oncologic radiology, St Louis, 1977, The CV Mosby Co.

75. Canalis RF et al: Nasopharyngeal rhabdomyosarcoma: a clinical perspective, Arch Otolaryngol Head Neck Surg 104:122-126, 1978.

76. Dito WR and Batsakis JG: Intra-oral, pharyngeal and nasopharyngeal rhabdomyosarcoma, Arch Otolaryngol Head Neck Surg 77:123-129, 1963.

77. McGill T: Rhabdomyosarcoma of the head and neck: an update, Otolaryngol Clin North Am 22(3):631-636, 1989.

78. Scotti G and Harwood-Nash DC: Computed tomography of rhabdomyosarcomas of the skull base in children, J Comput Assist Tomogr 6(1):33-39, 1982.

79. Som PM et al: Extracranial tumor vascularity: determination by dynamic CT scanning, Radiology 154:401-412, 1985.

80. Olsen W and Dillon WP: MR imaging of paragangliomas, AJR 148:201-204, 1987.

81. Som PM et al: Common tumors of the parapharyngeal space: refined imaging diagnosis, Radiology 161:81-85, 1988.

82. Stout AP: The peripheral manifestations of specific nerve sheath tumors (neurilemmomas), Am J Cancer 24:751-755, 1935.

83. Enzinger FM and Weiss SW: Soft tissue tumors, St Louis, 1983, The CV Mosby Co.

84. Geoffray A et al: Extracranial meningiomas of the head and neck, AJNR 5:595-604, 1984.

85. Hardin CW et al: Infection and tumors of the masticator space: CT evaluation, Radiology 157:413-417, 1985.

86. Yarington CT: Pathology of the oral cavity. In Paparella MM and Shumrick M, editors: Otolaryngology, Philadelphia, 1980, WB Saunders Co.

87. Batsakis JG: Tumors of the head and neck, ed 2, Baltimore, 1979, Williams & Wilkins Co.

88. Paparella MM and Shumrick DA: Otolaryngology, vol 3, Head and neck, Philadelphia, 1980, WB Saunders Co.

89. Enzinger FM and Weiss SW: Soft tissue tumors, St Louis, 1983, The CV Mosby Co.

90. Silverman SS et al: Oral findings in people with or at risk for AIDS: a study of 375 homosexual males, J Am Dent Assoc 112:187-192, 1985.

91. Lederman M: Cancer of the nasopharynx: its natural history and treatment, Springfield, Ill, 1961, Charles C Thomas.

92. Mancuso AA and Hanafee WN: Elusive head and neck carcinomas beneath intact mucosa, Laryngoscope 93:133-139, 1983.

93. Lederman M: Cancer of the pharynx: a study based on 2,417 cases with special reference to radiation treatment, J Laryngol Otol 81:151-172, 1967.

94. Ballantyne AJ: In Scott-Brown WG and Groves HJ, editors: Scott-Brown's diseases of the ear, nose and throat, London, 1979, Butterworths.

95. Harnsberger HR, Mancuso AA, and Muraki AS: The upper aerodigestive tract and neck: CT evaluation of recurrent tumors, Radiology 149:503-509, 1983.

96. Muraki AS, Mancuso AA, and Harnsberger HR: CT of the oropharynx, tongue base and floor of the mouth: normal anatomy and range of variations and applications in staging carcinoma, Radiology 148:725-731, 1983.

97. Million RR, Cassisi NJ, and Wittes RE: Cancer in the head and neck. In DeVita VT, Hellman S, and Rosenberg SA, editors: Cancer: principles and practice of oncology, Philadelphia, 1982, JB Lippincott Co.

98. Ballantyne AJ: Routes of spread. In Fletcher GH and MaComb WS, editors: Radiation therapy in the management of cancers of the oral cavity and oropharynx, Springfield, Ill, 1962, Charles C Thompson.

99. Million RR and Cassisi NJ: Oral Cavity. In Million RR and Cassisi NJ, editors: Management of head and neck cancer: a multidisciplinary approach, Philadelphia 1984, JB Lippincott Co.

100. Muraki AS, Mancuso AA, and Harnsberger HR: Metastatic cervical adenopathy from tumors of unknown origin: the role of CT, Radiology 152:749-753, 1984.

101. Mancuso AA and Hanafee WN: Computed tomography and magnetic resonance imaging of the head and neck, ed 2, Baltimore, 1985, Williams & Wilkins Co.

102. Russ JE, Applebaum EL, and Sisson CA: Squamous cell carcinoma of the soft palate, Laryngoscope 87:1151-1156, 1977.

103. Byrd SE et al: Computed tomography of palatine tonsillar carcinoma, J Comput Assist Tomogr 7:976-982, 1983.

104. Schaefer SD et al: Magnetic resonance imaging versus computed tomography: comparison in imaging oral cavity and pharyngeal carcinomas, Arch Otolaryngol Head Neck Surg 111:730-734, 1985.

105. Fletcher GH and Lindberg RD: Squamous cell carcinomas of the tonsillar area and palatine arch, Am J Roentgenol Radium Ther Nucl Med 96:574-587, 1977.

106. Unger JM: The oral cavity and tongue: magnetic resonance imaging, Radiology 155:151-153, 1985.

107. Gooding GA et al: Malignant carotid artery invasion: sonographic detection, Radiology 171:435-438, 1989.

108. Langman AW et al: Radiologic assessment of tumor and the carotid artery: correlation of MRI, US and CT with surgical findings, Head Neck Surg 11:443-449, 1989.

109. Iton K et al: MR imaging of cavernous hemangioma of the face and neck, J Comput Assist Tomogr 10:831-835, 1986.

110. Masson JK and Soule EH: Desmoid tumor of the head and neck, Am J Surg 112:615-622, 1966.

111. Braun IF et al: Computed tomography of benign masseteric hypertrophy, J Comput Assist Tomogr 9:167-170, 1985.

112. Som PM et al: Extracranial tumor vascularity: determination by dynamic CT scanning, Radiology 154:401-412, 1985.

113. Das Gupta TK: Tumors of the peripheral nerves. In Das Gupta TK, editor: Tumors of the soft tissues, East Norwalk, Conn, 1983, Appleton-Century-Crofts.

114. Kornbutt AD: Infections of the pharyngeal spaces. In Paparilla M and Shumrick M, editors: Otolaryngology, vol 3, Philadelphia, 1980, WB Saunders Co.

7 Parapharyngeal Space

PETER M. SOM

The parapharyngeal space is a difficult region to examine clinically because it is buried deep in the upper neck, beneath the ramus of the mandible, the parotid gland, and the sternocleidomastoid muscle. Only when a mass is sufficiently large does it displace the lateral pharyngeal wall towards the midline or cause fullness of the parotid gland, and only when a lesion is very large does it present a fullness near the angle of the mandible. In the era before CT and MRI, the only modalities the radiologist had available to investigate this region were the sialogram and the angiogram. If the tumor had a characteristic vascularity that suggested a paraganglioma, or if it had a specific sialographic appearance that suggested a parotid tumor, a preoperative diagnosis could be offered.[1-14] However, such a diagnosis was possible in only 20% to 40% of cases, and this approach necessitated performing angiograms and sialograms on virtually all patients (Fig. 7-1).

With the advent in the late 1970s of CT scanning for head and neck pathology, soft tissue masses in the parapharyngeal space could be directly visualized radiographically for the first time. The low resolution characteristics of the early CT scanners made the use of CT-sialography necessary to identify the parotid gland clearly and to distinguish it from the margins of a parapharyngeal space mass (Fig. 7-2).[15-18] With the development of high resolution CT scanners, however, CT-sialography was no longer required to accomplish this differentiation (Fig. 7-3).[19,20]

Concurrent with the technological developments of CT scanning, surgical techniques and approaches had advanced. Before the late 1970s, all parapharyngeal space masses were approached via a parotid incision, irrespective of whether the tumor was truly intraparotid in origin or not. This meant that there was facial nerve manipulation in all cases, accompanied by attendant morbidity.

However, in the late 1970s and early 1980s the surgical philosophy changed. If the surgeon could know preoperatively that a mass was extraparotid in origin, then a transcervical approach could be used without manipulation of the facial nerve (Fig. 7-4, A). Those patients with true intraparotid tumors would then be the only ones who had the transparotid approach (Fig. 7-4, B).[21] The information available from CT scanning led to the development of CT criteria to separate intraparotid from extraparotid masses, a distinction that could not be made clinically with confidence. Ultimately, therefore, the radiologic diagnosis has come to determine the surgical approach to the case.

The important CT observation in these cases is whether or not parapharyngeal space fat can be seen between the parotid gland and the posterolateral margin of the mass. If such fat is visible, the lesion is extraparotid in origin. Additionally, CT provides information about the consistency of lesions (whether solid or cystic) and identifies possible necrotic lymph nodes. CT examination with intravenous contrast may provide even more information. Enhancement may result either from the progressive extravascular accumulation of contrast material or from intravascular contrast media in a hypervascular mass. Although this distinction cannot be accomplished on routine postcontrast CT scans, it can be made by using CT dynamic scanning.[20,22,23] This approach is reliable, but necessitates an additional administration of contrast material and additional scanner time.

Using these CT techniques the radiologist can make a preoperative diagnosis in 80% to 90% of patients. The major remaining diagnostic problem is differentiating a neuroma from a minor salivary gland tumor.

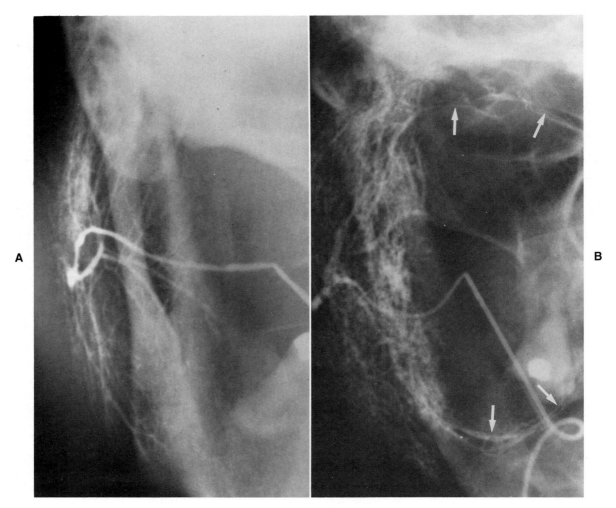

Fig. 7-1 **A,** Frontal view of a right parotid sialogram demonstrates a vaguely defined mass effect on the medial aspect of the parotid gland. This appearance could be from either a "deep lobe" parotid mass or an extra parotid lesion. **B,** Oblique frontal view of a right parotid sialogram shows a large mass *(arrows)* that smoothly displaces the parotid ducts almost entirely around it. When the ducts encircle more the half of the circumference of a mass, the lesion arises within the parotid gland. (**A** from Som et al: Radiology 135:387-390, 1980.)

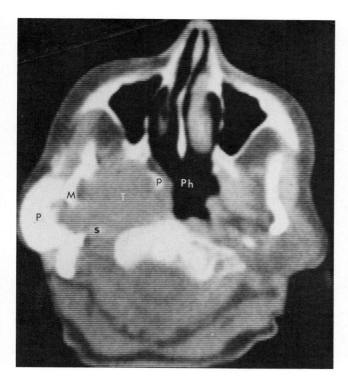

Fig. 7-2   Axial CT-sialogram scan shows a large "deep lobe" parotid benign mixed tumor *(T)*. The parotid gland *(P)* is filled with contrast material. *S,* styloid process, *M,* mandible, *p,* medially displaced contrast filled parotid gland, *Ph,* pharynx. (From Som et al: Ann Otol Rhinol Laryngol 88:590-595, 1979.)

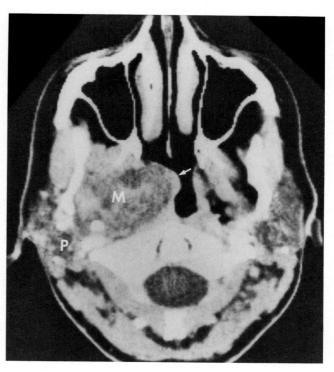

Fig. 7-3   Axial postcontrast CT scan shows a large "deep lobe" benign mixed tumor *(M)*, which displaces the right lateral pharyngeal wall *(arrow)* toward the midline. *P,* parotid gland. No fat plane is present between the mass and the parotid gland. (From Som et al: Radiology 153:149-156, 1984.)

With the development of MRI scanning, better soft tissue differentiation could be achieved and the parapharyngeal space fat could be better visualized.[24-28] In addition, the carotid arteries could be more reliably identified by their MRI signal flow voids than by their enhancement on CT, which often could not be clearly appreciated when a sizeable parapharyngeal space mass was present. Thus, MRI allows a more reliable distinction to be made between intraparotid and extraparotid lesions and allows most neuromas and minor salivary gland tumors to be differentiated: neuromas tend to displace the internal carotid artery anteriorly, whereas minor salivary gland tumors tend to displace this vessel posteriorly.[20,29] In addition, on MRI the contours of a tumor can be better identified; the smooth margins of a paraganglioma may help differentiate it from an invasive vascular metastasis.[28]

Presently, by using clinical and imaging information, a preoperative diagnosis can be made in over 90% of patients. This clearly reflects the great influence that CT and MRI have had on the diagnosis of these lesions.

ANATOMY AND CLINICAL FINDINGS

The general anatomy of the parapharyngeal space is discussed in Chapter 8. Worthy of specific mention are the following points: The *medial* wall of the parapharyngeal space is the most pliable, and therefore some degree of medial bowing of the lateral nasooropharyngeal wall and downward displacement of the soft palate can be seen with virtually all masses located in this area. This occurs with masses greater than 1.5 cm in diameter regardless of their parotid or extraparotid origin.

The only pliable portion of the *lateral* wall of the parapharyngeal space is the retromandibular portion of the parotid gland. This can be displaced laterally by almost any mass, irrespective of whether it is of intraparotid or extraparotid origin. When either of these lesions grows very large, a fullness can be noted near the angle of the mandible (Fig. 7-5).[9-14,18]

Lesions arising in the parapharyngeal space can be silent clinically until they are quite large. It is not unusual to find a 4 to 5 cm diameter mass at the time of initial clinical presentation. Most of these physical find-

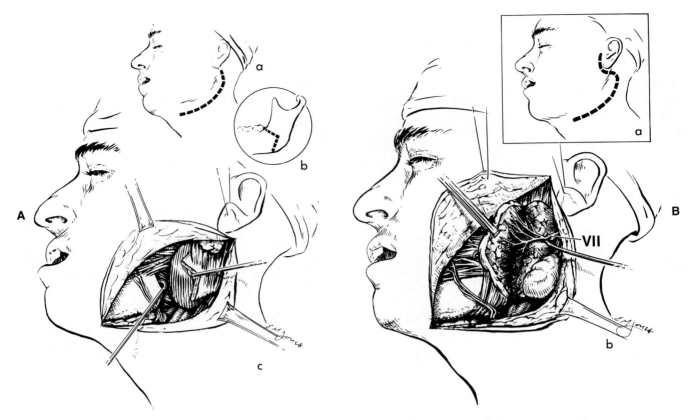

Fig. 7-4   A, Diagram of a transcervical surgical approach for removal of an extraparotid mass. *a,* skin incision, *b,* one of several types of mandibular sectionings that may be necessary in order to extirpate the tumor intact, and *c,* surgical exposure. **B,** Diagram of a transparotid surgical approach for removal of an intraparotid mass. *a,* skin incision and *b,* surgical exposure including isolation of the facial nerve. (From Som et al: Ann Otol Rhinol Laryngol [suppl 80] 90:1-15, 1981.)

ings are usually discovered incidently (either by the patient or the clinician). However, patients with parapharyngeal space masses may also have a variety of other complaints, including sore throat, change in voice quality, dysphagia, nasal obstruction, and sensation of aural fullness. With neuromas, paragangliomas, and malignant lesions, deficits of any or all of the last four cranial nerves often occur.[7,30,31]

PATHOLOGY

Although metastatic lymph nodes in the internal jugular chain are commonly found in the parapharyngeal space, most reported clinical series do not include them since they are not primary lesions. They are occasionally listed as incidental lesions. The general imaging appearances of lymph nodes are discussed in Chapter 8; metastatic nodes are mentioned in this chapter only as they pertain to the differential diagnosis of other parapharyngeal space masses.

Salivary Gland Tumors

Overall, the most common primary lesions to arise in the parapharyngeal space are salivary gland tumors. These include both major and minor salivary gland lesions and together they account for 40% to 50% of all parapharyngeal space primary masses. Between 80% to 90% of these tumors are benign pleomorphic adenomas (benign mixed tumors) and the most common malignancies encountered are mucoepidermoid carcinomas, adenoid cystic carcinomas, and acinic cell carcinomas.*

The parotid lesions arise in the deep or retromandibular portion of the parotid gland and their lateral growth is usually limited by the relatively narrow stylomandibular tunnel. The margins of this tunnel are the posterior edge of the ramus of the mandible, the undersurface of the middle cranial fossa, and the styloid pro-

---

*References 9, 11, 13, 14, 28, 30, 32-34.

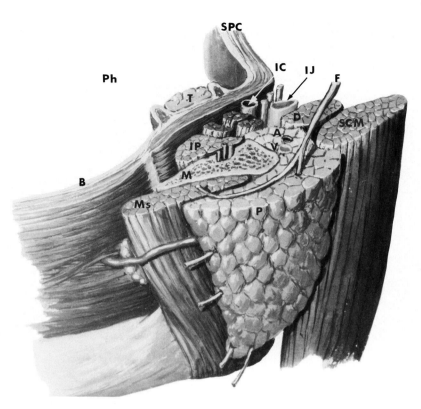

Fig. 7-5 Normal anatomic relationships of the left parapharyngeal space as viewed obliquely and from above. *Ph,* pharynx; *SPC,* superior pharyngeal constrictor muscle; *T,* tonsil; *B,* buccunator muscle; *Ms,* masseter muscle; *SCM,* sternocleidomastoid muscle; *D,* posterior belly of the digastric muscle; *IP,* internal pterygoid muscle; *M,* mandible; *IC,* internal carotid artery; *IJ,* internal jugular vein; *P,* parotid gland; *F,* facial nerve; *A,* external carotid artery; *V,* posterior facial vein. (From Som et al: Ann Otol Rhinol Laryngol [suppl 80] 90:1-15, 1981.)

cess and stylomandibular ligament. Most parotid tumors are ovoid masses (Figs. 7-2 and 7-3); however, occasionally, a dumbbell-shaped tumor is seen, with the waist of the dumbbell in the plane of the stylomandibular tunnel (Figs. 7-6 and 7-7). In the vast majority of cases, the benign lesions and low-grade malignancies are sharply delineated from the adjacent soft tissues, whereas the high-grade malignancies have infiltrative, unsharp margins. Because the retromandibular portion of the parotid gland lies in the prestyloid compartment of the parapharyngeal space, the tumors that arise from this portion of the gland all lie anterior to the internal carotid artery. Thus, these "deep lobe" tumors either push the internal carotid artery posteriorly, or do not displace it at all.[20,29]

Because these tumors arise within the parotid gland, a portion of their posterolateral margin is at some point in direct contact with the gland and no intervening parapharyngeal space fat is present at this tumor contour (Fig. 7-8). Careful attention, therefore, must be paid to this interface between a parapharyngeal space tumor and the parotid gland. *If fat is seen in this interface on all of the axial images through the tumor, the lesion is not of parotid origin.* But if no fat is seen on any of the axial scans through this area, the tumor either arises from, abuts, or infiltrates the parotid gland. In some patients, fat can be seen at this interface on all but one or two axial images through the tumor. The explanation lies in the fact that these lesions are pedunculated masses originating in the parotid but connected to it by only a small isthmus; if this narrow connection to the gland (the sections at which no fat is identified) is overlooked by the radiologist, an erroneous diagnosis of an extraparotid tumor will be made (Fig. 7-9). To avoid this problem, thin section (5 mm), contiguous axial scans must be taken through the tumor. This soft tissue detail is better seen on MR images than it is on CT scans.[28,29]

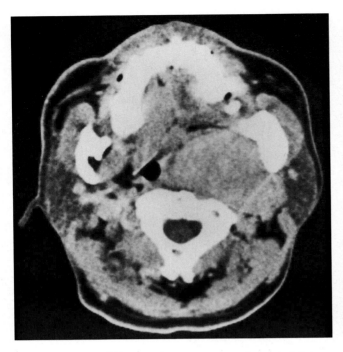

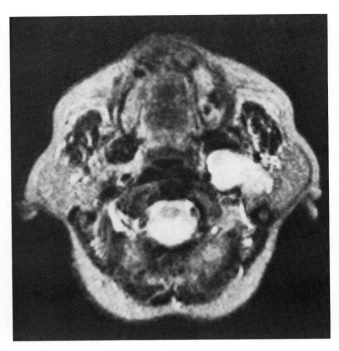

Fig. 7-6 Axial CT scan demonstrates a large left "deep lobe" parotid tumor that is slightly dumbbell shaped with its waist in the plane of the stylomandibular tunnel.

Fig. 7-7 Transverse T$_2$-weighted MRI scan (0.5T, TR = 2,500 msec, TE = 100 msec) shows a left "deep lobe" parotid tumor with a dumbbell shape. The waist of the tumor is in the plane of the stylomandibular tunnel. (From Som et al: Radiology 164:823-829, 1987.)

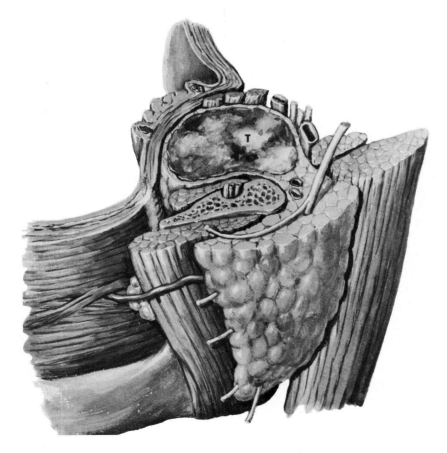

Fig. 7-8 Diagram of a large "deep lobe" tumor *(T)* of the left parotid gland as viewed obliquely and from above. The tumor displaces the lateral pharyngeal wall toward the midline, and the mass lies anterior to the internal carotid artery. (From Som et al: Ann Otol Rhinol Laryngol [suppl 80] 90:1-15, 1981.)

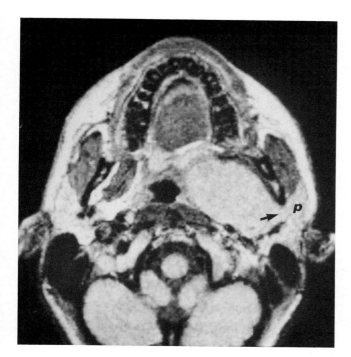

Fig. 7-9 Transverse mixed image MRI scan (0.5T, TR = 2000 msec, TE = 30 msec) demonstrates a large left parotid mass that has a narrow isthmus of tissue *(arrow)* that connects it to the parotid gland *(p)*. (From Som et al: Radiology 164:823-829, 1987.)

If the radiologist cannot clearly separate the mass from the parotid gland, the surgeon must use a transparotid approach to ensure surgical control of the facial nerve. One of three conditions can be present: the nonvisualized fat indicates (a) the tumor is truly of a parotid gland origin (80% of cases), (b) the tumor is extraparotid but is so large it compresses the fat so that it cannot be identified, or it is adherent to the gland's capsule (about 20% of cases), or (c) the tumor is extraparotid but invades the parotid gland (rare).

Medially, the fat of the parapharyngeal space may be identified separating the medial contour of the tumor from the pharyngeal musculature. Its identification is of equal importance to that of the lateral fat.

The classic teaching about parapharyngeal space minor salivary gland tumors is that these lesions develop in the minor salivary glands of the pharyngeal mucosa and submucosa[35] (Fig. 7-10). This now seems to be incorrect. Instead, the vast majority of minor salivary gland tumors arise from salivary rest tissue that lies within the prestyloid compartment. Presumably, these rests lie near the developmental tract of the parotid gland. These minor salivary gland tumors have fat on both their medial and their lateral margins (Figs. 7-11 to 7-15). They are almost always benign pleomorphic adenomas and thus are smooth, ovoid lesions. The rare

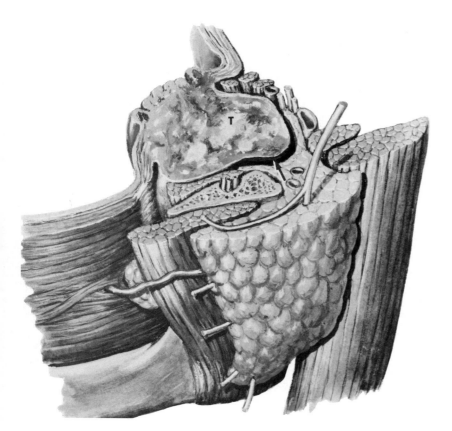

Fig. 7-10 Diagram of a large minor salivary gland tumor *(T)* that is arising from the pharyngeal mucosa as viewed obliquely and from above. Note the displaced parapharyngeal space fat *(arrow)* that lies between the posterolateral margin of the tumor and the parotid gland. (From Som et al: Ann Otol Rhinol Laryngol [suppl 80] 90:1-15, 1981.)

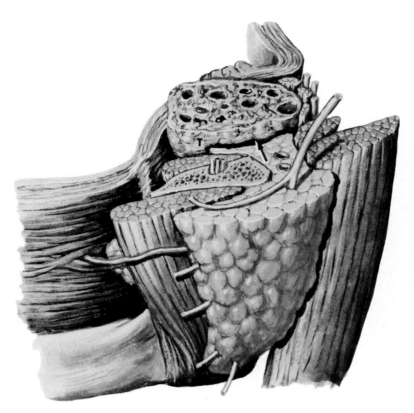

Fig. 7-11 Diagram of a large parapharyngeal space tumor *(T)* that arises within the space and has fat planes both on its medial side (separating it from the pharyngeal constrictor) and on its lateral side *(arrow)* separating it from the parotid gland. (From Som et al: Ann Otol Rhinol Laryngol [suppl 80] 90:1-15, 1981.)

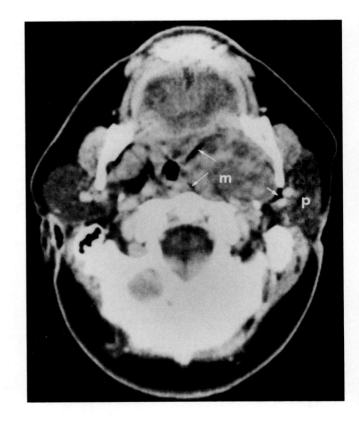

Fig. 7-12 Axial postcontrast CT scan demonstrates a left extraparotid benign mixed tumor *(m)* with fat planes both medially *(arrows)* and laterally *(short arrow)*. *P,* parotid gland. (From Som et al: Radiology 153:149-156, 1984.)

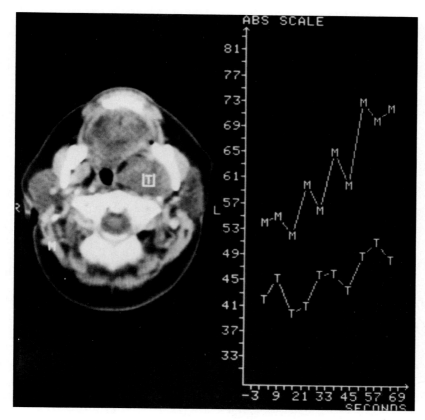

Fig. 7-13   CT dynamic scan shows a left extraparotid benign mixed tumor *(T)* with fat planes on both its medial and lateral margins. The lesion is hypovascular compared to a reference muscle *(M)*. (From Som et al: Radiology 153:149-156, 1984.)

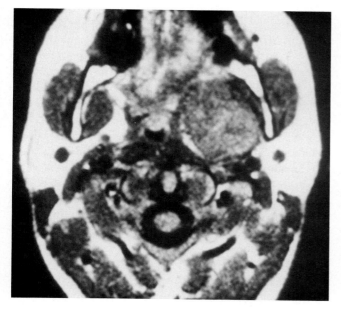

Fig. 7-14   Transverse T_1-weighted MRI scan (1.5T, TR = 500 msec, TE = 28 msec) demonstrates a left extraparotid benign mixed tumor with fat both on its medial and lateral margins. The left internal carotid artery is posteriorly displaced.

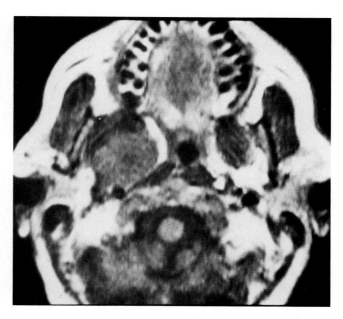

Fig. 7-15   Transverse mixed image (0.5T, TR = 1800 msec, TE = 27 msec) MRI scan demonstrates an ovoid right extraparotid benign mixed tumor with fat planes both on its medial and lateral aspects. (From Som et al: Radiology 164:823-829, 1987.)

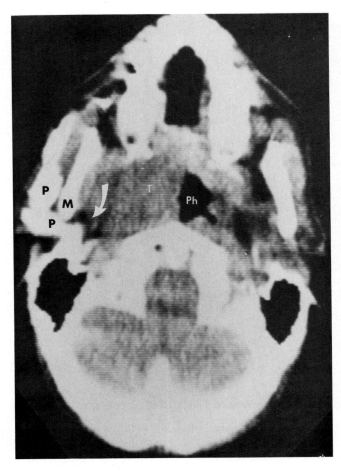

Fig. 7-16 Axial CT-sialogram scan shows a large right extraparotid benign mixed tumor *(T)* that is separated from the contrast filled parotid gland *(P)* by a zone of fat *(arrow)*. *M,* mandible; *Ph,* pharynx. (From Som et al: Ann Otol Rhinol Laryngol [suppl 80] 90:1-15, 1981.)

tumor that arises from the pharyngeal mucosa proper has fat only on its lateral contour and may have either a smooth or an infiltrative margin, depending primarily upon whether the lesion is benign or malignant. Because all of these minor salivary gland tumors develop anterior to the internal carotid artery, they displace this vessel posteriorly if they become large enough[29] (Fig. 7-16).

On CT, all of these tumors, when small, are homogeneous soft tissue attenuation masses that usually are clearly identified and separated from the adjacent muscles and fatty tissues, and, where appropriate, the parotid gland. On MRI, these small lesions are homogeneous. They usually have low-to-intermediate signal intensities on T_1-weighted and mixed images and high signal intensities on T_2-weighted sequences. When these tumors are large, they develop sites of cystic degeneration and hemorrhage. This results in a nonhomogeneous imaging appearance. On CT, the background

tumor matrix is soft tissue-muscle attenuation: lower attenuation areas represent sites of necrosis and cystic change; areas of increased attenuation correspond to regions of hemorrhage (Fig. 7-3). Calcifications are identified occasionally in the pleomorphic adenomas. A large solitary cystic region within the tumor, especially if it has nodular, variably thick walls, indicates a malignant process.[36]

On MRI, these large masses have nonhomogeneous signal intensities. On T_1-weighted and mixed images, most of the signals vary between low and intermediate signal intensities. Areas of high signal intensity usually correspond to sites of hemorrhage. On T_2-weighted images, high signal intensities most often represent sites of cystic degeneration and hemorrhage. Foci of low-to-absent signal intensity on all imaging sequences correspond to sites of calcification or fibrosis (Fig. 7-17).[36-39]

Neurogenic Tumors

The second most common type of primary lesions to arise within the parapharyngeal space are the neurogenic tumors. They represent 17% to 25% of all the lesions, and most are neuromas that arise from the vagus nerve.* Less commonly, a neuroma develops along the superior sympathetic chain, and rarely an isolated neurofibroma is found. Usually, neurofibromas involving this space are part of the neurofibromatosis syndrome and are multiple (Fig. 7-18). Those neuromas that arise from the vagus nerve and the sympathetic chain tend to displace the internal carotid artery anteriorly because these nerves are posterior to this vessel (Figs. 7-19 to 7-21).[29]

Most neuromas are otherwise indistinguishable on CT and MRI from minor salivary gland tumors (Figs. 7-22 to 7-24). However, about one third of the neuromas are enhanced significantly on postcontrast CT scans and can simulate a vascular process such as a paraganglioma (Fig. 7-25). Paradoxically, a CT dynamic scan reveals a flat, hypovascular curve and an angiogram reveals few, if any, tumor vessels (Figs. 7-26 and 7-27). The enhancement is believed to be caused by the extravascular accumulation of the contrast material as it leaks through the abnormally permeable tumor vessels. The hypovascular nature of these lesions also means that there are few, if any, veins to drain the extravascular contrast collections. As a result, the "leaked" contrast remains for a long time before eventually being eliminated (Fig. 7-28).[20,40]

Some neurofibromas can undergo considerable fatty degeneration and replacement, and often no capsule can be identified on imaging. In some cases, these neurofibromas mimic lipomatous lesions and are of low attenuation on CT. On MRI they also have a high non-

*References 9, 11, 13, 14, 28, 30, 32-34.

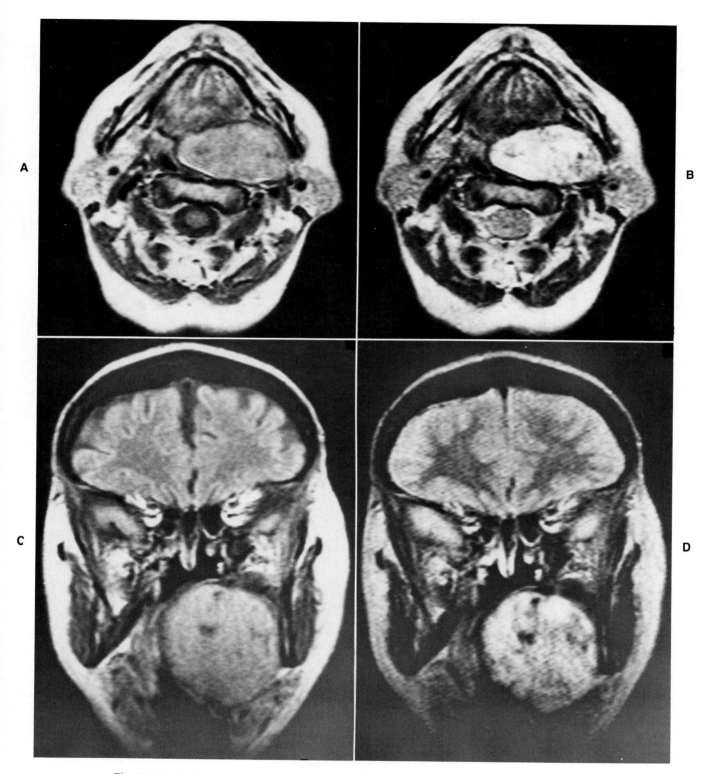

Fig. 7-17   A, Transverse mixed image and **B,** T$_2$-weighted MRI scans and **C,** coronal mixed image and **D,** T$_2$-weighted MRI scans demonstrate a large left parapharyngeal space benign mixed tumor. The mass has a slightly nonhomogeneous intermediate signal intensity on the mixed images and a nonhomogeneously high signal intensity on the T$_1$-weighted scans. The focal areas of low signal intensity correspond to sites of fibrosis and calcification. Because no fat could be identified between the mass and the parotid gland, this large minor salivary gland tumor was operated on via a transparotid approach.

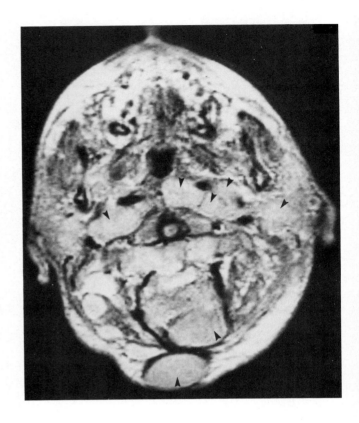

Fig. 7-18 Transverse mixed image (0.5T, TR = 2000 msec, TE = 30 msec) MRI scan shows multiple masses in both retropharyngeal spaces as well as in the posterior neck *(arrowheads)*. The lesions are homogeneous and of an intermediate signal intensity. Neurofibromatosis.

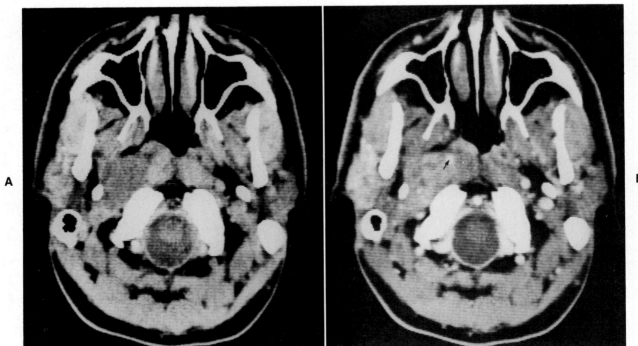

Fig. 7-19   **A,** Axial pre- and **B,** postcontrast CT scans show a right parapharyngeal space mass with minimal enhancement. The lesion displaces the internal carotid artery anteromedially *(arrow)*. Neuroma. (From Som et al: Ann Otol Rhinol Laryngol [suppl 80] 90:1-15, 1981.)

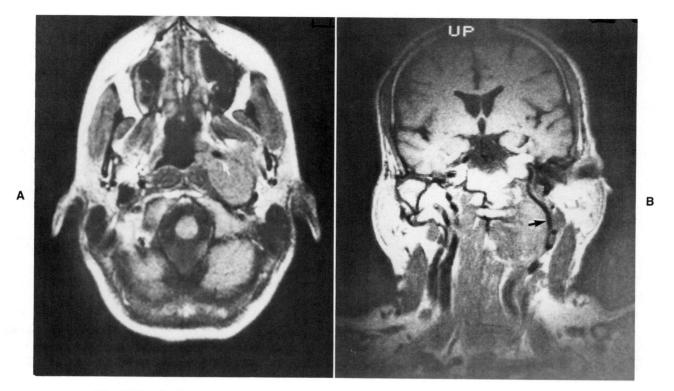

Fig. 7-20   A, Transverse and **B,** coronal T₁-weighted MRI scans (0.5T, TR = 500 msec, TE = 30 msec) demonstrate an intermediate signal intensity mass in the left parapharyngeal space that displaces the internal carotid artery *(arrow)* anterolaterally. Neuroma.

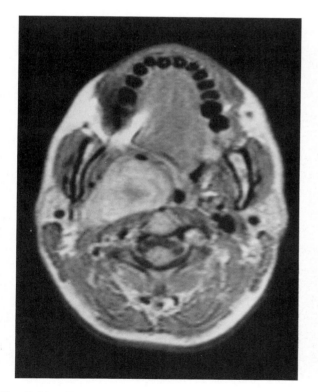

Fig. 7-21   Transverse mixed image (0.5T, TR = 1800 msec, TE = 30 msec) MRI scan demonstrates an intermediate signal intensity mass in the right parapharyngeal space that has displaced the internal carotid artery anteromedially. Neuroma.

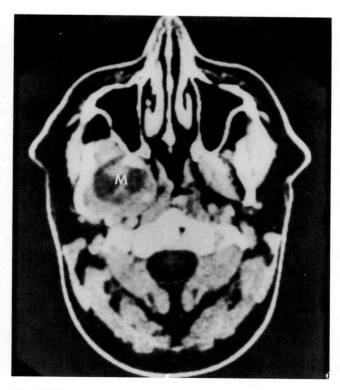

Fig. 7-22   Axial postcontrast CT scan shows a nonhomogeneous partially cystic right parapharyngeal space mass *(M).* Note the similarity to Fig. 7-12. Neuroma. (From Som et al: Radiology 153:149-156, 1984.)

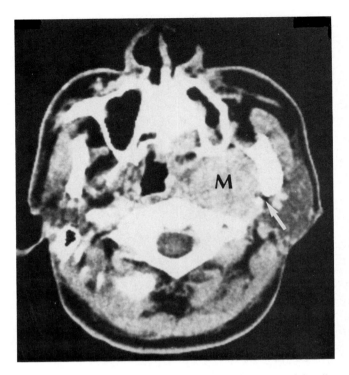

Fig. 7-23 Axial postcontrast CT scan shows a minimally enhancing mass (M) in the left parapharyngeal space. A zone of fat (arrow) is present between the mass and the parotid gland. Neuroma.

homogeneous T_1-weighted signal intensity and an intermediate T_2-weighted signal intensity.

Neurosarcomas are rare. These tumors either have the same imaging findings as a neuroma, or they have infiltrative margins.

Paragangliomas

The third most common group of tumors to arise within the parapharyngeal space are the paragangliomas. They represent 10% to 15% of all lesions and can be of three types, depending on their site of origin. Most commonly the tumor is a glomus vagale; it arises from paraganglionic cells about the nodose ganglion (below the skull base) of the vagus nerve. These tumors usually lie entirely within the parapharyngeal space, although in very large lesions some tumor extension can occur through the jugular fossa and into the posterior fossa. In such cases, the majority of the lesion lies below the skull base, and lateral destruction of the skull base is rare. In large tumors, the caudal tumor extension may splay the internal and external carotid arteries, but it does not fill the crotch of the carotid bifurcation, a differentiating point from large carotid body tumors, which fill in this area.[41] Carotid body tumors originate at the level of the carotid bifurcation. Only 8% of carotid body tumors are large enough to extend

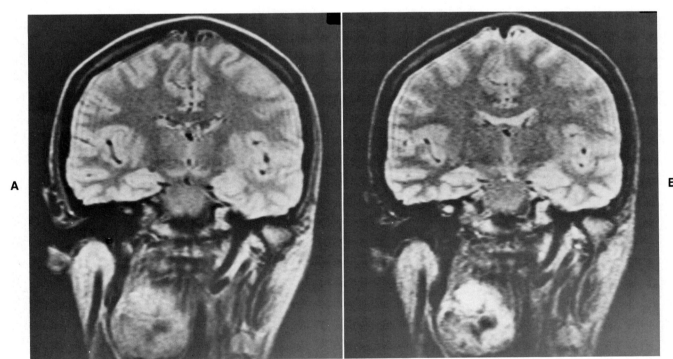

Fig. 7-24 **A,** Coronal mixed image and **B,** T_2-weighted MRI scans (0.5T, TR = 1800 msec, TE = 30 msec) demonstrate an ovoid nonhomogeneous mass in the right parapharyngeal space. Note the similarity to Fig. 7-17. Neuroma.

sufficiently upwards to appear as a parapharyngeal space mass. Glomus jugulare tumors arise from paraganglionic cells around the jugular ganglion (in the jugular bulb) of the vagus nerve and develop in the jugular fossa. Both intracranial and extracranial extension can occur, and spread above and below the skull base is usually nearly equal in bulk, distinguishing these lesions from the glomus vagale tumors. In addition, glomus jugulare lesions tend to erode the skull base laterally, extending into the middle ear cleft.[41]

These hypervascular tumors are enhanced on postcontrast CT scans; however, if there is a delay in imaging after the contrast is administered, the rich blood flow may "wash out" the contrast, and these tumors may appear not to be significantly vascular (Fig. 7-28). CT dynamic scanning reveals a hypervascular curve, differentiating it from a type of neuroma that is enhanced (Figs. 7-29 and 7-30).[20,22,23] In large lesions, areas of low attenuation can be seen on CT. These areas represent sites of hemorrhage and necrosis within the tumor (Figs. 7-31 and 7-32). The lesions tend to be ovoid and smoothly contoured. On MRI these tumors have an intermediate signal intensity background matrix on all imaging sequences, and scattered sites of high signal intensity can be seen on T_2-weighted sequences. The dominant MRI findings are serpentine or

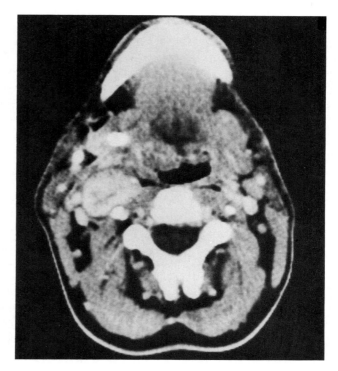

Fig. 7-25 Axial postcontrast CT scan demonstrates an enhancing right parapharyngeal space mass. On the basis of this single scan a vascular lesion could be considered as a diagnosis. Neuroma.

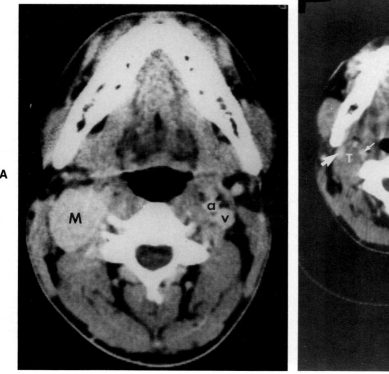

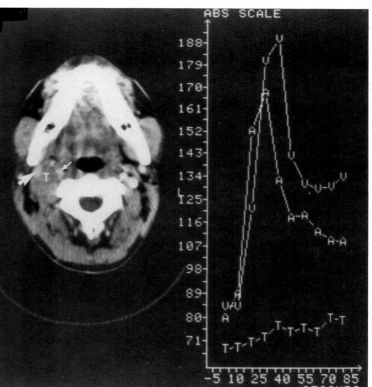

Fig. 7-26 **A,** Axial postcontrast CT scan demonstrates an enhancing mass *(M)* in the right parapharyngeal space. a = internal carotid artery, v = internal jugular vein. **B,** CT dynamic scan shows the tumor *(T)* to have a hypovascular curve *(T)*. A, left internal carotid artery (ICA) *(small arrow)* curve, V, left internal jugular vein (IJV) *(large arrow)* curve. Neuroma. (From Som et al: Radiology, 154:407-412, 1985.)

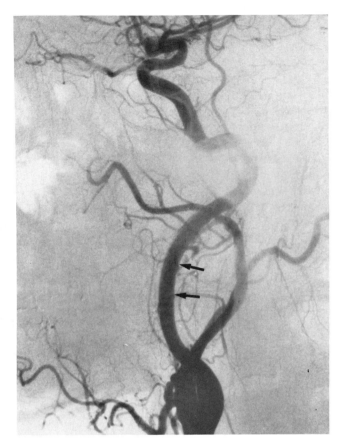

Fig. 7-27 Lateral subtraction angiogram film demonstrates an avascular mass that displaces the internal carotid artery anteriorly *(arrows)*. Neuroma. (From Som et al: Ann Otol Rhinol Laryngol [suppl 80] 90:1-15, 1981.)

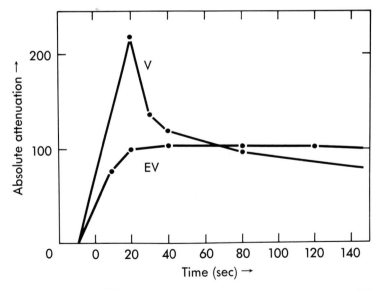

Fig. 7-28 Diagram of the CT dynamic scan curves for a vascular mass *(V)* and a hypovascular mass that has extravascular accumulation of contrast within it *(EV)*. Note that at 20 secs into the dynamic scan, the difference in vascularity between these lesions is most evident. However, if the CT scans are observed at 120 secs, the degree of enhancement of the hypovascular mass may appear greater than that of the vascular lesion.

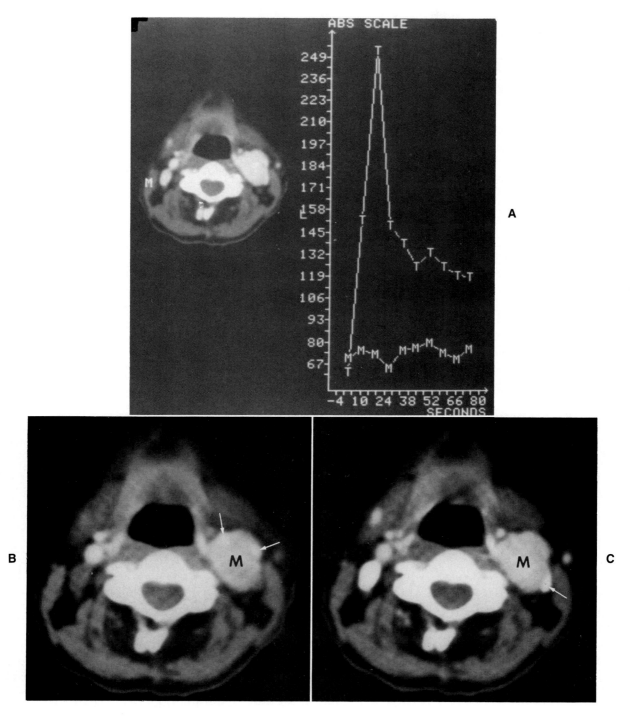

Fig. 7-29 **A,** CT dynamic scan reveals an enhancing left lower parapharyngeal space mass *(T)*. The tumor has a highly vascular flow curve *(T)*. *M*, reference muscle and flow curve. **B,** Early axial CT scan from dynamic study reveals the enhancing left neck mass *(M)* and the splayed carotid arteries *(arrows)*. **C,** Late axial CT scan from a dynamic study reveals "washout" of the arteries and visualization of the internal jugular vein *(arrow)*. *M*, tumor mass. Carotid Body Tumor. (From Som et al: Radiology 154:407-412, 1985.)

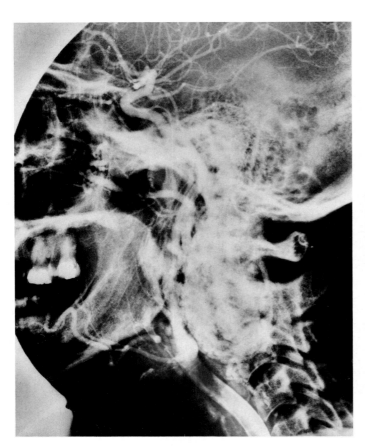

Fig. 7-30 Lateral angiogram film shows hypervascular mass in the parapharyngeal space that displaces the internal carotid artery and bifurcation anteriorly. Glomus Vagale Tumor. (From Som et al: Ann Otol Rhinol Laryngol [suppl 80] 90:1-15, 1981.)

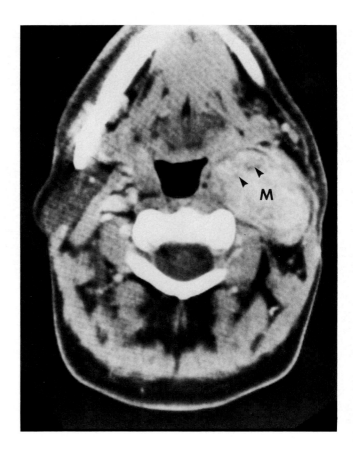

Fig. 7-31 Axial postcontrast CT scan shows large enhancing left parapharyngeal space mass *(M)*. There are focal nonenhancing areas *(arrowheads)* that represent sites of necrosis and clot. Glomus Vagale Tumor. (From Som et al: Radiology 153:149-156, 1984.)

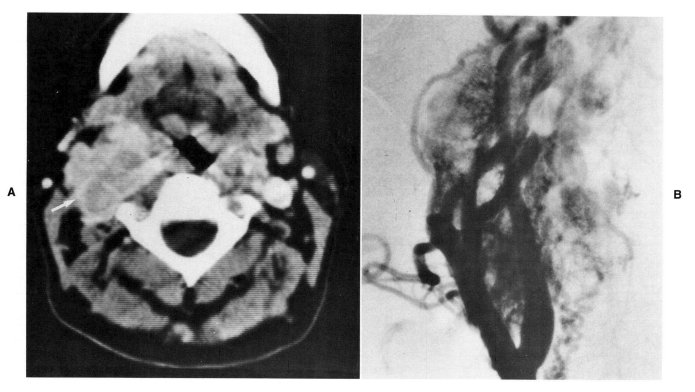

A   B

Fig. 7-32   A, Axial postcontrast CT scan shows partially enhancing right parapharyngeal space mass that has multiple low attenuation areas within it *(arrow).* The CT appearance simulates that of a conglomerate mass of necrotic lymph nodes. **B,** Lateral subtraction angiogram film shows hypervascular glomus vagale tumor with multiple avascular areas of clot and necrosis.

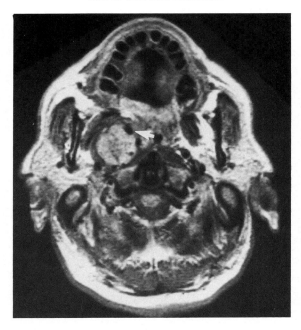

Fig. 7-33   Transverse mixed image (0.5T, TR = 1800 msec, TE = 28 msec) MRI scan shows a right parapharyngeal space mass of overall intermediate signal intensity that has multiple focal and serpentine areas of low signal intensity within it. The internal carotid artery *(arrow)* is displaced anteromedially. Glomus Vagale Tumor.

channel-like areas of signal void within the tumor seen on all imaging sequences. These represent the vascular flow voids of the dominant vessels of the tumor and approximate the characteristic large vascularity found on angiograms (Figs. 7-33 and 7-34).[28,29,42] Because the glomus vagale and glomus jugulare tumors arise around the vagus nerve, they displace the internal carotid artery anteriorly. The carotid body tumors also usually displace the internal and external carotid arteries anteriorly while splaying them at the bifurcation.[29]

The imaging appearance of a hypervascular, smoothly contoured, usually ovoid parapharyngeal space mass is sufficiently characteristic to establish the diagnosis of a paraganglioma in virtually all cases. This means that diagnostic angiograms need be performed only on the few cases whose diagnosis remains in question after appropriate imaging. In general, the only angiograms that need be done on these patients are on small tumors that do not have large enough vessels to give flow voids on MRI or as therapeutic angiograms in which preoperative embolization of the tumor is accomplished in order to reduce blood loss at surgery.

The presence of a hypervascular tumor on imaging studies does not always indicate that a paraganglioma is present. If the lesion's contours are irregular and inva-

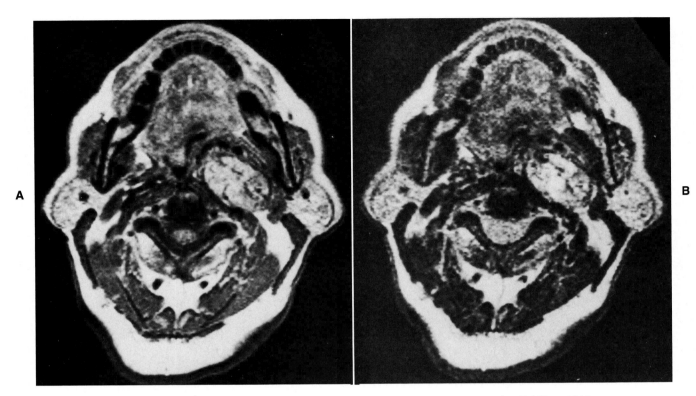

Fig. 7-34   A, Transverse mixed image and **B,** T$_2$-weighted MRI scans (0.5T, TR = 1800 msec, TEs 27, 80 msec) demonstrate an ovoid left parapharyngeal space mass that has a background intermediate signal intensity with focal areas of high signal on the T$_2$-weighted scans. Serpentine and focal areas of low signal intensity are seen on both sequences and represent vascular flow voids. Glomus Vagale Tumor. (From Som et al: Radiology 164:823-829, 1987.)

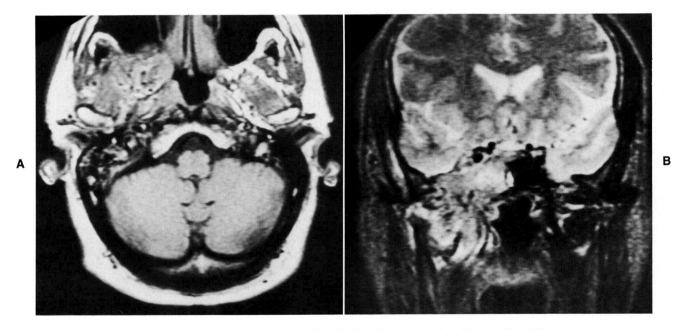

Fig. 7-35   A, Transverse T$_1$-weighted (1.5T, TR 600 msec, TE = 20 msec) and **B,** coronal T$_2$-weighted (1.5T, 2,500 msec, TE = 100) MRI scans show an infiltrating mass of the right parapharyngeal space with an intermediate signal intensity background and multiple vascular flow voids within it. The lesion has eroded the skull base and spread to involve the right cavernous sinus. Metastatic Hypernephroma. (From Som et al: Radiology 164:823-829, 1987.)

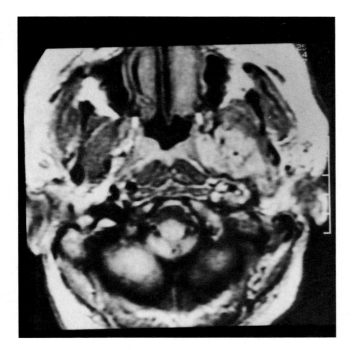

Fig. 7-36   Transverse mixed image (1.5T, TR 2500 msec, TE = 50 msec) MRI scan demonstrates an infiltrating left parapharyngeal space mass with multiple vascular flow voids within it. The tumor is invading the posterior margin of the left pterygoid muscles. Metastatic Thyroid Carcinoma. (From Som et al: Radiology 164:823-829, 1987.)

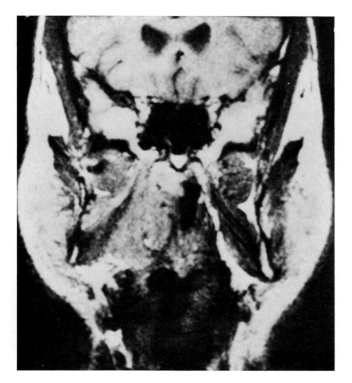

Fig. 7-37   Coronal T$_1$ weighted (0.5T, TR 722 msec, TE = 32 msec). MRI scan shows an intermediate signal intensity mass in the right parapharyngeal space. There are a few areas of vascular flow voids within the mass. The lesion is invading the right pterygoid muscles. Venous Hemangioma. (From Som et al: Radiology 164:823-829, 1987.)

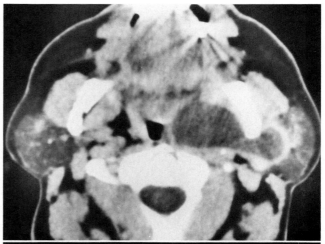

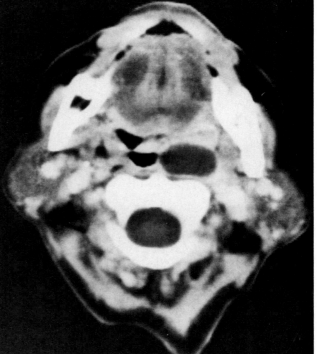

Fig. 7-38   **A,** Axial postcontrast CT scan show a dumbbell-shaped low attenuation mass in the right parapharyngeal space and parotid gland. The mass has a homogeneously thin, minimally enhancing rim. Branchial Cleft Cyst. **B,** Axial postcontrast CT scan demonstrates a low attenuation mass in the left parapharyngeal space and retropharyngeal space. The mass has a smooth, uniformly thin, minimally enhancing rim. Branchial Cleft Cyst. (From Som et al: Radiology 153:149-156, 1984.)

sive, a vascular metastasis should be diagnosed. The primary lesions in such cases may be in the kidney or thyroid gland (Figs. 7-35 and 7-36). Venous hemangiomas may also have a similar imaging appearance, although the flow voids may not be as dominant a feature as in the other tumors (Fig. 7-37).[28]

Miscellaneous Lesions

The remaining tumors that occur in the parapharyngeal space are rare and together represent about 10% to 33% of all the cases. The higher of these numbers results from the series that include metastatic nodes. These lesions can be grouped into three general categories: cystic masses, infiltrative masses, and tumors that extend down into the parapharyngeal space from the skull base.*

Cystic Lesions. The cystic lesions include branchial cleft cysts, abscesses, cystic lymphangiomas (cystic hygroma), and necrotic nodes. On CT, lesions possibly simulating a cyst with a thin or nonvisualized capsule include lipomas and neurofibromas. The branchial cleft cysts usually have a homogeneous low-attenuation (10 to 20 HU) central region with a thin, uniformly smooth wall. They most often are located in the medial aspect of the parapharyngeal space, near the retropharyngeal space, or laterally, adjacent to or involving the parotid gland (Fig. 7-38). On MRI the cyst's watery contents dominate the images, which have low T_1-weighted signal intensities and high T_2-weighted signal intensities.

If the cyst becomes infected, its wall thickens and the surrounding soft tissue planes become obliterated. On CT the cyst wall is enhanced on postcontrast CT scans and the central low density region of the cyst increases in attenuation, often approaching that of muscle. This increased density results from the increased protein concentration in the infected cyst contents. The overall imaging appearance is similar to that of an abscess; however, most such abscesses that arise in the parapharyngeal space are secondary to a primary infection in the soft tissues surrounding this space. Usually, the seeding source is the palatine tonsil (Fig. 7-39).

In some cases of a tonsillar or peritonsillar abscess, the only manifestation of the infection is a cellulitis in the parapharyngeal space. This is identified as a poorly defined infiltration of the fat and soft tissue planes in and immediately about this space. The primary tonsillar abscess usually is well seen on the scans (Fig. 7-39). Differentiation of a parapharyngeal space abscess (demonstrable mass with low attenuation central region) and cellulitis is important because an abscess must be drained expeditiously. Mycotic aneurysms of the carotid artery have been reported to occur in as few as 10 days after the development of a parapharyngeal space

abscess. On the other hand, surgical explorations of cellulitis in the vain pursuit of a nonexistent abscess are inadvisable.

Cystic hygromas are found rarely in adults, and when they involve the parapharyngeal space they usually are multicystic extensions of a posterior triangle mass. The cyst walls in noninfected lesions are usually so thin that they are not identified on imaging (Fig. 7-40). If infection is present, the cyst wall thickens and is enhanced on postcontrast films, and the normally sharp contours of noninfected cysts may become blurred with inflammatory infiltration and effacement of the surrounding fat planes. Areas of increased attenuation within the cyst contents usually reflect either infection or hemorrhage. On MRI the signal intensities are dominated by water and are those of low T_1- and high T_2-weighted signal intensities (Fig. 7-41).[43-46]

On CT, necrotic lymph nodes usually have low attenuation central regions with nodular, irregularly thick walls (Fig. 7-42). Effacement of surrounding fat planes implies extracapsular tumor extension. On MRI, the central necrotic areas usually have high signal intensity on T_2-weighted studies; this is not invariably the case, however, and low-to-intermediate signal intensities

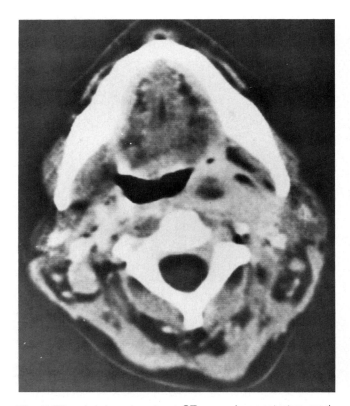

Fig. 7-39 Axial postcontrast CT scan demonstrates moderately enhancing left parapharyngeal space and tonsillar mass with a low attenuation area near the tonsil. Tonsillar abscess with cellulitis of the parapharyngeal space.

---

*References 9, 11, 13, 14, 20, 28, 30, 32-34.

may be present on all imaging sequences. Often, metastatic nodes are multiple and the primary tumor in the head and neck is visualized on the scans.[47]

Although not truly cystic, lipomas and fatty neurofibromas may mimic the CT appearance of a lymphangioma (Figs. 7-43 and 7-44).[46] The MRI findings, however, are quite different, with the fat-dominated lesions having high T_1- and intermediate T_2-weighted signal intensities.

On CT, a thrombosed internal jugular vein or an occluded carotid artery may simulate a cystic mass on a single scan (Fig. 7-45). However, the tubular configuration of the vessel is easily identified once all of the scans are examined serially. By using gradient echo and short flip angle techniques, slow flow through a partially occluded vessel can be identified on MRI (Fig. 7-46). The resulting high signal intensity of the blood can be helpful in diagnosing aneurysms in the parapharyngeal space. Most jugular vein thrombosis is secondary to iatrogenic causes: the introduction of a catheter or a needle either for medical reasons or by an IV drug abuser. Carotid artery occlusions usually are secondary to atherosclerotic disease or surgical trauma.

Medial displacement of the internal carotid artery is

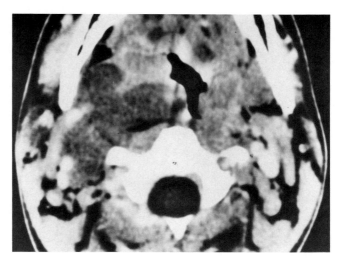

Fig. 7-40 Axial postcontrast CT scan shows multilobulated low attenuation right parapharyngeal space mass. No definite cyst wall is seen, yet the mass is fairly sharply defined. Cystic Hygroma.

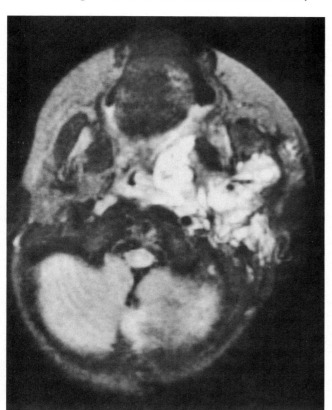

Fig. 7-41 Transverse T_2-weighted (1.5T, TR 2,500 msec, TE = 100 msec) MRI scan shows a multilobulated, partially infiltrating mass of the left parapharyngeal space with a high signal intensity. Cystic Hygroma.

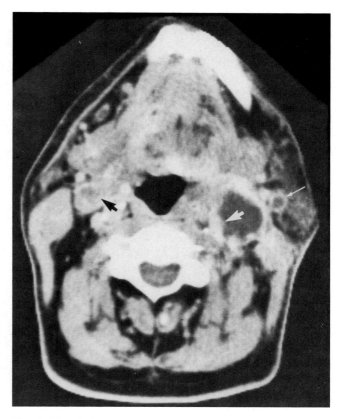

Fig. 7-42 Axial postcontrast CT scan demonstrates multiple necrotic masses *(arrows)* bilaterally in the parapharyngeal spaces. The larger masses have thick, irregular or nodular walls with areas of extension into the adjacent fat planes. Metastatic Squamous Cell Carcinoma. (From Som et al: Radiology 153:149-156, 1984.)

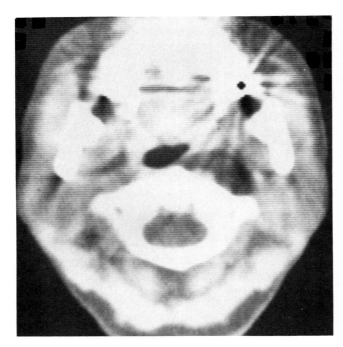

Fig. 7-43   Axial CT scan demonstrates a low attenuation mass in the parapharyngeal space. Lipoma.

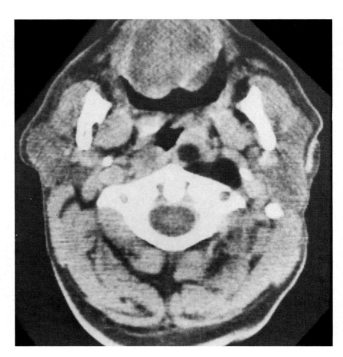

Fig. 7-44   Axial postcontrast CT scan shows two low attenuation masses in the left retropharyngeal and parapharyngeal spaces. The attenuation of the masses is that of fat. Neurofibromas. (From Som et al: Radiology 153:149-156, 1984.)

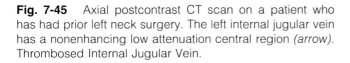

Fig. 7-45   Axial postcontrast CT scan on a patient who has had prior left neck surgery. The left internal jugular vein has a nonenhancing low attenuation central region (arrow). Thrombosed Internal Jugular Vein.

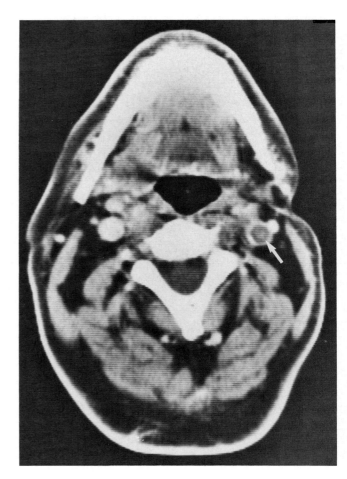

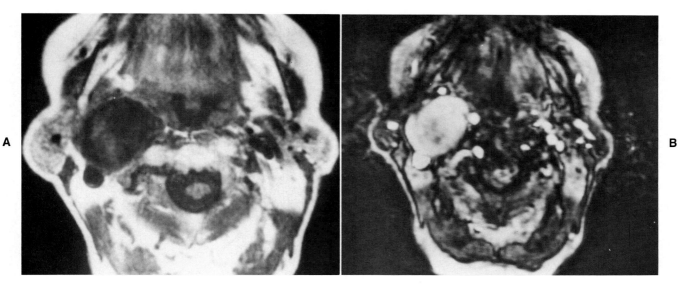

Fig. 7-46   A, Transverse T_1-weighted (0.5T, TR 500 msec, TE = 20 msec) and **B,** gradient echo MRI scans demonstrate a somewhat nonhomogeneous low signal intensity mass in the right parapharyngeal space on the T_1-weighted study. This mass and the normal cervical blood vessels have high signal intensities on the gradient echo image indicating the presence of flowing blood. Aneurysm Right Carotid Artery.

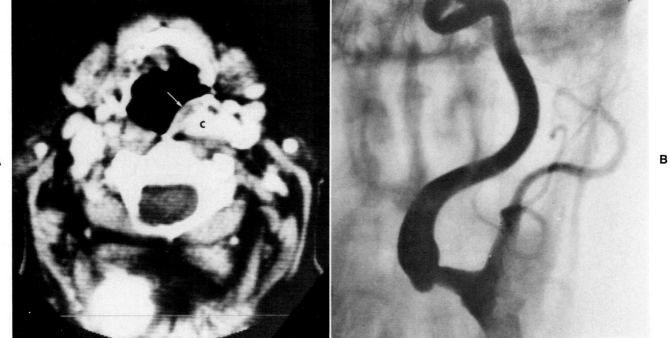

Fig. 7-47   A, Axial postcontrast CT scan demonstrates an enhancing structure *(C)* in the left parapharyngeal space. The mass bulges the left pharyngeal wall anteromedially *(arrow)*. **B,** Frontal subtraction film from a left carotid angiogram shows the medial positioning of the tortuous left internal carotid artery. (**A** from Som et al: Radiology 153:149-156, 1984.)

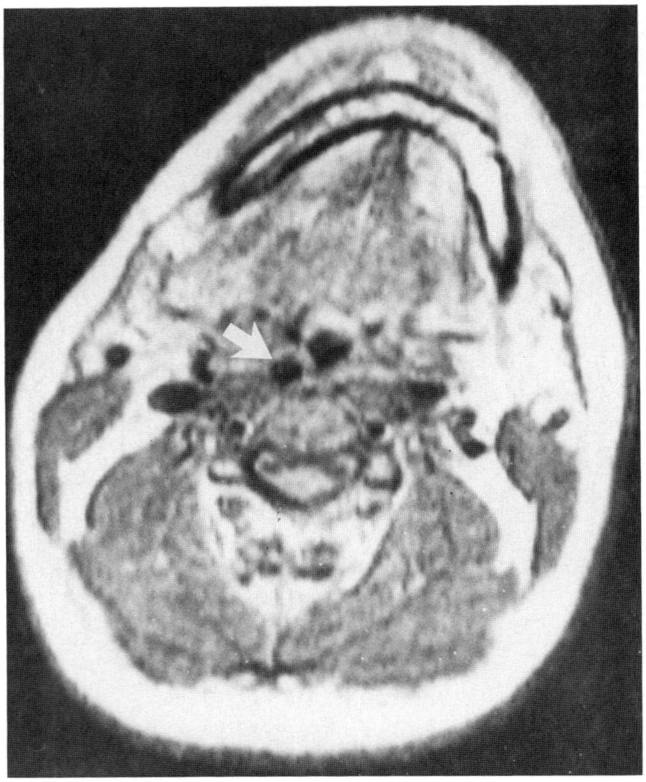

Fig. 7-48 Transverse mixed image (0.5T, TR 1800 msec, TE = 30 msec) demonstrates a vascular flow void *(arrow)* in the right retropharyngeal and parapharyngeal spaces. Aberrant Right Internal Carotid Artery.

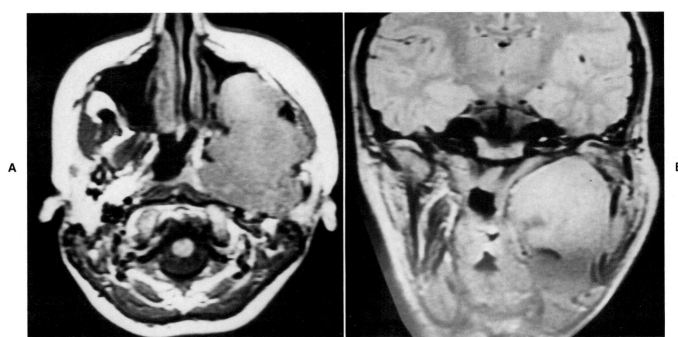

Fig. 7-49 A, Transverse and **B,** coronal T$_1$-weighted (1.5T, TR = 600 msec, TE = 20 msec) MRI scans demonstrate a homogeneous, intermediate signal intensity mass in the left parapharyngeal space and infratemporal fossa. The mass has destroyed the left mandible and posterior antral wall. Rhabdomyosarcoma. (**A** from Som et al: Radiology 164:823-829, 1987.)

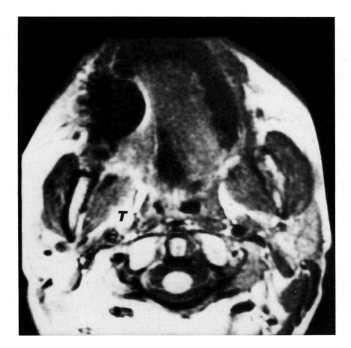

Fig. 7-50   Transverse mixed image (1.5T, TR 1000 msec, TE 20 msec) MRI scan demonstrates a high signal intensity mass in the right parapharyngeal space mass *(T)*. The lesion is invading the right pterygoid musculature. Liposarcoma. (From Som et al: Radiology 164:823-829, 1987.)

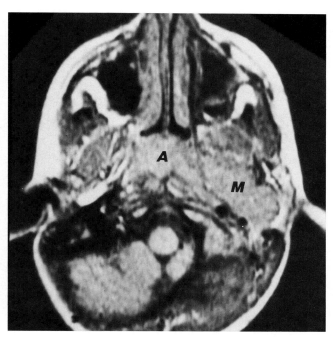

Fig. 7-51   Transverse T$_1$-weighted (1.5T, TR 800 msec, TE 20 msec) MRI scan shows a homogeneous signal intensity mass *(M)* in the left parapharyngeal space. The mass displaces the left parotid gland laterally and also has the same signal characteristics as the hyperplastic adenoidal tissue *(A)*. Lymphoma. (From Som et al: Radiology 164:823-829, 1987.)

an uncommon cause of a parapharyngeal or retropharyngeal fullness. Although such medial positioning can occur from atherosclerotic disease, aberrancy in an otherwise normal vessel is the most common imaging finding. This abnormal positioning of the artery can be well seen on either postcontrast CT scans or MRI studies (Figs. 7-47 and 7-48).

Infiltrative Masses. Infiltrative masses involving the parapharyngeal space are sarcomas of a fatty, muscular, vascular, or fibrous origin. They are rare and are usually highly cellular tumors that have a homogeneous, infiltrative appearance on CT and MRI. Usually there are associated areas of bone destruction (Figs. 7-49 and 7-50). On CT they are most often of an attenuation similar to that of muscle, and on MRI they have intermediate signal intensities on all imaging sequences. Lymphoma is similar in appearance because of its homogeneous nature, but it is less infiltrative, usually causing relatively little bone erosion. Its CT and MRI characteristics are otherwise similar to those of the sarcomas. Often a direct parallel of MRI signal intensities with those of normal adenoidal tissue can be seen, suggesting the possible diagnosis (Fig. 7-51).[20,28]

Skull Base Tumors. Tumors that extend down into the parapharyngeal space from the skull base are un-

common and include meningiomas, chordomas, carcinomas, and some rare osseous or fibroosseous lesions. The meningiomas are enhancing, homogeneous tumors that may have calcifications either in a localized portion of the lesion or scattered throughout the tumor. Once they extend below the skull base, they can grow at a rapid rate and become bulky masses. They usually cause a hyperostotic bony reaction in the skull base, but localized areas of erosion can occur (Figs. 7-52 and 7-53).[20,21,28] On MRI they usually have signal intensities similar to brain, and often the full intracranial component is better appreciated on CT. Most of these tumors are in the posterior fossa and extend down through the petrous apex, jugular fossa, and central skull base. Despite their vascularity on angiography, vascular flow voids are rarely seen on MRI.

Chordomas can extend down into the parapharyngeal space from the skull base. It is usually the central skull base that is involved, although the medial petrous apex can also be the site of origin. Both intracranial and extracranial extension can occur. On CT, most tumors have a nonhomogeneous enhancing appearance, with multiple scattered areas of calcification that presumably represent residual skull base fragments. On MRI, these tumors can have a variable signal intensity on all imag-

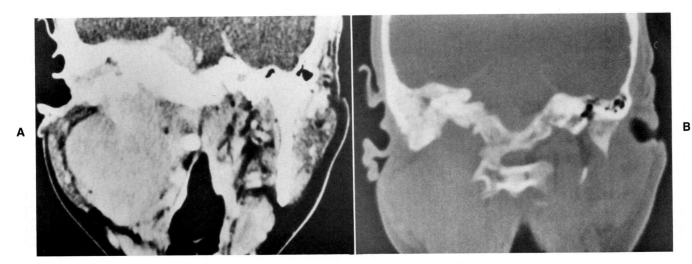

Fig. 7-52 Coronal postcontrast CT scans viewed at **A,** narrow window and **B,** wide window settings demonstrate a large enhancing mass in the right parapharyngeal space and posterior cranial fossa. The intervening skull base is thickened and hyperostotic. Meningioma.

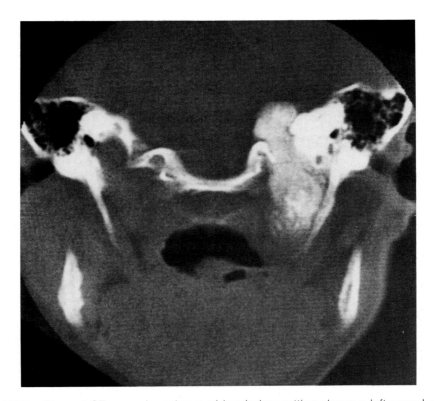

Fig. 7-53 Coronal CT scan viewed at a wide window setting shows a left parapharyngeal space mass that extends up through the jugular fossa to the posterior fossa. The mass is extensively calcified. Meningioma. (From Som et al: Radiology 153:149-156, 1984.)

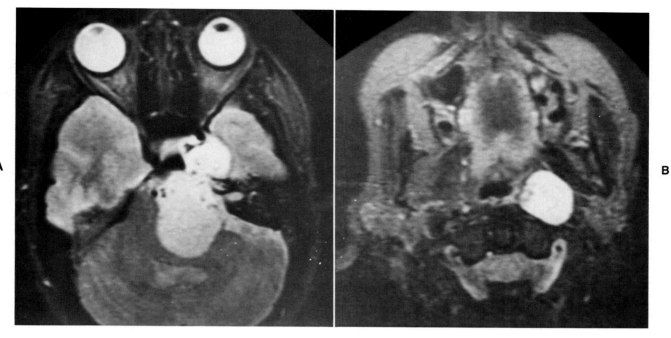

Fig. 7-54   A, Transverse mixed image (1.5T, TR 2000 msec, TE = 35 msec) and **B,** T_2-weighted (1.5T, TR = 2000 msec, TE = 75 msec) MRI scans demonstrate a mass with a high signal intensity on all imaging sequences. The mass arises from the left skull base in the petrous apex and basisphenoid and extends caudally into the left parapharyngeal space. Chordoma. (From Som et al: Radiology 164:823-829, 1987.)

ing sequences, depending upon the histologic makeup of the particular tumor (Fig. 7-54).[28]

Nasopharyngeal carcinomas usually are mucosal tumors that may have extensive submucosal and parapharyngeal space tumor extension, often with skull base erosion and intracranial spread. Rarely, the mucosal component is barely noticeable and the tumor appears as an unknown primary. Most are squamous cell carcinomas and as such are nonenhancing muscle attenuation masses on CT and have an intermediate signal intensity on all MRI sequences (Fig. 7-55).[25]

Osseous and fibroosseous lesions of the skull base are very rare. They are, in general, better visualized on CT than on MRI studies.

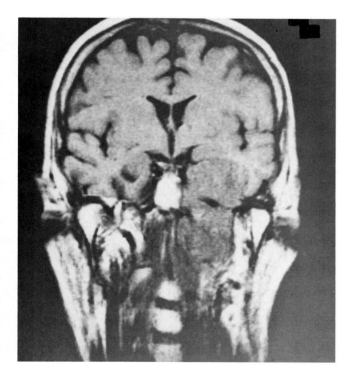

Fig. 7-55   Coronal T_1-weighted (0.5T, TR = 350 msec, TE = 28 msec) MRI scan reveals an intermediate signal intensity left parapharyngeal space mass that erodes through the skull base and extends intracranially to involve the cavernous sinus and temporal lobe. Squamous Cell Carcinoma.

REFERENCES

1. Einstein RAJ: Sialography in the differential diagnosis of parotid masses, Surg Gynecol Obstet 122:1079, 1966.
2. Meine FJ and Woloshen HJ: Radiologic diagnosis of salivary gland tumors, Radiol Clin North Am 8:475, 1970.
3. White IL: Sialoangiography: x-ray visualization of major salivary glands, Laryngoscope 82:2032, 1972.
4. Potter GD: Sialography and the salivary glands, Otolaryngol Clin North Am 6:509, 1973.
5. Calcaterra TC et al: The value of sialography in the diagnosis of parotid tumors, Arch Otolaryngol 103:727, 1977.
6. Work WP and Johns ME: Symposium on salivary gland diseases, Otolaryngol Clin North Am 10:261, 1977.
7. Som PM and Biller HF: The combined CT-sialogram, Radiology 135:387, 1980.

8. Tsai FY, Goldstein JC, and Parhad IM: Angiographic features of lateral cervical masses, ORL 84:840, 1977.

9. Work WP: Tumors of the parapharyngeal space, Trans Am Acad Ophthalmol Otolaryngol 73:389, 1969.

10. Baker D and Conley J: Surgical approach to retromandibular parotid tumors, Ann Plast Surg 3:304, 1979.

11. Work WP and Hybels R: A study of tumors of the parapharyngeal space, Laryngoscope 84:1748, 1974.

12. McLean WC: Differential diagnosis and management of deep lobe parotid tumors, Laryngoscope 86:28, 1976.

13. Lawson V: Unusual parapharyngeal lesions, J Otolaryngol 8:241, 1979.

14. Heeneman H and Maran A: Parapharyngeal space tumors, Clin Otolaryngol 4:57, 1979.

15. Carter BL et al: Cross-sectional anatomy: computed tomography and ultrasound correlation, New York, 1977, Apple-Century-Crofts, Sections 11, 13, 15.

16. Carter BL and Karmody CS: Computed tomography of the face and neck, Semin Roentgenol 13:257, 1978.

17. Mancuso A, Rice D, and Hanafee W: Computed tomography of the parotid gland during contrast sialography, Radiology 132:211, 1979.

18. Som PM and Biller HF: The combined CT-sialogram: a technique to differentiate deep lobe parotid tumors from extra parotid pharyngomaxillary space tumors, Ann Otol Rhinol Laryngol 88:590, 1979.

19. Bryan RN et al: Computed tomography of the major salivary glands, AJR 139:547, 1982.

20. Som PM et al: Parapharyngeal space masses: an updated protocol based upon 104 cases, Radiology 153:149, 1984.

21. Som PM, Biller HF, and Lawson W: Tumors of the parapharyngeal space: preoperative evaluation, diagnosis, and surgical approaches, Ann Otol Rhinol Laryngol 90(suppl 80):3, 1981.

22. Mafee M: Dynamic CT and its application to otolaryngology: head and neck surgery, J Otolaryngol 11:307, 1982.

23. Shugar MA and Mafee MF: Diagnosis of carotid body tumors by dynamic computerized tomography, Head Neck Surg 4:518, 1982.

24. Lloyd GAS and Phelps PD: Demonstration of tumours of the parapharyngeal space by magnetic resonance imaging, Br J Radiol 59:675, 1986.

25. Dillon WP et al: Magnetic resonance imaging of the nasopharynx, Radiology 152:731, 1984.

26. Dillon WP: Applications of magnetic resonance imaging to the head and neck, Semin Ultrasound CT MR 7:202, 1986.

27. Mancuso AA and Hanafee WN: Nasopharynx and parapharyngeal space. In Computed tomography and magnetic resonance imaging of the head and neck, ed 2, Baltimore, 1985, Williams & Wilkins, pp 428-497.

28. Som PM et al: Tumors of the parapharyngeal space and upper neck: MR imaging characteristics, Radiology 164:823, 1987.

29. Som PM et al: Common tumors of the parapharyngeal space: refined imaging diagnosis, Radiology 169:81, 1988.

30. Heeneman H, Gilbert JJ, and Rood SR: The parapharyngeal space: anatomy and pathologic conditions with emphasis on neurogenous tumors, Alexandria, Va, 1980, American Academy of Otolaryngology.

31. Lederman M: Cancer of the nasopharynx: its natural history and treatment, Springfield, Ill, 1961, Charles C Thomas.

32. McIlrath DC et al: Tumors of the parapharyngeal region, Surg Gynecol Obstet 116:88, 1963.

33. Batsakis JG: Tumors of the head and neck, clinical pathological considerations, ed 2, Baltimore, 1979, Williams & Wilkins, pp 1-75.

34. Peel RZ and Gnepp DR: Diseases of the salivary glands. In Barnes L, editor: Surgical pathology of the head and neck, vol 1, New York, 1985, Marcel Dekker, Inc, pp 533-645.

35. Batsakis JG: Tumors of the head and neck, clinical pathological considerations, ed 2, Baltimore, 1979, Williams & Wilkins, pp 76-99.

36. Som PM et al: Benign and malignant parotid pleomorphic adenomas: CT and MR studies, JCAT 12:65, 1988.

37. Mandelblatt SM et al: Parotid masses: MR imaging, Radiology 163:411, 1987.

38. Teresi LM et al: Parotid masses: MR imaging, Radiology 163:405, 1987.

39. Mirich DR, McArdle CB, and Kulkarni MV: Benign pleomorphic adenomas of the salivary glands: surface coil MR imaging versus CT, JCAT 11:620, 1987.

40. Kumar AJ et al: Computed tomography of extracranial nerve sheath tumors with pathological correlation, JCAT 7:857, 1983.

41. Zak FG and Lawson W: The paraganglionic chemoreceptor system: physiology, pathology, and clinical medicine, New York, 1982, Springer-Verlag, pp 287-411.

42. Olsen WL et al: MR imaging of paragangliomas, AJNR 7:1039, 1986.

43. Som PM: Cystic lesions of the neck, Postgrad Radiol 7:211, 1987.

44. Harnsberger HR et al: Branchial cleft anomalies and their mimicks: computed tomographic evaluation, Radiology 152:739, 1984.

45. Reede DL, Whelan MA, and Bergeron RT: CT of the soft tissue structures of the neck, Radiol Clin North Am 22:239, 1984.

46. Reede DL, Whelan MA, and Bergeron RT: Computed tomography of the infrahyoid neck. II, Pathol Radiol 145:397, 1982.

47. Som PM: Lymph nodes of the neck, Radiology 165:593, 1987.

8 The Neck

WENDY R.K. SMOKER
H. RIC HARNSBERGER
DEBORAH L. REEDE
ROY A. HOLLIDAY
PETER M. SOM
R. THOMAS BERGERON

SECTION FOUR
THORACIC INLET AND LOWER NECK
Phrenic nerve
Vagus nerve
Brachial plexus

SECTION ONE

NORMAL ANATOMY OF THE NECK

WENDY R.K. SMOKER
H. RIC HARNSBERGER

Currently, the way surgeons describe the clinical location of a neck lesion and plan their surgical approach differs from the way radiologists, as imaging specialists, localize and describe a pathologic condition on cross-sectional images. Clinicians usually refer to *triangles,* whereas radiologists usually describe *spaces.* For example, the clinician describes a lesion that is just above the clavicle and posterior to the sternocleidomastoid muscle as being in the subclavian triangle; the radiologist may localize it to the anteroinferior aspect of the posterior cervical space. Obviously imagers must become fluent in both languages to communicate effectively with referring clinicians; a way must be found to bridge the terminology gap between triangles and spaces. Thus the radiologist must have a thorough knowledge of the normal gross anatomy, including the triangles of the neck, before he or she can extrapolate these triangles into spaces.

Conversion of the triangles into spaces is the principal goal of this section on normal anatomy of the neck. After a discussion of pertinent embryology, the normal gross anatomy of the neck is presented, including the triangles and their contents. This is followed by a discussion of the cervical fascia and the spaces they create. A discussion of imaging techniques includes a section on special clinical situations and indications that require tailored imaging. The final section on imaging anatomy includes CT and MRI techniques and covers each of the characteristic levels in the suprahyoid and infrahyoid regions.

The larynx and cervical lymph nodes are discussed separately in subsequent sections. Also, since the suprahyoid region of the neck is functionally related to the oropharynx and oral cavity, some structures in those regions are of necessity included in this section. In the discussion of the fascia and spaces of the neck, the fascial attachments to the skull base and the spaces

they create above the suprahyoid region of the neck are included for completeness. These spaces (the oropharynx and nasopharynx) are detailed elsewhere in this book.

PERTINENT EMBRYOLOGY

The structures of the neck derive primarily from the branchial apparatus, which consists of the branchial (pharyngeal) arches, pharyngeal pouches, branchial clefts, and branchial, or closing, membranes. Most congenital malformations of the neck originate during the transformation of the branchial apparatus into adult derivatives[1] (Fig. 8-1).

At about 4 weeks of gestation, the *branchial arches* appear as rounded ridges on each side of the future head and neck. Four well-defined pairs of arches are visible by the end of the fourth week, whereas the fifth and sixth arches are rudimentary. The arches are separated from each other by prominent *branchial clefts.* The inner aspects of the branchial arches are lined by the endoderm of the primitive pharynx, which forms a number of outpocketings, the *pharyngeal pouches.* Four well-defined pairs of pouches develop in a craniocaudad sequence between the branchial arches. The fifth pair is absent or rudimentary. The endoderm of the primitive pharynx transiently contacts the ectoderm of the branchial clefts, forming thin, double-layered *branchial* (closing) *membranes* at the bottoms of the branchial clefts. Mesoderm soon separates the ectoderm and endoderm of the membranes. Only the first branchial membrane forms a structure in the human embryo, namely, the tympanic membrane.

Derivatives of the Branchial Arches

Each branchial arch has its own mesodermal core, externally covered by ectoderm and internally lined by endoderm. A typical branchial arch contains an artery,

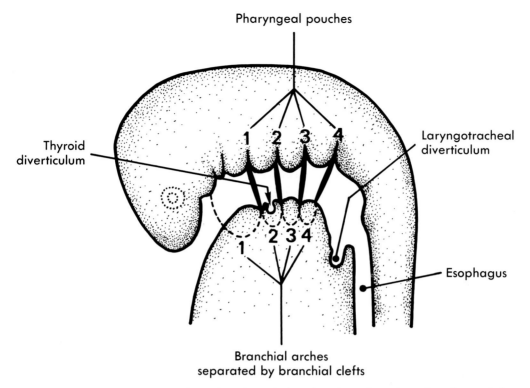

Fig. 8-1   Schematic sagittal section through head and neck region of embryo at 4 weeks of gestation. Note how pharyngeal pouches develop between branchial arches. Thyroid diverticulum originates at level between first and second pharyngeal pouches.

Table 8-1   Derivatives of branchial arch components

Arch	Skeletal structures	Ligaments	Muscles	Nerves
First (mandibular)	Upper portions of the malleus and incus	Anterior ligament of the malleus; sphenomandibular ligament	Muscles of mastication; mylohyoid; anterior belly of the digastric muscle; tensor tympani; tensor palati	Trigeminal (V) (maxillary and mandibular divisions)
Second (hyoid)	Lower portion of the malleus and incus; stapes crura; Styloid process of the temporal bone; lesser horns and upper part of body of hyoid bone	Stylohyoid ligament	Muscles of facial expression; stapedius; stylohyoid; posterior belly of the digastric muscle	Facial (VII)
Third	Greater horns and lower part of body of hyoid bone	None	Stylopharyngeus	Glossopharyngeal (IX)
Fourth, fifth, and sixth	Thyroid cartilage; arytenoid cartilage; corniculate cartilage; cuneiform cartilage; cricoid cartilage	None	Pharyngeal and laryngeal muscles	Vagus (X) (superior laryngeal and recurrent laryngeal branches)

a cartilaginous bar, muscle elements, and a nerve. Except for the nerve, which grows in from the developing brain, all these components derive from branchial arch mesoderm. The muscles of the various arches do not always attach to bony or cartilaginous components of their own arches; they may migrate to the surrounding regions. However, the origins of these muscles can always be established, since their nerve supply comes from the arch of origin (Table 8-1).

First (Mandibular) Branchial Arch. The first, or mandibular, arch consists of a small dorsal portion (the maxillary process) and a large ventral portion (the mandibular process). The cartilage of the first arch, known as Meckel's cartilage, arises between the forty-first and forty-fifth days of gestation and primarily provides the template of the mandible. Persistent portions of the cartilage also form the upper portions of the incus and malleus and the anterior ligament of the malleus and the sphenomandibular ligament.[1] The mandible is formed secondarily by intramembranous ossification of the mesodermal tissue surrounding Meckel's cartilage. The nerve of the first arch is the trigeminal nerve (V). The muscles of the first arch include the muscles of mastication and the mylohyoid, the anterior belly of the digastric, the tensor tympani, and the tensor palatini muscles. These muscles are innervated by the mandibular division of the trigeminal nerve. Only the maxillary (V2) and the mandibular (V3) divisions supply derivatives of the first branchial arch.

Second (Hyoid) Branchial Arch. The cartilage of the second arch, known as Reichert's cartilage, appears between the forty-fifth and forty-eighth days of gestation. It gives rise to the lower segments of the incus and malleus, the stapes crura, the styloid process of the temporal bone, the stylohyoid ligament, and the lesser cornuae (horns) and upper portion of the body of the hyoid bone. The muscles of the second arch are the posterior belly of the digastric, the stylohyoid, the stapedius, and the muscles of facial expression, all of which are supplied by the nerve of the second arch, the facial (VII) nerve.

Third Branchial Arch. The cartilage of the third arch ossifies to form the greater horns and lower portion of the body of the hyoid bone. The musculature of this arch is limited to the stylopharyngeus muscle, which is innervated by the glossopharyngeal (IX) nerve. Because the mucosa of the posterior third of the tongue is also derived from the third arch, its sensory innervation is supplied in part by the glossopharyngeal nerve.

Fourth, Fifth, and Sixth Branchial Arches. The cartilages of the fourth, fifth, and sixth branchial arches fuse to form the laryngeal cartilages. The precise arch or arches of origin of the laryngeal cartilages are uncertain. The fourth and fifth arch cartilages probably form the thyroid, arytenoid, corniculate, and cuneiform cartilages. The sixth arch cartilage probably contributes to the cricoid cartilage.[1] The muscles of the fourth arch are the cricothyroid and constrictor muscles of the pharynx, which are innervated by the fourth arch nerve, the superior laryngeal branch of the vagus (X) nerve.[2] The intrinsic laryngeal muscles are supplied by the nerve of the sixth arch, the recurrent laryngeal branch of the vagus (X) nerve.

Derivatives of the Pharyngeal Pouches

The first and second pharyngeal pouches give rise to structures associated with the ear and oropharynx (palatine tonsil) and are not germane to our discussion of the neck.

Third Pharyngeal Pouch. The third pharyngeal pouch expands into a solid dorsal portion and a hollow ventral portion. By 6 weeks of gestation, each dorsal bulbar portion begins to differentiate into an inferior parathyroid gland. The ventral portions of the two pouches migrate medially and eventually fuse to form the thymus, which then migrates in a caudal direction, pulling the inferior parathyroid glands with it. The inferior parathyroid glands later separate from the thymus and come to lie on the dorsal surface of the thyroid gland, which descends from the foramen cecum of the tongue (see discussion of thyroid gland). Occasionally the inferior parathyroid glands are pulled down too far and may be found at the lower pole of the thyroid or even in the thorax, close to the thymus.

Fourth Pharyngeal Pouch. The fourth pharyngeal pouch also expands into dorsal and ventral portions. Each dorsal portion develops into a superior parathyroid gland, which comes to lie on the dorsal surface of the thyroid gland. The parathyroid glands derived from the third pouch lie at a more inferior level than do those derived from the fourth pouch because of the former's caudal migration with the thymus gland. The ventral portion of each fourth pouch develops into an ultimobranchial body, which fuses with the thyroid gland.[1] This structure contains the parafollicular, or C, cells that secrete calcitonin; these secretory cells are of neural crest origin.

Fifth Pharyngeal Pouch. The fifth pharyngeal pouch is the last of the pharyngeal pouches to develop. It usually disappears or is incorporated into the fourth pouch, appearing as a diverticulum from the fourth pouch's ventral surface. Some believe that this caudal pharyngeal complex gives rise to the ultimobranchial body.[1]

Thyroid Gland

The thyroid gland appears at about 3 weeks of gestation as an epithelial proliferation in the floor of the primitive pharynx, between the first and second pharyngeal pouches, at a point later indicated by the foramen cecum[2] (see Fig. 8-1). This thyroid diverticulum penetrates the underlying mesoderm and descends in front of the pharyngeal gut as a bilobed diverticulum, passing through the tongue musculature and the mylohyoid muscle, deep to the platysma muscle but superficial to the hyoid bone. At the inferior margin of the hyoid bone, the thyroid transiently assumes a superior course, coming to lie either in the developing hyoid bone or in the concavity on the posterior surface of the hyoid bone.[3] Continuing its inferior course, the thyroid passes anterior to the thyrohyoid membrane, deep to the strap muscles, and comes to lie in front of the trachea by 7 weeks of gestation. Throughout its descent, the thyroid is connected to the tongue by a narrow epithelial-lined tubular structure, the thyroglossal duct. By 8 to 10 weeks of gestation, the duct normally undergoes involution and atrophy and disappears.[3] The pyramidal lobe, which is present about half the time, is derived from the lower portion of the thyroglossal duct.[1] The original opening of the thyroglossal duct persists as the midline foramen cecum, located in the terminal sulcus between the body (anterior two thirds) and root (posterior third) of the tongue.[1]

NORMAL GROSS ANATOMY

Covering the anterior and lateral aspects of the neck just below the skin is the platysma muscle, which is contained within the superficial fascia of the neck. (The origins, insertions, and motor innervations of the muscles discussed in this chapter are described in Table 8-2.)

Deep to the platysma muscle traditional anatomic descriptions divide the neck into a variety of triangles that are defined by various muscles and osseous structures (Fig. 8-2). The large sternocleidomastoid muscle runs obliquely across the neck, subdividing it into *anterior* and *posterior triangles*. These two large triangles thus share a common side. Structures located anterior to the sternocleidomastoid muscle lie within the anterior triangle; structures that lie deep to and posterior to this muscle fall within the posterior triangle.[4] Because of its oblique course, the sternocleidomastoid muscle is visualized in a progressively more anterior location when axial imaging is performed in a craniocaudad direction.

Anterior Triangle

The *anterior triangle* is bordered by the sternocleidomastoid muscle posterolaterally, the mandible superiorly, and the midline of the neck anteromedially. This triangle is subdivided by the hyoid bone into the suprahyoid and infrahyoid regions. The contents of the suprahyoid region are functionally related to the oropharynx and oral cavity.

Suprahyoid Compartment. The suprahyoid region of the anterior triangle is further subdivided by the anterior and posterior bellies of the digastric muscle into *submental* and *submandibular triangles*.

Submental Triangle. The submental triangle is a midline triangle outlined laterally by the anterior bellies of the digastric muscles and inferiorly by the hyoid bone (Figs. 8-3 and 8-4). The symphysis of the mandible is the submental triangle's superior margin; the mylohyoid muscles and their fibrous median raphe define the floor of the triangle and separate it from the floor of the mouth. The submental triangle contains small submental lymph nodes and small branches of the facial artery and vein.

Submandibular Triangle. The submandibular (digastric) triangle is bounded superiorly by the lower body of the mandible and inferiorly by the anterior and posterior bellies of the digastric muscle (Figs. 8-3 to 8-5). The floor of the submandibular triangle is formed by parts of the mylohyoid muscle anteriorly and the hyoglossus muscle posteriorly. The submandibular triangle is in broad communication with the sublingual space at the posterior margin of the mylohyoid muscle via the gap between the mylohyoid and hyoglossus muscles[5] (see Figs. 8-3 and 8-5). The submandibular triangle is almost completely filled by the superficial portion of the submandibular gland. Three to five submandibular lymph nodes 3 to 10 mm in size lie within this region, superficial to the gland, as do portions of the posterior (retromandibular) and anterior facial veins.[6] Between the deep surface of the superficial portion of the gland and the external surface of the mylohyoid muscle lie the mylohyoid nerve and the submental branch of the facial artery.[7] Posterior to the border of the mylohyoid muscle the deep surface of the submandibular gland is in contact with the hypoglossal nerve (see Fig. 8-5).

The smaller, deep portion of the submandibular gland enters the posterior aspect of the sublingual space at the posterior border of the mylohyoid muscle via the gap between it and the hyoglossus muscle (see Fig. 8-5). The hyoglossus muscle is a key landmark separating the superficially located duct and nerves from the lingual artery, which lies deep to the muscle.[8] The hypoglossal nerve also enters the sublingual space via this gap, medial to the deep portion of the submandibular gland. The submandibular duct (Wharton's duct), which is approximately 5 cm in length, arises from the deep portion of the gland and courses anteromedially in intimate relation with the lingual nerve.[9] Initially the duct lies between the mylohyoid and hyoglossus muscles, then between the mylohyoid and genioglossus muscles. (The genioglossus muscle is one of the extrinsic muscles of the tongue.) In its terminal course, the submandibular duct courses between the genioglossus

Table 8-2   Muscles of the neck

Muscle	Origin	Insertion	Motor innervation
Platysma	Fascia and skin over the upper part of the pectoralis major and deltoid muscles	Lower border of the mandible and muscles of the lips	Facial nerve (VII)
Sternocleidomastoid	Sternum and medial third of the clavicle	Mastoid process of the temporal bone and the superior nuchal line	Spinal accessory nerve (XI)
Anterior belly of the digastric muscle	Lower border of the mandible near the symphysis	Into an intermediate tendon, where it is united with the posterior belly	Mylohyoid branch of the mandibular division of the trigeminal nerve (III)
Posterior belly of the digastric muscle	Digastric notch of the temporal bone	Into an intermediate tendon, where it is united with the anterior belly	Facial nerve (VII)
Stylohyoid	Styloid process of the temporal bone	Distally it splits to surround the intermediate tendon of the digastric muscles before inserting on the hyoid bone	Facial nerve (VII)
Mylohyoid	Entire length of the mylohyoid line of the mandible	Into a midline fibrous raphe extending from the mandibular symphysis to the hyoid bone	Mylohyoid branch of the mandibular division of the trigeminal nerve (III)
Hyoglossus	Body and greater horn of the hyoid bone	Posterior half of the side of the tongue	Hypoglossal nerve (XII)
Superior belly of the omohyoid	Body and greater horn of the hyoid bone	United with the inferior belly by a tendon deep to the sternocleidomastoid muscle	Branches of the ansa cervicalis
Inferior belly of the omohyoid	Upper border of the scapula	United with the superior belly by a tendon deep to the sternocleidomastoid muscle	Branches of the ansa cervicalis
Sternohyoid	Manubrium of the sternum and medial third of the clavicle	Lower border of the hyoid bone	Branches of the ansa cervicalis
Sternothyroid	Posterior aspect of the manubrium and the first costal cartilage	Oblique line on the lateral surface of the thyroid cartilage	Branches of the ansa cervicalis
Thyrohyoid	Oblique line on the lateral surface of the thyroid cartilage	Lower border of the greater horn of the hyoid bone	Fibers from C1
Trapezius (upper and middle fibers)	Medial portion of the superior nuchal line, the external occipital protuberance, the ligamentum nuchae, and the spine of C7	Upper fibers: lateral third of the clavicle Middle fibers: acromion and spine of the scapula	Spinal accessory nerve (XI)

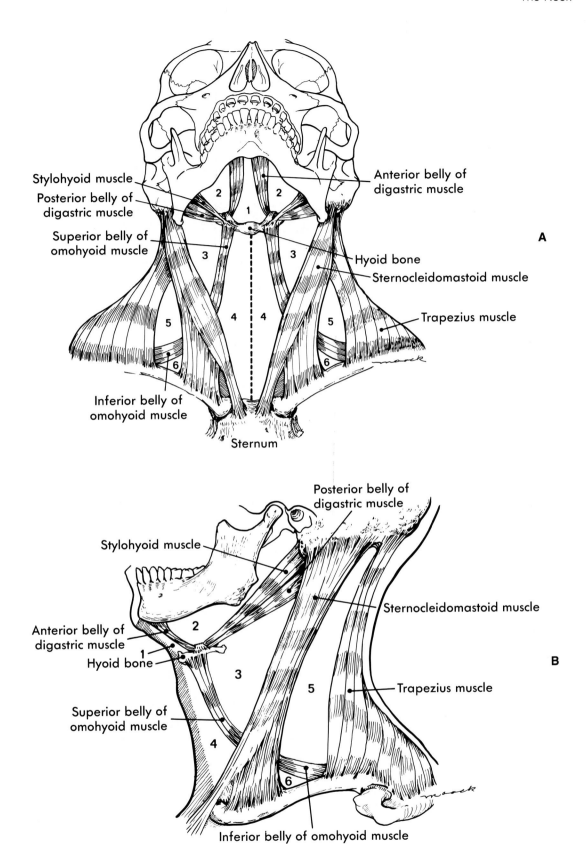

Fig. 8-2 Triangles of neck. **A,** Anterior view. **B,** Lateral view. Submental triangle *(1)* and submandibular triangle *(2)* make up suprahyoid portion of anterior triangle; carotid triangle *(3)* and muscular triangle *(4)* make up infrahyoid portion of anterior triangle; occipital triangle *(5)* and subclavian triangle *(6)* make up posterior triangle.

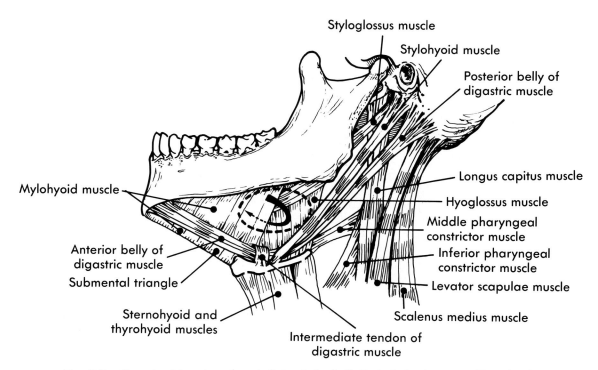

Fig. 8-3 Suprahyoid region of neck (lateral view). *Dotted circle* shows position of submandibular gland. Note gap between posterior margin of mylohyoid and hyoglossus muscles *(curved arrow)*.

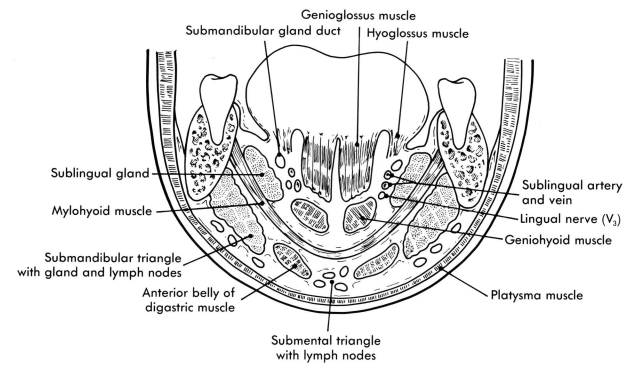

Fig. 8-4 Suprahyoid region of neck (coronal view). Note muscular sling provided by mylohyoid muscles. Submandibular and submental triangles lie below this muscular sling, the floor of the mouth above it.

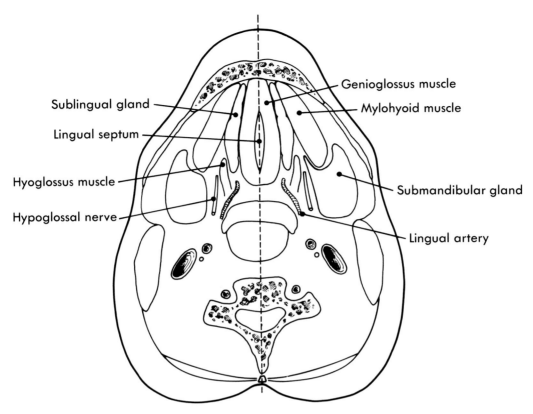

Fig. 8-5 Suprahyoid region of neck (axial view). Note how deep portion of left submandibular gland gains access to posterior aspect of sublingual space via gap between mylohyoid and hyoglossus muscles. Hypoglossal nerve lies just medial to gland, traversing same gap; lingual artery courses deep to hyoglossus muscle.

muscle and the sublingual gland before it drains into the floor of the mouth just to the side of the frenulum of the tongue at the sublingual caruncle (see Fig. 8-4).

Infrahyoid Compartment. The infrahyoid region is descriptively subdivided by the superior belly of the omohyoid muscle into *muscular* and *carotid triangles*.

Muscular Triangle. The paramedian *muscular triangle* is bounded by the superior belly of the omohyoid muscle posterosuperiorly, by the sternocleidomastoid muscle laterally and posteroinferiorly, and by the midline of the neck anteromedially (see Fig. 8-2). These bilateral triangles contain the strap muscles; larynx; hypopharynx; cervical trachea; esophagus; thyroid and parathyroid glands, along with their vascular supplies; and the recurrent laryngeal nerves, running in the tracheoesophageal grooves (Figs. 8-6 and 8-7).

The strap muscles include the superior belly of the omohyoid muscle and the sternohyoid, sternothyroid, and thyrohyoid muscles. Because of their muscular attachments the sternothyroid and thyrohyoid strap muscles lie in a deeper plane than do the more superficial sternohyoid and omohyoid (superior belly) muscles (see Table 8-2).

The recurrent laryngeal nerves arise from the vagus nerves at different levels on each side of the body (see Fig. 8-7). On the right side the recurrent laryngeal nerve arises anteriorly just below the subclavian artery, crosses under this vessel, and ascends deep to the subclavian and bracheocephalic vessels in the right tracheoesophageal groove. On the left side the recurrent laryngeal nerve arises anteriorly below the level of the aortic arch, crosses under it, and ascends in the left tracheoesophageal groove. Because of the nerve's low origin on the left side, imaging of the patient with paralysis of the left recurrent laryngeal nerve must be extended below the level of the aortopulmonary window.

The thyroid gland lies below and on the sides of the thyroid cartilage, covered by three of the four infrahyoid strap muscles. (The thyrohyoid muscle does not cover the thyroid gland.) The thyroid gland has two lateral lobes, located on either side of the upper trachea and lower larynx, and an interconnecting isthmus, which overlies the second to fourth tracheal rings just below the cricoid cartilage.[10] The gland varies greatly in size and is always relatively larger in women and children than in men.[10] Arising from the upper margin

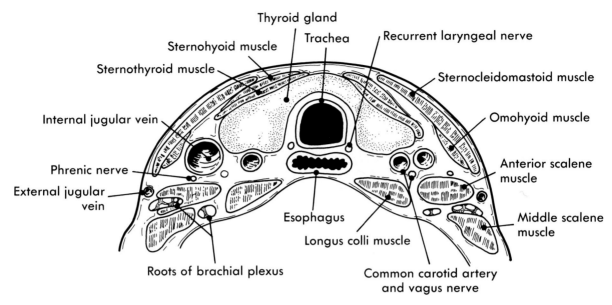

Fig. 8-6 Infrahyoid region of neck—thyroid gland level (axial view). Superior belly of omohyoid muscle often can be seen as separate structure on deep surface of sternocleidomastoid muscle. Recurrent laryngeal nerves lie in tracheoesophageal grooves. Posterior aspect of thyroid gland is in intimate contact with common carotid artery. Note locations of vagus and phrenic nerves.

of the isthmus but not always in a midline location is a variably sized process of thyroid tissue that projects superiorly. This is the pyramidal lobe, which is present in about 40% of the population. It may be represented either by a small stump of tissue or by a discrete large lobe.[7] A fibrous strand or a fibromuscular band (levator glandulae thyroideae) may attach the thyroid gland to the body of the hyoid bone. This fibrous strand is a remnant of the thyroglossal duct. The parathyroid glands are embedded in the posterior surface of the capsule of the thyroid gland, one pair in each lobe. The posterior aspect of each lobe is just medial to the common carotid artery (see Fig. 8-6).

Carotid Triangle. The *carotid triangle* is bounded by the superior belly of the omohyoid muscle anteroinferiorly, a portion of the sternocleidomastoid muscle posterolaterally, and the posterior belly of the digastric muscle superiorly. In the posterolateral aspect of the carotid triangle the carotid sheath envelopes the carotid arteries, the internal jugular vein, the vagus nerve, and sometimes the roots of the ansa cervicalis (ansa hypoglossi).[7,10] Within the carotid sheath the carotid artery lies anteromedially to the internal jugular vein, whereas the vagus nerve lies posterior and between these two vessels (see Fig. 8-6). The carotid triangle also contains the cervical sympathetic trunk, which is embedded in the posteromedial wall of the sheath. Nu-

merous lymph nodes from the internal jugular chain are entwined in the superficial aspects of the carotid sheath about the internal jugular vein. The ansa cervicalis is an arch of fibers that supplies motor innervation to three of the four strap muscles. Following its exit from the skull, the hypoglossal nerve is joined by fibers from the first cervical nerve that course with the hypoglossal nerve until it crosses the internal carotid artery. At this point many of the cervical fibers separate from the main trunk and descend as the superior ramus of the ansa cervicalis (descending hypoglossal ramus). The ramus runs inferiorly on the internal carotid artery to unite with the inferior ramus of the ansa cervicalis (descending cervical ramus), formed by fibers from the second and third cervical nerves.[11] The ansa supplies motor innervation to the sternohyoid, omohyoid, and sternothyroid muscles. The thyrohyoid and geniohyoid muscles are supplied by the few C1 fibers that course with the hypoglossal nerve beyond the origin of the superior ramus.

Posterior Triangle

The *posterior triangle* of the neck is bounded by the sternocleidomastoid muscle anterolaterally, the trapezius muscle posteriorly, and the clavicle inferiorly (Fig. 8-8). From above downward and from posteriorly to anteriorly, the floor of the posterior triangle is formed by

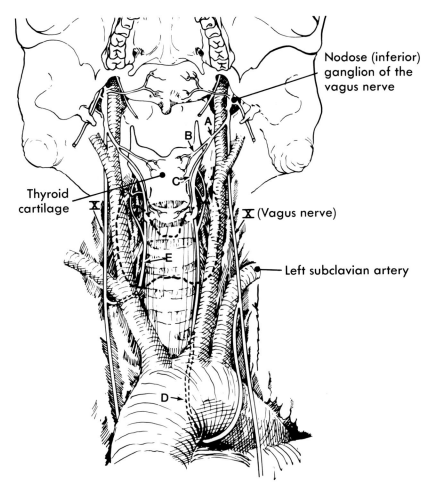

Nodose (inferior) ganglion of the vagus nerve

Thyroid cartilage

X (Vagus nerve)

Left subclavian artery

Fig. 8-7 Anterior triangle of neck (strap muscles have been removed). Note difference in levels of origin of recurrent laryngeal nerves: Left recurrent laryngeal nerve arises below level of aortic arch, which it loops under in region of aortopulmonary window. *A,* Superior laryngeal nerve; *B,* internal branch of superior laryngeal nerve; *C,* external branch of superior laryngeal nerve; *D,* left recurrent laryngeal nerve; and *E,* right recurrent laryngeal nerve.

the splenius capitus, levator scapulae, and posterior, middle, and anterior scalene muscles.

The anterior scalene muscle is an important landmark to the anatomy of the lower neck.[12] Arising from the anterior tubercles of the transverse processes of C3 to C6, this muscle runs inferiorly deep to the sternocleidomastoid muscle to insert onto the first rib. The anterior scalene muscle separates the subclavian vein, which lies superficial to the muscle, from the roots of the brachial plexus and the subclavian artery, which lie deep to the muscle. The anterior scalene muscle also descriptively divides the subclavian artery into three portions. The first segment lies medial to the anterior scalene muscle, the second segment lies deep to it, and the third segment extends from the lateral border of

the muscle to the outer margin of the first rib, where this vessel then becomes the axillary artery (Fig. 8-9). If the radiologist is unaware of these relationships, the second segment of the subclavian artery and/or the brachial plexus, lying deep to the anterior scalene muscle in the root of the neck, may be mistaken for a pseudotumor on a CT scan. MRI allows differentiation between the vessels and nerves.[12]

The brachial plexus is primarily formed by the ventral primary rami of the lower four cervical nerves and the first thoracic nerve, with small contributions from the fourth cervical and second thoracic nerves.[7,10] These ventral rami course between the anterior and middle scalene muscles, superior to the second portion of the subclavian artery. Close to the lateral margin of

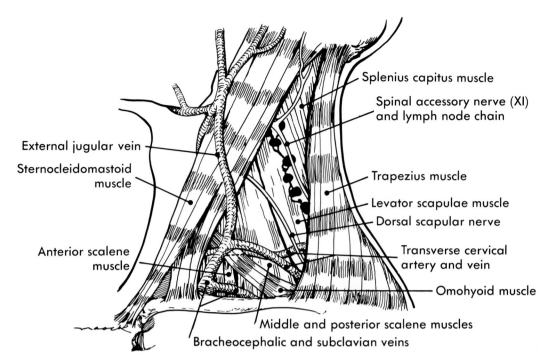

External jugular vein

Sternocleidomastoid muscle

Anterior scalene muscle

Splenius capitus muscle

Spinal accessory nerve (XI) and lymph node chain

Trapezius muscle

Levator scapulae muscle

Dorsal scapular nerve

Transverse cervical artery and vein

Omohyoid muscle

Middle and posterior scalene muscles

Bracheocephalic and subclavian veins

Fig. 8-8   Posterior triangle of neck. Inferior belly of omohyoid muscle subdivides posterior triangle into smaller subclavian and larger occipital triangles. Note superficial relationship of veins to anterior scalene muscle. External jugular vein lies superficial to sternocleidomastoid muscle.

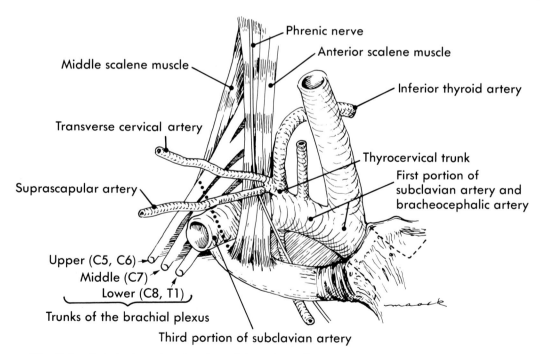

Phrenic nerve

Middle scalene muscle

Anterior scalene muscle

Inferior thyroid artery

Transverse cervical artery

Suprascapular artery

Thyrocervical trunk

First portion of subclavian artery and bracheocephalic artery

Upper (C5, C6)

Middle (C7)

Lower (C8, T1)

Trunks of the brachial plexus

Third portion of subclavian artery

Fig. 8-9   Subclavian triangle, viewed from front. Sternocleidomastoid muscle, clavicle, and veins have been removed to illustrate relationship of anterior scalene muscle to brachial plexus and subclavian artery. Second portion of subclavian artery and trunks of brachial plexus lie deep to anterior scalene muscle, between anterior and middle scalene muscles. At outer margin of first rib, subclavian artery becomes axillary artery. Note course of phrenic nerve as it descends on anterior surface of anterior scalene muscle.

the anterior scalene muscle, the ventral rami of C5 and C6 (and possibly a twig from C4) join to form the upper trunk. The ventral ramus of C7 forms the middle trunk. The ventral rami of C8 and T1 (and possibly a twig from T2) combine to form the lower trunk. Each trunk divides into an anterior and a posterior division. The three posterior divisions combine to form the posterior cord, the anterior divisions of the upper and middle trunks form the lateral cord, and the anterior division of the lower trunk forms the medial cord. The brachial plexus extends from the lateral border of the anterior scalene muscle to the lower border of the pectoralis minor muscle, where the cords divide into their terminal branches[7] (see Fig. 8-9).

The phrenic nerve chiefly arises from the fourth cervical nerve, with contributions from the third and fifth cervical nerves.[13] It courses inferiorly on the anterior scalene muscle, deep to the transverse cervical and suprascapular branches of the thyrocervical trunk (see Fig. 8-9). It gains access to the medial surface of the pleura by crossing anterior to the first portion of the subclavian and internal mammary (thoracic) arteries (see Fig. 8-6).

The inferior belly of the omohyoid muscle subdivides the posterior triangle into the *occipital* and *subclavian* (omoclavicular) *triangles.*

Occipital Triangle. The *occipital triangle* is primarily a fat-filled triangle traversed by the spinal accessory (XI) and dorsal scapular nerves, with the spinal accessory chain of lymph nodes in its midportion and portions of the transverse cervical artery and vein in its lower portion (see Fig. 8-8). It should be emphasized that, with the exception of small vessels, nerves, and lymph nodes, the occipital triangle is a fat-filled structure providing a constant imaging landmark on every axial section throughout the neck.

Subclavian Triangle. Within the smaller *subclavian triangle* are the third portion of the subclavian artery, the trunks of the brachial plexus, and portions of the transverse cervical artery and vein (see Figs. 8-8 and 8-9).

FASCIAL LAYERS

Although subdivision of the neck into triangles may be useful for anatomic and surgical dissection, it is not particularly helpful from an imaging standpoint, because the triangles, which are superficial and primarily aligned in the craniocaudal axis, are not well appreciated in the axial images usually obtained on CT and MRI scans. More important from an imaging perspective is the subdivision of the neck into a variety of spaces that are created by three layers of the deep cervical fascia. Although the fascial layers cannot be radiographically identified, the usually symmetric fat and muscle-filled spaces they define can provide important imaging landmarks. Thus divided the fascial spaces are

also important from a clinical standpoint, because they help to explain the routes of spread of specific-space infections[14,15] and can be used as a basis for devising space-specific differential diagnoses.

Superficial Cervical Fascia

The superficial cervical fascia is a fat-filled layer of connective tissue that completely surrounds the head and neck, encircling the platysma muscle and superficial lymph nodes of the neck. The superficial fascia contains blood and lymph vessels, hair follicles, and cutaneous nerves. Its primary function is to allow the skin to glide easily over the deeper structures of the neck. The structures in this space that normally are visualized on CT and MRI scans include the platysma muscle and portions of the anterior and external jugular veins.

Deep Cervical Fascia

The deep cervical fascia consists of three layers: the superficial (investing) layer, the middle layer, and the deep or prevertebral layer (Fig. 8-10).

Superficial (Investing) Layer (Fig. 8-11). The superficial layer surrounds the entire neck deep to the skin and the superficial cervical fascial layer, which contains the platysma muscle. Although the superficial veins of the neck (anterior and external jugular veins) primarily lie external to this fascia, they also are embedded within it as they pass obliquely through it to join the internal jugular vein. Superoposteriorly, the superficial layer of the deep cervical fascia is attached to the external occipital protuberance, the mastoid process, and the base of the skull. Anteriorly it attaches to the body and symphysis of the mandible, splitting to enclose the submandibular gland and to define the *submandibular space.* The investing fascia then passes inferiorly to attach to the hyoid bone, sternum, and upper margin of the clavicle and then courses posteriorly to attach to the acromion process and spine of the scapula. As it passes posteriorly, the fascia splits to invest the sternocleidomastoid and trapezius muscles and attaches posteriorly to the ligamentum nuchae and the spinous processes of the cervical vertebrae. A localized portion of the investing layer of fascia also splits around the omohyoid muscle and forms a fascial sling that binds the midportion of this muscle to the sternocleidomastoid muscle.[16,17]

At the lower margin of the mandible the investing fascia splits into superficial and deep layers that envelope the mandible, thus forming the *masticator space.*[18-20] The deeper of the two layers runs along the medial surface of the medial pterygoid muscle and attaches to the skull, medial to the foramen ovale.[20] The superficial layer runs along the outer surface of the masseter muscle and attaches to the zygomatic arch before continuing cephalad on the outer surface of the temporalis muscle.

From the posterior margin of the mandible the in-

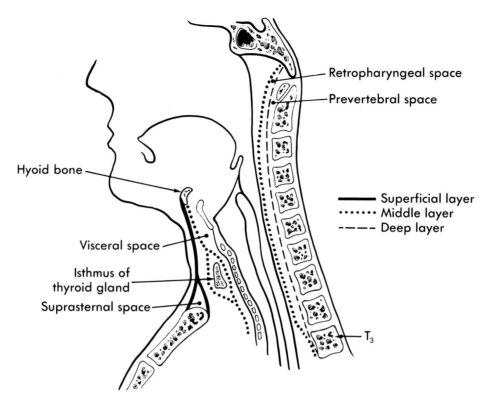

Fig. 8-10   Three layers of deep cervical fascia and spaces of neck (lateral view).

vesting fascia splits to enclose the parotid gland and defines the *parotid space*. A portion of the fascia posterior and deep to the parotid gland thickens to form the sty-lomandibular ligament, which separates the parotid gland from the submandibular gland[10,17] and extends from the styloid process to the posterior margin of the ramus of the mandible.

Slightly above the level of the sternum the investing fascia splits into two layers, one attaching to the anterior margin and one to the posterior margin of the sternum. The space thus created above the sternum is called the *suprasternal space* (of Burns), and it lies just anterior to the origins of the sternothyroid and sternohyoid muscles.[7,10,16,21] A communicating vein between the left and right anterior jugular veins runs in this space. Once an infection invades the suprasternal space, it may penetrate the thin posterior sheet of investing fascia overlying the strap (sternohyoid and sternothyroid) muscles and extend inferiorly, in front of the middle layer of the deep cervical fascia, finally manifesting itself in the upper intercostal spaces.

Middle Layer. The investing layer of fascia between the anterior borders of the sternocleidomastoid muscles forms an anterior fascial layer over the strap muscles; this is the middle layer of the deep cervical fascia (Fig. 8-12). This fascial layer also is called the visceral, pretracheal or buccopharyngeal fascia. The middle layer of the deep fascia lies deep to the strap muscles in the an-terior triangle of the neck and anterior to the thyroid and parathyroid glands, larynx, trachea, esophagus, and recurrent laryngeal nerves. The middle layer is continuous with the investing layer of fascia at the lateral border of the strap muscles and ends superiorly with the attachment of the strap muscles to the thyroid cartilage. Inferiorly, it ends with the attachment of the strap muscles to the deep surface of the sternum. The fascia then fuses with the fibrous pericardium as it is prolonged along the great vessels.

The loose, connective tissue surrounding the thyroid gland, trachea, and esophagus has been as a whole referred to as visceral fascia. It surrounds the pharynx above the esophagus (buccopharyngeal fascia) and extends with the pharynx to its attachment at the skull base.

The *visceral space* is contained by this visceral fascia and as such is a single space from the base of the skull down to the level at which the inferior thyroid artery enters the thyroid gland. From this point caudally, the space is divided into two compartments by dense fascia that extends from the lateral margins of the esophagus on each side to the deep layer of the cervical fascia. The anterior compartment lies around the trachea, abuts the anterior wall of the esophagus, and lies deep to the middle layer of the deep cervical fascia. The space is known as the pretracheal or previsceral space and extends above from the attachments of the strap muscles

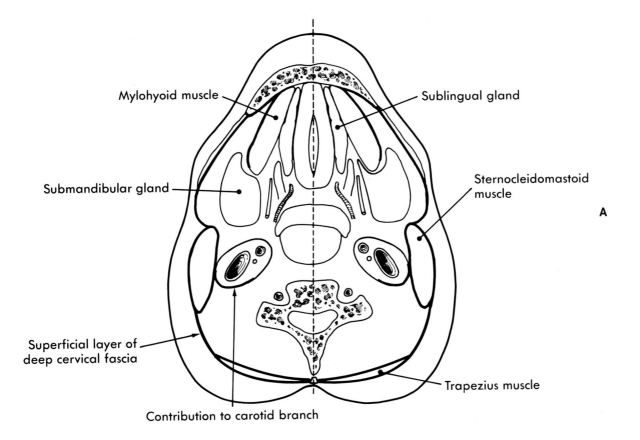

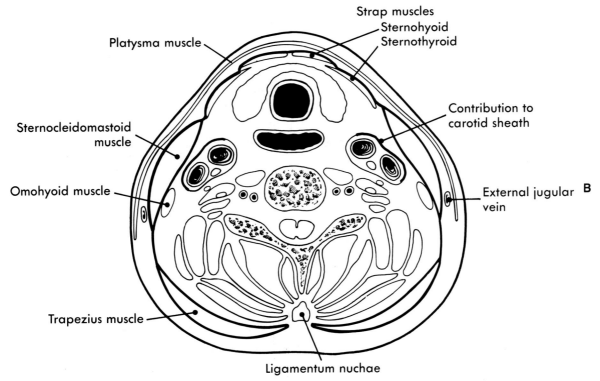

Fig. 8-11   Superficial layer of deep cervical fascia. **A,** Suprahyoid region of neck. **B,** Infrahyoid region of neck. Note how superficial layer splits to enclose sternocleidomastoid and trapezius muscles and contributes to carotid sheath. External jugular veins lie external to, or embedded within, this fascial layer.

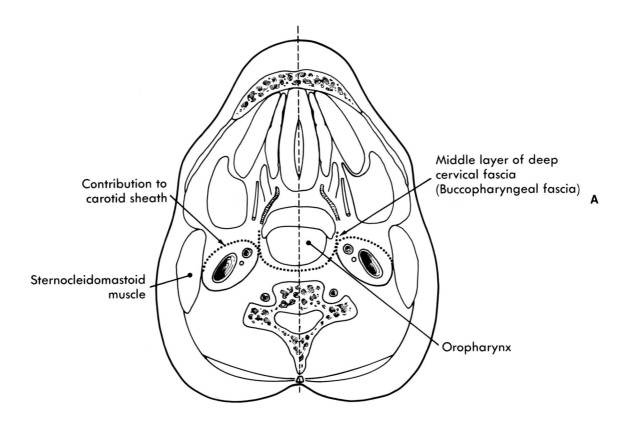

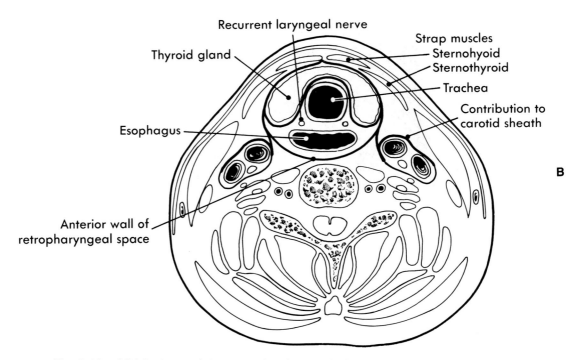

Fig. 8-12   Middle layer of deep cervical fascia. **A,** Suprahyoid region of neck. **B,** In-frahyoid region of neck. Middle layer contributes to formation of carotid sheath and blends with superficial layer covering deep surface of sternocleidomastoid muscle. In in-frahyoid region of neck, middle layer lies deep to strap muscles, fusing with superficial layer anteriorly, in midline. Posteriorly, middle layer forms anterior wall of retropharyngeal space.

and their fascia to the thyroid cartilage and hyoid bone down to the superior mediastinum and the upper border of the aortic arch at about the level of the fourth thoracic vertebra. The posterior compartment of the visceral space, called the retrovisceral or retroesophageal space, extends upward behind the pharynx to the skull base. Although this space often is called the retropharyngeal space, it is continuous below with the retroesophageal space. Inferiorly, behind the level of the inferior thyroid artery, the retrovisceral space extends down into the mediastinum and ends (according to various authors) either at the tracheal bifurcation or continues caudally with the esophagus to the diaphragm.

Infections thus can enter the pretracheal space by spread from the retrovisceral portion of the visceral space, by an anterior esophageal perforation, or around the sides of the esophagus and thyroid between levels of the inferior thyroid artery and the upper border of the thyroid cartilage. The retrovisceral space may be infected by means of posterior esophageal perforations, by infection that spreads from the adjacent deep cervical lymph nodes, or by infections originating about the pharynx in the head and upper portion of the neck. The medial and lateral retropharyngeal lymph nodes are in this space.[8,22]

Deep Layer. The deep layer of the cervical fascia can be thought of as beginning at the cervical vertebral spines and ligamentum nuchae and extending forward to cover the muscles of the upper back and of the floor of the posterior triangle. The deep layer then attaches to the transverse processes of the cervical vertebrae. As it covers these muscles, it invests the brachial plexus and subclavian artery as they extend through and lateral to the space between the anterior and middle scalene muscles. The phrenic nerve is also covered as it descends on the anterior surface of the anterior scalene muscle.[15-19]

The deep layer of the deep cervical fascia then extends from the transverse processes on one side, across the anterior surface of the vertebral bodies, to attach to the opposite transverse processes. This layer of fascia is called the prevertebral fascia. However, another sheet of fascia, the alar fascia, extends from the transverse processes on one side to those on the other but lies anterior to the prevertebral fascia. The space between them is filled with loose, connective tissue and often is called the danger space of Gradinsky and Holyoke. The space between the prevertebral fascia and the vertebra is called the prevertebral space. The danger space extends from the skull base to the level of the diaphragm, whereas the prevertebral space extends from the skull base to the level of the third thoracic vertebra, where the prevertebral fascia fuses with the anterior longitudinal ligament of the spine, below the termination of the longus colli muscles[15-19] (Fig. 8-13).

From an imaging point of view, since these fascial planes cannot be visualized, the retropharyngeal space, the danger space, and the prevertebral space may be grossly considered as representing one space; in these instances, it is loosely referred to as the prevertebral or retropharyngeal space.

Carotid Space

The carotid sheath is formed from fibers of the investing, middle, and deep layers of the deep cervical fascia. It has been suggested that this fascial sheath creates a space that extends from the skull base to the mediastinum and as such represents a route of potential spread of infection. However, such a space actually only exists between the level of the hyoid bone (the carotid bifurcation) and the root of the neck. Above the hyoid bone the fascia is so closely adherent to the vessels that a carotid space as such does not exist in all patients. Infections within the carotid space usually arise from thrombosis of the internal jugular vein or from the spread of infection from the deep cervical (internal jugular) chain of lymph nodes.[23,24]

In the suprahyoid portion of the neck the potential carotid space has been called the poststyloid space, the retrostyloid space, or the posterior or neurovascular compartment of the parapharyngeal space.[20,21,25-29]

At the level of the skull base the internal carotid artery lies anteromedial to the internal jugular vein. Near the level of the hyoid bone the vein is in the same coronal plane as the artery, whereas in the root of the neck the vein is anterolateral to the artery. This changing relationship of the artery and vein reflects the fact that the internal and common carotid arteries run almost in a direct craniocaudal axis, whereas the internal jugular vein follows the obliquity of the sternocleidomastoid muscle.

The vagus nerve lies posterior to these vessels, and in its superior extent portions of the glossopharyngeal, spinal accessory, and hypoglossal nerves are contained within the carotid sheath. The cervical sympathetic trunk lies posteromedially to the vessels and may be embedded with the fascia of the carotid sheath. Similarly, the ansa cervicalis may be within the carotid sheath or lie between it and the deep surface of the sternocleidomastoid muscle.[7]

Posterior Cervical Space

The *posterior cervical space* lies posterolaterally to the carotid space and corresponds to both the occipital and subclavian triangles of the posterior triangle of the neck (Fig. 8-14). The posterior cervical space is the only consistently visualized posterior fat-filled space in the neck and serves as a reliable imaging landmark. Laterally it is bordered by the superficial layer of the deep cervical fascia, which covers the sternocleidomastoid and trapezius muscles. Medially the posterior cervical space is bordered by the deep layer of the deep

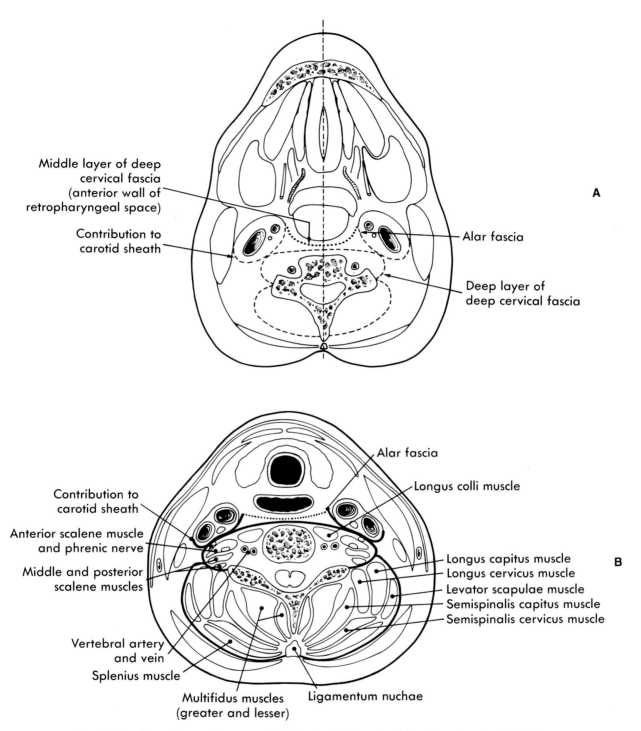

Fig. 8-13   Deep layer of deep cervical fascia. **A,** Suprahyoid region of neck. **B,** Infrahyoid region of neck. Two slips of deep layer (alar fascia) form lateral walls of retropharyngeal space and contribute to formation of carotid sheath. Attaching to transverse processes, deep layer subdivides prevertebral space into anterior and posterior compartments.

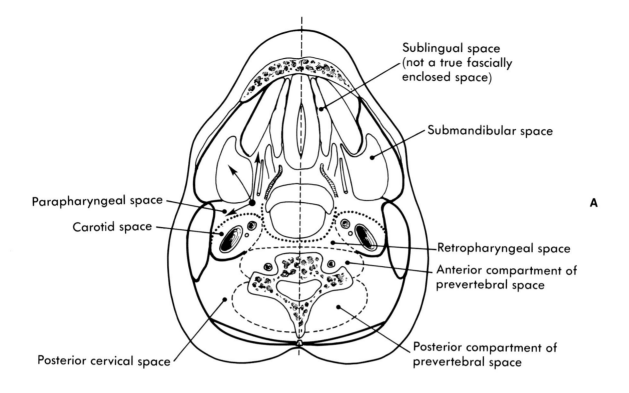

Sublingual space
(not a true fascially
enclosed space)

Submandibular space

Parapharyngeal space

Carotid space

Retropharyngeal space

Anterior compartment of
prevertebral space

Posterior compartment of
prevertebral space

Posterior cervical space

A

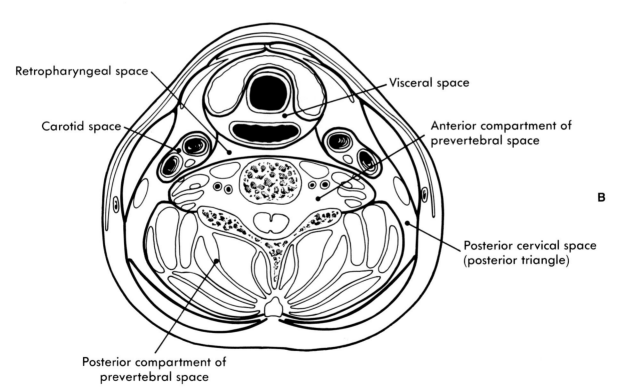

Retropharyngeal space

Carotid space

Visceral space

Anterior compartment of
prevertebral space

Posterior cervical space
(posterior triangle)

Posterior compartment of
prevertebral space

B

Fig. 8-14   Spaces of neck. **A,** Suprahyoid region of neck. **B,** Infrahyoid region of neck. Parapharyngeal space is a suprahyoid, fat-filled space. Characteristic compressions or displacements of this fat can help localize pathologic condition to one of surrounding spaces.

Table 8-3 Spaces of the neck

Space	Corresponding triangle(s)	Associated fascia	Extent	Contents
Submandibular	Submental, submandibular	Superficial layer of deep cervical fascia (DCF)	Suprahyoid compartment: floor of mouth (mylohyoid muscle) to hyoid bone	Submandibular gland, lymph nodes
Parapharyngeal	None	*Not* a fascially enclosed space; lies between layers of the deep cervical fascia. Laterally it contacts the superficial layer of the deep cervical fascia; medially it contacts the middle layer of the deep cervical fascia; posteriorly it contacts the carotid sheath.	Suprahyoid compartment: skull base to hyoid bone (inverted pyramid)	Fat
Carotid space	Carotid	Carotid sheath—composed of all three layers of the deep cervical fascia	Suprahyoid and infrahyoid compartments: skull base to mediastinum	Common carotid artery (infrahyoid); internal carotid artery (suprahyoid); vagus nerve (X); suprahyoid portion: portions of cranial nerves IX, XI, and XII; sympathetic chain; deep cervical lymph nodes; ansa cervicalis
Posterior cervical space	Occipital, subclavian	*Not* a fascially enclosed space; lies between layers of the deep cervical fascia. Anteriorly it contacts the carotid sheath; medially it contacts the deep layer of the deep cervical fascia Posterolaterally it contacts the superficial layer of the deep cervical fascia.	Suprahyoid and infrahyoid compartments: skull base to clavicle	Fat; spinal accessory nerve (XI); spinal accessory lymph nodes; small nerves and arteries
Visceral space	Muscular	Visceral fascia	Skull base to the mediastinum	Thyroid gland; parathyroid glands; larynx; pharynx; trachea; esophagus; recurrent laryngeal nerves; lymph nodes
Retropharyngeal space	None	Anterior wall—middle layer of the deep cervical fascia; lateral walls—alar slips from deep layer of the deep cervical fascia Posterior wall—deep layer of the deep cervical fascia	Suprahyoid and infrahyoid compartments: skull base to the mediastinum (approximately T3)	Fat; retropharyngeal lymph nodes

Table 8-3   Spaces of the neck—cont'd

Space	Corresponding triangle(s)	Associated fascia	Extent	Contents
Prevertebral space	None	Deep layer of the deep cervical fascia	Suprahyoid and infrahyoid compartments: skull base to mediastinum (approximately T3)	Anterior compartment: prevertebral muscles; scalene muscles; brachial plexus roots; phrenic nerve; vertebral artery and vein; vertebral body and pedicle. Posterior compartment: paraspinal muscles; vertebral laminae; and spinous processes.
Suprasternal space	Muscular (anterior-inferior portion)	Superficial layer of the deep cervical fascia	Infrahyoid compartment: 3 cm above sternum	Jugular arch; sternal heads of sternocleidomastoid muscles

cervical fascia, which is associated with the muscles of the floor of the posterior triangle and the anterior and posterior compartments of the prevertebral space. Anteriorly this space is associated with the carotid sheath. This space contains fat, the spinal accessory and dorsal scapular nerves, and the spinal accessory chain of lymph nodes.

Submandibular Space

The submandibular space actually comprises two spaces, the submaxillary and sublingual spaces, which communicate freely with each other around the posterior free edge of the mylohyoid muscles. The cranial limit of the submandibular space is the mucous membranes of the floor of the mouth; its floor is the superficial layer of the deep cervical fascia as it extends from the mandible to the hyoid bone. The mylohyoid muscle divides the submandibular space into an upper, sublingual space and a lower, submaxillary space. The submaxillary gland, which lies at the free edge of the mylohyoid muscle, is partly in the sublingual space and partly in the submaxillary space. The sublingual space contains the muscles of the tongue, the sublingual glands, the lingual arteries and nerves, the hypoglossal nerves, and a portion of the submaxillary glands and their ducts. The submaxillary space is divided into submental and submaxillary spaces by the fascial attachments to the anterior belly of the digastric muscles. The submaxillary space contains the submaxillary gland and submaxillary and submental nodes. The submandibular spaces are anterior extensions of the parapharyngeal spaces. Infections in the submandibular space thus may spread intraorally, superiorly into the parapharyngeal space or inferiorly into the mediastinum (Ludwig's angina).[16]

Parapharyngeal (Peripharyngeal) Space

The *parapharyngeal space* is a fat-filled suprahyoid space that extends from the base of the skull to the superior cornua of the hyoid bone. It encircles the pharynx and extends anteriorly into the submandibular spaces. In discussing the parapharyngeal space, the region described herein sometimes is called the prestyloid or anterior compartment of the parapharyngeal space; it is separated from the carotid space, or retrostyloid compartment, by the styloid process of the temporal bone and the muscles arising from it.[20,25-27] It is useful to consider only the prestyloid compartment as the parapharyngeal space, because it is the only anterior space consistently visualized on CT or MRI as a fat-filled space and is limited to the suprahyoid region of the neck, whereas the carotid space traverses the entire neck, being both suprahyoid and infrahyoid.[28] Although the fat within the lower parapharyngeal space is not always prominent, more superiorly (i.e., at the nasopharyngeal level) characteristic displacements of this fat-filled space are useful in localizing a pathologic condition as arising from the parotid gland, the pharyngeal mucosa and musculature, or from the structures within this space. Thus consideration of these fat planes helps limit the differential diagnostic considerations.[19,29-31]

Strictly speaking the parapharyngeal space is not defined by layers of the deep cervical fascia but rather lies between the layers. This space does not correspond to any of the triangles of the neck. Laterally and inferiorly the parapharyngeal space is in contact with the superficial layer of the deep cervical fascia, which is associated with the parotid, masticator, and submandibular spaces. Medially the parapharyngeal space is in contact with the visceral fascia, (often called the buccopharyngeal fascia in this region) which is associated with the pharyngeal mucosal space and the deglutitional muscles. Posteriorly the parapharyngeal space is in contact with the retropharyngeal space, and posterolaterally it is in continuity with the posterior cervical space and the carotid sheath structures (Table 8-3).

IMAGING TECHNIQUES
Computed Tomography

All dentures and nonfixed prostheses should be removed before CT scanning. The patient is placed in the supine position with the chin extended so that the horizontal ramus of the mandible is parallel to the localizing beam. Accurate alignment of the patient's head is critical, since asymmetry of structures on the scans may suggest a pathologic condition. A scanogram is obtained, and if necessary the gantry is angulated so that the plane of sectioning is parallel to the hyoid bone and vocal cords (for laryngeal pathologic conditions). Scanning usually proceeds according to one of two protocols. The first is a more tailored examination, which starts from just below the plane of the roots of the mandibular teeth (to avoid artifacts from dental amalgams) and extends to the level of the thoracic inlet (first rib). Alternately, the study can start at the level of the skull base and extend to the root of the neck. The scanning landmarks in the latter case are the external auditory canal above and the top of the manubrium below. Contiguous axial sections 4 to 5 mm thick are obtained, and 3-second scan times typically are employed. Patients are asked to breathe quietly; however, if significant motion artifact appears, breath-holding during scanning may produce the most motion-free images; this also usually prevents swallowing during scanning. Direct coronal CT scans are not used in neck imaging.

Contrast-enhanced scans better assure the accuracy of CT evaluation of the neck. If the patient has no major allergic history or significant renal impairment, intravenous contrast is given by means of a bolus-drip technique. With this method, 50 ml of 60% iodinated contrast medium is injected as a bolus, followed by rapid-drip infusion of 300 ml of 30% iodinated contrast medium. Scanning is begun immediately after the bolus has been injected. The bolus-drip technique produces maximum levels of intravascular contrast throughout the examination, permitting distinction between vascular structures and other soft tissue structures, especially muscles and lymph nodes.

In some cases rapid-sequence scanning, performed during bolus injection of contrast medium, may be helpful in assessing the vascularity of a neck lesion.[32] Attenuation/time curves for a specific region of interest may be calculated using this technique, thereby permitting differentiation between very vascular (paraganglioma) and slightly vascular (neuroma) lesions, both of which may enhance significantly on routine postcontrast CT studies albeit for different reasons.

Magnetic Resonance Imaging

The superior soft tissue discrimination, the multiplanar imaging capabilities, the demonstration of major vessels without the necessity of intravenous contrast, and the lack of ionizing radiation make MRI the preferred imaging technique for a variety of pathologic conditions of the neck. The beam-hardening artifacts from dental amalgams and the dense cortical bone of the mandible and from the shoulders—so problematic on CT images—are not a problem with MRI.[33]

Ideally a biopsy should be performed on a neck mass after the MRI study. However, if a biopsy already has been done, the MRI scan should be delayed at least 4 to 5 days until the edema and any hemorrhage have started to subside. The disruption of the mucosa and fascial planes by the biopsy procedure may mimic a pathologic condition on the MRI study.[33]

Specialized surface receiver (RF) coils, which improve the signal-to-noise response, are required for MRI scanning of the neck.[33,34] Circumferential surface coils are superior to planar surface coils in most instances, since they do not have the dramatic signal drop-off inherent in the use of planar coil imaging of the neck.[35] As an alternative we have found that the combination of a 5-inch planar surface coil placed behind the neck and a saddle-shaped surface neck coil placed anteriorly provides excellent visualization of all neck structures without deep-signal drop-off. The images are considerably better than those obtained by using either surface coil alone.

Because of the abundance of adipose tissue in the neck, T_1-weighted pulse sequences are most helpful, since they optimize contrast differences between fat and pathologic conditions. However, the relatively higher signal intensity of some neck tumors (e.g., squamous cell carcinoma) on T_2-weighted images is a disadvantage when the lesion is surrounded by the similar intensity signal of adipose tissue on these pulse sequences. The lower signal-to-noise of T_2-weighted sequences also limits the availability of thin-section scanning, which is required for proper evaluation of smaller areas of study such as the larynx.

As a general protocol a sagittal, T_1-weighted, 5 mm thick localizer scan is obtained first. If the patient has a known lesion on one side of the neck, the localizer scan is centered parasagittally toward the side of the lesion. Spin-echo, T_1-weighted axial, and coronal images are obtained. In most instances the coronal and sagittal images provide the most helpful information in assessing the craniocaudad extent of a lesion and its relationship to the base of the skull and great vessels.[36] The slice thickness usually is 5 mm with an interslice gap of 1 to 2 mm. Repetition times (TR) of 600 to 1000 msec and echo times (TE) of 20 to 30 msec commonly are used, with a 256 × 256 acquisition matrix. Depending on the area of interest and the type of lesion being evaluated (e.g., a suspected cystic lesion on the T_1-weighted sequence), proton density and T_2-weighted images may be obtained. Usually a TR of 2000 to 3000 msec with a first echo TE of 20 to 50 msec for proton density and a second echo TE of 80 to 120 msec for T_2-weighted images are employed. Additional sequences such as gradient refocused acquisition in the steady state (GRASS), fat-suppression sequences, or sequences obtained after administration of gadolinium are performed as needed, depending on the type and location of the lesion.

Special Situations Requiring Tailored Imaging

For routine CT or MR imaging of the cervical soft tissues, standard protocols are used that permit scanning without constant supervision by the radiologist. The routine tailored protocol generally extends from the mandibular fillings to the cervical-thoracic junction with contiguous axial images, not exceeding 5 mm in thickness. In most instances this approach suffices. However, in some clinical settings this standard protocol must be modified. This section highlights some of the situations in which special tailoring of the CT or MRI examination is required.

Cervical Adenopathy and the Unknown Primary Tumor. When an adult patient has a cervical neck mass that is clinically suspected of representing metastatic adenopathy, the radiologic examination must be extended from the standard tailored neck study to a more inclusive examination that searches the upper aerodigestive tract for a clinically occult submucosal primary tumor. Using this scanning approach the radiologist will not fail to image and thus identify the primary tumor, which often is not detected by the examining clinician.

The unknown or clinically occult primary tumor is most frequently hidden in the crypts of the lymphatic tissue of Waldeyer's ring (lingual, faucial, or adenoidal tonsils) or in the lower recess of the pyriform sinus. To comprehensively search for the unknown primary tumor, scanning should be extended to include the entire nasopharynx, oropharynx, and hypopharynx, and the scanning study should extend from the skull base to the rest of the neck.

Imaging is best completed before biopsy of the mass whenever possible. Biopsy-induced edema and hemorrhage surrounding malignant adenopathy may simulate the imaging appearance of extranodal tumor spread. Since the first attempt at treatment of squamous cell carcinoma of the upper aerodigestive tract has the best chance of success, the advantage of complete radiographic assessment before initial therapy is obvious.

Distal Vagal Neuropathy. When physical examination of a patient indicates isolated vocal cord paralysis and if no other cranial nerve dysfunction or oropharyngeal symptoms (normal proximal vagus nerve branch function) are present, a lesion affecting the distal vagus nerve trunk, or recurrent laryngeal nerve, is suspected.

If no mass is palpable, the neck should be imaged with specific attention to the carotid space (vagus nerve trunk) and the tracheoesophageal groove (recurrent laryngeal nerve). Scanning should begin superiorly at the lower oropharynx and should be extended inferiorly to the level of the aortopulmonary window for left vagal paralysis or to the level of the clavicle for right vagal paralysis. This approach directs attention to the levels at which the left and right recurrent laryngeal nerves loop cephalad to run in the tracheoesophageal grooves. In this way occult cervical-thoracic and mediastinal lesions are not overlooked.

Brachial Plexopathy. Two separate clinical situations involving the brachial plexus require tailored imaging of the neck and axillary apex. First, in the patient with arm or shoulder trauma suspected of sustaining proximal nerve root avulsion, axial CT with intrathecal contrast may demonstrate traumatic "pseudomeningoceles" and an absence of the nerve root in the neural foramen. T_1-weighted MRI scans in the sagittal plane permit identification of high-signal-intensity fat without the expected low-signal nerve root in the involved intervertebral foramen. T_2-weighted MRI scans may demonstrate high-signal-intensity cerebrospinal fluid extending outside the spinal canal and neural foramen, within the pseudomeningocele.

The second clinical setting requiring tailored imaging of the brachial plexus involves the patient with symptoms suggesting brachial plexus injury (arm pain, paresthesia, numbness) either with or without a cervical neck mass. In this situation complete imaging requires visualization of the entire brachial plexus. To achieve this axial CT scanning is begun at the level of the hyoid bone and extended inferiorly to the level of the aortic arch. When the cervical-thoracic junction is reached, the magnification factor must be decreased to allow visualization of the brachial plexus as it courses into the axillary apex. Contrary to the beliefs of some, the retroclavicular portion of the axillary apex is poorly examined by palpation. A modified protocol such as the one described prevents inadvertent exclusion of occult axillary apex lesions caused by overmagnification of the scan area.

Coronal MRI scans are ideal for the task of imaging the whole brachial plexus, since the images are acquired in the plane of the plexus. T_1-weighted coronal images obtained with a license plate–type coil placed at the base of the neck, permit one-step imaging in this second clinical setting.

In addition to lesions involving the brachial plexus, the above recommendations are applicable to any lesion of the cervical-thoracic junction. Both demagnified axial CT images or coronal T_1-weighted MRI scans give a clear view of this area and in so doing prevent overfocusing the study, which can lead to exclusion of the lesion from the scan. *Text continued on p. 530.*

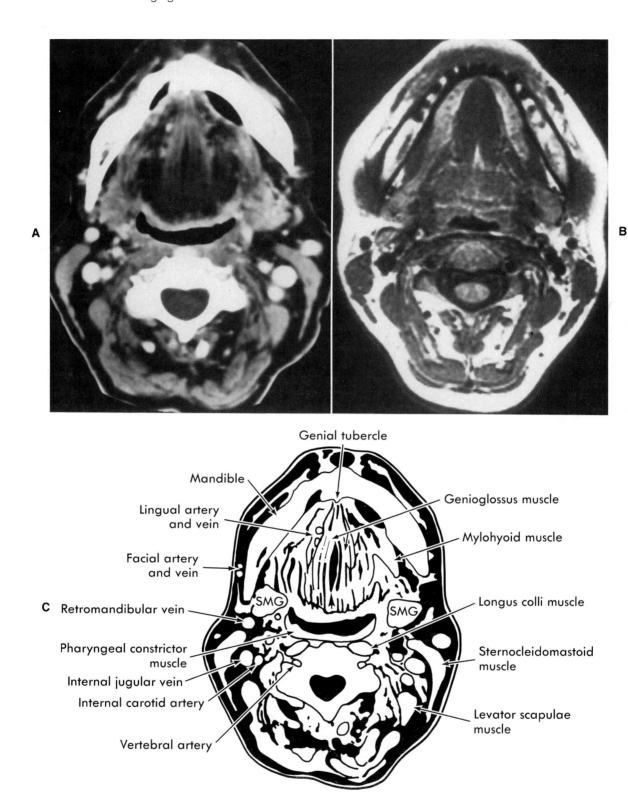

Fig. 8-15 Suprahyoid region of neck. Axial section through high floor of mouth. **A,** CT scan. **B,** MRI sequence. **C,** Line diagram. Arrow, lingual septum; *SMG,* submandibular gland.

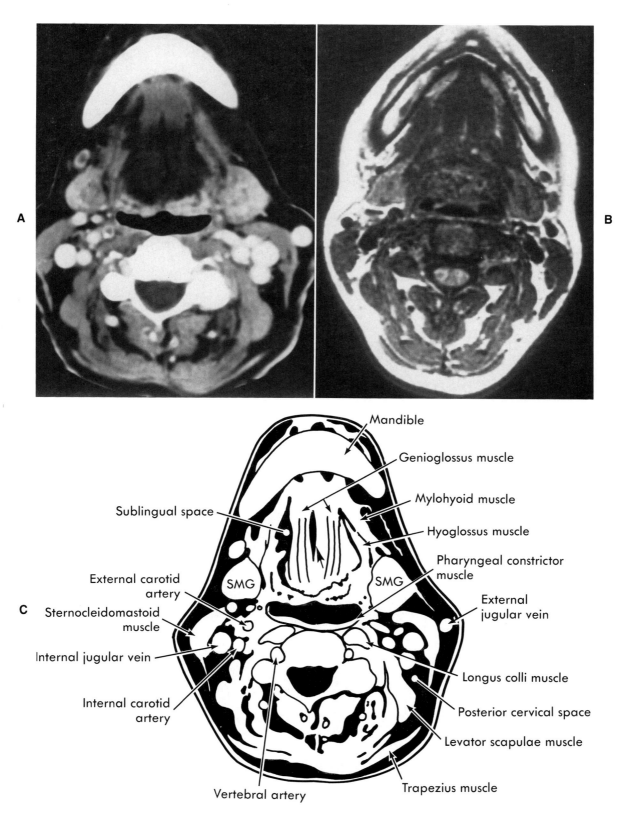

Fig. 8-16 Suprahyoid region of neck. Axial section through midfloor of mouth. **A,** CT scan. **B,** MRI sequence. **C,** Line diagram. *Arrow,* lingual septum; *SMG,* submandibular gland. Fat in posterior cervical space separates sternocleidomastoid muscle from levator scapulae. Fat-filled sublingual space lies between genioglossus and hyoglossus muscles.

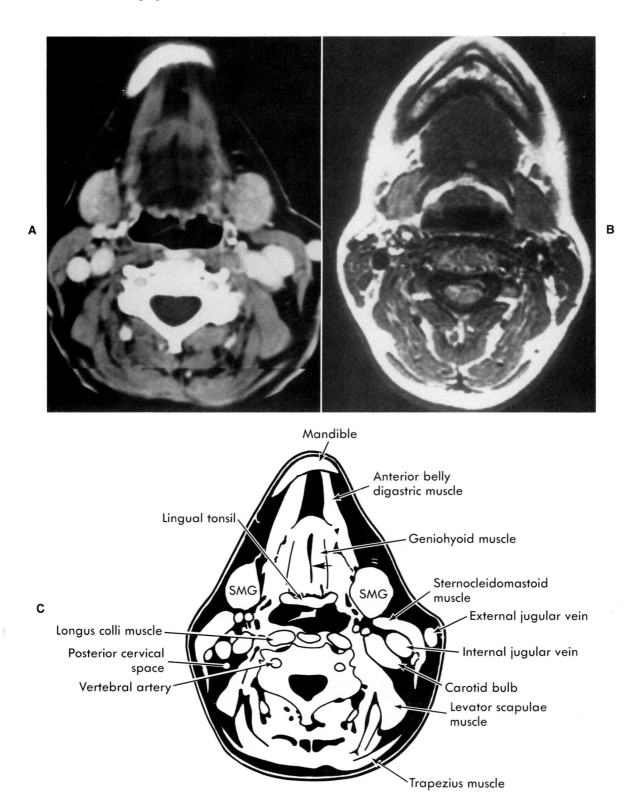

Fig. 8-17 Suprahyoid region of neck. Axial section through low floor of mouth. **A,** CT scan. **B,** MRI sequence. **C,** Line diagram . *Arrow,* lingual septum; *SMG,* submandibular gland. Some fibers of anterior belly of digastric muscle are visualized longitudinally. Uppermost fibers of geniohyoid muscle are visualized in cross-section.

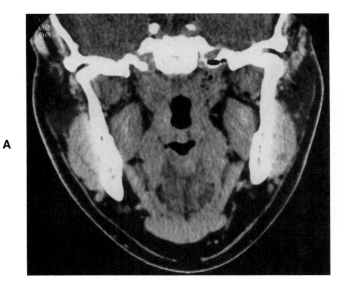

A

Fig. 8-18 Suprahyoid region of neck (coronal section). **A,** CT scan (angled coronal). **B,** Line diagram. **C** and **D,** MRI sequences (nonangled coronal). Muscular sling provided by mylohyoid muscles separates suprahyoid region of neck below from floor of mouth above. Fat-filled parapharyngeal spaces are well visualized on more posterior of MRI scan in **C,** whereas high-signal-intensity fat within sublingual spaces is seen on more anterior MRI scan in **D.**

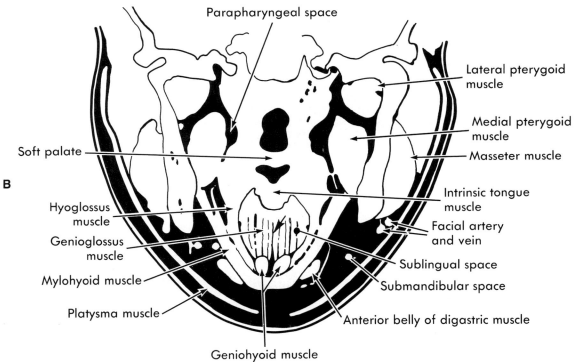

Parapharyngeal space

Lateral pterygoid muscle

Medial pterygoid muscle

Masseter muscle

Soft palate

B

Intrinsic tongue muscle

Hyoglossus muscle

Facial artery and vein

Genioglossus muscle

Sublingual space

Mylohyoid muscle

Submandibular space

Platysma muscle

Anterior belly of digastric muscle

Geniohyoid muscle

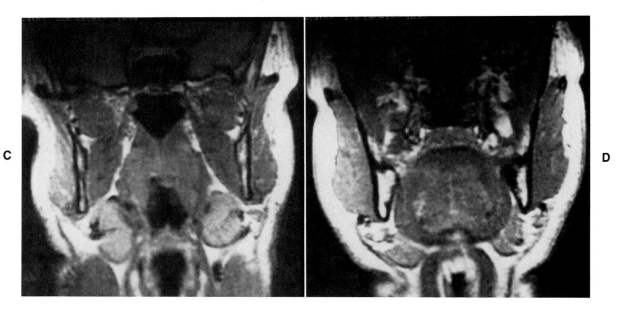

C

D

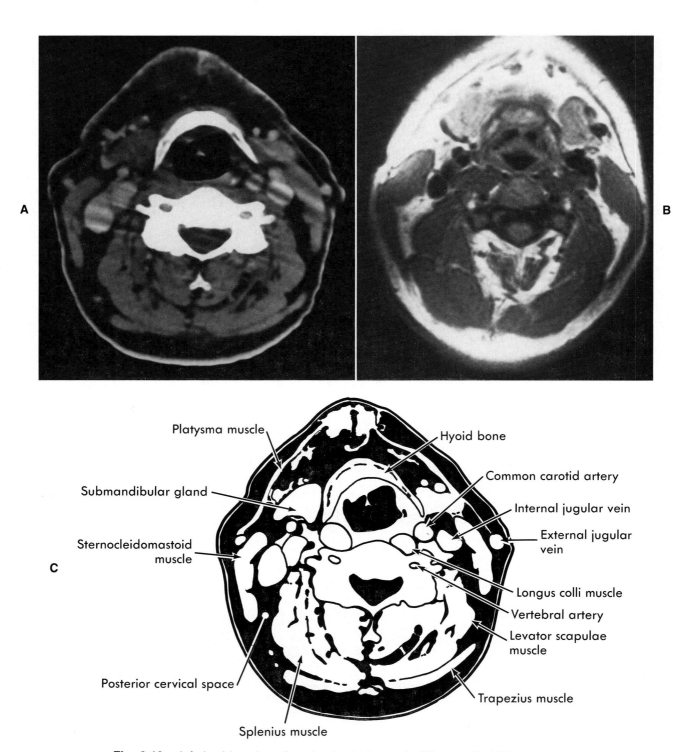

Fig. 8-19 Infrahyoid region of neck—hyoid level. **A,** CT scan. **B,** MRI sequence. **C,** Line diagram. Note fat-filled posterior cervical space. Thin fibers of platysma muscle are visible within subcutaneous fat.

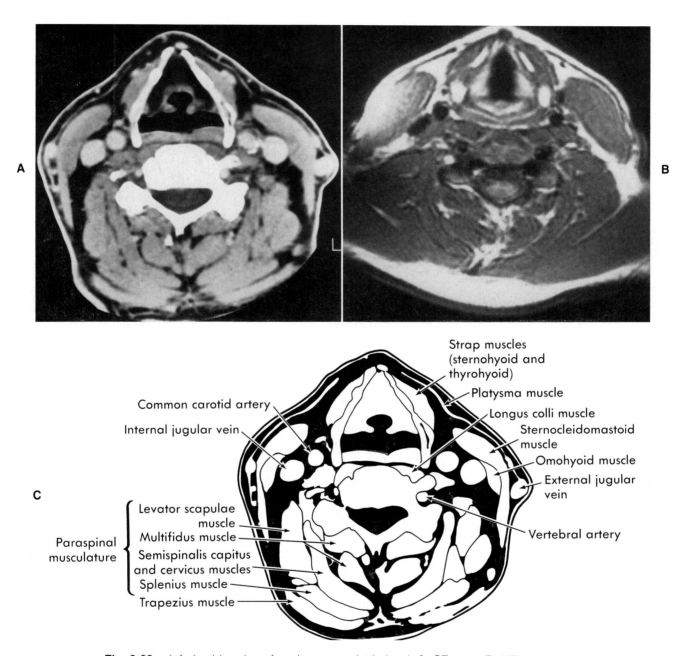

Fig. 8-20 Infrahyoid region of neck—supraglottic level. **A,** CT scan. **B,** MRI sequence. **C,** Line diagram. Various paraspinous muscles are exceptionally well visualized in this section. Fat-filled posterior cervical space separates these muscles from sternocleido-mastoid muscle, which is becoming progressively more anterior in location.

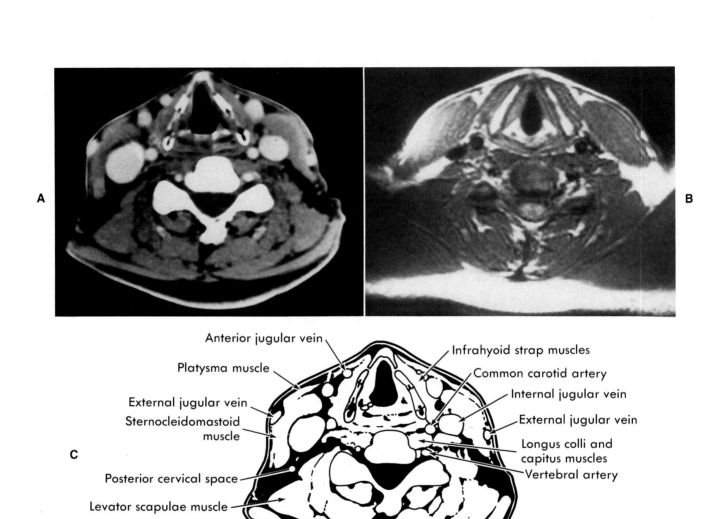

Fig. 8-21 Infrahyoid region of neck—glottic level. **A,** CT scan. **B,** MRI sequence. **C,** Line diagram. Internal jugular veins are becoming asymmetric in size, a normal variation.

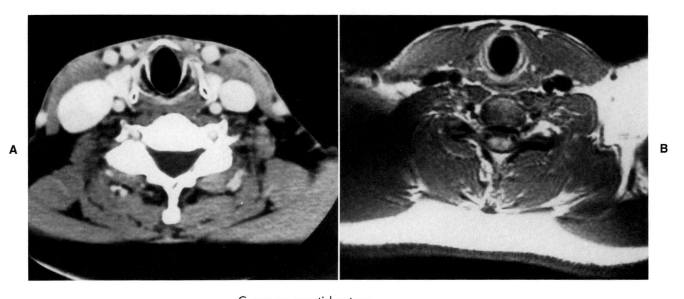

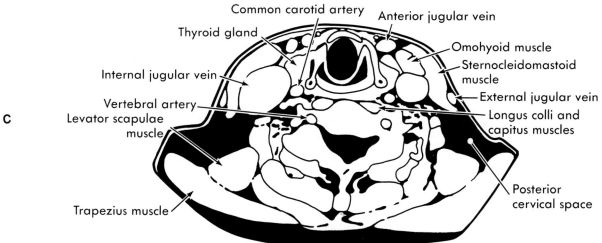

Fig. 8-22 Infrahyoid region of neck—cricoid level. **A,** CT scan. **B,** MRI sequence. **C,** Line diagram.

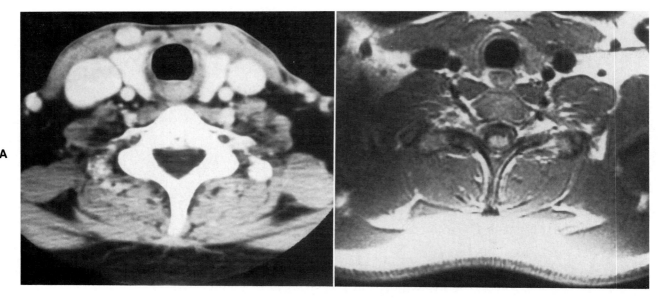

A   B

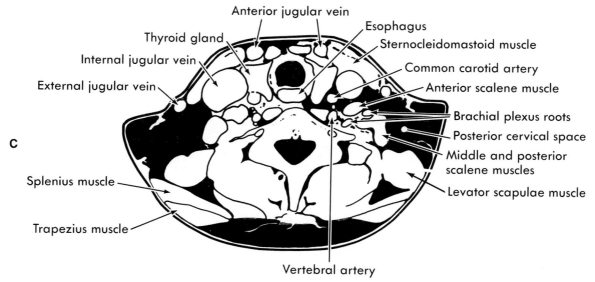

C

Fig. 8-23 Infrahyoid region of neck—first tracheal ring level. **A,** CT scan. **B,** MRI sequence. **C,** Line diagram. External jugular veins are coming to lie progressively more anterior in relation to common carotid arteries. Carotid arteries are in intimate contact with posterior aspect of thyroid gland.

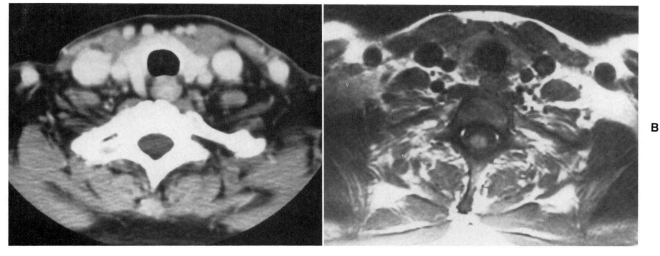

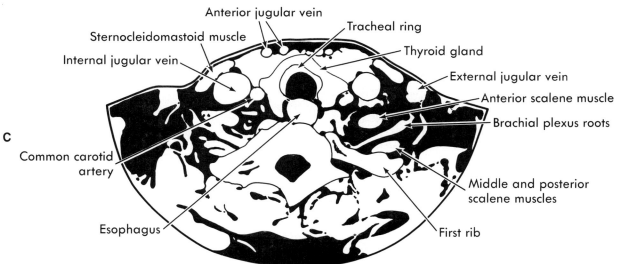

Fig. 8-24 Infrahyoid region of neck—first rib level. **A,** CT scan. **B,** MRI sequence. **C,** Line diagram. Roots of brachial plexus are well demonstrated bilaterally, coursing between anterior and middle scalene muscles. Sternocleidomastoid muscle is represented by thin band just above its origin from clavicle and sternum.

ATLAS OF NORMAL ANATOMY

Figs. 8-15 through 8-18 show the suprahyoid region of the neck, and Figs. 8-19 through 8-24 show the infrahyoid region of the neck.

REFERENCES

1. Moore KL: The developing human, Philadelphia, 1974, WB Saunders Co, pp 136-166.
2. Langman J: Medical embryology, Baltimore, 1969, Williams & Wilkins, pp 237-256.
3. Reede DL, Bergeron RT, and Som PM: CT of thyroglossal duct cysts, Radiology 157:121, 1985.
4. Reede DL, Whelan MA, and Bergeron RT: CT of the soft tissue structures of the neck, Radiol Clin North Am 22:239, 1984.
5. Coit WE et al: Ranulas and their mimics: CT evaluation, Radiology 163:211, 1987.
6. Mancuso AA et al: Computed tomography of cervical and retropharyngeal lymph nodes: normal anatomy, variants of normal, and applications in staging head and neck cancer, Radiology 148:709, 1983.
7. Montgomery RL: Head and neck anatomy with clinical correlations, New York, 1981, McGraw-Hill, Inc.
8. Larsson SG, Mancuso AA, and Hanafee W: Computed tomography of the tongue and floor of the mouth, Radiology 143:493, 1982.
9. Bryan RN et al: Computed tomography of the major salivary glands, AJR 139:547, 1982.
10. Romanes GJ: Cunningham's manual of practical anatomy, vol 3, Head, neck, and brain, London, 1971, Oxford University Press.
11. Smoker WRK, Harnsberger HR, and Osborn AG: The hypoglossal nerve, Semin Ultrasound CT and MR 8:301, 1987.
12. Kellman GM et al: MR imaging of the supraclavicular region: normal anatomy, AJR 148:77, 1987.
13. Reede DL and Bergeron RT: The CT evaluation of the normal and diseased neck, Semin Ultrasound CT and MR 7:181, 1986.
14. Nyberg DA et al: Computed tomography of cervical infections, J Comput Assist Tomogr 9:288, 1985.
15. Stiernberg CM: Deep-neck space infections. Diagnosis and management. Arch Otolaryngol 112:1274, 1986.
16. Hollinshead WH: Anatomy for surgeons, vol 1, The head and neck, ed 2, New York, 1968, Harper & Row, Publishers, Inc, pp 306-330.
17. Last RJ: Anatomy, regional and applied, New York, 1978, Churchill Livingstone, Inc.
18. Hardin CW et al: Infection and tumor of the masticator space: CT evaluation, Radiology 157:413, 1985.
19. Harnsberger HR: CT and MR of masses of the deep face, Curr Probl Diagn Radiol 16:147, 1987.
20. Curtin HD: Separation of the masticator space from the parapharyngeal space, Radiology 163:195, 1987.
21. Paff GH: Anatomy of the head and neck, Philadelphia, 1981, WB Saunders Co.
22. Som PM: Lymph nodes of the neck. Radiology 165:593, 1987.
23. Endicott JN, Nelson RJ, and Saraceno CA: Diagnosis and management decisions in infections of the deep fascial spaces of the head and neck utilizing computerized tomography, Laryngoscope 92:630, 1982.
24. Testut O and Latarjet A: Traite d'anatomie humaine, vol 2, Paris, 1928, Doin, pp 214-221.
25. Som PM, Biller HF, and Lawson W: Tumors of the parapharyngeal space. Preoperative evaluation, diagnosis, and surgical approaches, Ann Otol Rhinol Laryngol 90:1, 1981.
26. Lloyd GAS and Phelps PD: The demonstration of tumors of the parapharyngeal space by magnetic resonance imaging, Br J Radiol 59:675, 1986.
27. Unger JM: Computed tomography of the parapharyngeal space, CRC Crit Rev Diagn Imaging 26:265, 1987.
28. Silver AJ, Ganti SR, and Hilal SK: The carotid region. Normal and pathologic anatomy on CT, Radiol Clin North Am 22:219, 1984.
29. Silver AJ et al: Computed tomography of the carotid space and related cervical spaces. I. Anatomy, Radiology 150:723, 1984.
30. Hardin CW et al: CT in the evaluation of the normal and diseased oral cavity and oropharynx, Semin Ultrasound CT and MR 7:131, 1986.
31. Smoker WRK and Gentry LR: Computed tomography of the nasopharynx, Semin Ultrasound CT and MR 7:107, 1986.
32. Som PM et al: Parapharyngeal space masses: an updated protocol based upon 104 cases, Radiology 153:149, 1984.
33. Lufkin RB and Hanafee W: MRI of the head and neck, Magn Reson Imaging 6:69, 1988.
34. Kulkarni MV, Patton JA, and Price RR: Technical considerations for the use of surface coils in MRI, AJR 147:373, 1986.
35. Lufkin RB et al: Solenoid surface coils in magnetic resonance imaging, AJR 146:409, 1986.
36. Som PM et al: Tumors of the parapharyngeal space and upper neck: MR imaging characteristics, Radiology 164:823, 1987.

SECTION TWO

NONNODAL PATHOLOGIC CONDITIONS OF THE NECK

DEBORAH L. REEDE
ROY A. HOLLIDAY
PETER M. SOM
R. THOMAS BERGERON

CT and MRI have proved invaluable in evaluating neck masses. These imaging modalities are useful in defining the precise location of a lesion and its effect on adjacent structures. Correlation of the radiographic findings with the clinical history frequently enables the clinician to predict the tissue diagnosis with a high degree of accuracy. As a first step, however, the normal CT and MRI anatomy be mastered.

Most neck masses are located in the infrahyoid portion of the neck. Attentiveness to several facts leads to greater diagnostic accuracy: (1) As a general rule, neck masses in children tend to be benign. Reactive lymphadenopathy secondary to infection and congenital lesions accounts for most masses in this age group. Thyroglossal duct cysts, branchial cleft cysts, and cystic hygromas account for most of the benign congenital lesions. (2) Lymphoma is the most common head and neck malignancy in children; rhabdomyosarcoma is the second most common.[1] (3) If thyroid lesions are excluded, a unilateral neck mass usually is malignant in young and middle-aged adults (21 to 40 years of age). The most common disease in this age group is lymphoma. (4) Metastatic disease accounts for most neck masses in patients over 40 years of age.[2]

CONGENITAL LESIONS

Thyroglossal duct cysts, branchial cleft cysts, cystic hygromas, lymphangiomas, and dermoid cysts are common congenital lesions of the neck. The thyroglossal duct cyst is the most common nonodontogenic cyst that occurs in that area,[3] accounting for approximately 90% of congenital neck abnormalities.[4] Dermoid cysts are the rarest of "common" congenital lesions in the neck.

Thyroglossal Duct Cysts

Thyroglossal duct cysts usually are found in children, but they are not necessarily uncommon in adults. The embryology of the thyroid gland explains the location of this lesion and that of other lesions related to abnormal thyroid development (lingual thyroid and ectopic thyroid tissue).

The thyroid gland begins as a midline outgrowth from the floor of the pharynx between the first and second branchial pouches at about 3 weeks of gestation. The thyroid primordium forms an epithelial-lined tubular structure, the thyroglossal duct. The duct's site of origin is the foramen cecum, which is located behind the V-shaped row of circumvallate papillae in the base of the tongue. The duct penetrates the underlying mesoderm, enlarges, and descends as a bilobed diverticulum. En route from the base of the tongue to the lower neck, it passes through the tongue musculature, the mylohyoid muscle of the floor of the mouth, and the anterior triangle of the neck. It loops around the inferior border of the hyoid bone and extends upward either through the hyoid body or into the concavity of the posterior surface of the hyoid. From this point it renews its inferior course, coming to lie anterior to the thyrohyoid membrane and strap muscles before ending at what will be the level of the thyroid isthmus[5] (Fig. 8-25). By 7 weeks of gestation the thyroid gland has traversed the length of the duct and reached its final position, in front of and lateral to the trachea. The duct normally involutes, atrophies, and disappears by 8 to 10 weeks of gestation. The duct's caudal attachment may persist as the pyramidal lobe of the thyroid gland.[3,6]

The migration of the thyroid gland can be arrested anywhere along the course of the thyroglossal duct. A lingual thyroid results when the gland totally fails to migrate inferiorly from the level of the foramen cecum (Fig. 8-26). Even when the thyroid gland is located in its normal position in the lower neck, fragments of thyroid tissue may be found anywhere along the course of the thyroglossal duct.[7,8]

Because the duct is lined with secretory epithelium,[9-11] a cyst may form if any portion of the thyroglossal duct fails to involute. Two mechanisms have been proposed for the development of these cysts: (1) Inflammatory changes in the adjacent tissue stimulate the epithelial-lined remnant of the duct to secrete and then undergo cystic change. (2) Occasionally a persistent tract with secretory epithelium drains into the region of the foramen cecum. If this point of drainage becomes obstructed, secretions accumulate and a cyst forms, even without inflammation.[8]

As stated, these cysts can arise anywhere along the

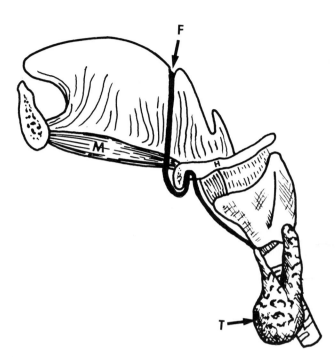

Fig. 8-25 Course of thyroglossal duct. *F*, Foramen cecum; *M*, mylohyoid muscle; *T*, thyroid gland; *H*, hyoid bone. (From Reede DL: CT of thyroglossal duct cyst, Radiology 157:123, 1985.)

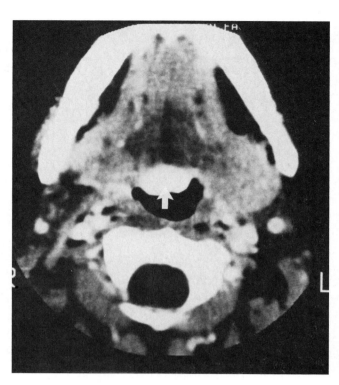

Fig. 8-26 Lingual thyroid. Enhancing mass is seen near base of tongue *(arrow)*.

course of the thyroglossal duct and may be midline or off-midline in location. However, most cysts are located below the level of the hyoid bone in the region of the thyrohyoid membrane. Batsakis[12] provides the following statistics for cyst location: suprahyoid region, 20%; at the level of the hyoid bone, 15%; and infrahyoid region, 65%.

Most patients with thyroglossal duct cysts have asymptomatic neck masses (unless there are local inflammatory changes) in the anterior triangles of the neck. Lesions above the thyroid cartilage usually are in the midline, whereas those at the level of the cartilage tend to be off the midline. Overall about 75% of thyroglossal duct cysts occur in the midline, making them the most common midline neck masses. Although the firmness of these lesions varies on physical examination, the lesions generally are mobile, regardless of their firmness. If an attachment persists between either the base of the tongue or the hyoid bone, the cyst moves when the tongue is protruded. Fistulas are uncommon but can occur secondary to infection, rupture of the cyst, or as a postoperative complication.

A carcinoma coexists in a thyroglossal duct cyst in fewer than 1% of patients, and invariably the carcinoma is of thyroid gland origin. Papillary carcinoma accounts for 85% of these carcinomas.[12] These carcinomas usually are discovered as incidental findings at the time of

surgery. They arise presumably in ectopic thyroid tissue along the course of the thyroglossal duct rather than from ductal tissue. The reported incidence of ectopic thyroid tissue along the thyroglossal tract varies widely, with figures ranging from 0.6% to 36.5%.[13,14] The low incidence of carcinoma developing within a cyst probably is the result of the observation that more than two thirds of patients who have residual thyroglossal duct tracts have no thyroid tissue within the tract.[15]

Surgery is the treatment of choice for these lesions, because they may become infected. Complete removal may be difficult. These cysts are more likely to recur when a sinus tract is present or if the patient has had previous surgery. Removing the entire tract of the duct, the midportion of the hyoid bone, and a portion of the base of the tongue (Sistrunk procedure) has decreased the rate of recurrence from 50% to 20%.[8]

Routine preoperative cross-sectional imaging is not performed in children who are thought to have a thyroglossal duct cyst, because the clinical presentation is so typical. However, adult patients with a similar clinical presentation are evaluated radiographically to rule out other lesions and to confirm the diagnosis. The radiographic characteristics of these lesions have been described: On a contrast-enhanced CT scan, the lesion appears as a low-density mass with a uniformly thin peripheral rim of enhancement (capsule). Septations occa-

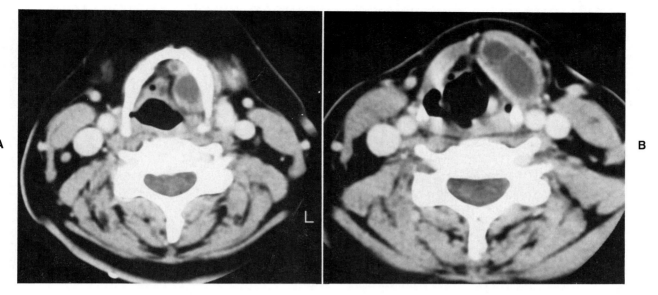

Fig. 8-27   Thyroglossal duct cyst. Contrast-enhanced CT scans at level of hyoid bone **(A)** and thyroid cartilage **(B)** show low-density mass with peripheral rim enhancement. Mass is posterior to hyoid bone in **A** and embedded in strap muscles. Note septation within mass in **B**.

sionally are seen (Fig. 8-27).[16] The adjacent soft tissues are normal unless the cyst is infected. An infected cyst may have a density approaching that of muscle because of the increased protein in the cyst's contents. Since these lesions can occur anywhere along the course of the thyroglossal duct, they can be found not only in the neck but also in the tongue (Fig. 8-28) and the floor of the mouth. On an MRI scan these lesions have an intermediate signal intensity on T_1-weighted images and a high signal intensity on T_2-weighted images (Fig. 8-29, A and B).

It should be noted that lesions located at or below the level of the hyoid bone invariably are *embedded* in the strap muscles adjacent to the outer margin of the thyroid cartilage (Fig. 8-30). This is an important observation that allows differentiation of thyroglossal duct cysts from other low-density lesions in this region, such as necrotic anterior cervical nodes (Fig. 8-31), a thrombosed anterior jugular vein, an abscess (Fig. 8-32), and lipoma (Fig. 8-33). Unlike the thyroglossal duct cyst, these other lesions are found *superficial* to the strap muscles.

A laryngocele with an external component may appear as an anterior lateral neck mass and may be filled with either air or fluid (obstructed laryngocele). An obstructed laryngocele can be mistaken for a thyroglossal duct cyst on a single cross-sectional image. However, careful assessment of sequential images resolves any confusion, because laryngoceles are located within the confines of the cartilaginous framework of the larynx and communicate with the laryngeal ventricle. Large

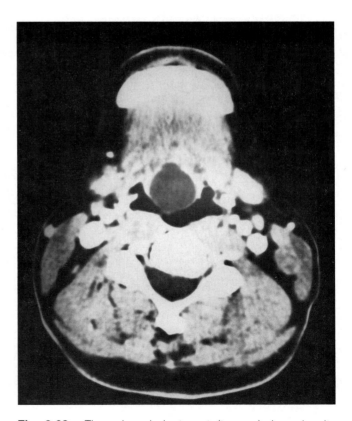

Fig. 8-28   Thyroglossal duct cyst (tongue). Low-density mass is seen in base of tongue.

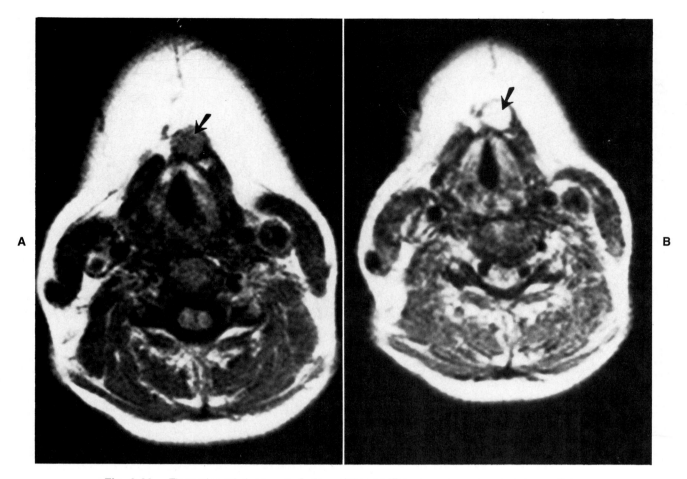

Fig. 8-29 Thyroglossal duct cyst. **A,** T$_1$-weighted MR image shows low-to-intermediate signal intensity mass *(arrow)* embedded in strap muscles. **B,** Lesion becomes hyperintense on T$_2$-weighted sequence.

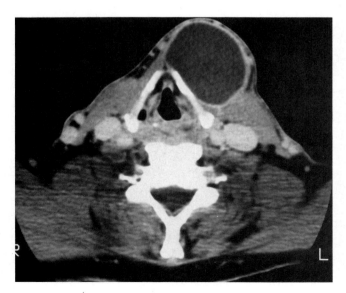

Fig. 8-30 Thyroglossal duct cyst. Low-density mass with peripheral rim enhancement is seen embedded in strap muscles on left.

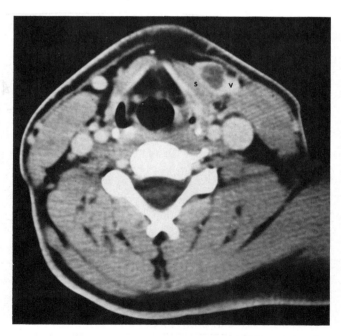

Fig. 8-31 Necrotic anterior cervical node. Low-density mass with peripheral rim enhancement is seen superficial to strap muscles *(S)* and anterior to anterior jugular vein *(V)* on left.

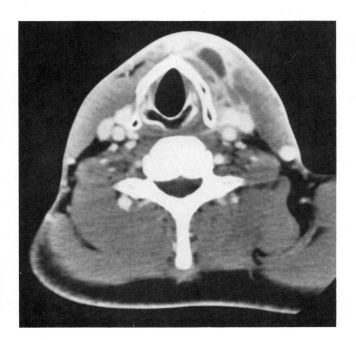

Fig. 8-32 Abscess. Contrast-enhanced CT scan shows low-density mass with peripheral rim enhancement. Fascial planes adjacent to mass are abnormal, and overlying skin is thickened.

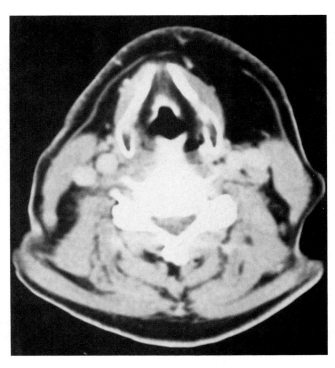

Fig. 8-33 Lipoma. Mass of same density as subcutaneous fat is seen adjacent to left strap muscles.

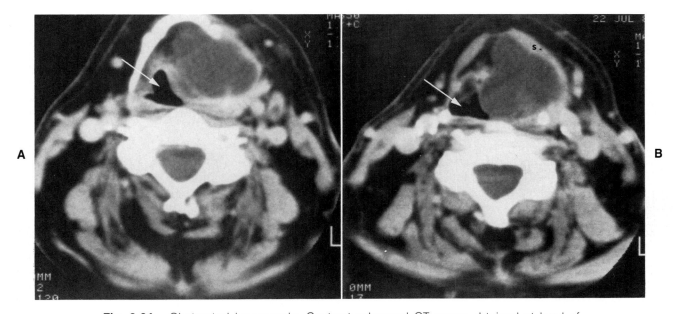

Fig. 8-34 Obstructed laryngocele. Contrast-enhanced CT scans obtained at level of hyoid bone **(A)** and below **(B)** demonstrate low-density mass in left preepiglottic and paraglottic spaces. Airway *(arrow)* is displaced to right, and strap muscles *(S)* are bowed laterally. Portion of lesion extends lateral to hyoid bone into neck. Lesion lies deep to strap muscles and displaces them but is not embedded in them. (From Reede DL: CT of thyroglossal duct cyst, Radiology 157:125, 1985.)

laryngoceles grow through the thyrohyoid membrane and are found *deep* to the strap muscles, neither approaching them from the superficial surface nor lying embedded within them (Fig. 8-34).

Branchial Cleft Cysts

The face and neck structures are derivatives of the branchial apparatus. They develop and differentiate between 4 and 7 weeks of gestation. These structures are described in the first section of this chapter, but specific points of interest that are germane to this discussion include the following:

1. The first branchial cleft gives rise to a definitive structure in the embryo, the external auditory canal. This cleft is unique in that respect.
2. The mesoderm in the second branchial arch proliferates and fuses caudally with the epicardiac ridge in the lower neck, obliterating the communication of the second through fourth clefts with the skin's surface. The second through fourth clefts fuse to form an epithelial-lined cavity called the *cervical sinus*. Subsequently this sinus (normally) disappears.

A branchial cleft cyst, sinus, or fistula may develop if one of the following occurs:

1. Failure of the second arch to proliferate.
2. Incomplete caudal migration of the arch.
3. Failure of the cervical sinus to obliterate.
4. Failure of the pouch remnants to obliterate. The second arch gives rise to the platysma muscle; this explains why abnormalities of the branchial apparatus usually are located deep to the platysma.
5. The mesoderm from which the sternocleidomastoid muscle develops is just behind the second branchial cleft. This relationship accounts for the fact that small second cleft cysts and their sinuses or fistulas occur just anterior to this muscle.

Sinuses are tracts with or without a cyst that communicate with either the skin or the gut. A fistula is a communication between the gut and the skin. There are a number of theories about the pathogenesis of these abnormalities in the neck. The generally accepted theory holds that sinuses are vestigial branchial pouches or clefts, and that fistulas arise from remnants of either pouches or clefts with rupture of the interposing branchial plate. Cysts arise from entrapped remnants of either the branchial clefts or pouches.[17]

Branchial abnormalities can arise from any of the pouches or clefts. Based on the pouch or cyst of origin, the precise location of these abnormalities often can be predicted.

Two types of sinuses arise from the first branchial apparatus. Type I cysts are located inferomedially and posterior to the pinna and concha of the ear. However, they can drain anterior to the ear. In other cases they are superior to the main trunk of the facial nerve and are parallel to and/or terminate in the external auditory canal, or mesotympanium. Type II lesions appear as superficial cysts or sinuses in the anterior triangle of the neck below the angle of the mandible. These lesions pass through the parotid and over the angle of the mandible in close proximity to the facial nerve and terminate in the bony or cartilaginous portion of the external auditory canal.

Only 8% of all branchial abnormalities arise from the first branchial apparatus; cysts and sinuses occur with equal frequency.[18]

Sinuses arising from the first branchial cleft should be suspected if persistent aural discharge is present without middle ear disease. Such a history, in conjunction with the presence or history of a mass or abscess in the neck, should increase suspicion that a type I sinus is present.

Lesions of the second branchial apparatus are the most common type of lesion and account for 95% of all branchial abnormalities. Cysts are more common than sinuses or fistulas in this group.[17] Second branchial apparatus lesions appear as either a mass or a sinus anterior to the middle to lower portion of the sternocleidomastoid muscle. The path of this lesion begins at the base of the tonsillar fossa; near the level of the hyoid bone, it passes superiorly between the stylohyoid ligament and hypoglossal nerve and then extends inferiorly between the internal and external carotid arteries. The course then is lateral to the carotid sheath structures. Although a cyst can occur anywhere along this path, the most common location is lateral to the internal jugular vein at the level of the carotid bifurcation.

A third branchial apparatus sinus tract is a rare lesion that passes from the pyriform sinus laterally between the common carotid artery and vagus nerve and then appears in the lateral part of the neck along the anterior margin of the lower third of the sternocleidomastoid muscle.

Fourth branchial pouch sinuses are even rarer than third branchial apparatus lesions. The fourth arch tract arises in one apex of the pyriform sinuses, passes caudally on the left side behind the aortic arch, under this vessel, and then courses superiorly in the neck, posterior to the common carotid artery. The tract then courses downward, looping over the hypoglossal nerve to open in the skin along the lower anterior edge of the sternocleidomastoid muscle. The lesion is found on the left side in 93% of cases. On the right side the tract passes behind, then under the right subclavian artery to ascend in the neck.[19]

As stated, most branchial cysts arise from the second branchial apparatus. These lesions may be associated with a sinus or fistula tract. If so, the opening on the skin is adjacent to the anterior border of the sternoclei-

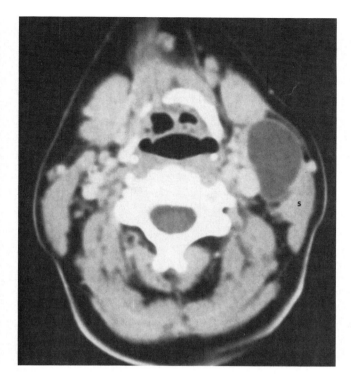

Fig. 8-35 Second branchial cleft cyst. Contrast-enhanced CT scan at level of hyoid bone shows low-density mass on left. No peripheral rim enhancement is noted. Mass is located adjacent to anterior border of sternocleidomastoid muscle *(S)* and anterolateral to carotid sheath structures.

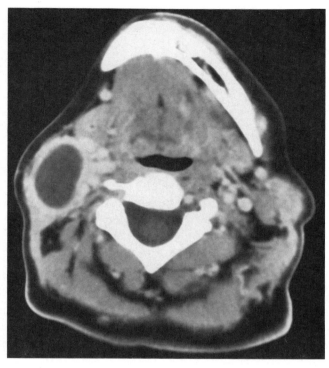

Fig. 8-36 Infected second branchial cleft cyst. Contrast-enhanced CT scan obtained at angle of mandible shows low-density mass with peripheral rim enhancement on right. Fascial planes adjacent to mass are abnormal.

domastoid muscle in its middle or lower portion. The usual clinical presentation is that of a painless neck mass just below the angle of the mandible along the anterior border of the sternocleidomastoid muscle. These cysts are lined with squamous epithelium with subepithelial lymphoid tissue. The initial presentation or enlargement of these cysts often is associated with an upper respiratory tract infection or trauma.[20] The patient usually is between 10 and 40 years of age when these lesions appear. Coexisting carcinomas in these lesions are rare.

Cysts arising from the branchial apparatus are readily identified on cross-sectional imaging. On a CT scan these lesions are low density and have a well-circumscribed rim. Peripheral rim enhancement may not be present (Fig. 8-35); however, the presence of peripheral rim enhancement usually indicates a coexisting infection (Fig. 8-36). Displacement of adjacent structures is a characteristic feature. The sternocleidomastoid muscle is displaced posterolaterally or posteriorly, the carotid sheath structures are displaced posteromedially or medially, and the submandibular gland is displaced anteriorly.[21] When the cysts are large, they may be located almost entirely deep to the sternocleidomastoid

muscle, lying in the posterior triangle of the neck. The fascial planes adjacent to these lesions usually are preserved and well defined unless the cyst is infected or a recent needle aspiration has been performed. Occasionally septations are seen in these lesions (Fig. 8-37). Necrotic nodes (Fig. 8-38), abscesses, cystic neural lesions, and thrombosed vessels may mimic a branchial cleft cyst on cross-sectional imaging.

MR imaging of a branchial cleft cyst demonstrates a cyst with quite variable wall thickness, depending on whether there has been a previous infection. The signal characteristics of these cysts vary considerably on T_1-weighted sequences. The cysts may be hypointense or slightly hyperintense to muscle on T_1-weighted sequences (Fig. 8-39, *A* and *B*). These cysts are hyperintense on T_2-weighted images. Inflammatory changes in the adjacent soft tissues often are hyperintense to fat on T_2-weighted images[22] (Fig. 8-40, *A* and *B*).

Cystic Hygromas and Lymphangiomas

Cystic hygromas are benign, nonencapsulated lesions that arise from lymphoid tissue. These lesions are classified into three groups, based on the size of the abnormal lymphatic spaces: (1) *lymphangioma simplex*, com-

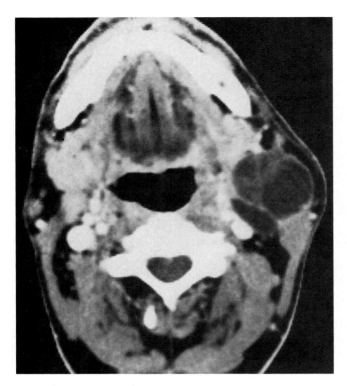

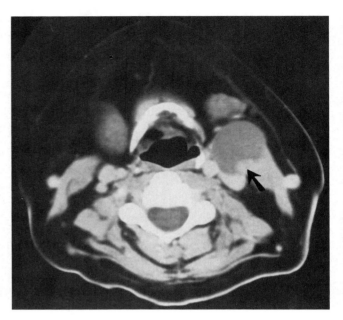

Fig. 8-37 Septated second branchial cleft cyst. Low-density septated mass without peripheral rim enhancement is seen on left side of neck. Location is similar to that of other branchial cleft cysts shown.

Fig. 8-38 Low-density node—metastatic thyroid carcinoma. Mass is seen on left side of neck in location similar to that of type II branchial cleft cyst. However, note soft tissue mass *(arrow)* in posterior aspect of low-density mass.

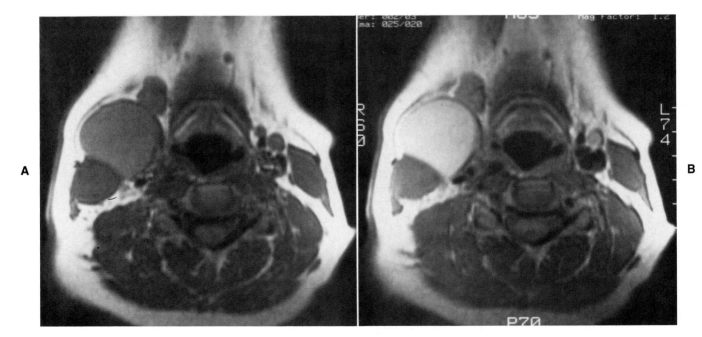

Fig. 8-39 Second branchial cleft cyst. **A,** T_1-weighted MRI shows lesion that is hypointense to muscle on right side of neck. Lesion is anterior to sternocleidomastoid muscle and carotid sheath structures. **B,** On T_2-weighted MRI, mass becomes hyperintense.

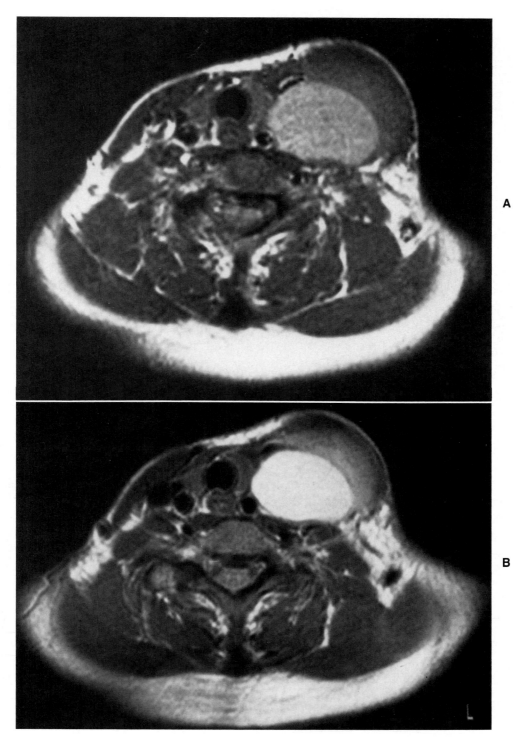

Fig. 8-40 Infected third branchial cleft cyst. **A,** T_1-weighted MRI at level of thyroid gland shows hypointense mass deep to left sternocleidomastoid muscle and posterolateral to carotid sheath structures. Left sternocleidomastoid muscle is enlarged. **B,** Mass and left sternocleidomastoid muscle become hyperintense on T_2-weighted MRI sequence.

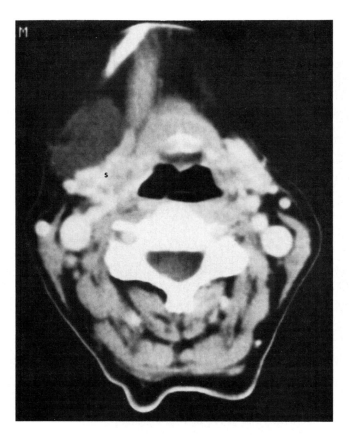

Fig. 8-41 Cystic hygroma—submandibular triangle. Nonenhancing low-density mass is seen in right submandibular triangle. Mass is compressing submandibular gland *(S)*.

posed of small, capillary-sized, thin-walled lymphatic channels; (2) *cavernous lymphangiomas*, composed of dilated lymphatics with a fibrous adventitia; and (3) *cystic hygromas*, composed of cysts that range in size from a few millimeters to several centimeters in diameter.[23] All three of these histologic types can be found in any lesion. The preponderance of one type dictates how the lesion is classified. Cystic hygromas are filled with either straw-colored fluid or milky chylous fluid. Most (75%) occur in the neck, and 20% occur in the axilla, and the remaining 5% arise in rare locations such as the mediastinum, retroperitoneum, bone, kidney, colon, liver, spleen, and scrotum.[24,25] Only 3% to 10% of neck lesions extend into the mediastinum.[26]

The most widely accepted theory about the development of these lesions is that they arise from sequestrations of the primitive embryonic lymph sacs. The lymphatic system develops from primitive sacs that are derived from the venous system. There are five sacs: two jugular, two posterior, and one retroperitoneal. At approximately 6 weeks of gestation the jugular lymphatic sacs into which the lymphatic channels in the upper extremities drain open into the jugular vein.[27] The jugu-

lar sacs become the terminal portions of the right lymphatic duct and thoracic ducts. If the communication between the jugular sac and the jugular vein fails to develop, the jugular sac dilates and fills with lymph, resulting in a host of consequences referred to as a "jugular lymphatic obstruction sequence."[27] Distension of the jugular sac causes excess growth of skin in the region of the distended sac, alters the zone of hair growth, and occasionally causes a protrusion of the lower auricle of the developing ear. Peripheral edema also develops. This may be incompatible with life, but if a communication between the lymphatic and venous systems develops before intrauterine death occurs, the cystic hygroma decreases in size and the amount of peripheral edema also decreases. This sequence of events accounts for the clinical features of patients with Turner's syndrome, that is, webbed neck, peripheral lymphedema, and low-set ears. A local defect in the communication between the lymphatic and venous systems, produces an isolated cystic hygroma. Extensive defects in this communication result in fetal hydrops.

A number of congenital malformation syndromes besides Turner's syndrome have been seen in association with fetal cystic hygromas, webbed neck, or redundant skin over the posterior aspect of the neck. These syndromes include fetal alcohol syndrome, Noonan's syndrome, familial pterygium colli, distichiasis-lymphedema syndrome, and several chromosomal aneuploidies.[28]

Most lymphangiomas occur in early childhood, because the greatest lymphatic development occurs between birth and 2 years of age. Of these lesions, 50% to 60% are present at birth, and 80% to 90% are detected by 2 years of age. A few cases have been reported in the fourth and fifth decades of life.[12,29] In adults, solitary cystic hygromas have been found in the submandibular and posterior triangles of the neck. These lesions may be the result of trauma rather than of congenital origin.

Cystic hygromas appear as painless neck masses that are compressible and, if large, they will transilluminate. The lesions commonly occur in the posterior triangle of the neck, although large lesions may extend into the anterior triangle. Cystic hygromas also can be found in the floor of the mouth and in the submandibular triangles (Fig. 8-41).

Prenatal and postnatal diagnosis of cystic hygromas can be made using ultrasound (Fig. 8-42). Sonographically these lesions are multiloculated, predominantly cystic masses with septa of variable thickness. Solid components related to the cyst wall or septa are seen in these cysts. Pathologic correlation shows that the echogenic components comprise abnormal clusters of lymphatic channels that are too small to be resolved on ultrasound.[30]

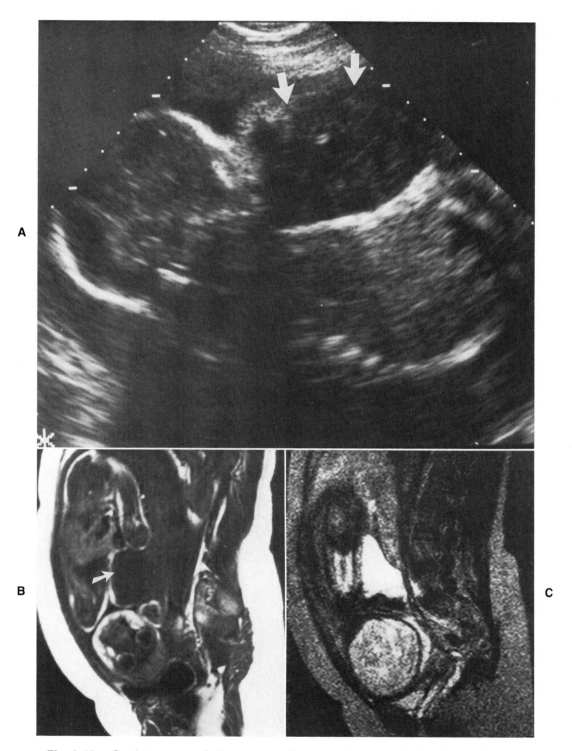

Fig. 8-42 Cystic hygroma. **A,** Intrauterine ultrasound shows predominantly cystic mass with scattered internal echoes, inferior to face of fetus *(arrows)*. **B,** T$_1$-weighted MRI of fetus in utero shows mass that is isointense to muscle *(arrow),* which becomes hyperintense on **C,** T$_2$-weighted sequence.

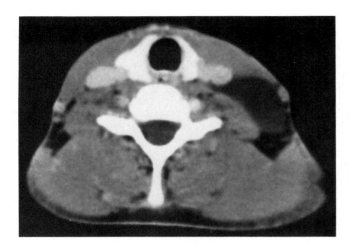

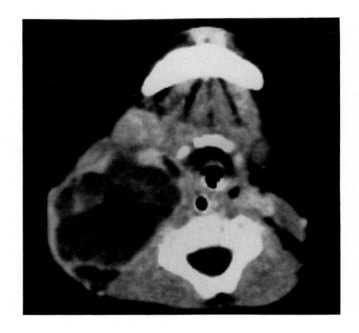

Fig. 8-43 Cystic hygroma. Contrast-enhanced CT scan at level of thyroid gland shows nonenhancing low-density mass in posterior triangle on left side of neck. Adjacent soft tissues are normal.

Fig. 8-44 Cystic hygroma. Multiloculated low-density mass is demonstrated on right side of neck. Fascial planes adjacent to mass are poorly defined. Mass displaces carotid sheath structures anteriorly.

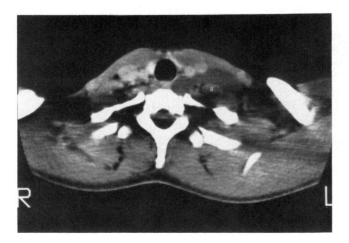

Fig. 8-45 Cystic hygroma. Well-circumscribed, nonenhancing, low-density mass is seen in left posterior triangle. Note that anterior scalene muscle (S) and carotid sheath structures are making indentations on lesion.

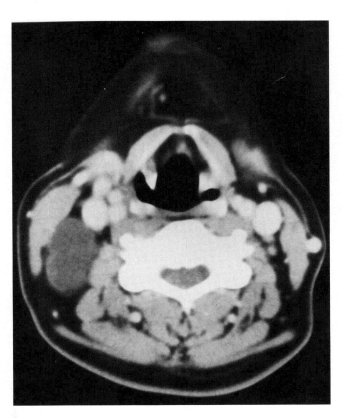

Fig. 8-46 Lymphoma. Low-density mass is seen in right posterior triangle; this is an enlarged lymph node. Adjacent structures are not compressing lesion.

Cross-sectional imaging either with CT or MRI is superior to ultrasound in mapping out the extent of the lesions. On a contrast-enhanced CT scan, cystic hygromas are low density in appearance without peripheral rim enhancement. Smaller lesions tend to be unilocular and well circumscribed (Fig. 8-43). Larger lesions are multiloculated and may be poorly circumscribed (Fig. 8-44).[24,31,32] Since the lesions are compressible, they do not displace adjacent soft tissue structures (muscles and blood vessels); instead, those structures often compress the lesion (Fig. 8-45). This observation may allow differentiation of a cystic hygroma from other low-density, nonenhancing lesions such as low-density lymph nodes (Fig. 8-46), neural tumors, and a branchial cleft cyst with a posterior triangle component. Some cystic lymphangiomas can infiltrate adjacent nerves, vessels, and muscle, making it difficult or impossible to extirpate the lesion without sacrificing major normal function.

On T$_1$-weighted MRI sequences cystic hygromas usually are hypointense to muscle unless there has been previous surgery, hemorrhage, or infection (Fig. 8-47, *A*). As with other cystic lesions, cystic hygromas usually are hyperintense on T$_2$-weighted sequences (Fig. 8-47, *B*).[22]

These lesions can enlarge rapidly if hemorrhage into the lesion occurs. Such hemorrhage produces a fluid-fluid level that can be seen on CT or MRI. MRI, however, is more sensitive for detecting hemorrhage (Fig. 8-48, *A* and *B*). If the lesion involves the parotid gland and if hemorrhage occurs within the cyst, compression of the facial nerve can result in facial nerve paralysis.

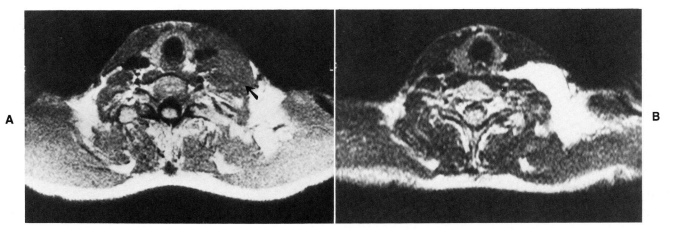

Fig. 8-47 Cystic hygroma. **A,** Lesion *(arrow)* slightly hypointense to muscle is seen posterior to carotid sheath structures and deep to sternocleidomastoid muscle on left. **B,** Lesion becomes hyperintense on more T$_2$-weighted MRI sequences.

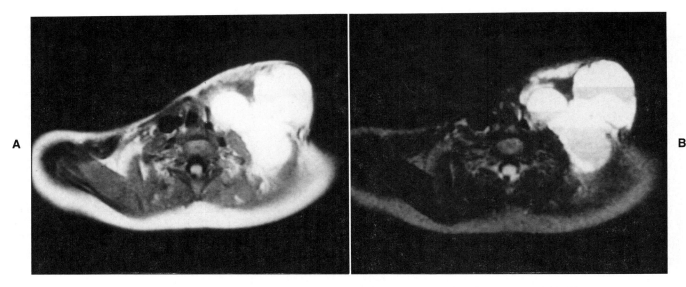

Fig. 8-48 Cystic hygroma with hemorrhage. **A,** T₁-weighted MRI scan and **B,** T₂-weighted image show multiloculated mass in anterior and posterior triangles on left side of neck. Fluid-fluid levels are seen secondary to hemorrhage. Hemorrhage is hyperintense on both T₁- and T₂-weighted MRI sequences; cyst fluid is hyperintense on T₁-weighted image and hypointense on T₂-weighted sequence.

Dermoid Cysts

The term "dermoid cyst" is used to describe a number of cystic lesions that occur in the body. New and Erich cataloged three types of dermoid cysts[33]:

1. A congenital dermoid cyst of the teratoma type found primarily in the testes and ovaries.
2. A dermoid cyst acquired by implantation.
3. A congenital inclusion cyst found along lines of embryologic fusion.

In the head and neck, the term *dermoid cyst* is used to describe three histologically different types of cyst[33]:

1. An epidermoid or epidermal cyst, which has an epithelial lining surrounded by a fibrous capsule and no skin appendages.
2. A dermoid cyst, which has an epithelial lining with skin appendages.
3. A teratoid cyst, which has an epithelial lining and a fibrous capsule and contains skin appendages and connective tissue derivatives.

In the head and neck the epidermal variety is the most common and the teratoid type is the rarest.

Only 7% of all dermoid tumors occur in the head and neck; 80% of these tumors occur in the orbit, oral, and nasal regions.[33] Those found in the oral region are located in the sublingual or submental spaces. Although the lesions found in the oral region are thought to be present at birth, they usually are not identified clinically until the second or third decade of life. In contrast, the epidermoid variety is more common in infants. Cervical dermoid lesions usually are present at birth and rarely are encountered after 1 year of age.[12]

Dermoid cysts usually are located in the midline or slightly off-midline. They have a doughy texture on palpation and may show pitting after pressure is applied. Unlike thyroglossal duct cysts, dermoid cysts have no attachment to the tongue or hyoid bone and therefore do not move when the tongue is protruded. Patients with dermoid cysts often show no symptoms unless the airway or other adjacent structures have been compressed.

On CT or MRI, these lesions may be difficult to distinguish from other low-density lesions such as thyroglossal duct cysts, ranulas, cystic hygromas, or abscesses. Fat detected within the lesion differentiates dermoid cysts from other low-density lesions.[34] If fat is not identified in the lesion, the diagnosis often cannot be made on the basis of imaging characteristics alone (Figs. 8-49 and 8-50).

INFECTION

Antibiotic therapy has reduced the incidence of inflammatory disease in the neck. Most patients who develop abscesses or cellulitis involving the soft tissue structures of the neck are either immunosuppressed or drug abusers. Other causes of neck infections include skin infections, dental disease, trauma, endocarditis, and systemic infections such as tuberculosis.

It often is difficult to determine by clinical examination alone if a patient with a painful, tender, swollen neck has an abscess or merely cellulitis. However, con-

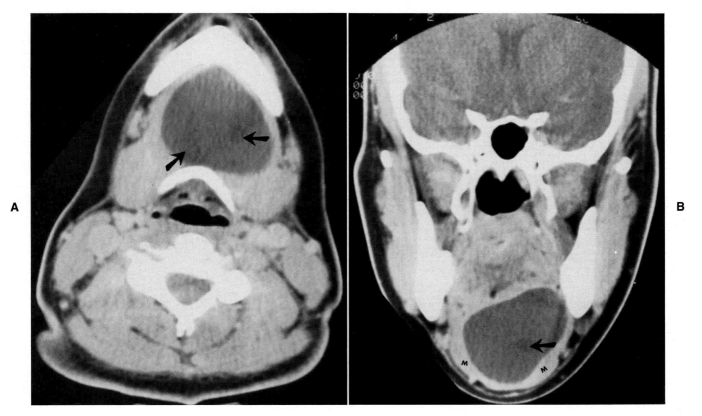

Fig. 8-49 Dermoid. **A,** Contrast-enhanced axial CT scan and **B,** coronal CT scan show low-density lesion with minimal peripheral rim enhancement in floor of mouth. Mass is located above mylohyoid muscle *(M).* Small globules of fat are identified in lesion *(arrows).*

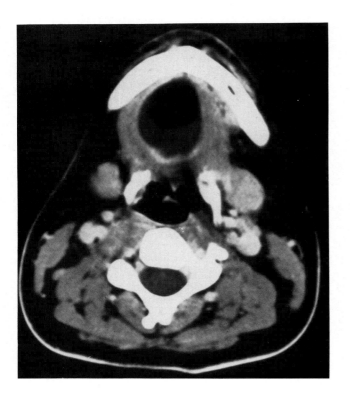

Fig. 8-50 Dermoid. Mass with peripheral rim enhancement and fat-fluid level is seen in submental triangle. Midportion of hyoid bone is absent because of previous surgery to remove thyroglossal duct cyst.

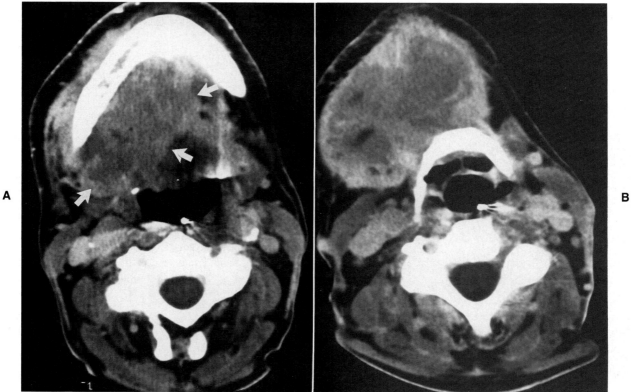

Fig. 8-51 Abscessed tooth. CT scans at level of mandible **(A)** and below **(B)** show low-density mass with septations and peripheral rim enhancement on left side of face and submandible triangle. Platysma muscle is thickened *(arrow),* as is overlying skin. Linear areas of increased density are seen in subcutaneous fat.

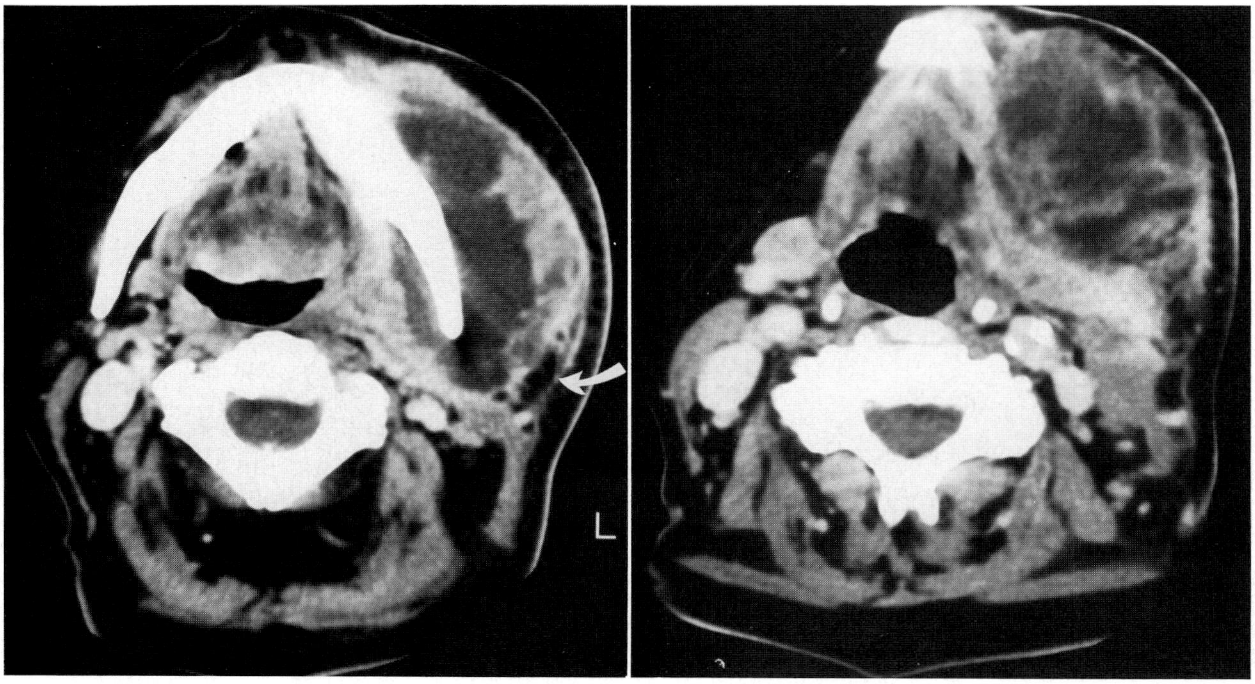

Fig. 8-52 Squamous cell carcinoma of tongue and floor of mouth. CT scan at level of mandible, **A,** shows large mass involving tongue and floor of mouth on right *(arrows).* Soft tissues lateral to mandible are involved at level of hyoid bone, **B;** tumor is seen in submental and right submandibular triangles. Skin and subcutaneous fat adjacent to mass are abnormal and may be mistaken for abscess.

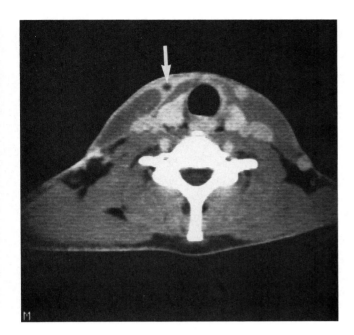

Fig. 8-53   Cellulitis. Right anterior jugular vein is throm-bosed *(arrow)*. Note enhancement of fascial planes around right sternocleidomastoid muscle and strap muscles.

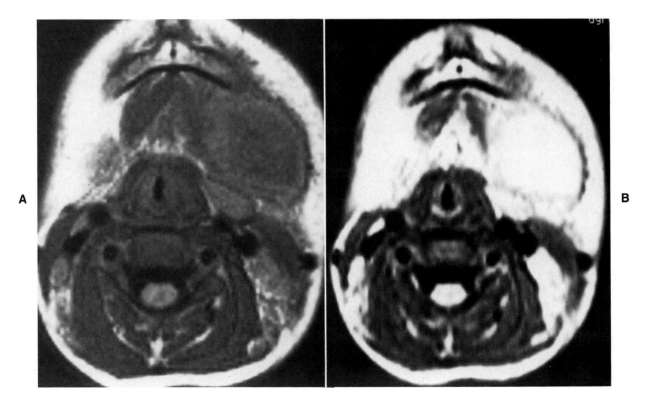

Fig. 8-54   Abscess. **A,** On T_1-weighted MRI, hypointense mass with thick rim that is slightly hyperintense to center of mass is identified in left submandibular triangle. **B,** On T_2-weighted sequence, entire mass becomes hyperintense. Although linear densities are seen in subcutaneous fat adjacent to mass in **A,** thickening of overlying skin could not be appreciated on these scans.

trast-enhanced CT has increased diagnostic acumen in these cases. With CT, cellulitis can be differentiated from an abscess, and complications of infection (venous thrombosis, airway compression, and osteomyelitis) can be detected. Occasionally CT findings can suggest the cause of an infection.

The CT characteristics of neck infections have been described.[35,36] Abscesses are seen as single or multiloculated low-density masses with peripheral rim enhancement that conform to fascial spaces. Cutaneous and subcutaneous manifestations of infection are also seen. Such manifestations include enlargement of adjacent muscles (myositis), thickening of the overlying skin, abnormal increased attenuation of the subcutaneous fat with visualization of small engorged veins and lymphatics, and enhancement of fascial planes (Fig. 8-51). Radiographically, a necrotic tumor, nodal disease with extension into the adjacent soft tissues, an infected branchial cleft cyst, and a thrombosed vessel all may mimic an abscess on cross-sectional imaging (Fig. 8-52).

The presence of cutaneous or subcutaneous findings of infection without a low-density collection is consistent with cellulitis (Fig. 8-53).

No studies currently compare CT and MRI in the evaluation of neck infection. Several possible problems have been mentioned in using MRI to evaluate inflammatory disease:

1. T_1-weighted images should be able to distinguish an abscess from fat (Fig. 8-54); however, an abscess can be isointense with the adjacent musculature.
2. Areas of abscess formation and cellulitis both tend to be hyperintense on T_2-weighted images; thus distinguishing between an abscess and accompanying cellulitic changes may be difficult or impossible.
3. The use of Gd-DTPA should demonstrate an enhancing rim in a mature abscess.
4. The cutaneous manifestations of infection are not obvious on MRI.
5. Subcutaneous manifestations of infection may be obscured on MRI if the imaging parameters are not monitored carefully.

Understanding the fascial planes and spaces in the neck enables the practitioner to better understand the patterns of spread of infection. Spread of infection is limited by the fascial compartments, and for this reason inflammatory processes in the neck rarely cross the thoracic inlet into the mediastinum.

It is worthwhile to consider the reason for this phenomenon. The fascial spaces within the neck and mediastinum are completely separate with only *two* exceptions: the visceral space anteriorly and the prevertebral space posteriorly.[11,37] These two spaces have components that cross the thoracic inlet.

The boundaries of these spaces are discussed in detail in the section on normal anatomy. The visceral space can be divided into two components: the pretracheal space and the retrovisceral space. Since the pretracheal component of the visceral space extends from the hyoid bone to the level of the aortic arch in the anterior mediastinum, infections in this region can extend into the anterior mediastinum (Fig. 8-55). Radiographically, it is difficult to differentiate the retrovisceral and prevertebral spaces. Both of these spaces extend from the base of the skull superiorly to the posterior mediastinum inferiorly. Therefore infections in these regions can extend inferiorly into the posterior mediastinum (Fig. 8-56). Infections in the retropharyngeal region (prevertebral and retrovisceral spaces) are uncommon in adults and usually are secondary to tuberculosis.

VASCULAR ABNORMALITIES

Major blood vessels in the neck (carotid arteries and jugular veins) are readily identified on CT, ultrasound, or MRI. The size, location, and patency of these vessels can be assessed with these imaging modalities.

Normal Variants

Nonpathologic variations in the vasculature of the neck may be mistaken for a mass clinically and radiographically. Asymmetry of the internal jugular veins is the most common variation in the vascular anatomy of the neck. An internal jugular vein that is significantly larger than its counterpart is not uncommon. The right internal jugular vein usually is larger than the left, presumably reflecting the predominance of right cerebral venous drainage. It is important to be aware of this potential variation so as not to mistake the larger vein for an enhancing mass. If no other abnormalities are present, enlargement of the internal jugular vein is of no significance. Duplication of the internal jugular veins has been reported in rare cases but usually is of no clinical significance. However, if phlebectasia of a large vein occurs, it may appear clinically as a fullness in the neck that is present when the patient is supine but that vanishes when the patient is erect. Tortuous arteries may be present as a submucosal pulsatile mass in the pharynx (Fig. 8-57). This variation in normal anatomy may be identified on CT or MRI, thus obviating the need for further diagnostic workup unless a posttraumatic aneurysm of the neck is a clinical consideration.

Venous Thrombosis

Venous thrombosis can be diagnosed on contrast-enhanced CT, ultrasound, or MRI,[38-44] thereby providing a noninvasive means of making the diagnosis. Venous thrombosis in the neck is not as common today as it was before the discovery of antibiotics, when the condition

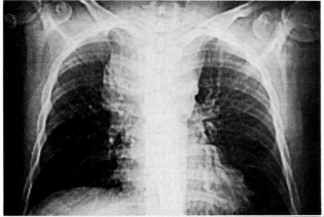

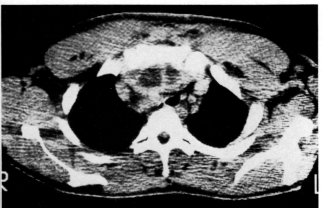

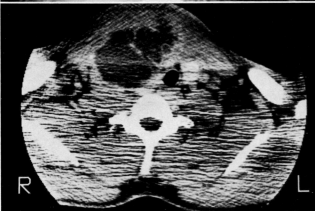

Fig. 8-55 Abscess. **A,** Scout image from chest CT scan shows widening of mediastinum with a shift of trachea to left. **B,** Low-density mass with peripheral rim enhancement is seen in visceral space on right side of neck. **C,** Mass extends into anterior mediastinum. Note obliteration of fascial planes and thickening of overlying skin in **B.**

usually was associated with aerobic infections.[45] Nowadays, venous thrombosis is seen primarily as a complication of central venous catheterization and intravenous drug abuse. Intravenous drug abusers may develop venous thrombosis as a consequence of injecting drugs directly into the vein or from an associated infection. Other less common causes of venous thrombosis include venous compression from benign or malignant tumors, hypercoagulable states, or infection.

The CT characteristics of venous thrombosis have been described:

1. The central portion of the vessel usually is less dense than contrast-enhanced blood (Fig. 8-58). However, a fresh thrombosis may be as dense as contrast-enhanced blood and escape detection.
2. Occasionally the thrombosed vein may be enlarged.[38-41]
3. There is enhancement of the blood vessel wall around the thrombus as a result of flow through the vasa vasorum.[41]
4. Contrast in collateral venous channels may also be identified (Fig. 8-59).
5. Abnormal density in the adjacent soft tissues often indicates coexisting fasciitis and cellulitis.

A number of lesions may mimic a venous thrombosis on one or two adjacent CT scans. Such lesions include an infected branchial cleft cyst, an abscess, a necrotic lymph node, and a thrombosed carotid artery (Fig. 8-60). In most cases careful analysis of sequential images and correlation with clinical history can distinguish venous thrombosis from other lesions.

Ultrasound also can be used to diagnose venous thrombosis. A thrombosed vessel appears dilated with intraluminal echoes. Additional ultrasound findings such as absence of venous pulsations, lack of normal changes with the Valsalva maneuver, and assessment of luminal compression in two planes can be detected with real-time scanning.[42] An acute thrombosis may escape detection on routine ultrasound[46-48] because of the low inherent echogenicity of a fresh thrombus. Adjusting gain settings enhances these low-amplitude signals and enables the practitioner to make the diagnosis. Doppler ultrasound allows this diagnosis to be made in cases of recent thrombus.

The advantages of using ultrasound to diagnose venous thrombosis include low cost, lack of ionizing radiation, and availability of portable units. A major disadvantage is a limited ability to evaluate disease in the

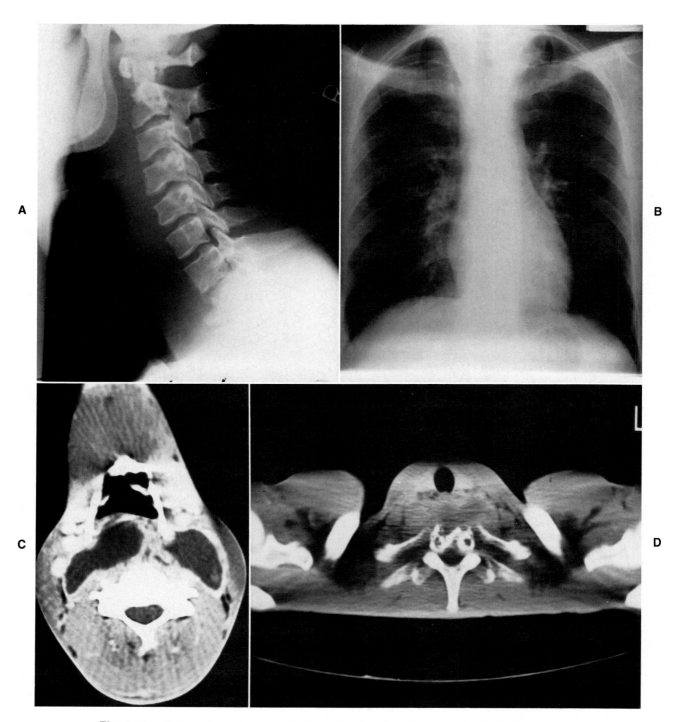

Fig. 8-56 Tuberculous abscess. **A,** There is widening of prevertebral soft tissues from base of skull to thoracic inlet, and T_1 vertebral body has been destroyed anteriorly. **B,** Superior mediastinum is widened on routine chest roentgenogram. **C,** CT scan at level of hyoid bone shows bilateral low-density masses with peripheral rim enhancement in prevertebral area. **D,** Scan at level of thoracic inlet shows mass in prevertebral area and destruction of anterior aspect of T_1 vertebral body.

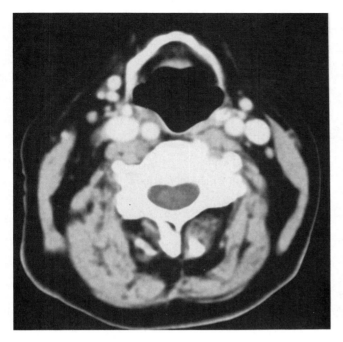

Fig. 8-57   Tortuous vessels. Right common carotid artery and internal jugular vein are displaced medially. Note anterior displacement of posterior pharyngeal wall caused by these displaced vessels.

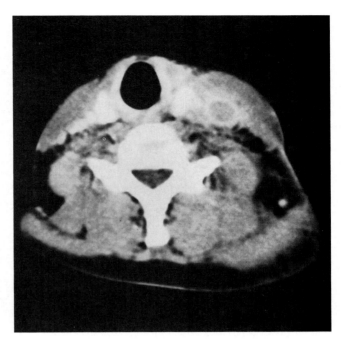

Fig. 8-58   Internal jugular vein thrombosis. No contrast enhancement is seen in center of left internal jugular vein. Vessel wall adjacent to thrombosis is enhanced.

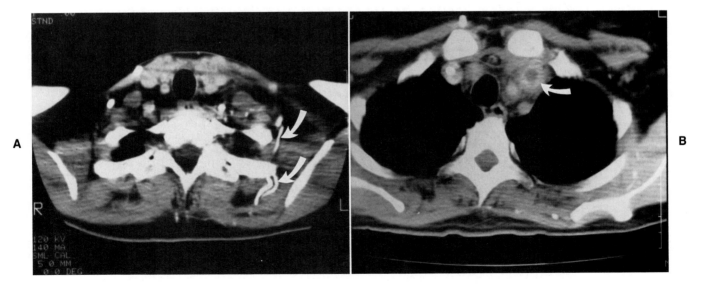

Fig. 8-59   Jugular vein thrombosis. **A,** Collateral vessels *(arrows)* are seen in left paraspinal area in this patient with thrombosis of left jugular vein **(B).** Arrow points to the area of abnormality.

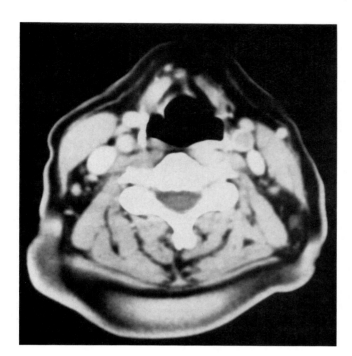

Fig. 8-60 Thrombosed common carotid artery. No contrast enhancement is seen in left common carotid artery.

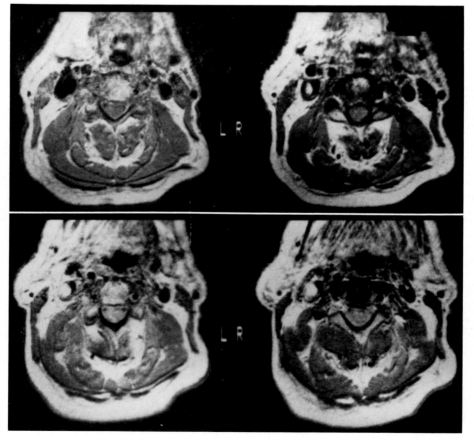

Fig. 8-61 Jugular vein thrombosis. Bright signal is seen in right internal jugular vein. Presence of intraluminal thrombus was confirmed on phase imaging.

retromandibular and infraclavicular regions.

Venous thrombosis can be diagnosed on MRI,[43,44] although this technique is far more expensive than CT or ultrasound. Also, the actual scanning time may be longer when compared with the other modalities.

Flowing blood may have a high or low signal intensity on MRI, depending on a number of factors such as flow velocity and direction, geometric factors, and pulse sequences.[49] The absence of signal (dark) in the region of a blood vessel is secondary to time-of-flight phenomena or dispersion properties. A high signal intensity seen in the region of a blood vessel may be secondary to flow-related enhancement or a thrombus (Fig. 8-61). Flow-related enhancement can be distinguished from a thrombus in a number of ways, including obtaining alternate pulse sequences, gradient echo imaging, or evaluation of the phase shift properties of the signal.[44,50-52] Occasionally differentiation may be difficult even when these techniques are performed.

PARAGANGLIOMAS

Paragangliomas arise from neural crest cell derivatives. In the head and neck, these tumors commonly are located in the carotid body in the region of the carotid bifurcation (carotid body tumor), along the nodose ganglion of the vagus nerve (glomus vagale), along the jugular ganglion of the vagus nerve (glomus jugulare), and around Arnold's and Jacobson's nerves in the middle ear (glomus tympanicum).

Both carotid body and glomus vagale tumors may appear as neck masses. This discussion deals primarily with carotid body tumors. Although glomus vagale tumors occur primarily in the parapharyngeal space, they may extend inferiorly into the lower neck. Therefore both carotid body and glomus vagale lesions should be considered if a patient has a pulsatile lateral neck mass.

The average age when a carotid body tumor appeared was 45 years in one series, with an age range of 6 months to 79 years.[53] There is a slight female predominance. Also, the evidence of several tumors (carotid body) is significant if a family history of these tumors exists; multiple tumors were been reported in 25% to 33% of patients with such a family history.[54,55] Paragangliomas other than carotid body tumors also have been reported in patients with a family history of these lesions.[56]

Typically a carotid body tumor appears as a painless, slow-growing mass just below the angle of the mandible at approximately the level of the carotid bifurcation. The mass may be pulsatile, and a bruit often can be heard over the mass. The history and physical findings often strengthen the suspicion that a patient has a carotid body tumor.

Angiographically, these lesions cause splaying of the internal and external carotid arteries, because the ca-

rotid body is located in the region of the carotid bifurcation. Well-defined nutrient vessels are seen in the arterial phase, and a dense, nonhomogeneous tumor blush is identified in the capillary phase of the angiogram.

Identification of an enhancing mass in the region of the carotid bifurcation and splaying of the internal and external carotid arteries enables the practitioner to make this diagnosis on contrast-enhanced CT.[57-60] However, several problems may be encountered when using contrast-enhanced CT. If a significant amount of thrombosis has occurred within the lesion, little if any enhancement is seen on CT. The same is true on angiography. Occasionally it is also difficult to distinguish the displaced vessels from the enhancing mass. Dynamic CT scanning or MRI can be used to help identify these vessels.[60-61]

Many paragangliomas are readily identified on MRI because of the signal voids (blood vessels) seen within them. These lesions have an intermediate signal intensity background and signal voids on all imaging sequences (Fig. 8-62). Focal areas of high signal may be seen in these lesions on T_2-weighted images.[61] It should be noted that not all paragangliomas have this appearance on MRI, because the vessels may have thrombosed or they are too small. This MRI pattern of multiple signal voids is not pathognomonic for paragangliomas and has been seen in other vascular lesions.[62]

Neuromas may mimic paragangliomas on contrast-enhanced CT, because they may enhance significantly on postcontrast studies. These lesions can be differentiated in several ways:

1. On dynamic CT, paragangliomas have a vascular flow curve and neuromas do not.[60]
2. Neuromas and paragangliomas differ in their angiographic appearance. Neuromas displace adjacent vessels but are hypovascular.
3. No signal voids are identified in neuromas on MRI.

LIPOMAS

Lipomas are benign, encapsulated lesions that usually are subcutaneous or submucosal. Although common throughout the body, they are relatively uncommon in the head and neck; only 13% of these lesions occur there. In the neck they are commonly located in the posterior triangle or in the midline posterior portion of the neck.

Lipomas are more common in obese people and tend to increase in size during periods of rapid weight gain.[12,63] However, they do not decrease in size during periods of weight loss. Based on sex, the location and age of presentation of lipomas vary. Lipomas tend to occur in obese women over 40 years of age and usually are found below the clavicles. In men, lipomas occur

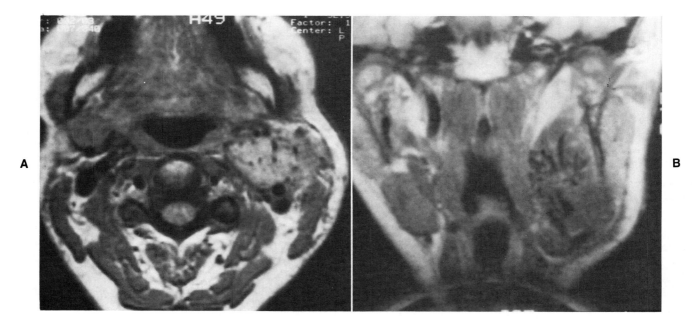

Fig. 8-62 Carotid body tumor. **A,** Axial T_1-weighted MRI scan and **B,** coronal T_1-weighted image show mass with intermediate signal background and signal voids on left side of neck. Relationship of mass and carotid arteries is best appreciated on coronal image, in which mass is seen in carotid bifurcation.

primarily in the head and neck region after the seventh decade of life.[12,63]

Clinically these lesions appear as painless neck masses, although compressing adjacent structures may produce symptoms. Although rare, neurologic disturbances have been reported as a result of compression of neural structures; these disturbances usually are reversible after the lesion is removed.[64-67] The incidence of recurrence in ordinary benign lipomas is less than 50%.[12] Infiltrating lipomas have a recurrence rate as high as 62.5%[64,68]; however, this type of lipoma is rare in the neck.

The CT appearance of lipomas is rather characteristic. These lesions are homogeneous and nonenhancing and have the same density as subcutaneous fat (Figs. 8-63 and 8-64). CT attenuation values range from −65 to −125 HUs.[69-71] The lesions often displace and compress adjacent structures but rarely infiltrate them. Gross infiltration of adjacent structures can be appreciated on CT. Microscopic areas of infiltration are not identifiable on sectional imaging and probably account for most recurrences.[64,65,68,72]

Because lipomas are composed of the same cells as normal fat; they should have the same signal as subcutaneous fat on all MRI sequences.[73] These lesions are hyperintense on T_1-weighted images and decrease in intensity on T_2-weighted images. The CT appearance of lipomas is specific. However, MRI does not have the same specificity because old hematomas may have the

same appearance. Using calculated relaxation times may help, since the calculated T_1 and T_2 values of old hematomas usually are longer than those of fat.[74] Chemical shift imaging also may be useful.[75] An additional problem is the not uncommon occurrence of hemorrhage within a benign lipoma. This increases the CT attenuation and confuses the MRI findings, often preventing an imaging diagnosis.

LIPOSARCOMA

Like their benign counterparts (lipomas), liposarcomas are rare in the head and neck but are common in the retroperitoneum and peripheral soft tissues. They originate from lipoblasts or totipotential mesenchyme either within or adjacent to fascia or intramuscular areas, but they do not arise from preexisting lipomas and rarely from subcutaneous fibroadipose tissue.[12]

On CT they are inhomogeneous, demonstrating a combination of fat and soft tissue elements (Figs. 8-65 and 8-66). Dynamic scanning may show subtle areas of enhancement in these lesions.[76] The density of the fat within the lesion is higher than that of normal subcutaneous fat. It should be noted, however, that use of attenuation coefficients may be meaningless in lesions of less than 2 cm because of partial voluming.[77] Infiltration of adjacent structures may or may not be demonstrated.

Based on a limited experience of two cases,[74] it has been suggested that the MRI signal intensity of liposar-

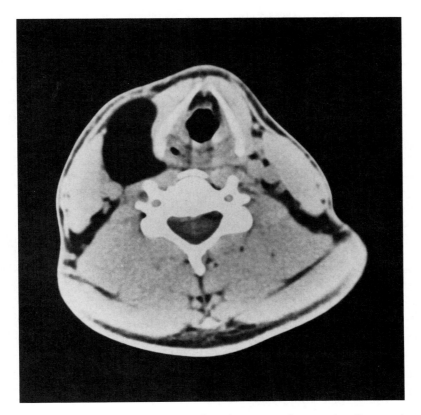

Fig. 8-63 Lipoma. Homogeneous, nonenhancing mass of same density as subcutaneous fat is identified in right anterior triangle.

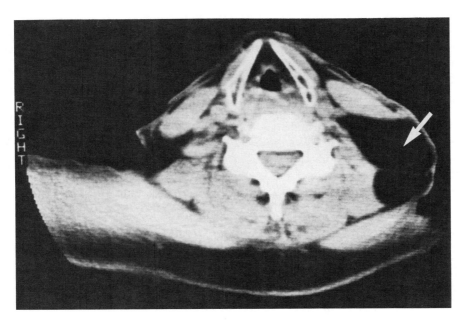

Fig. 8-64 Lipoma. Fat-density mass *(arrow)* is seen in left posterior triangle.

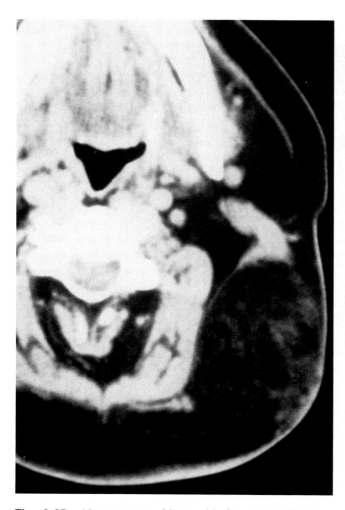

Fig. 8-65 Liposarcoma. Mass with fat and soft tissue components is shown posterior to sternocleidomastoid muscle.

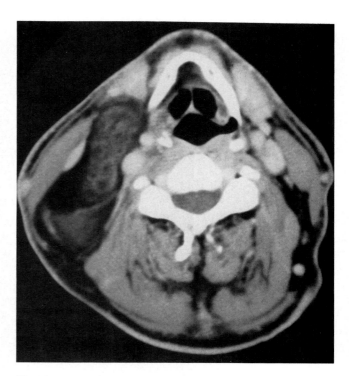

Fig. 8-66 Liposarcoma. Mass with fatty and soft tissue components is seen in anterior and posterior triangles on right side of neck.

comas may differ from that of subcutaneous fat. Two different TR sequences were needed to differentiate lipomas and liposarcomas. On short TR sequences the signal intensity of liposarcomas is lower than that of subcutaneous fat, but on long TR sequences it is similar to that of subcutaneous fat. Calculated T_1 values were longer for liposarcomas than for normal fat, and the T_2 values of liposarcomas varied from slightly to significantly longer than those of normal fat. The spin density in this series was greater for the tumors than for normal fat.[74]

REFERENCES

1. Healy G: Malignant tumors of the head and neck in children: diagnosis and treatment, Otolaryngol Clin North Am 13(3):483, 1980.
2. Shumrick DA: Biopsy of head and neck lesions. In Paperrella MN and Shumrick DA, editors: Otolaryngology, vol 1, Philadelphia, 1973, WB Saunders Co, pp 674-681.
3. Allard RHB: The thyroglossal cyst, Head Neck Surg 5:134, 1982.
4. Thomas JR: Thyroglossal duct cyst, Ear Nose Throat J 58:512, 1979.
5. Pounds LA: Neck masses of congenital origin, Pediatr Clin North Am 28(4):841, 1981.
6. Putney FJ: The diagnosis of head and neck masses in children, Otolaryngol Clin North Am 3:277, 1970.
7. Hawkins DB, Jacobsen BE, and Klatt EC: Cysts of the thyroglossal duct, Laryngoscope 92:1254, 1982.
8. Noyek AM and Friedberg S: Thyroglossal duct and ectopic thyroid disorders, Otolaryngol Clin North Am 14(1):187, 1981.
9. Telander RL and Deane SA: Thyroglossal and branchial cleft cysts and sinuses, Surg Clin North Am 57:779, 1977.
10. Paff GH: Anatomy of the head and neck, Philadelphia, 1981, WB Saunders Co.
11. Hollinshead WH: Anatomy for surgeons. vol 1: The head and neck, New York, 1968, Harper & Row, Publishers, Inc.
12. Batsakis JG: Tumors of the head and neck. Clinical and pathological considerations, Baltimore, 1979, Williams & Wilkins.
13. Hays LL and Marlow SF Jr: Papillary adenocarcinoma arising in a thyroglossal duct cyst, Laryngoscope 78:2189, 1968.
14. Butler EC et al: Carcinoma of the thyroglossal duct remnant, Laryngoscope 79:264, 1969.
15. Choy FS, Ward R, and Richardson R: Carcinoma of the thyroglossal duct, Am J Surg 108:361, 1964.
16. Reede DL, Bergeron RT, and Som PM: CT of thyroglossal duct cyst, Radiology 157:121, 1985.
17. Moran AG and Buchanan PR: Branchial cysts, sinuses and fistulae, Clin Otolaryngol 3:77, 1978.
18. Liston SL and Siegel LG: Branchial cyst, sinuses and fistulas, Ear Nose Throat J 58:504, 1979.
19. Godin MS et al: Fourth branchial pouch sinus: principles of diagnosis and management, Laryngoscope 100:174, 1990.

20. Proctor B: Lateral vestigial cysts and fistulas of the neck, Laryngoscope 65:355, 1955.
21. Harnsberger HR et al: Branchial cleft anomalies and their mimics: computed tomographic evaluation, Radiology 152:739, 1984.
22. Mancuso AA and Dillon WP: The neck, Radiol Clin North Am 27(2):407, 1989.
23. Bill AH Jr and Sumner DS: A unified concept of lymphangioma and cystic hygroma, Surg Gynecol Obstet 120:79, 1965.
24. Pilla TJ et al: CT evaluation of cystic lymphangiomas of the mediastinum, Radiology 144:841, 1982.
25. Siegel MJ, McAlister WH, and Askin FN: Lymphangiomas in children: report of 121 cases, Can Assoc Radiol 30:99, 1979.
26. Singh S, Baboo ML, and Pathak LC: Cystic lymphangioma in children: report of 32 cases including lesions at rare sites, Surgery 69:947, 1971.
27. Smith DW: Recognizable patterns of human malformation: genetic, embryologic and clinical aspects, Philadelphia, 1982, WB Saunders Co. pp 472-473.
28. Chervenah FA et al: Fetal cystic hygroma, N Engl J Med 309:822, 1983.
29. Leipzig B and Rabuzzi DD: Recurrent massive cystic lymphangioma, Otolaryngol 86:758, 1978.
30. Sheth S et al: Cystic hygromas in children: sonographic-pathologic correlation, Radiology 162(3):821, 1987.
31. Som PM, Zimmerman A, and Biller HF: Cystic hygroma and facial nerve paralysis: a rare association, JCAT 8(1):110, 1984.
32. Silverman PM, Korobkin M, and Moore AV: CT diagnosis of cystic hygroma of the neck, JCAT 7(3):519, 1983.
33. New GB and Erich JB: Dermoid cyst of the head and neck, Surg Gynecol Obstet 65:48, 1937.
34. Hunter TB et al: Dermoid cyst of the floor of the mouth: CT appearance, AJR 141:1239, 1983.
35. Nyber DA et al: Computer tomography of cervical infections, Comp Assist Tomog 9(2):288, 1985.
36. Holt GR et al: Computer tomography in the diagnosis of deep-neck infections, Arch Otolaryngol 108:693, 1982.
37. Paonessa DF and Goldstein JC: Anatomy and physiology of head and neck infections (with emphasis on the fascia of the face and neck), Otolaryngol Clin North Am 9:561, 1976.
38. Zerhouni EA et al: Demonstration of venous thrombosis by computed tomography, AJR 134:753, 1980.
39. Patel S and Brennan J: Diagnosis of internal jugular vein thrombosis by computed tomography, JCAT 5(2):197, 1981.
40. Albertyn LE and Alcock MK: Diagnosis of internal jugular vein thrombosis, Radiology 162:505, 1987.
41. Fishman EK et al: Jugular venous thrombosis: diagnosis by computed tomography, JCAT 8(5):963, 1984.
42. Wing V and Scheible W: Sonography of jugular vein thrombosis, AJR 140:333, 1983.
43. Braun IF et al: Jugular venous thrombosis MR imaging, Radiology 157:357-360, 1985.
44. McArdle CB et al: MR imaging of transverse/sigmoid dural sinuses and jugular vein thrombosis, JCAT 11(5):831, 1987.
45. Bartlett JG and Gorbach SL: Anaerobic infections of the head and neck, Otolaryngol Clin North Am 9:655, 1976.
46. Humber PR et al: Ultrasonic imaging of the carotid arterial system, Am J Surg 140:199, 1980.
47. Anderson JC, Baltaxe HA, and Wolf GL: Inability to show clot and limitations of ultrasonography of the abdominal aorta, Radiology 132:693, 1979.
48. Leopold GR: Ultrasonography of superficially located structures, Radiol Clin North Am 18:161, 1980.
49. Bradley WG and Waluch V: Blood flow: magnetic resonance imaging, Radiology 159:611, 1986.
50. Von Schulthess GK and Agustiny N: Calculation of T_2 values versus phase imaging for the distinction between flow and thrombus in MR imaging, Radiology 164:549, 1987.
51. Rumancik WM et al: Cardiovascular disease: evaluation with MR phase imaging, Radiology 166:63, 1988.
52. Dinsmore RE et al: Phase-offset techniques to distinguish slow blood flow and thrombus on MR images, AJR 148:634, 1987.
53. Fletcher WE and Arnold JN: Carotid body tumors: review of the literature and report of unusual cases, Am J Surg 87:617, 1954.
54. Pratt LW: Familial carotid body tumors, Arch Otolaryngol 97:334, 1973.
55. Rush BF Jr: Familial carotid body tumors, Ann Surg 157:633, 1963.
56. Lack EE et al: Paragangliomas of the head and neck region: a clinical study of 69 patients, Cancer 39:397, 1977.
57. Duncan AW, Lack EE, and Deck MF: Radiological evaluation of paragangliomas of the head and neck, Radiology 132:99, 1979.
58. Shugar MA and Mafee MF: Diagnosis of carotid body tumors by dynamic computed tomography, Head Neck Surg 4:518, 1987.
59. Mafee MF: Dynamic CT and its application to otolaryngology head and neck surgery, J Otolaryngol 11:307, 1982.
60. Som PM et al: Parapharyngeal space masses: an updated protocol based upon 104 cases, Radiology 153:149, 1984.
61. Olsen WL et al: MR imaging of paragangliomas, AJNR 7:1039, 1986.
62. Som PM et al: Common tumors of the parapharyngeal space: refined imaging diagnosis, Radiology 169:81, 1988.
63. Enzinger FM and Weiss SW: Soft tissue tumors, St Louis, 1983, The CV Mosby Co, pp 199-241.
64. Kindblom LG et al: Intermuscular and intramuscular lipomas and hibernomas: a clinical, roentgenologic, histologic and prognostic study of 46 cases, Cancer 33:754, 1974.
65. Schimmel J and Heckler FR: Extensive benign infiltrating lipoma with spinal cord compression and paraparesis, Ann Plast Surg 9:425, 1982.
66. Goynal RN: Epidural lipoma causing compression of the spinal cord, Surg Neurol 14:77, 1980.
67. Phalan GS, Kendrick JJ, and Rodriguez JM: Lipomas of the upper extremity, a series of fifteen tumors in the hand and wrist and six tumors causing nerve compression, Am J Surg 121:298, 1971.
68. Mattel SF and Persky MS: Infiltrating lipoma of the sternocleidomastoid muscle, Laryngoscope 93:205, 1983.
69. Reede DL, Whelan MA, and Bergeron RT: Computed tomography of the infrahyoid neck. II, Radiology 145:397, 1982.
70. Enzi G et al: Computed tomography of deep fat masses in multiple symmetrical lipomatosis, Radiology 144:121, 1982.
71. Egund N et al: CT of soft tissue tumors, AJR 137:725, 1981.
72. Bennhoff DF and Wood JW: Infiltrating lipomata of the head and neck, Laryngoscope 88:839, 1978.
73. Adair FE, Pack GT, and Farrior JH: Lipomas, Am J Cancer 16:1104, 1932.
74. Dooms GC et al: Lipomatous tumors and tumors with fatty component: MR imaging potential and comparison of MR and CT results, Radiology 157:479, 1985.
75. Rosen BR et al: Proton chemical shift imaging: an evaluation of its clinical potential using an in vivo fatty liver model, Radiology 154:469, 1985.
76. Friedman AC et al: Computed tomography of abdominal fatty masses, Radiology 139:415, 1981.
77. Hansen GE et al: Computed tomography diagnosis of renal angiomyolipoma, Radiology 128:789, 1978.

SECTION THREE
LYMPH NODES

DEBORAH L. REEDE
PETER M. SOM

Before the era of cross-sectional imaging, lymphangiograms were used to visualize the cervical lymph nodes. These studies were performed either by direct instillation of a contrast agent into the lymphatics[1,2] or by injection of a contrast agent into the perilymphatic tissues.[3-5]

Although direct instillation provided better visualization of regional lymphatics and nodes, it was technically more difficult. It also had interpretive limitations, because filling defects in cervical lymph nodes may be caused by reactive changes as well as by malignant implants. Thus the highly specific lymphangiographic criteria used to assess abdominal lymph node disease were not as applicable in the evaluation of cervical lymph node disease. In addition, groups of metastatic or hyperplastic nodes proximal to an area of interest could prevent the injected contrast agent from filling any distal nodes or even entire nodal groups. This could preclude a satisfactory study from being performed or even result in a false negative study. Radiation therapy, surgery, or inflammatory disease also may alter lymphatic pathways by creating lymphaticolymphatic or lymphaticovenous shunts.[2,6] Thus because cervical lymphangiography is both technically difficult and diagnostically unreliable in detecting occult cervical metastases, this examination never gained wide acceptance.

CT was well established as a means to evaluate mediastinal and abdominal adenopathy before it came into use for evaluating cervical nodal disease. It was not until 1981 that Mancuso et al first reported that CT could be used to detect cervical nodal metastasis.[7] They showed that CT could be used to detect clinically palpable and occult nodal metastasis. Subsequently, numerous articles have shown the utility of CT in detecting regional metastatic disease and staging head and neck tumors.[8-12]

A knowledge of the location of the cervical lymph node chains and the usual modes of spread of head and neck disease are prerequisites to successful analysis of cross-sectional images in patients with head and neck lesions. Since normal lymph nodes are not commonly visualized on CT or MRI, enlarged reactive or pathologic nodes are used to demonstrate the locations of the various lymph node chains.

NORMAL ANATOMY

The French anatomist Rouviere (1938) divided the nearly 300 lymph nodes of the head and neck into 10 principal groups[13]:

1. Occipital
2. Mastoid
3. Parotid
4. Submandibular
5. Facial
6. Submental
7. Sublingual
8. Retropharyngeal
9. Anterior cervical
10. Lateral cervical

The first six groups represent a "pericervical lymphoid ring," because they form a collar that may be likened to a garland at the junction of the head and neck.[13] Within this lymphoid ring are the retropharyngeal and sublingual nodes. The anterior and lateral cervical nodes descend respectively in the anterior and lateral regions of the neck (Fig. 8-67).

For purposes of discussion, the lymph nodes of the head and neck may be classified as those located primarily in the suprahyoid region of the neck and those situated in the infrahyoid region.

Infrahyoid Nodes

The lymph node chains in the infrahyoid region of the neck include the following:

1. Lateral Cervical Chains
   Deep
       Internal jugular
       Spinal accessory
       Transverse cervical
   Superficial
       External jugular
2. Anterior Cervical
   Juxtavisceral chains
       Prelaryngeal (Delphian nodes)
       Pretracheal
       Prethyroid
       Lateral tracheal (paratracheal nodes)

The *lateral cervical* and *anterior cervical* chains are the major infrahyoid nodes. Of all the cervical lymph

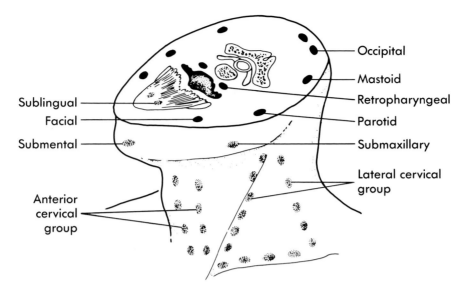

Sublingual

Facial

Submental

Anterior
cervical
group

Occipital

Mastoid

Retropharyngeal

Parotid

Submaxillary

Lateral cervical
group

Fig. 8-67 Location of cervical lymph nodes. Diagram of neck in left anterior oblique projection with transverse section made at level of floor of mouth. Pericervical ring of lymph nodes is seen at junction of head and neck (occipital, mastoid, parotid, submandibular, facial, and submental nodes). (From Som PM: Lymph nodes of the neck, Radiology 165:593, 1987.)

nodes, pathologic conditions are most commonly encountered in the lateral cervical chain, since it serves as a common route of drainage for all major regional structures from the nasopharynx superiorly to the thyroid gland inferiorly.

The lateral cervical chain is divided into *deep* and *superficial* portions. The deep portion has three components: the internal jugular chain, the spinal accessory chain, and the transverse cervical chain. This subgroup of nodes forms a triangle that lies within both the anterior and posterior muscular triangles of the neck (Fig. 8-68). Most of the nodes in the deep cervical (internal jugular) chain are located between the levels where the posterior belly of the digastric muscle above and the omohyoid muscle below cross this lymph node chain. The omohyoid muscle in turn divides the deep cervical nodes into two clinically important groups, the supraomohyoid nodes and the infraomohyoid nodes. The supraomohyoid nodes lie primarily anterolaterally to the internal jugular vein, whereas the infraomohyoid group may be anterior, medial, or posterior to the vein.

Lateral Cervical Chain

Internal Jugular Nodes. The internal jugular (deep cervical) nodes are located in the anterior and posterior triangles, lying deep to the sternocleidomastoid muscle and adjacent to its anterior border. They lie on the outer surface of the carotid sheath, and because they follow the course of the internal jugular vein, they have

an oblique craniocaudal course. These nodes may be identified in close apposition to the carotid sheath when they are pathologically enlarged (Fig. 8-69). Where the posterior belly of the digastric muscle crosses this chain (near the level of the hyoid bone), one node usually is larger then the others. This node, called the jugulodigastric, sentinel, or tonsillar node, receives lymph from one tonsil and from the oral cavity, pharynx, and submandibular nodes. Similarly, the juguloomohyoid node is found where the omohyoid muscle crosses the internal jugular chain of nodes; the juguloomohyoid node receives all of the lymph from the tongue. One inferior portion of the internal jugular chain contains Virchow's nodes (Troisier's or signal nodes), which may receive metastatic tumor from neoplasms originating in the thoracic and abdominal cavities.

Drainage

Afferent vessels. Vessels from the parotid, submandibular, submental, retropharyngeal, and some anterior cervical nodes constitute the afferent drainage. The supraomohyoid nodes also receive lymph from the arm and the superficial aspect of the thorax.

Efferent vessels. Each chain forms a jugular lymphatic trunk. On the right side, this trunk enters the right lymphatic duct, the subclavian vein, or the internal jugular vein. On the left side, the trunk enters the arch of the thoracic duct, the subclavian vein, or the internal jugular vein.

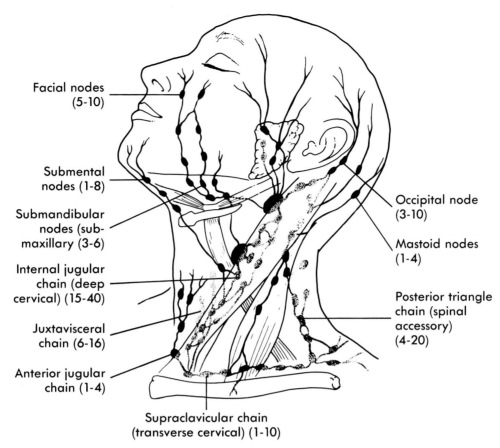

Facial nodes
(5-10)

Submental
nodes (1-8)

Submandibular
nodes (sub-
maxillary (3-6)

Internal jugular
chain (deep
cervical) (15-40)

Juxtavisceral
chain (6-16)

Anterior jugular
chain (1-4)

Occipital node
(3-10)

Mastoid nodes
(1-4)

Posterior triangle
chain (spinal
accessory)
(4-20)

Supraclavicular chain
(transverse cervical) (1-10)

Fig. 8-68 Location of cervical lymph nodes. Diagram shows cervical lymph node chains. Note that nodes in lateral cervical chain (internal jugular, transverse cervical, and spinal accessory nodes) form triangle of lymphoid tissues that is superimposed on portions of anterior and posterior triangles. Numbers represent approximate number of nodes found in each chain. (From Som PM: Lymph nodes of the neck, Radiology 165:593, 1987.)

Spinal Accessory Nodes. Following the course of the spinal accessory nerve, the spinal accessory (posterior triangle) chain crosses the posterior triangle obliquely, superoinferiorly and anteroposteriorly. When enlarged, the spinal accessory nodes appear in the posterior triangle, deep to the sternocleidomastoid muscle (Fig. 8-70). It should be emphasized that the posterior triangle is a fat-filled cleft spanning the entire length of the neck except where it is altered by a number of small structures of soft tissue attenuation, which represent nerves, tiny, inconsequential lymph nodes, and small nutrient vessels. The superior-most portions of the internal jugular and spinal accessory chains join just below the base of the skull.

Drainage

Afferent vessels. These vessels drain from the occipital and mastoid nodes, the parietal and occipital regions of the scalp, the nape, and the lateral portions of the neck and shoulders.

Efferent vessels. Efferent vessels drain to the transverse cervical and internal jugular chains.

Transverse Cervical Nodes. The transverse cervical (supraclavicular) chain joins the inferior limbs of the internal jugular and spinal accessory chains. These nodes travel along the course of the transverse cervical artery in the inferior aspect of the posterior triangle. The supraclavicular location of these nodes may be identified on CT (Fig. 8-71).

Drainage

Afferent vessels. The afferent vessels include the spinal accessory nodes, subclavicular nodes, anterior chest wall, and anterolateral portion of the neck.

Efferent vessels. These nodes drain in a manner similar to that of the internal juglar nodes.

External Jugular Nodes. The superficial lateral cervical chain follows the course of the external jugular vein. Enlarged nodes in this group can be seen superficial to the sternocleidomastoid muscle (Fig. 8-72).

Anterior Cervical Chain. The anterior cervical chains are located toward the midline, between the two carotid sheaths in the infrahyoid region of the neck. This lymph node chain has superficial and deep compo-

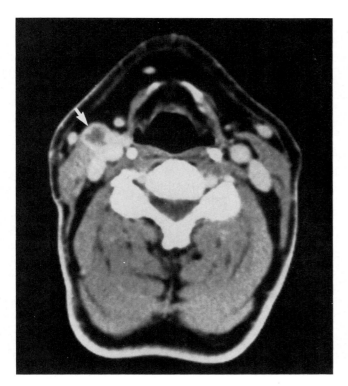

Fig. 8-69 Internal jugular node. On right side of neck necrotic node with peripheral rim enhancement is seen anterior to carotid sheath structures and adjacent to anterior border of sternocleidomastoid muscle *(arrow).*

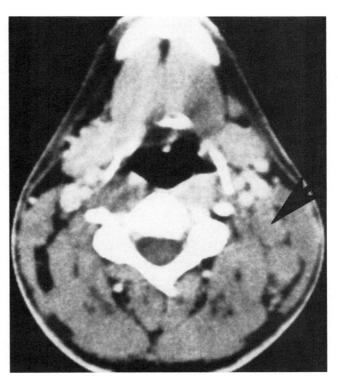

Fig. 8-70 Spinal accessory node. Enlarged nodes *(arrow)* are shown deep to sternocleidomastoid muscle on left side of neck in patient with Hodgkin's lymphoma.

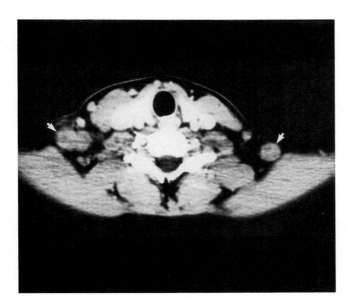

Fig. 8-71 Transverse cervical nodes. Bilateral, enlarged, nonnecrotic nodes are identified in supraclavicular regions *(arrows).*

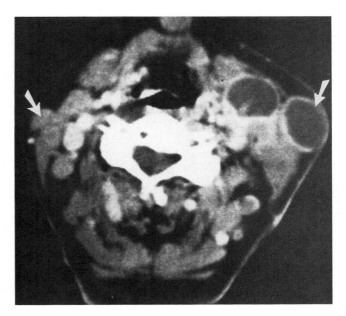

Fig. 8-72 External jugular nodes. Several enlarged lymph nodes are seen bilaterally. Note enlarged external jugular nodes *(arrows).*

nents. The superficial portion lies on the outer surface of the strap muscles and follows the course of the anterior jugular veins. The deep components (also known as the *juxtavisceral* nodes) take their names on the basis of their relationship to the major anterior midline structures:

1. Prelaryngeal nodes (Delphian nodes)
2. Prethyroid nodes
3. Pretracheal nodes
4. Lateral tracheal nodes (paratracheal or tracheo-esophageal nodes)

These nodes drain into the thoracic duct or anterior mediastinal nodes on the left side and into the internal jugular chain or highest intrathoracic nodes on the right side. Of these the Delphian node lies on the cricothyroid membrane of the larynx and draws the subglottic portion of the larynx. The tracheoesophageal nodes extend from the level of the thyroid glands down into one upper mediastinum. They drain the larynx and the pyriform sinuses. These nodes behind the thyroid gland may be confused on CT and MRI with a thyroid or parathyroid nodule.

Suprahyoid Nodes

The lymph node chains in the suprahyoid region include the following:

1. Occipital chain
2. Mastoid chain
3. Parotid chain
4. Submaxillary chain
5. Fascial chain
6. Submental chain
7. Sublingual chain
8. Retropharyngeal chain
9. Superior portions of the internal jugular and spinal accessory chains

Occipital Nodes. Occipital nodes are located at the junction of the neck and skull. They are divided into three groups based on their location: superficial nodes, subfascial nodes, and submuscular or subsplenius (deep occipital) nodes.

Drainage

Afferent vessels. These vessels drain from the occipital region.

Efferent vessels. These drain primarily to the spinal accessory chain and lateral cervical nodes.

Mastoid Nodes. The mastoid nodes are located behind the ear.

Drainage

Afferent vessels. These vessels drain from the parotid region, the parietal area, and the skin of the auricle.

Efferent vessels. These vessels drain to the inferior parotid nodes and superior internal jugular nodes.

Parotid Nodes. The parotid nodes are located superficial to and within the parotid gland. These nodes may

be enlarged in benign processes such as granulomatous disease (sarcoid and tuberculosis) as well as in metastatic disease and lymphoma. The most common neoplasms to metastasize to this area are melanoma and squamous cell carcinoma from a primary tumor in the head or neck (Fig. 8-73). As such, enlarged parotid nodes may be confused both on imaging and clinically with primary parotid lesions.

Drainage

Afferent vessels. Drainage is from the midline, anteriorly over the forehead and upper face to the postauricular region.

Efferent vessels. Either directly or indirectly, drainage is to the jugular chain.

Submandibular Nodes. The submandibular nodes are located in the submandibular triangle along the inferior border of the mandible. They can be situated anywhere laterally from the insertion of the anterior belly of the digastric muscle anteriorly to the angle of the mandible posteriorly (Fig. 8-74). Based on their location, they can be divided into three groups: preglandular, prevascular, and retrovascular nodes.

Drainage

Afferent vessels. These vessels drain from the lateral chin, lower lip, cheeks, nose, mucosa of the ante-

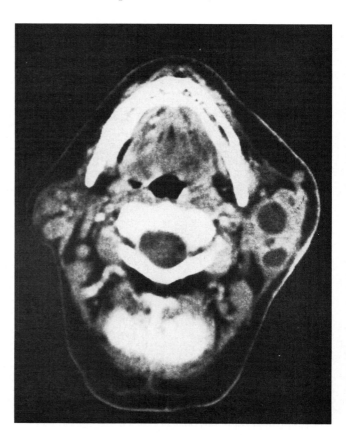

Fig. 8-73 Parotid nodes. Necrotic and nonnecrotic nodes are seen in parotid glands in patient with metastatic squamous cell carcinoma, from a primary tumor in the head or neck.

rior part of the nasal fossae, gums, teeth, soft and hard palate, tongue anterior to the lingual vein, submandibular gland, sublingual gland, and floor of the mouth.

Efferent vessels. These vessels drain to the internal jugular chain.

Facial Nodes. Facial nodes lie in the subcutaneous tissues of the face and generally follow the course of the facial artery and vein.

Drainage

Afferent vessels. These vessels drain from the upper and lower lids, nose, upper and lower lip, entire cheek, and in rare cases the gums and palate.

Efferent vessels. These vessels drain to the submandibular nodes.

Submental Nodes. The submental nodes lie between the anterior bellies of the digastric muscles. Small, clinically insignificant nodes often are seen here (Fig. 8-75).

Drainage

Afferent vessels. These vessels drain from the chin, middle of the lower lip, cheek, incisor region of the gums, anterior floor of the mouth, and tip of the tongue.

Efferent vessels. These vessels drain to the subman-

dibular nodes and internal jugular chains; they may cross to the opposite side.

Sublingual Nodes. The sublingual nodes have two components, a lateral group and a median group. The lateral nodes follow the course of the lingual vessels; the median nodes are located between the genioglossus muscles. Enlargement of these nodes rarely is identified on cross-sectional imaging.

Drainage

Afferent vessels. These vessels drain from the tongue and floor of the mouth.

Efferent vessels. These vessels drain to the submandibular, submental, and internal jugular nodes.

Retropharyngeal Nodes. The retropharyngeal chain consists of a median and lateral group on each side. The lateral retropharyngeal nodes are located along the lateral border of the longus capitis muscles (Figs. 8-76 and 8-77). They are almost always enlarged in infants but usually are not identified on CT or MRI on one side or the other in adults. These nodes are close to cranial nerves IX, X, XI, and XII in their extracranial course and lie medial to the carotid artery. These nodes can extend along the entire length of the pharynx. The median group is located near the midline in direct continuity with the posterior wall of the nasopharynx, at the

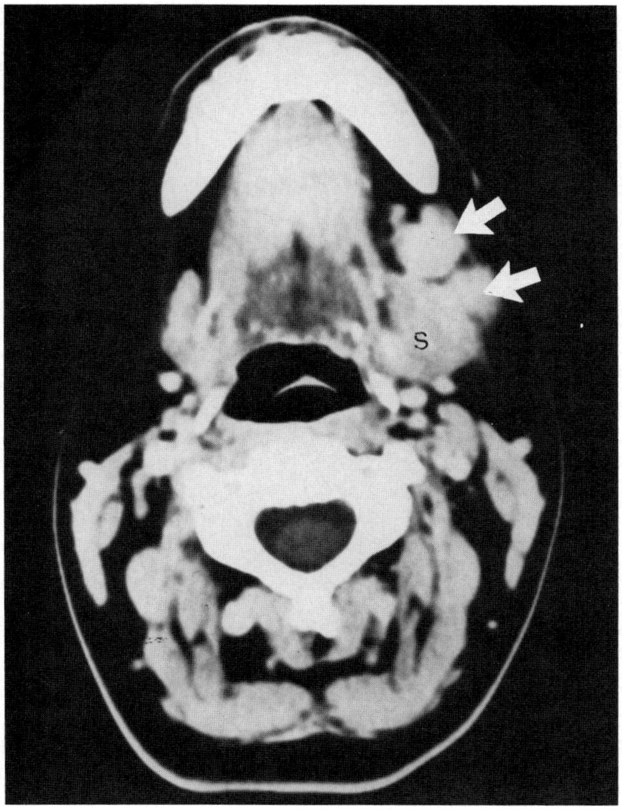

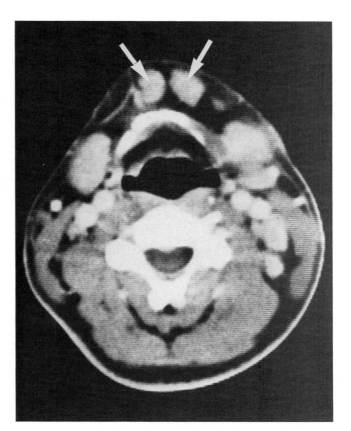

Fig. 8-74 Submandibular nodes. Two enlarged nodes *(arrows)* are identified in left submandibular triangle. These nodes are located anterolateral to submandibular gland *(S)*.

Fig. 8-75 Submental nodes. Several enlarged nodes are shown. Note enlarged submental nodes *(arrows)* anterior to the hyoid bone.

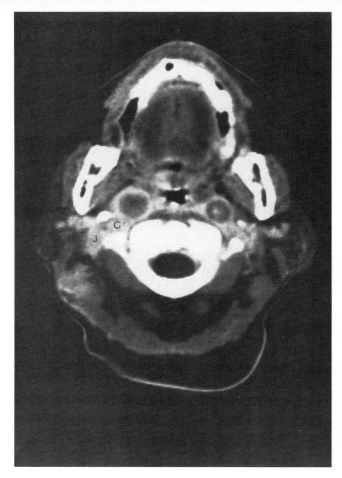

Fig. 8-76 Lateral retropharyngeal nodes. Patient has enlarged bilateral lateral retropharyngeal nodes, which are medial to carotid sheath structures. (*C*, Carotid artery; *J*, jugular vein.)

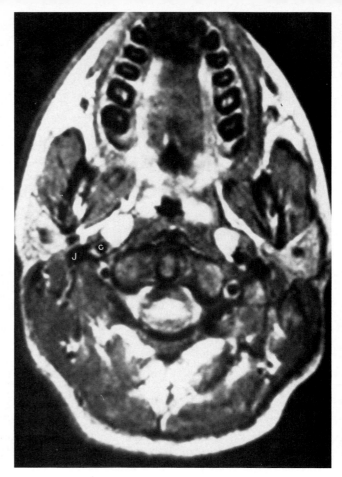

Fig. 8-77 Retropharyngeal nodes. T$_2$-weighted MRI scan shows bilateral enlarged retropharyngeal nodes, which have high signal intensity. Carotid sheath structures are readily identified because of flow voids in vessels. (*C*, Carotid artery, *J*, jugular vein.)

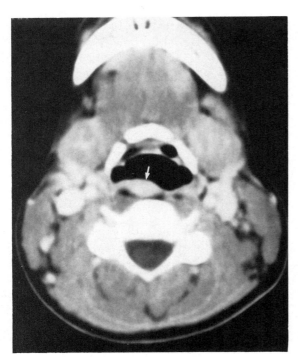

Fig. 8-78 Median retropharyngeal nodes. Enhancing hyperplastic node is seen adjacent to posterior wall of hypopharynx *(arrow)*.

Table 8-4 Simplified nodal classification*

Level	Location
I	Submandibular and submental nodes
II	Internal jugular chain from the skull base to the level of the carotid bifurcation (hyoid bone)
III	Internal jugular chain from the carotid bifurcation to the level of intersection of the omohyoid muscle (cricoid cartilage) with the internal jugular vein
IV	Infraomohyoid portion of the internal jugular chain
V	Posterior triangle nodes
VI	Nodes related to the thyroid gland
VII	Tracheoesophageal groove nodes and superior mediastinal nodes

*From Som PM: Lymph nodes of the neck, Radiology 165:595, 1987.

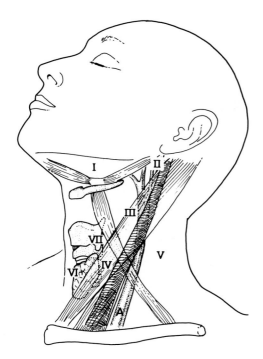

Fig. 8-79 Simplified nodal classification. Diagram of head and neck in left anterior oblique projection. Palpable nodes are indicated using a simplified nomenclature of Roman numerals I through VII (see Table 8-4). Retropharyngeal nodes are not included in this system and should be referred to separately. *A,* Carotid artery. (From Som PM: Lymph nodes of the neck, Radiology 165:596, 1987.)

Table 8-5 Primary sites of nodal metastasis in squamous cell carcinoma of the upper aerodigestive tract*

Lip and oral cavity
Deep cervical nodes, including jugulodigastric, juguloomohyoid, submental, and submaxillary nodes

Pharynx
(Nasopharynx, oropharynx, hypopharynx, soft palate, and uvula) Deep cervical nodes, including jugulodigastric, juguloomohyoid, submental, and submaxillary nodes

Larynx
Deep cervical nodes, including jugulodigastric, juguloomohyoid, submental, and submaxillary nodes

Maxillary sinus
Deep cervical nodes, including jugulodigastric, juguloomohyoid, submental, submaxillary, and parotid nodes

Salivary glands
Nodes immediately adjacent to the salivary glands (parotid, submandibular, and submental nodes) and deep cervical nodes

Thyroid gland
Juxtavisceral, internal jugular, and retropharyngeal nodes

*From Beahrs OH et al, editors: Manual for staging of cancer, ed 3, Philadelphia, 1988, JB Lippincott Co.

level of the C1-C2 articulation. Nodes in this group can extend down to the level of the hyoid bone (Fig. 8-78).

Drainage

Afferent vessels. These vessels drain from the nasal fossae, sinuses, nasopharynx, oropharynx, palate, and middle ear.

Efferent vessels. These vessels drain to the internal jugular chain.

As is obvious from the preceding discussion, the communication between the various lymph node groups is complicated. A simplified nomenclature for classification was suggested in 1981[14] (Fig. 8-79, Table 8-4). This method of nodal classification divides clinically palpable cervical nodes into seven groups or levels, designated by a Roman numeral. Retropharyngeal nodes, which are not readily identified on physical examination, are not included in this classification.

Using this system, the radiologist can assign a level number to a node seen on the cross-sectional images. If retropharyngeal nodes are identified, they should be referred to as such.

PATHOLOGIC CONDITIONS OF THE LYMPH NODES

A knowledge of the sites of nodal metastasis from various head and neck tumors is essential in both the clinical and imaging staging of these lesions. The primary and secondary locations of nodal metastasis in squamous cell carcinoma of the upper aerodigestive tract, based on the location of the primary neoplasm, are summarized in Table 8-5. This information is derived from the American Joint Committee on Cancer.[15]

It is well-known that cervical lymph node metastasis in squamous cell carcinoma of the aerodigestive tract is accompanied by a diminished cure rate.[16-21] The cure rate decreases progressively as the extent of lymph node involvement increases from solitary ipsilateral nodes to multiple ipsilateral, solitary contralateral, and finally bilateral nodes.[18] Since nodal metastasis may alter the treatment plan, its detection is of paramount importance.

The CT imaging protocols for patients with known and unknown primary lesions are discussed in the section on normal anatomy. MRI protocols used to evaluate lymphadenopathy vary, depending on the magnet field strength and the surface coils used. Axial images often are the most useful for detecting cervical lymph nodes; however, coronal scans also provide an excellent overview of the cervical nodes. Sections 5 mm thick provide excellent visualization of these nodes. Thicker sections are not used, because they may obscure visualization of small nodes. Primarily because of time constraints, usually only the area of interest is imaged. However, as MRI technology improves, such constraints may no longer present a problem.[12]

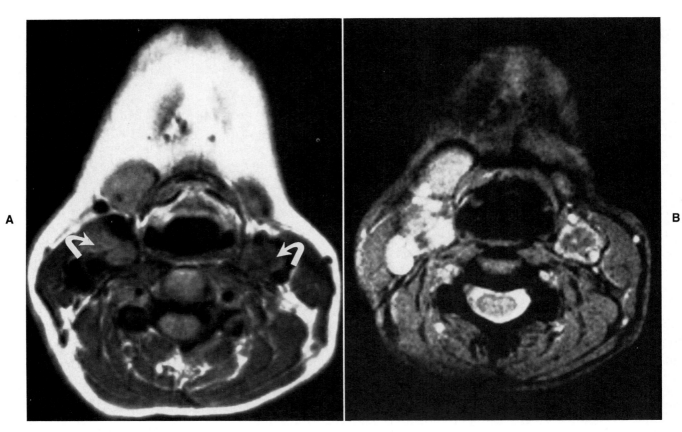

Fig. 8-80 Metastatic nodes. **A,** T$_1$-weighted MRI scan and **B,** T$_2$-weighted image show bilateral cervical lymphadenopathy. Nodes have low-to-intermediate signal intensity on T$_1$-weighted sequence *(arrows)* and become primarily hyperintense on T$_2$-weighted sequence. Nodes show some nonhomogeneity in signal intensity on T$_2$-weighted scans, suggesting metastatic disease.

T$_1$-weighted images provide good differentiation between most lymph nodes that have intermediate signal intensity and the high-signal-intensity fat (Fig. 8-80, *A*). Similar findings are observed on proton density (mixed) images. On strongly T$_2$-weighted images, pathologic nodes usually show an increase in signal intensity, and the surrounding fat has an intermediate signal intensity (Fig. 8-80, *B*). Focal areas of high signal seen on T$_2$-weighted images may represent sites of tumor necrosis.[12] More recently, MRI using Gd-DTPA in combination with gradient echo sequences or fat suppression techniques has shown promise in detecting areas of metastasis and necrosis.

Criteria for determining abnormal lymph nodes are well established on CT but are still in the process of being determined on MRI.[12] Large well-documented studies correlating the MRI and pathologic findings in lymph nodes need to be performed before radiographic criteria for nodal disease can be established for this imaging modality.

Before the era of cross-sectional imaging, physicians relied on physical examination to detect nodal disease. Such palpation depends on the size, location, and consistency of the lymph node. In a patient with an average-sized neck, the lower limit of palpability is approximately 0.5 cm for superficial nodes (submandibular or submental) and 1 cm for those in deeper areas.[22] Based on clinical and radiographic studies, the criteria for abnormal cervical nodes include size, density, extranodal extension, and fixation.

Size

Nodes larger than 1.5 cm in diameter in the submandibular (level I) and jugulodigastric regions of the internal jugular chain (low level II and high level III) should be considered abnormal. Nodes in other areas of the neck should be considered abnormal if they are more than 1 cm in diameter. If these criteria are used, approximately 80% of the enlarged nodes are secondary to metastatic disease and 20% are caused by hyperplasia. These statistics are similar to those reported by clinicians.[22-24]

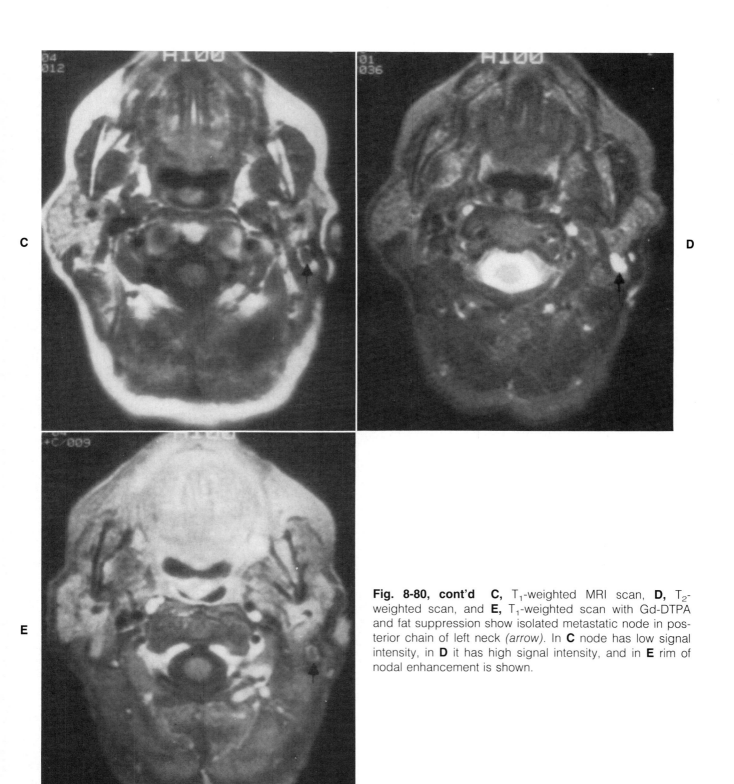

Fig. 8-80, cont'd **C,** T_1-weighted MRI scan, **D,** T_2-weighted scan, and **E,** T_1-weighted scan with Gd-DTPA and fat suppression show isolated metastatic node in posterior chain of left neck *(arrow)*. In **C** node has low signal intensity, in **D** it has high signal intensity, and in **E** rim of nodal enhancement is shown.

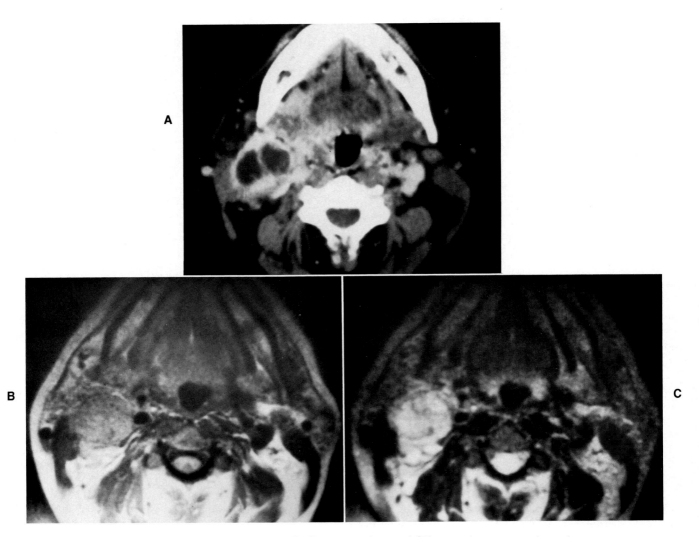

Fig. 8-81 Extranodal extension. **A,** Contrast-enhanced CT scan shows necrotic nodes with peripheral rim enhancement on right side of neck. Fascial planes adjacent to nodes are poorly defined, particularly where they abut carotid sheath and sternocleidomastoid muscle. Nodes are readily identified on T_1-weighted MRI sequence **(B)** and T_2-weighted image **(C).** No definite cleavage plane is seen between nodes, carotid sheath structures, and sternocleidomastoid muscle. Surgery revealed extranodal extension, but adjacent structures were free of disease.

Density

A lymph node with central lucency (not fat density) is abnormal, regardless of size. The central lucency in these nodes is secondary to necrosis and tumor infiltration. It should be noted that fatty replacement can occur in nodes following inflammation and irradiation. The area of decreased attenuation in these nodes usually is peripheral in location near the hilum and should not be mistaken for the more central low attenuation associated with metastatic disease.[10]

Cancer cells enter lymph nodes via the afferent lymphatics and lodge in the reticulum of marginal sinuses of the nodal cortex. As the malignant cells proliferate, they invade the medullary portion of the node, block the flow of lymph, and allow cancer cells to spread to other nodal chains. The nodal medulla eventually undergoes necrosis. Although metastatic nodal necrosis can occur at any time, it usually occurs late in the evolution of tumor within the lymph nodes.[25,26]

Extranodal Extension

When metastatic disease is confined to a lymph node, a sharp interface is seen between the node and the adjacent soft tissue structures. If disease extends beyond the nodal capsule, the margins of the node become ill-defined and ultimately lead to edema and infiltration of the surrounding fibroadipose tissues[10] (Fig. 8-81, *A*, *B*, and *C*). Since surgery and radiation therapy may produce similar alterations in the adjacent nodal soft tissues, the radiologist should know the clinical history before rendering a radiographic interpretation.[7] Also, an abscess with associated inflammatory infiltration and cellulitis of the skin and subcutaneous tissues may mimic nodal disease with extranodal extension on CT or MRI.

Fixation

When the extranodal changes extend to obliterate the fascial planes between the involved lymph node and adjacent structures (e.g., muscles, carotid sheath, nerves), there *may be* clinical fixation of the node to these structures. Since to a degree clinical detection of fixation is subjective and depends on the examiner, fixation recently was dropped from the new nodal staging system.

It is difficult at times to predict solely on the basis of CT or MRI findings whether clinical fixation exists. The only sure sign of nodal fixation is if the structure in question is completely surrounded by a nodal mass (Fig. 8-82). However, if the structure is not entirely surrounded, the node may or may not be fixed.

This point is particularly important in evaluation of extranodal tumor infiltration of the carotid artery, since such fixation may alter the treatment plan.[27] If this determination cannot be made confidently on CT or MRI,

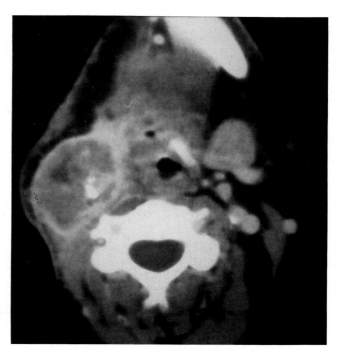

Fig. 8-82 Fixation. Axial contrast-enhanced CT scan shows large necrotic node that completely encircles right carotid artery. Arteriosclerotic calcifications show position of artery.

ultrasound can be used. On ultrasound the blood vessel wall appears as an isolated, echo-dense band separate from adjacent soft tissue structures. Loss of definition of the blood vessel wall, with visualization of an otherwise normal lumen, is consistent with infiltration of the blood vessel wall.[28] However, currently tumor infiltration of the adventitia of the artery cannot be detected by CT, MRI, or ultrasound and must be determined through surgery.

Unknown Primary Tumor

Cervical nodal metastasis may appear without evidence of a primary neoplasm. Approximately 5% of all patients with carcinoma and 12% of patients with head and neck carcinomas have cervical metastasis as the sole presenting sign.[29] If thyroid neoplasms are excluded, 90% of cervical masses in patients over 40 years of age are found to represent metastatic disease.[30] The number of patients in whom the primary neoplasm cannot be found after physical examination and thorough diagnostic testing is estimated to be fewer than 5%.[31] The nasopharynx, pyriform sinus, base of the tongue, and thyroid gland are the most common sites of occult primary tumors in patients with cervical nodal metastasis.

The location of the nodal metastasis, as well as its histology, may give a clue to the location of the primary site. This also has a bearing on the prognosis. In gen-

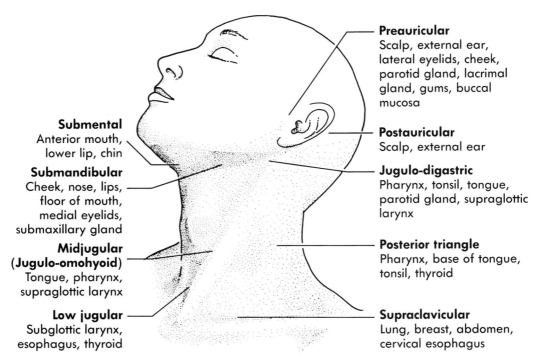

Submental
Anterior mouth,
lower lip, chin

Submandibular
Cheek, nose, lips,
floor of mouth,
medial eyelids,
submaxillary gland

**Midjugular
(Jugulo-omohyoid)**
Tongue, pharynx,
supraglottic larynx

Low jugular
Subglottic larynx,
esophagus, thyroid

Preauricular
Scalp, external ear,
lateral eyelids, cheek,
parotid gland, lacrimal
gland, gums, buccal
mucosa

Postauricular
Scalp, external ear

Jugulo-digastric
Pharynx, tonsil, tongue,
parotid gland, supraglottic
larynx

Posterior triangle
Pharynx, base of tongue,
tonsil, thyroid

Supraclavicular
Lung, breast, abdomen,
cervical esophagus

Fig. 8-83   Diagram of probable primary tumor sites, based on lymph node location.

eral, the lower in the neck the nodal metastasis, the worse the prognosis. Also, patients with adenocarcinoma tend to have a poorer prognosis then those with squamous cell carcinoma.

Based on the location of the enlarged lymph node, the following primary sites should be suspected:

1. Upper cervical nodes: nasopharynx, base of the tongue, tonsil, and pyriform sinus.
2. Middle and lower jugular nodes: larynx, pharynx, esophagus, and thyroid.
3. Midline and paratracheal nodes: thyroid, larynx, and lung.
4. Submandibular nodes: tongue and floor of the mouth.
5. Supraclavicular nodes: may be metastatic from any part of the body, especially lung, breast, stomach and esophagus.

The sites are summarized in Fig. 8-83.

If the primary site is not identified on physical examination, CT may be useful. CT is capable of detecting submucosal disease when mucosal changes are absent,[11,32] and MRI probably also will prove useful in this regard.

Lymphomas

Lymphomas are classified as being either Hodgkin's or non-Hodgkin's lymphomas. Both types occur in the head and neck region, with Hodgkin's lymphoma accounting for 25% of cases.[33]

Patients with Hodgkin's lymphoma in the head and neck region usually have painless neck masses (nodes). This disease spreads to contiguous lymph node groups via lymphatic channels,[34] and extranodal involvement is rare. Non-Hodgkin's lymphoma, however, frequently involves extranodal sites in the head and neck[35,36] and occurs in three sites: (1) nodal sites, (2) extranodal, lymphatic (Waldeyer's ring) sites, and (3) extranodal, extralymphatic sites. Of these three sites, nodal involvement is the most common, followed by extranodal, extralymphatic involvement and then extranodal, lymphatic involvement.[37]

Lymph node enlargement is the common presentation for both types of lymphoma. Nodes in the middle and lower portions of the internal jugular chain commonly are involved; however, isolated involvement of nodes in the superior portion of the internal jugular chain, as well as of the superficial nodes, also occurs. Disease may be present unilaterally or bilaterally. Disease in the superficial nodes or nodes in the superior portion of the internal jugular chain is in contrast to carcinomatous nodal involvement from unknown primary sites, which rarely involves nodes in these portions of the neck.[38]

The size of lymphomatous nodes varies, ranging from 0.5 cm to larger than 1 cm in diameter. On CT and MRI these nodes usually are homogeneous in density. On CT, peripheral rim enhancement may occur, but central necrosis is rare (Fig. 8-84, *A*, *B*, and *C*). Necro-

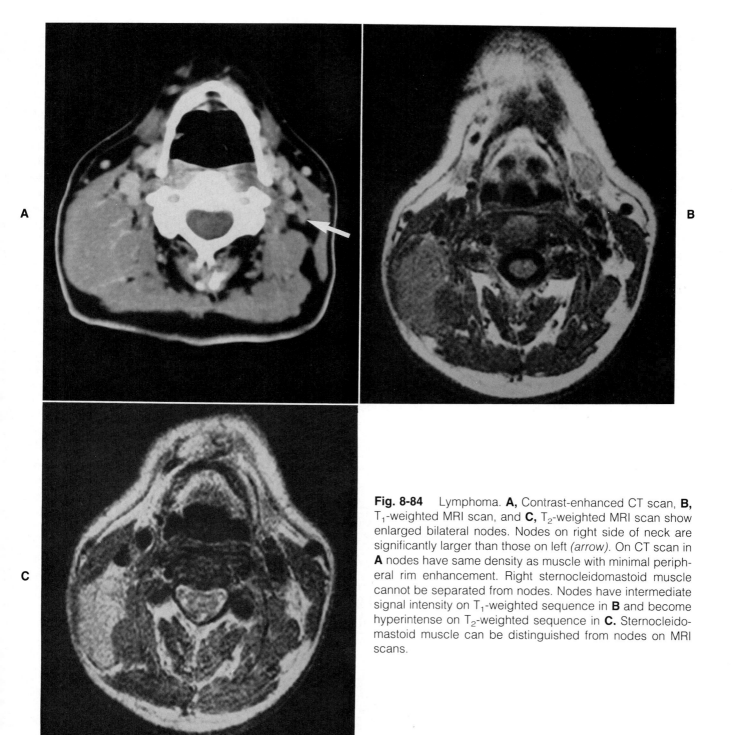

Fig. 8-84   Lymphoma. **A,** Contrast-enhanced CT scan, **B,** T_1-weighted MRI scan, and **C,** T_2-weighted MRI scan show enlarged bilateral nodes. Nodes on right side of neck are significantly larger than those on left *(arrow).* On CT scan in **A** nodes have same density as muscle with minimal peripheral rim enhancement. Right sternocleidomastoid muscle cannot be separated from nodes. Nodes have intermediate signal intensity on T_1-weighted sequence in **B** and become hyperintense on T_2-weighted sequence in **C.** Sternocleidomastoid muscle can be distinguished from nodes on MRI scans.

sis is more common in non-Hodgkin's lymphoma.[38,39]

Calcification in lymphomatous nodes is uncommon unless the patient has had previous irradiation or chemotherapy.[40-42] Such calcification occurs in approximately 2% of patients with lymphoma and usually is not detected until at least 8 months after the completion of therapy.[42-45] A few cases have been reported in which calcification was identified in nodes before therapy.[45-47] Calcification before and after treatment has been seen in both forms of lymphoma, but it appears to be more common in the nodular sclerosing form of Hodgkin's lymphoma probably because of the intensive collagen fibrosis and areas of cellular degeneration, which may serve as a substrate for the formation of dystrophic calcification.[45]

Based on the CT or MRI appearance, it is impossible to differentiate nodal disease secondary to Hodgkin's lymphoma from non-Hodgkin's lymphoma or metastatic disease. However, the ultrasonographic appearance of non-Hodgkin's lymphoma differs from that of Hodgkin's lymphoma and metastatic disease. Non-Hodgkin's lymphoma nodes are homogeneous and slightly echogenic or pseudocystic in appearance.[48] Metastatic and Hodgkin's lymphoma nodes tend to have a heterogeneous appearance.[49]

Lymphoma involving the structures of Waldeyer's ring (adenoids and palatine and lingual tonsils) cannot be differentiated from squamous cell carcinoma. The diagnosis of lymphoma, however, should be considered when a large lesion in the nasopharynx is not associated with bone destruction or when lymph nodes are seen in atypical locations for squamous cell carcinoma.[38,39] Infectious mononucleosis may have similar findings, that is, enlargement of the structures in Waldeyer's ring and peripheral lymphadenopathy (Fig. 8-85, *A* and *B*). When these findings are present, infectious mononucleosis should be included in the differential diagnosis, particularly in children and young adults.

Extranodal, extralymphatic lymphoma may mimic squamous cell carcinoma on cross-sectional imaging. The presence of more than one mass in extralymphatic sites suggests the diagnosis of lymphoma, since it is unusual to encounter two separate primary squamous cell carcinomas.[39]

Tuberculous Adenitis (Scrofula)

Tuberculous adenitis accounts for approximately 5% of cases of cervical lymphadenopathy.[50] The disease is uncommon in the United States, with only occasional cases being seen in rural areas. Most cases are found in

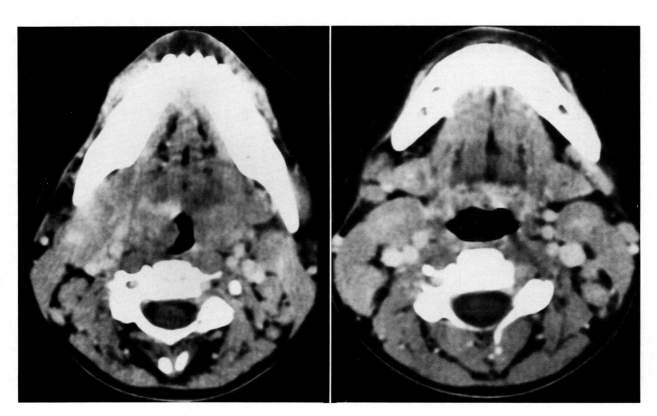

Fig. 8-85 Infectious mononucleosis. Right palatine tonsil is enlarged. Bilateral cervical lymphadenopathy is present. Nodes are homogeneous in density. Some nodes show areas of central enhancement, probably in region of hilum of node.

patients who have emigrated from endemic areas, primarily Southeast Asia.[51-54]

Classically, *Mycobacterium bovis* has been implicated as the cause of scrofula. However, in the United States *Mycobacterium tuberculosis* and atypical mycobacterium are the most common causes. Three species of atypical mycobacterium can cause lymphadenitis: *M. kansasii*, *M. avium intracellulare*, and *M. scrofulaceum*. Of these, *M. scrofulaceum* is most commonly associated with cervical lymphadenitis. Although these different organisms (*M. tuberculosis* and atypical mycobacterium) cause histologically indistinguishable tuberculous adenitis, the clinical presentations differ. These distinctions should be appreciated because treatments differ.

Atypical Mycobacterium. Most reported cases of cervical lymphadenitis secondary to atypical mycobacterium have occurred in children. The precise pathogenesis of this disease has not been established; however, most investigators believe that the peripheral lymphadenitis seen in these patients is secondary to direct lymphatic drainage of the primary complex.[55,56] The common portals of entry in children are the oropharynx and conjunctiva, accounting for the overwhelming involvement of the tonsillar tissue and submandibular, parotid, preauricular, and upper cervical nodes.

Clinically, these patient have unilateral involvement of a group of nodes. Few if any constitutional symptoms are present, and there usually is no evidence of old or active tuberculosis. A tuberculous skin test performed with intermediate-strength purified protein derivative of tuberculin (PPD) is usually negative or weakly positive.

Surgery is the treatment of choice, with the involved nodes and overlying skin being removed. Since these organisms are resistant to antituberculous therapy, such medication is not used.[57] However, antibiotics are used if *M. tuberculosis* is present in addition to atypical mycobacterium.[55]

Mycobacterium Tuberculosis. Cervical tuberculous adenitis secondary to *M. tuberculosis* is a manifestation of a systemic disease. A history of previous tuberculosis is present in approximately half of the patients. This condition is seen primarily in patients between 20 and 30 years of age; however, it can occur at any age. Clinically, patients often have an asymptomatic neck mass and few if any constitutional symptoms. The nodes are firm and nontender. Local inflammatory changes (tenderness and erythemia) are not present unless there is a coexisting (bacterial) infection or a previous biopsy has been performed. The duration of symptoms varies, ranging from less than 2 weeks to longer than 5 years, with an average duration of 1 to 6 months.[58]

Involvement of bilateral posterior triangle nodes is commonly seen in this form of tuberculous adenitis.

The more inferior the location of the involved cervical nodes, the higher the incidence of concomitant pulmonary tuberculosis.[58] The tuberculosis skin test performed with intermediate-strength PPD is strongly positive unless the patient is anergic.

If tuberculosis adenitis is suspected, an excisional biopsy should be performed. This is the preferred method of biopsy because of the high complication rate (fistula formation and poor wound healing) associated with an incisional biopsy in these patients. A presumptive diagnosis is made when caseating granulomas are identified in the biopsy specimen. Acid-fast bacilli are not identified in all specimens and may fail to grow in cultures.

Triple-drug antituberculin therapy is the treatment of choice. Surgery is reserved for patients who fail to respond to antibiotics or who develop complications.

Several patterns of nodal disease are encountered in this disease. On CT these nodes may have a homogeneous density (enhancing or nonenhancing), thick rims of peripheral enhancement with or without central necrosis, and calcifications[59] (Figs. 8-86 and 8-87, *A* and *B*). Any one or all of these patterns can be seen in any patient. The most common pattern of nodal disease is multiple, low-density nodes with thick rims of periph-

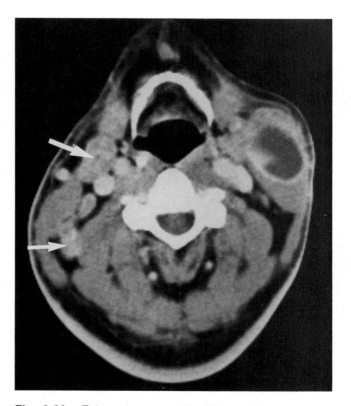

Fig. 8-86 Tuberculous adenitis. Enlarged lymph nodes are seen bilaterally. Low-density node with peripheral rim enhancement is seen on left anterior to sternocleidomastoid muscle. Enhancing nodes are seen on right *(arrows)*.

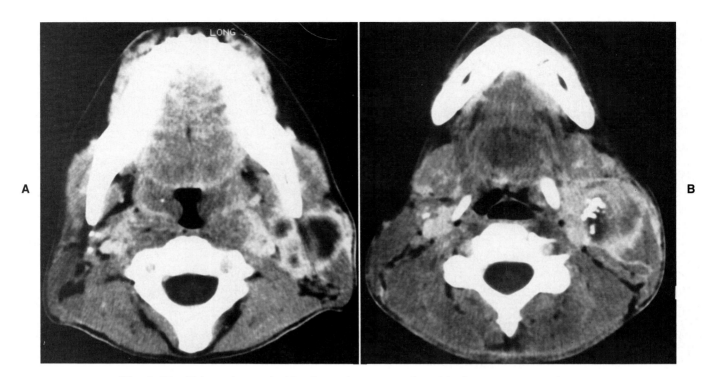

Fig. 8-87 Tuberculous adenitis. Several patterns of nodal disease are identified. **A,** Several low-density nodes with thick, irregular, enhancing rims are seen on left side of neck. Partly calcified nodes without central necrosis are demonstrated on right side of neck in **A** and **B.** Calcifications also are seen in partly necrotic node on left.

eral rim enhancement.[59] If the individual walls of the nodes break down, they coalesce to form a single necrotic mass; this is commonly called a "cold abscess," and the fascial planes adjacent to this mass are obliterated. Clinically and radiographically, the dermal and subcutaneous manifestations of inflammation (thickening of overlying skin, induration of the subcutaneous tissues, engorgement of the lymphatics and thickening of the adjacent muscles) are rarely observed. These findings are seen only if a superimposed nontuberculous infection or fistula is present (Fig. 8-88).

Since tuberculous adenitis shows several patterns of nodal disease, the disorder may mimic other diseases. For example, enhancement can occur in hyperplastic nodes (see Fig. 8-78), vascular metastases (thyroid, melanoma, and hypernephroma) granulomatous disease, and Castleman's disease.[60] Castleman's disease is a form of benign lymphoid hyperplasia that occurs primarily in the mediastinum but occasionally involves the cervical lymph nodes. Calcifications in lymph nodes are not pathognomonic for tuberculosis, because calcifications can occur in other forms of granulomatous disease, in lymphoma (primarily after irradiation or chemotherapy), and in metastatic disease (thyroid and mucin-producing carcinomas) (Fig. 8-89).

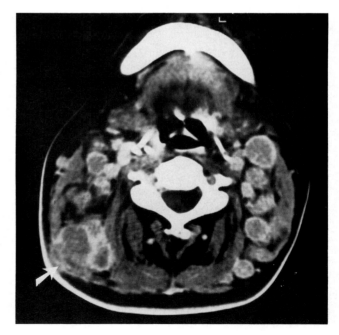

Fig. 8-88 Tuberculous adenitis—postincisional biopsy cutaneous fistula. Note bilateral nodes with minimal evidence of central necrosis. Fascial planes on right posterior aspect of neck are obliterated, and overlying skin is thickened *(arrow)* because of chronic draining fistula.

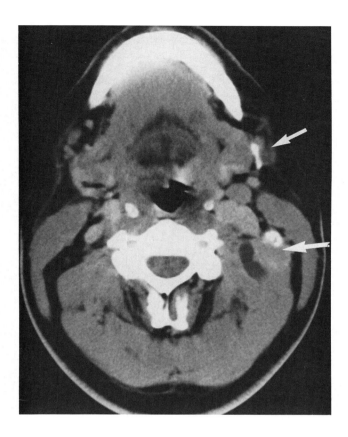

Fig. 8-89 Metastatic papillary thyroid carcinoma. Calcification is shown in enlarged lymph nodes *(arrows)* on left side of neck.

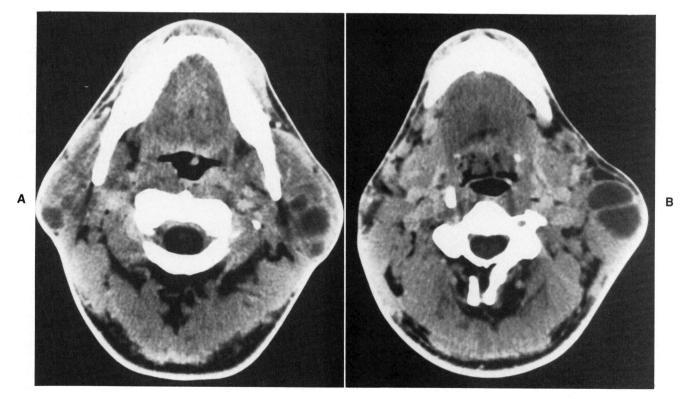

Fig. 8-90 Acquired immunodeficiency syndrome (AIDS). **A,** Bilateral intraparotid cystic masses with minimum peripheral rim enhancement and **B,** bilateral cervical lymphadenopathy are present in this HIV-positive patient.

Acquired Immunodeficiency Syndrome (AIDS)

Certain radiographic findings in the head and neck region may identify a patient who is at risk of developing AIDS. The presence of diffuse cervical lymphadenopathy in conjunction with several parotid cysts (lymphoepithelial cysts) should alert the radiologist that the patient may be human immunodeficiency virus (HIV) positive.[61] These CT findings may be seen before the patient tests positive for HIV.

Both hyperplastic intraparotid nodes and cysts have been found in patients who are HIV positive.[62-64] The cause of these cysts is uncertain, but two theories have been proposed: (1) The cysts are epithelial cysts that were trapped during embryologic development. This is similar to the pathogenesis suggested with papillary cystoadenoma lymphomatosum (Warthin's tumor).[65] (2) Cysts may develop as a result of partial obstruction of the terminal ducts by surrounding lymphocytic infiltration.[61]

Clinically these patients have painless facial swelling, and unilateral or bilateral parotid disease is seen in conjunction with cervical lymphadenopathy.

On CT the nodes are homogeneous in density with no necrosis and range in size from 0.5 to 2 cm in diameter; there is no clear predilection for a particular nodal group. The intraparotid cysts are low density in appearance with minimum peripheral rim enhancement. Several cysts usually are found; however a solitary cyst has been seen in some cases[61] (Fig. 8-90, *A* and *B*).

REFERENCES

1. Fisch VP and Sigel ME: Cervical lymphatic system as visualized by lymphography, Ann Otol Rhinol Laryngol 73:869, 1964.
2. Sigel ME: Cervical lymphangiography. In Paperrela MM and Shumrick DA, editors: Otolaryngology, vol I, Philadelphia, 1980, WB Saunders Co.
3. Gruart FJ, Yoel J, and Wagner A: Value of perilingual lymphography in cancer of the head and neck, Am J Surg 114:520, 1967.
4. Matoba N and Kikueli T: Thyroidolymphography, Radiology 92:339, 1967.
5. Sachdeva HS et al: Thyroid lymphography, Arch Surg 109:385, 1974.
6. Johner CH: The lymphatics of the larynx, Otolaryngol Clin North Am 3:439, 1970.
7. Mancuso AA et al: CT of cervical lymph node cancer, AJR 136:381, 1981.
8. Reede D and Bergeron RT: CT of cervical lymph nodes, J Otolaryngol 11(6):411, 1982.
9. Mancuso AA et al: Computed tomography of cervical and retropharyngeal lymph nodes: normal anatomy, variants of normal, and applications in staging head and neck cancer. I. Normal anatomy, Radiology 148:709, 1983.
10. Mancuso AA et al: Computed tomography of cervical and retropharyngeal lymph nodes: normal anatomy, variants of normal, and applications in staging head and neck cancer. II. Pathology, Radiology 148:715, 1983.
11. Muraki AS, Mancuso AA, and Harnsberger HR: Metastatic cervical adenopathy from tumors of unknown origin: the role of CT, Radiology 152:749, 1984.
12. Som PM: Lymph nodes of the neck, Radiology 165:596, 1987.
13. Rouviere H: Lymphatic system of the head and neck. In Tobias MJ, translator: Anatomy of the human lymphatic system, Ann Arbor, Mich, 1938, Edwards Brothers, pp 5-28.
14. Shah JP et al: Surgical grand rounds, neck dissection: current status and future possibilities, Clin Bull 11:25, 1981.
15. Beahrs OH et al, editors: Manual for staging of cancer, ed 3, Philadelphia, 1988, JB Lippincott Co.
16. Cachin U et al: Nodal metastasis from carcinoma of the oropharynx, Otolaryngol Clin North Am 12:145, 1972.
17. Kalnins IK et al: Correlation between prognosis and degree of lymph node involvement in cancer of the oral cavity, Am J Surg 134:450, 1977.
18. Spiro RH et al: Cervical nodal metastasis from epidermoid carcinoma of the oral cavity and oropharynx, Am J Surg 128:562, 1974.
19. Jesse RH: The philosophy of treatment of neck nodes, Ear Nose Throat J 56:58, 1977.
20. Jesse RH and Fletcher GH: Treatment of the neck in patients with squamous cell carcinoma of the head and neck, Cancer 39:868, 1977.
21. Ballantyne AJ: Significance of retropharyngeal nodes in carcinoma of the head and neck, Am J Surg 108:500, 1964.
22. Sako K et al: Fallibility of palpation in the diagnosis of metastasis to cervical nodes, Surg Gynecol Obstet 118:989, 1964.
23. Cinberg JZ et al: Cervical cysts: cancer until proven otherwise, Laryngoscope 92:27, 1982.
24. Stevens MH et al: Computed tomography of cervical lymph nodes: staging and management of head and neck cancer, Arch Otolaryngol 11:735, 1985.
25. Schuller DE: Management of cervical metastasis in head and neck cancer, No 82200, Washington, DC, American Academy of Otolaryngology, Head and Neck Surgery Foundation, 1982.
26. Som PM: An approach to tumors of the head and neck: the role of computed tomography in the staging and follow-up of patients. In Margulis RR and Gooding CA, editors: Diagnostic radiology, San Francisco, 1985, University of California, pp 347-352.
27. Ogura JH and Biller HF: Head and neck—surgical management, JAMA 221:77, 1972.
28. Hajek PC et al: Lymph nodes of the neck: evaluation with US, Radiology 158:739, 1986.
29. Simpson GT: The evaluation and management of neck masses of unknown etiology, Otolaryngol Clin North Am 13:489, 1980.
30. Winegar LK and Griffin W: The occult primary tumor, Arch Otolaryngol 98:159, 1973.
31. Jaques DA: Management of metastatic nodes in the neck from an unknown primary. In Apparella MM and Shumrick DA, editors: Otolaryngology, vol 3, Philadelphia, 1980, WB Saunders Co.
32. Mancuso AA and Hanafee WN: The radiographic evaluation of patients with head and neck cancer. RSNA Syllabus—Head and Neck Cancer (Categorical Course in Radiation Therapy), 1981.
33. Canellos GP: Malignant lymphomas. In Rubenstein E and Federman DD, editors: Scientific medicine, New York, 1986, Scientific American Books, pp 1-15.
34. Castellino RA: Hodgkin's disease: practical concepts for the diagnostic radiologist, Radiology 159:305, 1986.
35. Albada J et al: Non-Hodgkin's lymphoma of Waldeyer's ring, Cancer 56:2911, 1985.
36. Shidnia H et al: Extranodal lymphoma of the head and neck area, Am J Clin Oncol 8:235, 1985.
37. Batsakis JG: Tumors of the head and neck: clinical and pathological considerations, ed 2, Baltimore, 1979, Williams & Wilkins, pp 450-491.
38. Lee YY et al: Lymphomas of the head and neck: CT findings at initial presentation, AJNR 8:665, 1987.

39. Harnsberger et al: Non-Hodgkin's lymphoma of the head and neck: CT evaluation of nodal and extranodal sites, AJNR 8:673, 1987.
40. McLennan TW and Castellino RA: Calcification in pelvic lymph nodes containing Hodgkin's disease following radiotherapy, Radiology 115:87, 1975.
41. Brereton ND and Johnson RE: Calcification in mediastinal lymph nodes after radiation therapy of Hodgkin's disease, Radiology 112:705, 1973.
42. Bertrand M et al: Lymph node calcification in Hodgkin's disease after chemotherapy, Am J Roentgenol 129:1108, 1977.
43. Dolan PA: Tumor calcification following therapy, Am J Roentgenol 89:166, 1973.
44. DeGiuli E and DeGiuli G: Lymph node calcification in Hodgkin's disease following irradiation, Acta Radiol 16:305, 1977.
45. Shin MS, Branscomb BV, and Ho KJ: Massive mediastinal Hodgkin's disease with calcification masquerading as teratocarcinoma: differentiation by computed tomography, JCAT 9:321, 1985.
46. Panicek DM et al: Calcification in untreated mediastinal lymphoma, Radiology 166:735, 1988.
47. Wycoco D and Raval B: An unusual presentation of mediastinal Hodgkin's lymphoma on computed tomography, JCAT 7:187, 1983.
48. Callen PW and Marks WM: Lymphomatous masses simulating cyst by ultrasonography, J Can Assoc Radiol 30:244, 1979.
49. Bruneton JN et al: Ear, nose, and throat cancer ultrasound diagnosis of metastasis to cervical lymph nodes, Radiology 152:771, 1984.
50. Kent DC: Tuberculous lymphadenitis: not a localized disease process, Am J Med Sci 254:866, 1967.
51. Levin-Epstein AA and Lucente FE: Scrofula—the dangerous masquerader, Laryngoscope 92:938, 1982.
52. Summers GD and McNicul MW: Tuberculosis of superficial lymph nodes, Br J Dis Chest 74:369, 1980.
53. Newcombe J: Tuberculosis: tuberculosis glands in the neck, Br J Hosp Med 6:553, 1979.
54. Tomblin JL and Roberts FJ: Tuberculous cervical lymphadenitis, Can Med Assoc J 121:324, 1979.
55. Appling D and Miller RH: *Mycobacterium* cervical lymphadenopathy, 1981 update, Laryngoscope 91:1259, 1981.
56. Waldman RH: Tuberculosis and the atypical mycobacteria, Otolaryngol Clin North Am 15:581, 1982.
57. Domb GH and Chole RA: The diagnosis and treatment of scrofula (mycobacterial cervical lymphadenitis), Otolaryngol Head Neck Surg 88:338, 1980.
58. Wong ML and Jefek BW: Cervical mycobacterial disease, Trans Am Acad Ophthalmol Otolaryngol 78:75, 1974.
59. Reede DL and Bergeron RT: Cervical tuberculous adenitis: CT manifestations, Radiology 154:701, 1985.
60. Koslin DB et al: Cervical Castleman's disease: CT study with angiographic correlation, Radiology 160:213, 1986.
61. Holliday RA et al: Benign lymphoepithelial parotid cysts and hyperplastic cervical adenopathy in AIDS—risk patients: a new CT appearance, Radiology 168:439, 1988.
62. Smith F et al: Benign lymphoepithelial lesions of parotid gland in intravenous drug users, Lab Invest 56:74A, 1987 (abstract).
63. Iaochim HL, Ryan JR, and Blaugrund SM: AIDS-associated lymphadenopathies and lymphomas with primary salivary gland presentation, Lab Invest 56:33A, 1987.
64. Ryan JR et al: Acquired immune deficiency syndrome–related lymphadenopathies presenting in the salivary gland lymph nodes, Arch Otolaryngol 111:554, 1985.
65. Bernier JL and Bhaskar SN: Lymphoepithelial lesions of the salivary glands, Cancer 11:1156, 1958.

SECTION FOUR
THORACIC INLET AND LOWER NECK

DEBORAH L. REEDE

The thoracic inlet, which is located at the base of the neck, serves as a junction between the neck and the chest. It is delineated by Sibson's fascia, which extends on each side of the neck from the transverse process of the seventh cervical vertebra posteriorly to the medial border of the first rib anteriorly. Since the posterior attachment is more cranially located than the anterior aspect of the first rib, the plane of the thoracic inlet is tilted downward anteriorly and on each side it is higher medially than it is laterally. Because of this orientation, when axial images are obtained the apices of the lungs are seen posteriorly, whereas the soft tissue structures of the inferior neck are visualized anterolaterally. Several major neural and vascular structures are found in this region, and the key reference point for them is the anterior scalene muscle.

The subclavian vein is located just anterior to the anterior scalene muscle, and the subclavian artery runs just posterior to it. The phrenic nerve and vagus nerve cross the thoracic inlet anterior to the subclavian artery, with the phrenic nerve being lateral and the vagus nerve medial (Fig. 8-91). The brachial plexus is located just posterior and superior to the subclavian artery, and the sympathetic trunk is located in the lower neck along the anterior aspect of the longus capitis muscle (Fig. 8-92).

A knowledge of the location of these neural structures is important when looking for lesions that produce palsies of these nerves and when predicting what nerves will be affected by a mass in this region of the neck.

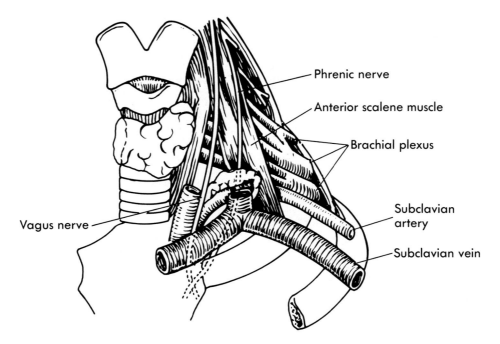

Fig. 8-91 Thoracic inlet. Neural and vascular structures are shown. Note relationship of these structures to anterior scalene muscle. (From Reede DL and Bergeron RT: The CT evaluation of the normal and diseased neck, Semin Ultrasound CT MR 7(2):181, 1986.)

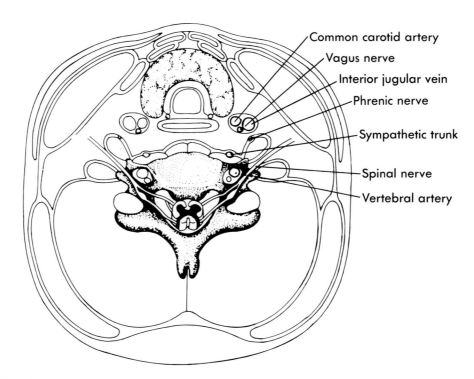

Fig. 8-92 Cross-sectional image showing location of major nerves in neck. (From Reede DL and Bergeron RT: The CT evaluation of the normal and diseased neck, Semin Ultrasound CT MR 7(2):181, 1986.)

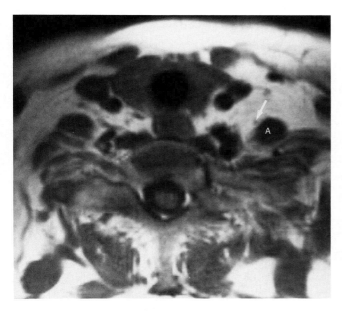

Fig. 8-93 Phrenic nerve—lower neck. Axial T₁-weighted MRI scan shows left phrenic nerve *(arrow)* adjacent to anterior border of anterior scalene muscle *(A)*.

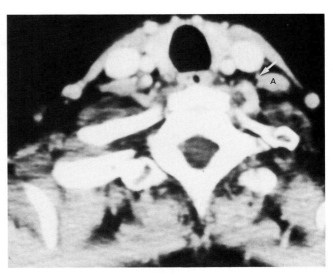

Fig. 8-94 Phrenic nerve—lower neck. Contrast-enhanced CT scan shows phrenic nerve *(arrow)* adjacent to anteromedial border of left anterior scalene muscle *(A)*.

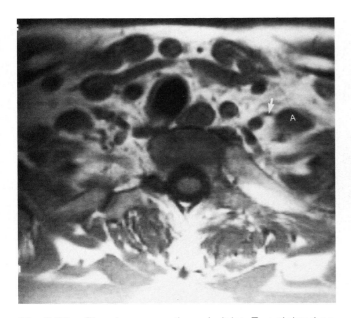

Fig. 8-95 Phrenic nerve—thoracic inlet. T₁-weighted axial MRI scan obtained at level of thoracic inlet shows left phrenic nerve *(arrow)*. In this region nerve is medial to anterior scalene muscle *(A)*.

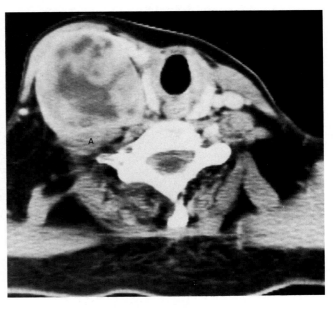

Fig. 8-96 Neurofibroma. Contrast-enhanced CT scan shows large nonhomogeneously enhancing neurofibroma pressing on anterior scalene muscle *(A)*. Patient had history of neurofibromatosis and paralyzed right hemidiaphragm.

PHRENIC NERVE

The phrenic nerve originates from the C3, C4, and C5 nerve roots. In the neck the phrenic nerve travels beneath the deep cervical fascia, which envelops the anterior scalene muscle (Figs. 8-92 through 8-94). The nerve runs obliquely downward along the outer aspect of this muscle, having a vertical course that crosses the muscle from superolaterally to inferomedially. Inferiorly the nerve passes medial to the muscle and thus comes to lie on the anterior surface of the subclavian artery (Figs. 8-91 and 8-95). After it crosses the thoracic inlet, the nerve travels in contact with the mediastinal pleura throughout its course to the diaphragm.

Paralysis of the diaphragm is a manifestation of phrenic nerve palsy. This diagnosis can be made when diaphragmatic motion is absent on inspiratory and expiratory roentgenograms or when paradoxical motion of the diaphragm is observed on fluoroscopy.

Phrenic nerve palsy has a number of causes, including viral neuritis, a mass pressing on the nerve, trauma, and iatrogenic causes (surgery). Radiologically, the goal is to identify any mass along the course of the nerve. Thus a mass that abuts the anterior border of the anterior scalene muscle in the neck (Fig. 8-96) or the anterior border of the subclavian artery at the thoracic inlet or that lies in the mediastinum in the chest can produce a phrenic nerve palsy.

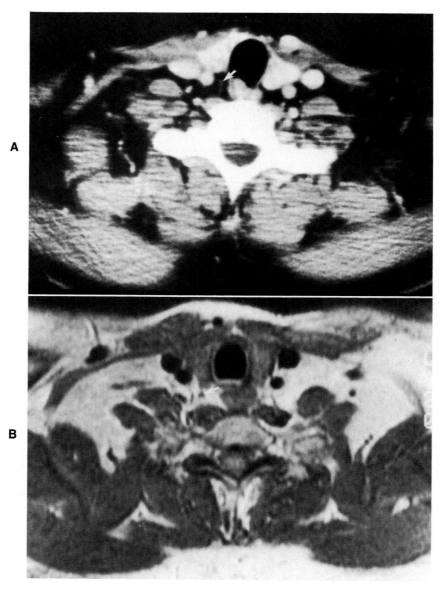

Fig. 8-97   Recurrent laryngeal nerve. **A,** Axial CT scan and **B,** axial MRI scan obtained at level of thyroid gland show right recurrent laryngeal nerve *(arrow)* in tracheoesophageal sulcus.

VAGUS NERVE

The vagus nerve is located in the posterior aspect of the carotid sheath between the carotid artery (medially) and the internal jugular vein (laterally) (see Fig. 8-92). On the right side the vagus nerve gives off the recurrent laryngeal nerve below the level of the right subclavian artery at the cervicothoracic junction. The right recurrent laryngeal nerve loops under and anterior to the subclavian artery and then travels superiorly in the tracheoesophageal sulcus (Figs. 8-92 and 8-97, *A* and *B*) en route to the larynx, where it terminates at the level of the cricoarytenoid junction. On the left side the recurrent laryngeal nerve arises from the vagus nerve in the mediastinum, not in the neck. The left recurrent laryngeal nerve travels between the aorta and the left pulmonary artery, passing first below and then anterior to the aortic arch and traversing the aortopulmonary window. The nerve travels posteriorly to reach the tracheoesophageal sulcus and then follows the same course as its counterpart on the right. Because the left recurrent laryngeal nerve has an intrathoracic course, it is susceptible to damage from mediastinal pathologic conditions as well as from disease in the neck.

The list of causes of recurrent laryngeal nerve palsy is lengthy and includes broad categories of disease such as inflammatory neuropathies, neoplasms of the neck and chest, trauma, cardiovascular disease (aortic aneurysm and left atrial enlargement) and idiopathic disorders. The nerve paralysis may be acute or chronic; in either case the patient has hoarseness and vocal cord paralysis.

An acute unilateral recurrent laryngeal nerve paralysis often is idiopathic, secondary to a toxic or infectious condition, or is the result of trauma. Most of these patients recover complete function of their vocal cords. This is especially true when the cause is inflammatory or idiopathic, with over 80% of these patients recovering function of their vocal cords. Function usually returns spontaneously within 6 months of the onset of paralysis; recovery is unlikely if function has not returned within 9 months.[1]

A chronic unilateral recurrent laryngeal nerve palsy usually is secondary to a neoplasm with extralaryngeal lesions, thyroid malignancies being the most common causes.[2,3]

The radiologist often is asked to evaluate patients with recurrent laryngeal nerve palsy. If a pulmonary lesion is suspected, a chest roentgenogram often is the initial study performed. By and large, however, CT or MRI is used to evaluate these patients.[4-6] By dividing vagal neuropathies into proximal and distal categories based on the clinical findings, it is possible to determine the region to be scanned and the preferred imaging modality.[6]

Lesions involving the proximal portion of the vagus nerve usually are accompanied by neuropathies of one or more associated cranial nerves (IX, XI, XII), since these nerves travel in close proximity to the vagus nerve both at their point of origin in the brainstem and below the skull base. MRI is the imaging modality of choice in these patients. The scans should be obtained through the levels of the brainstem and oropharynx. T_1-weighted images are most helpful in the extracranial region, whereas T_2-weighted images are more diagnostic in the brainstem.

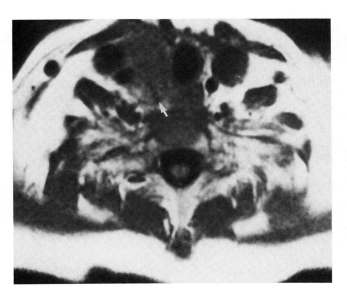

Fig. 8-98   Metastatic lung carcinoma. MRI study shows mass in paratracheal and tracheoesophageal regions on right. Mass is engulfing right recurrent laryngeal nerve *(arrow)*. Patient had lung carcinoma and right vocal cord paralysis.

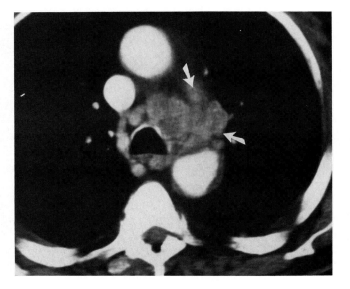

Fig. 8-99   Small cell carcinoma of the lung. In patient with left vocal cord paralysis, contrast-enhanced CT shows enlarged lymph nodes in aorticopulmonary window *(arrows)*.

If a patient presents with an isolated recurrent laryngeal nerve palsy (distal vagal neuropathy), CT is the preferred imaging modality. Scans should be obtained with intravenous contrast from the level of the hyoid bone to the level of the carina. Such a protocol includes the entire distal course of both recurrent laryngeal nerves. In the neck a lesion in the tracheoesophageal sulcus may produce a recurrent laryngeal palsy (Fig. 8-98). Both recurrent laryngeal nerves can be involved by lesions at the level of the thoracic inlet. Since the left recurrent laryngeal nerve has a longer intrathoracic course, it commonly is involved by mediastinal pathologic conditions (Fig. 8-99).

BRACHIAL PLEXUS

The brachial plexus is formed by the anterior nerve roots C5-T1 with occasional contributions from C4 and T2. The roots join to form nerve trunks, divisions, cords, and subsequently peripheral nerves (Fig. 8-100). Although the anatomic communication among these neural structures is complex, the components of the brachial plexus have a constant relationship to structures that are readily identified on both CT and MRI. Although direct visualization of the nerves can be routinely achieved with MRI, occasionally the nerves are identified on CT. Regardless of the imaging modality used, a knowledge of the location of the components of the brachial plexus is necessary when cross-sectional imaging is used to evaluate patients with brachial plexopathies.

The cervical nerve roots in the upper neck are located in a posteromedial position adjacent to the neural foramina. Because of the lordotic curvature of the cervical spine, the more superior nerve roots are located anterior to the inferior roots. The superior nerve roots run inferiorly, laterally, and anteriorly to pass between the anterior and middle scalene muscles (Fig. 8-101, A and B). The C5 and C6 cervical nerves unite adjacent to the lateral border of the anterior scalene muscle to form the upper trunk of the brachial plexus, whereas the seventh nerve emerges by itself as the middle trunk. In the lower neck the C8 and T1 nerves join behind the anterior scalene muscle to form the lower trunk (Fig. 8-102, A and B). Each trunk has an anterior and posterior division. The divisions of the superior and middle trunks form a little lateral to the anterior scalene muscle, whereas the lower trunk divides either behind the clavicle or in the axilla.

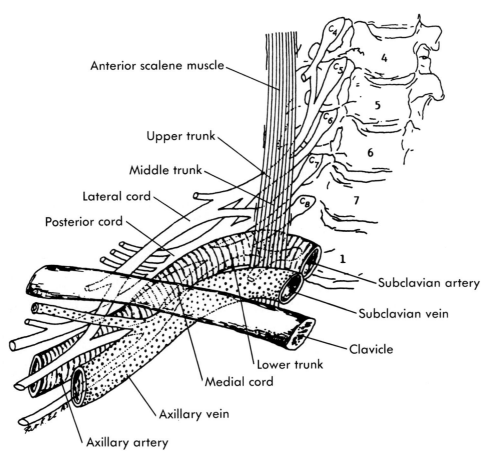

Fig. 8-100 Brachial plexus. Diagram shows brachial plexus and its relationship to anterior scalene muscle and axillary artery.

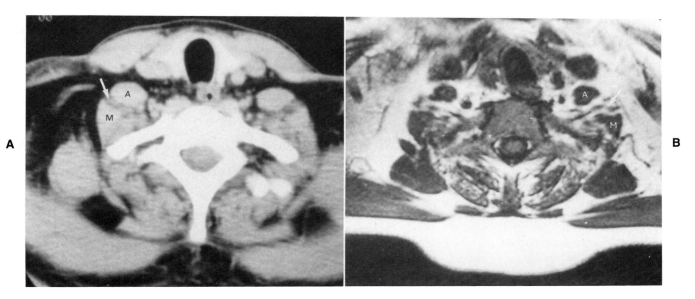

Fig. 8-101   Brachial plexus nerve roots. **A,** Axial CT scan and **B,** axial MRI scan obtained at level of thyroid gland show cervical nerve roots *(arrow)* passing between anterior scalene muscle *(A)* and middle scalene muscle *(M)*.

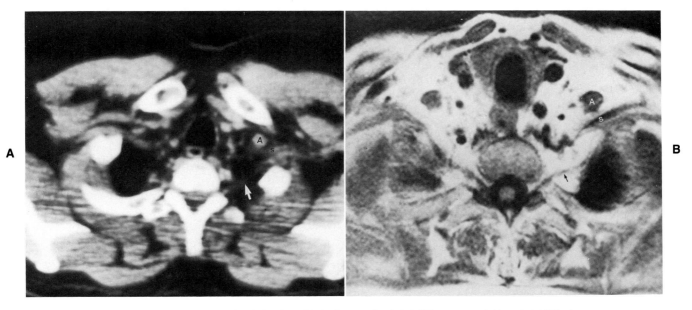

Fig. 8-102   Lower trunk of the brachial plexus. **A,** Axial CT scan and **B,** axial MRI obtained at level of thoracic inlet show T1 nerve root *(arrow)* traveling over apex of lung to join C8 nerve root behind subclavian artery *(s)*. Note that anterior scalene muscle *(A)* is anterior to artery at this level.

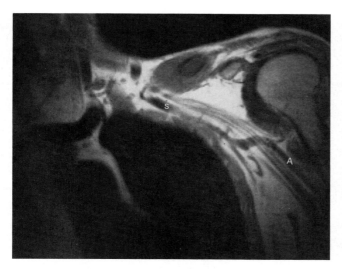

Fig. 8-103 Brachial plexus—supraclavicular and axillary region. Components of brachial plexus are nicely demonstrated above subclavian artery (s) in supraclavicular region and surrounding axillary artery in axilla (A) on coronal T₁-weighted MRI.

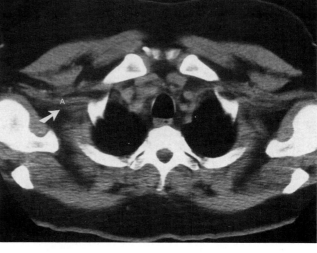

Fig. 8-104 Brachial plexus—axilla. CT scan obtained at level of thoracic inlet shows components of brachial plexus (arrow) posterior to axillary artery (A) in axilla.

Three cords are formed from the divisions as follows:
1. The lateral cord is formed by the anterior division of the upper and middle trunks, which unite in the lower neck (i.e., the anterior divisions of the C5, C6, and C7 nerves).
2. The medial cord is derived from the anterior division of the lower trunk in the lower neck (i.e., the C8 and T1 nerves).
3. The posterior cord is formed by the posterior divisions of all three trunks in the axilla (it has components of all the nerves that form the brachial plexus).

These three cords enter the axilla by traveling between the clavicle and first rib. As they pass over the rib, the cords are found around the axillary artery and are named for their location in reference to this vessel (lateral, medial, and posterior) (Figs. 8-103 and 8-104). After traveling a short distance in the axilla, the cords form peripheral nerves (musculocutaneous, median, and ulnar nerves).[7,8]

Patients with brachial plexopathies may have pain, numbness, and sensory and motor deficits in the upper extremity. Pain, if present, may increase with neck traction, shoulder movement, or deep inspiration. Palpation or percussion in the supraclavicular fossa often elicits tenderness. Occasionally a mass is palpated in the lower neck or axilla. Locating the precise site of involvement may be difficult, since several sites of disease can produce similar signs and symptoms.

Electromyography (EMG) may aid in distinguishing a root avulsion from a plexus level injury. EMG abnormalities in the paraspinal muscles indicate that a lesion is proximal to the plexus trunks. EMG abnormalities in peripheral muscles show which are abnormal and thus define which peripheral nerve territories are involved.[9]

Brachial plexopathy has a number of causes, which can be categorized as being traumatic or nontraumatic. Trauma accounts for approximately 50% of the cases. Injuries caused by trauma, with or without fractures, can cause compression, stretching, or avulsion of the nerve roots. The upper trunk is most frequently involved; the middle trunk is traumatized infrequently.[9] Nontraumatic causes of brachial plexopathy include metastatic disease, injury caused by irradiation, primary neoplasms (nerve sheath tumors), and idiopathic disease. With nontraumatic cases an attempt should be made to determine if the plexopathy is idiopathic, since this is a benign, self-limited condition that usually resolves within 3 years. A mass should be suspected as causing the brachial plexopathy if Horner's syndrome, lower plexus symptoms, and/or a history of a neoplasm is present.

Patients with known neoplasms who have had previous radiation therapy may develop brachial plexopathies, which may be caused by recurrent disease or radiation fibrosis. A study of 100 such cases showed that the clinical findings in these two entities were different.[10] Radiation fibrosis is unlikely to occur with doses of less than 60 Gy. If neurologic symptoms occur in less than a year after a dose of 60 Gy or greater, radiation damage is the most likely diagnosis. If the symptoms occur after a year, the plexopathy may be secondary to tumor recurrence or radiation damage. Pain and weakness in the distribution of the lower

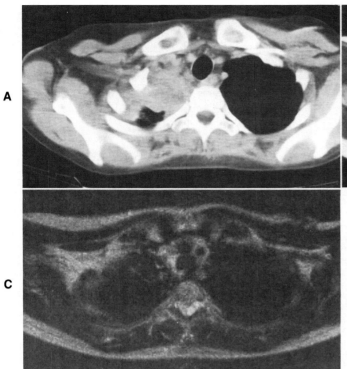

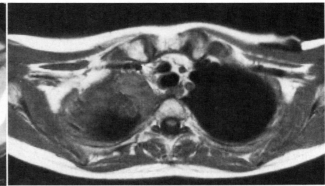

Fig. 8-105   Radiation fibrosis. Patient had surgery and radiation therapy for Pancoast tumor of right lung. He had mass in right lung apex and right brachial plexopathy. **A,** CT scan obtained at level of thoracic inlet shows mass in right lung apex that abuts posterior border of subclavian artery. **B,** T_1-weighted MRI and **C,** T_2-weighted scan show mass as having same density as muscle.

plexus and Horner's syndrome suggest metastatic disease. Patients with a postradiation plexopathy usually have painless weakness of the shoulder abductors, arm flexors, and lymphedema.[10]

MRI may be useful in distinguishing between radiation fibrosis and recurrent disease. Radiation fibrosis has a signal intensity similar to that of muscle on T_1- and T_2-weighted sequences[11]; fibrous tissue has calculated long T_1- and short T_2-relaxation times.[12] Although a tumor and radiation fibrosis may have a similar appearance on T_1-weighted sequences, their signal intensities on T_2-weighted sequences are different; tumors are hyperintense to muscle, whereas radiation fibrosis is isointense to muscle on T_2-weighted sequences (Fig. 8-105, *A, B,* and *C*). It should be noted, however, that infection and hemorrhage may have a high signal intensity on T_2-weighted images and thus may simulate tumor recurrence.[11]

A number of imaging modalities, including plain film roentgenograms of the cervical spine and shoulder girdle, myelography, CT, and MRI can be used to evaluate patients with brachial plexopathies. The initial imaging study used should be determined by the clinical setting. CT and MRI protocols for imaging of the brachial plexus are discussed in the section on normal anatomy of the neck.

The primary concern in patients who have suffered a traumatic injury and who have a brachial plexopathy is whether there is a fracture (cervical spine or clavicle) or

an avulsion of a nerve root. It should be noted, however, that soft tissue swelling and/or hematomas in the region of the brachial plexus can produce the same symptoms.

If a fracture is suspected, a plain film examination of the area is the initial radiographic study. However, if an avulsion of a nerve root and pseudomeningoceles are suspected, these neurogenic findings can be readily confirmed with myelography. This latter study can be augmented by a CT scan done afterward (Fig. 8-106, *A* and *B*).

MRI also can be used to make these diagnoses. Absence of the low-signal-intensity nerve root in the fat of the neural foramen on T_1-weighted images is consistent with a nerve root avulsion. This is best appreciated on sagittal images. Increased T_1-weighted signal intensity has been observed in traumatized nerves.[13,14] The cause of this high signal intensity is uncertain, but it is believed to be the result of neural edema.[13] Small pseudomeningoceles may not be detected on MRI. A pseudomeningocele appears as an extraarachnoid CSF-intensity mass extending outside the spinal canal (Fig. 8-106, *C*). Axial and coronal scans offer the best visualization of such lesions.

Either CT or MRI can be used to evaluate patients in the nontraumatic category of brachial plexopathy.[13-18] MRI is the imaging modality of choice because of its ability to directly visualize nerves and blood vessels, its lack of artifacts, and its multiplanar capabilities. One of

Text continued on p. 591.

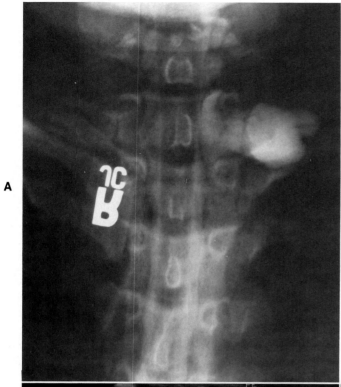

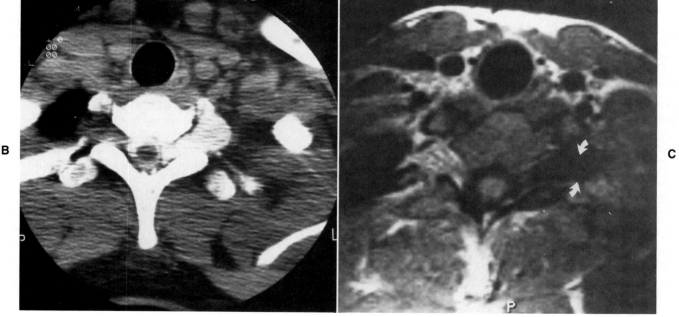

Fig. 8-106 Pseudomeningoceles. **A,** Myelogram shows pseudomeningoceles at C6, C7, and T1 on left; largest pseudomeningocele at C7 level. **B,** CT scan done after myelogram shows contrast in pseudomeningocele at C7 level *(left).* **C,** On T_1-weighted MRI scan, pseudomeningocele *(arrows)* has same signal intensity as cerebrospinal fluid.

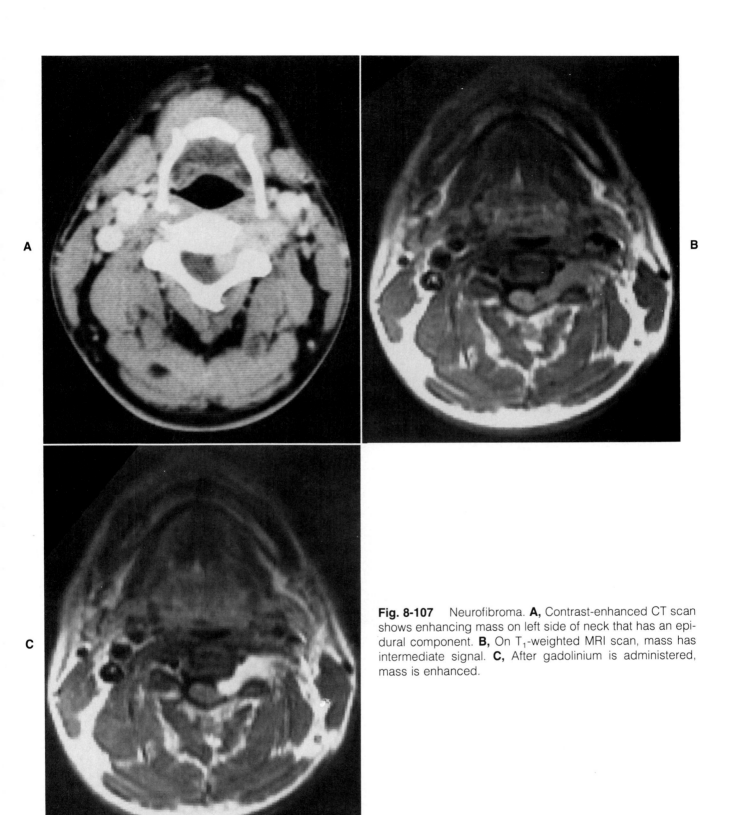

Fig. 8-107 Neurofibroma. **A,** Contrast-enhanced CT scan shows enhancing mass on left side of neck that has an epidural component. **B,** On T_1-weighted MRI scan, mass has intermediate signal. **C,** After gadolinium is administered, mass is enhanced.

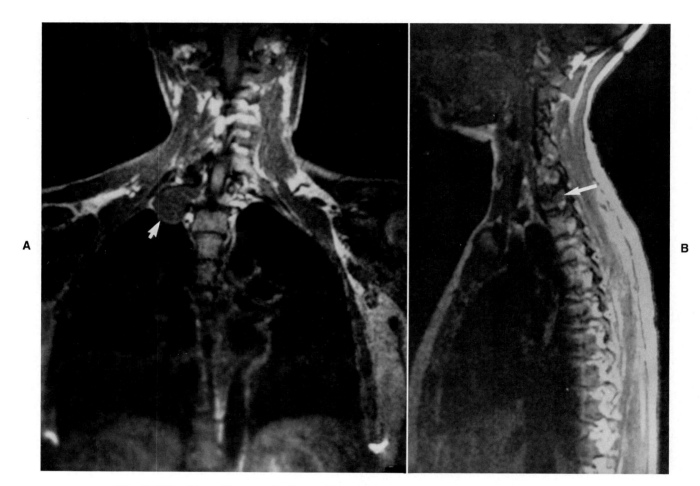

Fig. 8-108 Neurofibroma. **A,** Coronal T_1-weighted MRI scan shows mass arising from right C8 nerve root *(short arrow)*. Mass extends into soft tissues of neck and is causing extrensic compression of right lung apex. **B,** Sagittal T_1-weighted MRI scan shows enlargement of C8 nerve root *(arrow)*. Note that nerve roots are located in superior aspect of neurofibroma.

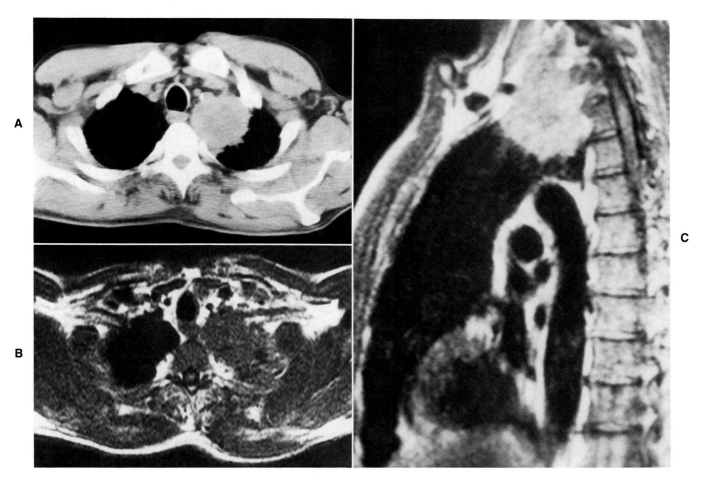

Fig. 8-109   Pancoast tumor. **A,** CT scan obtained at level of thoracic inlet shows mass in left lung apex. Mass abuts posterior wall of subclavian artery and therefore should involve brachial plexus. **B,** Similar findings are observed on axial T_1-weighted MRI scan in same region. **C,** Extension of tumor into base of neck is best appreciated on sagittal T_2-weighted MRI scan. Tumor becomes hyperintense on the T_2-weighted imaging sequence. Note irregular borders between mass and normal parenchyma.

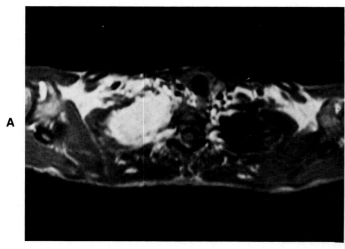

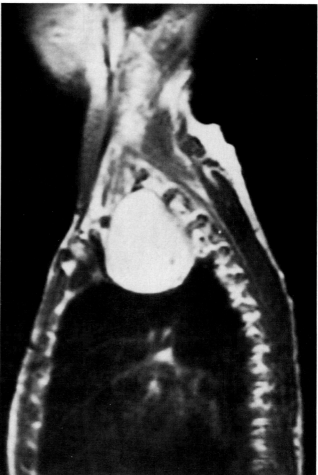

Fig. 8-110 Neurofibroma. **A,** Axial and **B,** sagittal T$_1$-weighted MR images after gadolinium administration show enhancing mass in right thoracic inlet region. Mass has sharp interface with lung and adjacent soft tissue structures.

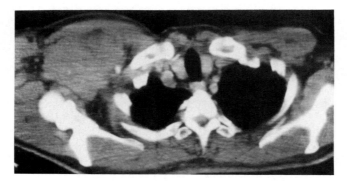

Fig. 8-111 Metastatic melanoma. Large metastatic nodes are seen in right axilla in patient with melanoma. Since nodes surround axillary vessels, it is easy to understand why patient developed brachial plexopathy.

the major disadvantages of CT in evaluating the lower neck is that only axial scans can be obtained directly. Additionally, beam-hardening artifacts are encountered at the level of the thoracic inlet, and contrast administration is required to visualize blood vessels. Regardless of which of these imaging modalities is used, a knowledge of the location of the components of the brachial plexus allows diagnosis of a mass or anatomic alteration that likely is the cause of a brachial plexopathy. To achieve this goal the following discussion covers examples of lesions located along the course of the brachial plexus on both CT and MRI.

Neural tumors, posttraumatic injuries, and metastatic disease are the common causes of disease in the region of the nerve roots. Since the nerve roots pass between the anterior and middle scalene muscles, they could be affected by a lesion in this region. Axial CT and MRI images are ideal for the evaluation of this area (Fig. 8-107, A, B, and C). Coronal and sagittal images may also be used (Fig. 8-108, A and B). Sagittal images are particularly useful when looking for an absent nerve root (avulsion) in the neural foramen.

Lesions involving the trunks and divisions of the brachial plexus occur in the lateral aspect of the posterior triangle and supraclavicular region. Metastatic disease and Pancoast tumors are primarily encountered in this region (Fig. 8-109, A, B, and C). Occasionally neural tumors are seen in the supraclavicular region and near the apex of the lung. These tumors tend to be well circumscribed and have a sharp interface with adjacent structures (Fig. 8-110). By comparison, metastatic disease and primary neoplasms tend to have irregular infiltrating borders.

The cords and proximal portions of the peripheral nerves formed by the brachial plexus are located in the axilla, where they are found adjacent to the axillary artery. Thus a lesion that abuts the axillary artery any-where in the axilla may produce brachial plexus symptoms. Metastatic disease is commonly encountered in this region (Fig. 8-111). Primary soft tissue tumors and trauma also may affect the brachial plexus in this area.

REFERENCES

1. Ballenger JJ: Disease of the nose, throat, ear, head and neck, ed 13, Philadelphia, 1985, Lea & Febiger, pp 513-548.
2. Clerf LH: Unilateral vocal cord paralysis, JAMA 151:900, 1953.
3. Tiche LL: Causes of recurrent laryngeal nerve paralysis, Arch Otolaryngol 102:259, 1976.
4. Glazer HS and Aronberg DJ: Extralaryngeal causes of vocal cord paralysis: CT evaluation, AJR 141:527, 1983.
5. Frisa J, Bellin M, and Laval-Jeantet M: CT mediastinal examination in recurrent nerve paralysis, JCAT 8:901, 1984.
6. Jacobs CJM et al: Vagal neuropathy: evaluation with CT and MR imaging, Radiology 164:97, 1987.
7. Hollinshead WH: Anatomy for surgeons. Vol I, The head and neck, New York, 1968, Harper & Row, Publishers, Inc.
8. Montgomery RL: Head and neck anatomy with clinical correlations, New York, 1981, McGraw-Hill, Inc.
9. Swanson PD: Signs and symptoms in neurology, New York, 1984, JB Lippincott Co.
10. Kori SH, Foley KM, and Posner JB: Brachial plexus lesions in patients with cancer: 100 cases, Neurology 31:45, 1981.
11. Glazer HS et al: Radiation fibrosis: differentiation from recurrent tumor by MR imaging, Radiology 156:721, 1985.
12. Farmer DW et al: Calcific fibrosing mediastinitis: demonstration of pulmonary vascular obstruction by magnetic resonance imaging, AJR 143:1189, 1984.
13. Rapoport S et al: Brachial plexus: correlation of MR imaging with CT and pathologic findings, Radiology 167:161, 1988.
14. Kneeland JB et al: Diagnosis of disease of the supraclavicular region by use of MR imaging, AJR 148:1149, 1987.
15. Kellman GM et al: MR imaging of the supraclavicular region: normal anatomy, AJR 148:77, 1987.
16. Castagno AA and Shuman WP: MR imaging in clinically suspected brachial plexus tumor, AJR 149:1219, 1987.
17. Armington WG et al: Radiographic evaluation of brachial plexopathy, AJNR 8:361, 1987.
18. Gebarski KS, Glazer GM, and Gebarski SS: Brachial plexus: anatomic, radiologic and pathologic correlation using computed tomography, JCAT 6:1058, 1982.

9 The Larynx

HUGH D. CURTIN

Although evaluation of the larynx uses many of the currently available imaging modalities, interest recently has centered on computed tomography (CT) and magnetic resonance imaging (MRI).[1-9] With these techniques the radiologist can visualize the deeper tissues directly. The information thus obtained, combined with the surface visualization of modern laryngoscopy, gives the referring clinician a much better understanding of the extent of the lesion than was previously possible.

In most cases the otolaryngologist has evaluated the mucosal surface and, in the case of carcinoma, has no question about the diagnosis. The radiologist's role, then, as is so often the case in head and neck radiology, is to show the deeper extent, defining the tumor margin in relation to precise anatomic landmarks. These determinations can make the difference between a total laryngectomy and a voice-sparing partial resection. Therefore the radiologist must know the anatomy from an otolaryngologist's perspective.

This chapter begins with the normal anatomy as seen using various imaging modalities. The discussion of the alterations of this anatomy as a result of various types of pathology follows. Some processes in which imaging is seldom helpful are included for completeness. The laryngopharynx is included because of its intimate relationship with the posterior aspects of the larynx.

593

SECTION ONE
ANATOMY

All the anatomy is important, but certain structures become key landmarks, either because of their surgical importance or because they provide orientation to the radiologist. The significance of these anatomic points is elaborated on later in the chapter.

Essentially the larynx is composed of a mucosal surface and a supporting cartilaginous skeleton. The mucosal surface, familiar to any otolaryngologist, has typical landmarks, including the epiglottis, true and false cords, aryepiglottic folds, and pyriform sinuses (Figs. 9-1 and 9-2). Between the mucosal surface and the cartilaginous skeleton lie the paraglottic and preepiglottic spaces, which contain loose areolar tissues, lymphatics, and key muscular structures.

The skeleton of the larynx is primarily made up of cartilage and fibrous bands (Figs. 9-3 and 9-4). The foundation is the cricoid, the only complete cartilaginous ring in the respiratory system. The cricoid is shaped like a signet ring, with the larger "signet" part facing posteriorly. This broader "signet" segment is called the quadrate lamina. The narrower arch extends

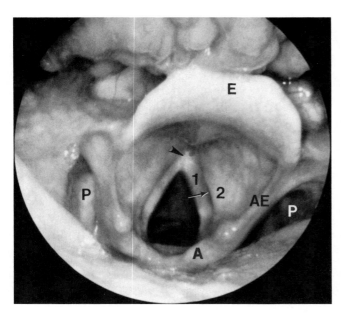

Fig. 9-1 Endoscopic view of the larynx. *1,* True vocal cord; *2,* false vocal cord; *E,* epiglottis; *AE,* aryepiglottic fold; *A,* arytenoid prominence; *P,* pyriform; *arrowhead,* anterior commissure. Arrow points to the entrance of the ventricle. (From Hanafee W: Hypopharynx and larynx. In Valvassori GE et al: Head and neck imaging, New York, 1988, Thieme Medical Publishers.)

anteriorly from the margins of the lamina to complete the ring. On each side at the junction of the arch and lamina is a small facet for the articulation of the inferior horn of the thyroid cartilage.

On the upper margin of the lamina are two paired facets, on which are perched the arytenoid cartilages (Figs. 9-3 to 9-5). Each arytenoid is pyramidal in shape and is important not only as a surgical landmark but also as a key guide to the radiologist in determining the level of the slice in an axial plane. The base of the arytenoid has a lateral bump called the muscular process. The vocal process projects from the anterior surface of the lower arytenoid. The vocal process forms a point to which the posterior vocal cord attaches (see Figs. 9-3 and 9-5).

The largest supporting cartilage is the double-winged thyroid cartilage, with the superior and inferior horns projecting from the posterior margins of the thyroid ala. The lower horn articulates with the lateral facets of the cricoid cartilage. The superior horn is connected to the hyoid by the thyrohyoid ligament. The anterior thyroid cartilage is marked by a deep notch on the superior margin. The thyroid and cricoid cartilages act as the external protection for the inner larynx. Because the cricoid, thyroid, and arytenoid cartilages are made of hyaline cartilage, they can calcify to varying degrees.

The flexible epiglottis is formed by yellow elastic fibrocartilage which, unlike the thyroid, cricoid, and arytenoid cartilages, seldom shows significant calcification. The epiglottis has a flattened teardrop shape that extends to a point inferiorly, the petiole of the epiglottis. Most of the epiglottis extends down behind the protective shield of the thyroid cartilage, and only a small portion of this cartilage extends above the hyoid bone, the so-called suprahyoid portion of the epiglottis. The epiglottic cartilage is held in place by the hyoepiglottic and thyroepiglottic ligaments.

Three smaller pairs of cartilage are found in the upper larynx. They are less significant radiologically but are occasionally visualized. The corniculate cartilages are small structures sitting immediately superior to the arytenoids (see Fig. 9-3). Slightly lateral and above the corniculate cartilages are the thin cuneiform cartilages, which are almost never visualized on sectional imaging. These cartilages help give shape to the upper margin of the larynx, the aryepiglottic fold. The triticeous cartilage is found in the posterior ligamentous connection between the thyroid cartilage and the hyoid bone.

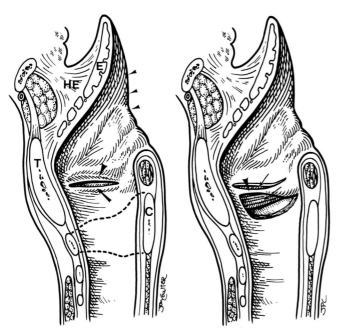

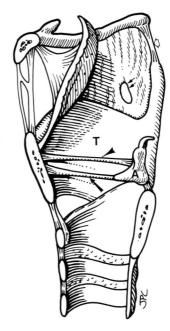

Fig. 9-2 **A,** Lateral wall of the airway. The larynx has been sectioned sagittally in midline. True cord *(arrow)* and the false cord *(large arrowhead)* are separated by the slit-like ventricle. AE fold *(small arrowheads); T,* thyroid cartilage; *C,* lamina of the cricoid cartilage (the projection of the arch of the cricoid is seen as a dashed line); *HE,* hyoepiglottic ligament; *E,* epiglottis. **B,** The mucosa of the true cord has been excised showing the thyroarytenoid muscle *(arrows)* paralleling the margin of the true cord *(arrowhead).*

Fig. 9-3 The mucosa, laryngeal muscles and paraglottic fat have been removed to show the skeleton of the larynx. The vocal ligament *(arrow)* stretches from the vocal process of the arytenoid *(A)* to the anterior thyroid cartilage. The ventricular ligament *(arrowhead)* stretches from the upper arytenoid to the thyroid cartilage. The small structure at the upper tip of the arytenoid is the corniculate cartilage. The lamina of the thyroid cartilage is represented by the letter T. The small hole *(double small arrows)* in the thyrohyoid membrane transmits the internal branch of the superior laryngeal nerve and accompanying vessel. The posterior thyrohyoid ligament *(open arrow)* represents the posterior margin of the thyrohyoid membrane.

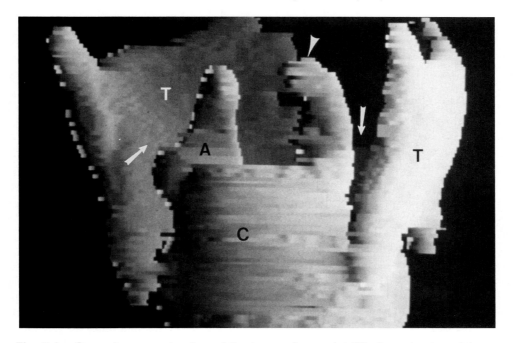

Fig. 9-4 Computer reconstruction of the larynx, from axial CT slices, is viewed from posteriorly and slightly to the right. The arytenoid *(A)* is perched on the lamina of the cricoid cartilage *(C).* Thyroid cartilage is represented by the letter T. Arrows show the thyroarytenoid gap representing the position of the apex of the pyriform sinus. Arrowhead shows the corniculate cartilage.

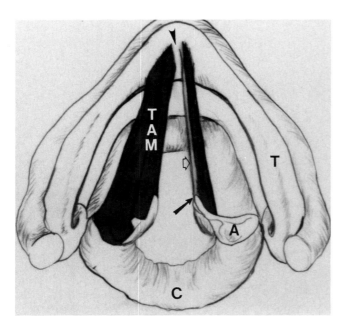

Fig. 9-5 View from above with mucosa and most of the soft tissue removed to show the relationship of arytenoid *(A)*, cricoid ring *(C)*, and thyroid cartilage *(T)*. The vocal ligament *(open arrow)* stretches from the vocal process *(arrow)* of the arytenoid to the anterior commissure *(arrowhead)*. TAM, Thyroarytenoid muscle. Only the medial muscle bundle *(vocalis)* is seen on the right.

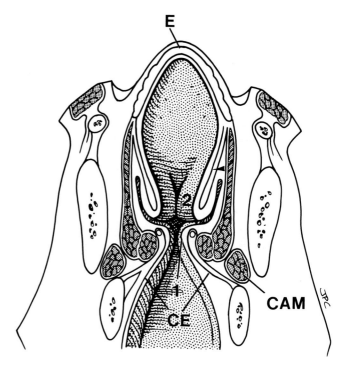

Fig. 9-6 Diagram of the coronal section through the larynx. The thyroarytenoid muscle forms the mass of the cord. The lateral cricoarytenoid muscle *(CAM)* is also seen slightly laterally and inferiorly. The conus elasticus *(CE)* extends from the vocal ligament at the cord level to the upper margin of the cricoid. On the right side of the diagram, the conus terminates at the upper margin of the cricoid cartilage. On the left side of the diagram some fibers of the conus continue along the medial surface of the cricoid as described by some. *E*, Epiglottis; *1*, true cord; *2*, false cord; quadrangular membrane *(arrowhead)*.

The hyoid bone is the rafter from which the larynx is suspended. Muscles acting on the hyoid elevate the larynx and by so doing provide the primary protection from laryngeal aspiration on swallowing. The hyoid bone is U shaped, having an anterior body, two small superior horns (or cornua), and two large horns that project posteriorly.

The ligaments and fascial layers are important not only for their role in structural support but also because they tend to organize certain disease processes. The cricothyroid membrane and thyrohyoid membrane close the gaps, respectively, between the cricoid and thyroid cartilage and between the thyroid cartilage and the hyoid bone. These membranes thus complete the external supportive architecture of the larynx and define the external anatomic limits of the larynx.

Two parallel ligaments extend from the arytenoid cartilages posteriorly to the inner lamina of the thyroid cartilage anteriorly (see Fig. 9-3). The more inferior vocal ligament stretches from the vocal process of the arytenoid cartilage to the thyroid cartilage and forms the medial and upper support of the true vocal cord. The ventricular ligament, on the other hand, attaches to the superior aspect of the arytenoid cartilage and stretches across the larynx (parallel to the vocal ligament) to attach to the inner lamina of the thyroid cartilage just above the attachment of the vocal ligament. This ligament is actually the lower free margin of the

quadrangular membrane and forms the edge of the false cord, or plica ventricularis.

The quadrangular membrane attaches posteriorly to the upper arytenoid and corniculate cartilages, then sweeps across the upper larynx to attach to the lateral margin of the epiglottis (Fig. 9-6). The lower margin is essentially free and therefore becomes the ventricular ligament. The upper margin forms the support of the aryepiglottic fold, which is the upper edge of the lateral wall of the inner larynx.

A similar membrane or fibrous layer stretches downward from the true cord to attach to the upper margin of the cricoid cartilage; this is the conus elasticus (see Fig. 9-6). Some fibers of this structure may reflect along the inner margin of the cricoid, but for the purposes of this discussion we can say it is attached to the superior cricoid margin. The conus elasticus is a thickened, more clearly defined structure than the quadrangular membrane. Anteriorly the conus fuses with the inner surface of the anterior cricothyroid membrane or ligament.

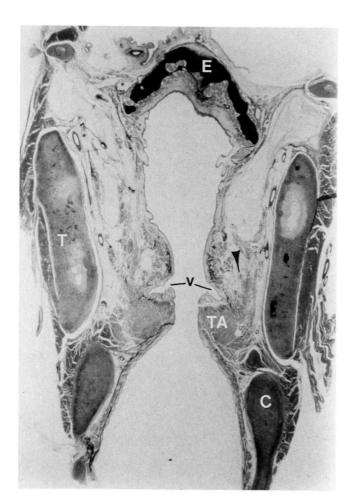

Fig. 9-7 Coronal section of the larynx. The bulk of the true cord is made up of the thyroarytenoid muscle *(TA)*. The ventricle *(v)* is seen between true and false cords. The paraglottic space *(arrowhead)* at the level of the false cord contains small slips of muscle but is predominantly filled with fat. *T,* Thyroid cartilage; *C,* cricoid cartilage; *E,* epiglottic cartilage.

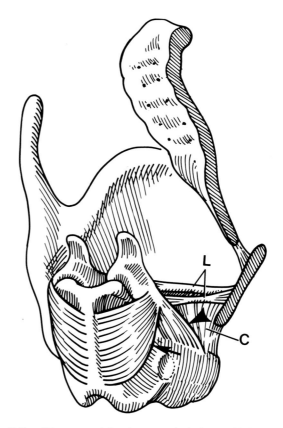

Fig. 9-8 Diagram of the laryngeal skeleton (right thyroid lamina has been removed) showing the posterior *(arrow)* and lateral *(arrowhead)* cricoarytenoid muscles. The posterior cricoarytenoid muscle is totally responsible for abduction of the true cord as the muscle pulls posteriorly on the lateral muscular process of the arytenoid. *C,* Conus elasticus; *L,* vocal ligaments.

As was previously mentioned, the epiglottis is supported partially by the quadrangular membrane. The epiglottis is also supported by ligaments or bands connecting the cartilage to the hyoid bone and to the pharyngeal wall and tongue base. The hyoepiglottic ligament is a definite fibrous structure extending from the vertical midline of the epiglottis anteriorly to the central hyoid (see Fig. 9-2). The midline (or median) glossoepiglottic fold and the more lateral pharyngoepiglottic folds are more mucosal reflections than true ligaments. Inferiorly, the thyroepiglottic ligament extends from the petiole to the midline inner surface of the thyroid cartilage, just above the level of attachment of the vocal ligaments.

The laryngeal muscles are described in terms of their origin and insertion. The most important muscle to the radiologist is the thyroarytenoid muscle because of its role as a landmark defining the level of the true vocal cord (see Figs. 9-2 and 9-5 to 9-7).

Each thyroarytenoid muscle stretches from the anterior lower surface of the arytenoid cartilage to the thyroid cartilage, thus paralleling the vocal ligament. The thyroarytenoid muscle is responsible for most of the bulk of the true cord. The thyroarytenoid muscle on each side can be separated into two bellies, medial and lateral, which run parallel to each other. The medial portion is often called the vocalis muscle. The mass of the lateral portion of the muscle is at the level of the true cord but variably some few fibers can extend superiorly to insert high on the thyroid cartilage. Thus a narrow slip of the thyroarytenoid muscle may be present above the level of the true cord.

Of equal importance to the function of the larynx but not as crucial to the radiologist are the cricoarytenoid muscles (Fig. 9-8). The lateral cricoarytenoid muscle stretches from the muscular process of the arytenoid to the upper lateral cricoid cartilage. The posterior cricoarytenoid muscle stretches from the posterior surface of the cricoid and attaches to the posterior surface of the lateral muscular process of the arytenoid. These small muscles can be seen occasionally on computed tomography or magnetic resonance imaging. The posterior cricoarytenoid muscle is the only muscle that directly swings the vocal cord laterally (abduction). The interarytenoid muscles stretch from arytenoid to arytenoid, completing the midline posterior wall of the larynx above the cricoid. These interarytenoid muscles have bilateral neural innervation. The cricothyroid muscle extends from the lower thyroid cartilage to the upper cricoid cartilage; it is the only external muscle of the larynx and the only muscle supplied by the superior laryngeal nerve (CN X) (external branch) rather than the recurrent laryngeal nerve (CN X).

The pharyngeal constrictors attach posteriorly to a midline raphe and then sweep obliquely downward around the lumen of the pharynx to attach to the hyoid bone above and more inferiorly to the sides of the cricoid and thyroid cartilages. Notably, the more inferior fibers attach to the lateral ala of the thyroid cartilage, not along the posterior margin of the cartilage but slightly more anteriorly along the lateral surface on the oblique line of this cartilage. This becomes important in tumor evaluation, as described in a later section. The pharyngeal constrictors are innervated by cranial nerve X, possibly with some influence from cranial nerve IX.

The lower fibers of the inferior constrictors are more parallel than are the more superior fibers and have been given a separate name: the cricopharyngeus muscle. The cricopharyngeus acts as a sphincter between the pharynx and the esophagus, stretching continuously from the lateral cricoid cartilage circumferentially around the gullet. There is a relatively weak point in the pharyngeal wall between the undersurface of the oblique fibers of the inferior constrictor and the upper surface of the cricopharyngeus muscle. This area is called Killian's dehiscence; it is discussed later with respect to Zenker's diverticula.

Discussion now returns to the various folds and recesses of the mucosal surface of the larynx. The inner larynx is marked by two prominent parallel bands, the true and false cords (see Figs. 9-1 and 9-2). Both are in the horizontal plane and run from posterior to anterior. The true cord is the more inferior and is separated from the false cord by a slitlike ventricle. The relationship of pathologic conditions to these three parallel structures is significant in evaluation of the larynx.

Each true cord attaches just slightly lateral to midline, leaving a very small "bare" area in the midline where the mucosa of the larynx is immediately adjacent to the thyroid cartilage and not separated from the cartilage by muscle, ligament, or a significant layer of fat. This region, called the anterior commissure, is slightly below the attachment of the petiole to the thyroid cartilage (see Fig. 9-3).

Above the false cords the mucosa reflects upward toward the free edges of the aryepiglottic folds, which form the lateral margins of the vestibule (supraglottic airspace), or entrance to the larynx. Each aryepiglottic fold stretches from the upper margin of the arytenoid to the lateral margin of the epiglottis. Within the aryepiglottic fold are the small corniculate and cuneiform cartilages that support the edge of the fold.

Lateral to the aryepiglottic fold is the pyriform sinus of the pharynx (Fig. 9-9). This mucosal recess pushes between the thyroid cartilage and the aryepiglottic fold. The extreme lower aspect of the pyriform sinus, called the apex, is actually situated between the mucosa-covered arytenoid and the mucosa-covered thyroid cartilage and is at the level of the true vocal cord. Anteriorly the pyriform sinus protrudes into the paraglottic space.

The epiglottis projects superiorly toward the oropharynx, causing several small folds and recesses to be defined. The valleculae are small recesses between the free margin of the epiglottis and the base of the

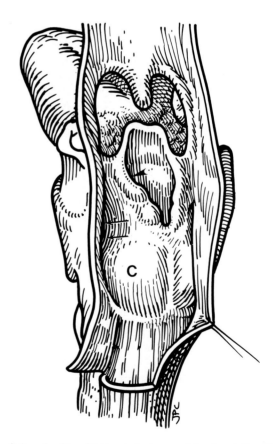

Fig. 9-9   A view from posterior and to the left with the pharynx open. The arrows show the pyriform sinus. *arrowhead*, aryepiglottic fold; *C*, cricoid. (Modified from Berman JM: Surgical anatomy of the larynx. In Bailey BJ and Biller HF: Surgery of the larynx, Philadelphia, 1985, WB Saunders Co, p. 20.)

tongue. The valleculae are crossed by a small fold in the midline called the median glossoepiglottic fold. More laterally the pharyngoepiglottic folds form the posterior aspect of the valleculae.

The paraglottic space (referred to by some authors as the paralaryngeal space) refers to the tissues between the mucosal surface of the inner larynx and the thyroid cartilage (see Figs. 9-6 and 9-7). Thus the paraglottic space is the region deep to the mucosal surface of the true and false cords. At the false cord level the paraglottic space is almost entirely composed of the fat between the quadrangular membrane and the thyroid cartilage. As previously stated, small slips of muscle may cross the space, but no bulky muscle mass is present. At the level of the true cord, the thyroarytenoid muscle fills almost all of the paraglottic space. The ventricle cleaves into the space just above the thyroarytenoid muscle but does not quite reach the thyroid cartilage (see Fig. 9-7). Thus the paraglottic space is continuous from true to false cords along the lateral aspect of the ventricle.

A small recess can project superiorly from the ventricle into the paraglottic fat at the level of the false cord. The small saccule, or appendix, of the ventricle is thus between the quadrangular membrane and the thyroid cartilage.

The posterior margin of the upper paraglottic space is the anterior mucosal surface of the pyriform sinus.

The preepiglottic space is between the epiglottis and the thyrohyoid membrane. Laterally on each side the space communicates with each paraglottic space. The preepiglottic space is composed predominantly of fat.

INNERVATION AND BLOOD SUPPLY

The larynx is innervated by the vagus nerve. The recurrent laryngeal nerves (after looping around the aortic arch on the left side and the subclavian artery on the right side) travel in the tracheoesophageal grooves at the lateral margins of the esophagus. The nerve passes medial to the lower margin of the cricopharyngeus muscle before entering the larynx in the sulcus between the thyroid cartilage and the cricoid cartilage. The recurrent laryngeal nerve innervates all of the intrinsic muscles of the larynx. The only extrinsic laryngeal muscle is the cricothyroid muscle; it is innervated by the external branch of the superior laryngeal nerve, which never actually enters the inner larynx. The internal branch of the superior laryngeal nerve does perforate the posterior lateral portion of the thyrohyoid membrane and provides sensation to the inner laryngeal mucosa.

The blood supply accompanies the nerves. The superior laryngeal artery is a branch of the superior thyroid artery and follows the internal branch of the superior laryngeal nerve. The inferior laryngeal artery is a branch of the inferior thyroid artery, which in turn is a branch of the thyrocervical trunk. The inferior laryngeal artery accompanies the recurrent laryngeal nerve into the larynx.

LYMPHATIC DRAINAGE

The upper and lower mucosal surfaces of the larynx have different lymphatic drainage. The true cord (mucosal surface) has almost no lymphatic drainage. The lymphatics of the supraglottic larynx drain to the upper jugular nodes. The preepiglottic and paraglottic spaces are particularly rich in lymphatics. The portion of the mucosal surface inferior to the cord (the subglottic region) drains to the paratracheal and pretracheal nodes and eventually into the lower jugular nodes. The Delphian node is situated anterior to the cricothyroid membrane. Tumor can reach this node either by direct extension or by lymphatic drainage from the region of the anterior commissure and subglottic larynx. The lymphatics of the paraglottic space drain superiorly, again to the upper jugular nodes. According to Pressman, Simon, and Monell, an injection of dye into the deep cord (thyroarytenoid muscle) also drains superiorly past the ventricle and through the thyrohyoid membrane into the upper jugular nodes along with the lymphatics of the upper larynx.[10] Thus the drainage of the deep larynx (as opposed to the mucosal surface) flows only in a superior direction.

REGIONS

Certain terms are important in the evaluation of the larynx, especially with regard to pathologic conditions involving tumors. Most surgery is described in reference to these terms. The free margin of the true cord defines the glottis. The glottic area extends from an imaginary horizontal plane that divides the laryngeal ventricle into upper and lower halves, down to an arbitrary line 1 cm below the apex of the ventricle. The subglottic area begins at this lower margin of the glottic region and extends down to the lower margin of the cricoid cartilage. The supraglottic larynx includes everything above the ventricle and extends to the free edge of the epiglottis and aryepiglottic folds.

The suprahyoid portion of the epiglottis is called the free segment. The anterior surface of the free margin of the epiglottis and the valleculae are often included in discussion of the base of the tongue and the pharynx. The postcricoid region is the mucosal covering of the posterior surface of the cricoid, representing the anterior wall of the pharynx at this level. The terms *junctional* and *marginal* are at times applied to the edge of the aryepiglottic fold because of its relationship to both the pharynx and the larynx.

REFERENCES

1. Castelijns JA et al: Invasion of laryngeal cartilage by cancer: comparison of CT and MR imaging, Radiology 166:199, 1987.
2. Castelijns JA et al: MR imaging of laryngeal cancer, JCAT 11(1):134, 1987.
3. Curtin HD: Current concepts of imaging of the larynx, Radiology 173:1, 1989.
4. Hanafee WN: Hypopharynx and larynx. In Valvassori GE et al: Head and neck imaging, New York, 1988, Thieme Medical Publishers, Inc, pp 311-338.
5. Lufkin RB and Hanafee WN: Application of surface coil to MR anatomy of the larynx, AJR 145:483, 1985.
6. Lufkin RB et al: Larynx and hypopharynx: MR imaging in surface coils, Radiology 158:747, 1986.
7. Mancuso AA and Hanafee WN: Larynx and hypopharynx. In Computed tomography and magnetic resonance of the head and neck, ed 2, Baltimore, 1985, Williams & Wilkins, pp 241-357.
8. McArdle CB, Bouley BJ, and Amparo EG: Surface coil magnetic resonance imaging of the normal larynx, Arch Otolaryngol Head Neck Surg 112:616, 1986.
9. Stark DD et al: Magnetic resonance imaging of the neck. I. Normal anatomy, Radiology 150:447, 1984.
10. Pressman JJ, Simon MB, and Monell C: Anatomic studies related to the dissemination of cancer of the larynx. Transactions of the American Academy of Ophthalmology and Otolaryngology 64:628, 1960.

SECTION TWO
IMAGING

In this section the various imaging modalities are discussed, along with the normal anatomy visible with each. A review of certain respiratory movements is also included, because these maneuvers can be used to accentuate different areas in the larynx during imaging.

RESPIRATORY MANEUVERS (Figs. 9-10 and 9-11)

In *quiet respiration* the vocal cord is off the midline but usually is not completely effaced against the lateral wall. In the coronal plane the cord has a slight triangular shape with the lower medial surface sloping downward to the lateral wall of the subglottic larynx and upper trachea. The upper surface of the cord is almost flat and horizontal. The ventricle may contain air or may be collapsed. With *slow inspiration* the true cords and false cords abduct, disappearing as they flatten against the now smooth lateral wall of the larynx. When the patient holds his or her breath and "bears down," *(Valsalva maneuver)* the cords go to the midline (adduct), squaring off the so-called subglottic angle (arch), which is the angle the undersurface of the true cord makes with the lateral wall of the subglottic airway. No airway is seen at the true cord level. The false cords may also approximate in the midline. The *modified Valsalva* maneuver is done with the cheeks puffed and the patient allowing the escape of only a small amount of air. This maneuver "puffs" not only the cheeks but also the pyriform sinuses and all the airway structures above the true cords. With *phonation* (the patient makes a high-pitched "eeee" noise), the cords tense and approach the midline, leaving a narrow airway. The cord now makes an angle with the lateral wall of the subglottis. The an-gle is variable but remains greater than 90 degrees. The ventricle may be expanded or collapsed in any maneuver. The *reverse or inspiratory "eeee"* usually expands the ventricle. The maneuver is difficult for many patients, but usually any noise made while breathing in will suffice.

Although these maneuvers are expected to produce the described effects, many times the particular structure the radiologist is trying to visualize shows up on the "wrong" maneuver.

PLAIN RADIOGRAPHS

Soft tissue technique uses a lower kilovolt (kV) than the cervical spine film. The soft tissue film of the neck is a very good survey study. Air is used as the natural contrast to visualize the lumen of the larynx and trachea (see Figs. 9-12 to 9-14). The retropharyngeal tissue thickness can be appreciated. Some information about the cartilages can be determined, depending on the degree of ossification. The epiglottis and the aryepiglottic folds are visualized. The ventricle often is seen marking the position of the upper margin of the true cord. The tracheal air column extends below the larynx.

The variability of calcification of the cartilage makes prediction of a pathologic condition from the radiographic appearance hazardous. Occasionally a fracture can be demonstrated. More often the partly calcified cartilages create a problem in diagnosing foreign bodies. This reflects the variable appearance of these cartilages. The radiologist should be familiar with the most common "pitfalls," or false foreign bodies.

The superior margin of the cricoid lamina often calcifies early, before the remainder of the signet portion

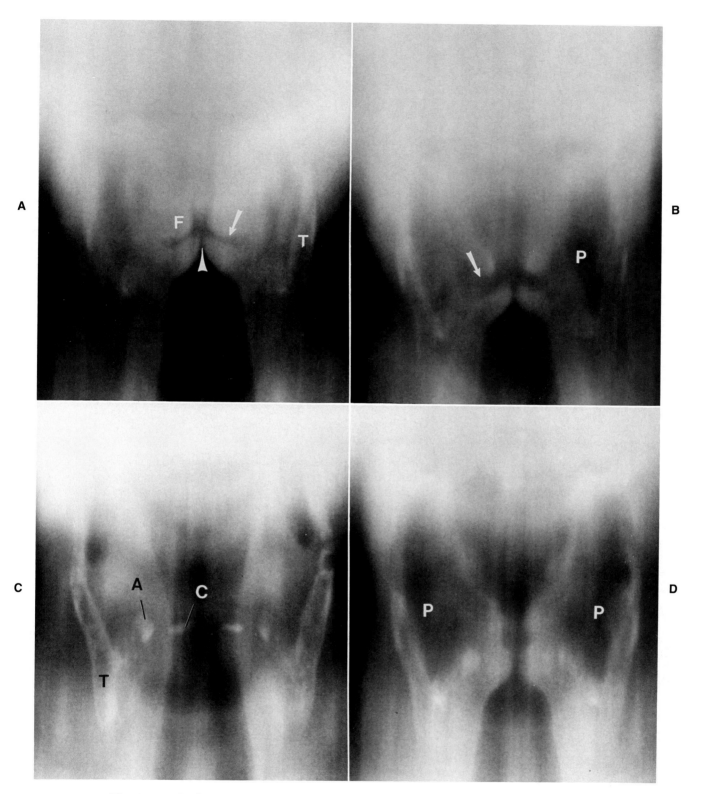

Fig. 9-10   A, Coronal tomograms during phonation. The true cords approximate with only a small residual airway *(arrowhead)*. The ventricle *(arrow)* is partially filled with air. *T,* Thyroid cartilage; *F,* false cord. **B,** Reverse phonation shows more dilatation of the ventricles *(arrow)*. *P,* Pyriform sinus. **C,** Coronal tomogram at inspiration shows flattening of the false and true cords against the lateral wall of the larynx. *T,* Thyroid cartilage; *A,* arytenoid; *C,* lamina of the cricoid (upper margin). **D,** Modified valsalva shows dilatation of the pyriform sinuses *(P)*.

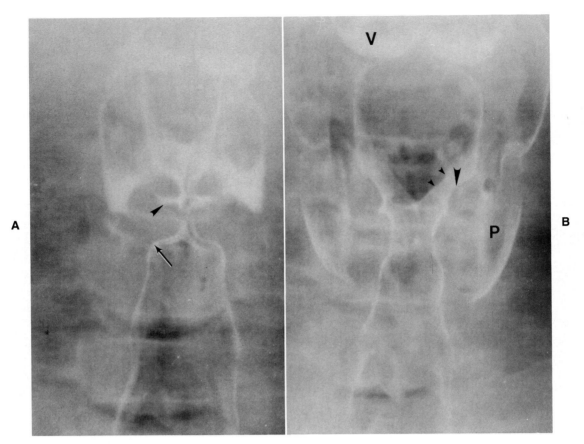

Fig. 9-11 **A,** Laryngogram, Valsalva maneuver. Note squaring of the subglottic angle *(arrow),* collapse of the ventricle *(arrowhead).* **B,** Laryngogram, puffed cheek. Modified valsalva. Pyriform sinuses *(P)* are distended. The AE fold *(small arrowheads)* and the inner wall of the larynx *(large arrowhead)* are well demonstrated. *V,* Valleculae.

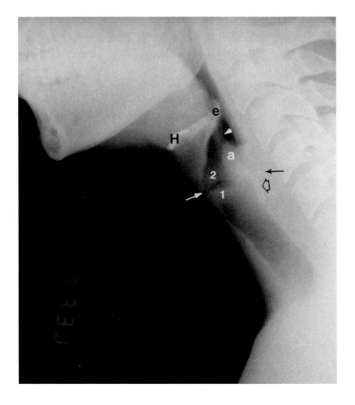

Fig. 9-12 Lateral plain film of the neck shows the true cord *(1)* and the false cord *(2)* separated by the black linear ventricle. The white arrow points to the anterior ventricle. The anterior commissure (junction of the true cords) is just inferior to this point. The black arrow shows the calcified superior margin of the cricoid lamina often mistaken for a foreign body. The open black arrow shows the calcified lower horn of the cricoid. *H,* Hyoid; *a,* arytenoid prominence; *e,* epiglottis; *arrowhead,* AE fold.

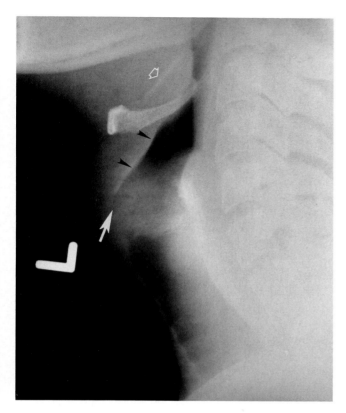

Fig. 9-13   Lateral plain film. The ventricle and cord cannot be well seen. The level of the true cord can be found by following the laryngeal surface of the epiglottis *(arrowheads)* to its lowest point *(arrow)*. This represents the level of the ventricle. Note the calcified stylohyoid ligament *(open arrow)* sometimes mistaken for a foreign body.

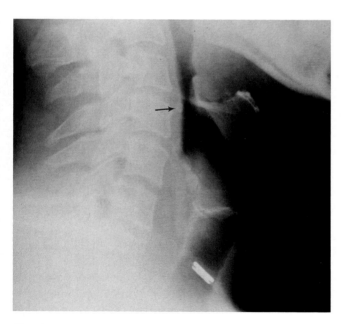

Fig. 9-14   Lateral soft tissue film with calcification of the cartilages including the triticeous cartilage *(arrow)* in the posterior margin of the thyrohyoid membrane (thyrohyoid ligament).

(see Fig. 9-12). This linear calcification is often misinterpreted as a foreign body. The triticeous cartilage in the posterior thyrohyoid ligament is another foreign body mimic (see Fig. 9-14). Less commonly the calcified arytenoid and the horns of the thyroid cartilage may be mistaken for a foreign body.

The frontal film is severely limited by superimposition of the spine. This problem is addressed by high-kilovolt filtered radiographs or tomography.

HIGH-KILOVOLT FILTERED RADIOGRAPH

High-kilovolt films are used to "soften" the spine, allowing visualization of the airway in the frontal projection[1,2]; 140 kV is used with 1 mm of copper placed between the tube and the patient to give a lowered film contrast.

XERORADIOGRAPHY

Xeroradiography uses edge enhancement to clearly show the anatomy of the airway, cartilages, and even muscle and fat planes (Fig. 9-15).[3] This technique is ideal for visualizing foreign bodies and for evaluation of the trachea (e.g., for subglottic stenosis, granuloma, and so forth). However, xeroradiography has an exposure three to five times that of the standard soft tissue film. In the routine case many radiologists do not think that the detail, although better than plain radiography, is worth the added exposure, especially in children.

TOMOGRAPHY

Conventional linear tomography is seldom done now, having been replaced by computed tomography and magnetic resonance imaging. Tomography provides the frontal view anatomy without the problems of the superimposed spine (Fig. 9-10). The lateral view with tomography offers little more than plain film radiography. Exposure can be made in several seconds, rapidly enough that the various maneuvers (e.g., phonation, Valsalva) can be used to show specific anatomic landmarks in the coronal plane.

Some detail of the mucosal surface is visible, but small lesions cannot be reliably excluded by this technique. One advantage of tomography over CT is the ability to show whether the ventricle can be filled with air during various maneuvers in the presence of a supraglottic tumor. However, this is seldom necessary because of the increased definition of the paraglottic space afforded by CT and MRI. On tomography, the general size of the false cord and true cord can be determined. Since the pyriform sinus protrudes between the thyroid cartilage and the inner wall of the larynx, the width of this wall can be estimated in an attempt to show tumor extending toward the true cord.

The subglottic angle is an important landmark that can be flattened or effaced by tumor extension or by a recurrent laryngeal paralysis.

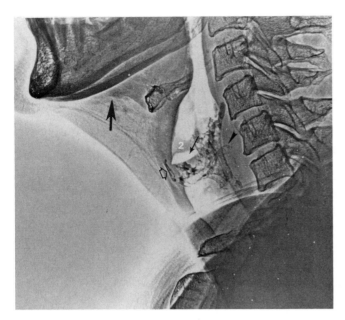

Fig. 9-15 Xeroradiogram shows the true cord, false cord and ventricle with better definition of the fat planes. Note the calcified upper margin of the cricoid lamina *(arrowhead)* more obviously calcified than in Fig. 9-12. Note how the muscles in the floor of the mouth *(large arrow)* can be seen against the fat. *2,* False cord; *small arrow,* ventricle; *open arrow,* partially calcified anterior thyroid cartilage.

Tomography is done with multiple slices and multiple maneuvers and thus has a fairly high radiation exposure. Every attempt should be made to place the airway in the plane of section that is parallel to the tabletop. Placing a bolster under the buttocks with additional support of the knees allows positioning without forcing the patient to straighten the natural angle between the thoracic and cervical spines.

FLUOROSCOPY

Fluoroscopy is helpful in the rare case in which the clinician cannot easily see the larynx. Vocal cord mobility must be assessed with the patient awake and able to follow commands. Some patients will not tolerate direct visualization without anesthesia, and in some patients a tumor may block the clinician's view. In these cases fluoroscopy can give some idea of cord mobility. The examination is recorded on videotape to allow review without additional exposure.

CONTRAST EXAMINATIONS

Laryngography was developed to define the mucosal irregularities of the larynx and to visualize areas that were a problem for the laryngologist.[4-6] The procedure is rarely done today because most of the information derived from the laryngogram is obtainable by endoscopy, and the submucosal region can be better seen with other imaging procedures. Laryngography is diffi-

cult for many patients and, in fact, contraindicated in those the clinician would most like to examine: patients in whom a tumor causes significant airway obstruction, thus limiting direct visualization.

The patient may be given atropine (0.4 mg) and codeine (60 mg) if no contraindication exists. Atropine decreases secretion and dries out the mucosa, enabling better coating, but it is not given to patients with glaucoma or prostate enlargement. Codeine limits coughing.

The anesthesia of the larynx is very important during laryngography. Initial anesthesia can be done with a spray or gargle using topical anesthetic. After initial anesthesia a curved cannula is placed over the back of the tongue and 2% xylocaine is dripped into the pyriform sinus as the patient is told to breathe in and out. Alternatively, a soft rubber tube can be passed through the nose and directed over the larynx.

Some radiologists have used 4% xylocaine, but this must be done with extreme caution since xylocaine is rapidly absorbed through the mucosa. This can precipitate cardiac arrhythmias and hypotension or central nervous system manifestations, either excitatory or depressant.

Contraindications include sensitivity to xylocaine. If atropine is contraindicated, it is simply not used. Significant respiratory compromise, either because of tumor size or poor pulmonary function, is also a contraindication.

Initially the patient will cough as the xylocaine drips into the laryngeal lumen, but as anesthesia occurs, the coughing stops. The procedure can then continue, with administration of the contrast medium. In the United States oily propyliodone (Dionosil) is the most common contrast agent used. The contrast is warmed and well mixed, then dripped by syringe and laryngeal cannula or nasal tube into the larynx. The patient is asked to breathe in slowly as the contrast is administered. The patient is asked to cough lightly to distribute the contrast. Administration can be monitored in the lateral projection with intermittent fluoroscopy. When sufficient coating has occurred, the patient is placed in different positions and asked to perform various maneuvers to distend the various parts of the larynx (see Figs. 9-11 and 9-16).

Historically the laryngogram has been considered especially helpful in certain important areas of the larynx. The ventricle and anterior commissure can be obscured from the clinician's view by overhanging tumor. If contrast fills the ventricle and the thin opaque contrast line reaches the anterior junction of ventricle and epiglottis, this is presumptive evidence that the region is clear of tumor. Phonation or inspiratory "eeee" may distend the ventricle. Problems can arise if the tumor overhangs to such a degree that the contrast does not fill the ventri-

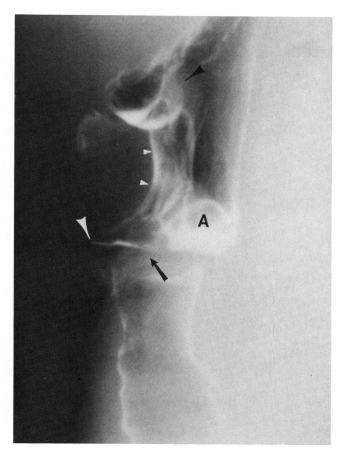

Fig. 9-16 Laryngogram, lateral view shows the linear, contrast filled, ventricle. The anterior limit of the ventricle *(large white arrowhead)* is just above the anterior commissure. *Black arrow,* true cord; *black arrowhead,* free margin of the epiglottis; *small white arrowheads,* laryngeal surface of the epiglottis; *A,* arytenoid.

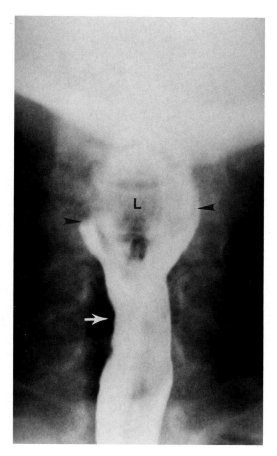

Fig. 9-17 Barium swallow. Normal. The barium is deflected around the larynx *(arrowheads)* with an apparent filling defect caused by the larynx *(L)*. The impression on the upper esophagus *(white arrow)* is caused by osteophytes.

cle well. Light coughing may help, but false-positive examinations can occur. The two ventricles are superimposed on the lateral projection, so the frontal projection must also be done to determine if the ventricle fills on both sides. With modern endoscopy this area usually can be visualized. The subglottic angle can be clearly defined with laryngography but is also well assessed by CT or MRI.

The pyriform sinus and postcricoid area are seen when coated with contrast. However, this area can be evaluated without anesthetizing the larynx merely by having the patient swallow thick barium or even propiliodone (Dionosil). After coating is accomplished, the patient does a modified Valsalva maneuver to distend the pyriform sinuses. Often the relationship of the tumor to the apex of the pyriform sinus can be shown.

BARIUM SWALLOW

The barium swallow is used to evaluate the pharyngeal wall. The barium column is followed through the

pharynx into the esophagus, and the motility of the pharynx and the mucosal surfaces are assessed. Demonstration of pliability of the pharyngeal wall suggests normal tissue. Tumors cause a lack of pliability or distensibility, as well as mucosal irregularity.

In the frontal view the pyriform sinuses fill as the epiglottis deflects the barium column to either side, around rather than over the vestibule of the larynx (Fig. 9-17). As the larynx elevates, the pyriform sinuses lose their sharply curved lower borders, become continuous with the remaining hypopharynx, and drain into the esophagus. As the barium column splits to pass through the pyriform sinuses, the larynx becomes a "filling defect" in the barium column and should not be mistaken for a mass.

On the lateral view the cricopharyngeus opens as the pharynx propels the bolus toward the pharyngoesophageal junction. The cricopharyngeus is inspected for late or incomplete relaxation and for the formation of an outpouching such as a Zenker's diverticulum. On the lateral film some irregularity is often seen on the anterior wall of the lower pharynx and the postcricoid area. This is thought to be a normal venous plexus; however, at times differentiation from a tumor may be impossible. The relationship of the posterior pharyngeal wall to the cervical spine and possible anterior vertebral osteophytes are well seen in the lateral view.

COMPUTED TOMOGRAPHY (CT) SCANNING

CT scanning allows evaluation of the laryngeal structures deep to the mucosa.[5,7,8] The scout view is made with the patient in the lateral position (Fig. 9-18). The slice orientation is selected parallel to the ventricle, which is seen as a dark air line crossing the laryngeal airway. If the ventricle is not seen well or if the airway is obscured by the shoulders in a patient with a short or thick neck, then the slice orientation is estimated as parallel to the intervertebral space or perpendicular to the axis of the spine at the level of the larynx. The axial images are made with a field of view corresponding to the size of the neck. Rapid scans (2 to 3 seconds) decrease respiratory or swallowing artifacts. The choice of slice thickness is arbitrary. Some use 1.5 mm every 3 mm, and some survey the larynx with 3 mm slices every 3 or 5 mm. Once the area of the ventricle is identified, thin slices (1.5 mm by 1.5 mm) can be taken if the relationship of the lesion to the ventricle is still in question.

The region covered should extend below the level of the cricoid cartilage. The starting point can be the tip of the epiglottis or the hyoid bone, depending on the origin of the lesion (see following discussions on squamous cell carcinoma, other tumors, and benign tumors).

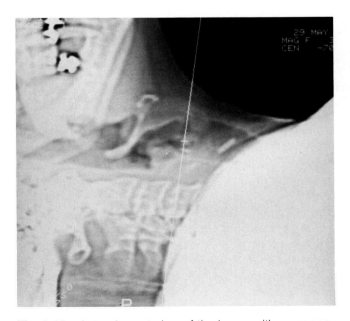

Fig. 9-18 Lateral scout view of the larynx with cursor positioned along the ventricle.

Nodal regions draining the area of the primary pathologic condition are also included. The examination can be done with the patient breathing quietly or by having the patient stop breathing for each slice. Before the actual scan the patient should practice, and the technologist should be confident that motion can be minimized during the scan. If the scan is done in quiet breathing, the patient should attempt to breathe with the abdominal muscles as much as possible.

Intravenous contrast helps distinguish lymph nodes from vessels and so is used in tumor cases, but it is not necessary in trauma evaluation. In the upper axial slices the epiglottis and connecting ligaments and folds are seen (Fig. 9-19). More inferiorly the lateral edges of the epiglottis begin to curve medially and posteriorly, forming the aryepiglottic folds. These converge toward the midline and unite posteriorly at an even lower level. At the upper levels the preepiglottic space is filled with fat except for a platelike density that represents a cross-section of the epiglottic cartilage. The hyoepiglottic ligament crosses the fat in the midline. At the level of the false cord the paraglottic region, lateral to the airway, is predominantly fat density. As the axial slice passes the ventricle, the paraglottic space changes from predominantly fat density to muscle density. Here the slice has entered the thyroarytenoid muscle. The shape of the airway narrows at the cord level, becoming more slitlike but then widening to a rounder appearance at the level of the subglottis. The paraglottic space, limited by the conus elasticus, stops at the upper margin of the cricoid. Thus there should be no tissue within the ring of the cricoid cartilage.

The appearance of the cartilage can vary considerably, depending on the degree of ossification or mineralization and the amount of fatty marrow in the medullary region of the cartilage. Both thyroid and cricoid cartilages are easily identified. The thyroid cartilage spans the level of true and false cord. The upper margin of the lamina of the cricoid is approximately the level of the ventricle or upper cord. The axial slice is ideal for evaluation of the thyroid and cricoid cartilages, slicing them in perfect cross-section. The arytenoid cartilages are important landmarks that can help identify the cord, ventricle, and false cord relationship. Approached superiorly, the upper arytenoid is first seen at the level of the false cord as a square or triangular shape. At the lower slice levels the pointed vocal process can be identified projecting anteriorly from the base. The vocal process identifies the level of the true cord. This is also seen when the arytenoid cartilages are seen with the upper posterior portion of the cricoid cartilage. Unfortunately, no definite landmark on any of the cartilages defines the exact level of the ventricle.

The appearance of the cord level varies on the phase of respiration. In quiet breathing the airway is open and the cord slightly abducted. If the patient stops

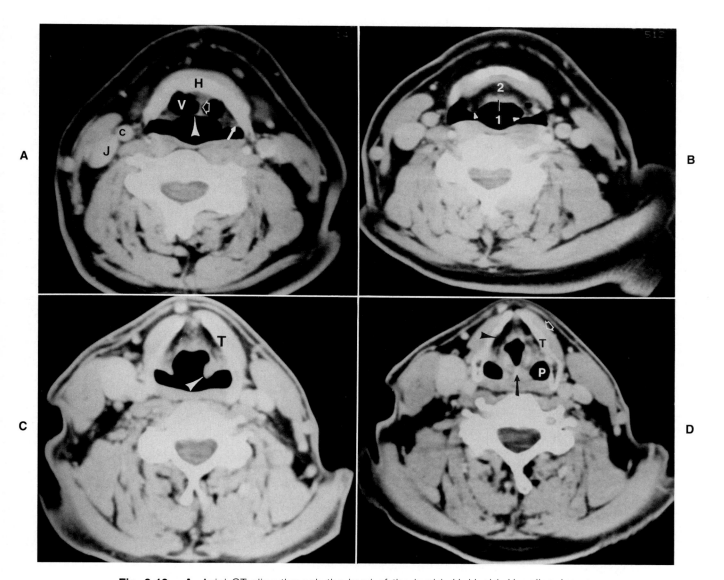

Fig. 9-19 **A,** Axial CT slice through the level of the hyoid. *H,* Hyoid; *V,* valleculae; *c,* carotid; *J,* jugular; *arrowhead,* epiglottis; *open arrow,* glossoepiglottic fold; *arrow,* pharyngoepiglottic fold. **B,** Slightly lower slice through upper AE fold *(arrowheads).* 1, Epiglottic cartilage; 2, preepiglottic space. **C,** CT slice, supraglottic larynx slightly lower than **B.** *T,* Thyroid cartilage; *(arrowhead),* aryepiglottic fold. Note the fat in the preepiglottic space. **D,** Slightly lower slice through the supraglottic larynx (male). The aryepiglottic folds have converged *(arrow).* *T,* Thyroid cartilage; *P,* pyriform sinus; *arrowhead,* fat in the paraglottic space *open arrow,* strap muscles. *Continued.*

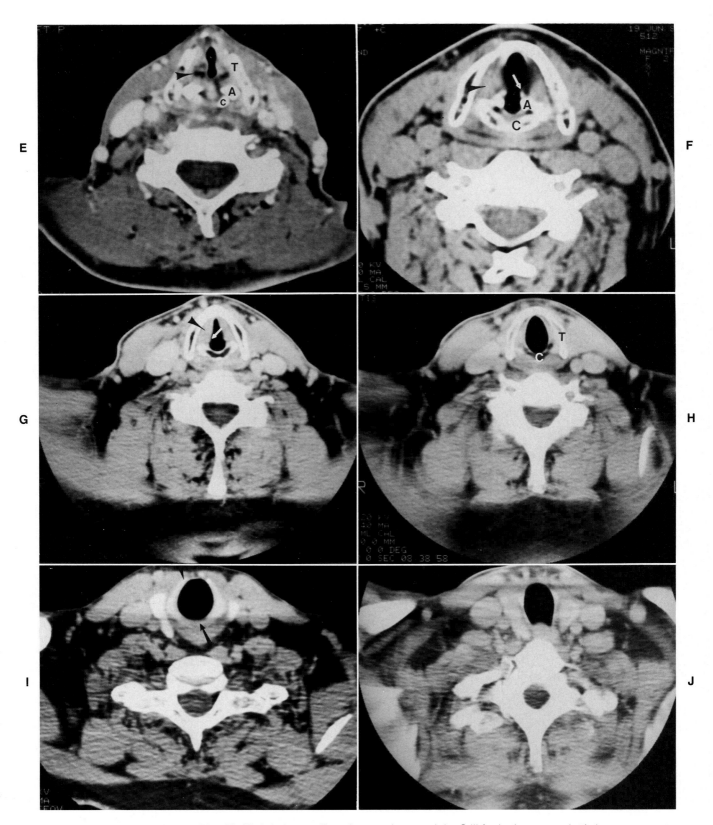

Fig. 9-19, cont'd **E,** Slightly lower slice close to the ventricle. Still fat in the supraglottic/paraglottic fat *(arrowhead)*. *T,* Thyroid cartilage; *A,* arytenoid cartilage; *C,* upper margin of the cricoid cartilage. **F,** Axial slice through the true cord. The paraglottic space now contains muscle *(arrowhead)*. Compare with Fig. 9-5. *A,* Arytenoid; *short arrow,* vocal process. **G,** Slice through the true cord slightly lower than previous slice. Thyroarytenoid muscle *(arrowhead)* fills the paraglottic space. Note the tip of the vocal process *(arrow)*. **H,** Slice through the lower true cord as the airway widens. *T,* Thyroid cartilage; *C,* cricoid. **I,** Slice through the lower cricoid showing the anterior arch *(arrowhead)* as well as the posterior lamina *(arrow)*. **J,** Slice through the trachea showing the U shaped tracheal cartilage with slight posterior indentation.

breathing for each slice, the cords usually come together (Fig. 9-20). This may actually give a slightly clearer visualization of paraglottic fat.

The anterior commissure between the true cords should have air approximating the cartilage, and if this is the case, the radiologist can confidently exclude disease. On CT, obliteration of the anterior airspace against the thyroid cartilage certainly can be seen with tumor but may also be artifactual as a result of minor cord position changes or cord edema. Repeating the slice at different phases of respiration may help, but re-

producing the exact level is difficult because the larynx moves slightly up or down, depending on the phase of respiration.

At the lower margin of the cricoid cartilage the appearance of the pharyngeal musculature changes from a flat, elongated appearance to a rounder shape (Fig. 9-21). This signifies the change from the pharynx to the esophagus and documents the level of the cricopharyngeus. The flatter shape of the pharynx musculature is the result of the attachment of these muscles to the lateral aspect of the thyroid and cricoid cartilages. In gen-

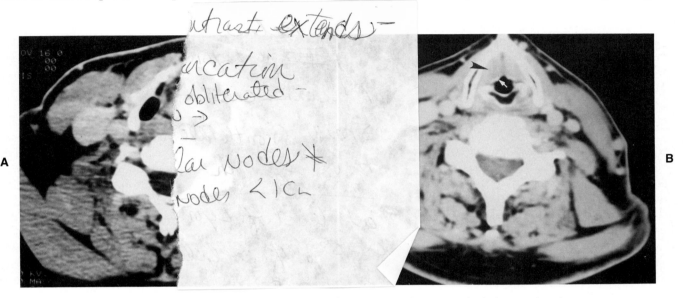

Fig. 9-20   Axial CT with breathholding. **A,** Slice through the supraglottic larynx showing closure of the airway and prominence of the paraglottic fat *(arrowhead)*. **B,** The true cords are opposed. *Arrowhead,* thyroarytenoid muscle; *arrow,* vocal process.

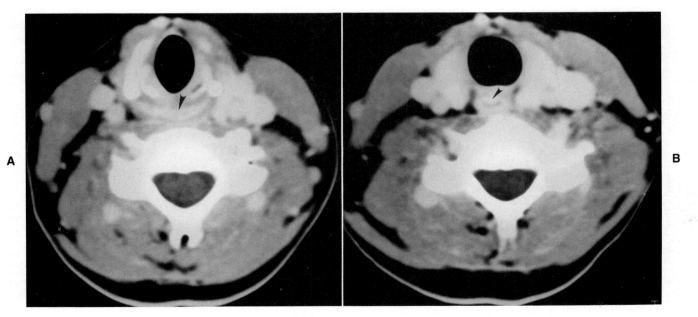

Fig. 9-21   **A,** Axial slice with bolus contrast showing enhancement of the mucosa of the pharynx at the level of the lower pharynx. Note its flattened configuration *(arrowhead)* due to the attachment of the pharyngeal musculature at the lateral aspect of the cricoid and thyroid. **B,** Lower slice showing the esophageal wall *(arrowhead)* with a rounder and narrower appearance than the wall of the pharynx.

eral, the angle made by the two thyroid alae is wider in women than in men (Fig. 9-22; compare with Fig. 9-19, *D*).

MAGNETIC RESONANCE IMAGING (MRI)

The larynx is a difficult target for magnetic resonance imaging that, nonetheless, has some potential advantages over CT. MRI enjoys the capability of multiplanar high-resolution imaging and the increased ability to separate various soft tissues.[7,9-16]

Precise pulse sequences vary considerably and certainly will change with evolution of this technology. As with CT the patient is positioned with the airway as parallel to the tabletop as possible. Our current methodology employs a sagittal, short TR/TE sequence (T_1-weighted) to localize and identify the axis of the larynx. This sequence is expanded laterally to cover from sternocleidomastoid to sternocleidomastoid muscle to include the major lymph node groups.

A sequence with coronal short TR / short TE images is done with thin sections (3 to 5 mm) from the anterior cord to the posterior larynx as perpendicular to the cord as possible. This may necessitate oblique off-axis imaging. An axial thin section short TR-TE sequence is then done encompassing the larynx from the midepiglottis to the lower cricoid. Short TR sequences are limited in the number of MR slices available in each study, so the anatomic level is chosen to cover the area of maximum interest (usually true cord, ventricle, and false cord). Finally, an axial, long TR / short and long TE sequence is done, usually with a TR of 2000 and TEs of 30 and 90 msecs. The long TR allows multiple slices to be obtained, and thus the node-bearing areas

can be covered. Usually the region from the midmandible to below the cricoid is covered in cases of a supraglottic lesion. In lower cord or subglottic lesions, the lower neck is evaluated.

The use of gadolinium is currently being assessed. After the basic sequences are performed, gadolinium-DTPA is injected and either an axial or a coronal short TR / short TE sequence is done, depending on whether cartilage invasion (axial) or the relationship of tumor to ventricle (coronal) is the major diagnostic question. Further experience may permit abbreviation of this protocol.

Because most pulse sequences are measured in minutes rather than seconds, motion artifacts from breathing, swallowing, and even pulsatile flow in the carotid arteries are a major problem. Various types of flow compensation, respiratory and cardiac gating, and presaturation pulses have all been tried with varying results. Phase encoding gradients are chosen in the anteroposterior direction to move flow artifact away from the larynx in the axial images. Nevertheless, patient education is even more important with MRI than with CT. The patient is instructed to breathe quietly and to practice doing so without moving the neck. Abdominal rather than chest breathing is encouraged, and the patient is instructed not to swallow or to swallow as seldom as possible during the sequence. The neck should not be hyperextended because this makes swallowing more difficult. The neck is kept in a more relaxed position.

A surface coil is used as a receiver.[13,14] Because the coil should move as little as possible, separating the coil from the chest wall while maintaining close approximation to the neck is desirable.

Sagittal images show the epiglottis, valleculae, and base of the tongue well (Fig. 9-23). The laryngeal surface of the epiglottis can be followed down to the petiole and anterior commissure. The postcricoid area is well seen, and the arytenoid cartilage often can be visualized perched on top of the cricoid cartilage. The preepiglottic fat is very obvious on T_1-weighted images.

The coronal view represents the ideal orientation for evaluation of the upper margin of the true cord (Figs. 9-24 and 9-25). The ventricle may not be seen, since the patient cannot maintain any particular maneuver during the entire time frame of the examination. The thyroarytenoid muscle makes up most of the true cord and, on the T_1-weighted image, can be seen contrasted against the high-signal-intensity fat of the false cord immediately above. The upper margin of the cord is considered to be the upper margin of the bulk of the thyroarytenoid muscle (TAM). Slips of the muscle do variably extend up into the false cord level of the paraglottic space but are very thin. Anteriorly, the petiole and the fat of the preepiglottic space are also visible just

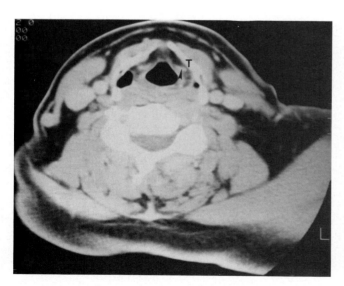

Fig. 9-22 Axial CT through the supraglottic larynx of a woman showing the wider angle of the thyroid cartilage *(T)*. The small soft tissue density *(arrowhead)* seen in the paraglottic fat represents a collapsed ventricular saccule.

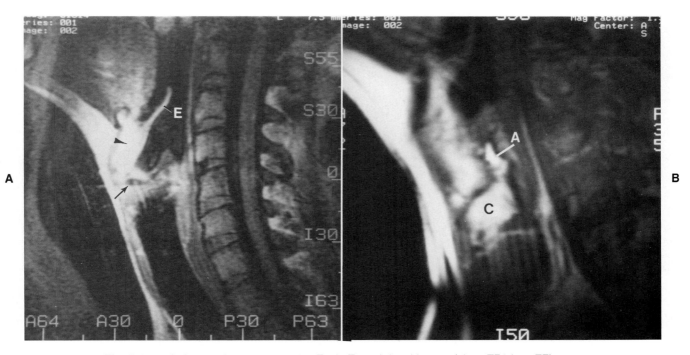

Fig. 9-23   **A,** Magnetic resonance 1.5 Tesla T$_1$-weighted image (short TR/short TE) sagittal, just off midline, shows the true cord and false cord separated by the dark air-filled ventricle *(arrow). Arrowhead,* Preepiglottic fat; *E,* epiglottis. **B,** More lateral slice shows the cricoid *(C)* and arytenoid *(A).*

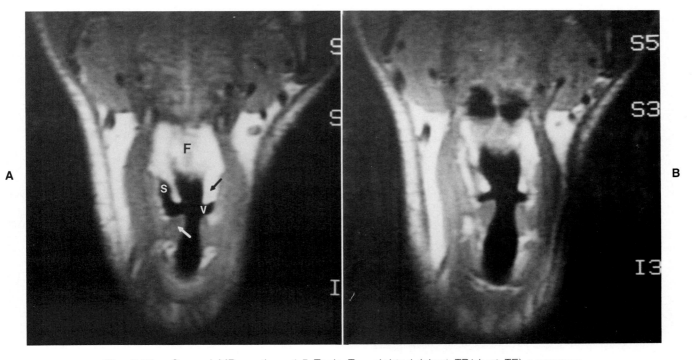

Fig. 9-24   Coronal MR sections 1.5 Tesla T$_1$-weighted (short TR/short TE) sequence from front to back. **A,** Anterior slice shows the muscle intensity *(white arrow)* of the thyroarytenoid muscle at level of the cord. The paraglottic space at the level of the false cord shows bright fat intensity *(black arrow). V,* Ventricle; *S,* saccule of the ventricle; *F,* preepiglottic fat. **B,** Slightly more posterior slice.   *Continued.*

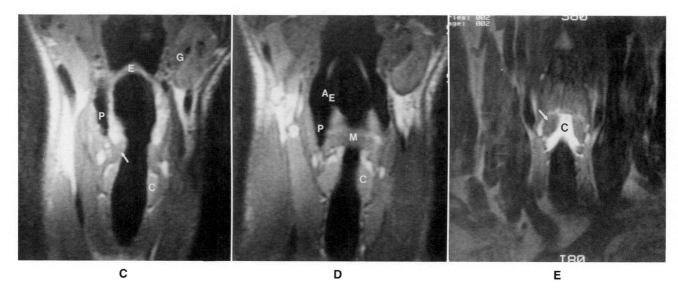

C   D   E

Fig. 9-24, cont'd   C, More posterior to **B.** *Arrow,* posterior thyroarytenoid muscle; *P,* pyriform sinus; *E,* epiglottis; *C,* cricoid; *G,* submandibular gland. **D,** Posterior to **C.** *C,* Cricoid lamina; *M,* interarytenoid muscle; *AE,* aryepiglottic fold; *P,* pyriform. **E,** Posterior larynx shows the posterior cricoid *(C).* The muscle intensity to either side *(arrow)* represents the posterior cricoarytenoid muscle. (From Curtin HD: Imaging of the larynx: current concepts, Radiology 713:1-11, 1989.)

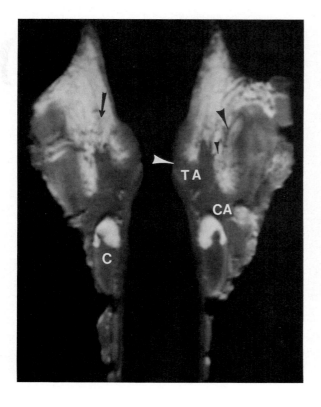

Fig. 9-25   Coronal MRI section 1.5 Tesla cadaver larynx (short TR/short TE). *TA,* Thyroarytenoid muscle; *CA,* lateral cricoarytenoid muscle; *C,* cricoid. The approximate upper margin of the cord *(large white arrowhead).* Fat at the false cord level paraglottic space *(black arrow).* Cortical margin of the inner cortex of the thyroid cartilage *(large black arrowhead).* Fat protruding towards the upper lateral margin of the thyroarytenoid muscle *(small black arrowhead).*

above the anterior commissure, whereas posteriorly the arytenoids again can be seen on the cricoid. The subglottic region and cricoid are seen on the same cut as the true cord.

The axial images represent slices perpendicular to the inner surface of the thyroid and cricoid cartilage, allowing assessment of cartilaginous erosion (Fig. 9-26). Again, the appearance of the cartilage is quite variable, depending on the degree of ossification. Ossified cartilage with fat in the medullary space is bright (high signal intensity) on T_1-weighted sequences and darkens on T_2-weighted sequences, whereas the nonossified cartilage tends to be dark on both sequences. The calcified cortex is black.

The cord level can be predicted on magnetic resonance imaging axial slices in much the same way as

with CT. The airway is narrow. A slice through the false cord level shows the high signal of fat in the paraglottic space on T_1-weighted imaging, whereas at the cord level the paraglottic region is filled with the lower signal intensity of muscle.

The carotid artery and jugular vein, along with the jugular lymph nodes, are seen in all slice orientations. The nodes are the same shape as the vessels on the axial view but can usually be differentiated on the basis of various flow phenomena. On the coronal and sagittal views the nodes often are more obvious because the nodes are still oval with superior and inferior margins, whereas the vessels are more linear.

Gradient echo images have been used with some success in decreasing imaging time, but experience is limited. Most laryngeal work in the literature has been

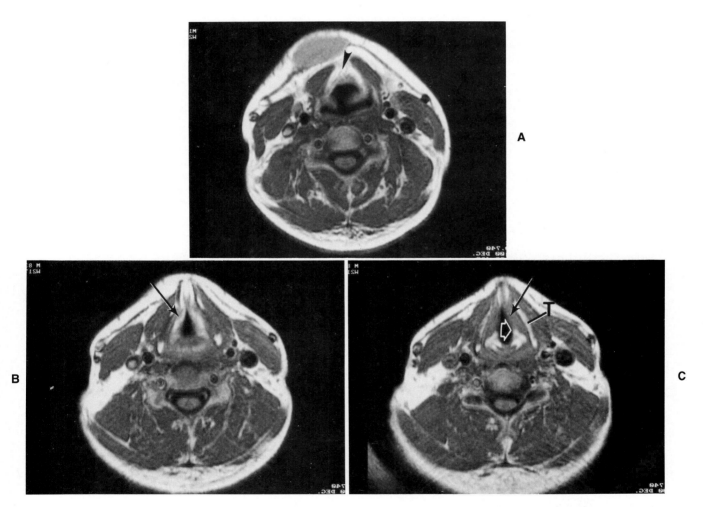

Fig. 9-26   Axial .35 Tesla axial images (short TR/short TE). **A,** Supraglottic larynx shows the preepiglottic fat *(arrowhead)*. **B,** Slice through the false cord shows the bright signal of the paraglottic fat *(arrow)*. **C,** Slice through the true cord shows the thyroarytenoid muscle intensity *(arrow)* in the paraglottic space. *Open arrow,* vocal process; *T,* fat in the medullary cavity of the ossified thyroid cartilage. (Courtesy of Robert Lufkin, MD and William Hanafee, MD.)

done with lower or midfield strength machines. The artifacts of motion tend to be less of a problem than on higher field strength magnets. Recent experience, however, has produced excellent laryngeal images on the larger magnets as well.

ULTRASONOGRAPHY, NUCLEAR MEDICINE, AND ANGIOGRAPHY[5]

Ultrasonography has little application in the larynx. The proximity of the larynx to the skin surface does allow use of very high-resolution, high-frequency 5 to 10 mHz probes.[17] Cartilage, when ossified, reflects most of the sound, thus limiting the ultrasonic access into the larynx to the cricothyroid or thyrohyoid membranes. The cystic nature of a laryngocele can conceivably be determined. Vocal cord mobility has been assessed, but this would have very limited applicability, since the cord is almost always accessible to direct visualization. Perichondritis or tumor extension through the thyroid cartilage has been evaluated with ultrasound,[18] but most centers would use computed tomography or magnetic resonance imaging. More experience may increase the applicability of ultrasound in the future.

Nuclear medicine likewise is seldom done specifically for pathologic conditions of the larynx. Increased uptake in inflammatory arthropathies or relapsing polychondritis occasionally has been mentioned in the literature.[5]

Arteriography can demonstrate the blood supply to the larynx. A primary glomus (paraganglioma) tumor or other vascular lesions can be evaluated by arteriography, but this is seldom necessary.[19]

REFERENCES

1. Maguire GH: The larynx: simplified radiological examination using heavy filtration and high voltage, Radiology 87:102, 1966.
2. Maguire GH and Beigue RA: Selective filtration: a practical approach to high kilovoltage radiography, Radiology 87:102, 1966.
3. Doust DB and Ting YM: Xeroradiography of the larynx, Radiology 110:727, 1974.
4. Momose KJ and MacMillan AS: Roentgenologic investigation of the larynx and trachea, RCNA 16:321, 1978.
5. Noyek A et al: The larynx. In Bergeron RT, Osborne AG, and Som PM, editors: Head and neck imaging: excluding the brain, St Louis, 1983, The CV Mosby Co, pp 402-490.
6. Powers WE, McGee HH, and Seaman WB: The contrast examination of larynx and pharynx, Radiology 68:169, 1957.
7. Mancuso AA and Hanafee WN: Computed tomography and magnetic resonance of the head and neck, ed 2, Baltimore, 1985, Williams & Wilkins, pp 241-357.
8. Mafee MF et al: Computed tomography of the larynx: correlation with anatomic and pathologic studies in cases of laryngeal carcinomas, Radiology 147:123, 1983.
9. Castelijns JA et al: Invasion of laryngeal cartilage by cancer: comparison of CT and MR imaging, Radiology 166:199, 1987.
10. Castelijns JA et al: MR imaging of laryngeal cancer, JCAT 11(1):134, 1987.
11. Hanafee WN: Hypopharynx and larynx. In Valvassori GE et al: Head and neck imaging, New York, 1988, Thieme Medical Publishers, Inc, pp 311-338.
12. Lufkin RB and Hanafee WN: Application of surface coil to MR anatomy of the larynx, AJR 145:483, 1985.
13. Lufkin RB et al: Larynx and hypopharynx: MR imaging in surface coils, Radiology 158:747, 1986.
14. McArdle CB, Bouley BJ, and Amparo EG: Surface coil magnetic resonance imaging of the normal larynx, Arch Otolaryngol Head Neck Surg 112:616, 1986.
15. Stark DD et al: Magnetic resonance imaging of the neck. I. Normal anatomy, Radiology 150:447, 1984.
16. Castelijns JA et al: MRI of normal or cancerous laryngeal cartilage: histopathologic correlation, Laryngoscope 97:1085, 1987.
17. Raghavendra BN et al: Sonographic anatomy of the larynx, with particular reference to the vocal cords, J Ultrasound Med 6:225, 1987.
18. Rothberg R et al: Thyroid cartilage imaging with diagnostic ultrasound: correlative studies, Arch Otolaryngol Head Neck Surg 112:503, 1986.
19. Konowitz PM et al: Laryngeal paraganglioma: update on diagnosis and treatment, Laryngoscope 98:40, 1988.

SECTION THREE
PATHOLOGIC CONDITIONS

Congenital, inflammatory, neoplastic, and traumatic abnormalities affect the larynx, as they do any other part of the body.[1,2] Imaging has a definite place in evaluating and diagnosing lesions and in assessing the extent of an abnormality. The clinician usually has a good idea of the basic problem and seeks the radiologist's help in determining the extent of the particular pathologic condition. Because most modern imaging has been directed toward evaluation of neoplasms, the chapter begins with and emphasizes tumors. Evaluation of congenital, traumatic, and inflammatory lesions follows. Some pathologic conditions are not often evaluated by radiology, but they are included here for completeness.

SQUAMOUS CELL CARCINOMA

The tumors of the larynx that are imaged by the radiologist are more likely malignant than benign. Cancer of the larynx essentially means squamous cell carcinoma (SCCa), and the diagnosis is seldom in doubt. The larynx is accessible to direct visualization, and these cancers arise on the mucosal surfaces. Small polyps never get to the radiologist for evaluation. Even with malignancy, the laryngoscopist may obtain all the information needed for treatment planning without the help of radiology. However, the endoscopist does have problems defining the deeper extent of a lesion relative to precise landmarks that determine whether the patient is a candidate for speech conservation surgery. Many times a tumor can cross the acceptable limits of a conservative resection by growing deeply through the paraglottic space, completely invisible to the laryngoscopist. Specific landmarks that are the keys to surgical staging are stressed in this chapter.

Clinically, tumors are staged by the *TNM classifications* developed by the American Joint Committee on Cancer.[3] ("T" stands for primary tumor, "N" for regional lymph nodes, and "M" for metastasis.) This classification is based on endoscopic and other clinical findings alone, and in that sense it is out of date. Nonetheless, the radiologist should be aware of this classification system, which is presented in Table 9-1, even though it does not take into consideration the abilities of contemporary imaging.

Several additional points deserve to be made regarding the relationship of radiology and endoscopy. First, whenever possible, CT or MRI should be done before biopsy to avoid a confusing appearance stemming from the trauma of the biopsy. Usually the diagnosis is strongly suspected after mirror examination, and the clinician can help direct the radiologist by an initial localization of the lesion. Second, the mucosal surface is the realm of the endoscopist. The radiologist should not do MRI or CT as a substitute for direct visualization. It

Table 9-1   Tumor staging by TNM* classification

Primary tumor	
TX	Primary tumor cannot be assessed
TO	No evidence of primary tumor
Tis	Carcinoma in situ
SUPRAGLOTTIS	
T1	Tumor limited to one subsite of supraglottis with normal vocal cord mobility
T2	Tumor invades more than one subsite of supraglottis or glottis, with normal vocal cord mobility
T3	Tumor limited to larynx with vocal cord fixation and/or invades postcricoid area, medial wall of pyriform sinus, or preepiglottic tissues
T4	Tumor invades through thyroid cartilage and/or extends to other tissues beyond the larynx (e.g., to oropharynx, soft tissue of neck)
GLOTTIS	
T1	Tumor limited to vocal cord(s) (may involve anterior or posterior commissures) with normal mobility
	T1a Tumor limited to one vocal cord
	T1b Tumor involves both vocal cords
T2	Tumor extends to supraglottis and/or subglottis and/or with impaired vocal cord mobility
T3	Tumor limited to the larynx with vocal cord vfixation
T4	Tumor invades through thyroid cartilage and/or extends to other tissues beyond the larynx (e.g., oropharynx, soft tissues of the neck)
SUBGLOTTIS	
T1	Tumor limited to the subglottis
T2	Tumor extends to vocal cord(s) with normal or impaired mobility

Primary tumor, cont'd	
SUBGLOTTIS, cont'd	
T3	Tumor limited to larynx with vocal cord fixation
T4	Tumor invades through cricoid or thyroid cartilage and/or extends to other tissues beyond the larynx (e.g., oropharynx, soft tissues of the neck)
Regional lymph nodes	
LARYNX	
NX	Regional lymph nodes cannot be assessed
NO	No regional lymph node metastasis
N1	Metastasis in a single ipsilateral lymph node, 3 cm or less in greatest dimension
N2	Metastasis in a single ipsilateral lymph node, more than 3 cm but not more than 6 cm in greatest dimension, or in multiple ipsilateral lymph nodes, none more than 6 cm in greatest dimension, or in bilateral or contralateral lymph nodes, none more than 6 cm in greatest dimension
	N2a Metastasis in a single ipsilateral lymph nodes, more than 6 cm in greatest dimension
	N2b Metastasis in multiple ipsilateral lymph nodes, none more than 6 cm in greatest dimension
	N2c Metastasis in bilateral or contralateral lymph nodes, none more than 6 cm in greatest dimension
N3	Metastasis in a lymph node more than 6 cm in greatest dimension
Distant metastasis	
MX	Presence of distant metastasis cannot be assessed
MO	No distant metastasis
M1	Distant metastasis

*T = primary tumor; N = regional lymph nodes; M = metastasis.

is impossible to exclude cancer of the larynx by imaging alone.

The clinical presence or pathologic detection of diseased *lymph nodes* is accompanied by a lowered rate of survival. Even more ominous is detection of extension through the capsule of a node, so-called extracapsular spread (ECS). Detection of large nodes by palpation is reliable, but detection of smaller nodes is unreliable, with many false positives and false negatives. Specifically, clinically occult nodes exist, and although CT is more sensitive than palpation, small positive nodes still go undetected on CT. These nodes are found histologically. The precise significance of CT- or MRI-detected nonpalpable lymphadenopathy relative to survival has not been assessed in any prospective study.

Currently, treatment of nodes is controversial.[4] Most discussions are based on studies that compare the size and site of origin of a lesion, the histologic findings, and the presence of palpable nodes to the rate of recurrence or survival. Physician bias has a definite impact on treatment technique.

Although the importance of CT or MRI detection of lymphadenopathy cannot be precisely determined at this time, the evaluation is worth doing. Accumulated experience certainly has an impact on physician bias, and hopefully randomized studies will clarify the question. Further comments are found in the section dealing with specific regions of the larynx and in a separate section on the lymph nodes.

As stated in the preceding section on anatomy, the larynx is subdivided into the supraglottic, glottic, and subglottic areas. This is based on embryologic derivation and the lymphatic drainage of the mucosa. The division is important to surgical statistics, but for our purposes the glottic and subglottic lesions can be discussed together. Because of the proximity of the hypopharynx and pyriform sinuses to the larynx, the discussion of carcinoma of one region necessitates discussion of carcinoma of the other; therefore hypopharyngeal carcinoma is covered as well. As previously stated, radiologists should be aware of the TNM classification system put forth by the American Joint Commission for Cancer (Table 9-1).[3] However, this system has less direct applicability to radiologists than to endoscopists. Radiologists should concentrate on the specific anatomic landmarks that make the difference in surgical planning.

Voice conservation therapy includes anything short of a total laryngectomy. The most common voice conservation surgeries are the (horizontal) supraglottic laryngectomy and the vertical hemilaryngectomy. The supraglottic laryngectomy is done for supraglottic carcinoma, whereas the vertical hemilaryngectomy is done for a lesion isolated to the true vocal cord. These procedures are described in the appropriate following sections and are emphasized regarding landmarks for limits of resectability. Recently larger segments of the larynx have been removed in the so-called extended or near-total laryngectomies, but the following discussion stresses the more standard procedures.

Speech conservative surgery allows the patient to maintain the function of speech using the residual portion of the larynx. However, in addition to vocalization, the larynx serves two more critical functions: maintenance of the airway and protection of the airway from aspiration. After speech conservative surgery the patient goes through a retraining process, learning to swallow again without aspiration. The patient must have both the desire to go through this retraining phase and an adequate pulmonary reserve. Some degree of aspiration almost certainly will occur until the patient learns to swallow again.

Radiation therapy also conserves voice. In this case the size of the lesion is, of course, important. Cartilage involvement usually limits the use of radiation therapy because of the higher incidence of radiation perichondritis and necrosis or treatment failure that eventually may necessitate a total laryngectomy. In general, radiation for superficial lesions is more successful than for more deeply invasive ones, so the radiologist may image these patients to detect evidence of deep soft tissue invasion as well as cartilage invasion. Radiation may still be used in these more extensive lesions because of patient preferences or medical contraindications to surgery. Finally, radiation may be tried as a first-treatment modality, with surgery remaining an option if the result is not adequate.

Supraglottic Larynx

The supraglottic larynx is the upper larynx, including the false cords, aryepiglottic folds, and epiglottis. The lower border is the ventricle. The speech conservation surgery related to the supraglottic larynx is the supraglottic laryngectomy (see box below).[5-7] Essentially all

---

CONTRAINDICATIONS TO SUPRAGLOTTIC LARYNGECTOMY

1. Tumor extension onto the cricoid cartilage.
2. Bilateral arytenoid involvement.
3. Arytenoid fixation.
4. Extension onto the glottis or impaired vocal cord mobility.
5. Thyroid cartilage invasion.
6. Involvement of the apex of the pyriform sinus or postcricoid region.
7. Involvement of the base of the tongue more than 1 cm posteriorly to the circumvallate papillae.

From Lawson W, Biller HF, and Suen JY: Cancer of the larynx. In Suen JY and Myers E, editors: Cancer of the head and neck, New York, 1989, Churchill Livingstone, pp 533-591.

of the larynx above the ventricle is removed (Fig. 9-27). A horizontal cut is made through the upper thyroid cartilage. The soft tissue incision line is along the ventricle and just above the anterior commissure. The cut moves upward over the aryepiglottic fold just anterior to the arytenoid before passing along the medial wall of the pyriform sinus to complete the resection. The hyoid may or may not be removed.

Almost all carcinoma of the supraglottic region is squamous cell carcinoma.[1,2] There is an association with ethanol use and tobacco smoking. Because the false cords are not directly used in vocalization, these tumors do not cause early hoarseness and appear somewhat later; they therefore often are larger than tumors of the true cord. The patients are not usually hoarse unless there is significant extension onto the arytenoids or down into the true cord.

The supraglottic larynx may be subdivided into the suprahyoid and infrahyoid regions. Many tumors involve both regions, but some are small enough to be localized to one area. Suprahyoid lesions include those of the free margin of the epiglottis. Small tumors in this area can be resected without removing the entire supraglottic larynx. The base of the tongue is often more of a problem, since these lesions tend to extend anteriorly (Fig. 9-28). The criteria for a partial resection or a supraglottic laryngectomy can be expanded to include lesions that extend less than 2 cm into the tongue base.

The suprahyoid or upper supraglottic larynx is well seen on axial CT or MRI. The lesion can extend laterally along the pharyngoepiglottic folds to reach the pharyngeal wall or along the glossoepiglottic fold in the floor of the valleculae to reach the tongue base. The extension into the tongue base is best seen on magnetic resonance imaging, especially with sagittal views (Fig. 9-28).[8] In the region of the valleculae there can be normal lymphoid tissue, called the lingual tonsil, that at times can be difficult to differentiate from a tumor. Deeper tumor extension can bring the lesion into the infrahyoid larynx and the preepiglottic fat. The preepiglottic fat is ideally seen on either CT or MRI (T_1-weighted). The size of these lesions is difficult for the endoscopist to appreciate unless the lesion is very small. The lesion may indeed be the tip of a silent lesion extending deep into the tongue.

The infrahyoid supraglottic larynx is bordered by the easily visualized aryepiglottic (AE) folds. Lesions of the margin of the AE fold can spill over onto the pharyngeal wall. Anterior extension from midline lesions is into the preepiglottic fat (Fig. 9-29). Grossly, the appearance of the epiglottis has been likened to a sieve, and the epiglottis is a poor barrier to tumor spread. Lesions extending into the preepiglottic fat replace the characteristic fat density on CT or the high signal intensity of fat on the short TR / short TE MRI. The fact that

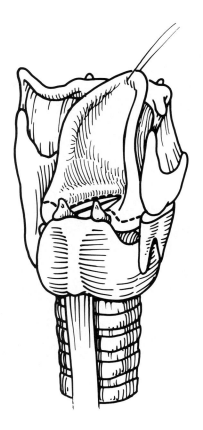

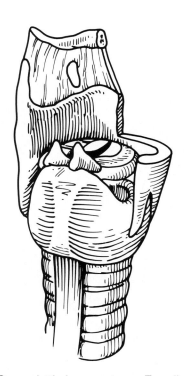

Fig. 9-27 Supraglottic laryngectomy. Top diagram shows the incision through the ventricle (the mucosa over the arytenoid has been removed for illustration). The bottom diagram shows the post surgical state. (From Curtin HD: Imaging of the larynx: current concepts, Radiology, 173:1-11, 1989.)

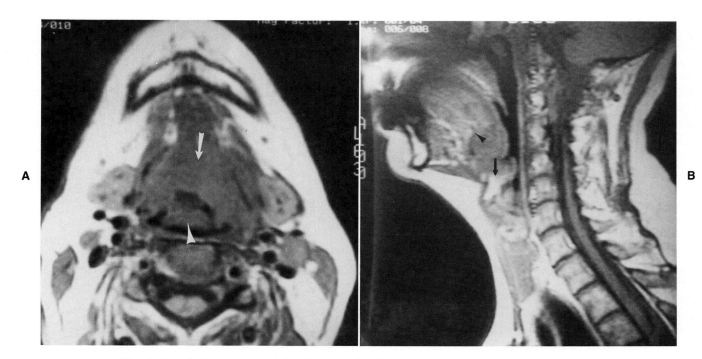

Fig. 9-28 **A,** Carcinoma of the free margin of the epiglottis, valleculae, and base of tongue. Axial (short TR/short TE) shows thickened tip of the epiglottis *(arrowhead)* and infiltration of the tongue base *(arrow)*. 1.5 Tesla. **B,** Sagittal view shows the margins of the lesion with the tongue *(arrowhead)* and with the fat-filled high signal intensity of the preepiglottic space *(arrow)*.

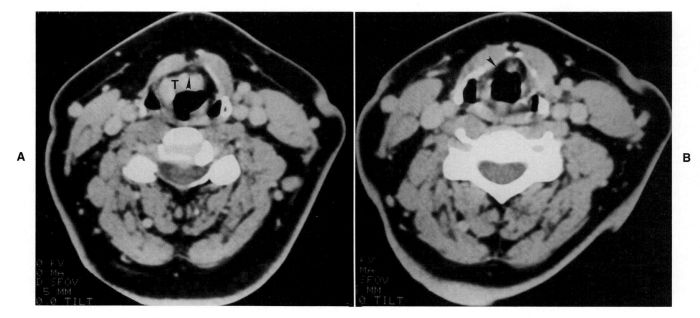

Fig. 9-29 **A,** Supraglottic carcinoma (rare adenocarcinoma) CT superior slice shows the tumor *(T)* as it extends *(arrowhead)* into the preepiglottic fat. **B,** Slightly lower slice shows no tumor. This slice is still at the level of the supraglottic larynx, well above the true cord as evidenced by the paraglottic fat *(arrowhead)*.

the lesion has entered the preepiglottic fat does not preclude a supraglottic laryngectomy but does modify the surgical approach.

Since the resection line of supraglottic resection is through the ventricles, the key to the feasibility of a supraglottic laryngectomy is the inferior tumor extension. The ventricle, arytenoids, and the anterior commissure are the critical landmarks to evaluate. The most important of these, from the radiologist's perspective, is the *ventricle.*

The ventricle is best evaluated in coronal sections. Because the slitlike structure is actually in the axial plane, it is poorly seen on the axial slices. The appearance of the arytenoid cartilage and the soft tissues in the paraglottic space helps determine the level of the ventricle as previously described. The midportion of the arytenoid actually spans the ventricle.

The upper arytenoid is at the level of the false cord, and the vocal process pointing anteriorly from the base of the arytenoid is a clearly identifiable marker for the

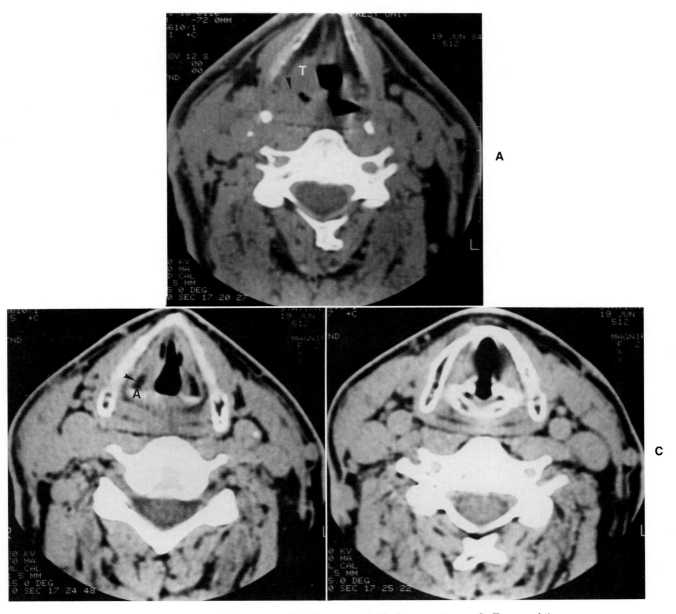

Fig. 9-30 Supraglottic lesion resectable by supraglottic laryngectomy. **A,** Tumor of the aryepiglottic fold extending onto the pharyngeal side of the fold *(arrowhead). T,* Tumor. **B,** Slightly inferior slice, free of tumor, but still above the ventricle. *A,* Upper arytenoid; *arrowhead,* paraglottic fat. **C,** Slightly inferior slice through the level of the true cord; no tumor. (From Curtin HD: Imaging of the larynx: current concepts, Radiology 173:1-11, 1989.)

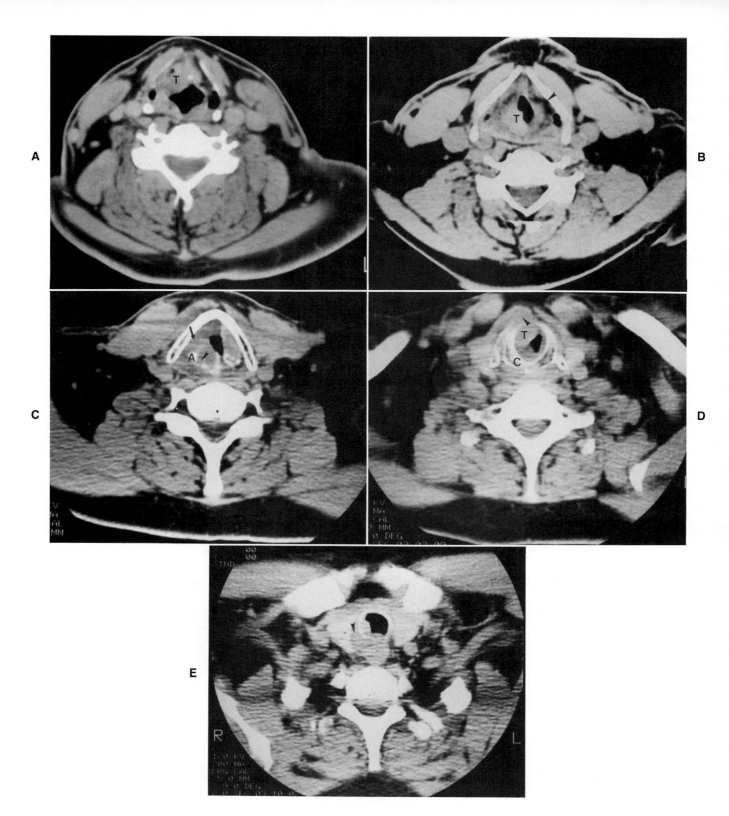

Fig. 9-31 Supraglottic/transglottic lesion involving false cord and true cord. **A,** Tumor seen at the level of the lower epiglottis. *T, Tumor.* **B,** Level of the false cord slightly inferior to **A**. Fat *(arrowhead)* in the paraglottic space. *T, Tumor.* **C,** Slice at the level of the true cord/ventricle. Lesion is seen involving the cricoarytenoid joint *(arrowhead)* and true cord *(arrow). A, Arytenoid.* **D,** Tumor *(T)* seen within the ring of the cricoid *(C)*. Note also tumor extending anteriorly *(arrowhead)* into the strap muscle. **E,** Further inferior slice shows lesion within the upper trachea and also in the tracheoesophageal groove posterolateral to the trachea *(arrowhead)*. (From Curtin HD: Imaging of the larynx: current concepts, Radiology 173:1-11, 1989.)

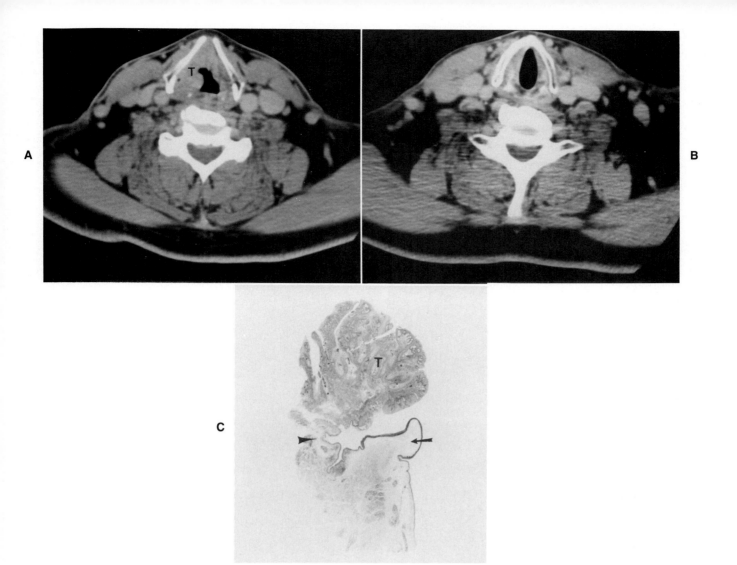

Fig. 9-32 Supraglottic lesion, which cannot be separated from the true cord by CT. **A,** Slice through the supraglottic level shows the tumor *(T).* **B,** The slice through the true cords is normal. **C,** Histological section of the laryngectomy specimen shows the tumor *(T)* in the false cord but the lateral margin of the ventricle *(arrowhead)* is free. *Arrow,* true cord.

true cord. As stated previously, the false cord is made up predominantly of fat, whereas the cord level is marked by the thyroarytenoid muscle. Thus the change from fat to muscle density marks the transition across the ventricle.

In axial imaging the radiologist tries to show a slice without tumor between the slice showing the lesion and the slice showing the upper margin of the cord (Figs. 9-29 and 9-30). If this is possible, the supraglottic laryngectomy is feasible. If, on the other hand, the lesion is seen both above and below the ventricle, then the lesion is transglottic (crosses the ventricle), and a supraglottic resection is not possible because the surgical line through the ventricle would go through the tumor (Fig. 9-31).

A major problem with axial imaging occurs in a patient with a tumor that is close to the ventricle. In this

circumstance a normal slice may not be found between the tumor and the true vocal cord (Fig. 9-32). In this case the decision on the feasibility of a supraglottic resection cannot be made based on the axial images. Similarly, an exophytic lesion can hang down over the cord but actually be attached only at the false cord level. This phenomenon is also difficult to exclude on axial imaging.

Coronal images are ideal for showing the vertical extent of a tumor, as the coronal orientation shows the true cord, ventricle, and false cord in cross-section. Conventional tomography gives a coronal view and indeed can adequately show a significant amount of inferior extension if the cord is disfigured by the lesion (Fig. 9-33). However, the tomogram does not adequately assess the paraglottic space (Figs. 9-34 and 9-35).

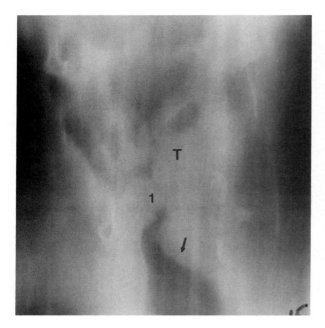

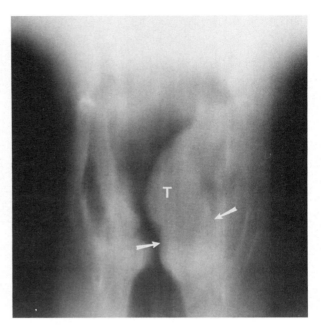

Fig. 9-33 Coronal tomogram of a transglottic lesion shows tumor *(T)* involving the supraglottic larynx extending well below the level of the true cord into the subglottic angle *(arrow)*. *1,* Normal cord.

Fig. 9-34 Coronal tomogram of a transglottic tumor *(T)*. The supraglottic component was obvious. Thickening of the wall of the larynx between arrows suggests but does not demonstrate tumor extending into the lateral margin of the true cord.

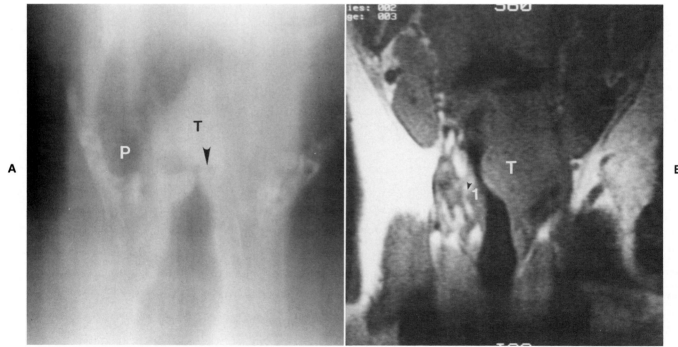

Fig. 9-35 **A,** Predominantly supraglottic lesion extending into the lateral margin of the true cord. Tomogram shows the tumor *(T)*. The ventricle *(arrowhead)* is filled with air. The pyriform sinus on the involved side does not fill (compare with normal side *P*). **B,** Coronal T_1-weighted MRI (short TR/short TE) in same patient. Tumor *(T)* extends into and widens intermediate signal intensity of the thyroarytenoid muscle. Compare with the normal thyroarytenoid muscle *(1)* on the opposite side. Normal fat at the upper lateral margin of the normal muscle is represented by the arrowhead. 1.5 Tesla.

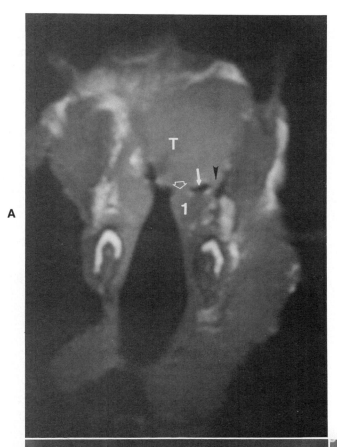

A

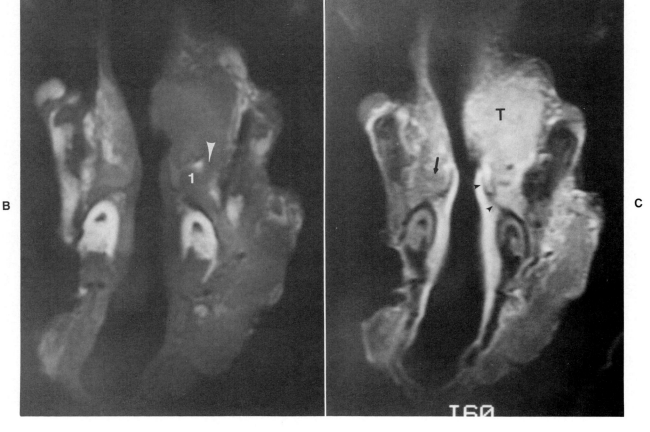

B

C

Fig. 9-36   Magnetic resonance image of a total laryngectomy specimen. Supraglottic lesion extending just lateral to the ventricle into the upper margin of the true cord. 1.5 Tesla, T_1-weighted. **A,** Tumor *(T)* with the lower margin at the lateral aspect *(arrowhead)* of the ventricle *(arrow)*. The tumor is not crossing the ventricle at the open arrow but has merely fallen onto the upper surface. It could easily be separated. *1,* Thyroarytenoid muscle. **B,** Slightly posterior slice shows tumor extension *(arrowhead)* into the lateral aspect of the thyroarytenoid muscle *(1)*. **C,** T_2-weighted image shows the tumor *(T)* with relatively increased signal intensity compared with the normal thyroarytenoid muscle opposite side *(arrow)*. There is some brightening of the thyroarytenoid muscle on the abnormal side. This was not tumor involvement histologically. Conus elasticus *(arrowheads)* is well seen. (From Curtin HD: Imaging of the larynx: current concepts, Radiology 173:1-11, 1989.)

A tumor growing from the false cord to the true cord does not usually "leap" the ventricle.[9-10] Although this is possible in very large tumors in which the ventricle has been destroyed, usually the tumor extends along the outside (lateral portion) of the ventricle to reach the lateral aspect of the true cord (Fig. 9-36). Here the lesion may travel through the paraglottic space.

MRI visualizes the paraglottic space and can provide a coronal image.[11] The ventricle is not usually seen except in very cooperative patients, but the upper margin of the cord is again marked by the upper margin of the bulk of the thyroarytenoid muscle (Figs. 9-35 and 9-37 to 9-39). A small amount of fat is seen at the upper outer margin of the thyroarytenoid muscle. As tumor extends into the lateral aspect of the cord, the fat is obliterated. If the fat is intact, this is good evidence that the tumor has not crossed into the cord. MRI is the best method for visualizing this important boundary zone, which is invisible to the clinician.

MRI signal characteristics using multiple sequences may also help define the relationship of the tumor to the ventricle and the thyroarytenoid muscle. A tumor has approximately the same CT appearance as muscle and has approximately the same signal intensity as muscle on a T_1-weighted MR image. However, on T_2-weighted images (long TR / long TE) the tumor has a relatively higher signal intensity (Fig. 9-40) than normal muscle. Again, this would be useful in regard to the upper margin of the thyroarytenoid muscle. Relative brightening of the muscle may indicate tumor invasion, but caution must be exercised. Other pathologic processes, such as edema, may cause such brightening (Fig. 9-41). More experience is needed to evaluate this aspect of laryngeal MR imaging. Currently we feel that a muscle of normal signal intensity is uninvolved, and one that is bright must be considered abnormal but not necessarily involved by a tumor.

In the midline a lesion growing down along the laryngeal surface of the epiglottis reaches the anterior

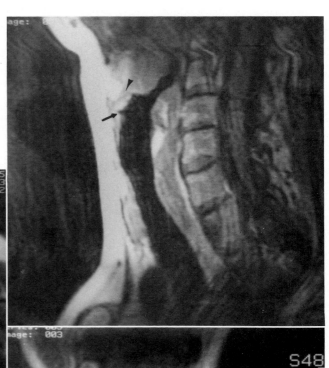

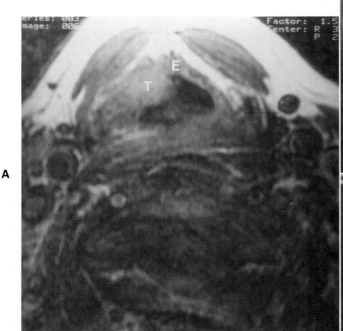

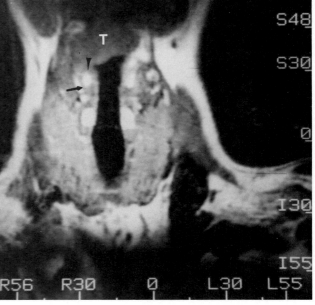

Fig. 9-37 Supraglottic tumor which does not reach the ventricle. A supraglottic laryngectomy is allowed. **A,** Axial slice showing the tumor (T) involving the epiglottic cartilage (E). **B,** Sagittal T_1-weighted image (short TR/short TE). The lower margin (arrowhead) is clearly separated from the anterior commissure (arrow). **C,** Coronal (short TR/short TE) T_1-weighted image. The lower margin of the tumor (arrowhead) is separated by the high intensity fat of the paraglottic space from the upper margin (arrow) of the thyroarytenoid muscle. T, Tumor.

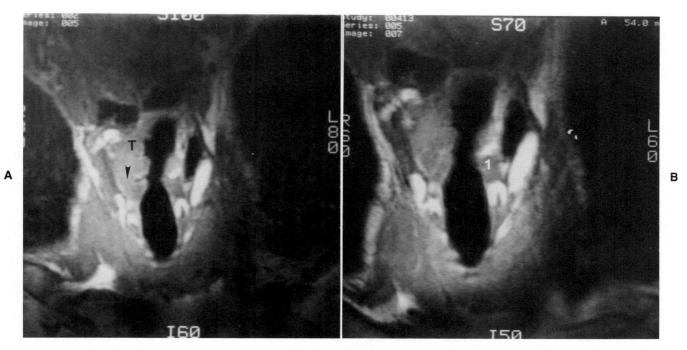

Fig. 9-38 A, Predominantly supraglottic tumor *(T)* obliterating the fat *(arrowhead)* at the upper outer margin of the thyroarytenoid muscle. Resection through the ventricle would intersect tumor so a partial resection is not possible. The ventricle is well seen partially due to fixation and therefore lack of movement of the true cord. 1.5 Tesla. **B,** Slightly posterior slice again showing thickening of false cord and true cord by the tumor: compare with normal thyroarytenoid muscle *(1)* on the uninvolved side. (**A** from Curtin HD: Imaging of the larynx: current concepts, Radiology 173:1-11, 1989.)

commissure rather than the ventricle (Fig. 9-42). This region is described more extensively in the following section on glottic carcinoma. In a supraglottic midline lesion, 2 to 3 mm should separate the tumor from the anterior commissure if a supraglottic laryngectomy is to be done. If assessing this region with axial slice orientation, the radiologist must be very careful to make the slice parallel to the ventricle. If the slice is oblique to the ventricular line, the orientation almost always slopes downward from anterior to posterior relative to the long axis of the larynx. Usually the head is propped up slightly for patient comfort, angulating the larynx out of the plane parallel to the tabletop. In this angle of obliquity the anterior false cord level is imaged on the same slice as the posterior segment of the true cord; thus miscalculation of the closeness of the tumor to the anterior commissure is possible.

MRI does show the fat on either side of the petiole and does have the capability of giving a sagittal orientation (Fig. 9-43). On a sagittal image air against the lower epiglottis is a reliable sign excluding extension to the anterior commissure (see Fig. 9-37). Partial volume effects of the anterior true cord / false cord can give a false-positive indication that tumor has reached the anterior commissure. Once again, the negative finding is more reliable than the positive one.

In the posterior supraglottic larynx the arytenoids are almost always assessed by direct visualization. Part of one arytenoid can be removed surgically if the upper level is only minimally involved by tumor. Involvement of the interarytenoid area is a contraindication to supraglottic resection because the surgeon would have to remove both arytenoids to attain a margin, and the patient would have no true cords with which to phonate. Thus primary lesions, even though small, of the interarytenoid area are almost always treated by total laryngectomy (Figs. 9-44 and 9-45). The interarytenoid region is not usually a problem for the radiologist, as this area can be clearly seen by the endoscopist. Involvement of the thyroid cartilage is also a contraindication and is discussed later in the chapter.

Lymph node involvement is common in supraglottic carcinoma. Nodal involvement is most common in lesions of the aryepiglottic fold and epiglottis (margin), which also involve contiguous regions such as tongue or pharynx.[4] The incidence of nodal disease gradually diminishes with lesions involving the margins of the larynx without contiguous spread and is lowest with those small tumors that are isolated to the more central supraglottic larynx (those tumors on the laryngeal surface of the epiglottis or the false cord that do not involve the margin of the AE fold). Deeper extension into the

Text continued on p. 632.

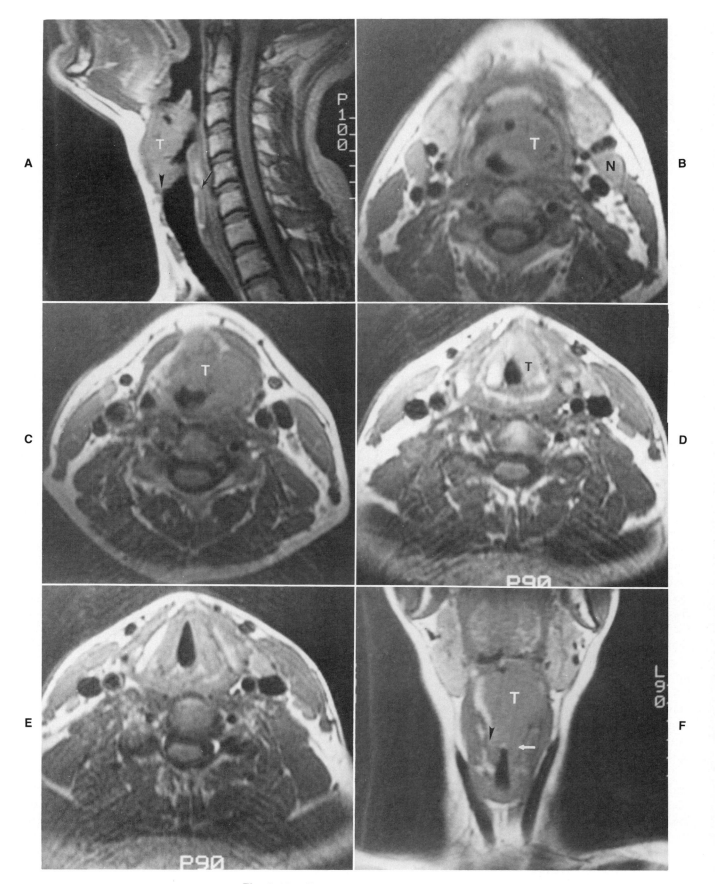

Fig. 9-39 For legend see opposite page.

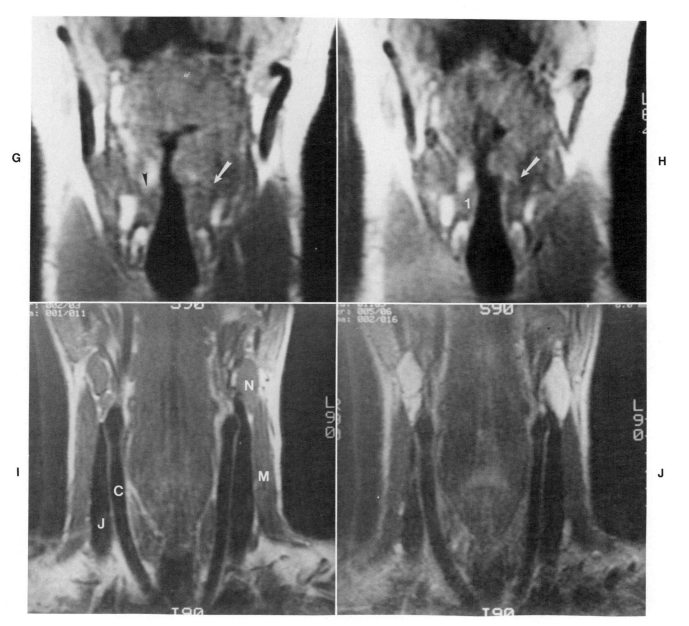

Fig. 9-39 Predominantly supraglottic tumor extending into the lateral aspect of the true cord; a supraglottic laryngectomy is not possible. 1.5 Tesla. **A,** Sagittal section. Tumor *(T)* obliterating the preepiglottic fat. The inferior margin *(arrowhead)* is well defined. Upper margin of the cricoid lamina *(arrow)*. **B,** Axial slice through the level of the supraglottic larynx shows the tumor *(T)*. Note the metastatic lymph nodes *(N)*. **C,** Slightly lower slice shows the tumor *(T)* obliterating the preepiglottic fat. **D,** Tumor is still seen at the false cord level. *T, Tumor.* **E,** The true cord level is normal. **F,** Coronal T₁-weighted (TR 500, TE 20) slice through the tumor *(T)*. Note the normal fat at the upper outer margin of the thyroarytenoid muscle on the normal side *(arrowhead)*. Approximate level of the lower margin of tumor *(arrow)*. **G,** Slightly more posterior slice again shows the tumor *(arrow)* close to the upper lateral margin of the true cord. Note the normal fat of the upper lateral margin of the normal side *(arrowhead)*. **H,** Inversion recovery image (TR 2000, TE 20, TI 20). Coronal through the tumor again shows the involvement of the upper lateral margin of the true cord *(arrow)*. The tumor is crossing the lateral aspect of the ventricle therefore disallowing a supraglottic laryngectomy. *1, Normal thyroarytenoid muscle.* **I,** More posterior slice T₁-weighted image shows the carotid *(C)*, jugular *(J)*, metastatic nodes *(N)*, and sternocleidomastoid muscle *(M)*. **J,** T₂-weighted (long TR/long TE) image through the nodes showing relative brightening of the nodes.

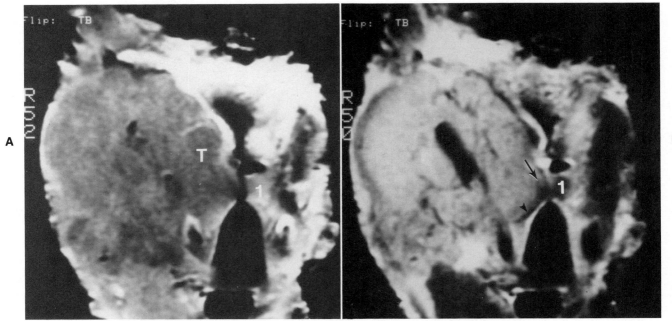

Fig. 9-40 **A,** Specimen MRI (1.5 Tesla) of a large tumor of the pharynx invading the larynx. Tumor *(T)* has the same signal intensity as the thyroarytenoid muscle and cannot be differentiated on the T_1-weighted image. *1,* Normal thyroarytenoid muscle. **B,** On a T_2-weighted image (long TR/long TE) the tumor brightens compared to the thyroarytenoid muscle *(1)*. Part of the thyroarytenoid muscle *(arrow)* can be seen pushed medially as the tumor invades from the lateral aspect. Note the tumor is limited in extent by the conus elasticus *(arrowhead)*.

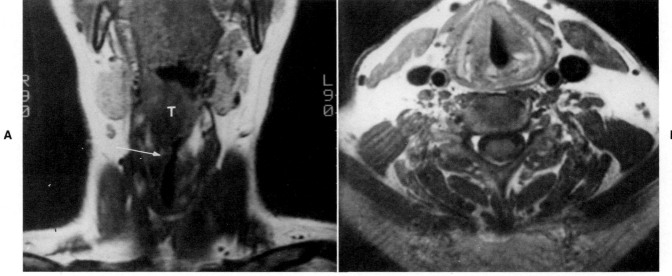

Fig. 9-41 Supraglottic tumor without extension into the true cord but with relative brightening of the atrophic cord on T_2-weighted image. **A,** Coronal image shows a supraglottic tumor. The lower margin of the tumor cannot be clearly defined on a T_1-weighted image. *T,* Tumor; *arrow,* approximate level of the upper margin of the cord. **B,** Axial T_1-weighting. The level of the true cord is fairly symmetrical.

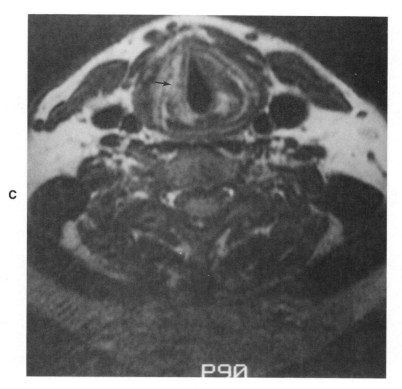

Fig. 9-41, cont'd   C, Axial T$_2$-weighting. There is brightening of the lateral aspect of the true cord *(arrow)* suggesting tumor invasion. Histology showed edema and atrophy but no evidence of tumor extension.

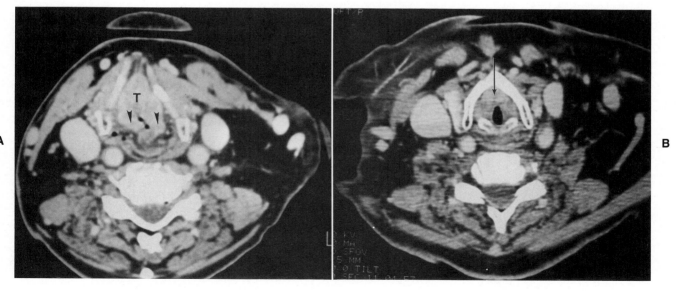

Fig. 9-42   A, Supraglottic tumor extending to the anterior commissure. Supraglottic tumor *(T)* crosses the midline and involves both aryepiglottic folds *(arrowheads).* **B,** More inferior slice at the level of the true cord shows involvement of the anterior commissure *(arrow).*

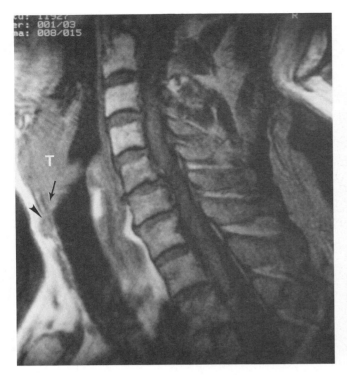

Fig. 9-43 Supraglottic tumor *(T)* with extension to the anterior commissure *(arrow)*. Submucosal extension through the cricothyroid membrane involves the region of the Delphian node *(arrowhead)*. Sagittal T$_1$-weighted image. 1.5 Tesla.

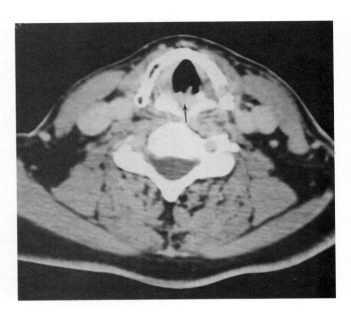

Fig. 9-44 Tumor of the inter-arytenoid area *(arrow)*.

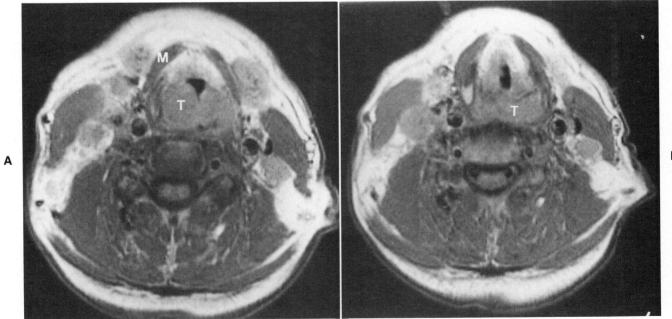

Fig. 9-45 For legend see opposite page.

C

D

E

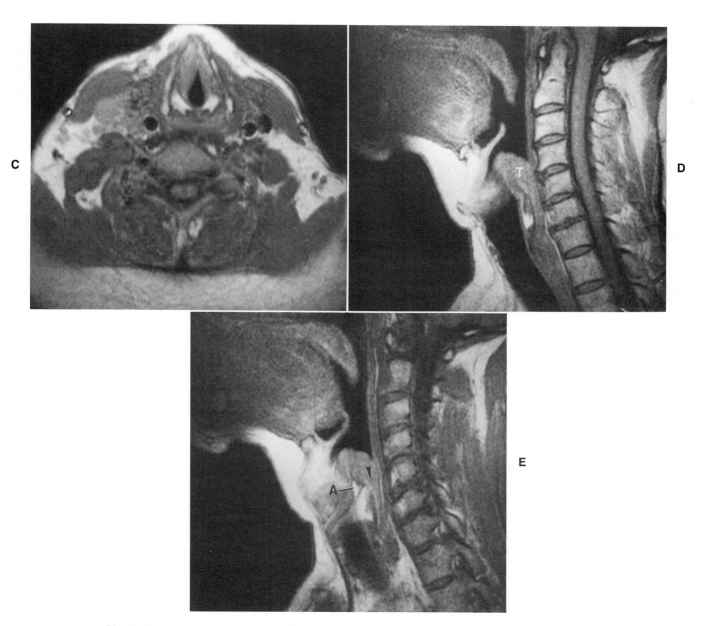

Fig. 9-45   Interarytenoid tumor .35 Tesla. **A,** Slice through the supraglottic larynx shows the tumor *(T). M,* Strap muscle. **B,** Slightly lower slice through the level of the false cord shows tumor *(T).* **C,** Level of the cricoid, tumor is no longer seen. **D,** Sagittal (near midline) T$_1$-weighted image shows the tumor *(T)* just superior to the cricoid. **E,** Slightly lateral slice shows the tumor extending behind *(arrowhead)* the arytenoid *(A).* Lower margin of the tumor is at the level of the upper margin of the cricoid lamina. (Courtesy of Robert Lufkin, MD.)

preepiglottic and paraglottic spaces would be expected to have a higher incidence of lymph node metastasis.

The lymphatic drainage of the supraglottic larynx is to the upper jugular chain. Bilateral involvement of the nodes is common, especially if the lesion crosses the midline. Therefore at least the upper nodes must be imaged, usually by extended axial slices. With MRI, coronal or sagittal imaging also visualizes these nodes.

Glottic and Infraglottic Regions

The region inferior to the ventricle is divided into the glottic and infraglottic regions. The division is somewhat arbitrarily placed at a line 1 cm below the lateral extent of the apex of the ventricle. Again, lesions are almost all squamous cell carcinoma and are associated with smoking. Unlike supraglottic lesions, tumors of the true cord usually appear fairly early because of interference with vocalization. Patients become hoarse with very small lesions of the true cord. If only the infraglottic area is involved and the free margin of the cord is not, the patient may not have hoarseness, but these lesions are very rare.

The speech conservation surgical procedure applicable in this region is the vertical hemilaryngectomy.[5,12,13] The resection removes one false cord, one true cord, and the intervening ventricle, as well as most of the ipsilateral thyroid ala (Fig. 9-46). The outer perichondrium of the thyroid ala is retained. If the tumor is close to or minimally involving the vocal process, the process can be resected, leaving most of the arytenoid. Slightly greater involvement necessitates re-

moval of the arytenoid. If there is deep extension, especially involving the cricoarytenoid joint, the procedure is not done. Similarly, if the lesion is deeply invasive with total fixation of a cord, vertical hemilaryngectomy is not done.

The key points for assessment are the inferior extension, the anterior commissure, the arytenoid, the thyroid cartilage, and the paraglottic space at the level of the ventricle (see box below). Nodes are less of a problem than with supraglottic carcinoma but they

---

CONTRAINDICATIONS TO VERTICAL FRONTOLATERAL HEMILARYNGECTOMY

1. Tumor extension from the ipsilateral vocal cord across the anterior commissure to involve more than one third of the contralateral vocal cord.
2. Extension subglottically greater than 10 mm anteriorly and more than 5 mm posterolaterally.
3. This technique can still be used if the vocal process and anterior surface of the arytenoid are involved, but involvement of the cricoarytenoid joint, interarytenoid area, opposite arytenoid, or rostrum of the cricoid is a contraindication.
4. Extension across the ventricle to the false cord.
5. Thyroid cartilage invasion.
6. Impaired vocal cord mobility is a relative contraindication.

From Lawson W, Biller HF, and Suen JY: Cancer of the larynx. In Suen JY and Myers E, editors: Cancer of the head and neck, New York, 1989, Churchill Livingstone, pp. 533-591.

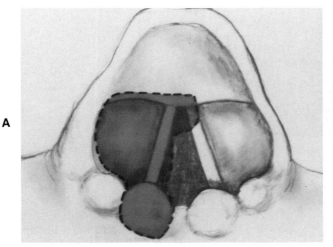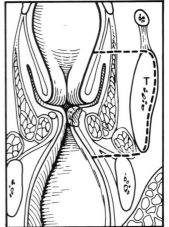

Fig. 9-46 Vertical hemilaryngectomy. **A,** View from above. Diagram of tissue removed in a vertical hemilaryngectomy involving the true cord and false cord. One arytenoid can be resected. **B,** Coronal diagram showing the tissue resected in a vertical hemilaryngectomy. Note that the outer perichondrium of the thyroid cartilage *(T)* is retained. (**A** from Curtin HD: Imaging of the larynx: current concepts, Radiology 173:1-11, 1989.)

should be sought in the paratracheal and lower jugular nodes.

The most important discussion for the radiologist concerns inferior extension. Inferior extension is easily assessed in axial and coronal orientation (Figs. 9-47 to 9-49). If the lesion reaches the upper margin of the cricoid, then a routine vertical hemilaryngectomy cannot be done. Some surgeons have resected the upper margin of the cartilage, and work is being done on "near-total" laryngectomies. However, the cricoid is the structural foundation of the larynx, and reconstruction of a usable larynx after partial removal of the cricoid is difficult; with total removal of the cricoid, it has proved impossible.

The conus elasticus is also considered an important landmark (see Figs. 9-6 and 9-40). This membrane, which is the lower boundary of the paraglottic space, extends from the free edge of the true vocal cord to the upper margin of the cricoid cartilage. The membrane does limit the extension of a tumor somewhat. Mucosal

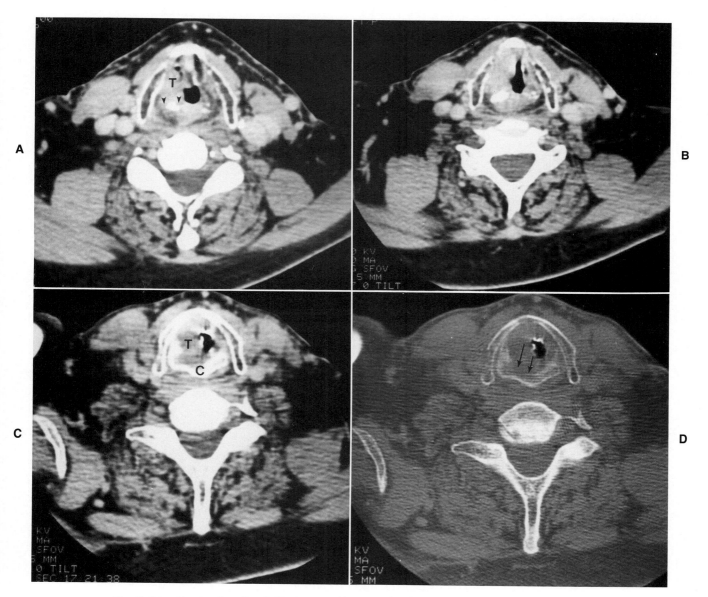

Fig. 9-47 Predominantly glottic tumor with extension into the false cord and subglottic extension. **A,** Supraglottic level shows tumor *(T)* with involvement of the anterior surface of the upper arytenoid *(arrowheads).* **B,** Lower slice shows the tumor at approximately the level of the ventricle. **C,** Inferior slice through the level of the cricoid shows tumor *(T)* within the ring. *C,* Cricoid. **D,** Bone algorithm shows loss of the cortical margin of the inner surface of the cricoid *(arrows).*

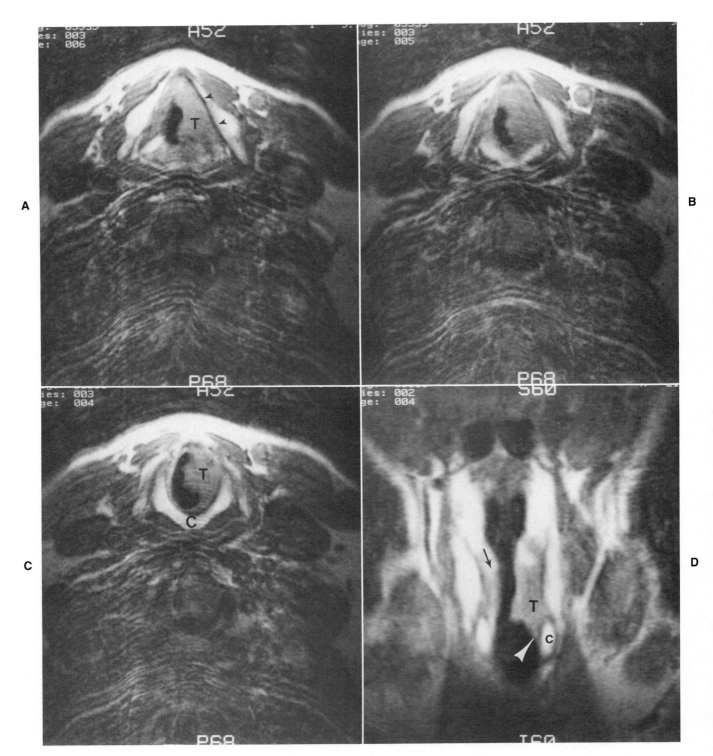

Fig. 9-48 Tumor of the cord with subglottic extension. **A,** Tumor *(T)* at the level of the cord. Note that the cortical line of the thyroid cartilage is intact *(arrowheads)*. **B,** Inferior slice shows tumor at the subglottic level. **C,** Inferior slice shows tumor *(T)* definitely within the cricoid ring *(C)*. **D,** Coronal T₁-weighted image shows the tumor *(T)* extending along the inner cortex of the cricoid arch *(arrowhead)*. *C,* Cricoid; *arrow,* approximate level of the upper margin of the cord. (**D** from Curtin HD: Imaging of the larynx: current concepts, Radiology 173:1-11, 1989.)

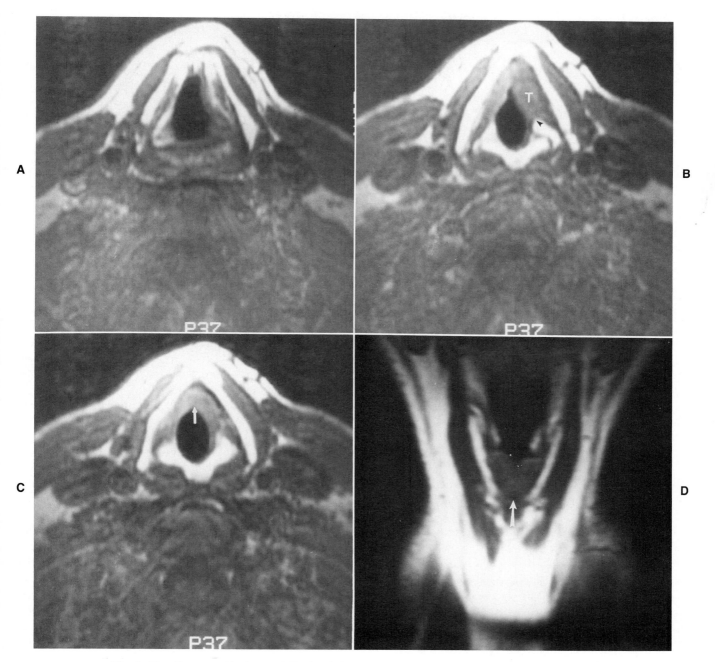

Fig. 9-49   True cord lesion. 1.5 Tesla. **A,** Level of the false cord is relatively normal. T_1-weighting. **B,** Tumor *(T)* at the level of the true cord. *Arrowhead,* vocal process. **C,** Level of the lower true cord. The tumor crosses the midline *(arrow)*. **D,** Coronal image shows increased tissue *(arrow)* beneath the anterior commissure. **E,** Slightly posterior slice shows only slight thickening of the right true cord. **F,** Sagittal T_1-weighted image shows small amount of tumor *(arrow)* immediately inferior to the anterior commissure *(arrowhead)*. Evaluation of tumor in this anterior part of the cord can be unreliable because of partial volume artifact.   *Continued.*

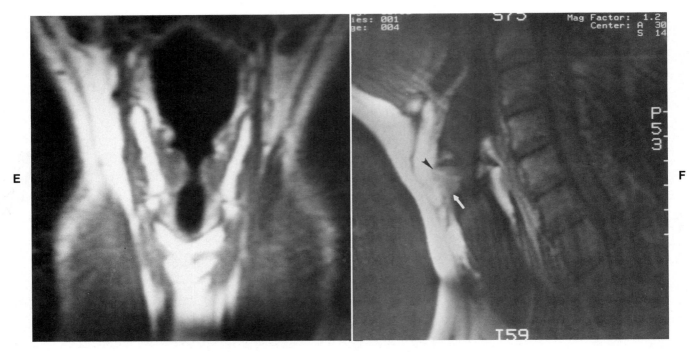

Fig. 9-49, cont'd   For legend see previous page.

tumors at the level of the conus elasticus are separated from cartilage by the thick ligamentous conus and by the thyroarytenoid muscle. Below the conus, a tumor invading the mucosa immediately reaches the cartilage. If a tumor has extended deep to the mucosa into the true cord (thyroarytenoid muscle), the conus elasticum becomes a barrier to inferior growth and directs the tumor laterally. Radiologically, the key concept is demonstration of whether the tumor has reached the upper margin of the cricoid, a structure that cannot be easily sacrificed.

Because of the cricoid's shape, the extent of tolerable inferior growth varies from anterior to posterior. Anteriorly 1 cm of mucosal extension is acceptable. More posteriorly only 0.5 cm is allowed before the cartilage margin is reached. The cartilage is easily recognizable on an axial scan. If the lesion extends "into the ring," a total laryngectomy is required. The cricoid is easily identified on coronal scans on magnetic resonance imaging, and tumor extending along the inner cortex is an ominous sign.

Although inferior extension is the most important information sought by the radiologist, other findings can also alter surgical planning. The true vocal cords converge anteriorly, reaching the thyroid cartilage at the anterior commissure (Figs. 9-49 and 9-50). At this midline point there is only mucosa between the airway and thyroid cartilage. Thus a lesion at this position can easily involve the cartilage early. If air is seen against the inner lamina of the cartilage, tumor is excluded. The finding of "tissue" against the cartilage is less reliable because the cords may come together, obliterating the airway, depending on the phase of respiration or breath-holding during the imaging procedure or as a result of any cord edema.

Even if the lesion crosses the anterior commissure, an extended vertical hemilaryngectomy may be done as long as the posterior half of one true cord is free of tumor and the cartilage is not eroded. The surgeon alters the cut through the thyroid cartilage, depending on the amount on the opposite cord that must be resected.

Superficial extension along the cord or across the anterior commissure is best evaluated by direct visualization if possible. Some estimate can be made on imaging. If the finding is crucial in deciding the feasibility of voice-sparing surgery, confirmation by direct inspection is necessary, even though the anterior commissure may at times be difficult to visualize directly.

In the proximity of the anterior commissure, the radiologist's role is once again to search for deep extension. Cartilage invasion may be assessed by CT or MRI (see following section on cartilage involvement). Mineralization of the thyroid cartilage varies, but demonstration of the tumor anterior to the cartilage is reliable evidence of cartilage involvement. Many times the anterior extent is through the cricothyroid membrane just below the inferior margin of, rather than directly through, the thyroid cartilage (see Figs. 9-43 and 9-50). In some cases both processes are seen. This anterior extension can be undetectable to the examining clinician.

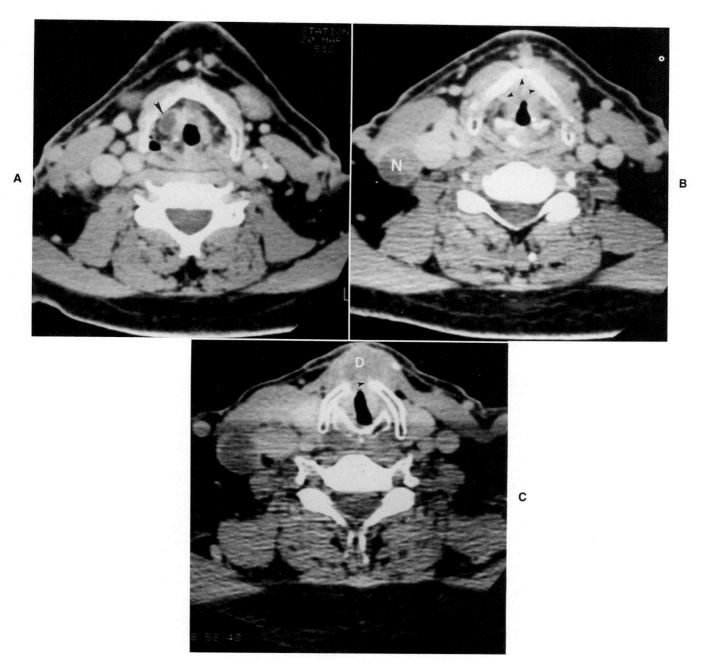

Fig. 9-50   Tumor of the anterior commissure and anterior ventricles. **A,** Slice through the supraglottic larynx shows a small saccular cyst (laryngocele) as the tumor obstructs the ventricle. *Arrowhead,* saccular cyst. **B,** Level of the anterior commissure and ventricles shows the tumor crossing the midline but no definite erosion of the thyroid cartilage. *Arrowheads,* tumor margins; *N,* node. **C,** Slice through the level of the cricothyroid membrane shows very small mass within the airway but large tumor mass in the region of the delphian node *(D).* There is some erosion of the thyroid cartilage *(arrowhead)* but most of the tumor extends through the cricothyroid membrane. (**C** from Curtin HD: Imaging of the larynx: current concepts, Radiology 173:1-11, 1989.)

The region just anterior to the cricothyroid membrane is the so-called Delphian node region. Some authors have described lymphatic extension from the anterior commissure region and subglottis to this node. In our experience more cases seem to involve the area by direct extension through the ligamentous membrane.

Posteriorly the lesion cannot involve an entire arytenoid cartilage if a vertical hemilaryngectomy is to be done. The vocal process can be involved, and in these cases the arytenoid is sacrified. However, if a large portion of the arytenoid is involved, the lesion would either be touching or in close proximity to the cricoid cartilage, thus disallowing the standard resection on that basis alone (see Figs. 9-31, *C,* and 9-47).

The degree of arytenoid involvement is usually assessed by endoscopy. However, deep extension to the region of the cricoarytenoid joint may be submucosal and thus best established by CT or MRI.

Superior extension of a glottic tumor brings the tumor into the false cord (Fig. 9-51). Currently, significant extension disallows vertical hemilaryngectomy. Presumably a significant supraglottic tumor would re-quire a supraglottic resection, which cannot easily be combined with a vertical hemilaryngectomy.

Lymph node involvement is seldom a problem with a true cord lesion. However, if the lesion extends significantly below the cord or is primarily in the infraglottic area, nodal involvement can occur in the paratracheal and pretracheal areas, eventually draining to the lower jugular or upper mediastinal nodes. Thus the lower neck should be examined if a significant subglottic tumor is present.

Pharynx

The lower pharynx (hypopharynx, laryngopharynx) has rather simple lateral and posterior walls and a more complex anterior wall formed by the pyriform sinuses, postcricoid area, and the posterior wall of the upper larynx. The superior limit of the hypopharynx is the hyoid bone or valleculae, and the inferior margin is the lower edge of the cricopharyngeus, where the pharynx meets the esophagus.

The pyriform sinus invaginates between the thyroid cartilage and the aryepiglottic fold. As such the para-

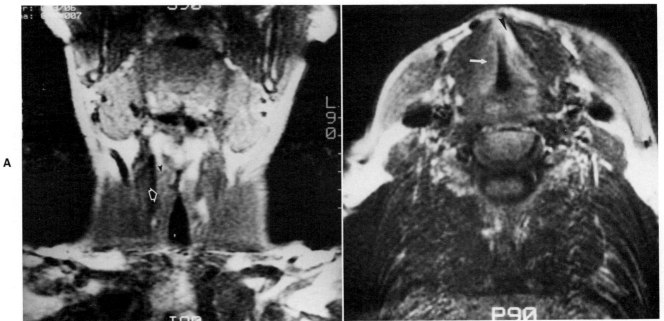

Fig. 9-51 Tumor of the ventricle involving the upper margin of the true cord and the lower margin of the false cord. 1.5 Tesla. **A,** Coronal image. Tumor extends around the ventricle involving the false cord *(arrowhead)* and the upper margin of the true cord *(open arrow).* T_1-weighting. **B,** Axial T_1-weighted image with tumor at the level of the false cord *(arrow).* Normal fat indicating false cord level *(arrowhead).* **C,** Same level as **B,** T_2-weighted image (long TR/long TE) showing relative brightening of the tumor *(arrow)* only appreciated by comparison with the T_1-weighted image. **D,** Lower slice, level of the true cord, no definite asymmetry of the cord. **E,** Same level as **D,** T_2-weighted image shows brightening of the involved cord *(arrow).* Note the normal intermediate signal intensity of the thyroarytenoid muscle on the normal side *(arrowhead).*

glottic space of the larynx is just anterior to the pyriform sinus mucosa. A lesion of the anterior wall of the pyriform sinus extending through the mucosa involves the paraglottic space at the level of the false cord (Figs. 9-52 and 9-53). On CT or MRI the lesion can be seen extending between the thyroid and arytenoid cartilages through the "thyroarytenoid gap." The tumor may then extend further inferiorly into the vocal cord via the paraglottic pathway. Primary tumors of the lower false cord and ventricle can extend through the thy-roarytenoid gap toward the pharyngeal mucosa, but they usually do not ulcerate this mucosa.

The apex of the pyriform sinus extends deeply into the thyroarytenoid gap and thus is very close to the cricoid cartilage. Lesions of the pyriform apex usually require a total laryngectomy for complete resection. If a lesion is confined to the upper lateral aspect of the aryepiglottic fold or the upper pyriform sinus, a partial pharyngectomy can be done with a supraglottic laryngectomy (Fig. 9-54).

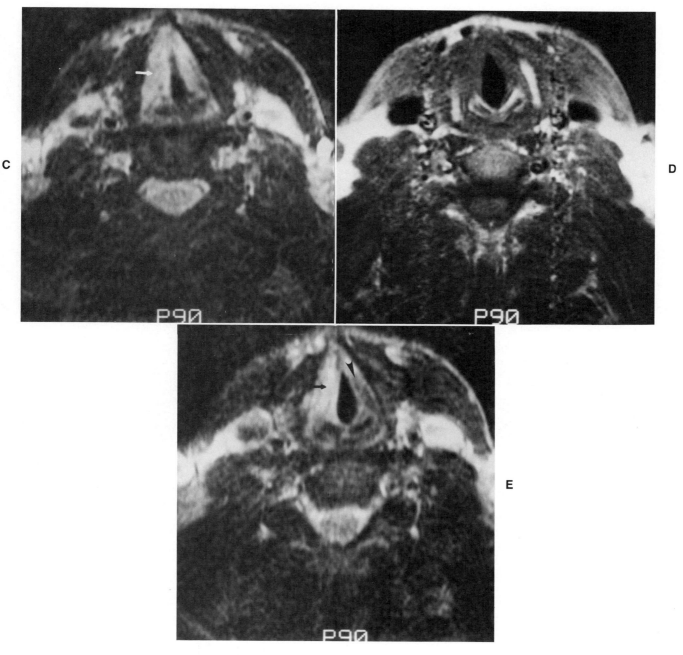

Fig. 9-51, cont'd   For legend see opposite page.

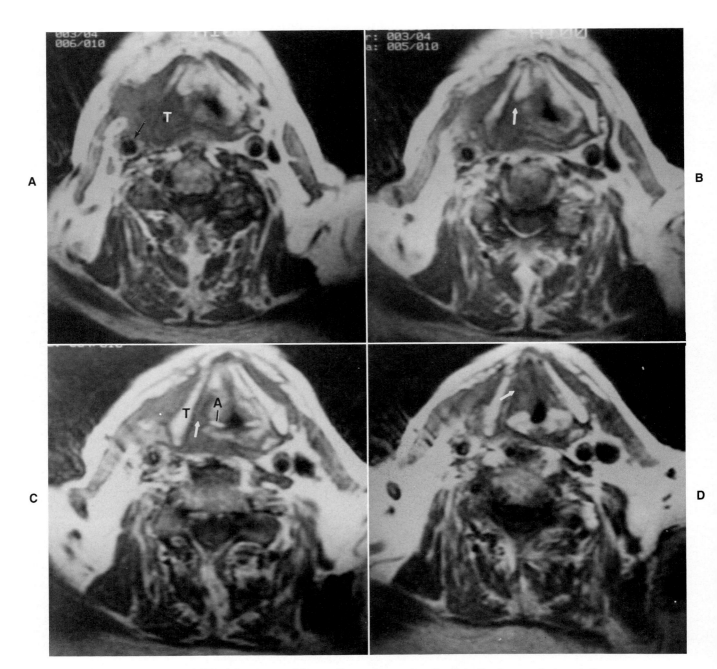

Fig. 9-52 MRI of the tumor of the pyriform sinus extending into the larynx. **A,** Level of a supraglottis tumor *(T)*. The tumor touches the carotid artery *(arrow)*. **B,** Slightly inferior slice shows tumor impinging on the paraglottic fat *(arrow)*. **C,** Tumor in the thyroarytenoid gap *(arrow)*. *T,* Thyroid cartilage; *A,* arytenoid cartilage. **D,** Slight thickening of the cord *(arrow)* as tumor invades via the paraglottic space.

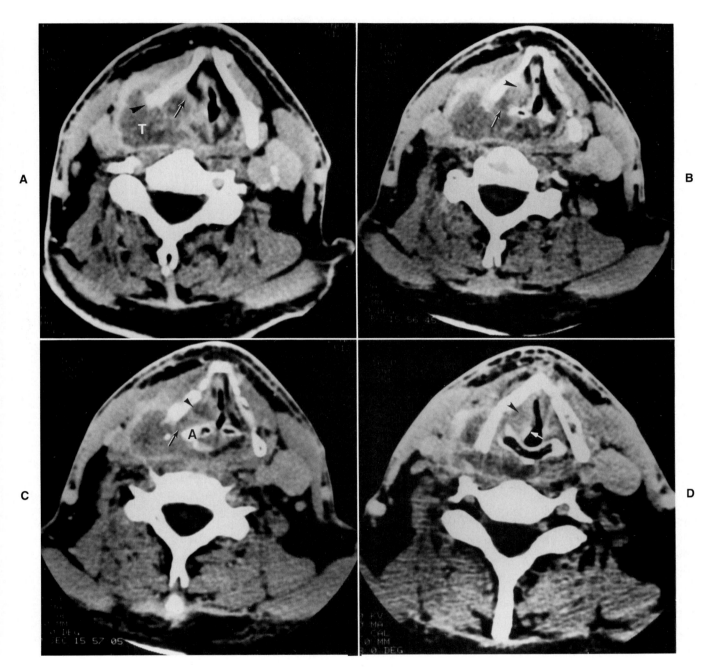

Fig. 9-53 CT of the pyriform sinus tumor invading the larynx and eroding the thyroid cartilage. **A,** Tumor *(T)* extending into the paraglottic fat *(arrow)*. There is erosion of the posterior margin of the thyroid cartilage *(arrowhead)* and tumor extending along the outer aspect of the thyroid cartilage. This phenomenon is due to the attachment of the pharyngeal muscle to the outer cortex of the thyroid cartilage rather than to the posterior margin. **B,** Tumor in the thyroarytenoid gap *(arrow)* and obliterating the paraglottic fat *(arrowhead)*. **C,** Lower slice still with tumor in the thyroarytenoid gap *(arrow)* and paraglottic space *(arrowhead)*. Again note the erosion of the thyroid cartilage. *A,* Arytenoid. **D,** Lower slice showing tumor in the paraglottic space at the level of the true cord *(arrowhead)* widening the cord. Vocal process *(short white arrow)*.

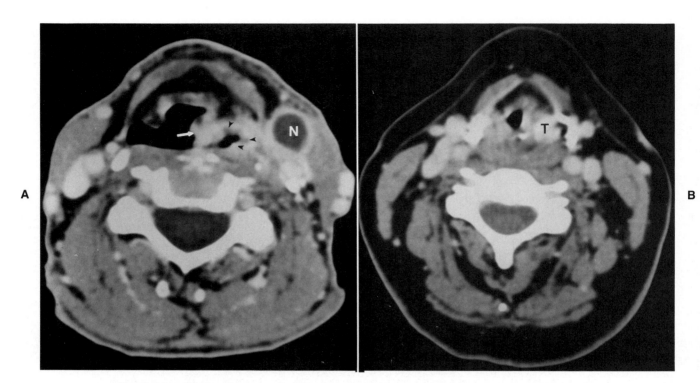

Fig. 9-54 CT of a pharyngeal tumor limited to the level of the supraglottic larynx. **A,** The lesion *(arrowheads)* extends around the lateral wall of the pharynx onto the posterior wall. The aryepiglottic fold *(arrow)* is involved. Typical appearance of a metastatic node *(N).* **B,** Lower margin of the tumor *(T)* is seen on the axial slice at the level of the supraglottic fat. The slice immediately inferior to this was normal.

The involvement of the pyriform apex can be visualized on axial CT or MRI as obliteration of the fat within, or a widening of, the thyroarytenoid gap (see Figs. 9-52 and 9-53). A pharyngogram done with thicker barium or propyliodone (Dionosil) will coat the mucosal surface and help define the inferior margin of a pyriform lesion. As with a laryngogram, the patient puffs out the cheeks (modified Valsalva maneuver) to distend the pyriform apex. Unlike the laryngogram, no anesthesia or aspiration of contrast is necessary.

The postcricoid region is the anterior wall of the pharynx at the level of the cricoid (Fig. 9-55). A lesion here calls for a total laryngectomy because resection would necessarily include the cricoid. The surgical question becomes the lower extent of the lesion relative to the pharyngoesophageal junction, and the cricopharyngeus marks this transition zone. This definition of the lower tumor margin helps make the decision of whether the surgical wound can be closed primarily or whether reconstruction (e.g., with a jejunal interposition) will be necessary.

The definition of the lower tumor margin is usually made on a barium swallow. On axial CT or MR images, the level of the cricopharyngeus muscle is approximately at the lower margin of the cricoid cartilage (see Fig. 9-21). Lack of esophageal involvement by a tumor is suggested on axial images if the thickness of the pharyngeal wall at the lower margin of the cricoid cartilage returns to normal. However, minimum submucosal tumor spread into the esophagus will go undetected on these images. The sagittal slice available on MRI gives improved visualization of the lower margin of the lesion (Fig. 9-56).

The actual mucosal surface in the postcricoid region can be difficult to evaluate on barium swallow because of the normal irregularity of the anterior wall. This irregularity is caused by a submucosal venous plexus. The fluoroscopist should attempt to make a judgment on the pliability of the surface. However, the pliability of the postcricoid area is more difficult to assess than the pliability of the lateral or posterior pharyngeal walls.

The pharyngeal constrictors, a relative barrier to tumor spread, attach to the lateral aspect of the thyroid cartilage 1 cm anterior to the posterior cartilage border. This allows a tumor "wraparound" effect, since the lateral pharyngeal wall lesion extends along the outer surface of the thyroid cartilage or erodes the posterior margin of the thyroid ala (see Fig. 9-53).

Further lateral extent brings a lesion to the carotid artery (see Fig. 9-52). Involvement of the artery is an important and ominous finding. Reports of the use of

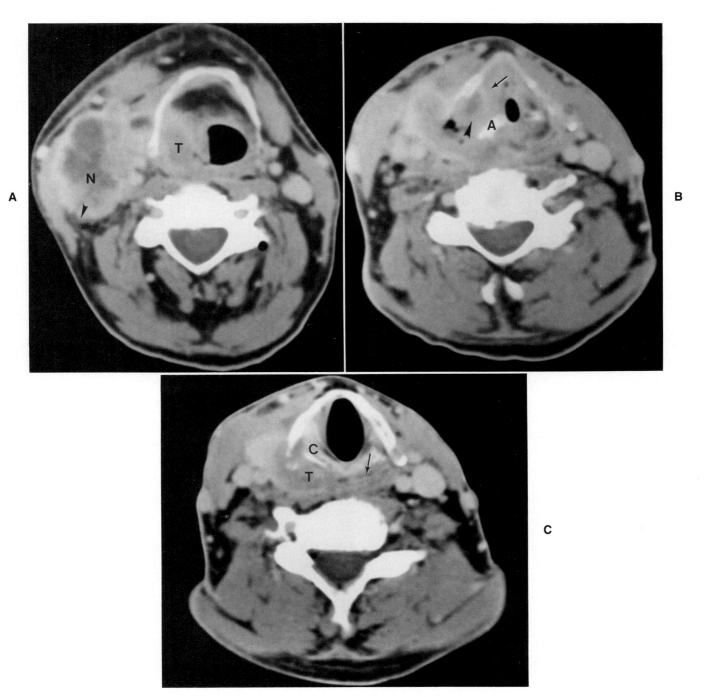

Fig. 9-55 Pharyngeal/pyriform sinus lesion extending onto postcricoid area. **A,** Superior slice shows tumor *(T)* in the pharyngeal wall. Metastatic nodes *(N)* with irregular margins *(arrowhead)* suggested extracapsular spread. **B,** Slice through the level of the thyroarytenoid gap and false cord shows tumor in the paraglottic space *(arrow)* after passing through the thyroarytenoid gap *(arrowhead)*. Note sclerosis of the arytenoid *(A)*. **C,** Tumor *(T)* is seen along the posterior aspect of the cricoid *(C)*. Note the normal fat lines on the opposite side *(arrow)*.

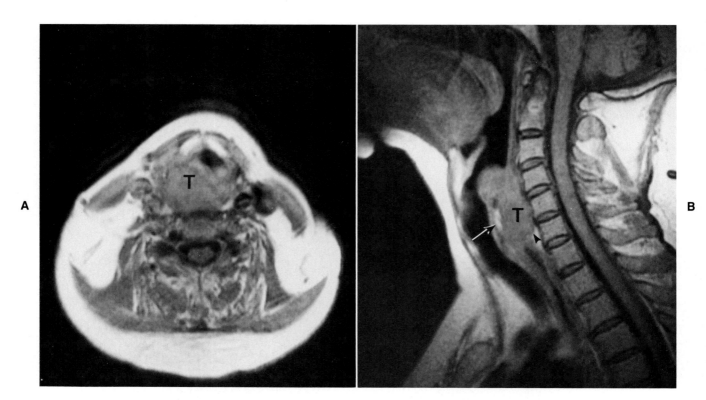

Fig. 9-56 MRI of postcricoid tumor. **A,** Axial slice shows tumor *(T)* in the posterior aspect of the larynx (T$_1$-weighted .35 Tesla). **B,** Sagittal view shows the tumor *(T)*. The inferior margin *(arrowhead)* is best defined in this sagittal view. Bright signal is fat in the medullary cavity of the cricoid lamina *(arrow)*. (**A** courtesy of Robert Lufkin, MD.)

ultrasound or MRI to assess actual involvement or fixation of the tumor to the carotid have not provided signs of consistent reliability. The radiologist should report the degree to which the tumor encircles the vessel.

Direct posterior extension of the lesion involves the posterior pharyngeal wall and brings the tumor to the prevertebral fascia and muscles. Fixation of the fascia worsens the prognosis and limits the surgical possibilities. If the lesion is ulcerative, there is often invasion of the fascia. If a lesion is predominantly exophytic, however, the fascia may not be involved. This can be assessed on lateral fluoroscopy during barium swallow, since a lesion that is not fixed to the fascia can slide up and down relative to the spine as the barium passes (Fig. 9-57).

Pharyngeal lesions spread initially to the high jugular nodes, which are easily seen on axial images. Occasionally a lesion arising in the lower pharynx can spread superiorly to the high lateral retropharyngeal nodes (nodes of Rouviere), which are immediately beneath the skull base. These areas should be carefully evaluated both at the time of initial diagnosis and on follow-up examinations.

Cartilage Involvement

Involvement of the cricoid or thyroid cartilage not only disallows the standard partial laryngeal resection but also is a relative contraindication to radiation therapy. Thus cartilage involvement is extremely important in a patient considered for radiation therapy or any surgery short of total laryngectomy.

The epiglottis is not as crucial. This cartilage is an elastic yellow cartilage and a poor barrier to tumor extension. However, as discussed before, supraglottic resection can still be done if the epiglottis is involved. The epiglottis is removed with the specimen. Similarly, minimum involvement of the vocal process of the arytenoid does not necessarily exclude a partial resection.

The mineralization of the cartilages is nonuniform and may be asymmetric. By the age that most patients develop carcinoma, however, much of both the cricoid and the thyroid cartilage is ossified. The thyroid cartilage usually ossifies from the inferior margin superiorly and from the posterior margin anteriorly. Small islands of ossified and nonossified cartilage are frequently seen in the thyroid cartilage's broad, flat alar surfaces. Three possible normal materials can be present in these laryngeal cartilages: cortical bone, fatty marrow, and unossified cartilage.

On CT, a tumor usually has the same attenuation as unossified cartilage (soft tissue density). Since the degree of cartilage ossification is extremely variable, cartilage involvement can be very difficult to assess (Fig. 9-

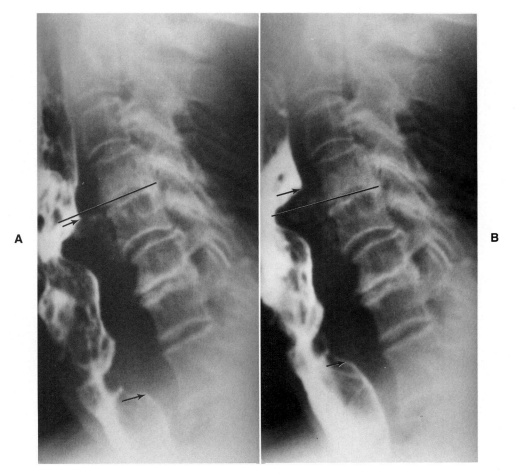

Fig. 9-57 Exophytic lesion of the posterior wall of the pharynx. The lesion is not fixed to the prevertebral fascia. Compare the position of the upper and lower margin of the lesion *(arrows)* compared to the cervical spine interspace C-4–C-5 line. **A,** At rest. **B,** During swallow.

58). Gross destruction, of course, can be easily determined; however, the only truly reliable CT sign of cartilage destruction is the demonstration of a tumor on the opposite side of the cartilage from the primary lesion.

Sclerosis seen on CT is a reactive phenomenon and does not mean actual invasion of the cartilage (Fig. 9-59). A tumor close to the perichondrium can cause sclerosis within the cartilage without tumor cells actually being in the area of the sclerosis. More experience is needed to clarify this relationship.

On MRI the most reliable sign is still demonstration of a tumor on the outer side of the cartilage (Fig. 9-60), but some hope exists that lesser degrees of tumor involvement may be detectable. Early reports indicate that MRI will offer an advantage in cartilage evaluation because of the variability in the appearance of both normal and abnormal cartilages afforded by different pulse sequences.[11,14,15]

MRI shows the cortex of ossified cartilage as a black signal void. The fatty marrow is bright on short TR / short TE (T_1-weighted) sequences but darkens somewhat on the long TR / long TE (T_2-weighted) sequence. The unmineralized cartilage is relatively dark on T_1-weighted images and remains dark on the T_2-weighted images. The unmineralized cartilage is not as black as cortical bone but is much darker, obviously, than the fat (Fig. 9-61).

A tumor is intermediate in intensity or relatively dark on T_1-weighted (short TR / short TE) sequences (Fig. 9-61). Thus if a segment of a cartilage is relatively dark on a T_1-weighted image, the radiologist cannot reliably distinguish between a tumor and unmineralized cartilage on this sequence alone. The long TR sequences are helpful (Figs. 9-61 and 9-62).

According to Castelijns et al, a tumor (squamous cell carcinoma) brightens on the later echo of a long TR sequence, whereas the unmineralized cartilage does not.[11,14,15] On T_2-weighted images, the involved and uninvolved cartilage may actually look the same. The tumor is relatively bright, and a fatty medullary area may "retain" a significant amount of signal because of

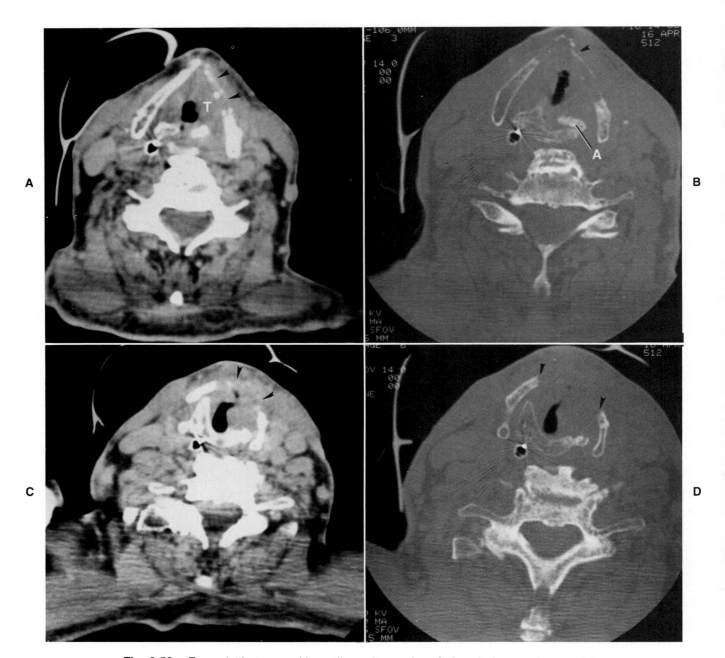

Fig. 9-58 Transglottic tumor with cartilage destruction. **A,** Level close to the ventricle shows the tumor *(T)*. There is definite demineralization of the thyroid ala *(arrowheads)* but no significant thickening of the strap muscles on the outer surface of the thyroid. **B,** Bone algorithm shows the demineralization of the cartilage strongly suspicious of tumor invasion. There has actually been slight buckling *(arrowhead)* of the thyroid ala due to the weakening of the cartilage. The arytenoid *(A)* is sclerotic. **C,** Slice through the cricoid shows tumor within the ring of the cricoid and, at this level, tumor extending outside of the larynx *(arrowheads)*. **D,** Bone algorithm showing destruction of the thyroid cartilage *(arrowheads)*.

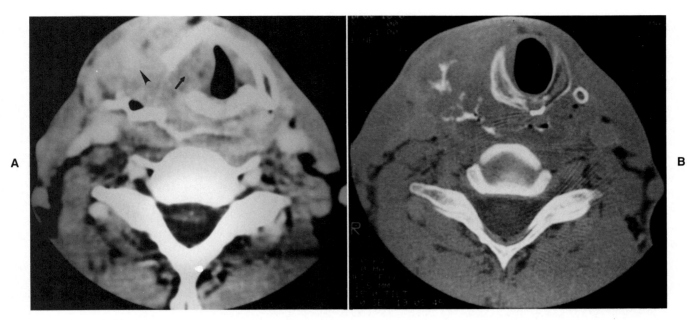

Fig. 9-59 Extensive pharyngeal tumor invading the larynx. **A,** Tumor of the pyriform sinus extending into the true cord level *(arrow)* as well as laterally *(arrowhead).* **B,** Lower level shows marked sclerosis of the cartilage on the involved side. The uninvolved side is normal. Tumor did not extend into the cartilage. The sclerotic reaction was definitely free of tumor histologically.

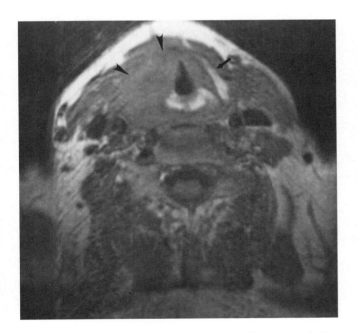

Fig. 9-60 Tumor of the true cord extending through the thyroid ala. Tumor *(arrowheads)* is demonstrated outside of the normal position of the larynx as noted by the elevation of the strap muscle. This tumor *(arrowheads)* is beyond the normal limit of the thyroid cartilage. Compare with the normal low signal of the cortical bone and the high signal of the medullary cavity of the uninvolved thyroid ala opposite side *(arrow).*

the proximity to the surface coil. The important finding is the *change* in appearance, with *relative brightening* between T_1- and T_2-weighted images suggesting a tumor.

Castelijns et al actually used a midfield strength unit and an earlier echo because of the diminishing signal on the later echo images. Still, they demonstrated the tumor involvement as relative brightening *compared to the T_1-weighted appearance.* Again, nonmineralized cartilage remained dark. Early experience using high-field units and later echoes are encouraging. More experience is needed for verification, but if reliable, this finding will certainly be helpful.

Gadolinium also increases the signal of the tumor but presumably not that of nonossified cartilage. This may eventually allow determination of cartilage involvement with the use of the shorter imaging times of a T_1-weighted, short TR/TE sequence. Again, experience is not extensive at the time of this writing.

Further Workup in Squamous Cell Carcinoma

A patient with squamous cell cancer of the larynx, especially of the supraglottic larynx, has a relatively high chance (10% to 20%) of having or developing a second primary lesion.[16] This may be the result of the common exposure of certain areas to cigarette smoke or ethanol. The regions most likely involved are the oral cavity, lar-

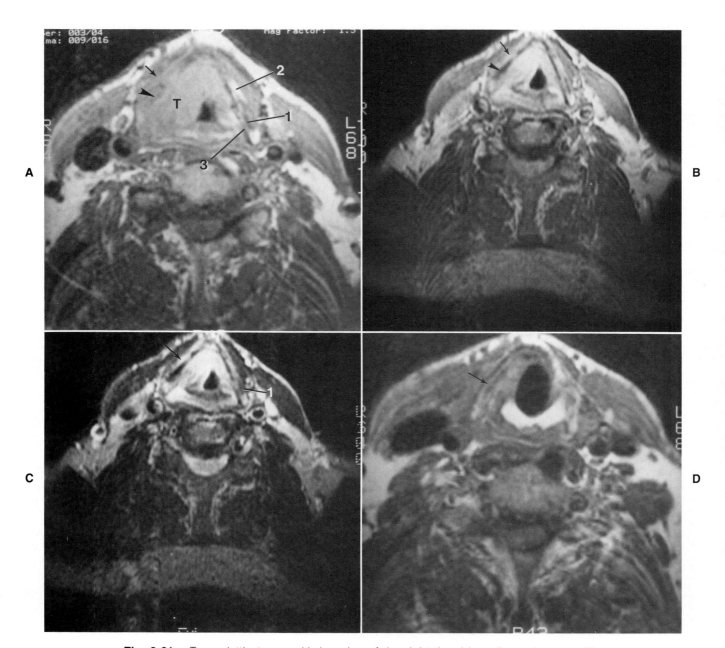

Fig. 9-61 Transglottic tumor with invasion of the right thyroid cartilage shown on T$_2$-weighted image. (1.5 Tesla.) **A,** Supraglottic level T$_1$-weighted (TR 600, TE 20). Tumor *(T)* has pushed the thyroid ala laterally. The entire right ala is of intermediate signal intensity. On the opposite side the cartilage is normal. *1,* Non mineralized cartilage; *2,* bright signal of fat in medullary cavity; *3,* low signal of cortex of ossified cartilage; *arrow,* outer tumor margin. *Arrowhead,* approximate position of inner cortex of the right thyroid ala. Compare with **B** and **C. B,** Same level as **A.** TR 2875, TE 30 early echo on a long TR sequence. The normal thyroid cartilage is essentially unchanged. The right side shows relative brightening of the involved cartilage *(arrow)* and accentuation of the residual nonossified cartilage *(arrowhead)* because of brighter signal both medially and laterally. **C,** Same level as **A** and **B.** TR 2875, TE 80 late echo in a long TR sequence showing further brightening of the tumor involved cartilage *(arrow)* compared with the normal side. The T$_2$-image cannot be interpreted alone. The two sides are relatively symmetric. The change in appearance between T$_1$- and T$_2$-weighted image is important. The nonossified cartilage *(1)* on the normal side remains dark. **D,** Subglottic level. T$_1$-weighted image (TR 600, TE 20) shows the lower thyroid cartilage. The central medullary area has an intermediate signal *(arrow),* which could represent nonossified cartilage or tumor. The cortex of the cartilage (low signal) does not appear to be eroded.

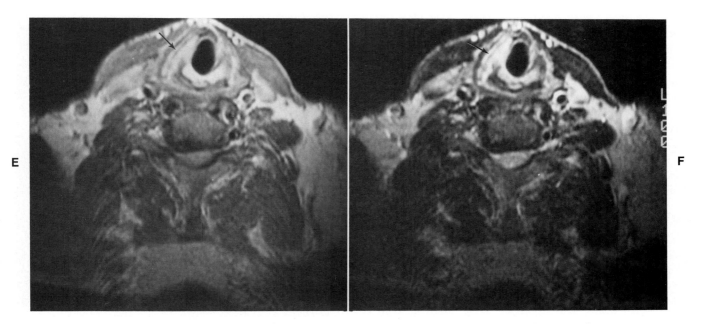

Fig. 9-61, cont'd   E, Long TR/short TE (TR 2875, TE 30) shows relative brightening of the medullary cavity of the cartilage *(arrow)*. **F,** Long TR/late TE (TR 2875, TE 80) shows definite relative brightening of the medullary cavity *(arrow)* strongly suggesting tumor involvement. (From Curtin HD: Imaging of the larynx: current concepts, Radiology 173:1-11, 1989.)

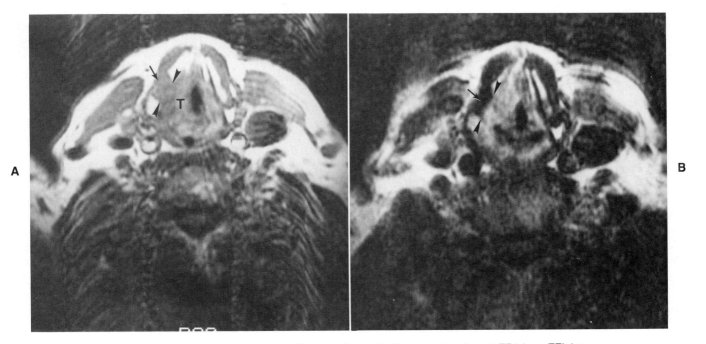

Fig. 9-62   Tumor against nonossified cartilage. **A,** T_1-weighted (short TR/short TE) image shows tumor *(T)* and nonossified cartilage *(arrow)* both have intermediate signal intensity and the tumor-cartilage junction between arrowheads cannot be defined. **B,** T_2-weighted (long TR/long TE) image shows brightening of the tumor. The nonossified cartilage does not brighten *(arrow)*. The margin between tumor and cartilage is now clearly defined *(between arrowheads)*.

ynx, pharynx, lung, esophagus, and, less often, the stomach (Fig. 9-63).

It is our practice to perform a barium swallow examination to search for second primary lesions in patients diagnosed with squamous cell carcinoma of the larynx. A truly negative barium swallow examination is a very reliable test. Any diminution of pliability or distensibility revealed by barium study is evaluated by endoscopy and biopsy.

A chest radiograph is used to seek a second primary lesion in the lung rather than to search for the extremely rare pulmonary metastases.

OTHER MALIGNANT TUMORS

Squamous cell carcinoma accounts for 95% of malignancies of the larynx. However, there are other diagnoses, both benign and malignant, that must be considered.[1,2] The pathologic diagnosis is still usually made by endoscopy and biopsy, but the radiologist may direct the clinician toward a diagnosis other than squamous cell carcinoma. This is especially true when there is no obvious mucosal lesion but rather a submucosal pathologic condition.

Other carcinomas of the larynx include adenocarcinoma (1%) arising in the minor salivary glands, verrucous carcinoma, and anaplastic carcinoma.[1]

Adenocarcinoma (see Fig. 9-29) has the same subtypes as salivary gland neoplasms elsewhere. Adenoid cystic carcinoma is slightly more common in the subglottic larynx. Mucoepidermoid and nonspecific adenocarcinoma (not otherwise categorized) are more common in the supraglottic larynx. Other subtypes of adenocarcinomas are rare.

Verrucous carcinoma refers to a primarily exophytic tumor that is wartlike and not very invasive. This lesion almost never metastasizes.

Anaplastic carcinoma, similar to oat cell carcinoma in the lung, is another rare carcinoma of the larynx. The prognosis is poor.

Spindle cell carcinoma is a rare lesion with squamous cell carcinoma and a spindle cell stroma. There is a difference of opinion as to whether this is a peculiar kind of squamous cell carcinoma or a combination of squamous cell carcinoma and a sarcoma.[1] Either or both components can metastasize. Other names for this lesion occasionally found in the literature are pseudosarcoma, carcinosarcoma, pleomorphic carcinoma, polypoid sarcoma, and pseudosarcomatous squamous cell carcinoma. The basic controversy depends on definition of the cell of derivation and the potential of the spindle cell stroma. Does the spindle cell develop directly from the squamous cell? Is the spindle cell truly of mesenchymal origin? A third theory holds that the spindle cell stroma is a reactive phenomenon.

Any type of *sarcoma* can be found in the larynx. As a group sarcomas make up only 0.3% to 1% of all laryn-

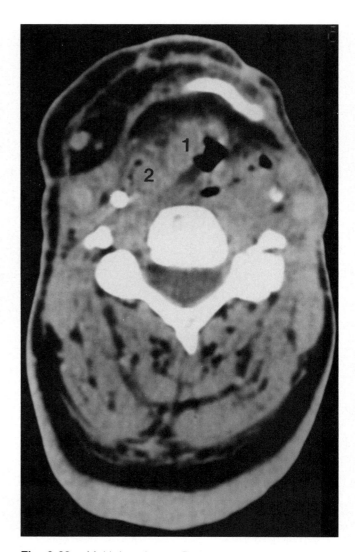

Fig. 9-63 Multiple primary. Patient with previous floor of the mouth and radical neck dissection now with three separate primaries in the pharynx/larynx. Slice through the supraglottic level shows an endolaryngeal lesion *(1)* and a lesion of the pyriform sinus *(2)*. These lesions were not connected directly. The patient also had a lesion of the opposite subglottic region.

geal malignancies. Although in rare cases they can be large or fungating, they are primarily submucosal. Usually the masses are somewhat nonspecific on imaging, but a smooth mucosal covering should direct the radiologist away from a diagnoses of squamous cell carcinoma.

Special mention should be made of chondrosarcoma because the calcification (often ringlike) can indicate a specific diagnosis to the radiologist. These calcifications may be suggested on MRI but are more obvious on CT (Figs. 9-64 and 9-65). The origin of the lesion in the cartilage is usually suspected because of the obvious defect in either the cricoid or the thyroid cartilage. It may be difficult or impossible to separate benign from malignant lesions.

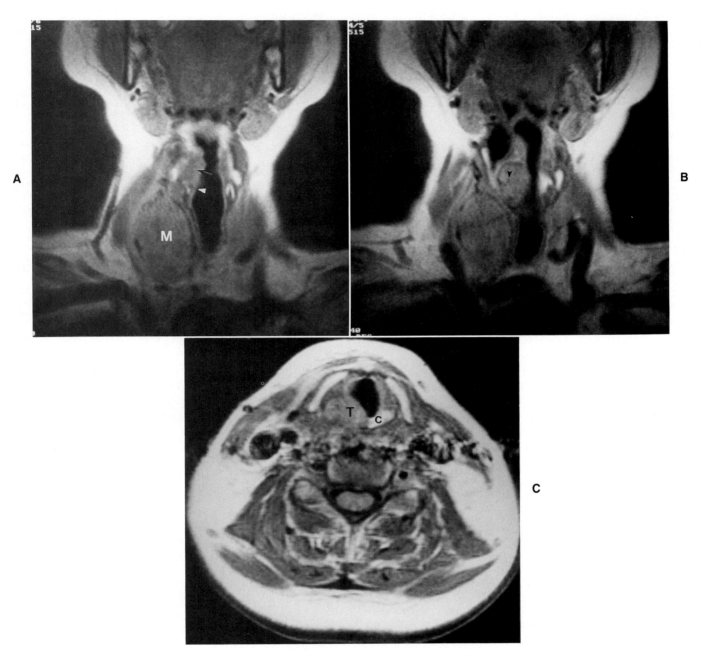

Fig. 9-64   Chondrosarcoma of the larynx (short TR/short TE .35 Tesla). **A,** Coronal slice shows thickening at the level of the true cord *(arrow)* extending and effacing the subglottic angle *(arrowhead)*. The etiology of the thyroid mass *(M)* is unknown. **B,** Slightly more posterior slice through the lamina of the cricoid shows the tumor mass on the right. The small dark areas within the mass *(arrowhead)* may represent calcification. **C,** T_1-weighted image (short TR/short TE) shows tumor *(T)* replacing the right side of the cricoid cartilage *(C)*. (Courtesy of William Hanafee, MD.)

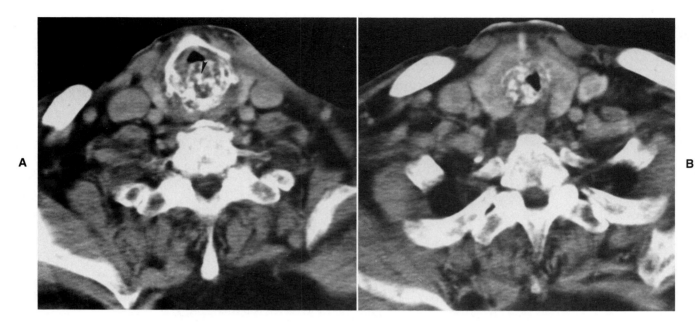

Fig. 9-65   Chondrosarcoma of the larynx. **A,** CT shows definite ring-like calcifications *(arrowhead)* within the tumor mass. **B,** Inferior extension shows similar calcifications.

Melanomas have been described in the supraglottic larynx and in the true cord and are extremely rare metastatic tumors.[1]

Secondary involvement of the larynx other than by direct extension from a malignancy near the larynx is rare. Metastatic deposits to the larynx from distant sites have been reported in rare cases.[1,17] Melanomas, renal cell cancer, and breast and lung metastases have been reported, as have involvement by leukemia and lymphoma. No characteristic imaging appearances have been described.

BENIGN TUMORS

Benign lesions of the larynx include vocal cord nodules, juvenile papillomatosis, and a variety of nonepithelial tumors.

Vocal cord nodules (nonneoplastic) represent a stromal reaction in patients with a history of vocal abuse. They may be seen incidentally by the radiologist but are usually diagnosed by the clinician with no radiologic investigation (Fig. 9-66). Vocal cord nodules occur on the free margin of the true vocal cord. Occasionally the clinician may confuse a vocal cord nodule with one of the other small lesions but imaging is not likely to be of much help in achieving clarification.

Papillomas, although benign and noninvasive, tend to recur after therapy.[1] The wartlike lesions, most often multiple, occur most often in children. Any part of the larynx can be affected, and involvement of the trachea and bronchial tree can occur in severe cases, especially if there is a history of tracheostomy. Currently the laser

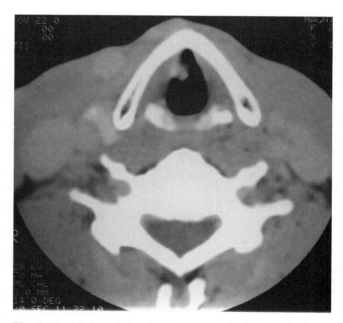

Fig. 9-66   Polyp of the right true cord. Incidental finding.

is used to excise the papillomas in children. Regrowth can be so rapid that many children require repeat procedures every few weeks. Most cases go into remission eventually, but some persist into adulthood. Although the lesions are benign, many deaths are caused by pneumonia or airway compromise. The high correlation between children with juvenile papillomatosis and mothers with venereal warts suggests a viral cause.

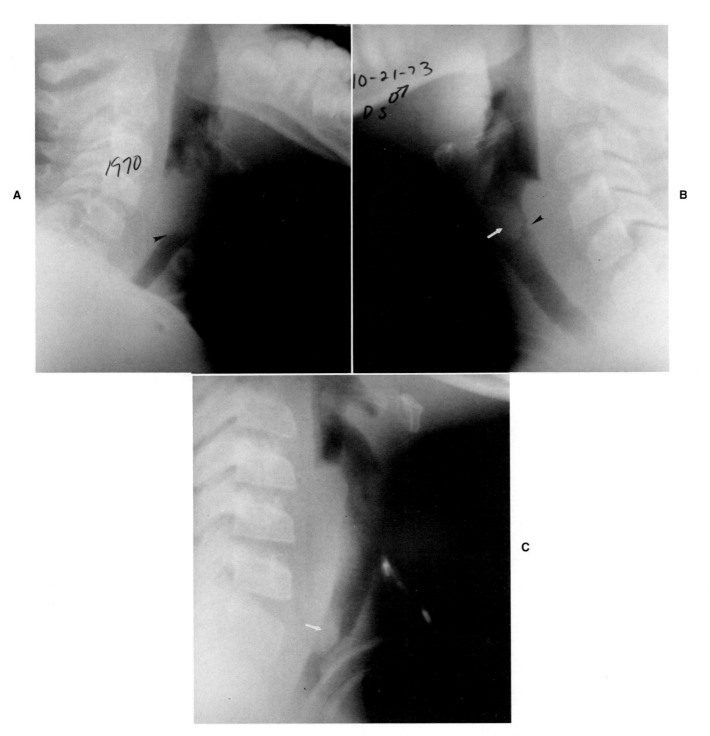

Fig. 9-67   Juvenile papillomas with multiple treatments. **A,** Nodular tumor mass completely obstructing the larynx. Note the slight nodularity of the inferior margin of the tumor *(arrowhead).* **B,** Later study shows small airway *(arrowhead)* with nodular mass in the anterior larynx *(arrow).* **C,** Later film in adolescence showing good laryngeal airway but nodular mass just above the tracheostomy. Mass *(arrow).*

Papillomas do occur in adults, usually in men, but in the adult they are less often multiple.

Radiologically the multiple nodules can be seen impinging on the airway on plain radiograph or tomography (Fig. 9-67). Chest films are used to evaluate possible pulmonary involvement when small nodules can be detected. The nodules may cavitate.

Benign nonepithelial or mesenchymal tumors include hemangiomas, neural tumors, lipomas, leiomyomas, rhabdomyomas, and chondromas, as well as a few other rare tumors.[1,2] Of these, lipomas have a characteristic appearance both on CT or MRI because of their high fat content (Fig. 9-68).[18] Chondromas can often be identified by the mineralized matrix and the relationship to the laryngeal cartilage. The lesion cannot reliably be established as benign or malignant unless there is a very aggressive appearance.

Hemangiomas deserve special mention. Hemangiomas are more common in adults than in children, but the pediatric type is more likely to cause airway obstruction and so has received more attention.[19]

Hemangiomas in adults are usually localized (Fig. 9-69) and tend to be glottic or supraglottic. They could be expected to enhance on CT, and on MRI probably behave as hemangiomas elsewhere in the body with a fairly bright T_2 appearance.

Hemangiomas of the young can occur anywhere in the larynx but have a predilection for the subglottic area (Figs. 9-70 to 9-72). This is a major problem because even though the hemangioma is expected to regress, airway compromise can force intervention. In a typical pediatric hemangioma the infant has partial airway obstruction within the first 6 months to a year. Subglottic hemangiomas may appear as recurrent croup because any inflammation further compromises an already narrowed subglottic area. Crying also exacerbates the problem because of venous engorgement. The larynx lesion is often associated with cutaneous or soft tissue hemangiomas. The diagnosis may be suggested by radiography but is usually made by endoscopy, when a compressible red or blue mass is seen. Topical epinephrine may cause the lesion to diminish in size.

Tracheostomy may be necessary while waiting for the tumor to diminish. Steroid therapy and surgery have been tried. Laser excision or reduction is now popular because of the lower bleeding tendency. Eventual tracheal stenosis is not uncommon, especially after surgery.

The most common radiographic appearance of a pediatric hemangioma is a localized or concentric narrowing of the airway just below the true cords (Fig. 9-72). This can be appreciated on CT or MRI with axial, coronal,

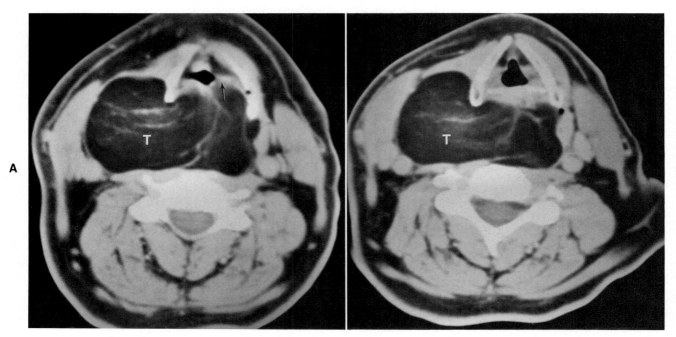

Fig. 9-68 **A,** Lipoma in the soft tissues of the neck and retropharyngeal space. Large tumor extending posterior to the larynx displacing the larynx anteriorly. Note how the fat appears to "bulge" into the supraglottic/paraglottic space *(arrow)*. The lesion at this level is actually retropharyngeal with the pharyngeal lumen going between the tumor and the larynx. The anterior wall of the pyriform sinus is being pushed anteriorly compressing the paraglottic fat but not invading. *T,* Tumor. **B,** Slightly lower level at the upper arytenoid. *T,* Tumor.

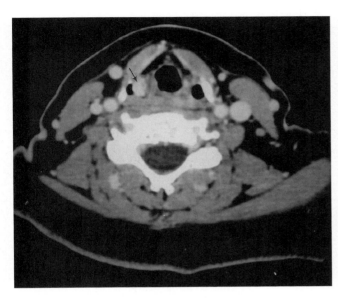

Fig. 9-69 Hemangioma of the pyriform sinus shows enhancement of the small lesion attached to the medial wall of the pyriform sinus just below the aryepiglottic fold. Tumor *(arrow)*.

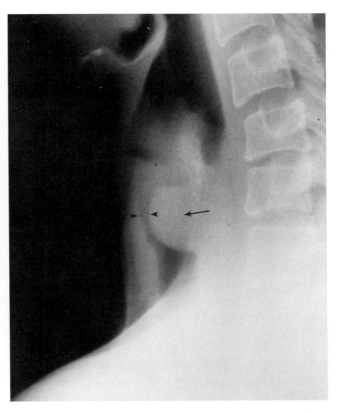

Fig. 9-71 Large subglottic hemangioma protruding from the posterior wall with significant narrowing of the airway *(arrowheads)*. Hemangioma *(arrow)*. This in an older patient than is typical for the infantile type of hemangioma.

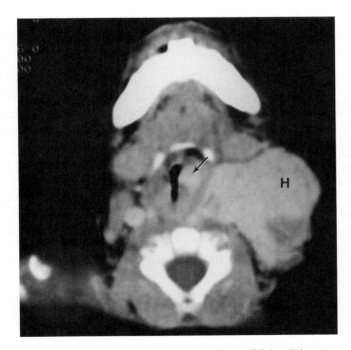

Fig. 9-70 Child with large hemangioma *(H)* involving the soft tissues of the neck with involvement of the aryepiglottic fold and supraglottis *(arrow)*.

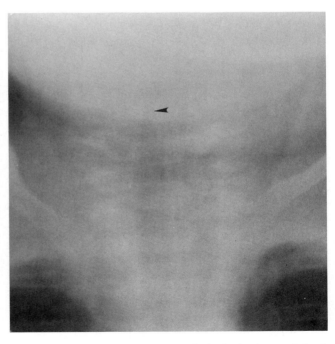

Fig. 9-72 Small hemangioma (subglottic in an infant) showing slight bulge *(arrowhead)* narrowing the airway from the left side.

or sagittal planes, but the actual airway configuration is most easily appreciated on plain films done in several projections. Conventional tomography can also show the airway well.

Occasionally phleboliths may be seen in a larger hemangioma, either with CT or with plain film (usually in somewhat older patients).

Paragangliomas (glomus tumors) have been reported in the larynx, usually in the supraglottic location[20] (Fig. 9-73). These lesions enhance on CT and, as might be expected from their vascular nature, tend to bleed if biopsied.

Neural lesions may be isolated tumors in the larynx. In neurofibromatosis, isolated localized lesions can occur or a more infiltrative abnormality can diffusely involve the paraglottic structures or other areas of the extralaryngeal neck.[21,22]

Granular cell tumor is a benign lesion of unknown origin that involves the mucosal membranes of the head and neck.[1] Most theories implicate either a Schwann cell or a more primitive mesenchymal cell as the cell of origin. The larynx can be involved. The epithelium over the granular cell tumor may be hyperplastic and thus mimic squamous cell carcinoma at direct inspection, but biopsy can establish the diagnosis. The most common site is the true cord. The age occurrence is usually 35 to 45 years, which is also younger than the usual age of squamous cell carcinoma.

CYSTS AND LARYNGOCELES

Cysts of the larynx can arise from obstruction of mucous gland ducts.[1] Symptoms include dysphagia or respiratory problems, depending on the location of the lesion. A laryngocele represents an abnormality of the laryngeal saccule. This small "diverticulum" extends superiorly from the anterior part of the ventricle. Thyroglossal duct cysts are primarily outside of the larynx but can protrude into it (see Fig. 9-73).

Mucosal cysts can arise anywhere there are glands.[1,23] Thus only the free margin of the true cord is spared, and almost any other location is a possible site of cyst development. These cysts are superficial, and submucosal and protrude into the airway while maintaining an intact mucosa. Deep extension is not seen. Vallecular cysts are seen as fluid-filled masses anterior to the epiglottis (Fig. 9-74). Often seen in children, vallecular cysts can be quite large but tend to have a smooth margin.

The saccule or appendix of the ventricle extends vertically into the paraglottic region of the false cord (Fig. 9-75). The saccule communicates with the ventricle through a very small channel. If the saccule enlarges, the *laryngocele or saccular cyst forms.*[24,25] Many authors refer to this abnormality as a laryngocele if it is air filled and as a saccular cyst if it is fluid filled. Some use laryngocele to mean either and differentiate by saying "air filled" or "fluid filled."

A laryngocele can be internal, external, or mixed. Internal refers to a laryngocele or cyst totally within the larynx and not extending through the thyrohyoid membrane. External laryngoceles protrude through the thyrohyoid membrane but with little dilation within the larynx itself. Mixed laryngoceles are those with both an internal and external component. In our experience almost all of these laryngoceles have some internal component, since the site of origin, the laryngeal saccule, is within the larynx.

The laryngocele and saccular cysts behave as supraglottic submucosal masses. A laryngocele can be diagnosed on CT, MRI, tomography or even plain films (Figs. 9-76 to 9-79). The internal consistency of the fluid-filled cysts may vary somewhat, depending on their protein content. This is only apparent on MRI or CT. The air-filled cysts can be appreciated on any form of imaging (Fig. 9-78).

A laryngocele, although always benign, can be associated with a malignancy in the region of the ventricle (Figs. 9-78 to 9-80). The tumor obstructs the outflow of the saccule, causing either trapping of air or retention of mucus. For this reason the ventricular area should be closely examined in patients with a laryngocele or saccular cyst. On CT or MRI, if the abnormality can be followed through the paraglottic area of the false cord to the level of the ventricle, the true cord is normal.

The term laryngopyocele refers to an infected laryngocele or saccular cyst (Figs. 9-81 and 9-82). Enlargement can cause airway compromise and increase swelling in the lateral neck.

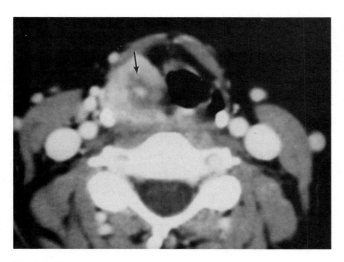

Fig. 9-73   Paraganglioma of the supraglottic larynx and pyriform sinus shows enhancing mass in the aryepiglottic fold and pyriform sinus *(arrow).* (Courtesy of Peter Som, MD.)

Text continued on p. 663.

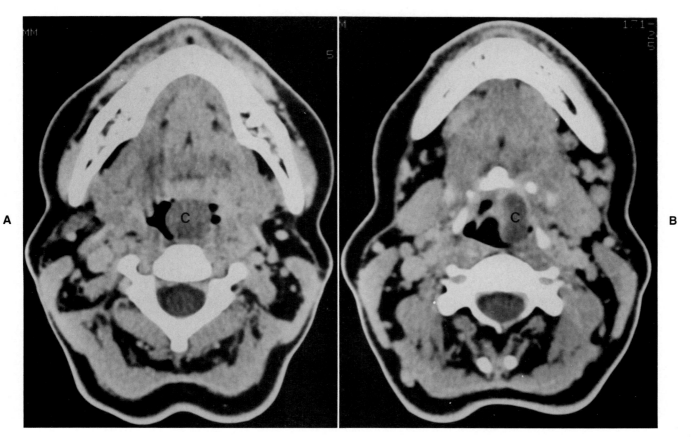

Fig. 9-74 **A,** Vallecular cyst on CT. Midline cyst *(C)* seen at the level of the base of the tongue. **B,** Slightly lower level shows the origin of the cyst in the left valleculae deforming the epiglottis. *C,* cyst.

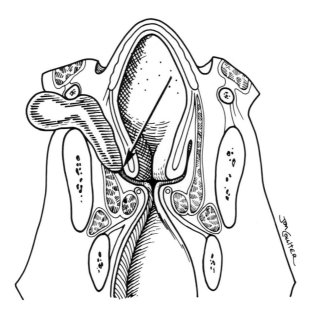

Fig. 9-75 Diagram showing a laryngocele protruding between hyoid and thyroid cartilage. The laryngocele is caused by a relative obstruction *(arrow)* at the level of the ventricle.

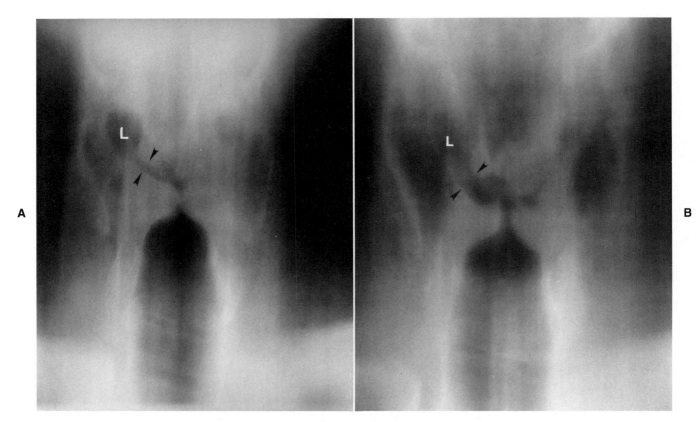

Fig. 9-76 Laryngocele. **A,** Tomography shows the air-filled laryngocele *(L)* with a narrow neck *(arrowheads)* communicating with the ventricle. **B,** Modified valsalva maneuver with distention of the laryngocele *(L)* and widening of the communication with the ventricles *(arrowheads)*.

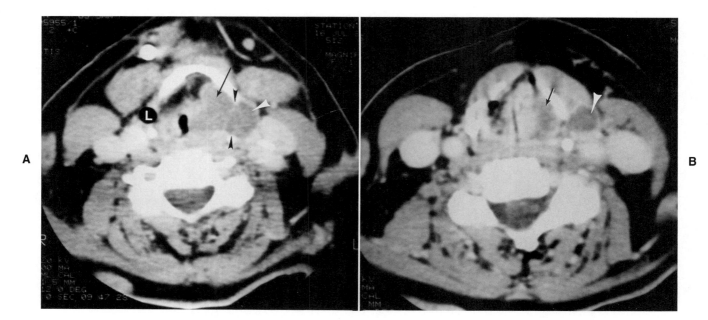

Fig. 9-77 Laryngocele (saccular cyst). **A,** There is both an internal *(arrow)* and external *(white arrowhead)* component. The position of the thyrohyoid membrane is signified by black arrowheads. A small air-filled external laryngocele *(L)* is seen on the opposite side. **B,** Lower slice through the supraglottic larynx shows the abnormality in the paraglottic space *(arrow)* and the external component *(arrowhead)*.

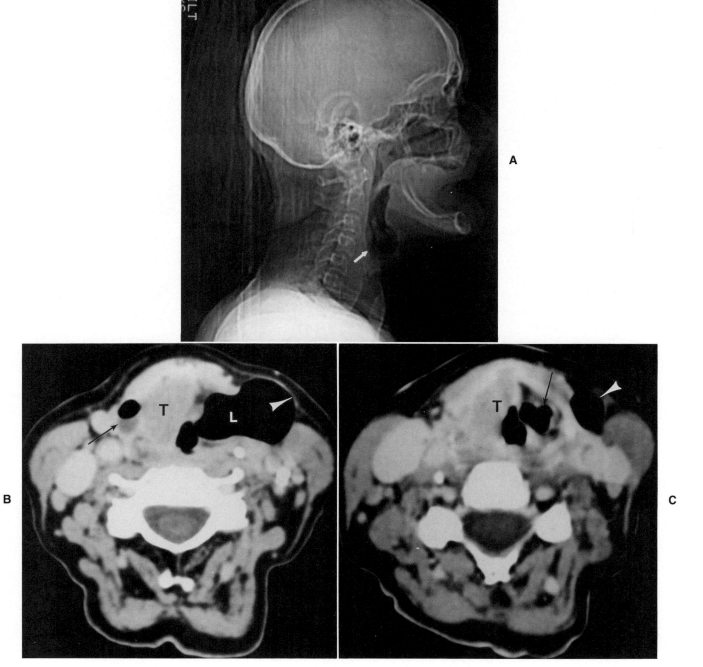

Fig. 9-78 Bilateral laryngocele with large supraglottic tumor on one side. **A,** Scout view shows the dilated air-filled sac *(arrow)*. **B,** Axial slice through the upper larynx shows the air-filled laryngocele *(L)* on the left protruding through the thyrohyoid membrane. The lateral aspect of the laryngocele *(arrowhead)* caused a significant bulge in the neck. Tumor fills the opposite supraglottis *(T)*. The smaller laryngocele *(arrow)* is seen on the side of the tumor with an air-fluid level. **C,** Lower slice shows the tumor *(T)*. Intralaryngeal segment (paraglottic space) of the laryngocele *(arrow)*. The external component *(arrowhead)*.

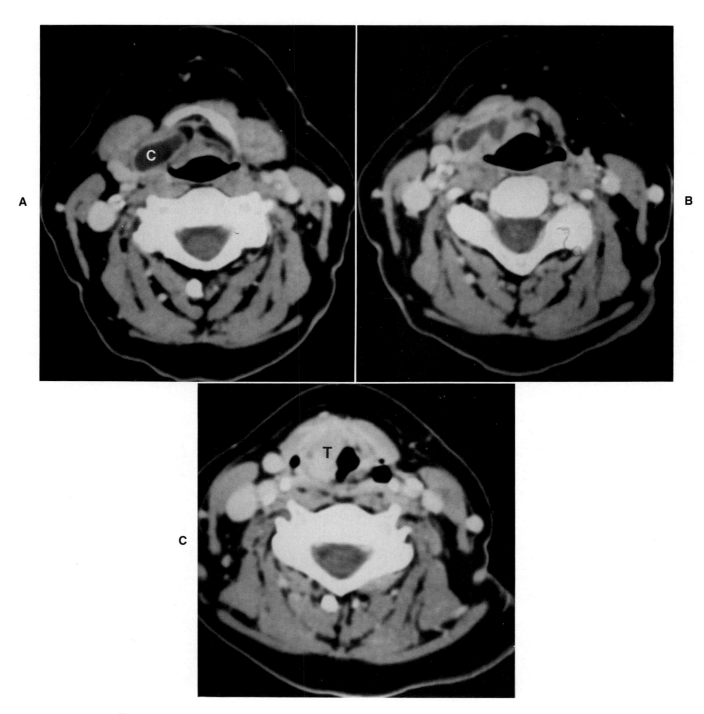

Fig. 9-79 Saccular cyst (laryngocele) with tumor of the lower false cord; CT and MRI. **A,** CT slice through the supraglottic larynx shows the saccular cyst *(C)* with smooth margins. **B,** Slightly lower slice shows the bilobular nature of the internal and external component. **C,** Lower slice through the lower false cord shows the tumor *(T).* **D,** T$_1$-weighted image shows the bilobular cyst at the supraglottic level. *C,* Cyst. **E,** T$_2$ (long TR/long TE) shows relative brightening of both the cyst *(arrow)* and the tumor *(arrowheads)* compared to the intermediate signal of the uninvolved thyroarytenoid muscle *(open arrow).*

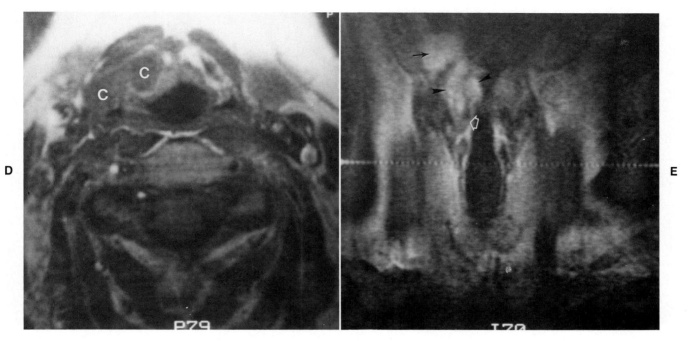

Fig. 9-79, cont'd   For legend see opposite page.

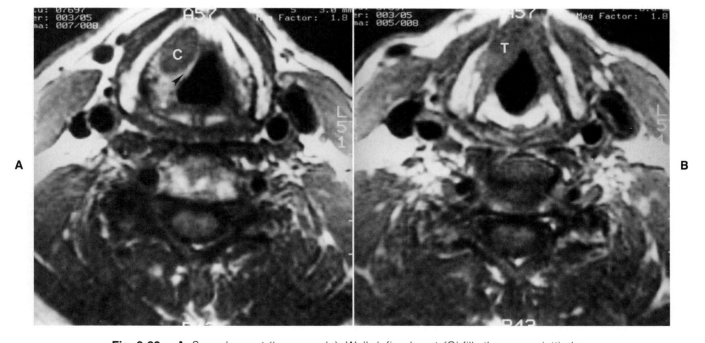

Fig. 9-80   **A,** Saccular cyst (laryngocele). Well defined cyst *(C)* fills the supraglottic larynx. Note the definite separation *(arrowhead)* from the mucosa. **B,** Slice inferior to **A**
shows a tumor at the level of the ventricle and true cord. *T,* tumor.   *Continued.*

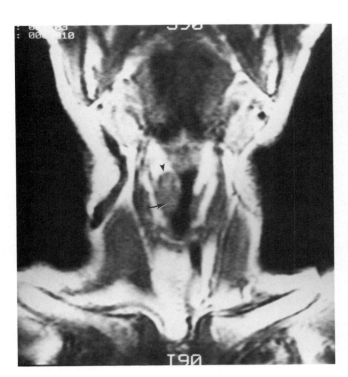

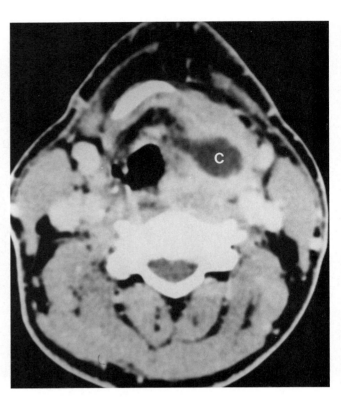

Fig. 9-80, cont'd **C,** Coronal T₁-weighted (short TR/short TE) image. Note the smooth upper margin *(arrowhead)* and the slight thickening *(arrow)* of the tumor involved true cord.

Fig. 9-81 Laryngopyocele with contrast enhanced CT shows the saccular cyst *(C).* There is irregular enhancement of the inflamed wall.

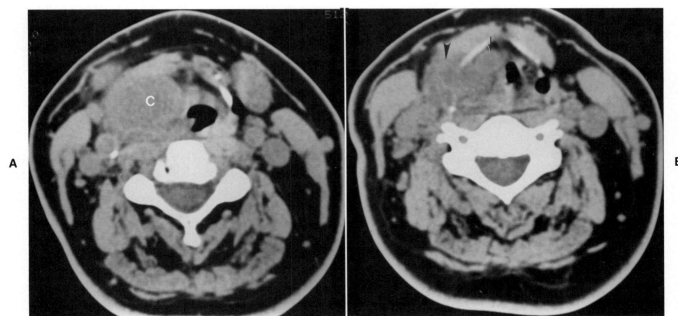

A   B

Fig. 9-82 Laryngopyocele, pre- and posttreatment, nonenhanced scans. **A,** Supraglottic slice shows a large mass representing the laryngopyocele *(C).* **B,** Slightly lower slice shows both internal components *(arrow)* and external components *(arrowhead).* **C,** Slightly lower slice through the false cord level shows the "neck" of the laryngocele *(arrow)* extending through the paraglottic fat. Note the small air-filled laryngocele *(arrowhead)* on the opposite side. **D,** Post antibiotic treatment (no surgery). The mass has resolved and there is air in the laryngocele *(arrow).*

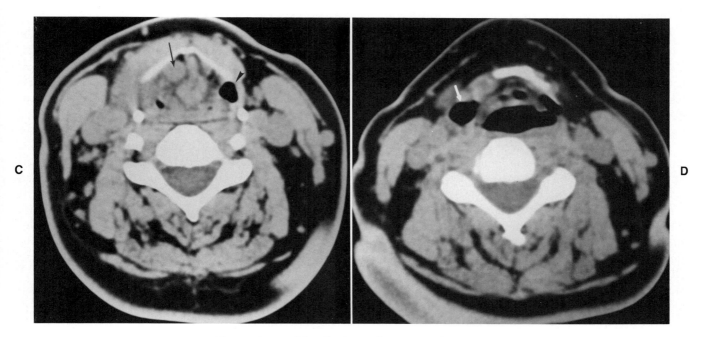

Fig. 9-82, cont'd   For legend see opposite page.

Treatment of a symptomatic laryngocele is surgical. A tracheostomy is often performed because of concern that even minor postoperative swelling or bleeding can compromise the airway.

Thyroglossal duct cysts are covered elsewhere in this volume but are briefly mentioned here (Fig. 9-83). During development the thyroid descends to the pretracheal region from the primordial tissue in the region of the developing tongue base. Any remnant of the tract along which the thyroid descends is referred to as the thyroglossal duct. This passes anterior to the hyoid bone before wrapping around the inferior margin extending to the posterior surface of the bone. The remnant then passes inferiorly along the anterior margin of the larynx. A cyst can form anywhere along this path. In the infrahyoid location, the cysts are intimately associated with the larynx. The cyst can protrude into the preepiglottic fat just above the notch of the thyroid cartilage or can lie anterior to the midline of the upper thyroid cartilage. Most cysts at the levels of the larynx insinuate themselves between the strap muscles anterior to the thyroid ala and off the midline. These cysts are easily distinguished from a laryngocele because of their more anterior location outside the larynx, and because the paraglottic fat at the false cord level is normal.

Treatment is excision. The midhyoid bone is resected in an effort to remove any remnant, and the tract is followed up to the tongue base as well.

INFECTION AND INFLAMMATION

Infections that may come to the attention of the radiologist are usually those of childhood: epiglottitis or

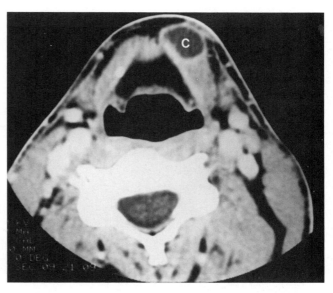

Fig. 9-83   Thyroglossal duct cyst *(C)*. Note that the fat within the larynx is normal. The paraglottic level would be normal as well.

croup. Tuberculosis or other granulomatous diseases are rare.[26] Perichondritis or infection of the laryngeal cartilages is most commonly associated with radiation therapy and is discussed later in this chapter, along with postradiation mucositis. Previously perichondritis and abscesses were caused by typhoid fever, measles, scarlet fever, erysipelas, anthrax, and mycoses.[27] Occasionally infections of the soft tissues of the neck can involve the larynx secondarily.[26] Other inflammatory processes include arthritis and the collagen vascular diseases.

Croup

Croup refers to an inflammation of the subglottic larynx with greater or lesser involvement of the trachea and bronchi. Occurring in younger children (6 months to 3 years of age), croup is usually caused by type 1 parainfluenza virus, but many other organisms have occasionally been implicated. Croup appears with a barking cough and stridor. The edema involves the mucosa of the subglottic larynx. Because this tissue is looser in children than in adults, the swollen wall can impinge upon the airway. This is usually appreciated on the frontal film as the "wine bottle" or "steeple-shaped" airway with loss of the subglottic angle (Fig. 9-84). If the film is taken at inspiration, there may be ballooning of the pharynx, including the pyriform sinus. In expiration, the trachea and subglottis may be distended. Usually, however, the diagnosis is made clinically, and the factors that determine more extensive treatment such as intubation or even tracheostomy are clinical rather than radiographic. Plain films are used to confirm the diagnosis and to exclude a foreign body.

Epiglottitis or Supraglottitis

Epiglottitis or *supraglottitis* occurs in a slightly older age group than croup and is caused by *Haemophilus influenzae*. A sore throat and inability to swallow are the key features, along with airway compromise. The epiglottis is swollen and has a typical "cherry red" appearance.

The lateral radiograph is characteristic and reflects the extent of the abnormality. The epiglottis is thickened, losing its normal sharp linear curve (Fig. 9-85). The epiglottis blends into the aryepiglottic folds, which are also enlarged. The arytenoid prominence may be swollen in severe cases. The radiograph is taken to document the disease and to exclude foreign bodies. Epiglottitis can advance quickly to severe airway compromise or occlusion. Thus manipulation is minimized, including attempts at direct visualization of the large epiglottis. The patient must never be out of an environment where there are personnel and equipment necessary for doing an emergency tracheostomy. Radiographs are usually done either in the emergency department or even in the operating room. At our institution the child is not submitted to the risk of transport to the radiology department.

Therapy includes intubation or even tracheostomy, as well as administration of antibiotics. Decannulization is usually possible in 24 to 36 hours.

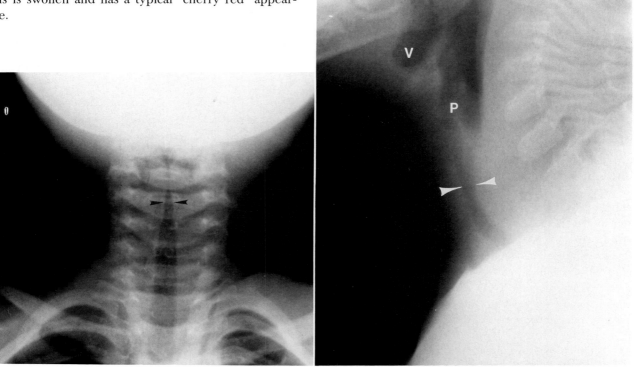

Fig. 9-84 Croup. **A,** Frontal film shows narrowing of the airway between arrowheads just beneath the cord. This is the so-called "steeple" or "winebottle" sign. **B,** Lateral film shows dilation of the pyriform sinuses *(P)* and the valleculae *(V)* with narrowing *(between arrowheads)* of the subglottic larynx.

Tuberculosis and Other Granulomatous Lesions

Tuberculosis of the larynx is exceedingly rare. In the past it was associated with pulmonary tuberculosis. Edema is present early, but with more severe involvement, ulceration and necrosis with a multinodular, irregular large epiglottis can be seen on a plain radiograph (Fig. 9-86). The cricoarytenoid joint can be involved, causing fixation. Perichondritis can also occur.

Rhinoscleroma (Fig. 9-87), Wegener's lethal midline granulomatosis, pemphigus, leprosy, and syphilis, as well as numerous mycotic infections, have been noted to involve the larynx but are rare.

Sarcoid can cause diffuse thickening, small nodular lesions, or localized infiltrative lesions. No radiographic finding is specific. The patients should be expected to have other systemic manifestations of this disease.

Neck Infection

Soft tissue infection rarely involves the larynx, and clinical findings should suggest the diagnosis (Fig. 9-88). The findings in the larynx reflect the area of involvement. Usually the soft tissues contiguous to the larynx show obvious inflammatory change.

Rheumatoid and Collagen Vascular Disease

The cricoarytenoid and cricothyroid joints are true synovial joints and can be affected by rheumatoid disease.[28] Swelling of the cricoarytenoid joint may cause hoarseness. Later sequelae include fixation. On CT this can be reflected by irregular sclerosis or erosions in the region of the cricoarytenoid joint. The soft tissues close to the arytenoid may be swollen.

On conventional tomography fixation of the arytenoid can be suggested when the cord does not move as well as the opposite side but does not show the typical findings of denervation atrophy (see the following section on vocal cord paralysis).

Relapsing polychondritis is a rare, nonsuppurative inflammatory condition affecting various cartilages.[29] The cause is unknown. The ear cartilages and nasal cartilages, as well as joint cartilages, can be involved. Airway involvement is present in about half of the patients afflicted. This can be quite significant because of airway compromise. The laryngeal cartilages can be involved, and generalized laryngeal edema can occur. Sclerosis of the cartilage can be present, with apparent enlargement of the cartilage. One report showed considerable calcification in the region of the arytenoid. Radionuclide bone scans can be positive over the region of the larynx as well as over other affected areas of the body.[30]

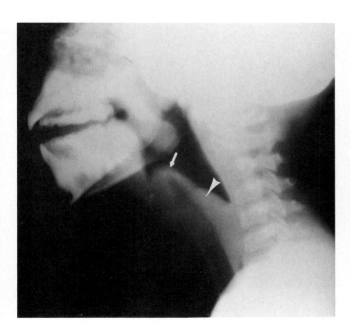

Fig. 9-85 Epiglottitis showing thickening of the epiglottis *(arrow)* and prominence of the arytenoid *(arrowhead)*.

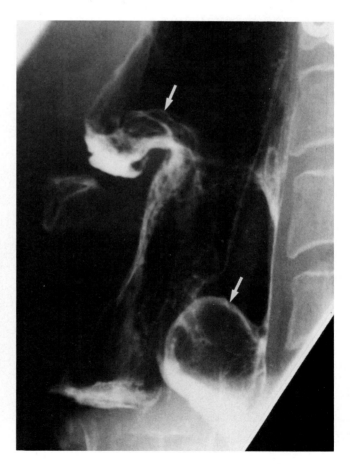

Fig. 9-86 Laryngeal tuberculosis. Lateral view of laryngogram shows nodular, thickened epiglottis *(upper arrow)*. The arytenoid mucosa is edematous *(lower arrow)*. (Courtesy of Peter Som, MD.)

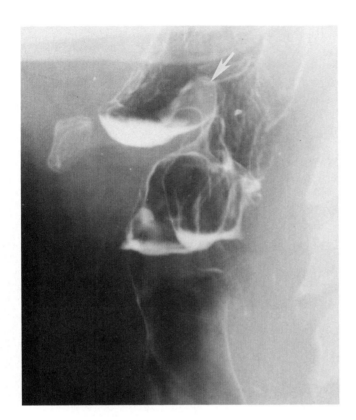

Fig. 9-87 Rhinoscleroma (Klebsiella rhinoscleromatis). There is polypoid thickening of the epiglottis *(arrow)*. (Courtesy of Peter Som, MD.)

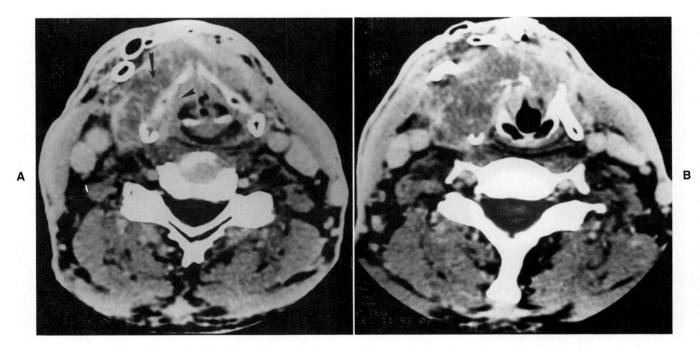

Fig. 9-88 **A,** Infection of the soft tissues of the neck showing obscuration of the fat plane *(arrow)* and extension into the paraglottic fat of the larynx *(arrowhead)*. The drains in the neck are from decompression of an abscess. **B,** Level of the cricoid showing considerable soft tissue thickening impinging on the airway.

TRAUMA

Vehicular accidents account for the most significant trauma to the larynx and upper trachea. The larynx is crushed against the spine. In children the larynx is higher in position relative to the mandible and is thus relatively protected. With adulthood the larynx descends into a more vulnerable position.

In many circumstances the radiologic examination cannot be performed acutely because compromise of the airway demands immediate attention. However, early, definitive surgical intervention for the trauma is associated with better end results, and thus the diagnostic evaluation should not be substantially delayed.

Fractures of the cartilage can be seen on plain radiographs if the cartilage is well-enough calcified. CT usually gives better visualization. The interpreter should seek fragments of cartilage that may impinge on the airway or perforate the mucosa. In significant airway compromise endoscopy is done for assessment of mucosal tears. If the airway is perforated, air can be seen in the adjacent soft tissues; soft tissue swelling is visible on either plain films or CT. Hematomas may appear as a mass or may cause obliteration of normal fat density in the upper larynx (Fig. 9-89).

Fractures of the larynx involve the thyroid cartilage, cricoid cartilage, or both.[31] Thyroid cartilage fractures are either vertical or horizontal. Vertical fractures are the result of the splaying action as the thyroid cartilage is pushed against the spine. A horizontal fracture crosses both thyroid alae and is usually seen in combination with a supraglottic soft tissue injury (Fig. 9-90). The superior fragments of the thyroid cartilage can be posteriorly displaced. The thyroepiglottic ligaments or petiole of the epiglottis may be torn, resulting in a dislocated epiglottis. The hyoid bone may also be fractured. Vertical fractures of the thyroid cartilage are best appreciated on computed tomography (Fig. 9-91). Horizontal fractures are in the plane of the axial CT slice and may be difficult to demonstrate on CT. Plain films or tomography may show the fracture and displacement of the thyroid ala because of the usual calcification of the posterior margins of the ala. Hyoid fractures are easily seen in axial CT slices.

Cricoid fractures cause collapse of the normal cricoid ring (Fig. 9-92). Small fragments again can be displaced into the airway, causing significant airway compromise. These fractures usually require surgical intervention with sutures or stent placement because of the cricoid's key role in the maintenance of the airway.

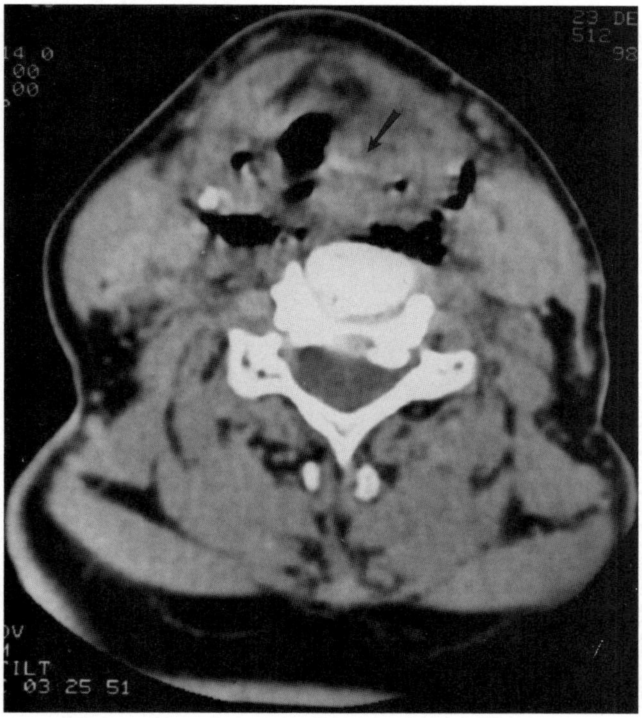

Fig. 9-89 Vehicular injury. Hematoma of the larynx and laceration of the pharynx. There is a hematoma *(arrow)* of the aryepiglottic fold. The gas in the soft tissues is from laceration of the pharyngeal wall.

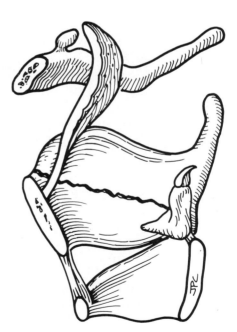

Fig. 9-90 Diagram of a horizontal fracture crossing the thyroid cartilage. These fractures can often involve the petiole and lower epiglottis causing dislocation of the upper epiglottis.

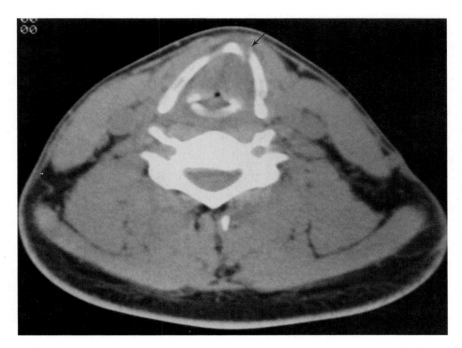

Fig. 9-91 Longitudinal (vertical fracture of the larynx) showing the defect in the ala *(arrow)*.

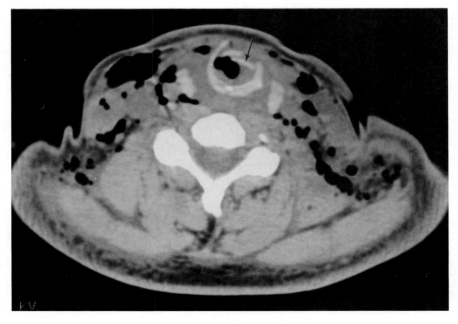

Fig. 9-92 Fracture of the cricoid with posterior positioning of the fragments *(arrow)* into the airway.

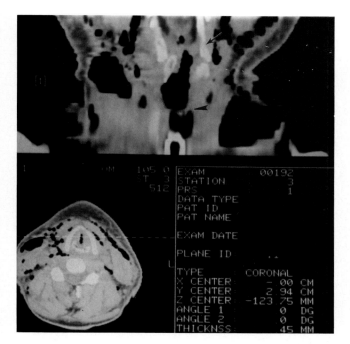

Fig. 9-93 Coronal reformat of a horizontal fracture of the thyroid cartilage *(arrow)* and laryngotracheal partial separation. Note the lack of alignment of the trachea *(arrowhead)*. This finding can be mimicked on reformatted CT slices by movement of the patient during the exam.

Laryngotracheal separation is a complete tear of the trachea and is usually fatal because of the loss of the airway (Fig. 9-93). Plain radiographs may show the malignment of an incomplete separation. Few of these cases get as far as the radiology department; those that do usually have already been tracheotomized.

Arytenoid dislocation usually results in an abnormal position of the arytenoid relative to the cricoid cartilage (Fig. 9-94). Often there is an associated fracture of one of the larger laryngeal cartilages. A dislocation of the cricothyroid joint is seen as a malalignment of the thyroid and cricoid cartilages (Fig. 9-95). The thyroid cartilage may be rotated to one side, while the cricoid retains normal orientation. These dislocations are usually seen with cartilage fractures as well.

Foreign bodies may be the result of trauma but are more commonly the result of ingestion or aspiration. The pyriform sinus is a common location for a foreign body. Most foreign bodies of the airway do not stay in the larynx but continue into the trachea or bronchi.

CONGENITAL LESIONS

Radiology can be helpful in assessing laryngeal congenital anomalies. Plain radiographs or conventional tomography can give an assessment of the size of the residual airway or the length of a stenosis. CT in the axial plane is less useful in demonstrating the length of the stenosis but can characterize the tissues deep to the mucosal surface.

Embryology[32,33]

An outpouching or bud initially extends from the primitive pharynx to form the respiratory system. The cells on either side of the entrance to this respiratory diverticulum pinch together to form the tracheoesophageal septum, thereby isolating the trachea from the food passageway. Later the central cells in the septum undergo necrosis, reopening the communication. The cartilages form from mesenchyme on either side of the primitive respiratory passage. The components from each side then fuse in the case of the cricoid and thyroid cartilages. Congenital abnormalities are related to problems of the development process or simply delays in normal maturation.

Laryngomalacia

Laryngomalacia represents delayed development of the laryngeal support system.[34] The structures are there but not firm enough to keep the larynx open. The supraglottic larynx is affected. The epiglottis may be floppy, or the entire supraglottic larynx may collapse. The infant outgrows the abnormality as the cartilages mature. Tracheostomy may be needed.

Subglottic Stenosis

Subglottic stenosis is a narrowing of the subglottic larynx from the true cord down to the lower cricoid.[34-36] The patient normally outgrows the abnormality, but a tracheostomy may be needed transiently. Plain radiographs can demonstrate the narrowing. The stenosis is usually the result of soft tissue thickening in the subglottis between a normal cricoid cartilage and the lumen of the airway. Less commonly, an abnormality of the cricoid has been described. In this anomaly the cricoid is elliptical rather than round and thus narrows the airway.[36] No radiologic cases of the abnormality have been described. Because the cricoid is not calcified at this age, imaging is unlikely to help. The diagnosis is suggested by endoscopy because of the consistency of the subglottic wall.

Webs and Atresia

Small webs can be seen at any level but are usually at the level of the true cords.[34] Subglottic webs may be associated with cricoid abnormalities. Webs are seldom evaluated radiographically, but radiographs may be done to exclude other abnormalities. Atresia of the larynx is a failure of complete recanalization, and no airway exists through the larynx. The trachea, however, is present, and a tracheostomy at birth is life saving.

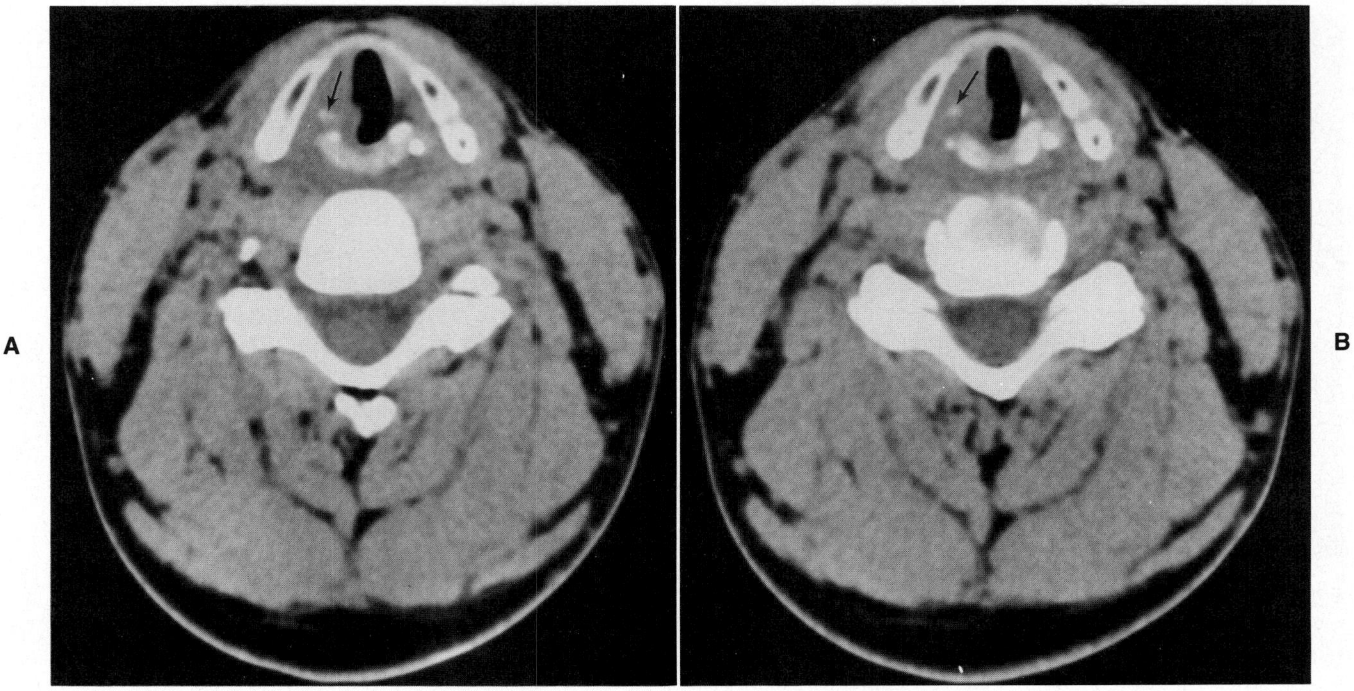

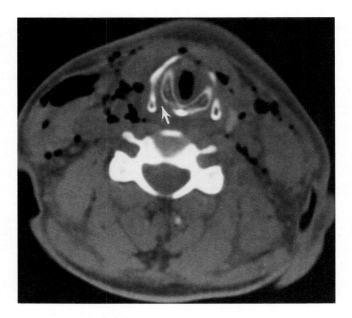

Fig. 9-94 **A,** Arytenoid dislocation shows the arytenoid anteriorly displaced *(arrow)*. **B,** Slightly lower slice again shows the abnormal position of the arytenoid *(arrow)*.

Fig. 9-95 Cricothyroid separation. The cricoid is rotated relative to the thyroid with widening of the space *(arrow)* between the lower thyroid and the cricoid. Compare with the opposite side.

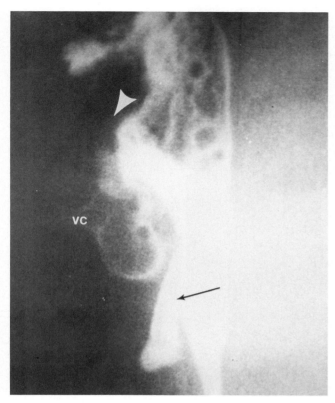

Fig. 9-96   Laryngeal cleft at the level of the cricoid. Barium swallow. Contrast is seen entering the lumen of the trachea via a defect on the posterior wall *(arrow)* at the level of the cricoid. Vocal cord level *(VC)*. Normal entrance to the larynx *(arrowhead)*. (From Ravich WJ, Donner MW, Kashima H, et al: The swallowing center: concepts and procedures, Gastrointest Radiol, July 1985, pp 255-263.)

Clefts

Laryngotracheal clefts are exceedingly rare and are presumed to be the result of failure of complete fusion of the tracheoesophageal septum as it grows to separate the trachea from the esophagus.[34] The cricoid cartilage is a fusion of cells from mesenchyma on either side of the airway and may be affected. Although an isolated cleft of the larynx does occasionally occur, the more likely case combines laryngeal and tracheal clefts. The child aspirates and may have multiple pneumonias (Fig. 9-96).[37]

Subglottic Hemangiomas

Subglottic hemangiomas were mentioned in the preceding section on benign tumors but are included here because they are vascular malformations as much as tumors. The lesion usually can be seen on a lateral neck radiograph as narrowing of the airway. Therapy is conservative, but tracheostomy may be necessary.

Other Anomalies

Other rare anomalies such as bifid epiglottis and duplication occasionally have been reported.

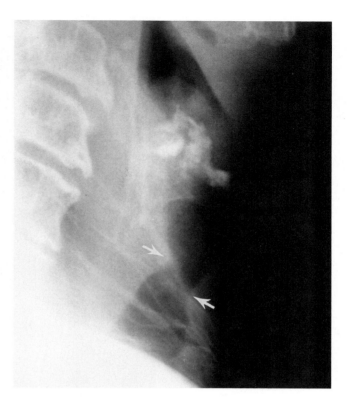

Fig. 9-97   Tracheal stenosis characteristic of tracheostomy site *(arrows)*.

STENOSIS

Stenosis of the larynx or upper trachea can be a congenital anomaly, or it can be the sequela of trauma or of therapy for a subglottic lesion. Most commonly the stenosis is the result of prolonged intubation (Figs. 9-97 and 9-98). Plain films, xeroradiographs, or conventional tomograms are the best methods for assessing the length of the stenosis or the extent of a "granuloma" (Fig. 9-99). Two projections are used, usually frontal and lateral. Tomography is not necessary for the lateral view.

MRI gives a good sagittal depiction of the airway, but accuracy is compromised by long imaging times. MRI and CT are occasionally useful as adjuncts to assess the soft tissues adjacent to the airway (Figs. 9-100 and 9-101), especially in trauma cases in which the position of cartilage fragments is important. The position of the stenosis secondary to tracheostomy or prolonged intubation is characteristic, but stenosis secondary to trauma is more variable. Ingestion of corrosive materials usually causes strictures of the supraglottic larynx, especially posteriorly.

VOCAL CORD PARALYSIS

Vocal cord paralysis is usually categorized as either a superior laryngeal nerve defect or a recurrent laryngeal nerve abnormality.

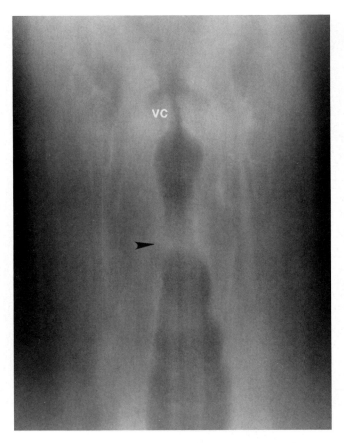

Fig. 9-98 Tomogram showing a narrowing of the tracheal lumen *(arrowhead)* just below the cricoid. Vocal cord *(VC)*. A narrowing resulting from prolonged intubation would be lower in position.

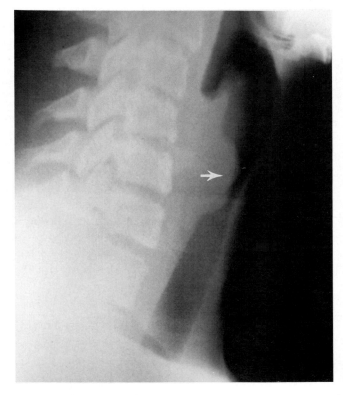

Fig. 9-99 Granuloma of the posterior wall of the upper trachea *(arrow)*.

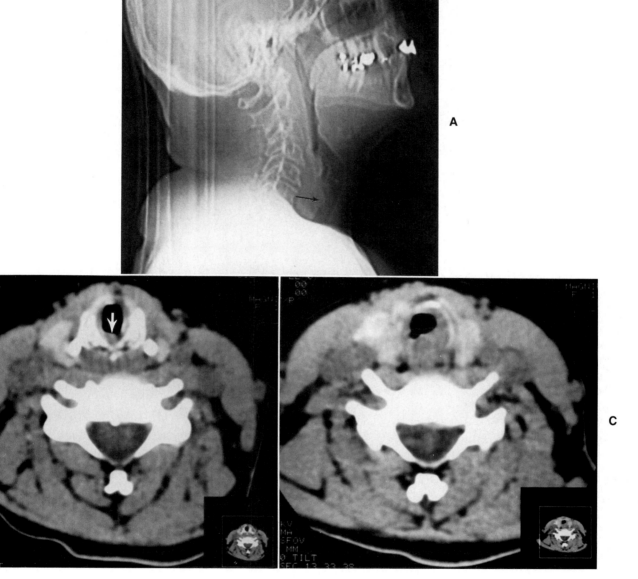

Fig. 9-100   A, CT scan. Scout view shows narrowing of the trachea with a granuloma *(arrow)* on the posterior wall. **B,** Axial CT shows slight soft tissue thickening *(arrow)* within the cricoid cartilage. **C,** Slightly lower slice gives good estimation of the size of the airway and the thickening within the tracheal ring. The actual distance between the lumen and the cartilage can be defined.

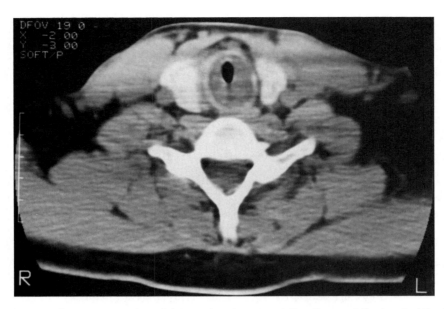

Fig. 9-101 Severe narrowing of the trachea by granulation tissue at the level of the thyroid shows an intact tracheal ring with soft tissue filling the space between the ring and the airway. No portion of the tracheal ring has been pushed into the lumen.

Superior Nerve

On laryngoscopy the posterior larynx (arytenoid) is deviated toward the side of the nerve lesion. The only muscle innervated by the superior laryngeal nerve is the cricothyroid muscle, which spans the gap laterally between these two cartilages. Contraction of the normal muscles pulls the anterior cricoid toward the lower margin of the thyroid cartilage. This rotates the upper margin of the posterior cricoid, and thus the arytenoid, posteriorly, putting tension on the true vocal cords. Contraction of one muscle rotates the posterior cricoid to the contralateral, paralyzed side.

With this history the radiologist should examine the skull base and upper neck for a lesion along the course of the upper vagus, which passes through the pars nervosa of the jugular foramen and follows the carotid artery to the level of the larynx. The radiographic findings in the larynx itself are usually normal, even with CT.

Recurrent Nerve

The more usual clinical case is paralysis of the *recurrent laryngeal nerve*.[38] All the muscles of the larynx other than the cricothyroid are innervated by this nerve. The classic findings of recurrent laryngeal palsy on tomography or plain radiograph are also seen on CT (Figs. 9-102 and 9-103).

Most of the findings are caused by atrophy of the thyroarytenoid muscle (the medial bundle of which is called the vocalis). As the muscle atrophies, the cord becomes thinner and more pointed, with loss of the subglottic angle. As the muscle diminishes in size, the ventricle enlarges. The pyriform sinus and vallecula also enlarge on the ipsilateral side. The changes in the shape of the cord are best appreciated by tomography. Different maneuvers show the lack of motion of the cord, whereas the contralateral side moves normally.

CT can show the enlarged ventricle. The vocal process of the arytenoid may remain in an anteromedial position because it is moored to the anterior thyroid cartilage by the vocal ligament. The actual atrophy of the muscle can be appreciated by the lack of muscle density in a CT slice just below the margin of the cord.

When an abnormality of the recurrent laryngeal nerve is suspected or when the type of paralysis is not specified, the radiologist must examine the pathway of the vagus and recurrent laryngeal nerves. The vagus follows the carotid artery and jugular vein, lying between the posterior margins of these two vessels. On the left the nerve passes around the aortic arch, passing anterior to the arch before curving through the arch and passing superiorly again. Ascending, the nerve travels in the tracheoesophageal groove, entering the larynx near the cricothyroid junction. On the right side the nerve curls around the right subclavian artery, passing first anteriorly and then looping underneath before ascending in the tracheoesophageal groove.

Adductor Paralysis

Cases of adductor paralysis have been described; however, they are rare. This paralysis affects muscles that bring the cords together but spares the posterior

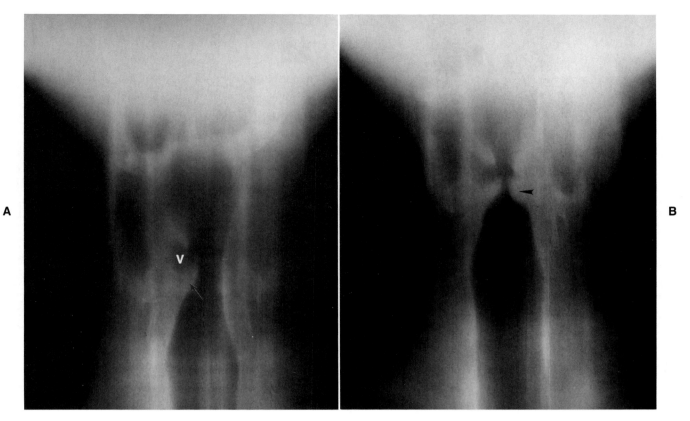

Fig. 9-102   A, Tomogram. Right cord paralysis. Inspiration. The true cord on the affected side remains in the paramedian position and is more pointed than usual *(arrow).* The ventricle *(v)* is enlarged. **B,** Phonation. There is no change in the affected cord or ventricle. The normal cord now moves to midline *(arrowhead).* Compare the size of the ventricle on the paralysed side to that on the opposite side.

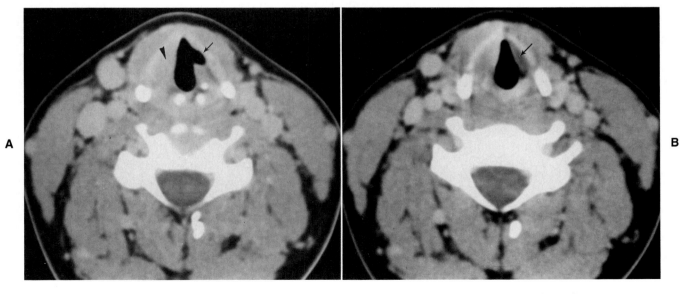

Fig. 9-103   Vocal cord paralysis. A, Level of the cord shows dilated ventricle *(arrow).* Thyroarytenoid muscle on the opposite side *(arrowhead)* is of the normal size. **B,** Inferior slice shows again decreased size of the thyroarytenoid muscle with decreased density *(arrow)* compared with the opposite side.

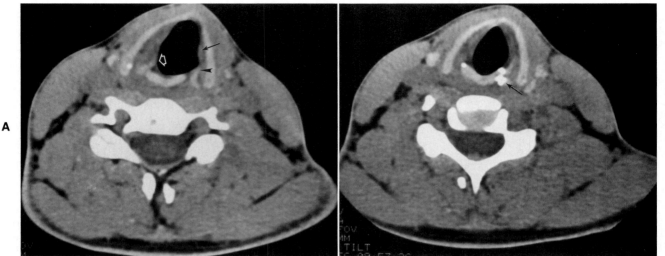

Fig. 9-104 **A,** Adductor paralysis. Left side shows almost no thyroarytenoid muscle *(arrow).* The vocal process *(arrowhead)* is pulled laterally as the posterior cricoarytenoid muscle rotates the arytenoid laterally and posteriorly. Compare the position of the vocal process on the normal side *(open arrow).* **B,** Slightly lower slice shows a portion of the arytenoid pulled posteriorly and downward *(arrow)* overlapping the posterior surface of the cricoid.

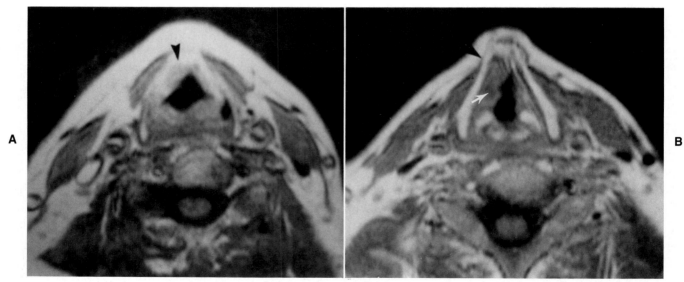

Fig. 9-105 **A,** Submucosal amyloid. Axial slice through the supraglottis shows thickening of the lateral epiglottis with soft tissue extending minimally *(arrowhead)* into the preepiglottic fat. (.35 Tesla.) **B,** Minor thickening of the true cord *(arrow).* (**A** courtesy of William Hanafee, MD.)

cricoarytenoid muscle. This muscle stretches from the posterior surface of the cricoid to the lateral aspect of the arytenoid (muscular process) and is the only muscle that rotates the cord outward. Because the posterior cricoarytenoid muscle is unopposed, the cord remains in a lateral position (Fig. 9-104). The lesion must affect only certain fibers of the recurrent laryngeal nerve while sparing others. The cause of this abnormality is poorly understood, although an intracranial abnormality has been postulated.[39]

MISCELLANEOUS

Amyloid can affect the larynx and produce nodules or small deposits deep to the mucosal surface.[40] The findings on CT may be mistaken for a tumor (Fig. 9-105).

Diverticula of the pharynx are herniations of mucosa through dehiscences in the muscular constrictors. These have been related to patients who play wind instruments. Most are just above or below the hyoid bone from the valleculae or from the upper pyriform sinus (Figs. 9-106 and 9-107). The diverticula are usually incidental findings on barium swallow examinations.

Zenker's diverticulum is an outpouching of mucosa through the inferior constrictors of the pharynx. Most of the diverticula herniate through a small gap between the cricopharyngeus muscle and the inferior fibers of the pharyngeal constrictors (Killian's area). Although the actual dehiscence or entrance to the diverticulum is in the midline, the diverticulum usually protrudes to the left side. The neck or the anterior wall of the diverticulum is appreciated on barium swallow, using oblique as well as frontal and lateral projections (Fig. 9-108). A second weak point occurs laterally between the

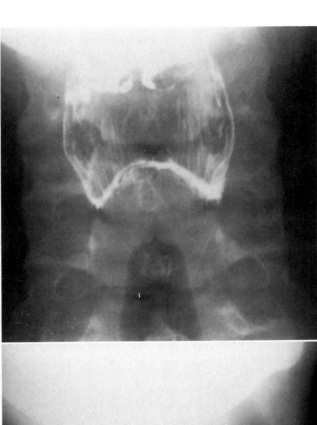

A

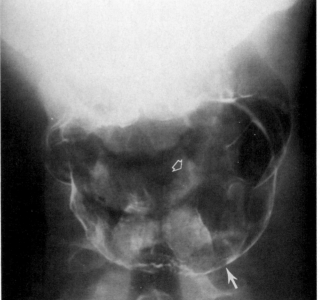

B

Fig. 9-107 Ballooning of the pharynx in a trumpet player. **A,** At rest the striated appearance of the pharynx is due to redundancy of the mucosa. **B,** On valsalva there is gross distention of the pharynx with bilateral ballooning. Lower margin of the pyriform *(arrow);* AE fold *(open arrow).*

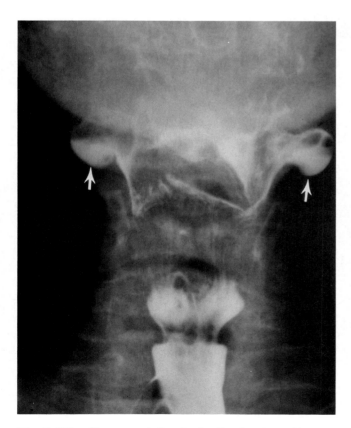

Fig. 9-106 Pharyngeal diverticula. Small outpouching extending through the pharyngeal wall.

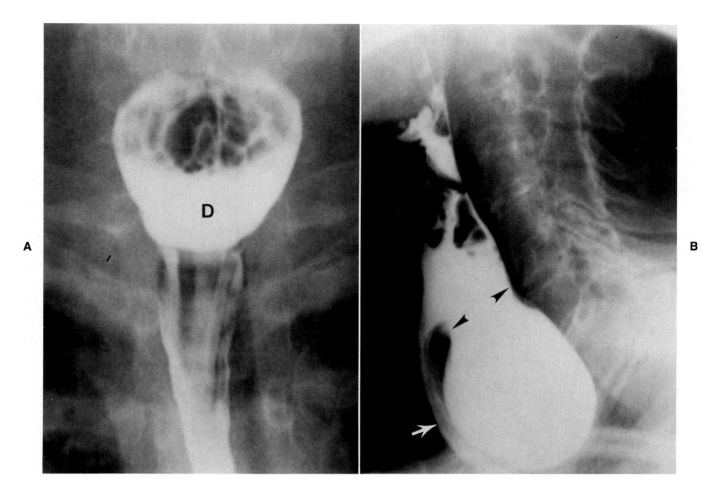

Fig. 9-108   A, Zenker's diverticulum. Frontal view shows large diverticulum *(D).* **B,** Lateral film shows a large diverticulum with a wide entrance *(arrowheads)* and the barium column of the true esophagus continuing anterior to the diverticulum *(arrow).* The level of the persistent cricopharyngeus is at the level of the anterior arrowhead. This diverticulum was somewhat unusual because of its midline rather than its left sided position.

cricopharyngeus and esophageal musculature, through the so-called Killian-Jamieson area at the margin of the cricoid. Herniations here have been reported but are extremely rare compared to the more typical posterior location.

The *cricopharyngeus* is prominent in Zenker's diverticula. The muscular band may also be prominent without a diverticulum (Fig. 9-109). Failure of the muscle to relax during swallowing can cause dysphagia. Occasionally a small collection of barium is seen just above the muscle after the barium column has passed. Some call this a primordial Zenker's diverticulum, but it does not necessarily go on to become a larger diverticulum.

Failure of relaxation of the cricopharyngeus has been associated with gastric reflux and other abnormal motility problems in the esophagus, as well as with neurologic pathologic conditions affecting the medulla.

Benign Cartilage Changes

The cartilage is a changeable tissue and can be remodeled by pressure or eroded by malignancy. This remodeling can be the result of either prominent osteophytes in the spine or benign tumors (Figs. 9-110 and 9-111).

Occasionally an ala of the thyroid cartilage can bow medially. This may be the result of old trauma, but many times no history can explain it. The abnormal shape may cause a bulge in the wall of the larynx that mimics a submucosal mass endoscopically. The lack of obliteration of the paraglottic fat on CT or MRI excludes the possibility of tumor (Fig. 9-112).

Osteophytes of the Spine

Large osteophytes arising from the anterior cervical spine can cause dysphagia.[41] These osteophytes cause a

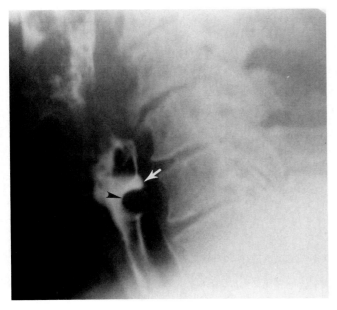

Fig. 9-109 Slightly prominent persistent cricopharyngeus *(arrowhead)*. There is a small collection of barium *(arrow)* just above the muscle band. This is sometimes referred to as a primordial Zenker's.

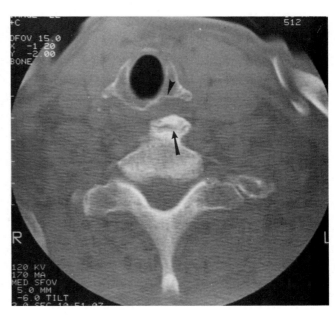

Fig. 9-110 Osteophyte *(arrow)* causing erosion *(arrowhead)* of the cricoid.

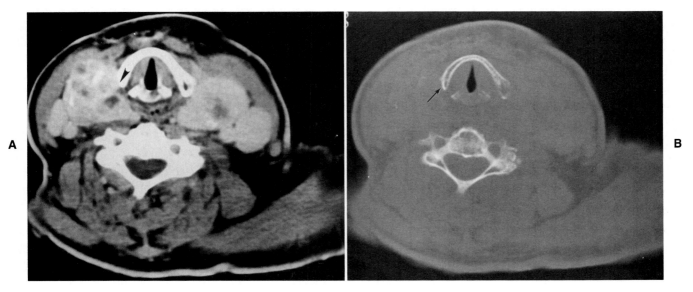

Fig. 9-111 **A,** Large multinodular goiter causing shortening and remodeling of the lateral aspect of the thyroid ala *(arrowhead)*. **B,** Bone algorithm showing the intact cortical line of the remodeled cartilage *(arrow)*.

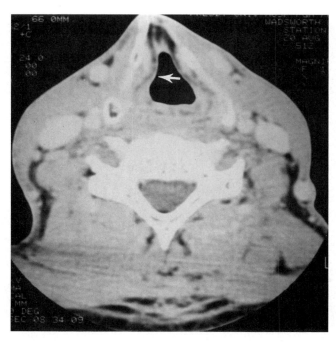

Fig. 9-112 Asymmetrical shape of the thyroid causing a slight bulge in the supraglottic larynx *(arrow)*, which could be confused with a submucosal tumor.

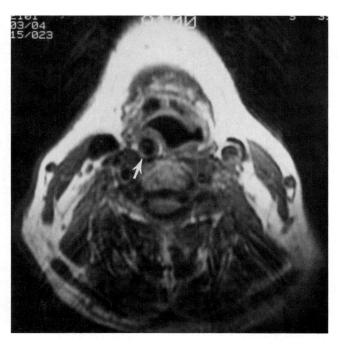

Fig. 9-113 Torturous carotid artery *(arrow)* causing a submucosal "mass" of the pharyngeal wall at the level of the epiglottis.

significant mass effect on the posterior pharyngeal wall or can even interfere with the normal movement of the larynx during swallowing.

A common related problem occurs when evaluating a barium swallow. An osteophyte causes an apparent mass effect seen on the frontal view of the barium swallow. This may appear to be at the lateral aspect of the pharynx but lateral and oblique positioning during repeat swallows usually shows the direct relationship of the defect to the offending osteophyte. These may be incidental findings, and the patient may have no symptoms related to the osteophyte.

Carotid Position

Not infrequently the carotid artery deviates medially between the pharynx and spine (Fig. 9-113). Although not likely to cause symptoms, the unusual position should be mentioned, especially in patients for whom surgery is contemplated.

Posttreatment Changes

The appearance of the neck after surgery varies, depending on the procedure performed. However, there are certain general postoperative appearances in the larynx and neck. Radiation changes are also fairly characteristic.

After *total laryngectomy,* the normal landmarks of the epiglottis, cords, and cartilage are no longer seen

on CT or MRI. As the fascial layers are disrupted during the surgical approach, the food tube or pharyngoesophageal remnant may migrate anteriorly and should not be mistaken for an airway. The esophagus may actually protrude between the lobes of the thyroid gland, mimicking the trachea (Fig. 9-114). The tracheostomy is seen just above the sternal notch, thus identifying the actual airway.

A *radical neck dissection* removes the sternocleidomastoid muscle and jugular vein, as well as the surrounding nodes.[42] The thyroid gland may assume a rounder shape because of the disruption of the bordering fascial layers. The gland may mimic a blood vessel because of the intrinsic high iodine content of the normally functioning thyroid tissue. Because the thyroid no longer has a characteristic shape, the appearance may also mimic a tumor recurrence.

The normal laryngeal structures are obviously missing on a barium swallow done after total laryngectomy.[43] At closure the mucosa is pulled together, often causing a ridge to form just posterior to the tongue base. The ridge can have an appearance that mimics the epiglottis (Fig. 9-115). This is also the area where most postoperative fistulas occur, extending either into the soft tissue or onto the surface of the neck.

At our institution a contrast swallow is performed 7 to 10 days after laryngectomy, before the patient is allowed to eat. Barium can be used, but if a fistula into

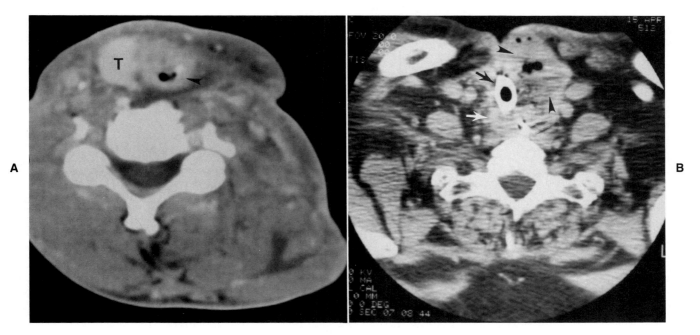

Fig. 9-114   **A,** Postoperative laryngectomy and bilateral radical neck dissection. The esophagus has migrated anteriorly *(arrowhead)* to lie in the usual position of the trachea next to the thyroid gland *(T)*. The sternocleidomastoid and jugular veins have been removed. **B,** Lower slice. The tracheostomy tube is seen documenting the position of the airway *(black arrow)*. The esophagus is seen immediately posteriorly *(white arrow)*. Note the large stomal recurrence *(arrowheads)*.

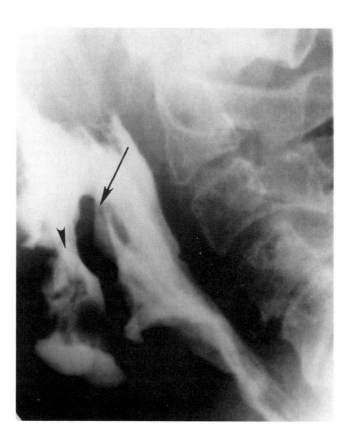

Fig. 9-115   Post laryngectomy with fistula *(arrowhead)* extending to a collection in the soft tissues anteriorly. Note the "pseudoepiglottis" *(arrow)* caused by the drawing up of mucosal folds at the closure.

the soft tissues is present, the residual barium can interfere with subsequent follow-up studies. If there is no concern that a fistula passes directly into the trachea, Gastrografin can be used with careful fluoroscopic control to exclude aspiration. If significant aspiration occurs, the hypertonic Gastrografin can cause pulmonary edema. Even if a sinus tract to the skin exists, Gastro-grafin can traverse along the surgical dressings into the tracheal stoma, so care must be taken. Before choosing a contrast material, the radiologist should determine whether the surgeon has purposely created a fistula or placed a valve between the trachea and esophagus; in such cases a small amount of contrast material may pass into the trachea, and Gastrografin should not be used.

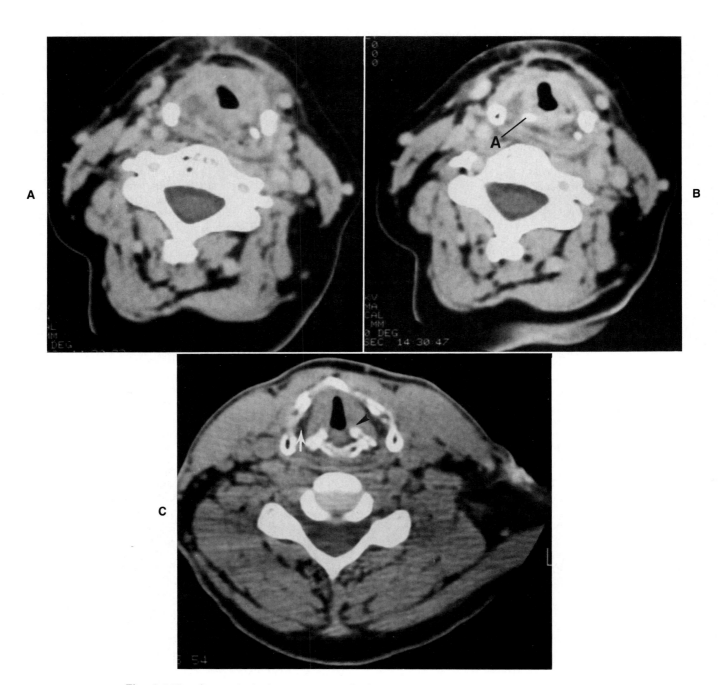

Fig. 9-116 Supraglottic laryngectomy. **A,** Supraglottic level. There is no evidence of epiglottis or paraglottic space. **B,** At the level of the upper arytenoid *(A)* most of the thyroid cartilage has been resected. **C,** At the level of the true cord the thyroid cartilage is present. There is actually prominence of the paraglottic fat *(arrow)* at the lateral margin of the thyroarytenoid muscle. Vocal process *(arrowhead)*.

Propyliodone (Dionosil) can also be used in questionable cases when connections between the trachea and esophagus are suspected.

In a *supraglottic laryngectomy* the normal supraglottic structures are removed, including epiglottis, false cords, aryepiglottic folds, and preepiglottic fat. The hyoid may or may not be removed. A CT slice through the true cords appears relatively normal, and the arytenoids usually remain (in rare cases, one arytenoid may be removed). The remaining tissues above the true cords appear slightly irregular (Figs. 9-116 and 9-117). A large portion of the thyroid cartilage is removed, but at the level of the cord the cartilage should look essentially normal.

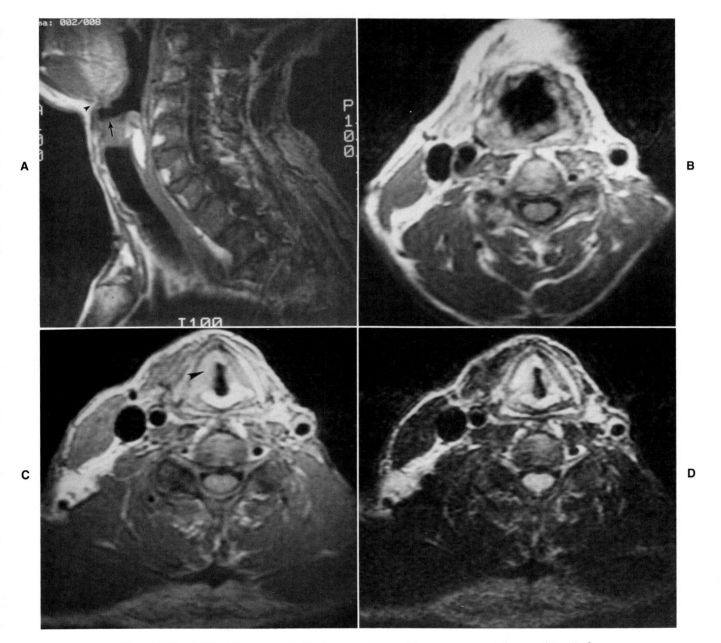

Fig. 9-117 MRI of the supraglottic laryngectomy with recurrence at the cord level. **A,** Sagittal T$_1$-weighted image shows the absence of supraglottic structures including the epiglottis. The upper margin of the larynx has taken on a rather square appearance *(arrow)*. The larynx has been sutured to the base of the tongue and mylohyoid *(arrowhead)*. **B,** Axial T$_1$-weighted slice, supraglottic level, shows the irregular appearance of the supraglottic defect above the cord. **C,** Long TR/short TE shows thickening of the involved cord *(arrowhead)*. **D,** Long TR/long TE shows brightening of the involved cord. This could be from tumor or from edema. In this case this represented recurrence.

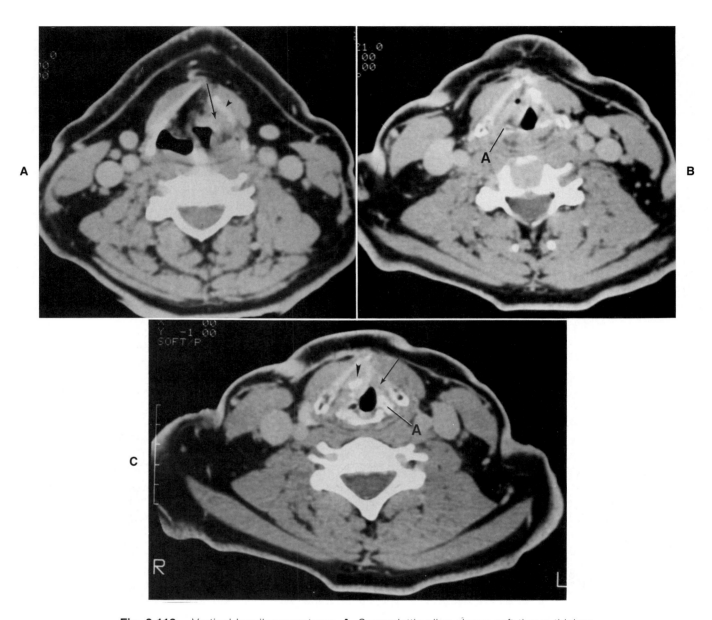

Fig. 9-118 Vertical hemilaryngectomy. **A,** Supraglottic slice shows soft tissue thickening of the supraglottic fat *(arrow)* due to the resection. The thyroid ala *(arrowhead)* has partially regenerated from the residual perichondrium. **B,** Lower slice through the upper arytenoid *(A)* again shows the loss of tissue on the affected side. **C,** Slice through the level of the true cord shows loss of tissue *(arrow)*. The arytenoid *(A)* has been retained. Teflon has been injected into the normal cord *(arrowhead)* to add bulk, bringing the cord across midline.

After a supraglottic laryngectomy, some aspiration is almost always present if a contrast swallow is done in the early postoperative period. Gastrografin is not used in the postoperative period. Barium swallow shows absence of the epiglottis, and usually some barium coats the vocal cords.

Vertical hemilaryngectomy removes the true and false cords on one side. Extended vertical hemilaryngectomy may take the anterior portion of the opposite cord. The soft tissue on the resected side of the larynx may be absent and flat in appearance. Some soft tissue may be present from an attempted reconstruction of the cord (Figs. 9-118 and 9-119), or from a resection of one contralateral vocal cord consistently hitting the operated mucosa. In some cases a strap muscle (sternohyoid) may be passed across the larynx and attached to the arytenoid, thus providing bulk against which the opposite cord can abut. In this instance the muscle outside the larynx is abnormal, and excess tissue is present at the level of the cord on the resected side.

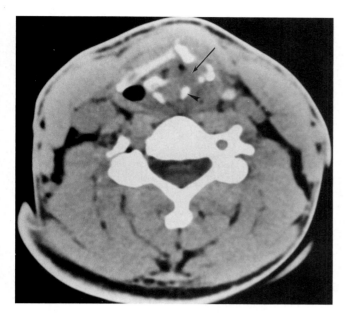

Fig. 9-119   Vertical hemilaryngectomy shows loss of soft tissue on the left side of the larynx *(arrow)*. The arytenoid has been removed. The small calcification is the upper margin of the cricoid *(arrowhead)*. Note the irregularity of the resected thyroid cartilage with partial calcification from the retained perichondrium.

The amount of thyroid cartilage that is resected also depends on the extent of the lesion. The resection extends at least to midline but usually extends a variable distance along the opposite side. The outer perichondrium is left intact, and some regeneration of the thyroid ala often occurs. One arytenoid may be removed if the tumor reaches the vocal process. The cricoid usually remains intact, although some surgeons remove the upper margin of this cartilage.

The variability of the postoperative appearance is greater with the vertical than with the supraglottic partial laryngectomy. Still, some statements can be made by the radiologist regarding deep recurrence, especially if a baseline scan is available that was performed after the surgery but before recurrence. However, this situation is rare.

Reconstruction of a *pharyngeal defect* can be done with primary closure of the remainder of the tissue, jejunal interposition, or various flaps (e.g., the deltopectoral flap). The jejunal interposition can have a tortuous appearance through the neck but is usually midline.[44] The flap reconstruction alters the appearance on the side of the neck. Replacing the normal neck soft tissues is the bulky mass of the flap, most of which is fat.[42] The muscle tends to atrophy.

Radiation Changes

Radiation is used to treat many laryngeal lesions, either as isolated therapy or in conjunction with surgery.

Radiation changes can confuse the postoperative imaging assessment for possible tumor recurrence.

Relatively low doses of radiation can cause mucositis and throat pain. Higher doses result in deeper edema and fibrosis and can be associated with perichondritis and chondronecrosis. Almost all patients receiving 60 Gy to 65 Gy will have definable changes in the larynx. Clinically the epiglottis thickens and the arytenoids swell, often before the course of radiation is complete. Although gradual improvement is probable, some degree of change persists because of fibrosis and damage to the microvasculature.[45]

CT scans show thickening of the epiglottis and prominence of the soft tissues in the aryepiglottic fold and around the arytenoids (Figs. 9-120 and 9-121). There is a streaky increased attenuation in the preepiglottic and paraglottic spaces (dirty fat). The true vocal cords are often less involved.

Perichondritis and chondronecrosis are much more significant clinical problems.[42] Perichondritis is an inflammation or infection of the cartilages. High doses of radiation can cause necrosis and collapse of the cartilages. In addition, radiated tissue is less resistent to infection. Deep biopsy of an irradiated larynx may have an association with so-called perichondritis. The CT findings are usually superimposed on the streaky changes in the fat mentioned previously. Perichondritis causes considerable edema around the cartilage, and at times gas bubbles can be seen (Fig. 9-122). The cartilage may collapse, assuming peculiar angles in the axial slices (Fig. 9-123).

Radiation may lead to collapse of a cartilage invaded by a tumor. This is not necessarily perichondritis or radiochondronecrosis. The tumor has replaced the cartilage and therefore actually becomes part of the support structure. As the tumor regresses, this support structure is lost and the eroded cartilage cannot support itself.

Stents, Tubes, and Teflon

Stents or bone grafts are most often seen in the anterior arch of the cricoid (Fig. 9-124). They are placed in an effort to maintain or improve the cricoid lumen as part of the treatment of laryngeal stenosis.

Tracheostomy tubes and speaking tubes are seen in the lower neck (Figs. 9-125 and 9-126). A tracheostomy tube is usually placed at the level of the trachea but occasionally can pass through the cricothyroid membrane if the tracheostomy was done as an emergency procedure. Secretions can accumulate above the tracheostomy, and there can be some mucosal swelling. This may be difficult to differentiate from a tumor, especially in the immediate subglottic area (Fig. 9-125).

The various *valves* used to force air from the trachea to the esophagus for use in esophageal speech are seen in the extreme lower neck. These are most often noted

Text continued on p. 691.

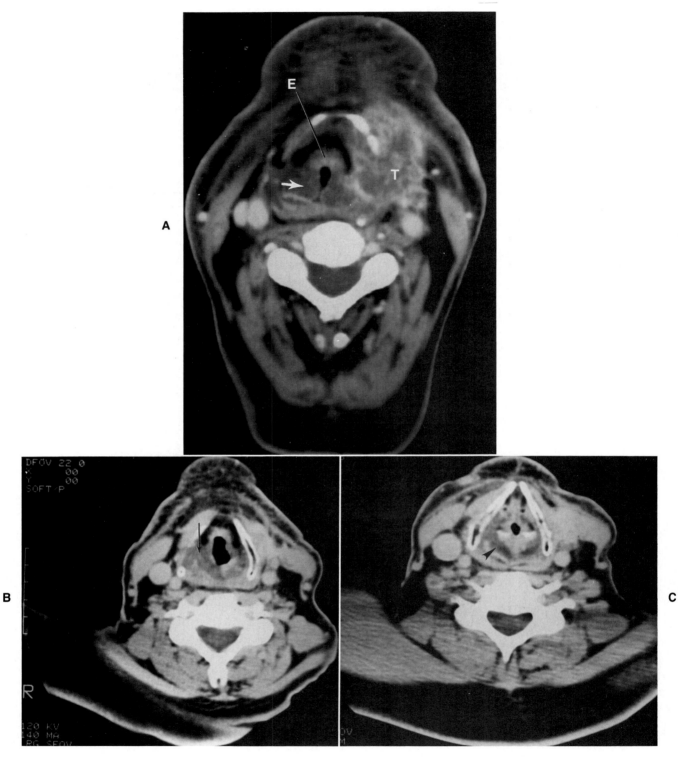

Fig. 9-120 **A,** CT of postradiation tumor recurrence *(T).* Note the swelling of the aryepiglottic fold *(arrow)* and apparent thickening of the epiglottic cartilage *(E).* **B,** Lower slice shows increased streaky density and thickening of the wall of the pyriform *(arrow).* Note also the streaky lymphedema ("dirty fat") in the fat anterior to the larynx. **C,** Slice through the upper arytenoid shows continued swelling in the soft tissues *(arrowhead)* posterior to the arytenoid.

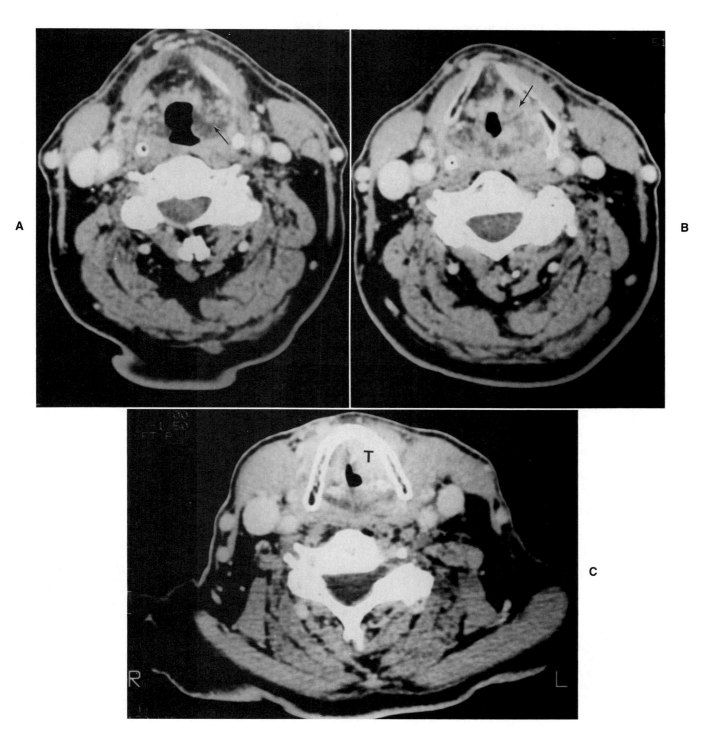

Fig. 9-121   Postradiation recurrent lesion of the true cord. **A,** Supraglottic slice shows spotty densities throughout the preepiglottic fat and thickening of the aryepiglottic fold *(arrow).* **B,** Slightly lower level again shows "spotty" densities throughout the paraglottic fat *(arrow)* representing post radiation change. **C,** Lower slice shows tumor *(T)* at the level of the ventricle.

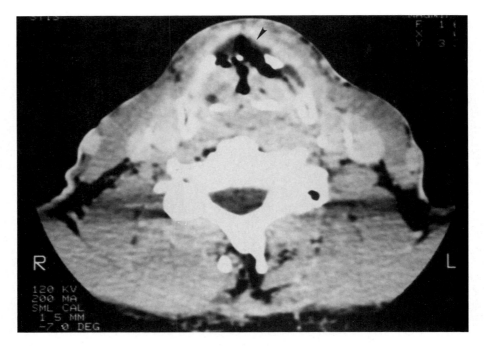

Fig. 9-122 Necrosis and perichondritis of the thyroid cartilage postradiation. Axial slice shows necrosis of the anterior thyroid cartilage with gas in the soft tissues *(arrowhead).*

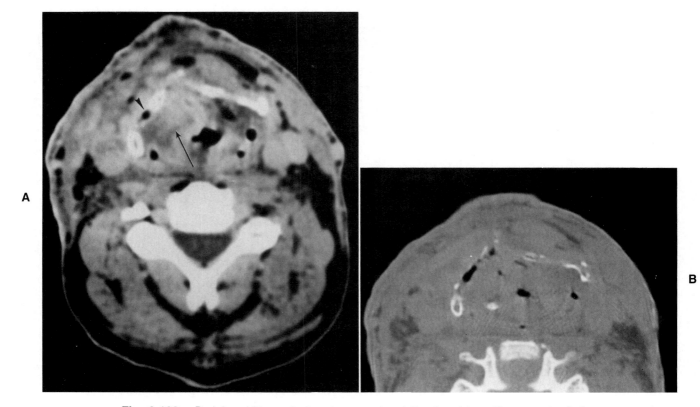

Fig. 9-123 Perichondritis and chondronecrosis of the thyroid cartilage postradiation therapy. **A,** Significant soft tissue swelling of the wall of the larynx *(arrow).* There are gas bubbles within the thyroid cartilage *(arrowhead).* **B,** Bone algorithm shows partial collapse of the thyroid cartilage due to demineralization and chondronecrosis.

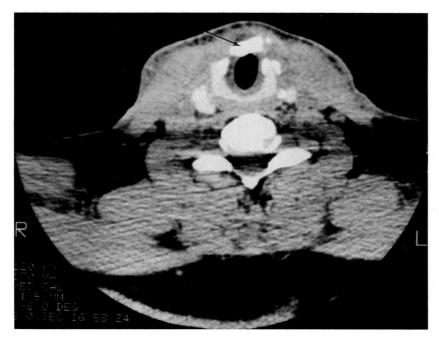

Fig. 9-124 Cartilaginous graft *(arrow)* placed in the anterior arch of the cricoid to support and maintain the lumen of the airway.

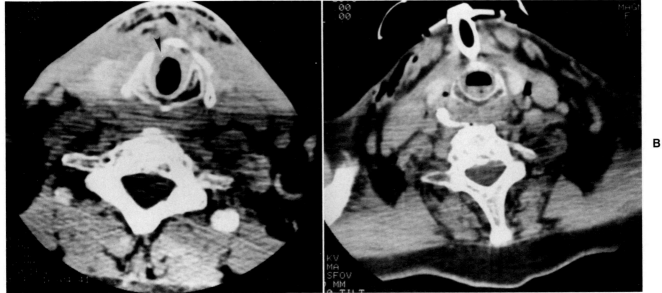

Fig. 9-125 **A,** Tracheostomy tube. Axial slice through the cricoid shows swelling in the subglottic region *(arrowhead)* due to recent tracheostomy placement. This can mimic tumor. **B,** Slice through the cricoid shows the extratracheal portion of the tracheostomy tube and an air-fluid level in the trachea.

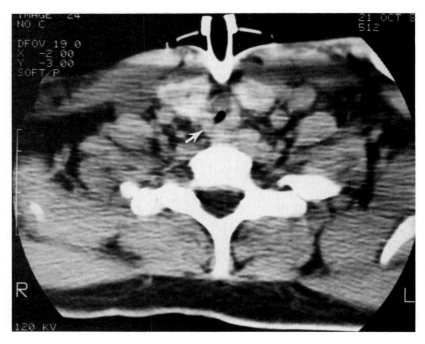

Fig. 9-126   Slice through the lower neck and tracheostomy tube. The air-filled structure represents the esophagus *(arrow)* in this patient postlaryngectomy. The airway and actual trachea would not be found until a more inferior slice.

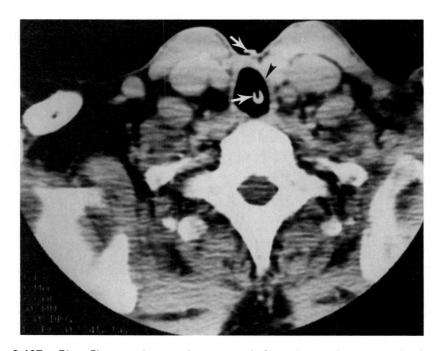

Fig. 9-127   Blom-Singer valve used to pass air from the tracheostomy site into the esophagus. The tube *(arrows)* is too small to be a tracheostomy tube. The apparent airway *(arrowhead)* is actually a gas-filled esophagus. The airway would be seen on a lower slice. If the air-filled structure were the airway, one would expect to show the esophagus just posteriorly.

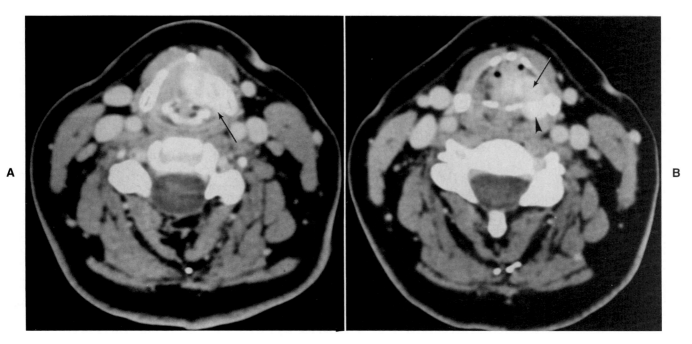

Fig. 9-128 **A,** Radiopaque teflon injected into the cord. Note the small amount of teflon *(arrow)* squeezing between the thyroid cartilage and the arytenoid. **B,** Supraglottic slice. The radiopaque teflon *(arrow)* again squeezes between the thyroid cartilage and the upper arytenoid *(arrowhead)*. This amount of teflon is more than is usually seen in a routine injection.

on CT or on barium swallow examinations. They can be aspirated into the lung and are much smaller than a tracheostomy tube (Fig. 9-127). Nasogastric tubes may traverse the neck, usually in a lateral pharyngeal position. The radiopaque marker can cause an artifact on CT, which can interfere with imaging near the larynx.

Teflon can be injected into the paraglottic space just lateral to the true cord (Fig. 9-128). This is done to add bulk to a paralyzed cord so that the cords can make contact near the midline and thereby improve voice quality. The procedure has also been performed to build up the resected side of a vertical hemilaryngectomy. The teflon is radiopaque and can easily be seen on CT in the region of the cord.

CONCLUSION

As with any facet of radiology, the choice of imaging techniques depends on the specific clinical information required. Plain film, fluoroscopy, CT, and MRI are the most frequently used imaging modalities. Currently CT and MRI are competitive in laryngeal imaging. Either can usually provide the necessary diagnostic information. MRI is more affected by artifacts, but further developments in technology will allow more widespread use of MRI, with its distinct advantage of multiplanar imaging.

REFERENCES

1. Barnes L and Gnepp DR: Disease of the larynx, hypopharynx, and esophagus. In Barnes L, editor: Surgical pathology of the head and neck, New York, 1985, Marcel Dekker, Inc, pp 141-226.
2. Batsakis JG: Tumors of the head and neck: clinical pathological consideration, ed 2, Baltimore, 1979, Williams & Wilkins.
3. American Joint Committee on Cancer: Manual for staging of cancer, ed 3, Philadelphia, 1988, JB Lippincott Co.
4. Johnson J: The role of neck and mediastinal dissection. In Fried MP, editor: The larynx: a multidisciplinary approach, Boston, 1988, Little, Brown & Co, pp 543-556.
5. Lawson W, Biller HF, and Suen JY: Cancer of the larynx. In Suen JY and Myers EN, editors: Cancer of the head and neck, New York, 1989, Churchill Livingstone, pp 533-591.
6. Lawson W and Biller HF: Supraglottic cancer. In Bailey BJ and Biller HF, editors: Surgery of the larynx, Philadelphia, 1985, WB Saunders Co, pp 243-256.
7. Thawley SE and Sessions DG: Surgical therapy of supraglottic tumors. In Thawley SE and Panje WR, editors: Comprehensive management of head and neck tumors, Philadelphia, 1987, WB Saunders Co, pp 959-990.
8. Lufkin RB, Larsson SG, and Hanafee WN: Work in progress: NMR anatomy of the larynx and tongue base, Radiology 148:173, 1983.
9. Kirchner JA: Pathways and pitfalls in partial laryngectomy, Ann Otol Rhinol Laryngol 93:301, 1984.
10. Kirchner JA: Two hundred laryngeal cancers: patterns of growth and spread as seen in serial section, Laryngoscope 87:474, 1977.
11. Castelijns JA et al: MR imaging of laryngeal cancer, JCAT 11(1):134, 1987.

12. Bailey BJ: Glottic carcinoma. In Bailey BJ and Biller HF, editors: Surgery of the larynx, Philadelphia, 1985, WB Saunders Co, pp 257-278.

13. Lawson W and Biller HF: Glottic and subglottic tumors. In Thawley SE and Panje WR, editors: Comprehensive management of head and neck tumors, Philadelphia, 1987, WB Saunders Co, pp 991-1015.

14. Castelijns JA et al: Invasion of laryngeal cartilage by cancer: comparison of CT and MR imaging, Radiology 166:199, 1987.

15. Castelijns JA et al: MRI of normal or cancerous laryngeal cartilage: histopathologic correlation, Laryngoscope 97:1085, 1987.

16. Wagenfeld DJH et al: Second primary respiratory tract malignant neoplasms in supraglottic carcinoma, Arch Otolaryngol 107:135, 1981.

17. Batsakis JG, Luna MA, and Byers RM: Metastases to the larynx, Head Neck Surg 7:458, 1985.

18. Johnson J and Curtin HD: Deep neck lipoma, Ann Otol Rhinol Laryngol 96:472, 1987.

19. Jones SR, Myers EN, and Barnes EL: Benign neoplasms of the larynx. In Fried MP, editor: The larynx: a multidisciplinary approach, Boston, 1988, Little, Brown & Co, pp 401-420.

20. Konowitz PM et al: Laryngeal paraganglioma: update on diagnosis and treatment, Laryngoscope 98:40, 1988.

21. Stines J et al: CT findings of laryngeal involvement in von Recklinghausen disease, JCAT 11(1):141, 1987.

22. Supance JS, Queneue DJ, and Crissman J: Endolaryngeal neurofibroma, Otolaryngol Head Neck Surg 88:74, 1980.

23. Henderson LH, Denneny JC III, and Teichgraeber J: Airway obstructing epiglottic cyst, Ann Otol Rhinol Laryngol 94:473, 1985.

24. Glazer HS et al: Computed tomography of laryngoceles, AJR 140:549, 1983.

25. Hubbard C: Laryngocele—a study of five cases with reference to radiologic features, Clin Radiol 38:639, 1987.

26. Michel JL and Weinstein L: Laryngeal infections. In Fried MP, editor: The larynx: a multidisciplinary approach, Boston, 1988, Little, Brown & Co, pp 237-247.

27. Souliere CR and Kirchner JA: Laryngeal perichondritis and abscess, Arch Otolaryngol 111:481, 1985.

28. Brageau-Lamontagne L et al: Cricoarytenoiditis: CT assessment in rheumatoid arthritis, Radiology 158:463, 1986.

29. Casselman JW et al: Polychondritis affecting the laryngeal cartilages: CT findings, AJR 150:355, 1988.

30. Noyek A et al: The larynx. In Bergeron RT, Osborne AG, and Som PM, editors: Head and neck imaging: excluding the brain, St Louis, 1983, The CV Mosby Co, pp 402-490.

31. Biller HF and Lawson W: Management of acute laryngeal trauma. In Bailey BJ and Biller HF, editors: Surgery of the larynx, Philadelphia, 1985, WB Saunders Co, pp 149-154.

32. Love JT: Embryology and anatomy. In Bluestone CD and Stool SE, editors: Pediatric otolaryngology, Philadelphia, 1983, WB Saunders Co, pp 1135-1140.

33. Tucker JA: Developmental anatomy of the larynx. In Bailey BJ and Biller HF, editors: Surgery of the larynx, Philadelphia, 1985, WB Saunders Co, pp 3-14.

34. Cotton R and Reilly JS: Congenital malformations of the larynx. In Bluestone CD and Stool SE, editors: Pediatric otolaryngology, Philadelphia, 1983, WB Saunders Co, pp 1215-1224.

35. McMillan WG and Duvall AJ: Congenital subglottic stenosis, Arch Otolaryngol 87:272, 1968.

36. Schlesinger AE and Tucker GF: Elliptical cricoid cartilage: a unique type of congenital subglottic stenosis, AJR 146:1133, 1986.

37. Ravich WJ, Donner MW, and Kashima H: The swallowing center: concepts and procedures, Gastrointest Radiol 10(3):255, 1985.

38. Farooq P: Recurrent laryngeal nerve paralysis: laryngographic and computed tomography study, Radiology 148:149, 1983.

39. Levine HL and Tucker HM: Surgical management of the paralyzed larynx. In Bailey BJ and Biller HF, editors: Surgery of the larynx, Philadelphia, 1985, WB Saunders Co, pp 117-134.

40. McAlpine JC and Fuller AP: Localized laryngeal amyloidosis: a report of a case with a review of the literature, J Laryngol 78:296, 1964.

41. Deutsch EC, Schlid JA, and Mafee MF: Dysphagia and Forrestier's disease, Arch Otolaryngol 111:400, 1985.

42. Som PM and Biller HF: Computed tomography of the neck in the postoperative patient: radical neck dissection and the myocutaneous flap, Radiology 148:157, 1983.

43. Niemeyer JH, Balfe DM, and Hayden RE: Neck evaluation with barium-enhanced radiographs and CT scans after supraglottic subtotal laryngectomy, Radiology 162:493, 1987.

44. Williford ME et al: Revascularized jejunal graft replacing the cervical esophagus: radiographic evaluation, AJR 145:533, 1985.

45. Perez CA and Marks JE: Radiation therapy for carcinoma of the larynx. In Bailey BJ and Biller HF, editors: Surgery of the larynx, Philadelphia, 1985, WB Saunders Co, pp 417-434.

10 The Orbit

MAHMOOD F. MAFEE
CHARLES J. SCHATZ

SECTION ONE
THE EYE

MAHMOOD F. MAFEE

Although computed tomography (CT) provided a major imaging advance over conventional films and tomography in examining the eye, the development of magnetic resonance imaging (MRI) technology has proved to be an even greater breakthrough in diagnostic medical imaging and biomedical research.[1,2] Intrinsic differences in proton density and the relaxation times of tissues allow excellent MRI contrast between various normal structures and provide a high sensitivity for detecting pathologic states.[3,4,5] This section discusses CT and MR imaging of the normal globe and the features of ocular pathology, with particular emphasis on the potential of MR imaging in the practice of ophthalmology.

IMAGING TECHNIQUES
MRI Technique

The MRI studies in this section were performed on a 1.5-T Signa unit (General Electric, Milwaukee) with 3 mm or 5 mm thick sections and with 0.6 to 1.5 mm intersection space. Single echo spin-echo (SE) pulse sequences, using a head coil as the receiver coil, were obtained with a repetition time (TR) of 300 to 800 ms and an echo time (TE) of 20 to 25 ms (TR/TE = 300 − 800/ 20 − 25 ms). Multiple SE pulse sequences were ob-

tained with a TR of 1500 to 2500 ms and a TE of 20 to 100 ms. The early echo (20 to 25 ms) yielded proton-weighted (PW) images, and the later echo (60 to 100 ms) yielded T_2-weighted (T_2W) images. The studies were most often performed with 1 excitation (NEX), a 256 × 256 matrix, and a 20 to 24 cm field of view. For a shorter TR (300 to 800 ms), the studies were often performed with 2 excitations. A 3-inch diameter surface coil (Medical Advance Corp., Milwaukee) and an experimental butterfly-type surface coil (General Electric) were used to improve spatial resolution per imaging tissue. For surface coil studies, a field of view of 12 or 16 cm, a matrix of 256 × 128, and 2 excitations were used.[5,6] For all ocular lesions, in addition to surface coil imaging an SE sequence (2000/20,80 ms) of the eye and head was obtained, using the head coil as a receiver, a 5 mm thick section, a 256 × 256 matrix, 1 excitation, and a 20 cm field of view. Because motion artifact is more pronounced on images obtained with the surface coil (because of the inherent increased sensitivity of the coil)[5] a lesion is sometimes better seen on images obtained with a head coil. With the surface coil a 3 mm thick section is used to reduce the problem of partial volume averaging. However, the thin section has the disadvantage of generating less signal (small volume) and this may result in a decreased amount of T_2 information in later echoes, particularly in rapidly decaying T_2 signal. Because of these factors, a uveal melanoma at times may be better seen on T_2W images obtained with a head coil rather than with a surface coil. This point is

ACKNOWLEDGMENT: I would like to thank Dr. Heraldo Belmont for his expert advice and Dale Peal and Mari Salazar for their secretarial assistance.

important, because the hypointensity of melanotic tissues in T_2W images is an important diagnostic feature of these lesions.[4,5,7]

CT Technique

The protocol for intraocular lesions includes 1.5 to 3 mm thick axial sections of the globe. For all foreign bodies and lesions at 6 and 12 o'clock, we also obtain additional direct 3 to 5 mm thick coronal sections. Additional 1.5, 3, or 5 mm thick axial sections (depending on the size of lesion) of the orbit are then obtained after administration of iodinated contrast material. In cases of suspected retinoblastoma and uveal melanoma, 5 to 10 mm thick axial sections of the head are also obtained to investigate the presence of any intracranial pathology.

MRI and Evaluation of Intraocular Foreign Bodies

Despite the many advantages of MRI, it may not be the primary imaging modality for evaluating a traumatized eye harboring a possible intraocular foreign body; using the technique may cause additional damage to the injured eye by inducing movement of ferromagnetic foreign bodies. In vitro and in vivo (rabbit) experiments[8] performed to study magnetic resonance imaging of intraocular foreign bodies revealed that diamagnetic and paramagnetic foreign bodies were imaged with neither artifacts nor movement during the imaging process. On the other hand, ferromagnetic foreign bodies produced large artifacts that often prevented meaningful images from being obtained. In addition, all ferromagnetic foreign bodies moved during in vitro imaging and in vivo studies, and this movement caused substantial retinal injury. These studies indicate that magnetic resonance imaging is contraindicated in trau-

matized eyes that are suspected of having ferromagnetic foreign bodies. For those patients with even a remote history of a traumatic foreign body or in metal workers, a high-resolution 1.5 mm thick CT study of the orbits and a 5 to 10 mm thick CT study of the head are recommended.

MRI Artifacts

Motion artifacts may result in marked degradation of MR images. To minimize this type of artifact, it is important to ask patients to close their eyes during the examination. Artifacts may also occur as a result of tattooing of eyelids with iron oxide and even from external application of certain eye cosmetics (Fig. 10-1). The artifacts arising from tattooing or related to eye cosmetics usually appear as distortions of the skin contour in the location of the iron oxide. The shape of the globe also may be distorted, and several hyperintense artifacts may be present around the contour of the eyelids.

NORMAL OCULAR ANATOMY

The globe (eye) is well examined by MRI, because it contains the most (vitreous) and least (lens) water-laden soft tissues in the human body.[9,10] The magnetic resonance appearance of the vitreous and lens is a function of the interaction between tissue proteins and water (see Fig. 10-2). The water content of the vitreous is 98% to 99%; the cornea, 80%; and the lens, 65% to 69%.[5,9]

The vitreous represents about two thirds of the volume of the eye, or approximately 4 ml.[11] The vitreous humor is a gel-like, transparent, extracellular matrix composed of a meshwork of 0.2% collagen fibrils interspersed with 0.2% hyaluronic acid, polymers, water, and a small amount of soluble proteins.[3,9] A number of

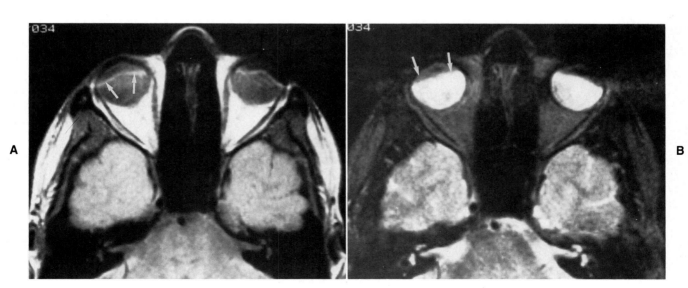

Fig. 10-1   **A,** PW MRI scan and **B,** T_2W MRI scan show makeup artifacts *(arrows).*

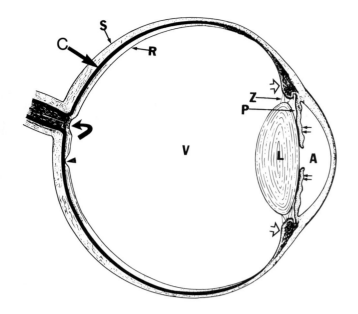

Fig. 10-2 Ocular coats and chambers. The three ocular coats consist of sclera *(S)*, middle layer; uvea *(black layer)*, consisting of choroid *(C)*, ciliary body *(hollow arrows)*, and iris *(double black arrows)*; and inner layer, the retina *(R)*. Note optic nerve disc *(curved arrow)*, fovea *(arrowhead)*, vitreous chamber *(V)*, lens *(L)*, zonule fibers *(Z)*, posterior chamber *(P)* and anterior chamber *(A)*.

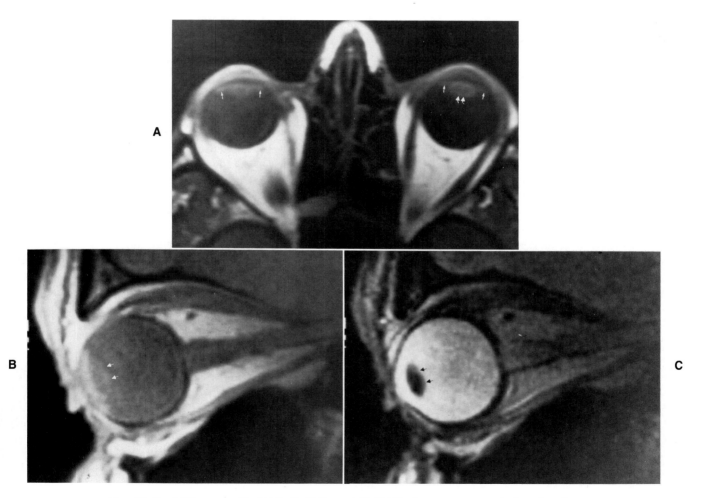

Fig. 10-3 MRI scans (**A**, T_1W; **B**, PW; and **C**, T_2W) show cornea, anterior chamber, lens, and vitreous chamber. The three ocular coats may not be distinguished as distinct individual layers. Lens capsule *(double arrows)* appears hyperintense relative to its nucleus in T_1- and proton-weighted images. Ciliary body and lens zonules appear slightly hyperintense in T_1W images *(arrows in **A**)* and usually hypointense in T_2W images (see Fig. 10-4). Lens nucleus appears hypointense in T_2W scan.

ocular diseases,[3,12] as well as the aging process, can cause it to degenerate to a liquid state devoid of collagen. The vitreous is both viscous and gel-like, characteristics associated with the hyaluronic acid and collagen components, respectively. In a manner similar to synovial fluid, vitreous serves as somewhat of a biologic shock absorber.[5,12] Because vitreous is a gel composed of long, fixed collagen fibrils bathed only with dilute dissolved proteins, just a fraction of its water content is in contact with the macromolecules.[9] Consequently, the bulk of the water in vitreous relaxes on MRI as free water, with only a small protein-water interaction (bound water) component.[5,9] As a result, the vitreous' relaxation times are longer than those of most tissues but shorter than those of water (Fig. 10-2).

The lens is approximately 9 mm in diameter and 4 to 4.5 mm thick. Anterior to the lens are the iris and the aqueous humor; posteriorly, the lens is bordered by vitreous humor (see Fig. 10-2). The zonular fibers (zonules of Zinn) are inserted on the outermost surface of the lens along the equatorial margin of the capsule and extend to the ciliary body (see Fig. 10-2). As previously mentioned, the chemical composition of the lens includes 66% water, making the lens the least hydrated soft tissue organ of the body.[9] The remaining bulk of the lens is composed of protein. On MRI the normal lens appears to have long T_1 and short T_2 relaxation times, and it is characteristically darker than the surrounding fluid-laden tissues on most pulse sequences[9] (see Fig. 10-3). The nucleus of the lens has both a lower water content and a shorter T_2 relaxation time than does the cortex.

MRI provides precise information about other ocular structures as well. For example, the anterior chamber is seen as a crescent of signal anterior to the lens; it is isointense with the vitreous humor on short TR studies and slightly hypointense to vitreous on longer TR images.[9]

The three ocular coats include the inner sensorineural layer, consisting of the sensory retina and retinal pigment epithelium (RPE); the middle layer (tunica vasculosa), which includes the uveal tract, consisting of the choroid, ciliary body, and iris; and the outer fibrous layer, consisting of the sclera and cornea. The ciliary body may be seen on T_2W MR images as a hypointense area running from the edge of the lens to the wall of the globe (Fig. 10-4). The individual layers of the sclera, choroid, and retina cannot be differentiated by MRI in the normal eye.[5]

The anterior chamber is the space lying between the cornea and the crystalline lens (see Figs. 10-2 and 10-3). The chamber contains aqueous fluid, which nourishes the corneal epithelium and the lens.[13] The iris, the most anterior extension of the uveal tract, lies at the anterior surface of the lens (see Fig. 10-2). The cil-

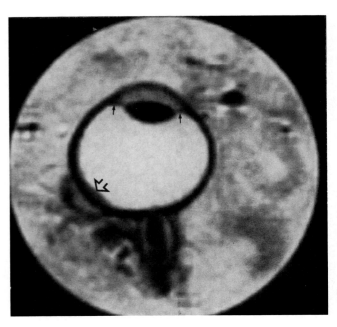

Fig. 10-4 Uveal melanoma. T_2W MRI scan of enucleated eye shows hypointense posterior uveal melanoma *(hollow arrow)*. Note hypointensity of lens and hyperintensity of vitreous humor. Ciliary body and lens zonules appear hypointense *(arrow)*.

iary body, which is just posterior to the iris, produces aqueous fluid. Aqueous fluid drains from the eyeball through the trabecular meshwork at the angle formed by the joining of the root of the iris, the anterior margin of the ciliary body, and the corneoscleral junction.[13] The ciliary body and the iris divide the globe into two compartments, or segments: the anterior segment and the posterior segment (vitreous chamber). The anterior chamber is anterior to the iris, and the posterior chamber is a small space that extends from the pigment epithelium at the posterior surface of the iris to the anterior surface of the vitreous. The posterior chamber is filled with aqueous.

Ocular Structures

The eye consists of three primary layers (Fig. 10-5): (1) the sclera, or outer layer, which is composed primarily of collagen-elastic tissue; (2) the uvea, or middle layer, which is richly vascular and contains pigmented tissue consisting of three components: the iris, ciliary body, and choroid; and (3) the retina, or inner layer, which is the neural, sensory stratum of the eye.

Tenon's Capsule

The sclera is covered by Tenon's capsule, a fibroelastic membrane that envelops the eyeball from the optic nerve to the level of ciliary muscle. Tenon's capsule is also called the bulbar fascia of the eyeball, or the episcleral membrane.[14] This fibroelastic socket encloses the

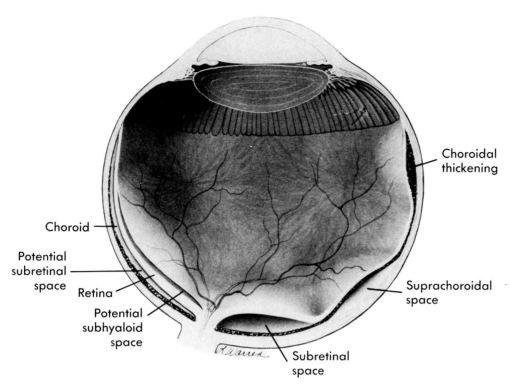

Fig. 10-5 Diagram demonstrates various intraocular potential spaces. Principal potential spaces include subretinal, suprachoroidal, and subhyaloid spaces.

posterior four fifths of the eyeball and separates it from the central orbital fat. Anteriorly, it blends with the sclera just behind the corneoscleral junction and fuses with the bulbar conjunctiva. The fascia is perforated behind by the optic nerve and its sheath, as well as by the ciliary nerves and vessels, and fuses with and extends to the sheath of the optic nerve and the sclera around the entrance of the optic nerve.[15] Septa of fibrous tissue are attached to the outer surface of Tenon's capsule.[15] Near the equator Tenon's capsule is perforated by the vorticose veins (the draining veins of the choroid and sclera). The inner surface of Tenon's capsule is smooth and is separated from the outer surface of the sclera by the episcleral space, or Tenon's space.[15] This is a potential space that is traversed by fibers of loose connective (areolar) tissue, which extend between the fascia and the sclera.[14] The episcleral space begins anteriorly between the bulbar conjunctiva and sclera near the sclerocorneal junction, extends posteriorly to the optic nerve, and continues with the subdural and subarachnoid spaces around the optic nerve.[14] The tendons of the extrinsic ocular muscles pierce Tenon's capsule to reach the sclera, and at the site of perforation, Tenon's sheath is reflected back along the muscles as a tubular sheath.[14] Because the connection between the muscle fibers and the sheath is especially strong at the point where the two fuse,[15] the muscles retain their attach-

ment to the capsule and do not extensively retract after enucleation (tenotomy).[15]

Inflammatory and intraocular neoplastic processes are the most common lesions to involve Tenon's space. In posterior scleritis, episcleritis, Tenon's fasciitis, and pseudotumor, inflammatory effusion in this space produces characteristic circular or semicircular distention of Tenon's capsule (Fig. 10-6). Retinoblastomas (Fig. 10-7) and melanomas (Fig. 10-8) also may invade Tenon's space.[16]

Sclera

The sclera is the globe's outer white, leathery coat. It extends from the limbus at the margin of the cornea to the optic nerve, where it becomes continuous with the dural sheath.[13] The external side of the sclera lies against Tenon's capsule; the internal surface of the sclera blends with the suprachoroidal tissues (see Fig. 10-5).[13] Posteriorly, the sclera is perforated by the vortex veins, the long posterior ciliary arteries and nerves, and the short posterior ciliary arteries and nerves. The sclera is predominantly cellular, composed mostly of extracellular bundles of collagen.

Uvea (Choroid, Ciliary Body, and Iris)

The uveal tract lies between the sclera and the retina. It comprises the choroid, ciliary body, and the

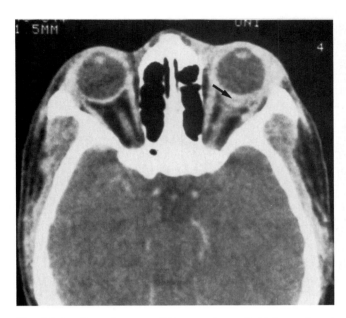

Fig. 10-6   Pseudotumor. CT scan shows fluid *(arrow)* and inflammatory infiltration in Tenon's space.

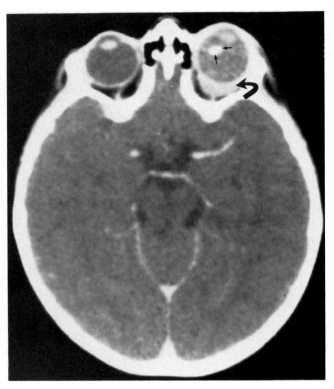

Fig. 10-7   Retinoblastoma with extension into Tenon's capsule. Mass with focal calcification *(arrows)* fills entire left globe and extends into Tenon's space *(curved arrow)*.

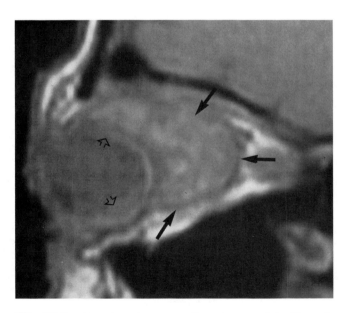

Fig. 10-8   Uveal melanoma with extension into Tenon's capsule. PW MRI scan shows large, well-capsulated retrobulbar mass *(arrows)* in this patient with uveal melanoma (not seen in this section). Note subretinal fluid *(open arrows)*. Surgery confirmed intraocular tumor and massive Tenon's capsule extension.

tract's most anterior extension, the iris. The choroid is the section of the uveal tract that lies between the sclera and the retinal pigment epithelium (RPE), the outer layer of the retina (see Figs. 10-1 and 10-5). The choroid forms a membrane of predominantly vascular tissue extending from the optic nerve to the ora serrata, beyond which it continues as the ciliary body.[13] The membrane's thickness varies from approximately 0.22 mm at the posterior pole to 0.10 mm near the ora, at the optic nerve where it forms part of the optic nerve canal, and at the point of internal penetration of the vortex veins. This accounts for the characteristic shape of the choroidal detachment, which shows valleys at the site of the vortex veins.[16] The choroid can be divided into four layers. Extending from internal to external, they are: Bruch's membrane, the choriocapillaris, the choroidal stroma, and the suprachoroidea.[13]

Bruch's Membrane.   Bruch's membrane is a tough, acellular, amorphous, bilamellar structure situated between the retina and the rest of the choroid (Fig. 10-9). Microscopically, Bruch's membrane consists of five layers: the basement membrane of the RPE, the inner collagenous zone, the elastic layer, the other collagenous zone, and the basement membrane of the choriocapillaris.[17]

Choriocapillaris.   The choriocapillaris is the capillary layer of the choroid lying immediately external to Bruch's membrane (see Fig. 10-1). The capillaries are drained by the vortex veins. The choriocapillaris is a visceral type of vasculature with fenestrations in the vessels.[18] These openings are covered by diaphragms, permitting a relatively free exchange of material between the choriocapillaris and the surrounding tissues. By contrast, the retinal capillaries show no fenestrations and present a strong barrier to the interchange of material from capillary to retinal tissue.[13]

Choroidal Stroma. The choroidal stroma lies external to the choriocapillaris and consists of blood vessels, nerves, melanocytes, fibroblasts, a collection of immunologic cells, macrophages, lymphocytes, mast cells, plasma cells, and collagenous supporting tissue. The blood vessels of the stroma are branches of the feeding arteries and draining veins.

Suprachoroidea. The suprachoroidea, approximately 30 μm in thickness, lies between the stroma and the sclera.[13] This layer displays pigmentation, fibroblasts, melanocytes, ganglion cells, and nerve plexuses within its collagen matrix.

Function. The uvea's most important function is to provide a vascular supply to the eye and to regulate the ocular temperature.[19] The choroid is also responsible for nourishing the pigment epithelium and the outer third of the retina.[13] The fenestrations in the choroid's capillaries permit proteins and other larger molecules to diffuse through Bruch's membrane. The selectivity of passage of these materials anterior to Bruch's membrane depends on the retinal pigment epithelium.[13]

Retina

The external surface of the retina is in contact with the choroid and the internal surface with the vitreous body. Posteriorly, the retina is continuous with the optic nerve. The optic nerve and the inner layer of the eye represent an anteriorly protruding portion of the brain. Grossly the retina has two layers: (1) the inner layer, which is the sensory retina and contains photoreceptors, the first and second order neurons (ganglion cells), and the neuroglial elements of the retina (Müller's cells or sustentacular gliocytes); and (2) the outer layer, which is the retinal pigment epithelium, consisting of a single lamina of cells whose nuclei are adjacent to the basal lamina (Bruch's membrane) of the choroid.[20,21]

The retina is very thin, measuring .056 mm near the disc to 0.1 mm anteriorly.[22] It is much thinner at both the optic disc and the fovea of the macula. The retina anteriorly creates a crenated margin, called the ora serrata (see Fig. 10-1). The sensory retina ends here, but a thin epithelium extends forward over the back of the internal portion of the ciliary body and iris. The macula, the center of the retina, lies 3.5 mm temporal to

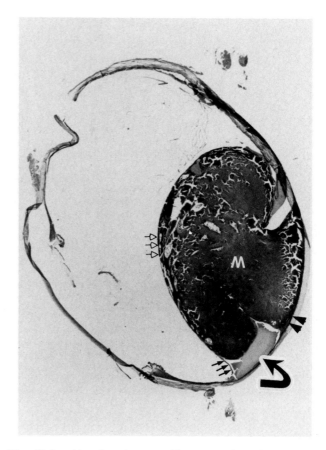

Fig. 10-9 Uveal melanoma. Tissue section shows mushroom-shaped uveal melanoma *(M)* arising from choroid *(arrowheads)* and breaking through Bruch's membrane *(curved arrows)*. Retina *(open arrows)* is elevated at top of tumor and is detached *(arrows)* at slope of tumor.

the margin of the optic nerve. The retina is attached tightly to the vitreous and loosely to the RPE[13]; it is nourished by the choroid and the RPE.

Vitreous

The vitreous body chamber, which occupies the space between the lens and the retina, represents about two thirds of the volume of the eye, or approximately 4 ml.[19,20] Its water component (98% to 99%) is bound with a fibrillar collagen meshwork and hyaluronic acid.[6,19,20] Any insult to the vitreous body may result in a fibroproliferative reaction (such as proliferative vitreoretinopathy), which subsequently can result in a tractional retinal detachment.[6]

Basically, three potential spaces—the posterior hyaloid space, the subretinal space, and the suprachoroidal space—can accumulate fluid, and result in detachment of the various coats of the globe (see Fig. 10-5).[23] The posterior hyaloid space is the potential space between the base (posterior hyaloid membrane) of the hyaloid and the sensory retina (see Fig. 10-5). A separation of the posterior hyaloid membrane from the sensory ret-

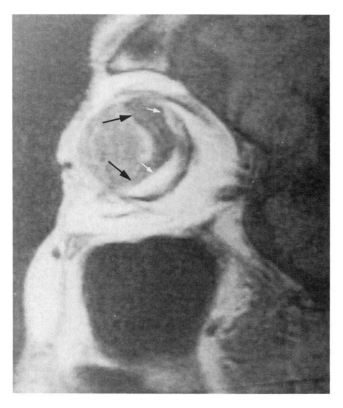

Fig. 10-10 Posterior hyaloid detachment and retinal detachment in patient with complicated macular degeneration. T₁W MRI scan shows two semilunar images; posterior image *(white arrows)* is caused by chronic subretinal hemorrhage, and anterior image *(black arrows)* is caused by posterior hyaloid detachment. Surgery confirmed findings.

ina is referred to as a posterior hyaloid detachment[20] (see Fig. 10-5). The subretinal space is the potential space between the sensory retina and the RPE. A separation of the sensory retina from the retinal pigment epithelium is referred to as a retinal detachment (see Fig. 10-5). The suprachoroidal space is the potential space between the choroid and the sclera. The RPE and Bruch's membrane are tightly adherent to the choroid and become separated when both layers are torn; however, the choroid is loosely attached to the sclera and can be separated rather easily, resulting in a choroidal detachment (see Fig. 10-5).

OCULAR PATHOLOGY
Posterior Hyaloid Detachment

A posterior hyaloid detachment usually occurs in adults over 50 years of age, but it may occur in children with persistent hyperplastic primary vitreous (PHPV).[20,23-25] This type of detachment in adults usually is caused by liquefaction of the vitreous and is often associated with macular degeneration (Fig. 10-10).

The posterior hyaloid membrane is very thin and is invisible on MRI or CT scans, but it can become visible if blood or other fluid fills the posterior hyaloid space, causing thickening of the membrane (see Fig. 10-10). Fluid in the retrohyaloid space is seen on CT and MRI as a layer that shifts its location in the lateral decubitus position (Figs. 10-11 and 10-12). The retrohyaloid layered fluid is shifted in the decubitus position, because it is not within the substance of the vitreous (Fig. 10-11, *B*). By comparison, hemorrhage within the vitreous

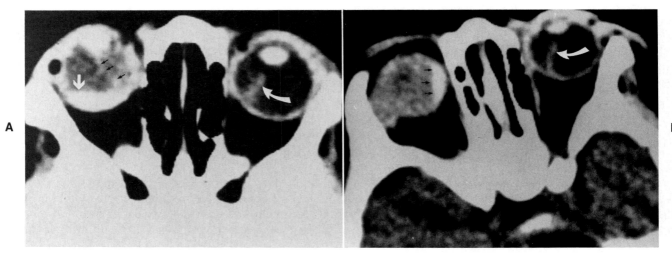

Fig. 10-11 Posterior hyaloid detachment and congenital nonattached retina. CT scans obtained without contrast in supine position **(A)** and decubitus position **(B)** show gravitational layering fluid *(white arrow in A)*, which is related to hemorrhage in subhyaloid space. Fluid shifts more freely in subhyaloid space than in subretinal space *(black arrows in B)*. Note congenitally nonattached retina of left eye *(curved arrows)*. Increased density, as well as retrolental soft tissue of right eye *(black arrows in A)*, are related to persistent hyperplastic primary vitreous (PHPV).

is mixed with the vitreous humor, which is a gel-like extracellular material, and therefore does not show intragel layering. Fluid within the retrohyaloid space and the subretinal space may be indistinguishable on both CT and MRI scans.[23]

Retinal Detachment

Retinal detachment occurs when the sensory retina is separated from the retinal pigment epithelium. The RPE has a barrier function, and if the barrier is damaged, fluid leaks into the potential subretinal space.[23] A retinal detachment caused by a hole (or tear) in the retina is referred to as a rhegmatogenous retinal detachment. Because the sensory retina is part of the central nervous system, a tear in the sensory retina cannot heal. On the other hand, a tear in the retinal pigment epithelium can possibly heal. In laser treatment for retinal detachment, the energy of the laser beam is absorbed by the RPE at the site of the retinal detachment, and the resultant heat heals and closes the tear. Fluid in the subretinal space can be detected by both CT and MR scans (Fig. 10-13).

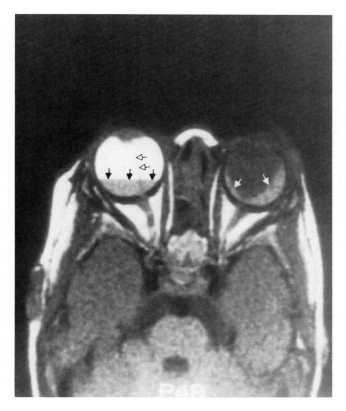

Fig. 10-12   Posterior hyaloid and retinal detachment. T_1W MRI scan shows fluid-fluid level *(black arrows)* in right vitreous chamber. This is thought to be caused by chronic (hyperintense) and acute (hypointense) hemorrhage in subhyaloid or subretinal space. Note detached leaves of retina of left eye *(white arrows)*. Patient was diagnosed as having Warburg's syndrome.

Rhegmatogenous retinal detachments are rare in children. Most retinal detachments in children are non-rhegmatogenous and secondary to other ocular diseases (Fig. 10-14). A retinal detachment may result from retraction caused by a mass or from a fibroproliferative disease in the vitreous, such as vitreoretinopathy of prematurity or vitreoretinopathy of diabetes. A detachment also may occur with an inflammatory process, such as endophthalmitis resulting from a larval granuloma caused by *Toxocara canis*.[23] Retinal detachment also may occur because of a retinal vascular leakage, as is seen in patients with Coats' disease, a primary vascular anomaly of the retina characterized by telangiectasis. The telangiectatic vessels leak serum and lipid, resulting in accumulation of a lipoproteinaceous exudate in the subretinal space (Fig. 10-15). Retinal detachment is sometimes the result of subretinal hemorrhage, which may be caused by trauma, senile macular degeneration, or persistent hyperplastic primary vitreous. Any choroidal lesion can cause retinal detachment (Figs. 10-16 and 10-17).

In an axial CT or MRI scan taken below or above the lens, the retinal detachment will appear, respectively, either as a homogeneous increased density or an increased signal intensity of the globe (see Fig. 10-15). Because the retina is very thin, it is beyond the limits of resolution of either CT or MRI scanners. However, it may be shown when outlined by a significant contrast difference between the density or signal intensity of the subretinal effusion and the vitreous cavity (Fig. 10-18). The appearance of a retinal detachment varies with the amount of exudation present (see Figs. 10-15 to 10-20) and the organization of the subretinal materials. In a section taken at the level of the optic disc, a retinal detachment has a characteristic indentation at the optic disc (Figs. 10-19 and 10-20). When total retinal detachment has occurred and the entire vitreous cavity is ablated, the leaves of the detached retina may not be clearly detected (see Fig. 10-15). A retinal detachment is seen on coronal MRI images as a characteristic folding membrane (Fig. 10-21). The subretinal fluid in the exudative retinal detachment is rich in protein, giving a higher CT attenuation and stronger MRI signal intensities than the subretinal fluid (transudate) that is seen in a rhegmatogenous detachment. A rhegmatogenous retinal detachment is caused by a retinal tear and subsequent ingress of fluid vitreous into the subretinal space.[23]

In many cases of retinal detachment the MRI and in particular the CT scans may not detect the detached retina. In these cases ultrasonography is superior to both MRI and CT. When visualized, retinal detachment is characteristically seen on CT or MRI scans as a V-shaped image with its apex at the optic disc and its extremities toward the ciliary body (see Figs. 10-18 to

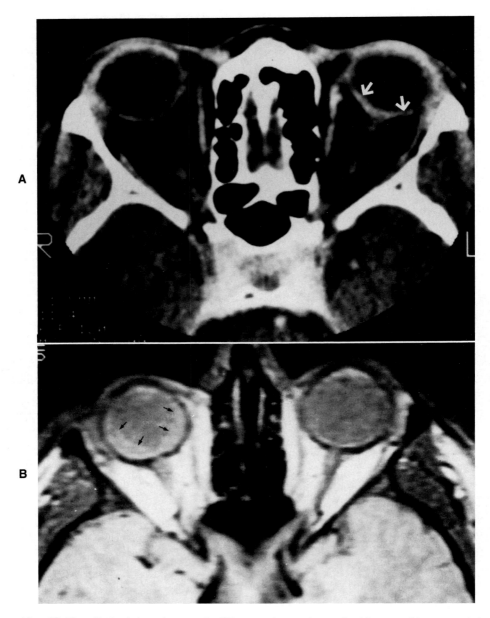

Fig. 10-13 Retinal detachment. **A,** CT scan shows dependent image of increased density *(arrows)* of left eye caused by retinal detachment. **B,** PW MRI scan shows dependent hyperintense image *(arrows)* of right vitreous chamber caused by subretinal exudate.

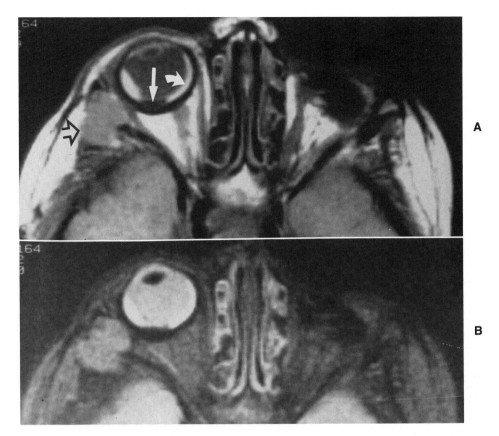

Fig. 10-14 Exudative retinal detachment and regressed retinoblastoma after radiation therapy. **A,** PW MRI scan and **B,** T$_2$W MRI scan show mass *(white arrow)* and hyperintense subretinal exudate *(curved arrow)*. Mass is hypointense in PW and T$_2$W MR images because of calcification. Note destructive lesion *(open arrow)*, presumably sarcoma that developed in field of radiation therapy. Left eye has been enucleated in this patient, who had bilateral retinoblastoma.

10-20). This appearance of a retinal detachment may be confused with the appearance of a posterior choroidal detachment; however, a posterior choroidal detachment, in the region of the optic disc and macula, involves detachment of the choroid that is restricted by the anchoring effect of the short posterior ciliary arteries and nerves.[26] This restriction usually results in a characteristic appearance in which the leaves of the detached choroid, unlike those of the detached retina, do not extend to the region of the optic disc (Fig. 10-22).[23]

Inflammatory diseases of the uvea are seldom limited to this vascularized layer of the eye. The sclera and retina usually are also involved, producing scleritis or chorioretinitis, respectively. Inflammation of the choroid can damage the retinal pigment epithelial cells, causing a breakdown of the ocular blood barrier and a subsequent outpouring of proteinaceous fluid (exudate) into the subretinal space. This produces an exudative retinal detachment,[23] and the sensory retina can subsequently detach. Interestingly, neoplastic diseases of the choroid may produce similar changes in the retinal pigment epithelium; however, these changes usually occur only in the more advanced stages of the lesion (see Figs. 10-16 and 10-17). Malignant melanomas and choroidal hemangiomas are the most common choroidal neoplasms that produce retinal detachments in adults (see Figs. 10-16 and 10-17).[4,21] These tumors produce various degrees of subretinal fluid accumulation, depending on the size and location of the tumor (see Figs. 10-16 and 10-17). The subretinal fluid often has a high density on CT scans and high signal intensity on MRI scans. MRI is superior to CT in differentiating choroidal lesions from subretinal exudate,[23] whereas ultrasonography is superior to MRI and CT in the evaluation of retinal detachment.

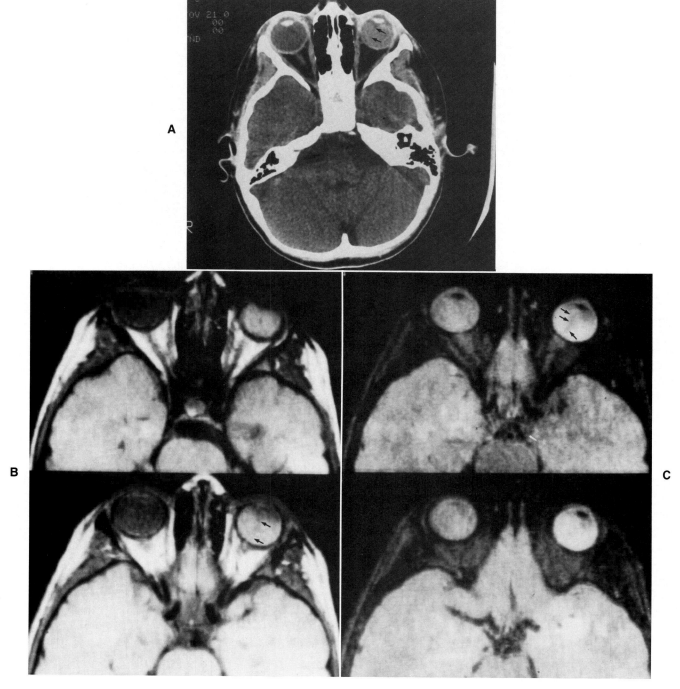

Fig. 10-15 Retinal detachment caused by Coats' disease. **A,** CT scan, **B,** PW MRI scan, and **C,** T$_2$W MRI scan show total retinal detachment *(arrows)*.

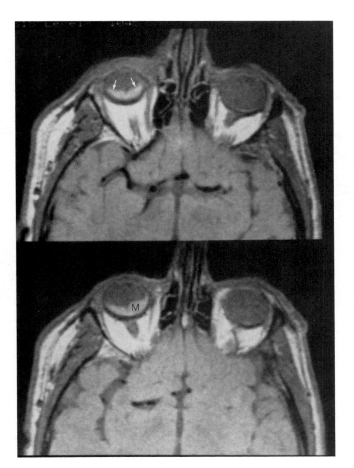

Fig. 10-16 Retinal detachment caused by uveal melanoma. PW MRI scans show mass *(M)* and exudative retinal detachment *(arrows)*.

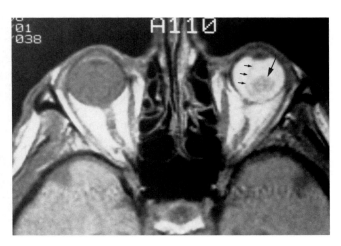

Fig. 10-17 Total retinal detachment. PW MRI scan shows mass *(arrow)* with total retinal detachment *(arrows)*. Subretinal exudate is hyperintense.

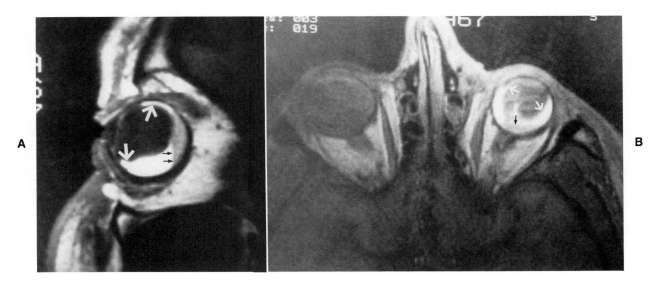

Fig. 10-18 Retinal detachment. **A,** T_1W sagittal MRI scan shows leaves of detached retina *(white arrows)*. Subretinal fluid is hyperintense because of either exudate or chronic hemorrhage. Note layered fluid *(black arrows)* caused by recent hemorrhage. **B,** PW MRI scan shows leaves of detached retina *(white arrows)* and layered recent hemorrhage *(black arrow)*.

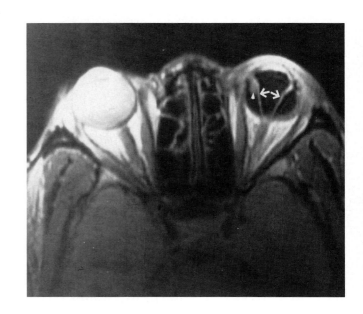

Fig. 10-19 Total retinal detachment. T₂W MRI scan shows detached retina *(arrows)* with characteristic V-shaped configuration with apex at optic disc. Hypointensity of left globe is caused by injection of silicone oil into vitreous, which also has escaped into subretinal space. Arrowhead points to residual subretinal fluid not replaced by silicone oil.

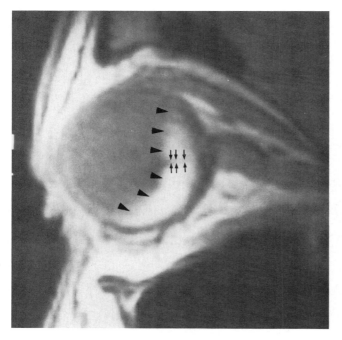

Fig. 10-20 Retinal detachment. PW MRI scan shows detached retina *(arrowheads)* with characteristic folding of retinal leaves *(arrows)* toward optic disc.

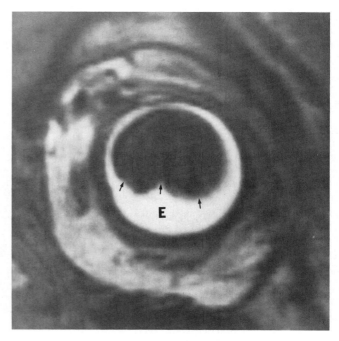

Fig. 10-21 Retinal detachment. T₁W coronal MRI scan shows characteristic appearance of retinal folds *(arrows)* and hyperintense subretinal exudate *(E)*.

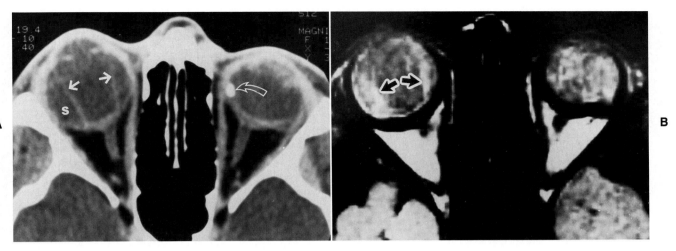

Fig. 10-22 Serous choroidal detachment. **A,** CT scan shows two prominent linear images *(solid arrows)* in right eye. Because of anchoring effect of posterior ciliary arteries and nerves, detached leaves of choroid usually do not appear to converge at disc, unlike retinal leaves in retinal detachment. Suprachoroidal space *(S)* is isodense with vitreous, indicating serous choroidal detachment. Enlarged right globe results from known congenital glaucoma. Note postsurgical changes in left eye and scleral-encircling silicone band *(curved arrow).* **B,** PW MRI scan shows choroidal detachment *(arrows)* with increased intensity in suprachoroidal space.

Choroidal Detachment, Choroidal Effusion, and Ocular Hypotony

Choroidal detachment is caused by the accumulation of fluid (serous choroidal detachment) or blood (hemorrhagic choroidal detachment) in the potential suprachoroidal space.[23,27-29] Serous choroidal detachment (see Fig. 10-22) frequently occurs after intraocular surgery, penetrating ocular trauma, or inflammatory choroidal disorders.[28] Hemorrhagic choroidal detachment often occurs after a contusion, after a penetrating injury, or as a complication of intraocular surgery. Such detachment significantly influences the prognosis of the involved eye.[28] In these cases ophthalmoscopic visualization of the fundus may be precluded by hyphema (blood in the anterior chamber) or by vitreous hemorrhage. A- and B-scan ultrasound, although useful, has certain shortcomings when examining a traumatized eye in the presence of an opaque medium. Contact B-scan ultrasound can expel the intraocular contents, is not tolerated by a patient with a painful eye, and increases the risk of inflammation.[30] The A-scan, although less traumatic, is not often used, because it is time-consuming and its interpretation requires greater expertise. The water bath B-scan carries the risk of infection in an open wound.[31] Evaluating a postoperative choroidal detachment is difficult if air or gas is present in the vitreous cavity. Although CT is the method best suited for evaluating lacerated globes if no ferromagnetic for-

eign body is suspected, MRI is probably preferable to CT.

Ocular hypotony is the essential underlying cause of serous choroidal detachment.[28] Ocular hypotony may be the result of inflammatory diseases (uveitis, scleritis), accidental perforation of the eyeball, ocular surgery, or intensive glaucoma therapy.[23,28,29,32] The pressure within the suprachoroidal space is determined by the intraocular pressure, the intracapillary blood pressure, and the oncotic pressure exerted by the plasma protein colloids.[27]

The capillaries of the choriocapillaris differ from other capillary beds in the body[13] in that the choriocapillaris is a visceral type of vasculature with fenestrations in the vessels.[18] These openings are covered by diaphragms, which permit the relatively free exchange of material between the choriocapillaris and the surrounding tissues.[13] Ocular hypotony causes increased permeability of the choroidal capillaries. This increased permeability leads to the transudation of fluid from the choroidal vasculature into the uveal tissue and causes diffuse swelling of the entire choroid (choroidal effusion). As the edema of the choroid increases, fluid accumulates in the potential suprachoroidal space, resulting in serous or exudative choroidal detachment.[23,28,29] Choroidal effusion, like choroidal hematoma, may be preceded by surgery or other types of trauma to the eye.[33] In fact, choroidal effusion may be a common, al-

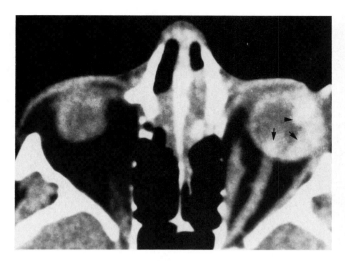

Fig. 10-23 Acute choroidal hemorrhage (detachment). CT scan shows choroidal hematomas *(arrows)*.

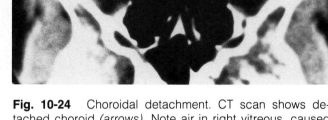

Fig. 10-24 Choroidal detachment. CT scan shows detached choroid *(arrows)*. Note air in right vitreous, caused by air-fluid exchange from detached choroid.

beit transient, occurrence after intraocular surgery.[34] Other causes of choroidal effusion include inflammatory disorders of the eyeball, myxedema, photocoagulation,[35] retinal cryopexy, Vogt-Koyanagi syndrome, Harada's syndrome, and uveal effusion syndrome.[36]

Clinically, the choroidal detachment appears as a smooth, grey-brown elevation of the choroid extending from the ciliary body to the posterior segment.[28,30] Even when the ocular media are clear in pigmented eyes, it is difficult to differentiate between a serous and a hemorrhagic choroidal detachment by ophthalmoscopy.[28,30] The appearance of a serous choroidal detachment on CT scans is that of a semilunar or ring-shaped area of variable attenuation. The degree of attenuation depends on the cause, but it is generally greater with the inflammatory disorders of the eyeball. Inflammatory diseases of the choroid (uveitis) seldom appear as a localized mounding of the choroid; rather, they generally produce a diffuse thickening with no localized area of mounding unless a choroidal abscess is present.[23]

A hemorrhagic choroidal detachment appears on a CT scan as a low or high moundlike image of high attenuation. The mound can be quite large and irregular (Fig. 10-23). In a fresh hemorrhagic choroidal detachment, the choroid and hemorrhage in the potential suprachoroidal space are both isodense. However, it may be possible to separate choroid and suprachoroidal fluid accumulations[28] in patients with chronic choroidal hematoma or a serosanguineous choroidal detachment (Fig. 10-24).

MRI is an excellent modality for evaluating the eye in patients with a choroidal detachment, particularly if ultrasound or CT, in conjunction with the clinical ex-

amination, have not provided sufficient information. The direct multiplanar imaging ability of MRI is very helpful, and MR imaging shows a choroidal hematoma as a focal, well-demarcated, lenticular mass in the wall of the eyeball (Fig. 10-25). This characteristic configuration usually does not change as the hematoma ages[29]; however, a decrease in the size of the choroidal hematoma may be observed. Occasionally several lesions may be seen (Fig. 10-25). The signal intensity of the choroidal hematoma depends on its age. Within the first 48 hours, the hematoma is isointense to slightly hypointense relative to the normal vitreous body on T_1W and PW MR images (Fig. 10-25, *A*), whereas it is markedly hypointense on T_2W images (Fig. 10-25, *B*). After 5 days its signal intensity characteristics change, becoming relatively hyperintense on T_1W and PW images (Fig. 10-26, *A*) but rather hypointense on T_2W images (Fig. 10-26, *B*).[4,23,29] At this stage the choroidal hematoma may be confused with a choroidal melanoma.[29] The hematoma usually continues to increase in signal intensity on T_1W, PW, and T_2W images (Fig. 10-26)[4,23,28] and by 2 weeks usually becomes markedly hyperintense on all MRI studies (Figs. 10-26 and 10-27).

A serous choroidal detachment (Figs. 10-28 and 10-29) and a choroidal effusion (Figs. 10-30 and 10-31) each have a different appearance on CT and MRI scans from that of a choroidal hematoma (see Figs. 10-23 and 10-25). Serous choroidal detachment is caused by a nonhemorrhagic accumulation of fluid in the suprachoroidal potential space. The choroidal detachment appears as a smooth elevation of the choroid (Figs. 10-28 and 10-29). The fluid in the suprachoroidal space is often hypodense on CT scans (Fig. 10-28), and its MRI appear-

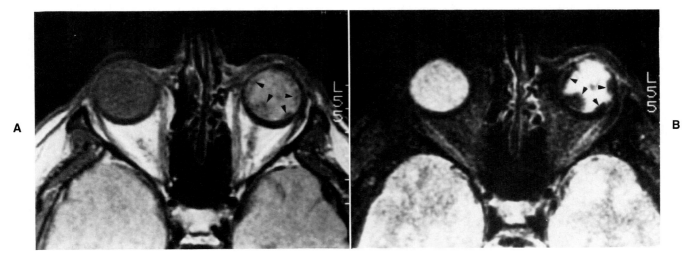

Fig. 10-25 Acute choroidal hemorrhage (detachment). **A,** PW MRI scan and **B,** T$_2$W MRI scan show choroidal hematomas *(arrowheads).* Increased intensity of left globe is probably caused by protein leaking into vitreous as a result of impaired retinal blood barrier.

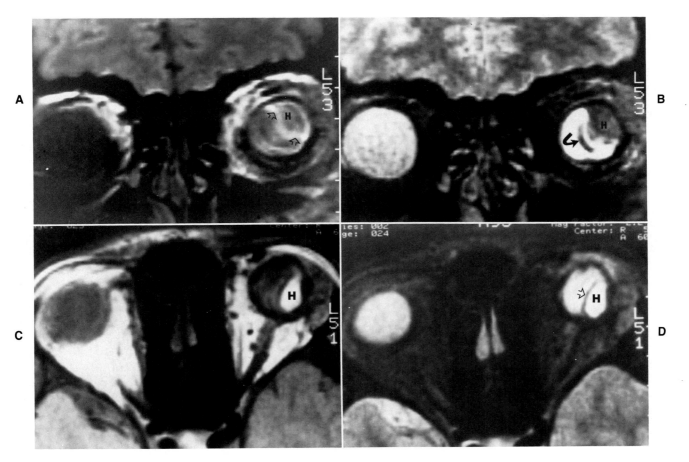

Fig. 10-26 Subacute and chronic hemorrhagic choroidal detachment. **A,** PW MRI scan shows choroidal hematoma *(H)* as area of mixed signal intensity. Peripheral part of hematoma is hyperintense *(arrows).* **B,** T$_2$W MRI scan shows choroidal hematoma *(H)* as hypointense image. Curved image *(curved arrow)* is thought to be caused by residual intravitreal silicone oil. **C,** PW and **D,** T$_2$W MRI scans obtained about 9 days after scans in **A** and **B** show that hematoma is markedly hyperintense.

ance is that of an exudate (Fig. 10-29). A choroidal effusion usually is seen as a crescentic or ring-shaped lesion on both CT scans[27] and MRI images[6,23,29] (Figs. 10-30 and 10-31). It does not resemble the lenticular appearance of a hematoma. Inflammatory choroidal effusions usually appear as increased signal intensity on all MRI images (Figs. 10-30 and 10-31). This high signal intensity is thought to be caused by the high protein content of the effusion fluid.[29] Posttraumatic effusions, although

also demonstrating increased signal on T_1W and T_2W images, are not as hyperintense as the inflammatory effusions.[29] A retinal detachment cannot always be differentiated from a choroidal detachment, because it may be impossible to distinguish between a choroidal effusion and a subretinal effusion.[23,29,30] However, because subretinal fluid shifts rapidly and suprachoroidal fluid shifts slowly,[6] rapidly shifting fluid within the wall of the eye, as demonstrated on either a CT or MRI scan, favors a retinal detachment.

Leukokoria

Leukokoria is a white, pink-white, or yellow-white pupillary reflex (cat's eye). It is a sign caused by any intraocular abnormality that reflects the incident light back through the pupil toward the observer. This reflection of light is the result of a white or light-colored intraocular mass, membrane, retinal detachment, or of a retinal storage disease.[25,37] The degree of leukokoria depends on the size, location, and pigmentation of the intraocular pathologic condition. When a child with leukokoria is being examined, the major diagnostic considerations are retinoblastoma, persistent hyperplastic primary vitreous (PHPV), retinopathy of prematurity (ROP), congenital cataract, Coats' disease, toxocariasis, total retinal detachment, and a variety of other nonspecific causes.

Leukokoria is the most common presenting sign of retinoblastoma, the highly malignant primary retinal cancer. Howard et al studied 500 consecutive patients in whom the diagnostic possiblity of retinoblastoma was raised.[38] Of these 500 patients, diagnoses other than retinoblastoma were made in 53% of the cases. Of 27

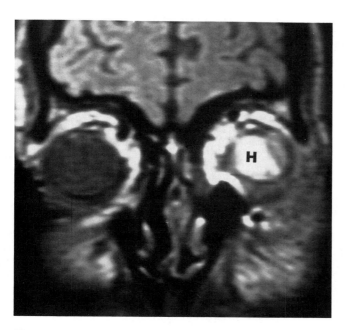

Fig. 10-27   Chronic hemorrhagic choroidal detachment. PW MRI scan shows hyperintense choroidal hematoma *(H)*.

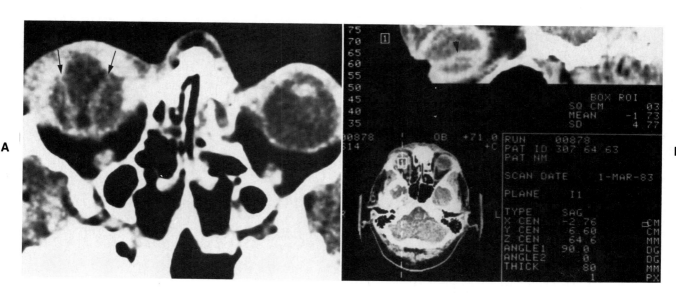

Fig. 10-28   Serous choroidal detachment. **A,** Axial CT scan and **B,** reformatted sagittal CT image show detached choroid *(arrows and arrowhead)*. Suprachoroidal space is isodense to vitreous compatible with serous fluid.

conditions, the most common was persistent hyperplastic primary vitreous (PHPV), followed by retinopathy of prematurity, posterior cataract, coloboma of the choroid or optic disc, uveitis, and larval granulomatosis. Prompt identification of the cause of the leukokoria is critical so that the appropriate treatment can be started immediately. Diagnostic accuracy is particularly important, because retinoblastoma is one of the few human cancers in which definitive treatment is carried out without a confirmed histopathologic diagnosis.[37]

Retinoblastoma

Retinoblastoma is the most common intraocular tumor of childhood. It is a highly malignant, primary retinal tumor that arises from neuroectodermal cells (the nuclear layer of the retina) that are destined to become retinal photoreceptors.[39,40-42] The manner of intraocular and extraocular extension, patterns of metastasis and recurrence, ocular complications, and associated malignancies make the diagnosis of retinoblastoma one of the most challenging problems of pediatric ophthalmology and radiology. Retinoblastoma must be differentiated from a host of benign lesions that simulate the disorder to assure that appropriate therapy is undertaken.[37] This diagnosis must be established rapidly to permit maximum ocular salvage and to minimize tumor-associated mortality.[37,43] When the disease extends beyond the eye, mortality approaches 100%.[43] With earlier diagnosis the 5-year survival rate is 92%.[44] Useful vision in the treated eye is attained in 90% of group I patients with a very favorable prognosis and overall in about 75% of eyes not enucleated.[44]

Retinoblastomas have been classified into five groups, with specific regard to the expected results of therapy. Group I includes tumors with a very favorable prognosis. These are either solitary tumors or multiple tumors of less than 4 disc diameters in size at or behind the equator. With group II lesions the prognosis is also favorable. This group includes tumors with one or several lesions measuring between 4 and 10 disc diame-

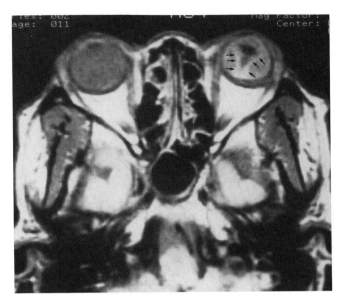

Fig. 10-29   Serous choroidal detachment. PW MRI scan shows kissing choroidal detachment *(arrows).* Suprachoroidal fluid is slightly hyperintense compared to normal right vitreous. Detached choroid *(arrows)* appears thick, and its hyperintensity is caused by accumulation of fluid in its interstitium.

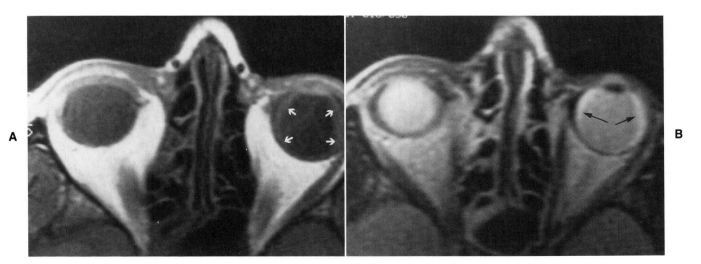

Fig. 10-30   Choroidal detachment. **A,** PW MRI scan and **B,** T$_2$W MRI scan show choroidal effusion of left eye as ring-shaped area of increased signal intensity *(arrows).*

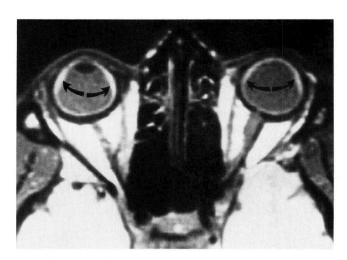

Fig. 10-31 Bilateral choroidal effusion. PW MRI scan shows bilateral ring-shaped areas of increased signal intensity *(arrows)*. This MR appearance may be difficult to differentiate from retinal detachment.

ters. Group III tumors are anterior to the equator, or a solitary tumor larger than 10 disc diameters is present. Group IV includes multiple tumors that extend up to the ora serrata. Group V includes tumors that involve half of the retina or in which vitreous seeds are also present. With group III lesions, the prognosis is doubtful; lesions in groups IV and V have unfavorable prognoses.

It is now well-known that retinoblastomas are derived from primitive embryonal retinal cells (either photoreceptor or neuronal retinal cells).[45] The tumor can be undifferentiated or well differentiated and may display evidence of photoreceptor differentiation in the form of Flexner-Wintersteiner rosettes and fleurettes.[39,40-42] The tumor is composed of small round or ovoid cells with scant cytoplasm and relatively large nuclei. The histologic features of retinoblastoma vary markedly. Some tumors display significant necrosis and prominent foci of calcification, and a few tumors show areas of glial differentiation.[42,46]

The occurrence of a second cancer arising outside the field of radiation was pointed out by Jensen and Miller[47] and by Abramson et al.[48] Abramson et al[48] demonstrated that patients with heritable retinoblastoma are highly susceptible to the development of other nonocular cancers, usually osteogenic sarcomas at sites of irradiation.

The worldwide incidence of retinoblastoma has been reported to be 1 in 18,000 to 30,000 live births.[49] The tumor is congenital in origin but is usually not recognized at birth.[50] Ocular involvement and metastasis may be present at birth. In the United States the average age of the child at diagnosis is 13 months.[51] In other countries the disease often is not detected until 4

years of age, when it is usually far advanced.[52] Over 90% of all diagnoses are made in children under 5 years of age. The sex distribution is equal,[53] and there is no preference for either the right or the left eye.[53]

Four types of retinoblastomas have been recognized: (1) those that are nonheritable and presumably caused by postzygotic retinoblast mutations[44]; (2) those that are inherited as an autosomal dominant trait; (3) those that are associated with the deletion of band 14 of the long arm of chromosome 13[54,55]; and (4) bilateral retinoblastoma and pinealoma (trilateral retinoblastoma).[55-58]

The tumor occurs in one eye in 66% to 75% of patients and in both eyes in 25% to 33%.[25,53] All patients with bilateral retinoblastoma harbor the germinal mutation.[53,55] Fifteen percent of patients with unilateral retinoblastoma also harbor the retinoblastoma gene.[53] Forty percent of retinoblastoma cases are hereditary.[59] However, 5% to 10% of the patients have a positive history of retinoblastoma.[53] A parent with bilateral retinoblastoma has about a 50% chance of passing retinoblastoma on to one child.[53] A parent with unilateral retinoblastoma has about a 50% chance of passing retinoblastoma on to one child if the tumor is truly unifocal.[53] When the parent's tumor is unifocal, about 15% of the children are affected.[53] Some affected children have been found to have an associated deletion of the long arm of chromosome 13 involving band 13q14.[60,61] The association between retinoblastoma and deletion of the q14 band of chromosome 13 j (13q14) has been convincingly documented.[60-63] Esterase D, an electrophoretically polymorphic human enzyme, has also been mapped to chromosomal band 13q14.[64] In several families with hereditary retinoblastoma without apparent chromosomal deletion, the gene for retinoblastoma has been shown to be closely linked to that for esterase D and assigned to chromose band 13q14.[64,65] Compilation of data from recent studies suggests an approximately 7% incidence of 13q-chromosomal deletion in patients with retinoblastoma.[66,67] Only a few of the patients with retinoblastoma have a sufficiently large chromosomal deletion to produce systemic dysmorphic features such as microcephaly, genital malformations, ear abnormalities, mental retardation, and toe and finger abnormalities.[67] Karyotype analysis of these children with congenital dysmorphic features may allow detection of chromosome 13 deletion involving band 13q14, prompting ophthalmic examination and therefore allowing early diagnosis of retinoblastoma.[67]

Trilateral Retinoblastoma. The occurrence of ectopic retinoblastoma in the pineal body or in a parasellar region (trilateral retinoblastoma) stemmed from reports by Jakobiec et al[56] and Bader et al.[57] The association of retinoblastoma-pinealoma suggests that these tumors may be related.[55] In addition to sharing a common neuroectodermal origin, it is well-known that in lower vertebrates the pineal gland has photoreceptor functions (similar to those seen in their retinas) and endocrine functions.[55] It is also well-known that the histologic appearance of retinoblastomas and pinealomas may be the same.[56,68] It is postulated that, because of their similar origin, the same mutations may be cancerogenic for both retinoblasts and pinealoblasts.[68]

Clinical Diagnosis. Retinoblastoma accounts for about 1% of all deaths from childhood cancer in the United States.[69] The diagnosis of retinoblastoma can usually be made by an ophthalmoscopic examination; however, detecting retinoblastoma and clinically differentiating it from a host of benign simulating lesions may be difficult.[20,24,70-72] The most common sign associated with retinoblastoma is leukokoria, which is present in 60% of patients.[53] Strabismus (deviation of the eye) is the second most common sign. Pain caused by secondary glaucoma, often with heterochromia (different colored irides), is the next most common sign leading to ophthalmologic evaluation. Ophthalmologic recognition of retinoblastoma is quite reliable. Small lesions are seen as gray-white intraretinal foci. Because of the difference in color from the surrounding retina and choroid, retinoblastomas can be seen when they are as small as 0.02 mm.[53] Other characteristic ophthalmoscopic findings include tumor calcification and vitreous seeding.

As tumors grow in size, they often assume a convex configuration and produce three forms of growth patterns: endophytic, exophytic, or diffuse. An endophytic retinoblastoma projects anteriorly, breaks through the internal limiting membrane of the retina, and grows into the vitreous. An exophytic retinoblastoma arises intraretinally and subsequently grows into the subretinal space, causing elevation of the retina.[37,72] With

growth of the tumor, associated exudation and in rare cases subretinal hemorrhage occur and a progressive retinal detachment develops. Exophytic tumors can simulate a traumatic retinal detachment on ophthalmoscopic examination. A diffuse retinoblastoma grows along the retina, appearing as a placoid mass. This diffuse form represents a perplexing diagnostic difficulty because it has an atypical ophthalmoscopic feature (which simulates inflammatory or hemorrhagic conditions), it characteristicly lacks calcification, and it usually occurs outside the typical age group of 3 to 4 years of age or younger.[37]

Diagnostic Imaging. Although ophthalmoscopic recognition of retinoblastoma is often reliable, imaging modalities should be used on all patients suspected of having a retinoblastoma to determine the presence of gross retrobulbar spread, intracranial metastasis, or a second tumor. In addition, imaging techniques may allow differentiation of retinoblastoma from lesions such as persistent hyperplastic primary vitreous, Coats' disease, retinopathy of prematurity, toxocariasis, retinal detachment, organized subretinal hemorrhage, organized vitreous, endophthalmitis, retinal dysplasia, retinal astrocytoma (hamartoma), retinal gliosis, myelinated nerve fibers, choroidal hemangioma, coloboma, morning glory anomaly, congenital cataract, choroidal osteoma, drusen of optic nerve head, and other so-called pseudogliomas and leukokorias. These lesions may have a clinical appearance similar to that of retinoblastoma. Ultrasonography, computed tomography, and magnetic resonance imaging are the most useful imaging techniques in the evaluation of these lesions.[25,37,69,72,73] The tumor and calcification can be diagnosed by ultrasonography. However, the accuracy of ultrasonography

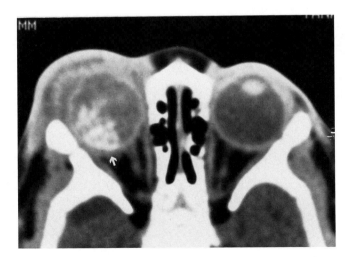

Fig. 10-32 Retinoblastoma. CT scan shows calcified mass *(arrows)* in right eye with involvement of eyelid and early invasion into Tenon's space *(arrow)*.

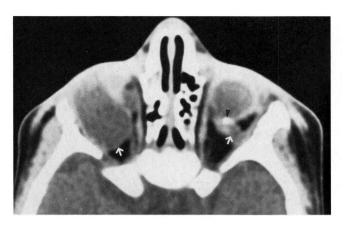

Fig. 10-33 Colobomatous cysts with calcification. CT scan shows bilateral microphthalmia with cysts *(white arrows)*. Note calcification *(arrowhead)*, most likely caused by dystrophic calcification within abnormal glial tissue.

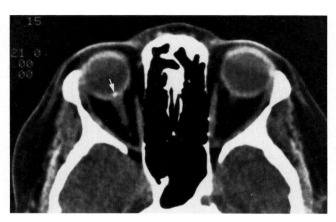

Fig. 10-34 Optic nerve head drusen. CT scan shows increased density at optic disc *(arrow)*.

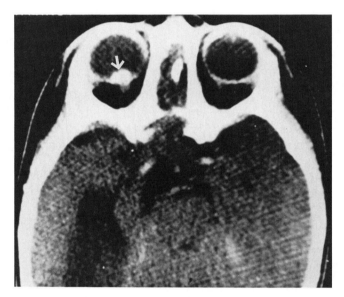

Fig. 10-35 Astrocytic hamartoma. CT scan shows mass *(arrow)* in posterior aspect of right eye.

for this condition is only 80%.[74] Diagnosis of tumor extension to the medial and lateral aspects of the orbit and extraocular extension is particularly limited with ultrasound.

High-resolution, thin section (1.5 mm) CT scanning can detect a tumor and calcification within it with a high degree of accuracy.[25,72,73] Over 90% of retinoblastomas show evidence of calcification on CT scan.[73] Cal-

cification may be small and single, large and single, multiple and punctate (Fig. 10-32), or appear as few to several fine speckled foci.[25] The deoxyribonucleic acid (DNA) released from necrotic cells in retinoblastoma has a propensity to form a DNA-calcium complex. It is the frequent presence of this calcified complex that allows the intraocular tumor to be identified by funduscopic, ultrasonic, and CT methods.[25,50,73,75] In the extraocular component of retinoblastoma, calcification is rarely present.[25] The presence of intraocular calcification in children under 3 years of age is highly suggestive of retinoblastoma.[25,73,75] None of the simulating lesions (except in patients with microphthalmos and colobomatous cyst [Fig. 10-33]) contain calcification in children (up to 3 years of age) in whom retinoblastoma is usually diagnosed (98% of cases present before 6 months of age). In children over 3 years of age, some of the simulating lesions, including retinal astrocytoma, retinopathy of prematurity, toxocariasis, and optic nerve head drusen (Fig. 10-34) can produce calcification.[25] The diffuse infiltrating form of retinoblastoma is rare and may have no calcification.[25,72]

Retinal astrocytoma (astrocytic hamartoma) initially may resemble retinoblastoma.[25,53] It may be present before any neurologic or dermatologic manifestations of tuberous sclerosis appear[25] (Fig. 10-35). The CT appearance of myelinated nerve fibers may also be similar to that of retinoblastoma.[25]

Magnetic Resonance Imaging. MRI has been used to evaluate retinoblastoma and other simulating lesions.[25,69,72,76,77] In the diagnosis of retinoblastoma, MRI is not as specific as CT scanning (Fig. 10-36) because of its lack of sensitivity in detecting calcification.

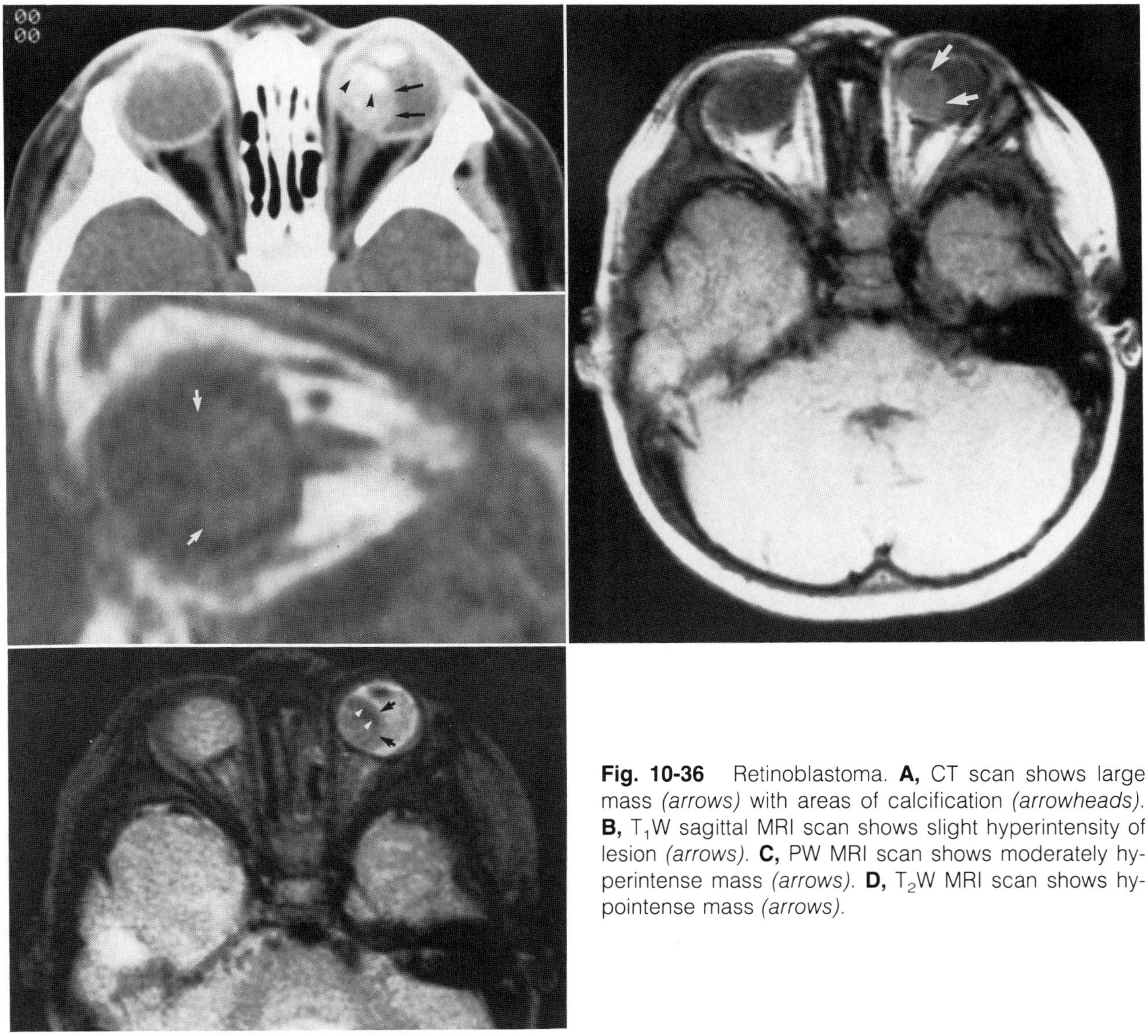

Fig. 10-36 Retinoblastoma. **A,** CT scan shows large mass *(arrows)* with areas of calcification *(arrowheads)*. **B,** T_1W sagittal MRI scan shows slight hyperintensity of lesion *(arrows)*. **C,** PW MRI scan shows moderately hyperintense mass *(arrows)*. **D,** T_2W MRI scan shows hypointense mass *(arrows)*.

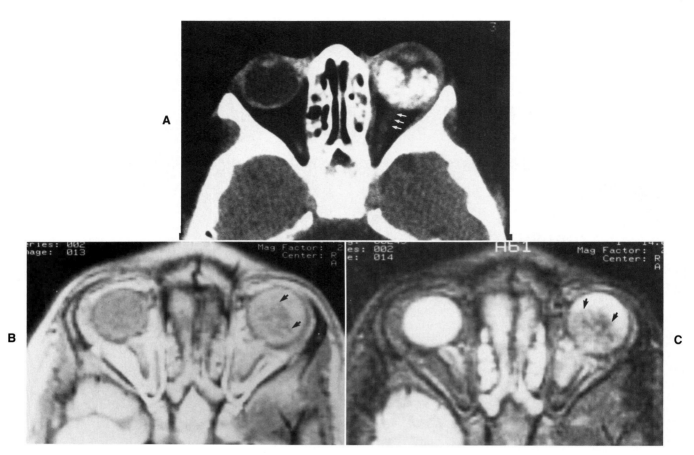

Fig. 10-37 Retinoblastoma. **A,** CT scan shows large calcified retinoblastoma of left eye. Note enlargement of optic nerve *(arrows),* caused by tumor involvement. **B,** PW MRI scan shows mass *(arrows)* being isodense relative to normal right vitreous chamber. **C,** T₂W MRI scan shows that mass is very hypointense *(arrows).*

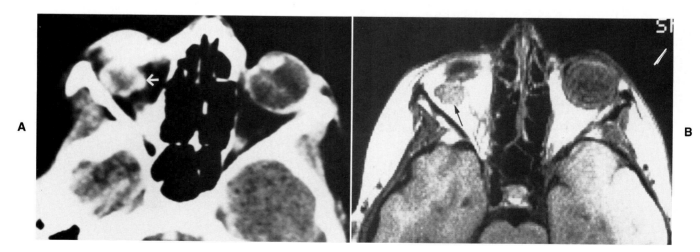

Fig. 10-38 Recurrent retinoblastoma. **A,** CT scan and **B,** T₁W MRI scan show recurrent disease *(arrow)* after enucleation. Note right false eye. (Courtesy Dr. G. Schullman.)

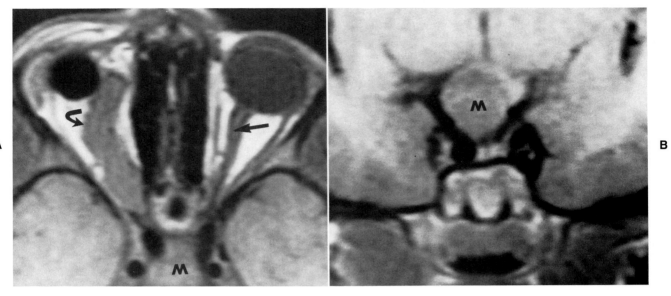

Fig. 10-39   Recurrent retinoblastoma. **A,** PW MRI scan shows right false eye and marked tumor along right optic nerve *(curved arrow).* Note normal left optic nerve *(arrow)* and tumor mass *(M)* in sellar region. **B,** Coronal PW MRI scan shows marked tumor mass *(M)* in sellar and suprasellar region.

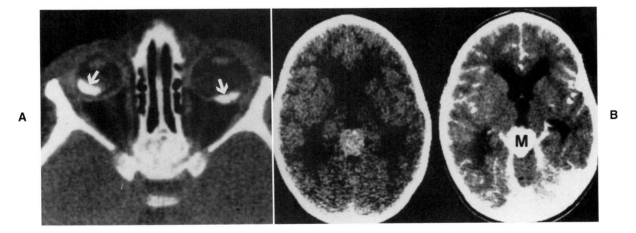

Fig. 10-40   Presumed trilateral retinoblastoma. **A,** CT scan shows bilateral calcified retinoblastomas *(arrows).* **B,** CT scans with and without contrast enhancement show large mass *(M)* in region of pineal gland with associated moderate hydrocephaly. This presumed pinealoma (retinoblastoma?) developed 2 years after external radiation to both eyes through lateral ports.

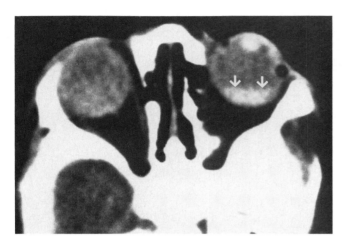

Fig. 10-41   PHPV. CT scan shows increase in density of both vitreous chambers with gravitational layering of high density fluid in left eye *(arrows)*. The high density fluid is most likely caused by blood in the subhyaloid space.

However, the MRI appearance of retinoblastoma may be specific enough to differentiate retinoblastoma from simulating lesions.[77,78] Retinoblastomas appear slightly or moderately hyperintense in relation to normal vitreous on T_1W (Fig. 10-36, *B*) and PW (Fig. 10-36, *C*) MRI scans. On T_2W MRI scans the tumors appear as areas of markedly (Fig. 10-36, *D*) to moderately (Fig. 10-37, *C*) low signal intensity. Tumors elevated 3 to 4 mm in height may not be definitely identified on MRI scans.[25,78] Lesions less than 3 mm in height are not recognized by present MRI technology. Calcifications on MRI scans may be seen as varied degrees of hypointensity in all pulse sequences (Fig. 10-37). In contrast to CT scanning, which is highly specific for calcification, MRI may be nonspecific. In many cases a calcification may not be recognized on MRI scans (Figs. 10-36, *B* and 10-37, *B*). In the diagnosis of retinoblastoma, CT is the study of choice because of its superior sensitivity for detecting calcifications; deposits as small as 2 mm can be reliably detected.[78] MRI, however, has superior contrast resolution and provides more information for the differentiation of leukokoric eyes.[78]

In a study of 27 patients with leukokoria, MRI in all retinoblastomas (17 cases) showed a mass.[78] These masses had a relatively short T_1 and short T_2. All retinoblastomas were seen as mildly to moderately hyperintense lesions on T_1W and PW MRI scans (Figs. 10-36

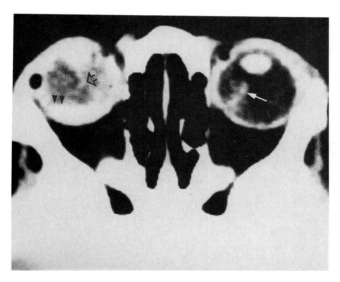

Fig. 10-42   PHPV. Noncontrast CT scan shows increased density of right vitreous with gravitational layering fluid *(arrowheads)*. Note triangular density *(hollow arrow)* posterior to right lens caused by persistence of primary vitreous (hyaloid vascular system). Left globe shows congenitally nonattached retina *(arrow)*.

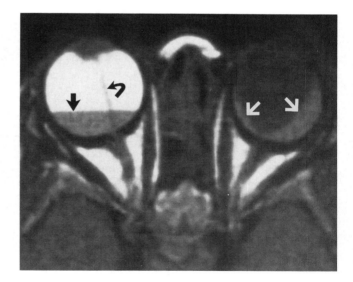

Fig. 10-43   PHPV. This 5-month-old girl was diagnosed as having Warburg's Syndrome (congenital oculocerebral disorder). T_1W MRI scan shows hyperintense subretinal fluid in left eye with detached retina *(arrows)*. Note fluid-fluid level in right vitreous *(solid arrow)*. This is thought to be caused by chronic (hyperintense) and acute (hypointense) hemorrhage in subhyaloid or subretinal space. Note tubular image *(curved arrow)*, which suggests congenital nonattached retina or Cloquet's canal.

and 10-37). This appearance is very similar to the MRI characteristics of uveal melanoma.[7,21] None of the patients with persistent hyperplastic primary vitreous, retinopathy of prematurity, Coats' disease, or toxocariasis demonstrated MRI characteristics similar to retinoblastomas.

In the study of eyes suspected of having retinoblastoma, the protocol includes plain CT of the eyes and MRI of the eyes and brain. Optic nerve involvement (Figs. 10-37, *B* and *C*), extracranial involvement (Figs. 10-38 and 10-39, *A*), and intracranial involvement (Figs. 10-39, *B* and 10-40) may be better evaluated by MRI than by CT scanning. Both techniques can detect the intraocular and extraocular lesions; however, MRI often gives more information in the differentiation of pathologic intraocular conditions responsible for leukokoria (Figs. 10-41 to 10-49) and other lesions such as medulloepithelioma and mesoectodermal leiomyoma.

Persistent Hyperplastic Primary Vitreous

Persistent hyperplastic primary vitreous (PHPV) is caused by the failure of the embryonic hyaloid vascular system to regress normally. The basic lesion is caused by a persistence of various portions of the primary vitreous and tunica vasculosa lentis with hyperplasia and extensive proliferation of the associated embryonic connective tissue.[20] In a study by Howard and Ellsworth[38] of 500 children with leukokoria, PHPV accounted for 51 of the 265 nonretinoblastoma cases. Howard and Ellsworth concluded that other than retinoblastoma, PHPV is the most frequent cause of leukokoria in childhood. The nosology of PHPV is extremely complex.[79,80] The ocular malformation can reflect either an isolated congenital defect or a manifestation of more extensive ocular or systemic involvement. The term PHPV, therefore, is a marked oversimplification that offers no etiologic precision and only the grossest of prognostic implications.[24]

The embryonic intraocular vascular system may be divided into two components: an anterior system in the region of the iris and a posterior (retrolental) component within the vitreous. The anterior system is composed of the pupillary membrane, which is formed by small vascular buds that grow inwardly to vascularize the iris mesoderm anterior to the lens.[81] The posterior system includes the main hyaloid artery, vasa hyaloidea propria, and tunica vasculosa lentis.[20,81] The first vessels to undergo regression are the vasa hyaloidea propria, followed by the tunica vasculosa lentis and eventually by the the main hyaloid artery.[11,14,20] During the first month of gestation, the space between the lens and the retina contains the primary vitreous. It consists of two parts: mesodermally derived tissue, including the hyaloid vessel and its branches, and a fibrillar meshwork of ectodermal origin.[81] In the second month of embryonic development, collagen fibers and a ground substance or gel component consisting of hyaluronic acid are produced. They form the secondary vitreous and begin to replace the vascular elements of the primary vitreous. By the 14th gestational week, the secondary vitreous begins to fill the vitreous cavity.[20,81] By the fifth to sixth month of development, the cavity of the eye is filled almost exclusively with the secondary vitreous, which represents the adult vitreous. The primary vitreous is thus reduced to a small central space, Cloquet's canal, which runs in an S-shaped course between the optic nerve head and the posterior surface of the lens.[14,20]

Clinical Diagnosis. Diagnosis of PHPV is often difficult because of its broad array of clinical manifestations,[24,79,82] etiologic heterogeneity, and frequently opaque ocular media.[24] Complete inspection of the interior of the eye may be precluded not only by cataract but also by vitreous hemorrhage or by opaque retrolental fibrovascular tissue. This condition usually manifests clinically as unilateral leukokoria in a microphthalmic eye. At birth the lens is clear with a white to pinkish fibrovascular mass behind it; later the lens usually becomes swollen and cataractous.[83] In the natural course of untreated PHPV, the eye often develops glaucoma and eventually buphthalmos or phthisis, sometimes leading to loss of the globe.[83] The clinical presentation of PHPV varies. Its main features include a unilateral (in rare cases bilateral) presentation, usually with leukokoria; microphthalmos; lens opacity; retinal detachment; and vitreous hemorrhage. In severe forms elongated ciliary processes, elongated radial iris vessels, shallow anterior chamber, and phthisis may occur. The diagnosis of the different types or causes of PHPV can sometimes be inferred from the family and birth histories, as well as from the details of the clinical examination.[24] Direct visualization of remnants of the fetal hyaloid vascular system offers the best evidence. Direct visualization, however, by ophthalmoscopy or microscopy is sometimes impossible because of the opaque media. In these circumstances indirect visualization by CT and MRI can be useful diagnostically.[20,24]

The CT findings of PHPV were first reported by Mafee[20] and Goldberg.[24] The maximum information derived from the use of CT is gained after use of intravenous contrast media and by repeating CT scanning in the lateral decubitus position.[20] The CT findings include the following: (1) microphthalmos is usually detectable, although it may be minimal or absent; other deformities in the globe configuration are also demonstrable even when undetectable by physical examination or ultrasonography[24]; (2) calcification is absent within or around the globe; (3) generalized increased density of the entire vitreous chamber may be visible (see Fig. 10-41), although minimally affected cases may

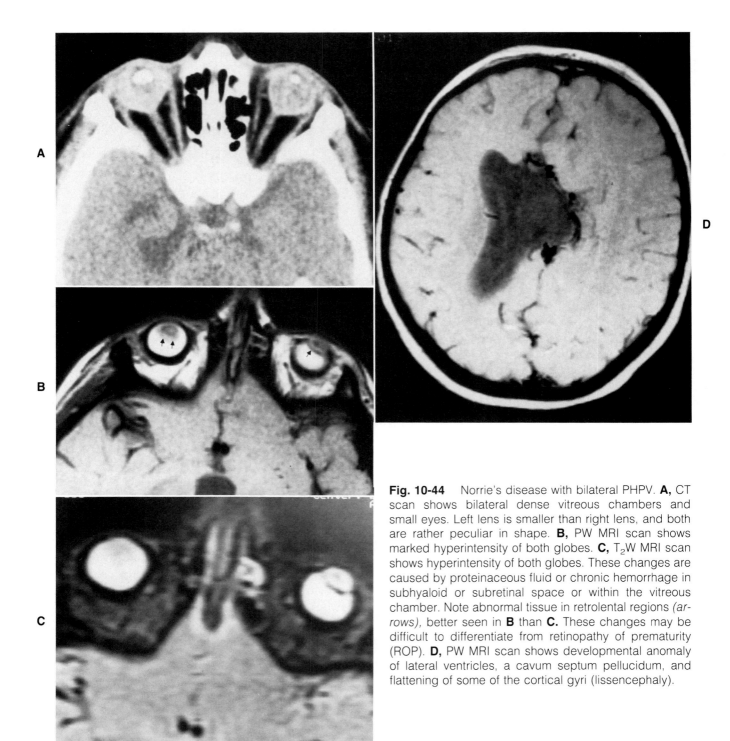

Fig. 10-44 Norrie's disease with bilateral PHPV. **A,** CT scan shows bilateral dense vitreous chambers and small eyes. Left lens is smaller than right lens, and both are rather peculiar in shape. **B,** PW MRI scan shows marked hyperintensity of both globes. **C,** T₂W MRI scan shows hyperintensity of both globes. These changes are caused by proteinaceous fluid or chronic hemorrhage in subhyaloid or subretinal space or within the vitreous chamber. Note abnormal tissue in retrolental regions (arrows), better seen in **B** than **C.** These changes may be difficult to differentiate from retinopathy of prematurity (ROP). **D,** PW MRI scan shows developmental anomaly of lateral ventricles, a cavum septum pellucidum, and flattening of some of the cortical gyri (lissencephaly).

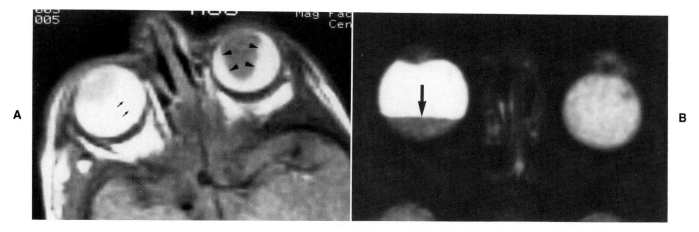

Fig. 10-45   Warburg's Syndrome. **A,** T$_1$W MRI scan shows subretinal effusion with detached retina *(arrows)* of left eye. Hyperintensity of right globe is caused by chronic hemorrhage in subhyaloid or subretinal space. Note congenitally nonattached retina or Cloquet's canal and abnormal retrolental soft tissue. **B,** T$_1$W MRI scan obtained 4 months later reveals progression of disease in both eyes with fluid-fluid level *(arrows)* caused by chronic (hyperintense) and acute (hypointense) hemorrhage in subhyaloid or subretinal space.

show normal attention values in the vitreous chambers; (4) enhancement of abnormal intravitreal tissue may be seen after intravenous administration of a contrast media; (5) the presence of tubular, cylindrical, triangular, or other discrete intravitreal densities suggests the persistence of fetal tissue along Cloquet's canal or the congenital nonattachment of the retina (see Figs. 10-42 and 10-43) (it is almost impossible to differentiate a hyaloid remnant from an organized retinal detachment[72]); (6) decubitus positioning may show a gravitational effect on a fluid level within the vitreous chamber (see Fig. 10-42, *B*), reflecting a serosanguineous fluid in either the subhyaloid space or the subretinal space; and (7) the lens may be small and irregular and the anterior chamber may be shallow.

Magnetic Resonance Imaging. The MRI appearances of the different of causes of PHPV may also be different. Early experience with MRI in patients with PHPV revealed marked hyperintensity of the vitreous chamber on T$_1$W, PW, and T$_2$W images.[23,25] In a patient with bilateral PHPV caused by Norrie's disease, MRI scanning revealed microphthalmos and hyperintense vitreous chambers on all pulse sequences (see Fig. 10-44).[23,25] In another patient with bilateral PHPV caused by Warburg's syndrome, MRI scanning revealed bilateral retinal detachment with hyperintensity of the subretinal fluid and layered blood in the vitreous chamber (see Fig. 10-45). The MRI appearance of retinopathy of prematurity may be identical to that of PHPV (see Fig. 10-46). The appearance of retinal detachment in PHPV has two forms: retinal elevation into the vitreous from the optic nerve, resembling acquired forms of retinal detachment (see Figs. 10-42 and 10-43), and retinal elevation from a point in the wall of the eye that was eccentric to the optic nerve, suggesting a falciform fold or congenital nonattachment of the retina (see Figs. 10-42 and 10-43).[24,79]

PHPV is often associated with severe malformations of the optic nerve and retina.[24] The ocular malformation usually reflects a manifestation of more extensive disease such as Norrie's disease, Warburg's syndrome, primary vitreoretinal dysplasia, or other congenital defects. Nonetheless, the clinical or imaging detection of PHPV alerts the clinician to the appropriate diagnostic and prognostic possibilities. CT and MRI scanning are certainly not indicated if the diagnosis and management of PHPV can be determined easily by conventional techniques. On the other hand, any procedure, including CT or MRI, that aids in the complex diagnostic and therapeutic decision-making that often is required for such affected children should be considered clinically useful and employed in these selected circumstances. In a CT study by Goldberg and Mafee[24] of eight children referred with several diagnoses, including retinoblastoma, congenital cataract, and microphthalmos, PHPV (which was not the initial diagnosis in any case) proved to be the most acceptable diagnosis for all patients, after collation of data from clinical examinations under anesthesia and from CT scanning. MRI provides even more information in the diagnosis of PHPV. In none of the patients with PHPV were we able to visualize the hypointensity (T$_2$-weighted) of the vitreous chamber mass that is characteristic of retinoblastoma (see Figs. 10-36, *D* and 10-37, *B*). However, a retinoblastoma is not always easily differentiated from PHPV by CT scanning.

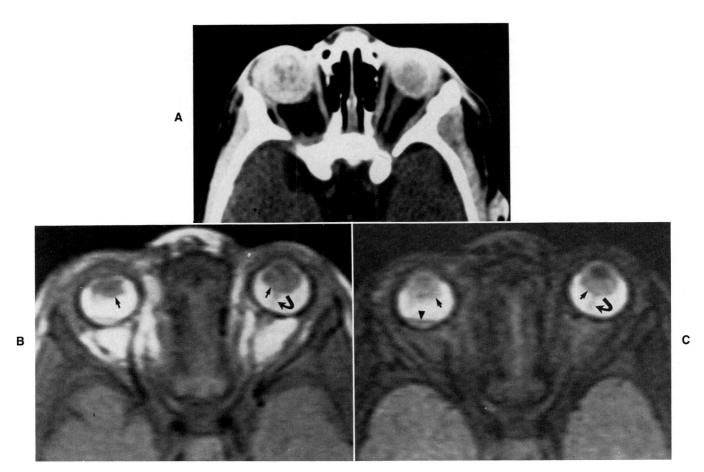

Fig. 10-46   Retinopathy of prematurity. **A,** CT scan shows increased density of globes and left microphthalmos. **B,** PW MRI scan shows hyperintensity of both globes, presumably caused by subretinal hemorrhage. Note retrolental abnormal tissues *(arrows)* and detached retina *(curved arrow)*. **C,** T$_2$W MRI scan shows hyperintensity of globes and abnormal retrolental soft tissues *(arrows)*. Note detached retina *(curved arrow)* and layered acute hemorrhage in right subretinal space *(arrowhead)*.

Norrie's Disease

Norrie's disease, or congenital progressive oculo-acoustico-cerebral degeneration, is a rare X-linked recessive syndrome of retinal malformation, deafness, and mental retardation and/or deterioration.[84] In 1927 Norrie described seven cases in two families with the same hereditary blindness.[85] In 1961 Warburg described the disease, coined the eponym Norrie's disease,[86] and later added the features of hearing loss and mental retardation, describing the disorder as "congenital progressive oculo-acoustico-cerebral degeneration."[87,88] Warburg established that Norrie's disease has an X-linked recessive pattern of inheritance, affecting only males, with completely unaffected female carriers.[87,88] Ophthalmologically, affected males exhibit ocular changes, including partial or complete retinal detachments, vitreoretinal hemorrhage (which can be present

in the early neonatal period[84]), retrolental mass, cataract, glaucoma, optic nerve atrophy, choroidal hypercellularity, and phthisis bulbi, which after varying periods of time leads to bilateral blindness.[84] Other findings include progressive high-tone sensorineural hearing loss,[87,89] congenital nystagmus,[84] mild to severe mental retardation, and psychotic symptoms.[84,87,89]

The pathogenesis of Norrie's disease is unknown. Warburg[88] postulated that the basic lesion is a genetically determined biochemical defect that causes a primary arrest in the development of the embryonic neuroectodermal structures of the retina, with consequent changes within the primary and secondary vitreous. Neuroectodermal changes also occur in the cerebral cortex.

Histopathologically, the early stage of the condition is characterized by the absence of retinal ganglion cells and of normal nerve fiber layer structures in the retina.[90] Most authors have been impressed with the similarity between Norrie's disease in its advanced stages and Coats' disease.[91] However, Apple et al[90] felt that in the earlier stages it was possible to differentiate between Norrie's disease and Coats' disease. Associated changes in Norrie's disease that may be present include optic nerve atrophy, atrophy of visual pathways, incomplete stratification of the brain cortex, and abnormalities of the brain.[87]

Diagnostic Imaging. The CT findings of Norrie's disease were first reported by Mafee[20] and Goldberg.[24] These findings include bilaterally dense vitreous chambers (see Fig. 10-44), a retrolental mass, retinal detachment, microphthalmia, optic nerve atrophy, a shallow anterior chamber, and a small lens.[25] There was no evidence of intraocular or extraocular calcification or of any gravitational layering of intravitreal fluid. The MRI findings of Norrie's disease include bilateral hyperintense vitreous caused by chronic vitreous or subretinal hemorrhage (see Fig. 10-44). Persistence of the primary vitreous may also be present, the optic nerves may be hypoplastic, and associated developmental anomalies of the brain may also be detected (see Fig. 10-44, *D*).

Warburg's Syndrome

Complex syndromes with congenital malformations of the central nervous system, microphthalmia, and congenital unilateral or bilateral retinal nonattachment have been described in a number of disorders such as Meckel syndrome,[92] a disorder with malformations of the central nervous system (including encephalocele), cleft palate, polydactyly, cysts of the liver and kidneys, genital malformations, and microphthalmia.

In 1971 Warburg[93] suggested that such patients might suffer from a nosologically distinct syndrome. She described an autosomal recessive disorder consisting of profound mental retardation with death in infancy, hydrocephaly, microphthalmia, and congenital nonattachment of the retina.[93] Subsequent postmortem studies[94,95] confirmed these clinical observations and noted the coexistence of lissencephaly in these patients.

In 1978 the syndrome was redescribed, and the mnemonic HARD±E was coined to point out the characteristic features: hydrocephaly, agyria, and retinal dysplasia (detachment) with or without encephalocele.[96] The HARD±E, or Warburg's, syndrome is a congenital oculocerebral disorder caused by a genetic defect that simultaneously affects ocular and cerebral embryogenesis and specifically involves the retina and the brain.[97] The syndrome emphasizes the developmental and morphologic similarities between the cerebral cortex and retina. It is characterized by congenital bilateral leukokoria.

The ophthalmic findings associated with this syndrome include microphthalmos and retinal dysplasia with congenital retinal nonattachment.[93,98] Associated anomalies may include vitreous hemorrhage, large intravitreal vessel, opaque retrolental tissue, persistent hyperplastic primary vitreous, and hypoplastic optic disc.[97] The lens may have a pear-shaped configuration because of a posterior bulge (posterior lenticonus).[97] Postmortem studies of the brain[94,95,97] attested to the poor growth of the cerebral hemispheres with disorganization and dysgenesis of the cerebral and cerebellar gray and white matter.[97]

Clinical Diagnosis. Microphthalmia and hydrocephaly may be seen in children with congenital toxoplasmosis, rubella syndrome, congenital syphilis, herpes and cytomegalic virus (CMV) infections. In toxoplasmosis characteristic chorioretinal scars may be present, and a positive serologic test for toxoplasmosis is very supportive evidence. The presence of significant serum antibody titers against rubella, CMV, herpes, and syphilis should serve to distinguish Warburg's syndrome from these simulating disease entities.

Diagnostic Imaging. The ocular CT and MRI findings in patients with Warburg's syndrome include bilateral retinal detachment (see Fig. 10-45, *A*), subretinal hemorrhage, vitreous hemorrhage, and gravitational intravitreal fluid (see Fig. 10-45, *B*). Persistence of the primary vitreous may also be present.[97] The congenital nonattached retina or the totally detached retina exhibits a characteristic narrow, funnel-shaped or triangular intravitreal image adjacent to Cloquet's canal (see Fig. 10-45, *B*).

Retinopathy of Prematurity (ROP) Retrolental Fibroplasia (RLF)

The essential feature of retinopathy of prematurity (ROP) appears to be prematurity. The smaller the infant, the greater the risk of developing this disease. ROP usually develops as a response to prolonged exposure to supplemental oxygen therapy. However, excessive oxygen may play only a participating role in the development of ROP. Eller et al[99] noticed that 14 patients had an associated persistent hyaloid vascular system, and a massive persistent hyaloid vascular system was found in seven of their patients. The authors concluded that ROP may be related to a combination of developmental and environmental factors that prevent normal retinal vasculogenesis outside the womb.

Ophthalmoscopic Picture. The ophthalmoscopic findings of ROP have been divided into active, regressive, and cicatricial phases.

Active Phase. The initial, or active, phase is characterized by arteriolar narrowing caused by a spastic response of the vessels to hyperoxia.[100] The vessels then start to dilate and become tortuous. The subsequent sign is the presence of a fine delicate neovascularization in the periphery. These changes are most marked in the temporal periphery, because this is the region where the retinal vascularization develops last. Commonly, as long as premature infants are in oxygen, there is no vascular dilation or tortuosity, both of which occur 24 to 48 hours after the infants are removed rapidly from the oxygen incubator.[101] Gradually, strands containing new vessels pass into the vitreous from the retina. There may be vitreous hemorrhage, and the retina may become detached. The detachment of the retina may become complete, and occasionally there may be massive vitreous hemorrhage.[101]

Regressive Phase. A characteristic of the disease is a tendency to show spontaneous regression during the early stage; the neovascularization and even a detachment of the retina may disappear.[101] However, the detached retina may not always become reattached. About 85% to 90% of cases show spontaneous regression.[101]

Cicatricial Phase. Finally, a dense membrane or a grey-white vascularized mass will be left as permanent evidence of the active phase. The lens always remains clear, and the retina is detached with associated retinal scars. The growth of the eye is often inhibited, with microphthalmus as the final outcome.

Diagnostic Imaging. The early stage of ROP may have no specific CT or MRI findings except that the eyes may be microphthalmic. In more advanced cases the differential CT and MRI diagnosis may be difficult between ROP (see Fig. 10-46), PHPV, retinoblastoma, endophthalitis,[101] or a number of pathologic conditions in which retinal detachment is a common feature.[6,98] The history of incubator treatment, the birth weight, bilaterality, and ophthalmoscopic, ultrasound, and CT findings are usually sufficient to establish the diagnosis. Calcification is rare in ROP but may be present in the more advanced stage. In the most advanced case of ROP, both eyes are microphthalmic with very shallow anterior chambers. Calcification in a microphthalmic eye is less in favor of retinoblastoma, although retinoblastoma rarely has been reported in microphthalmic eyes with and without ROP or PHPV.[6] ROP on occasion may resemble unilateral leukokoria; however, in most cases ROP appears as a bilateral but often markedly asymmetric disease.[82] A persistent hyaloid vascular system may be an associated finding in patients with ROP.[99] Recognition of a massive, persistent hyaloid vascular system on clinical, MRI, CT, or ultrasound examination is of prognostic importance. In these cases surgical dissection of the retrolental membrane in the presence of a persistent hyaloid vascular system is more difficult, because these vessels tend to bleed, and the retrolental membrane is tightly adherent to the detached retina.[99]

Coats' Disease

Coats' disease is a primary vascular anomaly of the retina characterized by idiopathic retinal telangiectasis and exudative retinal detachment (exudative retinopathy).[13,102-105] The condition occurs more frequently in juvenile males than in juvenile females. The condition is also seen in adults, and it is almost always unilateral.[13,102-104] The formation of retinal telangiectasia and the breakdown in the blood-retinal barrier at the telangiectasia are the essential underlying causes for the changes that occur in Coats' disease.[13] The blood-retinal barrier breakdown causes the leakage of the lipoproteinaceous exudate that accounts for the pathologic changes in Coats' disease. The primary cause for the telangiectasia, the leakage of serum and lipid, and the eventual closure of the retinal vessels in the area of the telangiectasia is unknown.[13] The degree of lipoproteinaceous subretinal exudation in Coats' disease appears to be proportional to the extent of the retinal telangiectasis.[106] Intraretinal or subretinal exudation, hemorrhages, lipid and fibrin deposition, phagocytic proliferation (ghost cells), and ultimately glial and fibrous tissue organization of the retina are the spectrum of pathologic changes in Coats' disease.[13] The vascular anomaly of Coats' disease, although present at birth, usually does not cause symptoms until the retina detaches and central vision is lost.[107]

The ophthalmoscopic findings in Coats' disease vary with the stages of progression. Telangiectasia can be observed in the early stages. In the later stages, when the retina is filled with and detached by a mass of cholesterol exudate (total bullous exudative retinal detachment), the telangiectasia can be seen only on fluorescein angiography.[13] In the early stage of the disease, when the retinal disease is not too extensive and the retinal detachment is shallow, photocoagulation, cryotherapy, or both usually obliterate the telangiectatic vessels and reduce or eliminate the exudative retinal detachment.[106] When there is extensive retinal telangiectasis and a total bullous exudative retinal detachment, cryotherapy and photocoagulation may not be sufficient to obliterate leaking vessels. Such eyes commonly progress to secondary angle closure or iris neovascularization, become blind, and become painful as a result of acute congestive (neovascular) glaucoma.[105,106]

Diagnostic Imaging. The ophthalmoscopic and biomicroscopic features of eyes with advanced Coats' disease may closely resemble findings in eyes with exophytic retinoblastoma and leukokoria.[108] It is important to distinguish retinoblastoma from Coats' disease since many eyes with advanced Coats' disease have been enucleated because retinoblastoma could not be excluded.[105] In a study at the Armed Forces Institute of Pathology,

62 eyes that satisfied the histologic diagnostic parameters of Coats' disease were researched. Chang et al[109] found that 52 eyes (84%) had been enucleated with the diagnosis of retinoblastoma or to rule out retinoblastoma. Coats' disease is almost always unilateral, and it usually appears in boys slightly older (4 to 8 years of age) than those who have retinoblastoma.[53] CT and MRI have proved to be very valuable in the diagnosis of Coats' disease.[25]

The CT and MRI findings in Coats' disease vary with the stages of progression of the disease. In the early stages both techniques may yield little information. In later stages retinal detachment accounts for all of the pathologic findings on CT and MRI scans. Sherman et al[107] reported two children with Coats' disease. They concluded that CT could not differentiate between Coats' disease and unilateral noncalcifying retinoblastoma. Haik et al[76] reported the CT findings in 14 patients with Coats' disease. A total retinal detachment (see Fig. 10-47) was routinely seen in advanced Coats' disease. Our experience with CT in patients with Coats' disease[25] would agree with those of Haik et al.[76] MRI is superior to CT in differentiating Coats' disease from retinoblastomas and other leukokoric eyes.[7,25,78] The subretinal exudation of Coats' disease is usually seen as a hyperintense image on T_1W, PW, and T_2W MRI scans (see Fig. 10-47, *A* and *B*). In retinoblastomas the MRI characteristically shows a mass that can be easily differentiated from associated subretinal exudate. The retinoblastoma is relatively hyperintense in T_1W and PW MRI scans (see Figs. 10-36, *B* and *C* and 10-37, *B*) and becomes hypointense in T_2W scans (see Figs. 10-36, *C* and 10-37, *C*). The subretinal fluid of associated retinal detachment will be seen as various degrees of hyperintensity in all pulse sequences. Although Coats' disease can produce a subretinal mass re-

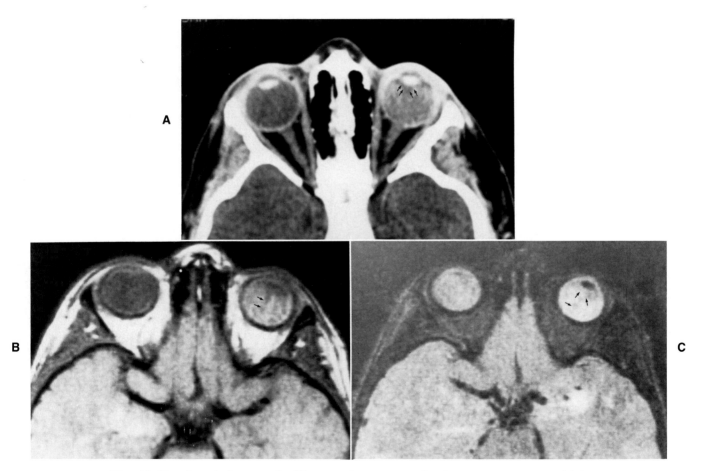

Fig. 10-47   Coats' disease. **A,** CT scan shows generalized increased density of left globe, caused by bullous retinal detachment. Leaves of detached retina are faintly seen, as shown by arrows. **B,** PW MRI scan shows hyperintensity of left globe caused by subretinal lipoproteinaceous effusion. Note leaves of detached retina *(arrows)*. **C,** T_2W MRI scan shows detached retina *(arrows)*.

sembling retinoblastoma, the mass in Coats' disease is caused by cholesterol, organized hemorrhage, and fibrosis and therefore is presumed to be inhomogeneous in signal character. We studied four patients with Coats' disease. In one patient the MRI findings were compatible with retinal detachment without the presence of an intraocular mass. The MRI findings in the other patients with early stages of the disease were normal.

In general, if an ophthalmologist suspects advanced Coats' disease but is uncertain as to the correct clinical diagnosis and is unable to rule out retinoblastoma conclusively, a diagnostic imaging study should be requested.[105] When retinoblastoma presents with what appears to be total retinal detachment, three other basic diagnoses should be considered: persistent hyperplastic primary vitreous (PHPV), Coats' disease, and retinopathy of prematurity (ROP). In the appropriate clinical setting, the MRI and CT findings of Coats' disease, PHPV, and ROP should be helpful in establishing a correct diagnosis.[6,25]

Ocular Toxocariasis (Sclerosing Endophthalmitis)

The granuloma of *Toxocara canis* is actually an eosinophilic abscess with the second-stage larva of *Toxocara* within the abscess.[53] The infection results from ingestion of eggs of the nematode *Toxocara canis*. In these patients the death of the larva results in a wide spectrum of intraocular inflammatory reactions,[110] the more severe of which has a characteristic pathologic appearance.[111,112] In most instances the anterior segment is uninvolved. A funnel-shaped retinal detachment is typically associated with an organized vitreous.[110] The histologic changes of the globe are characterized by an infiltration with lymphocytes, plasma cells, eosinophils,

and giant cells. Retinal, subretinal, and vitreous hemorrhages may occur frequently.

Remnants of the secondary larval stage of *Toxocara canis* are often difficult to find. The larva was present in 24 of 46 cases originally reported by Wilder.[111] In many cases the diagnosis of ocular nematode infection is presumptively based on the characteristic histopathologic features of sclerosing endophthalmitis. An enzyme-linked immunosorbent assay (ELISA) for *Toxocara* is now available that has sufficient specificity and sensitivity to be diagnostic.

Diagnostic Imaging. Margo et al[110] reported the CT findings in three cases of histopathologically proven sclerosing endophthalmitis. These findings consisted of

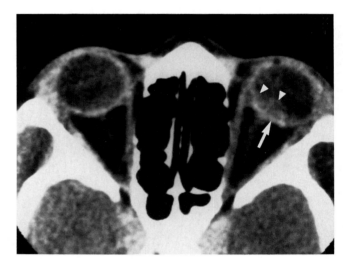

Fig. 10-48 Ocular toxocariasis. CT scan shows irregular, moderately enhancing mass *(arrowheads)* with irregularity of uveoscleral coat *(arrow)*.

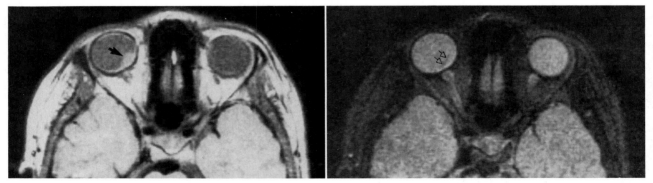

Fig. 10-49 Ocular toxocariasis. **A,** PW MRI scan and **B,** T₂W MRI scan show hyperintense mass *(black arrow)* with associated minimum subretinal effusion. Mass remains hyperintense in T₂W MRI scan, unlike retinoblastoma, which is almost always hypointense in T₂W scans. Note ill-defined image of hypointensity *(open arrows)*, which may represent scar tissue. Clinical and ophthalmologic findings were most compatible with granuloma of *Toxocara canis*.

a homogeneous intravitreal density that corresponded to detached retina, organized vitreous, and inflammatory subretinal exudate. These investigators concluded that the findings are similar to those seen in Coats' disease and noncalcified retinoblastoma. We reported[6,25,78] on three cases of toxocariasis in young adults that appeared on CT scans as a localized or diffuse, ill-defined mass with no significant enhancement (see Fig. 10-48). Clinical examination in these patients frequently shows vitreous, retinal, or choroidal signs of previous inflammation.[53] This inflammatory process (chronic abscess) is seen on CT scans as an irregularity of the uveoscleral coat with a diffuse or locally thickened, slightly enhanced uveoscleral coat. This CT appearance favors a diagnosis of *Toxocara canis* or other granulomatous disease of the globe and is caused by diffuse inflammatory infiltration of the choroid and sclera[6] (see Fig. 10-48).

In the appropriate clinical setting, the CT findings of the granuloma of *Toxocara canis* should be relied upon to establish a presumptive diagnosis of ocular toxocariasis.[6] MRI scanning has been reported to have the ability to detect the site of the larval granuloma.[72,76] The MRI scans of a patient with a presumptive diagnosis of toxocariasis are shown in Fig. 10-49. In general, the proteinaceous subretinal exudate produced by the inflammatory response to the larval infiltration is seen as a variable hyperintense image on T_1W, PW, and T_2W MRI scans. These MRI characteristics were found in two of our cases with suspected toxocariasis. Further studies are needed to establish the spectrum of MRI characteristics of this relatively uncommon ocular disease. It should be noted that the MRI appearance, as well as the CT appearance, of chronic retinal detach-

ment and organized vitreous may be difficult to differentiate from *Toxocara* granuloma, Coats' disease, ROP, PHPV, and retinoblastoma.[6,23,25]

Ocular Hamartoma

Although retinoblastoma constitutes the major life-threatening cause of leukokoria in children, a host of other simulating conditions (pseudogliomas) can cause diagnostic confusion.[20,38,110] In some cases of leukokoria, it is exceedingly difficult to exclude the possibility of retinoblastoma without having to resort to enucleation.[110] Retinal astrocytomas are rare tumors seen in patients with tuberous sclerosis and neurofibromatosis or as an isolated finding.[113] Early retinal astrocytoma (astrocytic hamartoma) may look exactly like early retinoblastoma (Fig. 10-50)[53] and may be present before any neurologic or dermatologic manifestations of tuberous sclerosis appear. These tumors may appear in the retina or in the optic nerve. The usual appearance is that of a single nodule or multiple nodules elevated 1 or 2 mm above the surface of the retina. At this stage CT and MRI cannot visualize the lesions. Tumors elevated more than 3 mm can be demonstrated by CT and MRI. The CT appearance of astrocytic hamartomas is similar to that of a retinoblastoma (see Fig. 10-50). If typical tuberous sclerosis features are not present, differentiating between astrocytic hamartomas and other ocular lesions may be very difficult. The CT appearance of myelinated nerve fiber also may be similar to retinoblastoma (Fig. 10-51).

Coloboma and Morning Glory Anomaly

A coloboma is a notch, gap, hole, or fissure, either congenital or acquired, in which a tissue or portion of a

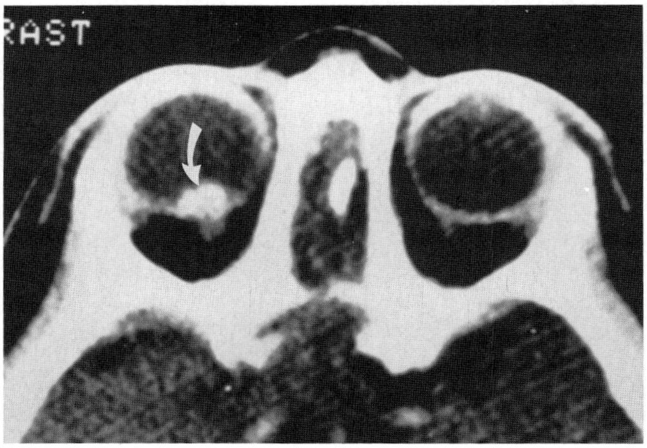

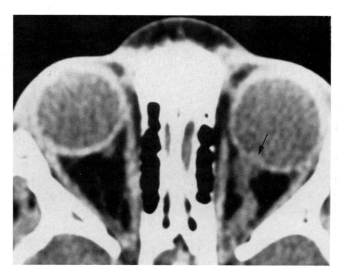

Fig. 10-50 Retinal astrocytic hamartoma. CT scan shows enhancing mass *(arrow)* at right optic disc.

Fig. 10-51 Myelinated nerve fiber (retinal gliosis). CT scan shows tortuous left optic nerve and soft tissue density at optic disc *(arrow)*.

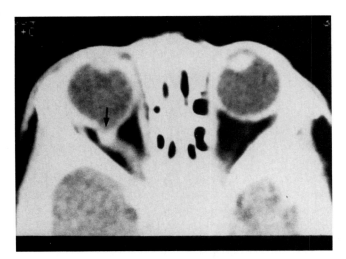

Fig. 10-52 Typical coloboma of optic disc. CT scan shows large posterior global defect *(arrow)* with optic disc excavation on right side. Defect appears surrounded by enhancing, deformed sclera and seems to have direct connection with vitreous body.

tissue is lacking. When examining a child with leukokoria, the major diagnostic considerations are retinoblastoma, congenital cataract, and a variety of other nonspecific causes of leukokoria, including coloboma of the choroid or optic disc.[38]

Three types of optic nerve colobomas occur[114-116]: isolated coloboma of the optic nerve, retinochoroidal coloboma, and Fuchs' coloboma. The congenital optic pit has also been considered by some[117] to be a coloboma of the optic nerve, as has the morning glory disc anomaly.[115] A variety of ocular and systemic abnormalities may be seen with an optic nerve coloboma.[115,116] For example, microphthalmos with a cyst is an anomaly in which an eye with a retinochoroidal coloboma has an associated cyst, which is usually attached to the inferior aspect of the globe.[118] Fuchs' coloboma (tilted disc syndrome, nasal fundus ectasia syndrome) involves a congenital, inferiorly tilted optic disc in conjunction with an inferonasal crescent or conus along the border of the disc in the direction of the tilt. Myopia and astigmatism accompany these changes.

Ophthalmoscopically, optic nerve colobomas characteristically show enlargement of the papillary areas with partial or total excavation of the disc. A brief review of the embryonic ocular derivation is important in understanding the origin of optic nerve colobomas. This is discussed on p. 768.

Isolated optic nerve colobomas arise only when the most superior end of the embryonic fissure fails to close.[115,116,119] Failure of other parts of the fissure to close causes iridic, lenticular, ciliary body, and retin-

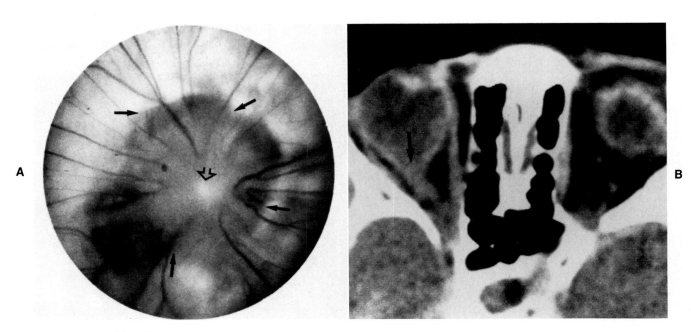

Fig. 10-53 Morning glory anomaly. **A,** Disc is enlarged *(solid arrows)* and has central core of white glial tissue *(open arrows)*. **B,** CT scan shows funnel-shaped deformity of posterior globe *(arrows)*.

ochoroidal colobomas.[120] The visual acuity in eyes with optic nerve colobomas varies and may range from normal to no light perception.[115] Nonrhegmatogenous or rhegmatogenous retinal detachment has been well described in association with optic nerve coloboma.[115,120] Optic nerve colobomas have been observed in association with ocular abnormalities, including a congenital optic pit, a cyst of optic nerve sheath, posterior lenticomas, and remnants of the hyaloid artery.[115,116] Systemic abnormalities, including cardiac defects, dysplastic ears, facial palsy, and transsphenoidal encephaloceles,[121] also have been reported in these patients.

Morning glory disc anomaly was first characterized by Kindler in 1970.[122] He described a unilateral congenital anomaly of the optic nerve head in 10 patients. Because of the similarity in appearance between the nerve head and a morning glory flower, he referred to

the anomaly as the morning glory syndrome. Ophthalmoscopically, the abnormal nerve head has several characteristic findings. The disc is enlarged and excavated and has a central core of white tissue. It is surrounded by an elevated annulus of light but also by variably pigmented subretinal tissue.

Diagnostic Imaging. The CT and MRI appearance of an optic disc coloboma includes a posterior global defect with optic disc excavation (Fig. 10-52). The CT and MRI appearance of the morning glory anomaly is quite characteristic (Fig. 10-53) and corresponds to its clinical appearance of a large, funnel-shaped disc.[116] The colobomatous cyst associated with coloboma of the optic disc can be easily identified on CT and MRI scans (Fig. 10-54). Any retroglobal cyst associated with a microphthalmic eye should be suspected of being a colobomatous cyst (Figs. 10-54 and 10-55).

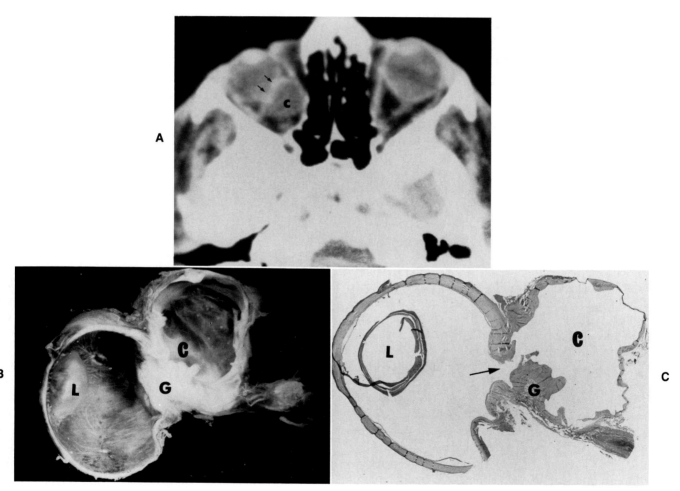

Fig. 10-54 Colobomatous cyst. **A,** CT scan shows bilateral microphthalmia and large cyst *(C)*, separated from right globe by band of enhancement *(arrows)*, which is related to abnormal gliotic tissue. **B,** Anatomic section of enucleated right eye. Note small eye, large colobomatous defect, abnormal white tissues, gliotic tissues *(G)*, and large cyst *(C)*. Note lens *(L)* and optic nerve. **C,** Histologic section of eye shows large retinochoroidal coloboma *(arrow)*, gliotic tissue *(G)*, cyst *(C)*, and lens *(L)*.

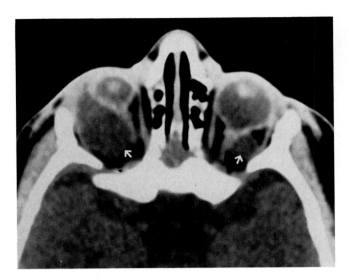

Fig. 10-55 Colobomatous cyst. CT scan shows microphthalmic eyes with large cysts *(arrows).*

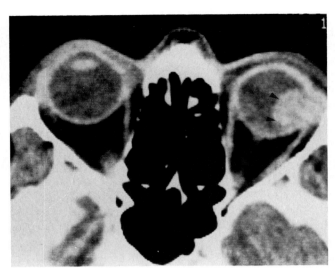

Fig. 10-56 Malignant melanoma of choroid. CT scan shows mushroom-shaped mass with increased density in temporal quadrant of left globe *(arrowheads).*

Malignant Uveal Melanoma

The uvea (iris, ciliary body) is derived from the mesoderm and neuroectoderm and may harbor tumors of both origins. Since it is the most highly vascular portion of the eyeball, it provides a suitable substrate for tumor cells. Most primary and metastatic ocular neoplasms involve the choroid, the most common being primary malignant melanoma.[123] Malignant melanomas of the uvea are unusual in blacks; the white-to-black ratio is about 15:1.[124] Those tumors involving the ciliary body and choroid are thought to originate from preexisting nevi.[123]

Callender's classification of melanotic lesions,[125] which is based on cellular features, offers the best indication of prognosis.[125] Spindle-A tumors are composed of spindle cells with elongated nuclei that characteristically lack nucleoli; these tumors have the best prognosis. Spindle-B tumors are composed of cells that have the same shape as those of spindle-A tumors but are slightly larger and have a nucleus containing a prominent nucleolus. Their prognosis is worse than that of spindle-A tumors. Epithelioid-cell tumors are composed of larger, more pleomorphic cells than spindle-cell tumors and carry the worst prognosis. Mixed-cell tumors are made up of both spindle and epithelioid cells.[123,126] Some tumors may be amelanotic, especially the amelanotic spindle-cell tumors.[126] The tumor initially grows flat within the choroid, then later elevates Bruch's membrane and finally ruptures through it so that the tumor assumes the characteristic mushroom shape, which grows toward the vitreous cavity. The retina over the surface of the tumor becomes elevated and detached (solid retinal detachment). This detachment gradually extends as a serous detachment over the slopes of the tumor.

Ophthalmoscopically, the lesion is seen as a circumscribed mass of varied pigmentation along with a solid retinal detachment. The retinal vessels over the surface of the mass are elevated. The retina usually is attached to the mass and does not float easily, as is seen in rhegmatogenous retinal detachments. If the tumor is not treated, secondary glaucoma may develop, and the tumor may eventually break through the eye into the retrobulbar region. Metastases occur primarily to the liver.

Management of clinically suspected choroidal melanomas has been the subject of increasing controversy in recent years.[127] Enucleation has been a standard treatment for more than a century.[128] However, enucleation has not been proved to prevent metastasis. Furthermore, Zimmerman et al have hypothesized a potentially harmful effect from intraoperative dissemination of tumor cells.[129] The controversy over the efficacy of enucleation remains unresolved.[127]

In general, relatively small choroidal melanomas (less than 10 mm in diameter and 3 mm in thickness) have a relatively favorable prognosis, with an 85% to 90% survival rate after 5 years.[130] Biologic aggressiveness has been judged by a clinically visible increase in the size of the tumor. Clinically stable choroidal melanomas are managed with longitudinal observations by clinical examination, echography, CT, and MRI and no other therapeutic procedures. Nevertheless, visibly stationary melanomas have been known to have considerable extraocular extension[131] and possibly even distant metastasis.[132] Furthermore, it has been suggested that tu-

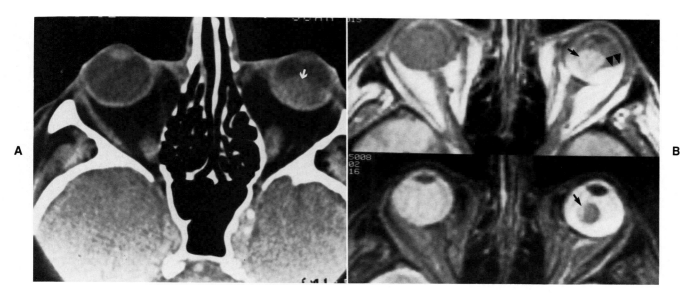

Fig. 10-57 Malignant melanoma of choroid. **A,** CT scan shows mass *(arrow)*. **B,** PW MRI scan *(top)* and T₂W MRI scan *(bottom)* show mass *(arrow)* and exudative retinal detachment *(arrowheads)*. Retinal detachment is better distinguished on MRI scans than on CT scan.

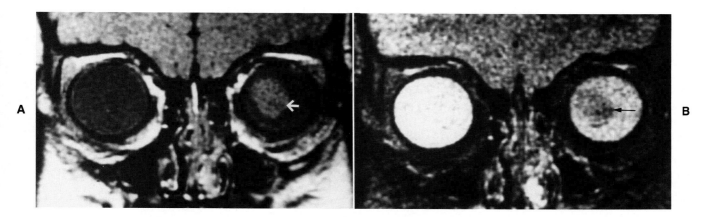

Fig. 10-58 Retinoblastoma. **A,** PW MRI scan and **B,** T₂W MRI scan show retinoblastoma *(arrows)*.

mor cell dissemination may occur early in the course of the disease, with distant metastasis appearing many years later.[133] Thus the clinical management of even small and relatively stable choroidal melanomas warrants careful consideration and the use of all reasonable clinical aids.[127]

If there is evidence of tumor growth, enucleation, local excision,[134] or other modes of therapy such as photocoagulation and radiation therapy are indicated.[130,134] Some advocate early enucleation of all melanomas to prevent metastasis.[133] Metastatic sites of primary uveal melanoma include the liver, lungs, bones, kidneys, and brain, in order of decreasing frequency.[127] A thorough search for metastasis is important to save the patient an unnecessary enucleation.

Diagnostic Imaging. Although uveal melanomas can be accurately diagnosed by ophthalmoscopy, fluorescein angiography, or ultrasonography, misdiagnosis continues to occur,[135] particularly when opaque media preclude direct visualization.[135-137] CT scanning has proved to be highly accurate in demonstrating uveal melanoma and a wide variety of pathologic conditions.[21] In addition, dynamic CT can provide information about the vascularity and perfusion of intraocular lesions and can help distinguish uveal melanomas from other lesions such as choroidal hemangiomas.[21] A uveal melanoma usually is seen on CT scans as an elevated, hyperdense, sharply marginated lesion (Figs. 10-56 and 10-57, *A*).

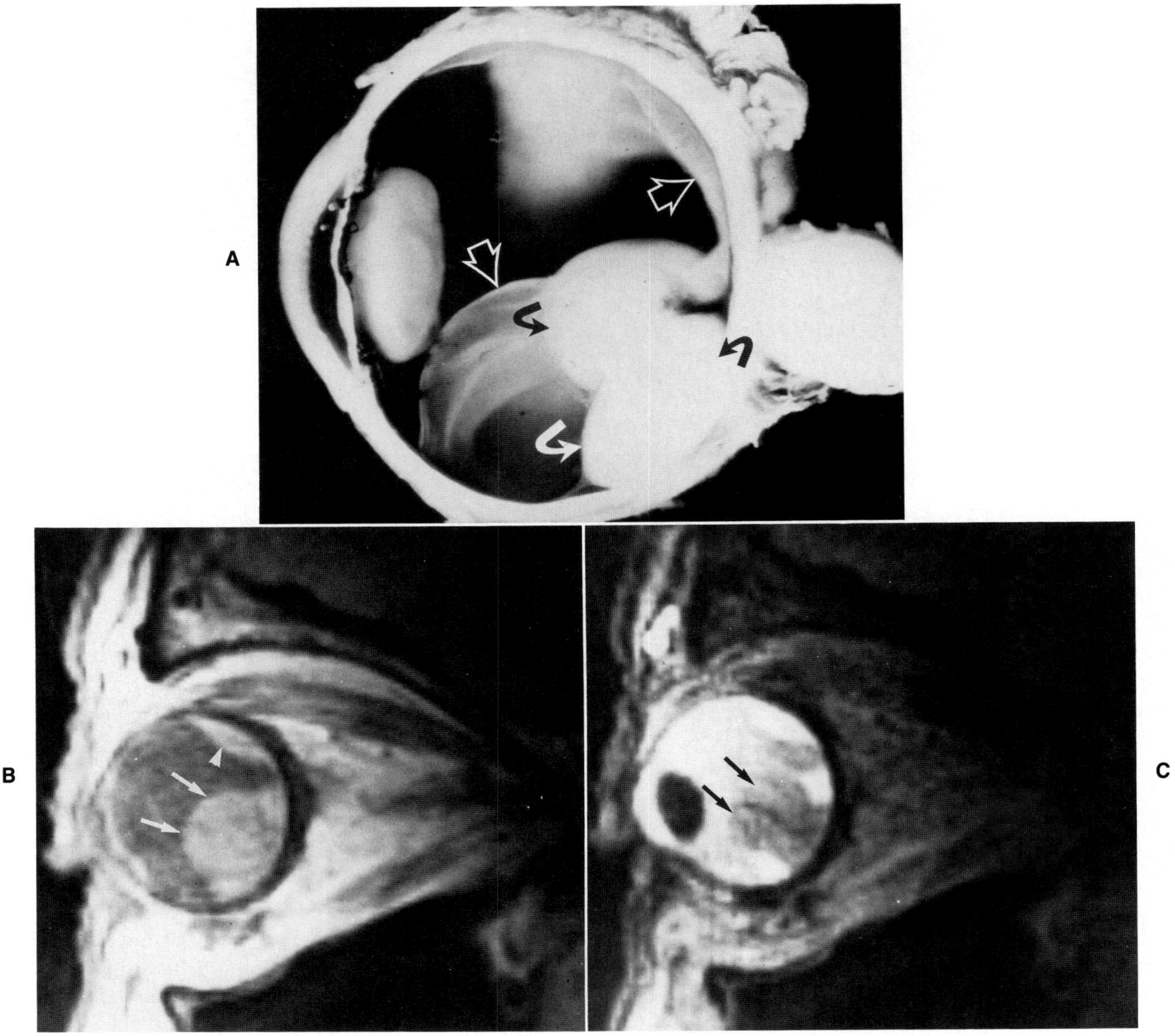

Fig. 10-59 Malignant uveal melanoma. Macroscopic section showing mushroom-shaped melanoma *(curved arrows)* and detached retina *(open arrows).* **B,** PW MRI scan of another patient shows hyperintense mass *(arrows)* and retinal detachment *(arrowhead).* **C,** T$_2$W MRI scan shows mushroom-shaped hypointense melanoma *(arrows).* Subretinal effusion remains hyperintense.

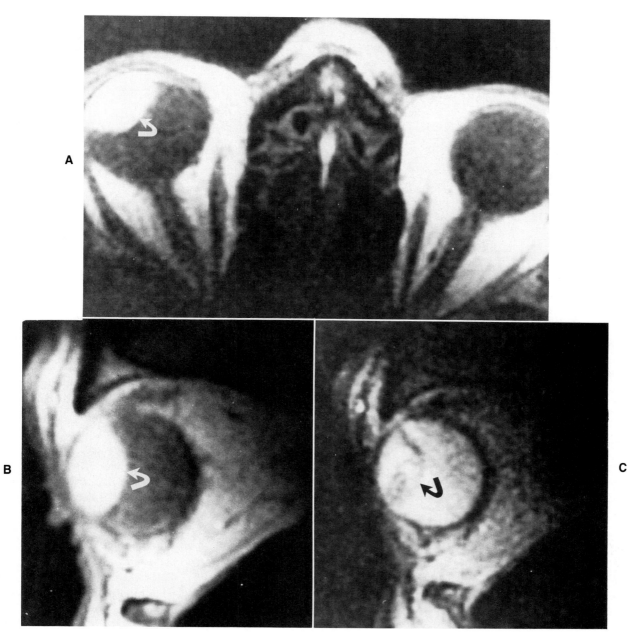

Fig. 10-60   Malignant uveal melanoma. **A,** T$_1$W MRI scan shows hyperintense mass *(arrow)*. **B,** Sagittal PW MRI scan shows hyperintense mass *(arrow)*. **C,** Sagittal T$_2$W MRI scan shows mixed signal appearance of lesion *(arrow)*. Anterior portion is hyperintense because of necrosis or hemorrhage.

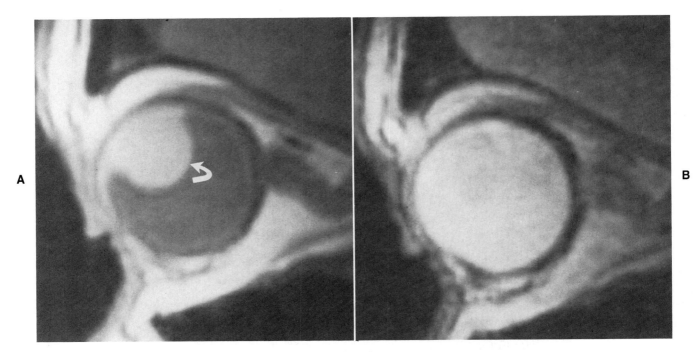

Fig. 10-61   Malignant uveal melanoma. **A,** PW MRI scan and **B,** T$_2$W MRI scan show mass *(arrow),* which is better seen in PW MRI scan. The lesion remains slightly hypointense in T$_2$W MR scan.

MRI has been used to diagnose intraocular lesions.[5,29,138,139] On T$_1$W and PW MRI scans, uveal melanomas are seen as areas of moderately high signal (greater signal intensity than vitreous) (Fig. 10-57, *B,* top). On T$_2$W images, melanomas are seen as areas of moderately low signal (lesser intensity than vitreous) (Fig. 10-57, *B,* bottom). These MRI characteristics of uveal melanomas are very similar to those of retinoblastomas (Fig. 10-58). Associated retinal detachment is better visualized by MR imaging than by CT scanning (see Fig. 10-57). Exudative retinal detachment is usually depicted on MR images as a dependent area of moderate to very high intensity in T$_1$W, PW, and T$_2$W images (see Figs. 10-57, *B* and 10-59). Total retinal detachment may be present. Chronic retinal detachment and hemorrhagic subretinal fluid have varied MRI appearances.

A uveal melanoma usually appears as a well-defined, solid mass (Fig. 10-60). At times atypical features of ocular melanoma may be present. When necrotic or hemorrhagic foci are present within the uveal melanoma, the inhomogeneity present within the tumor can cause diagnostic problems (Fig. 10-60). Some melanomas may be seen better in T$_1$W MR images (Fig. 10-61). Discoid melanomas or ring melanomas may not be detected on sectional imaging if they are flat. Organized subretinal exudate with or without associated hemorrhage may have MRI characteristics similar to those of uveal melanomas (Fig. 10-62). Invasion of the sclera, extension of the tumor into the optic disc and Tenon's capsule, and extraocular invasion are easily detected by MRI (Fig. 10-63).

Choroidal lesions elevated more than 3 mm usually are well visualized on MRI scans. Any lesion less than 3 mm is better studied with ultrasound.[21] The MRI characteristics of melanotic lesions are believed to be related to the paramagnetic properties of melanin.[140] Damadian et al reported that, unlike other tumors, melanomas have short T$_1$ values, which the authors attributed to paramagnetic proton relaxation by stable radicals in melanin.[140] Electron spin-resonance studies have shown that melanin produces a stable free radical signal under all known conditions.[141] These stable radicals cause a proton relaxation enhancement that shortens both T$_1$ and T$_2$ relaxation time values. Uveal melanomas, therefore, are rather unique among malignant tumors in that both T$_1$ and T$_2$ relaxation values are relatively shortened, owing to the paramagnetic property of melanin.[4,7,141]

Differential Diagnosis. A number of benign and malignant lesions of the eye may be confused with malignant uveal melanomas. The main fundal conditions that may be mistaken for a malignant uveal melanoma include metastatic tumors, choroidal detachment, choroidal nevi, choroidal hemangioma, choroidal cyst, neurofibroma and schwannoma of the uvea, leiomyoma, adenoma, medulloepithelioma, retinal detachment, and disciform degeneration of the macula.[4,21,101]

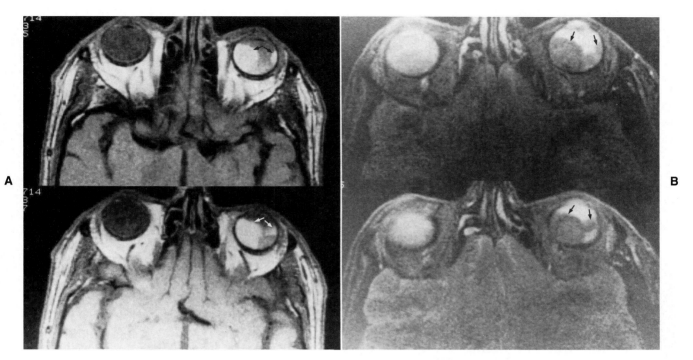

Fig. 10-62   Malignant uveal melanoma and postradiation retinal detachment simulating recurrent tumor. **A,** PW MRI scans show hyperintense masses *(arrows).* **B,** T_2W MRI scans show hypointense masses *(arrows).* Eye was enucleated, and masses were found to be caused by highly proteinaceous, organized subretinal fluid with some degree of hemorrhage as well. Uveal melanoma was seen as small, partially necrotic lesion. The MRI appearance of these subretinal changes is identical to MRI characteristics of melanotic lesions. Therefore, caution must be exercised in MRI interpretation of intraocular lesions. When highly proteinaceous lesions are present, such as in this case or in the case of mucin-producing metastatic adenocarcinoma, MRI may not differentiate them from uveal melanomas.

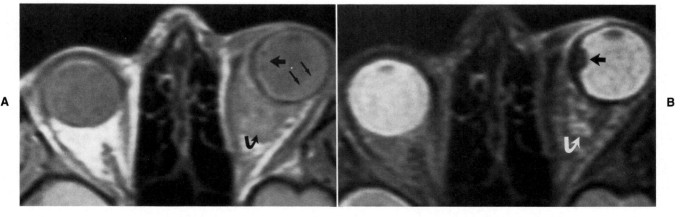

Fig. 10-63   Uveal melanoma with massive retrobulbar extension. **A,** PW MRI scan and **B,** T_2W MRI scan show uveal melanoma *(large arrow),* subretinal fluid *(small arrows),* and massive extraocular tumor extension *(curved arrow).*

Uveal Metastasis

On sectional imaging and clinically, uveal metastasis can be confused with uveal melanoma. Metastatic lesions of the uvea grow chiefly in the plane of the choroid and produce relatively little thickening of the uvea. Unlike uveal melanomas, which tend to form a protuberant mass, metastatic lesions often have a mottled appearance and diffuse outline.[101] The malignant cells (emboli) gain access to the eye via the bloodstream by means of the short posterior ciliary arteries, and this may be the reason why the site of most metastases is in the posterior half of the eye. The most common source of secondary carcinoma within the eye is from the breast or lung. Tumor metastasis may occur in both retina and choroid, both eyes being affected in about one third of the cases.[101] Unlike uveal metastasis, bilateral

uveal melanomas are rare. Metastatic growth in the retina is rare, with carcinoma of the pancreas and stomach probably being the most common primaries to have metastatic growths in the retina.[101] Uveal metastasis may be difficult to differentiate from uveal melanomas on CT scans.[21] A case with presumed bilateral ocular metastasis from a primary carcinoma of the prostate that demonstrated marked calcification is shown in Fig. 10-64. MRI has been shown to be superior to CT in differentiating uveal metastasis from uveal melanoma.[4] In our series, MRI in a patient with known metastatic breast carcinoma showed a hyperintense area on T_1W MR images that remained hyperintense on T_2W images. Metastatic lesions to the choroid may lead rapidly to prominent and widespread detachment of the retina[101] or choroid. In these cases a mottled MRI appearance and diffuse outline of the ocular coats help differentiate these lesions from uveal melanomas. At times uveal metastasis may not be distinct from uveal melanoma on MRI scans (Fig. 10-65). A mucin-producing metastatic lesion (adenocarcinoma) may also simulate a uveal melanoma, because the carcinoma's proteinaceous fluid tends to decrease the T_1 and T_2 relaxation times of the lesion.[5]

Choroidal Nevus

Choroidal nevi are congenital lesions, usually recognized late in the first decade of life and most frequently located in the posterior third of the choroid.[142] They appear clinically as flat or minimally elevated slate gray choroidal masses with slightly indistinct margins. The color of these lesions depends largely on the composition of the cell types within the nevus. Occasionally, choroidal nevi may be associated with a shallow serous retinal detachment with or without subretinal neovascularization.[134,142-144] Involvement of the macula may result in visual field defects, with decreased vision.[145] Under such circumstances a choroidal nevus may simu-

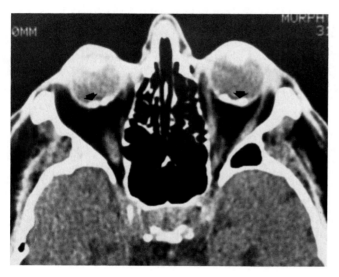

Fig. 10-64 Choroidal metastasis. CT scan shows presumed bilateral calcified choroidal metastases *(arrows)* from primary prostatic carcinoma. Ophthalmoscopic findings were most compatible with bilateral metastasis.

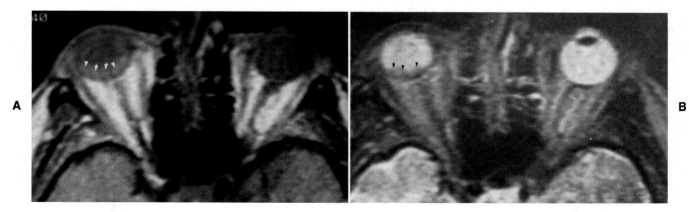

Fig. 10-65 Choroidal metastasis. **A,** PW MRI scan shows hyperintense lesion *(arrows)* consistent with ophthalmoscopic finding of choroidal metastasis. Note irregularity of lesion's surface. **B,** Lesion remained hyperintense in T_2W MRI scans.

late a choroidal melanoma, both ophthalmoscopically and angiographically. In fact, the choroidal nevus is one of the most commonly misdiagnosed lesions to be enucleated under the misdiagnosis of malignant melanoma.[108,136,137] It is sometimes extremely difficult to differentiate these two lesions, with long-term follow-up being the only possible solution.[145]

Diagnostic Imaging. Several patients have been examined by CT and MRI in whom a uveal nevus was considered the likely diagnosis upon ophthalmoscopic examination. In most cases the lesion could not be visualized because of the small size of the nevus. Most uveal nevi are less than 2 mm in size. In our series we were able to visualize one on CT and another on CT and MRI. The CT and MRI appearances of both were identical to those of a uveal melanoma. Both patients underwent an internal eye wall resection of the lesion. The histopathologic study revealed a diagnosis of a choroidal nevus. These two cases emphasize the inability of CT and MRI to differentiate uveal nevi from uveal melanomas. Internal eye wall resection may now provide an alternative approach to enucleation for suspicious lesions near the posterior pole, with the advantage of preserving the globe.

Choroidal and Retinal Hemangiomas

Choroidal hemangiomas usually are seen in association with Sturge-Weber disease (encephalotrigeminal syndrome). Retinal angiomas (angiomatosis retinae), on the other hand, are seen in patients with von Hippel-Lindau disease. The diagnosis of choroidal hemangiomas on clinical grounds presents some difficulty. In most cases the lesion was discovered in the course of a pathologic examination, and where an ophthalmoscopic examination had been made, the tumor was concealed by the detachment of the retina.[101] Conversely, the diagnosis of angiomatosis retinae of von Hippel-Lindau depends chiefly on the ophthalmoscopic appearance. Sturge-Weber disease and von Hippel-Lindau disease belong to the general class of disorders referred to as phakomatoses. The major syndromes include neurofibromatosis, tuberous sclerosis (Bourneville's disease), encephalotrigeminal syndrome (Sturge-Weber disease), cerebelloretinal hemangioblastomatosis (von Hippel-Lindau disease), and ataxia telangiectasia (Louis-Bar syndrome).

Sturge-Weber disease consists of capillary or cavernous hemangiomas with the cutaneous distribution of the trigeminal nerve and of predominantly venous hemangiomas of the leptomeninges.[146] The intracranial and cutaneous lesions may occur separately. The most familiar manifestation takes the form of the port-wine stain or capillary nevus of the face, which varies in extent and sometimes is limited to the skin of the eyelids and conjunctiva. The eye changes usually are ipsilateral to the changes elsewhere but may be bilateral and may be found without any surface angiomas. The ophthalmic changes consist of an angioma of the choroid, of buphthalmos, or of chronic glaucoma with atrophy and cupping of the optic nerve.[101] The glaucoma may be explained by the angiomatous changes in the ciliary body or angle of the anterior chamber.

Angiomatosis retinae and von Hippel-Lindau disease are interchangeable names for the phakoma of the retinal angioma.[13] This syndrome consists of a vascular malformation of the retina and cerebellum. The retinal lesion usually has the characteristics of a malformation; the cerebellar lesion consists of a slowly growing cystic tumor. The cerebellar lesions may be multiple and associated with one or more spinal hemangioblastomas. Von Hippel described the ocular changes in 1885 from the clinical perspective and in 1911 from the pathologic aspects. In 1926 Lindau described the frequent occurrence of von Hippel's medullary and spinal cord angiomas, with angiomas or cysts of the pancreas, liver, kidney, adrenals, epididymis, and ovaries.[13] This combination has been recognized as von Hippel-Lindau disease. Not all patients have a retinal lesion, the von Hippel part of the disease. Both eyes are affected in about 50% of cases.[101] Twenty-five percent of patients with retinal angiomas manifest systemic involvement.[13] Retinal angiomas are present at birth as hamartomatous collections of small nests of angioblastic and astroglial rest cells, but it is not until the second or third decade of life that an angioma grows sufficiently large to be detected clinically.[13] Among conditions that must be considered in the differential diagnosis of angiomatosis retinae of von Hippel-Lindau are Eales' disease, Coats' disease, multiple retinal aneurysm (Leber's disease), and capillary angiectasis of the retina.[13,101] Eales' disease, or retinal periphlebitis, occurs in young men (15 to 35 years of age) and is characterized by the vessel sheating in the retina and vitreous hemorrhage. The retinal veins show sheating with exudates, hemorrhage, and vasoproliferation.[101] There are recurrent vitreous hemorrhages from the affected veins.

Diagnostic Imaging. Although uveal hemangiomas can usually be diagnosed by ophthalmoscopy, fluorescein angiography, or ultrasound, this is a lesion that may present some difficulty in clinical diagnosis.[101] A choroidal hemangioma is seen on noncontrast CT scans as an ill-defined mass (Fig. 10-66, A) that demonstrates marked enhancement on contrast-infusion (Fig. 10-66, B and C) and dynamic CT scans (Fig. 10-66, D). In some cases the choroidal angioma may be concealed by the detachment of the retina (Fig. 10-66, C and D). On MRI, a choroidal hemangioma may be seen as a hypointense area on T_1-weighted images (Fig. 10-66, E) and as a hyperintense area on T_2-weighted images (Fig. 10-66, F). Some choroidal hemangiomas are seen as

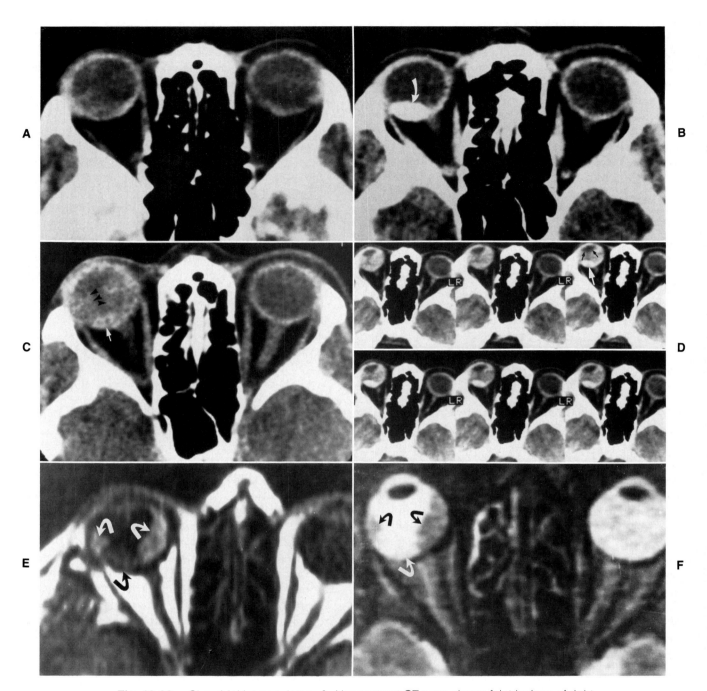

Fig. 10-66 Choroidal hemangioma. **A,** Noncontrast CT scan shows faint lesions of right globe. **B,** Contrast CT scan obtained with rapid injection of contrast shows marked enhancement of hemangioma *(arrow)*. This patient later developed total retinal detachment. **C,** Routine contrast enhancement shows mass *(arrow)* and retinal detachment *(arrowheads)*. **D,** Dynamic CT scans show hemangioma *(white arrow)*, differentiating it from total retinal detachment *(black arrows)*. **E,** T₁W MRI scan shows hemangioma *(black arrow)* and chronic subretinal effusion *(white arrows)*. **F,** T₂W MRI scan shows hemangioma as hyperintense image *(white arrow)* and chronic subretinal effusion as hypointense image *(black arrows)*. Hypointensity of subretinal effusion is thought to be caused by highly organized proteinaceous fluid.

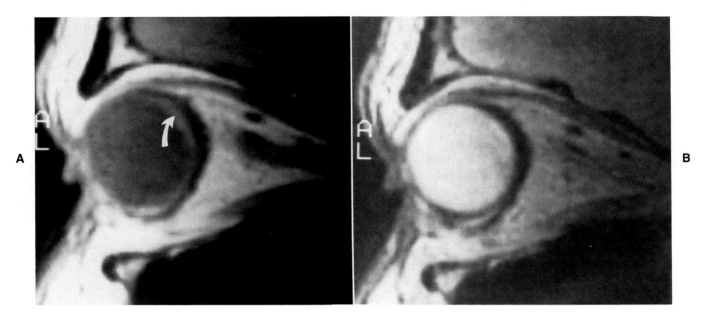

Fig. 10-67   Choroidal hemangioma. **A,** PW MRI scan shows hyperintense mass *(arrow)*. **B,** T$_2$W MRI scan shows that mass remains hyperintense. Ophthalmoscopic findings were most compatible with hemangioma. This MRI appearance may be difficult to differentiate from retinal detachment. Combined clinical and MRI findings should make the right diagnosis.

moderately intense areas in T$_1$W, PW, and T$_2$W images (Fig. 10-67).[5]

In one of our patients with Sturge-Weber disease and choroidal hemangioma, MRI demonstrated a mixed but predominantly hyperintense mass on proton-weighted MRI scans and a hypointense mass on T$_2$-weighted scans. In this patient CT demonstrated an intense contrast enhancement that is characteristic of choroidal hemangiomas.

Whenever a choroidal hemangioma cannot be definitely differentiated from uveal melanoma by MRI, we recommend contrast-enhanced CT scans using a combination of the infusion-bolus technique (see Fig. 10-66, *B*) or a dynamic CT technique (see Fig. 10-66, *C*) to differentiate hemangiomas from uveal melanomas.[4,21] Alternatively, gadolinium MRI may differentiate these entities. The diagnosis of angiomatosis retinae of von Hippel-Lindau disease depends chiefly on the ophthalmoscopic appearance.

Choroidal Hemorrhage and Choroidal Detachment

In discussing the differential diagnosis of uveal melanoma, choroidal hemorrhage and choroidal detachment may easily be mistaken for a choroidal tumor. A choroidal hemorrhage that has not ruptured the lamina of Bruch may simulate the ophthalmoscopic, CT, and MRI appearance of a choroidal tumor, because it forms a round, even globular, dark brown prominence that is opaque to transillumination (Figs. 10-68 and 10-69). The covering of pigmented choroid, if the hemorrhage is in the suprachoroidal space, and of the retinal pigment layer cause the color of the hemorrhage to be even darker than that of most melanomas.[101] Such hemorrhage may become encapsulated and subsequently absorbed, leaving behind a more or less dense membrane. Choroidal effusion (uveal effusion) is another pathologic entity that can be confused with a ring melanoma.[4,25] The CT and MRI appearances of choroidal hemorrhage (see Figs. 10-23 and 10-68), choroidal detachment (see Figs. 10-22, 10-28, and 10-29), and uveal effusion (see Fig. 10-30) were discussed earlier in this chapter.

Choroidal Cyst

A choroidal cyst is very rare; however, it could be mistaken for a choroidal tumor.[101] Choroidal cysts may be bilateral and may give rise to retinal detachment. A cyst may be treated by removing its fluid content.[101]

Other Tumors of the Uvea

Several types of tumors affect the choroid and ciliary body. Some are so rare that, when present, they may cause diagnostic confusion with uveal melanomas. Such tumors include neurofibroma and schwannoma of the choroid and ciliary body, adenoma, leiomyoma, and lymphoreticular proliferative disorders of the uveal tract.

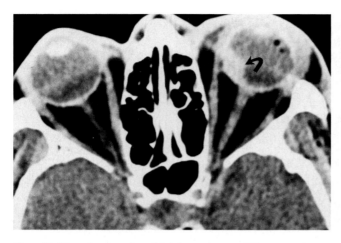

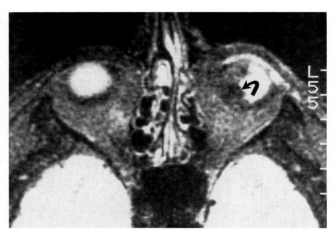

Fig. 10-68 Acute choroidal hematoma. CT scan shows hyperdense mass *(arrow)* related to traumatic choroidal hematoma. Note air bubbles in left globe.

Fig. 10-69 Acute choroidal hematoma. T₂W MRI scan shows hypointense fresh choroidal hematoma *(arrow)*.

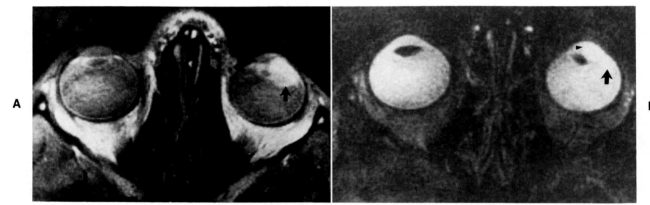

Fig. 10-70 Leiomyoma of ciliary body. **A,** PW MRI scan shows large, hyperintense mass *(arrow)*. **B,** T₂W MRI scan shows that lesion remains hyperintense *(arrow)*. Note extension into anterior chamber *(arrowhead)*.

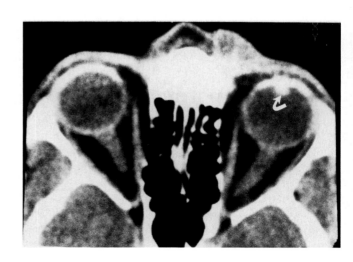

Fig. 10-71 Medulloepithelioma. CT scan shows hyperdense mass *(arrow)*.

Neurofibroma, Schwannoma, and Adenoma. In neurofibromatosis there may be small, pigmented nodules in the iris, ciliary body, and choroid. If the changes involve the trabecular meshwork, a severe glaucoma may develop. If these lesions are large enough, they may be depicted by CT and MRI.

Adenomas of the ciliary bodies are rare and may appear as small defined tumors.

Leiomyoma. Smooth muscle tumors of the ciliary body are extremely rare and must be distinguished from other spindle-cell tumors, especially the more common amelanotic spindle-cell melanoma.[147,148] Electron microscopic examination is necessary to prove the smooth muscle origin of these tumors.[147] Jakobiec et al[148] reported two benign tumors of the ciliary body (one in a 37-year-old woman and the other in a 20-year-old woman) that were diagnosed as neurogenic tumors by light microscopy, whereas electron microscopic examination revealed that the tumors were composed of smooth muscle cells with unusual morphologic features. The researchers concluded that the combined myogenic and neurogenic characteristics resulted from the neural crest origin of the smooth muscle of the ciliary body (mesectoderm) and suggested that the tumors constituted a new nosologic entity of myogenic neoplasia; they offered the term "mesectodermal leiomyoma of the ciliary body."[148] The cells of the neural crest that contribute to the formation of bone, cartilage, connective tissue, and smooth muscle in the region of the head and neck have been called "mesectoderm." The MRI appearance of a mesectodermal leiomyoma of the ciliary body has been reported.[25] The lesion appeared as a well-defined, noninfiltrative mass that demonstrated hyperintensity in T_1W, PW, and T_2W MR images (Fig. 10-70).

Medulloepithelioma

Medulloepithelioma, or dictyoma, is a rare tumor of the ciliary body usually seen in young children,[149] although it can be seen in adults.[21] The tumor arises from the primitive unpigmented epithelial lining of the ciliary body. Histologically, the tumor resembles embryonic retina and neural tissue.[149] From its point of origin on the ciliary body, the tumor may spread forward along the surface of the iris or backward along the surface of the retina.[101] In children medulloepithelioma should be considered in the differential diagnosis of retinoblastoma. In adults this tumor may simulate uveal melanoma on ophthalmoscopic evaluation, fluorescein angiography, ultrasonography, and CT scanning (Fig. 10-71).[21] We have studied an adult patient with medulloepithelioma in which MRI-depicted signal characteristics were identical to those of uveal melanoma.

Retinal Detachment in the Differential Diagnosis of Uveal Melanoma

The ophthalmoscopic smooth globular outline of the elevated retina characteristic of most cases of malignant uveal melanoma occasionally may be present in patients with a simple detachment of the retina. A retinal hole, however, is present in practically all cases of simple retinal detachment. The MRI appearance of a simple retinal detachment, on the other hand, is characteristic, and the absence or presence of a mass (provided that it is elevated more than 3 mm) can be readily assessed on MRI scans (see Fig. 10-16). Chronic organized or hemorrhagic subretinal fluid may have MRI characteristics identical to those of uveal melanoma (see Fig. 10-65, *A* and *B*).

Senile Macular Degeneration

Macular degeneration in the elderly is a leading cause of legal blindness. Arteriosclerosis of the choriocapillaries, dysfunction of the pigment epithelial cells, and loss of neuroepithelial cells are the fundamental causes of macular degeneration syndrome in the elderly.[13] The earliest change at the macula is hyalinization and thickening of Bruch's membrane. Later, ingrowth of choroidal neovascularization into the subpigment epithelial space occurs, resulting in detachment of the pigment epithelium. The serous fluid that accumulates in the subpigment space eventually finds its way into the subretinal space. One of the serious possible complications is hemorrhage, which is limited at first to the subpigment epithelial space; later the hemorrhage extends into the subretinal space and eventually forms an organized fibrous scar, with consequent

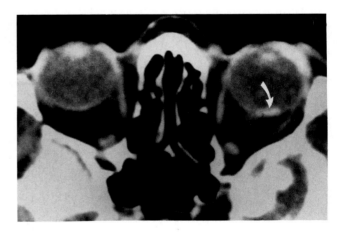

Fig. 10-72 Senile macular degeneration. PW MRI scan shows hyperintense mass *(arrow)* compatible with discoid macular degeneration. Lesion remained mixed in signal intensity in T_2W image with small, ill-defined area that appeared hypointense.

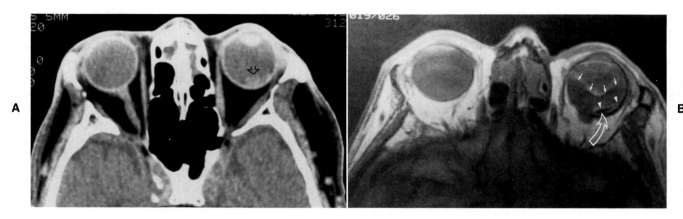

Fig. 10-73 Senile macular degeneration associated with complications. **A,** CT scan shows mass *(arrow)* and dependent image probably caused by effusion in subretinal space. **B,** T₁W MRI scan shows characteristic posterior hyaloid detachment *(arrows).* Unlike in retinal detachment, detached posterior hyaloid membrane does not extend toward optic disc. Note detached retina *(arrowheads)* and hypointense image *(curved arrow)* related to scar tissue in subretinal and retinal region. Surgery confirmed findings. Notice that information obtained by MRI is far superior to that obtained by CT.

loss of almost all function of the involved macula.[13] The process of senile macular degeneration may be associated with liquefaction of the vitreous, and this may cause posterior hyaloid detachment. The CT appearance of senile macular degeneration may be similar to that of uveal melanoma. However, more iodinated contrast enhancement is seen in macular degeneration than in uveal melanomas. The MRI appearance of macular degeneration varies, depending on the stage of the disease. The lesion may show hyperintensity on all pulse sequences because of fluid in the subretinal space (Fig. 10-72), or it may be seen to have varied MRI characteristics if it is associated with hemorrhage and other complications (Fig. 10-73).

REFERENCES

1. Wehrli, FW, MacFall, JR, and Newton, TH: Parameters determining the appearance of NMR images. In Newton TH and Potts DG, editors: Modern neuroradiology, vol 2, Advanced imaging techniques, San Anselmo, Calif, 1983, Clavadel Press, pp 81-117.
2. Wehrli FW et al: Time of flight MR flow imaging: selective saturation recovery with gradient refocusing, Radiology 160:781, 1986.
3. Aguayo JB et al: Study of vitreous liquifaction by NMR spectroscopy and imaging, Invest Ophthalmol Vis Sci 26:692, 1985.
4. Mafee MF et al: Malignant uveal melanoma and simulating lesions: MR imaging evaluation, Radiology 160:773, 1986.
5. Mafee MF et al: MRI and in vivo proton spectroscopy of the lesions of the globe, Semin Ultrasound CT MR 9:59-71, 1988.
6. Mafee MF and Peyman GA: Retinal and choroidal detachments: role of MRI and CT, Radiol Clin North Am 25:487, 1987.
7. Mafee MF et al: Magnetic resonance imaging in the evaluation and differentiation of uveal melanoma, Ophthalmology 94:341, 1987.
8. Lagouros PA et al: Magnetic resonance imaging and intraocular foreign bodies, Arch Ophthalmol 105:551, 1987.
9. Penning DJ et al: MR imaging of enucleated human at 1.4 Tesla, J Comput Assist Tomogr 10:551, 1986.
10. Aguayo JB et al: Nuclear magnetic resonance imaging for a single cell, Nature 322:190, 1986.
11. Anderson H and Apple D: Anatomy and embryology of the eye. In Peyman GA, Sanders DR, and Goldberg MF, editors: Principles and practice of ophthalmology, vol 1, Philadelphia, 1980, WB Saunders Co, pp 3-68.
12. Balaz EA: The molecular biology of the vitreous. In McPhearson A, editor: New and controversial aspects of retinal detachment, New York, 1968, Harper & Row, Publishers, Inc, pp 3-15.
13. Sigelman J, Jakobiec FA, and Eisner G, editors: Retinal diseases, pathogenesis, laser therapy and surgery, Boston, 1984, Little, Brown & Co, Inc, pp 1-66.
14. Mafee MF et al: Orbital space-occupying lesions: role of computed tomography and magnetic resonance imaging. An analysis of 145 cases, Radiol Clin North Am 25:529, 1987.
15. Reeh MF, Wobij JL, and Wirtschafter JD: Ophthalmic anatomy: a manual with some clinical applications, San Francisco, 1981, American Academy of Ophthalmology, pp 11-54.
16. Rutnin U: Fundus appearance in normal eye. I. The choroid, Am J Ophthalmol 64:821, 1967.
17. Nakaizumi Y: The ultrastructure of Bruch's membrane. II. Eyes with a tapetum, Arch Ophthalmol 72:388, 1984.
18. Wudka E and Leopold IM: Experimental studies of the choroidal blood vessels, Arch Ophthalmol 55:857, 1951.
19. Balaz EA: Physiology of the vitreous body. In Schepens CL, editor: Importance of the vitreous body in retinal surgery with special emphasis on reoperations, St Louis, 1960, The CV Mosby Co, pp 29-48.
20. Mafee MF et al: Computed tomography in the evaluation of patients with persistent hyperplastic primary vitreous (PHPV), Radiology 145:713, 1982.
21. Mafee MF, Peyman GA, and McKusick MA: Malignant uveal melanoma and similar lesions studied by computed tomography, Radiology 156:403, 1985.
22. Warwick R and Williams, PL, editors: Gray's anatomy, ed 35 (British), Philadelphia, 1973, WB Saunders Co.

23. Mafee MF and Goldberg MF: CT and MR imaging for diagnosis of persistent hyperplastic primary vitreous (PHPV), Radiol Clin North Am 25:683, 1987.

24. Goldberg MF and Mafee MF: Computed tomography for diagnosis of persistent hyperplastic primary vitreous (PHPV), Ophthalmology 90:442, 1983.

25. Mafee MF et al: Retinoblastoma and simulating lesions: role of CT and MR imaging, Radiol Clin North Am 25:667, 1987.

26. Weiter JJ and Ernest JT: Anatomy of the choroidal vasculature, Am J Ophthalmol 78:583, 1974.

27. Capper SA and Leopold IH: Mechanism of serous choroidal detachment, Arch Ophthalmol 55:101, 1956.

28. Mafee MF and Peyman GA: Choroidal detachment and ocular hypotony: CT evaluation, Radiology 153:697, 1984.

29. Mafee MF et al: Choroidal hematoma and effusion: evaluation with MR imaging, Radiology 168:781, 1988.

30. Peyman GA, Mafee MF, and Schulman JA: Computed tomography in choroidal detachment, Ophthalmology 91:156, 1984.

31. Iijima Y and Asanagi K: A new B-scan ultrasonographic technique for observing ciliary body detachment, Am J Ophthalmol 95:498, 1983.

32. Wing GL et al: Serous choroidal detachment and the thickened choroid sign detected by ultrasonography, Am J Ophthalmol 84:499, 1982.

33. Archer DB and Canavan YM: Contusional eye injuries: retinal and choroidal lesions, Aust J Ophthalmol 11:251, 1983.

34. Maumenee AE and Schwartz MF: Acute intraoperative choroidal effusion, Am J Ophthalmol 100:147, 1985.

35. Gole GA: Massive choroidal hemorrhage as a complication of krypton red laser photocoagulation for disciform degeneration, Aust N Z J Ophthalmol 13:37, 1985.

36. Schepens CL and Brockhurst RJ: Uveal effusion. I. Clinical picture, Arch Ophthalmol 70:189, 1963.

37. Haik BG et al: Current diagnostic techniques in retinoblastoma, American Academy of Ophthalmology, scientific exhibit, Nov. 9-13, 1986.

38. Howard GM and Ellsworth RM: Differential diagnosis of retinoblastoma: a statistical survey of 500 children. I. Relative frequency of the lesions which simulate retinoblastoma, Am J Ophthalmol 60:610, 1965.

39. Popoff NA and Ellsworth RM: The fine structure of retinoblastoma, in vivo and in vivo observations, Lab Invest 25:389, 1971.

40. Tso MOM et al: Photoreceptor elements in retinoblastoma: a preliminary report, Arch Ophthalmol 82:57, 1969.

41. Tso MOM, Zimmerman LE, and Fine BS: The nature of retinoblastoma: 1 photoreceptor differentiation. A clinical and histopathologic study, Am J Ophthalmol 69:339, 1970.

42. Tso MOM: Clues to the cells of origin of retinoblastoma, Int Ophthalmol Clin 20(2):191, 1980.

43. Kodilyne HC: Retinoblastoma in Nigeria: problems in treatment, Am J Ophthalmol 63:467, 1967.

44. Abramson DH et al: Treatment of bilateral groups I through III retinoblastoma with bilateral radiation, Arch Ophthalmol 99:1761, 1981.

45. Kyritsis AP et al: Retinoblastoma: origin from a primitive neuroectodermal cell? Nature 307:471, 1984.

46. Tso MOM et al: A cause of radioresistance in retinoblastoma: photoreceptor differentiation, Trans Am Acad Ophthalmol Otolaryngol 74:959, 1970.

47. Jenson RD and Miller RW: Retinoblastoma: epidemiologic characteristics, N Engl J Med 285:307, 1971.

48. Abramson DH, Ellsworth RM, and Zimmerman LE: Nonocular cancer in retinoblastoma survivors, Trans Am Acad Ophthalmol Otolaryngol 81:454, 1976.

49. Pendergrass TW and Davis S: Incidence of retinoblastoma in the United States, Arch Ophthalmol 98:1204, 1980.

50. Zimmerman LE and Bilaniuk LT: CT in the evaluation of patients with bilateral retinoblastomas, J Comput Tomogr 3:251, 1979.

51. Ellsworth RM: The management of retinoblastoma, Trans Am Ophthalmol Soc 67:462, 1969.

52. Lennox EL, Draper GJ, and Sanders BM: Retinoblastoma: a study of natural history and prognosis of 268 cases, Br Med J 3:731, 1975.

53. Abramson DH: Retinoblastoma: diagnosis and management, CA 32:130, 1982.

54. Knudson, AG: Retinoblastoma: a prototype heredity neoplasm, Semin Oncol 5:57, 1978.

55. Judisch GF and Patil SR: Concurrent heritable retinoblastoma, pinealoma and trisomy X, Arch Ophthalmol 99:1767, 1981.

56. Jakobiec FA et al: Retinoblastoma and intracranial malignancy, Cancer 39:2048, 1977.

57. Bader JL et al: Trilateral retinoblastoma, Lancet 2:582, 1980.

58. Bader JL et al: Bilateral retinoblastoma with ectopic intracranial retinoblastoma: trilateral retinoblastoma, Cancer Genet Cytogenet 5:203, 1982.

59. Knudson AG Jr: Mutation and cancer: a statistical study of retinoblastoma, Proc Natl Acad Sci USA 68:820, 1971.

60. Lele KP, Penrose LS, and Stallard HB: Chromosome deletion in a case of retinoblastoma, Ann Hum Genet 27:171, 1963.

61. Knudson AG Jr et al: Chromosomal deletion and retinoblastoma, N Engl J Med 295:1120, 1976.

62. Yunis JJ and Ramsey N: Retinoblastoma and subband deletion chromosome 13, Am J Dis Child 132:161, 1978.

63. Cavenee WK et al: Prediction of familial predisposition to retinoblastoma, N Engl J Med 314:1201, 1986.

64. Sparkes RS et al: Regional assignment of genes for human esterase D and retinoblastoma to choromosome band 13q14, Science 208:1042, 1980.

65. Sparkes RS et al: Gene for hereditary retinoblastoma assigned to human chromosome 13 by linkage to esterase D, Science 219:971, 1983.

66. Motegi T: High rate of detection of 13q14 deletion mosaicism among retinoblastoma patients (using more extensive methods), Hum Genet 61:95, 1982.

67. Seidman DJ et al: Early diagnosis of retinoblastoma based on dysmorphic features and karyotype analysis, Ophthalmology 94:663, 1987.

68. Stefanko SZ and Manschot WA: Pinealoblastoma with retinoblastomas differentiation, Brain 102:321, 1979.

69. Schulman JA et al: The use of magnetic resonance imaging in the evaluation of retinoblastoma, J Pediatr Ophthalmol Strabismus 23:144, 1986.

70. Robertson DM and Campbell RJ: Analysis of misdiagnosed retinoblastoma in a series of 726 enucleated eyes, Mod Probl Ophthalmol 18:156, 1977.

71. Char DH: Current concepts in retinoblastoma, Ann Ophthalmol 12:792, 1980.

72. Haik BG et al: Magnetic resonance imaging in the evaluation of leukokoria, Ophthalmology 92:1143, 1152, 1985.

73. Char DH, Hedges TR, and Norman D: Retinoblastoma: CT diagnosis, Ophthalmology 91:1347, 1984.

74. Goldberg BB, Kotler MN, and Ziskin MD: Diagnostic uses of ultrasound, New York, 1975, Grune & Stratton, Inc, p 100.

75. Danziger A and Price MI: CT findings in retinoblastoma, AJR 133:695, 1979.

76. Haik BG et al: Computed tomography of the nonrhegmatogenous retinal detachment in the pediatric patient, Ophthalmology 92:1133, 1985.

77. Mafee MF et al: Potential use of in vivo proton spectroscopy for head and neck lesions, Radiol Clin North Am 27:243, 1989.

78. Mafee MF et al: Magnetic resonance imaging versus computed tomography of Leukocoric eyes and use of in vitro proton magnetic resonance spectroscopy of retinoblastoma, Ophthalmology 96(7):965, 1989.

79. Warburg M: Retinal malformations: aetiological heterogeneity and morphological similarity in congenital retinal non-attachment and falciform folds, Trans Ophthalmol Soc UK 99:272, 1979.

80. Ohba N, Watanabe S, and Fujita S: Primary vitreoretinal dysplasia transmitted as an autosomal recessive disorder, Br J Ophthalmol 65:631, 1981.

81. Peyman GA and Sanders DR: Vitreous and vitreous surgery. In Peyman GA, Sanders DR, and Goldberg MF, editors: Principles and practice of ophthalmology, vol. 2, Philadelphia, 1980, WB Saunders Co, pp 1327-1401.

82. Katz NNK, Margo CE, and Dorwart RH: Computed tomography with histopathologic correlation in children with leukocoria, J Pediatr Ophthalmol Strabismus 21:50, 1984.

83. Caudhill JW, Streeten BW, and Tso MOM: Phacoanaphylactoid in persistent hyperplastic primary vitreous, Ophthalmology 92:1153, 1985.

84. Liberfarb RM et al: Norrie's disease: a study of two families, Ophthalmology 92:1445, 1985.

85. Norrie G: Causes of blindness in children: twenty-five years experience of Danish Institutes for the Blind, Acta Ophthalmol 5:357, 1927.

86. Warburg M: Norrie's disease: a new hereditary bilateral pseudotumour of the retina, Acta Ophthalmol 39:757, 1961.

87. Warburg M: Norrie's disease (atrophia bulborum hereditaria): a report of eleven cases of hereditary bilateral pseudotumour of the retina, complicated by deafness and mental deficiency, Acta Ophthalmol 41:134, 1963.

88. Warburg M: Norrie's disease: a congenital progressive oculo-acoustico-cerebral degeneration, Acta Ophthalmol (Suppl) 89, 1966.

89. Holmes LB: Norrie's disease: an X-linked syndrome of retinal malformation, mental retardation, and deafness, J Pediatr 79:89, 1971.

90. Apple DJ, Fishman GA, and Goldberg MF: Ocular histopathology of Norrie's disease, Am J Ophthalmol 78:196, 1974.

91. Blodi FC and Hunter WS: Norrie's disease in North America, Doc Ophthalmol 26:434, 1969.

92. Meckel S and Passarge E: Encephalocele, polycystic kidneys and polydactyly as an autosomal recessive trait simulating certain other disorders. The Meckel syndrome, Ann Genet (Paris) 14:97, 1971.

93. Warburg M: The heterogeneity of microphthalmia in the mentally retarded, Birth Defects 7:136, 1971.

94. Chemke J et al: A familial syndrome of central nervous system and ocular malformation, Clin Genet 7:1, 1975.

95. Chan CC et al: Oculocerebral malformations: a reappraisal of Walker's "lissencephaly," Arch Neurol 37:104, 1980.

96. Pagon RA et al: Hydrocephalus, agyria, retinal dysplasia, encephalocele (HARD+E) syndrome: an autosomal recessive condition, Birth Defects 14(6):233, 1978.

97. Levine RA et al: Warburg syndrome, Ophthalmology 90:1600, 1983.

98. Warburg M: Hydrocephaly, congenital retinal nonattachment, and congenital falciform fold, Am J Ophthalmol 85:88, 1978.

99. Eller AW et al: Retinopathy of prematurity: the association of a persistent hyaloid artery, Ophthalmology 94:444, 1987.

100. Ashton N, Ward B, and Sperpell G: Role of oxygen in the genesis of retrolental fibroplasia: a preliminary report, Br J Ophthalmol 37:513, 1953.

101. Michaelson IC: Retrolental fibroplasia. In Michaelson IC, editor: Textbook of the fundus of the eye, Edinburgh, 1980, Churchill Livingstone, Inc, pp 303-315.

102. Coats G: Forms of retinal disease with massive exudation, Royal London Ophthalmologic Hospital Reports 17:440, 1908.

103. Reese AB: Telangiectasis of the retina and Coats' disease, Am J Ophthalmol 42:1, 1956.

104. Woods AC and Duke JR: Coats' disease. I. Review of the literature, diagnostic criteria, clinical findings, and plasma lipid studies, Br J Ophthalmol 47:385, 1963.

105. Silodor SW et al: Natural history and management of advanced Coats' disease, Ophthalmic Surg 19:89, 1988.

106. Egerer I, Tasman W, and Tomer TL: Coats' disease, Arch Ophthalmol 92:109, 1974.

107. Sherman JL, McLean IW, and Brallier DR: Coats' disease: CT pathologic correlation in two cases, Radiology 146:77, 1983.

108. Shields JA: Diagnosis and management of intraocular tumors, St Louis, 1983, The CV Mosby Co, pp 497-533.

109. Chang M, McLean IW, and Merritt JC: Coats' disease: a study of 62 histologically confirmed cases, J Pediatr Ophthalmol Strabismus 21:163, 1984.

110. Margo CE et al: Sclerosing endophthalmitis in children: computed tomography with histopathologic correlation, J Pediatr Ophthalmol Strabismus 20:180, 1983.

111. Wilder HC: Nematode endophthalmitis, Trans Am Acad Ophthalmol Otolaryngol 55:99, 1950.

112. Zinkham WM: Visceral larva migrans: a review and reassessment indicating two forms of clinical expression: visceral and ocular, Am J Dis Child 132:627, 1978.

113. Reesner FH, Aaberg TM, and VanHorn DL: Astrocytic hamartoma of the retina not associated with tuberous sclerosis, Am J Ophthalmol 86:688, 1978.

114. Lyle DJ: Coloboma of the optic nerve, Am J Ophthalmol 15:347, 1932.

115. Brown G and Tasman W, editors: Congenital anomalies of the optic disc, New York, 1983, Grune & Stratton, Inc, pp 97-191.

116. Mafee MF et al: Computed tomography of optic nerve colobomas, morning glory anomaly, and colobomatous cyst, Radiol Clin North Am 25:693, 1987.

117. Tyson HH: Crater-like cavities in the optic disc, Am J Ophthalmol 10:239, 1927.

118. Makley TA Jr and Battles M: Microphthalmus with cyst, Surv Ophthalmol 13:200, 1969.

119. Mann I: Developmental abnormalities of the eye, ed 2, Philadelphia, 1957, JB Lippincott Co, pp 74-78.

120. Savell J and Cook JR: Optic nerve colobomas of autosomal dominant heredity, Arch Ophthalmol 94:395, 1976.

121. Pollock JA, Newton TH, and Hoyt WF: Transsphenoidal and transethmoidal encephaloceles, Radiology 90:442, 1968.

122. Kindler P: Morning glory syndrome: unusual congenital optic disc anomaly, Am J Ophthalmol 69:376, 1970.

123. McMahon RT: Anatomy, congenital anomalies, and tumors. In Peyman CA, Sanders DR, and Goldberg MF, editors: Principles and practice of ophthalmology, Philadelphia, 1980, WB Saunders Co, pp 1491-1553.

124. Yanoff M and Fine BS: Ocular pathology: a text and atlas, Hagerstown, Md, 1975, Harper & Row, Publishers, Inc, p 831.

125. Callender GR: Malignant melanotic tumors of the eye: a study of histologic types in three cases, Trans Am Acad Ophthalmol Otolaryngol 36:131, 1931.

126. McLean JW, Foster WU, and Zimmerman LE: Prognostic factors in small malignant melanomas of choroidal and ciliary body, Arch Ophthalmol 95:148, 1977.

127. Duffin RM et al: Small malignant melanoma of the choroid with extraocular extension, Arch Ophthalmol 99:1827, 1981.

128. Donders PC: Malignant melanoma of the choroid, Trans Ophthalmol Soc UK 93:745, 1973.

129. Zimmerman LE, McLean IW, and Foster WD: Does enucleation of the eye containing a malignant melanoma prevent or accelerate the dissemination of tumor cells? Br J Ophthalmol 62:420, 1978.

130. Char DH: The management of small choroidal melanomas, Surv Ophthalmol 22:377, 1978.

131. Canny CLB, Shields JA, and Kay ML: Clinically stationary choroidal melanoma with extraocular extension, Arch Ophthalmol 96:436, 1978.

132. Ruiz RS: Early treatment in malignant melanomas of the choroid. In Brockhurst RJ et al, editors: Controversy in ophthalmology, Philadelphia, 1977, WB Saunders Co, pp 604-610.

133. Manschot WA and VanPeperzeel HA: Choroidal melanoma: enucleation or observation? A new approach, Arch Ophthalmol 98:71, 1980.

134. Peyman GA et al: Ten years experience with eye wall resection for uveal melanomas, Ophthalmology 91:1720, 1984.

135. Mauriello JA Jr, Zimmerman LE, and Rothstein TB: Intrachoroidal hemorrhage mistaken for malignant melanoma, Ann Ophthalmol 15:282, 1983.

136. Ferry AP: Lesions mistaken for malignant melanoma of the posterior uvea: a clinicopathologic analysis of 100 cases with ophthalmoscopically visible lesions, Arch Ophthalmol 72S:463, 1964.

137. Shields JA and Zimmerman LE: Lesions simulating malignant melanoma of the posterior uvea, Arch Ophthalmol 89:466, 1973.

138. Mafee MF: Magnetic resonance imaging and its simplifications for ophthalmology. Reinecke RD, editor: Ophthalmology annual, New York, 1988, Raven Press, pp 193-264.

139. Peyster RG et al: Intraocular tumors: evaluation with MR imaging, Radiology 168:73, 1988.

140. Damadian R et al: Human tumors by NMR, Physiol Chem Phys 5:381, 1973.

141. Gomori JM et al: Choroidal melanomas: correlation of NMR spectroscopy and MR imaging, Radiology 158:443, 1986.

142. Naumann G, Yanoff M, and Zimmerman LE: Histogenesis of malignant melanomas of the uvea: histopathologic characteristics of nevi of the choroid and ciliary body, Arch Ophthalmol 76:784, 1966.

143. Peyman GA and Cohen SB: Ab interno resection of uveal melanoma, Int Ophthalmol 9:29, 1986.

144. Peyman GA and Schulman JA: Intravitreal surgery: principles and practice, Norwalk, Conn, 1986, Appleton & Lange, pp 338-364.

145. Gonder JR et al: Visual loss associated with choroidal nevi, Ophthalmology 89:961, 1982.

146. Adams RD and DeLong GR: Developmental and other congenital abnormalities of the nervous system. In Harrison's principles of internal medicine, ed 7, New York, 1974, McGraw-Hill, Inc, pp 1849-1863.

147. Meyer SI et al: Leiomyoma of the ciliary body: electron microscopic verification, Am J Ophthalmol 66:1061, 1968.

148. Jakobiec FA et al: Mesectodermal leiomyoma of the ciliary body: a tumor of presumed neural crest origin, Cancer 39(5):2102-2113, 1977.

149. Apt L et al: Dictyoma (embryonal medulloepithelioma): recent review and case report, J Pediatr Ophthalmol 10:30, 1973.

SECTION TWO
THE ORBIT PROPER

MAHMOOD F. MAFEE

ANATOMIC AND DEVELOPMENTAL CONSIDERATIONS

The orbits are two recesses that contain the globes, the muscles, the blood vessels, lymphatics, nerves (II, III, IV, V, and VI), adipose and connective tissues, and most of the lacrimal apparatus. The orbit is bordered by the periosteum and separated from the globe by Tenon's capsule. Anteriorly are the orbital septum and the lids. The orbital cavity is pyramidal; its apex is directed posteriorly and medially and its base is directed anteriorly and laterally as the orbital opening. Its bony walls separate it from the anterior cranial fossa superiorly, the ethmoid and sphenoid sinuses and nasal cavity medially, the maxillary sinus inferiorly, and the lateral surface of the face and temporal fossa laterally and posteriorly.

BONY ORBIT

Each orbit presents a roof, floor, medial and lateral walls, a base or orbital opening, and an apex (Figs. 10-74 and 10-75). The roof of the orbit comprises the orbital plate of the frontal bone and most of the lesser wing of the sphenoid bone (Fig. 10-75). Anteromedially, it is the frontal sinus; anterolaterally in the shallow hollow of the lacrimal fossa, lies the orbital part of the lacrimal gland. At the posterior end of the junction of the roof with the medial wall, the optic canal and optic foramen (Fig. 10-76) establish communication between the orbit and the middle cranial fossa. The optic canal contains the optic nerve, ophthalmic artery, and sympathetic fibers.

The medial wall is exceedingly thin, except at its most posterior part, and comprises a portion of the

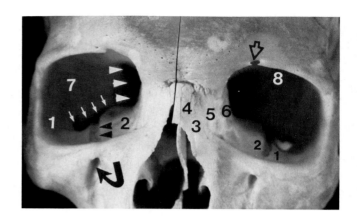

Fig. 10-74 Frontal view of orbits. *1,* Orbital process of zygomatic bone; *2,* orbital process of maxilla; *3,* frontonasal process of maxilla; *4,* nasal bone; *5,* lacrimal bone; *6,* orbital plate of ethmoid bone (lamina papyracea); *7,* orbital surface of greater wing of sphenoid bone; *8,* orbital surface of frontal bone. Note supraorbital foramen (notch) *(hollow arrow),* superior orbital fissure *(white arrowheads),* inferior orbital fissure *(white arrows),* infraorbital groove *(black arrowheads),* and infraorbital foramen *(curved arrow).*

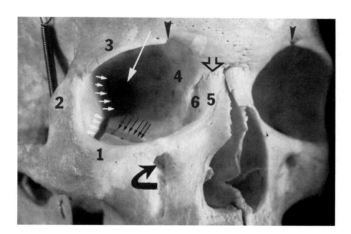

Fig. 10-75 Frontal and slightly oblique view of orbits. *1,* Zygomatic bone; *2,* frontal process of zygomatic bone; *3,* zygomatic process of frontal bone; *4,* orbital plate of ethmoid bone (lamina papyracea); *5,* nasal bone; *6,* lacrimal bone and lacrimal fossa. Note frontonasal suture *(hollow arrow),* supraorbital notch (foramen) *(black arrowheads),* optic canal *(white long arrow),* superior orbital fissure *(white short arrows),* inferior orbital fissure *(white arrowheads),* infraorbital groove *(black arrows),* and infraorbital foramen *(curved arrow).*

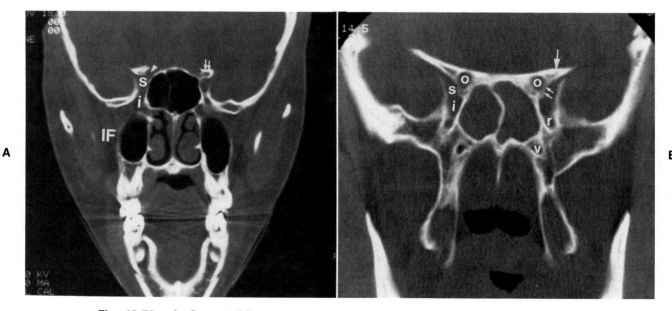

Fig. 10-76 **A,** Coronal CT scan shows anterior clinoid *(arrows);* optic canal *(arrowhead);* superior orbital fissure *(S);* inferior orbital fissure *(i);* and lateral extension of inferior orbital fissure into infratemporal fossa *(IF).* **B,** Coronal CT scan a few millimeters posterior to view in **A,** shows anterior clinoid *(arrow);* optic canal *(o);* optic strut *(two small arrows);* superior orbital fissure *(s);* inferior orbital fissure *(i);* foramen rotundum *(r);* and pterygoid (vidian) canal *(v).*

frontal process of the maxilla, the lacrimal, the ethmoid, and the body of the sphenoid bones (Figs. 10-74 and 10-75). The medial wall slopes gently downward and laterally into the orbital floor. Anteriorly is the lacrimal groove for the lacrimal sac. The groove communicates below with the nasal cavity through the nasolacrimal canal, which is about 1 cm long and contains the nasolacrimal duct, which opens into the inferior meatus of the nasal cavity.

The inferior wall or floor of the orbit is relatively thin, and in most of its extent forms the roof of the maxillary sinus (Figs. 10-74 and 10-75). The floor comprises the orbital part of maxilla, the orbital process of zygomatic bone, and the orbital process of palatine bone (Figs. 10-74 and 10-75). The orbital process of the palatine bone forms a small triangular area of the posteromedial corner of the orbital floor, where the floor meets the medial wall. The floor is not quite horizontal but faces upward and slightly laterally.[1] In front it is continuous with the lateral wall, but posteriorly the inferior orbital fissure separates the two walls (Figs. 10-74 and 10-75). This inferior orbital fissure leads into the orbit from the pterygopalatine fossa posteriorly, and anteriorly from the infratemporal fossa. The medial lip of the fissure is notched by the infraorbital groove (Figs. 10-74 and 10-75), which passes forward in the floor, sinking into it anteriorly and becoming the infraorbital canal, whose anterior opening is the infraorbital foramen (Figs. 10-74 and 10-75).[1] The groove, canal, and foramen transmit the infraorbital nerve, the continuation of the maxillary nerve.

The lateral wall of the orbit is the thickest wall and comprises the orbital surface of the greater wing of the sphenoid bone behind and the orbital surface of the frontal process of the zygomatic bone in front (Figs. 10-74 and 10-75). The two bones meet at the sphenozygomatic suture. This aspect of the zygomatic bone presents the two openings of minute canals for the zygomaticofacial nerve (near the junction of the floor and lateral walls) and (slightly more cranially) the zygomaticotemporal nerve.[1]

Orbital Apex

The apex of the orbit is basically formed by the optic canal and the superior orbital fissure.[2] The optic canal and the superior and inferior orbital fissures allow various structures to enter and leave the orbit. The optic canal, having virtually no length at birth, becomes 4 mm long by 1 year and increases up to 9 mm in adults. The optic canal, forming an angle of about 45 degrees with the sagittal plane of the head, is bounded medially by the body of the sphenoid bone (Figs. 10-76 and 10-77), superiorly by the superior root of the lesser wing of the sphenoid bone, and inferiorly and laterally by the inferior root (optic strut) of the lesser wing of the sphe-

noid bone.[3] Close to the superior, medial, and lower margins of the orbital opening of the optic canal, the common tendinous ring of Zinn is attached to the orbital walls for the origin of several of the extraocular muscles[1] (Fig. 10-77).

Superior Orbital Fissure

Just lateral and inferolateral to the optic canal and separated from it by the optic strut is the superior orbital fissure (Fig. 10-76). This fissure is somewhat comma-shaped, bulbous inferomedially, and thin superolaterally. Its long axis is directed medially, backward, and slightly downward. Where the fissure begins to widen, its lower border is marked by a bony projection, often sharp in character, which gives attachment to the lateral part of the common tendinous ring of Zinn. The superior orbital fissure in fact is bounded above by the lesser and below by the greater wings of the sphenoid and bounded medially by the sphenoid body.[1] It communicates with the middle cranial fossa and transmits the oculomotor, trochlear and abducens nerves, and the terminal branches of the ophthalmic nerve and the ophthalmic veins. The lacrimal and frontal nerves traverse the narrow, lateral part of the fissure, which transmits also the meningeal branch of the lacrimal artery and the occasional orbital branch of the middle meningeal artery. The trochlear nerve is situated more medially and lies just outside the common tendinous ring of Zinn.[1] The two divisions of the oculomotor nerve, the nasociliary (a branch of ophthalmic nerve) and the abducens nerves, pass within the tendinous ring and therefore traverse the wider, medial part of the fissure. They may be accompanied by the superior and inferior ophthalmic veins; but the superior ophthalmic vein may accompany the trochlear nerve, while the inferior ophthalmic vein may pass through the medial end of the fissure below the ring.[1]

Inferior Orbital Fissure

At the posterior aspect of the orbit the inferior and lateral walls of the orbit are separated by the inferior orbital fissure (Figs. 10-74 to 10-76). The fissure is bounded above by the greater wing of the sphenoid, below by the maxilla and the orbital process of palatine bone, and laterally by the zygomatic bone or the zygomaticomaxillary suture. In fact, the inferior orbital fissure extends obliquely as a gently curving continuation of the more medial pterygopalatine fossa (Fig. 10-78). The maxillary nerve is the most important structure traversing the inferior orbital fissure. In addition to the maxillary nerve, the inferior orbital fissure transmits the infraorbital vessels, the zygomatic nerve, and a few minute twigs from the pterygopalatine ganglion. Through the anterior part of the inferior orbital fissure, a vein passes to communicate the inferior ophthalmic

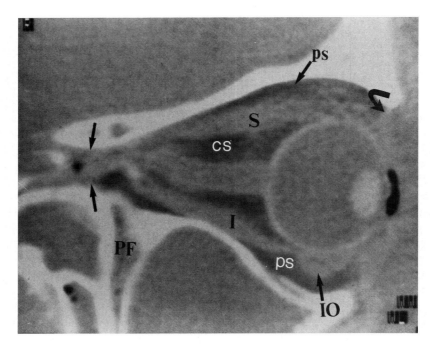

Fig. 10-77 Orbital CT anatomy. Direct parasagittal CT scan of cadaver head shows peripheral orbital space *(PS)*; central orbital (intraconal) space *(CS)*; optic nerve; superior rectus muscle *(S)* and inferior rectus muscle *(I)*; inferior oblique muscle *(IO)*; orbital septum *(curved arrow)*; and common tendon of Zinn *(arrows)*. Periosteum (periorbita) lines bony orbit as orbital fascia and is loosely attached to bony orbit. Periosteum is united with dura matter and sheath of optic nerve at optic canal. Normally periosteum cannot be differentiated from adjacent soft tissues. Periosteum is continuous with periosteum of bones of face and is also continuous with layer of dura at superior orbital fissure. Note continuity of periorbita with periosteum of pterygomaxillary fossa *(PF)*. Infection or infiltrative process of pterygomaxillary fossa may invade orbital subperiosteal space (periorbita) or vice versa. (CT scan courtesy FW Zonneveld.) (From Mafee MF et al: Orbital space-occupying lesions: role of CT and MR: an analysis of 145 cases, Radiol Clin North Am 25:529, 1987.)

vein with the pterygoid plexus in the infratemporal fossa.[1] The pterygopalatine fossa is a small, narrow, pyramidal space situated below the apex of the orbit and tapering inferiorly (Fig. 10-77). It is bounded above by the body of the sphenoid, in front by the maxilla, behind by the pterygoid processes and greater wing of sphenoid, and medially by the palatine bone (Fig. 10-77). It communicates with the infratemporal fossa through the pterygomaxillary fissure. Five foramina and canals open into the fossa: the rotundum, the pterygoid (vidian), the pharyngeal (palatovaginal) (Fig. 10-76, *B*), the sphenopalatine, and the pterygopalatine. The most important contents of the fossa are the maxillary nerve, the pterygopalatine (sphenopalatine) ganglion, and the terminal part of the maxillary artery.

Periorbita

The periosteum of the bony orbit is known as the periorbita. The periosteum is a specialized connective tissue structure that covers the bones. It consists of two strata: a superficial fibrous mantle and an active inner layer known as the *cambium*.[4] Duhamel[5] is credited with the first scientific investigation of the osteogenic properties of the periosteum. The periorbita (orbital fascia) is generally loosely adherent to the surrounding bones except at the anterior orbital margin, trochlear fossa, lacrimal crests, and the margins of the fissures and canals.[1,2,6,7] Posteriorly it is continuous with the dura of the optic nerve and the area surrounding the superior orbital fissure. Anteriorly it is continuous with the periosteum of the orbital margins (Fig. 10-77). Thus, surgery or trauma posteriorly may result in cerebrospinal fluid leaks.[2] The dura mater is composed of a meningeal layer and a periosteal layer; these two layers are so closely bound together at this point that they are separated only with difficulty.[7] However, after these layers pass through the optic foramen, they become separated. The meningeal layer continues as the sheath of the optic nerve, and the periosteal layer lines the bony orbit as the orbital fascia or periorbita. Numerous septa and fascial bands from various structures in the orbit are attached to the inner surface of the perios-

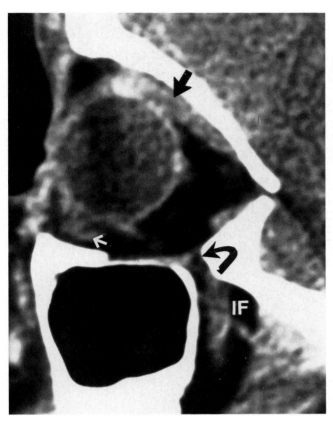

Fig. 10-78 Direct parasagittal CT scan shows lateral extension of inferior orbital fissure *(curved arrow)* into infratemporal fossa *(IF)*. Note inferior oblique muscle *(white arrow)* and superior rectus muscle *(black arrow)*.

teum.[7] In front the periorbita is fused with the orbital septum along the margins of the base of the orbit.[8] The orbital septum in fact is the continuation of the periosteum.

Orbital Septum and Eyelids

The orbital septum is a weak, membranous sheet that forms the fibrous layer of the eyelids and is attached to the margins of the bony orbit where it is continuous with the periorbita. In the upper lid it joins the tendon of the levator palpebrae muscle. In general, each eyelid or palpebra from without inwards consists of skin, subcutaneous areolar tissue without fat, fibers of the orbicularis oculi, tarsus and orbital septum, tarsal glands (meibomian), and conjunctiva. The conjunctiva is the transparent mucous membrane that covers the inner surfaces of the eyelids and is reflected over the front part of the sclera and cornea.[1] The line of reflexion of the conjunctiva from the eyelids on the eyeball is called the conjunctival fornix. The palpebral conjunctiva is highly vascular, and its deeper portion contains a con-

siderable amount of lymphoid tissue, especially near the fornices. It is intimately adherent to the tarsi.[1] The ocular conjunctiva is loosely connected to the eyeball. On reaching the cornea, the ocular conjunctiva continues as the corneal epithelium.[1] Anteriorly the orbit is closed by the orbital septum (Figs. 10-77 and 10-79), which forms the fibrous layer of the eyelids. Anterior to the septum lies the orbicularis oculi and the skin. Within each eyelid, the orbital septum is thickened to form a tarsal plate. The levator palpebrae superioris is attached to the upper edge of the superior tarsal plate. A few fibers of inferior rectus muscle are attached to the lower edge of the inferior tarsal plate.[9] Posteriorly each plate has meibomian glands (modified sebaceous glands embedded in the tarsi), and the plate is covered by conjunctiva.

Tenon's Capsule (Fascia Bulbi) and Tenon's Space

Tenon's capsule is a fibroelastic membrane that envelopes the eyeball from the optic nerve to the level of the ciliary muscle. Tenon's capsule, which is also called the *fascial sheath*, fascia bulbi, and the bulbar fascia of the eyeball, is discussed on pp. 698 and 699.

Orbital Fatty Reticulum

Within the orbit all structures are embedded in a fatty reticulum. The fibroelastic tissue that makes up the reticulum divides the fat into lobes and lobules.[7] The fatty reticulum is divided into (1) the peripheral orbital fat, which is outside the muscle cone, and its intermuscular membranes (Figs. 10-75, 10-77, and 10-79); and (2) the central orbital fat, which is within the muscle cone (Figs. 10-77 and 10-79).

The Extraocular Muscles

The six striated extraocular muscles, including the four recti and the two oblique muscles, control eye movement (Figs. 10-77 and 10-79). The rectus muscles arise from the annulus of Zinn, which is a funnel-shaped tendinous ring that encloses the optic foramen and the medial end of the superior orbital fissure,[6,10] where it is continuous with the dural sheath of the optic nerve and the periorbita.[2] The annulus has an upper common tendon of Lockwood and lower common tendon of Zinn. Because of this intimate relationship, apical disease frequently affects all of these structures simultaneously. In addition, surgical removal of the optic nerve must be done within the annulus, which is most safely entered superomedially after removing the orbital roof.[2] The inferior rectus muscle originates from the common tendon of Zinn below the optic foramen. It inserts into the inferior sclera 6.5 mm from the limbus. The superior rectus (the longest of the four recti) originates from the common tendon of Lockwood above the

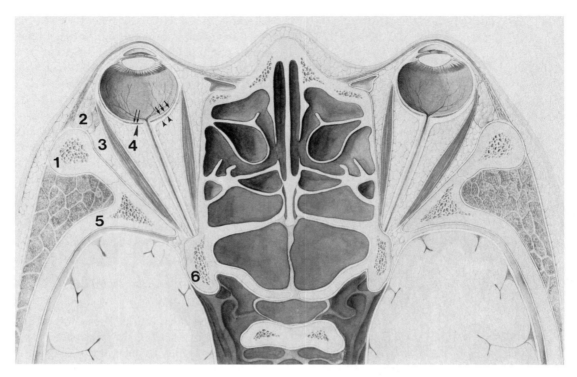

Fig. 10-79 Diagram of the orbital-cranial region showing the zygomatic bone, *(1)*; lacrimal gland, *(2)*; peripheral orbital fatty reticulum, *(3)*; central orbital fatty reticulum, *(4)*; greater wing of the sphenoid, *(5)*; lesser wing (anterior choroid) of the sphenoid, *(6)*. Notice the retina *(three arrows)*, choroid *(two arrows)*, sclera *(arrowhead)*, and tenon capsule *(two arrowheads)*.

optic foramen and from the sheath of the optic nerve. It passes below the levator aponeurosis and inserts into the upper sclera 7.7 mm from the limbus. The medial rectus muscle (the thickest of recti) arises from the upper tendon of Lockwood, the lower tendon of Zinn, and the sheath of the optic nerve[10,11] and inserts 5.5 mm from the limbus. The lateral rectus originates from the lower common tendon of Zinn and the upper common tendon of Lockwood and inserts 6.9 mm from the limbus.[11] The superior oblique (longest and thinnest of the extraocular muscles) originates from the periosteum of sphenoid bone above and medial to the annulus of Zinn and the origin of the medial rectus.[10,11] It passes anteriorly along the upper part of the medial orbital wall[10,11] as a slender tendon and enters the trochlea, a fibrocartilaginous ring lined with a synovial-type sheath.[12] The tendon slides through the trochlea and then turns sharply posterolaterally and downward beneath the superior rectus muscle to insert in the lateral sclera, behind the equator of the eye. The inferior oblique muscle is the only extrinsic eye muscle that originates not from the orbital apex but from the orbital plate of the maxilla just posterolateral to the orifice of the nasolacrimal duct. It passes under the inferior rectus and inserts to the posterior and inferolateral aspect of the globe.[13] All of the extraocular muscles are about 40 mm in length except for the 37 mm inferior oblique.[14] One important difference among the muscles is the ratio of tendinous tissue to muscle fibers. The inferior oblique muscle contains essentially no tendon, whereas the superior oblique muscle has 20 mm of tendon.[14]

The levator palpebrae is often called the *seventh extraocular muscle*. It originates from a thickening of the periosteum of the greater wing of the sphenoid bone, just above the annulus of Zinn, and passes between the roof of the orbit and the superior rectus muscle. Frequently the levator shows many attachments to the superior rectus and cannot be easily separated from it on CT and MRI sections. Both appear as thin structures in the posterior orbit but widen (the levator more than the superior rectus) as they pass anteriorly. Müller's muscle, a sympathetically innervated smooth muscle, is attached anteriorly to the levator muscle and aponeurosis.[2] The third cranial nerve (oculomotor) supplies the superior, inferior, and medial recti; the inferior oblique muscle; and the levator palpebrae. The lateral rectus is innervated by the sixth nerve (abducens), and the fourth cranial nerve (trochlea) innervates the superior oblique muscle.

Movements of Eyelid and Eyeball

The levator palpebrae superioris is the main, striated voluntary part of the levator muscle that elevates the upper eyelid. It is opposed by the orbicularis oculi.[1,9] The smaller, inferior stratum of the levator is the non-striated part of the muscle, the superior palpebral, tarsal, or Müller's muscle, which is responsible for ptosis in Horner's syndrome. The inferior rectus depresses the lower eyelid.

Within its fascial sheath, the eyeball is rotated by the extraocular muscles, which displace the gaze upward (elevation), downward (depression), medially (adduction), and laterally (abduction). Rotation about an anteroposterior axis (torsion) may also occur.[9] The actions of the medial and lateral recti are adduction and abduction, respectively. They are antagonists; and by reciprocal adjustment of their lengths, the visual axis can be swept through a horizontal arc. The primary action of the superior rectus is elevation; its secondary action is a less powerful medial rotation (adduction).[1,9] Its primary antagonist is the inferior rectus muscle, which depresses and adducts the eyeball and whose primary antagonist is the superior rectus muscle. The superior oblique muscle acts on the eyeball from the trochlea. Since the attachment of the inferior oblique is for practical purposes vertically inferior to this, both muscles approach the eyeball at the same angle, being attached in approximately similar positions in the superior and inferior posterolateral quadrants of the eyeball.[1] From these attachments it is easy to understand that the inferior oblique muscle elevates the gaze and the superior oblique muscle depresses it. Both oblique muscles produce abduction.[1,9] Like the superior and inferior recti, the two oblique muscles have opposed forces in respect to the other (antagonist). Acting together in concert, they could therefore assist the lateral rectus in abduction of the visual axis.[1]

INNERVATION
Optic Nerve

The optic nerve (Fig. 10-77) is a nerve fiber tract that conveys visual sensation. It traverses the optic canal with the ophthalmic artery, passes forward and laterally within the cone of rectus muscles, and enters the eyeball just medial to its posterior pole. The optic nerve is about 4.5 cm to 5 cm long and about 4 mm in diameter.[2] It is divided into four portions: intraocular (1 mm), intraorbital (3 cm), intracanalicular (5 to 6 mm), and intracranial (1 cm).[2] From the optic foramen the optic nerve takes a tortuous, S-shaped configuration to the back of the globe because the distance from the globe to the orbital apex is 20 mm. The optic nerve is covered by three layers: the pia mater, the arachnoid, and the dura, all which sheathe the nerve and extend from the canal forward to the globe. The pia mater is highly vascular and is attached tightly to the optic nerve.[15] The subarachnoid space is filled with CSF in continuity with the intracranial subarachnoid space. The subdural space surrounding the optic nerve, however, has no direct connection to the intracranial subdural space.[15] The optic nerve is fixed to the orbital apex by fusion of the dura mater to the periosteum at the optic canal.[15] The ophthalmic artery is encased by dura in the optic canal, where it lies inferolateral to the nerve. At the orbital end of the canal, it loses the dural coat and crosses medially in the intraconal space.[2]

Peripheral Nerves

Several nerves reach the orbit from the middle cranial fossa and pterygopalatine fossae. The optic nerve traverses the optic canal. Other nerves gain access to the orbit through the orbital fissures.

Sensory Innervation

The major sensory innervation of the orbit is by means of the ophthalmic (V_1) and maxillary (V_2) divisions of the trigeminal nerve. The cell bodies of the ophthalmic nerve are in the semilunar (gasserian) ganglion. From the ganglion the nerve courses along the lateral wall of the cavernous sinus, below the oculomotor and trochlear nerves, and enters the orbit through the superior orbital fissure. Before entering the orbit, the ophthalmic nerve divides into lacrimal, frontal, and nasociliary nerves, each of which enters the orbit through the superior orbital fissure.[2,9] The frontal (largest branch) and lacrimal (smallest branch) branches of the ophthalmic nerve enter the orbit outside the annulus of Zinn and run forward between the periorbita and the levator complex to supply the forehead and lacrimal gland. The nasociliary branch is intraconal, crosses medially over the optic nerve, continues forward along the medial wall of the orbit below the superior rectus and superior oblique muscles,[8] and terminates as the ethmoidal (anterior and posterior) and infratrochlear nerves. Its branches include one to the ciliary ganglion and two long ciliary nerves.[2,9] The long ciliary nerves carry sympathetic vasoconstrictor fibers to supply the vessels within the eyeball.[9]

Motor Innervation

Oculomotor Nerve (III). The nucleus of the oculomotor nerve is in the midbrain tegmentum. The nerve appears in the interpeduncular fossa and courses in the most cephalic, lateral wall of cavernous sinus to enter the orbit through the superior orbital fissure. It has superior and inferior divisions, which are often formed before entering the orbit.[9] The nerve enters the muscle cone within the annulus of Zinn as a superior division (supplying the levator and superior rectus) and an inferior division (supplying the medial and inferior rectus and inferior oblique). Just lateral to the optic nerve about 1.5 to 2 cm behind the globe is the ciliary ganglion.[2,9] It is chiefly a ganglion where the parasympathetic fibers from the inferior division of the oculomotor nerve form a synapse.[2] The sympathetic fibers to the smooth muscle in the levator palpebrae superioris (Müller's muscle) and inferior rectus (Müller's muscle) enter the oculomotor nerve in the cavernous sinus and travel with its branches to these muscles.[9]

Trochlear Nerve (IV). The nucleus of the trochlear nerve is in the midbrain tegmentum. Its fibers leave the central nervous system through the anterior medullary velum dorsally, cross to the opposite side, pass rostrally and caudally, and then run in the lateral wall of the cavernous sinus between the oculomotor (III) and ophthalmic (V_1) nerves. The trochlear nerve then crosses the oculomotor nerve, passes through the superior orbital fissure above the other nerves,[8] and enters the orbit via the superior orbital fissure, passing above the muscle cone to supply the superior oblique muscle.[9]

Abducens Nerve (VI). The nucleus of the abducens nerve is in the tegmentum of pons. Its fibers leave the central nervous system in the ventral groove between the medulla and pons, pass through the cavernous sinus between the internal carotid artery and the ophthalmic nerve (V_1), enter the orbit through the superior orbital fissure,[8] and then pass forward on the inner surface of the lateral rectus, which it supplies.[9]

Other Nerves. The seventh cranial nerve is the motor supply for the orbicularis oculi; and its sensory division, the nervus intermedius, gives the parasympathetic supply to the lacrimal gland. The facial nerve enters the parotid gland and then divides into upper and lower branches. It innervates the orbicularis from the upper division, by the temporofrontal and zygomatic branches.[2]

Autonomic Nerves. The ciliary ganglion lies 1.5 to 2 cm behind the eyeball, lateral to the optic nerve. It receives sensory fibers from the nasociliary nerve, parasympathetic fibers from the oculomotor nerve, and sympathetic fibers from the internal carotid plexus in the cavernous sinus (via the superior orbital fissure).[2,9] Only the parasympathetic fibers synapse in the ganglion. The sensory root subserves the cornea, iris, and ciliary body through short ciliary nerves that pass from the anterior part of the ciliary ganglion into the eyeball.[9] The parasympathetic fibers supply the ciliary muscle and the iris sphincter, which constricts the pupil. The preganglionic parasympathetic fibers to sphincter muscle arise in the Edinger-Westphall nucleus of midbrain, travel through the oculomotor nerve, run into its inferior division, and end by synapse in the ciliary body. The postganglionic fibers arise from the cells of ciliary ganglion, leave the ganglion by the short ciliary nerves piercing the sclera, and run to the iris. The sympathetic fibers supply the ocular vessels, the iris dilator (by means of the ciliary nerves), the lacrimal

gland, and the sympathetic muscles of the upper (Müller muscle) and lower lids. The sympathetic fibers to the dilator pupillae muscle pass through the ciliary ganglion without synapse and run with the short ciliary nerves.

The preganglionic fibers of the sympathetic to dilator pupillae arise in the intermediolateral gray column of the upper thoracic cord, enter the sympathetic trunk, and ascend in the cervical sympathetic trunk to end by synapses in the superior cervical ganglion.[8]

The postganglionic sympathetic fibers arise in cells of the superior cervical ganglion and ascend through the carotid and cavernous plexuses. Some fibers join the ophthalmic nerve to continue in its nasociliary branch and are carried to the eye with the long ciliary branches of this nerve; others from the cavernous plexus enter the sympathetic "root" of the ciliary ganglion, pass through without synapse, and run with the short ciliary nerves.[8] Other intraorbital sympathetic fibers travel in the oculomotor nerve to the smooth muscle components of the levator palpebrae superiosis and the inferior rectus (Müller's muscles).[9] Parasympathetic and sympathetic fibers reach the lacrimal gland via the fibers of the maxillary nerve, which communicate with the lacrimal branch of the ophthalmic nerve to reach the gland. The preganglionic parasympathetic fibers of the lacrimal gland arise from cells in the superior salivatory nucleus and run in the nervus intermedius (with facial nerve), then to the great superficial petrosal nerve, which becomes part of the nerve of the pterygoid (vidian) canal, to enter and synapse in the pterygopalatine ganglion. The postganglionic fibers arise from the cells of the pterygopalatine ganglion, pass through the pterygopalatine nerves to the maxillary nerve, and then through the zygomatic branch of the latter.[8] These fibers enter the zygomaticotemporal branch of the zygomatic nerve in the orbit and communicate with the lacrimal branch of ophthalmic nerve to reach the gland.

The preganglionic sympathetic fibers of the lacrimal gland arise in the intermediolateral gray column of the upper thoracic cord, enter the sympathetic trunk, and ascend in the cervical sympathetic trunk to end by synapses in the superior cervical ganglion.[8] The postganglionic sympathetic fibers of the lacrimal gland arise in cells of the superior cervical ganglion, pass through the carotid plexus, continue rostrally in the deep petrosal nerve, and join the superficial greater petrosal nerve to become the pterygoid (vidian) nerve. Then the fibers pass through the pterygopalatine ganglion without synapse and are distributed similar to the postganglionic parasympathetic fibers to reach the lacrimal gland.[8]

Vascular Anatomy

The major arterial supply of the orbit is from branches of the ophthalmic artery, which generally arises from the internal carotid artery at the end of the cavernous sinus. Rarely it may arise from the middle meningeal artery and enter the orbit through the superior orbital fissure.[2] In the optic canal it courses below and lateral to the optic nerve within the dural sheath, and at the orbital apex penetrates laterally through the dura and then crosses in 82.6% of subjects to the medial orbit over the optic nerve.[2] In the remaining 17.4% of subjects, the artery courses under the nerve.[2] The branches of the ophthalmic artery with some variations in origin are the lacrimal, supraorbital, anterior and posterior ethmoidal, nasofrontal, and dorsonasal arteries. Its branches for the eyeball include the central artery of the retina and the ciliary arteries. The central artery of the retina is the first branch of the ophthalmic artery.[9] It crosses the optic nerve, pierces it, and runs in its center to spread over the retina.[8] The ciliary arteries are arranged in three groups: the short posterior ciliary, the long posterior ciliary, and the anterior ciliary arteries.[8] The posterior ciliary arteries supply the globe by 15 to 20 short branches (to the choroid, ciliary processes, and the optic nerve head) and two long branches (to the ciliary muscle, iris, and the anterior choroid).[2] The long posterior ciliary arteries enter the sclera on either side of the optic nerve and run between the choroid and the sclera to the ciliary body, where their branches form an anterior major arterial circle. The anterior ciliary arteries arise from the muscular branches running with the tendons of the recti muscles to form a vascular zone under the conjunctiva. They pierce the sclera to join the major circle.[8] The lacrimal artery branches into recurrent meningeal, zygomatic, glandular, and lateral palpebral arteries (which form the arcades of the lid). The ophthalmic artery frequently has anastomotic branches to the external carotid system by means of the middle meningeal and lacrimal arteries, which pass through the superior orbital fissure, and by means of the anterior deep temporal, superficial temporal, and lacrimal arteries.[2]

Venous Drainage of Orbit and Eyeball. The venous blood from the eyeball and adjacent structures drains into the inferior and superior ophthalmic veins. The orbital veins are valveless, and the superior ophthalmic vein drains into the cavernous sinus by the superior orbital fissure. The inferior ophthalmic vein passes through the inferior orbital fissure into the pterygopalatine fossa.[2,9] Both superior and inferior ophthalmic veins communicate with the veins of the face.[9] The superior ophthalmic vein is the larger and is formed by the confluence of the angular, nasofrontal, and supraorbital veins. It has three sections, the first extending posterolaterally to the medial border of the superior rectus. The second section enters the muscle cone, passing to the lateral orbit beneath the superior rectus muscle. The third section extends posteromedially along the lateral border of the superior rectus muscle

into the superior orbital fissure.[2] The more variable inferior ophthalmic vein forms inferolaterally as a plexus and passes posteriorly adjacent to the inferior rectus muscle. It anastomoses with the superior ophthalmic vein, and it has a similar branch that connects with the pterygoid plexus through the inferior orbital fissure.[2]

Lacrimal Apparatus

The lacrimal gland lies in the superolateral angle of the orbit in a shallow fossa (lacrimal fossa) behind the upper eyelid and is deeply indented by the lateral border of the tendon of levator palpebrae superioris.[2,9] It weighs about 80 g and measures approximately 20 mm by 12 mm by 5 mm.[2] It is divided into palpebral and orbital (larger) lobes by the lateral border of the levator aponeurosis.[2] The orbital lobe is superior to the palpebral lobe. Ten to twelve small ducts open from the deep surface of the gland into the conjunctival sac. Resection of the palpebral lobe functionally destroys the gland.[2] The borders of the gland are related anteriorly to the orbital septum, posteriorly to the periorbital fat, and medially to the superior rectus, globe, and lateral rectus; the inferior surface rests on the lateral rectus.[2] The lacrimal gland is a serous gland having a nodular surface with a fine connective tissue pseudocapsule.[2] The gland is supported by Whitnall's ligament as well as by septal attachments to the superior periorbita. The lacrimal artery penetrates it posteriorly, and the vein from it drains into the superior ophthalmic vein. Its lymphatic drainage is by means of the lid and conjunctiva to the preauricular nodes.[2] The lacrimal nerve and sometimes branches of the zygomatic nerve carry the sensory afferents. The parasympathetic efferents are by the nervus intermedius, facial, greater superficial petrosal, vidian, sphenopalatine ganglion, infraorbital, and lacrimal nerves.[1,2] The sympathetic efferents are from the internal carotid plexus through the sphenopalatine ganglion. In addition to the main lacrimal gland, there are accessory glands (Krause's and Wolfring's) in the lids and conjunctiva. There are 20 to 40 glands of Krause in the upper fornix and six to eight in the lower fornix. The glands of Wolfring are fewer, consisting of three at the upper border of the superior tarsus and one at the lower border of the inferior tarsus.[2] Tears produced by the gland pass medially toward the lacrimal puncta across the surface of the cornea, assisted by blinking of the eyelids. Evaporation of the fluid is retarded by the oily secretion of the tarsal glands. The tears are drained into the lacrimal sac through the lacrimal canaliculi of the upper and lower lid. The canaliculi originate at the puncta and have a 2.0 mm vertical portion and an 8.0 mm horizontal portion, which join into a common canaliculus. The superior canaliculus first is directed upward, then medially and downward. The inferior canaliculus first descends and then is directed medially. The common canaliculus enters the lateral wall of the lacrimal sac by means of Rosenmüller's valve, which prevents reflux.[2] The lacrimal sac lies in the lacrimal groove, which is formed by lacrimal bone and frontal process of maxillary bone.[8] The lacrimal canaliculi are lined by squamous epithelium, whereas the sac and nasolacrimal duct are lined by columnar epithelium, goblet cells, and ciliated cells. The lacrimal sac is 13 to 15 mm in vertical length. The tears drain through the nasolacrimal duct just beneath the inferior turbinate through a fold in the duct (called the valve of Hasner) in the lateral wall of the nasal cavity.[2]

TECHNIQUE FOR ORBITAL CT AND MRI
General Considerations

CT and MRI are the two modalities commonly used for imaging the orbit. Each has advantages and disadvantages. In general CT is the modality of choice for bony details. MRI is superior to CT for soft tissue details. Radiation to the orbital structures is one of the disadvantages of CT. The radiation dose to the lens, although less than that of an orbital series of complex motion tomography, averages about 5 rad per imaging plane. MRI, on the other hand, has no known biological side effect. CT is superior to MRI for detecting calcification, and it is the study of choice for the evaluation of foreign bodies. MRI should not be used for the evaluation of the orbit whenever there is a suspicion of a ferromagnetic foreign body around the orbit.

Computed Tomography

A routine CT examination of the orbits includes contiguous axial and coronal sectioning with 5 mm slice thickness. If there is a suspicion of a smaller lesion, thinner sections should be obtained. Such 3 or 1.5 mm sections are essential for the optimal demonstration of the optic nerve and its pathology. Thin slices have the advantage of less volume averaging and thus provide finer spatial resolution. The radiologist should always tailor the examination according to the clinical information and the preliminary diagnosis on noncontrast CT examination. For foreign bodies it is important to obtain 1.5 mm axial sections to increase the index of detection for smaller objects. It is often unnecessary to obtain additional direct coronal sections for the localization of foreign bodies, since the use of computer reformatting is helpful in producing images in other planes, provided there is no motion in axial sections. For lesions of the globe, thin sectioning (1.5 mm) is exceedingly important,[16-18] since one can easily miss an ocular lesion on routine 5 mm sections. For primary bony lesions, orbital fractures, or when there is secondary involvement of the bony orbit, in addition to the routine study, we obtain retrospective high resolution, ex-

tended bone scale (4000 HU) images, similar to the technique for temporal bone (4000 window width, 700 to 800 window level).[6]

The need for intravenous (IV) contrast media administration for orbital CT scanning should be determined by the clinical information and the discretion of the radiologist. Contrast material uniformly increases the density of most intraorbital soft tissue structures.[16] Although it is not always an easy task to discriminate between orbital lesions based on their density patterns of enhancement, contrast material is often necessary to evaluate the degree of their vascularity, and more importantly, for the evaluation of any intracranial extension of orbital lesions. Not uncommonly an apical orbital mass may be an extension of an intracranial lesion such as a meningioma, which can be readily missed in noncontrast CT scans. In general, one should not use contrast media in the following cases: foreign bodies, uncomplicated orbital fractures, thyroid ophthalmopathy, for evaluating the morphologic changes or variations of extraocular muscles, dermoid cyst (unruptured), and bony lesions such as osteoma, osteoid osteoma, fibrous dysplasia and Paget's disease. Contrast enhanced CT study is necessary in patients with osteogenic or chondrogenic sarcomas or metastatic bone disease.

Technique. The axial sections are normally obtained roughly parallel to the infraorbital-meatal line.[17] This can be easily determined by obtaining a lateral digital scout view. The inferior section should include the upper portion of the maxillary sinuses, and the upper section should include the sella and the entire frontal sinuses. For all orbital and ocular tumors it is our practice to routinely obtain additional postcontrast 10 mm axial sections of the remainder of the head. Although brain metastasis from orbital and ocular tumors is uncommon, the additional six to eight sections may provide information about unsuspected lesions (meningioma, aneurysm, and AVM). The coronal sections are obtained roughly perpendicular to the infraorbital-meatal line. In many instances, the angle of the coronal sections is made more oblique (semicoronal) when the patient has many dental fillings or other metallic prosthesis. Patient positioning for the coronal plane can be in either prone or supine positions. As for axial sections, the coronal plane can be easily determined by obtaining a lateral digital scout view of the orbit.

Coronal examination of the orbits should be tailored according to the clinical information and the findings on the axial sections. In patients suffering from visual loss and for evaluation of the intracranial extension of an apical lesion, coronal sections should be extended posteriorly to include at least the optic chiasm. For lesions involving the anterior ethmoid air cells, the nasal cavity and those arising from the nasolacrimal sac and duct, coronal sections should be extended anteriorly enough to include the nasal bones.

In general, axial and coronal sections are complementary to each other. The bony orbital floor and roof, and ocular lesions in the 6 or 12 o'clock positions in particular require coronal sections for evaluation.

Sagittal Plane. Almost all CT scanners are capable of performing computer reformation of compiled data from axial sections into coronal, sagittal, or oblique planes. Although the quality of the images is inferior to direct scanning, in many instances additional information can be obtained, particularly if high quality thin (1.5 to 3 mm) direct axial or coronal sections are available. Direct sagittal scanning of the craniofacial structures can be achieved by laying the patient on a separate support and using a special head holder, which is fitted to the standard tabletop.[18]

MRI Techniques

Almost all MRI presented in this section was performed with a 1.5 Tesla Signa unit (General Electric, Milwaukee). Using a head coil, single echo spin-echo (SE) pulse sequences were obtained with a repetition time (TR) of 300 to 800 ms and an echo time (TE) of 20 to 25 ms (TR/TE = 300-800/20-25 ms). Multiple echoes SE pulse sequences were obtained with a TR of 1500 to 2500 ms and a TE of 20 to 100 ms. The early echo (20 ms) in this sequence yielded proton-weighted (PW) images, and the later echo (40 to 100 ms) yielded T_2-weighted (T_2W) images. The single echo SE pulse sequences with short TR and short TE (TR/TE = 300-800 ms/20-25 ms) yielded T_1-weighted (T_1W) images. Although individual examinations should always be specifically tailored according to the problems of individual patients, for orbital lesions our routine MRI orbital examination consisted of a short TR, short TE, sagittal images 5 mm in thickness with 1 to 1.5 mm intersection spacing, using the routine head coil. The studies were most often performed with one excitation, a 256×256 matrix, and a 20 to 24 cm field of view. Following the sagittal T_1W scans, an axial SE sequence (TR/TE 2,000/ 20, 80 ms) was obtained to include the entire orbital structures. An additional single echo or multiple echo, SE sequence in the coronal plane was also obtained according to the findings on sagittal and axial sections. The T_1W images provide the most spatial resolution; therefore, if more anatomic details are essential, coronal T_1W images are preferred. The T_2W images, on the other hand, provide more contrast resolution. In case more pathologic detail is needed, coronal multiple SE pulse sequences are obtained (TR/TE, 2000/20, 80 ms). It is our practice to routinely obtain an SE sequence (2,000/20, 80 ms) axial sections of the remainder of the supraorbital head. The parameters remain the same except we use a 256×128 matrix to cut the scan time in half (usually 4 minutes) of the orbital axial scans (8 minutes). For optic nerve lesions additional parasagittal images are obtained by using a head coil. For some of the orbital lesions, additional images were obtained using a surface coil. Images with a surface coil provide better spatial resolution; however, the apical lesions and intracranial extension of the orbital lesions cannot be fully evaluated because of signal dropout proportional to the distance from the surface coil. Paramagnetic contrast material should be used for suspected orbital meningiomas, schwannomas, hemangiopericytomas, lacrimal gland tumors, metastases, lymphomas, pseudotumors, other specific or nonspecific orbital masses and optic nerve lesions including optic neuritis.

Inversion Recovery and Application of Fat-Suppression Technique

Short Time Inversion Recovery (STIR) results in very high lesion conspicuity by suppressing the signal from fat and by adding T_1 and T_2 together. Since most pathology has long T_1 and T_2 relaxation times, pathology appears with a high signal intensity on STIR. Darkening (suppressing) the fat signal intensity further makes any pathology stand out. The optimal TI (time of inversion) for fat suppression may vary from one individual to another, depending on coil loading and the fat composition. The optimal TI for fat suppression at 1.5 Tesla is in the 145 to 170 ms range. We usually use a TR of 2000 and TI of 150 to 160 and TE of 20 msec for obtaining STIR images. We use a STIR pulse sequence for optic neuritis, as well as in other pathologic conditions.

Normal CT and MRI Anatomy

Axial, coronal, sagittal, and oblique views are complementary for showing bony and soft tissue anatomy.

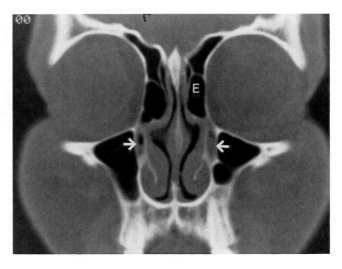

Fig. 10-80 Nasolacrimal canals. Coronal CT scan shows nasolacrimal canals *(arrows)*. Note anterior ethmoid cells *(E)*.

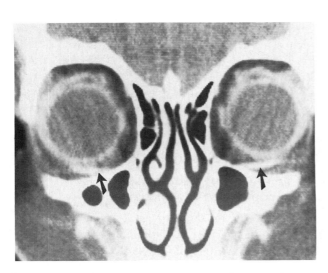

Fig. 10-81 Inferior oblique muscles. Coronal CT scan shows inferior oblique muscles (arrows).

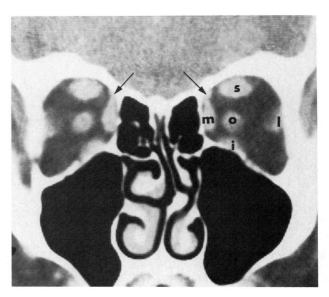

Fig. 10-82 Extraocular muscles. Coronal CT scan shows inferior rectus muscle (i); lateral rectus muscle (l); medial rectus muscle (m); and superior rectus muscle (s). Note superior oblique muscles (arrows) and optic nerve (o).

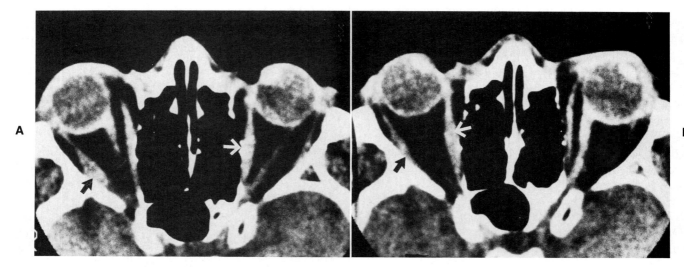

Fig. 10-83 Demonstration of Sherrington's law of reciprocal innervation. **A,** Axial CT scan obtained during right lateral gaze demonstrates Sherrington's law of reciprocal innervation. Note that right lateral rectus muscle (black arrow) and left medial rectus muscle (white arrow) contract, and that right medial and left lateral rectus muscles relax (lengthen). **B,** Axial CT scan obtained during left lateral gaze. Right medial rectus muscle (white arrow) and left lateral rectus muscle are contracted, and right lateral rectus muscle (black arrow) and left medial rectus muscle are relaxed (lengthened). (From Mafee MF et al: CT in the evaluation of Brown's superior oblique tendon sheath syndrome, Radiology 154:691, 1985.)

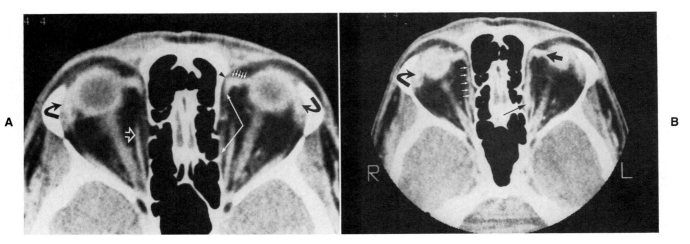

Fig. 10-84 Normal superior oblique muscles. **A,** Axial CT scan demonstrates superior oblique tendon *(crossed arrows);* trochlea *(arrowhead);* reflected portion of superior oblique muscles tendon *(white arrows);* medial rectus *(hollow arrow);* and lacrimal glands *(curved arrow).* **B,** Scan obtained 1.5 mm superior to view in **A** demonstrates entire course of both superior oblique muscles *(long arrow)* and their tendons *(white arrows),* including their reflected portion *(short thick arrow).* Partially volumed medial rectus is just lateral to superior oblique muscles. Note lacrimal glands *(curved arrow).*

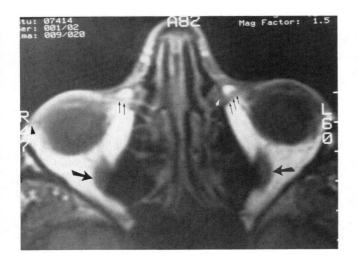

Fig. 10-85 Normal MRI anatomy. T₁W (800/20) MRI scan shows medial palpebral ligament *(black arrows);* lateral palpebral ligament *(small black arrowhead);* nasolacrimal duct *(white arrowhead);* and inferior rectus muscles *(large black arrows).*

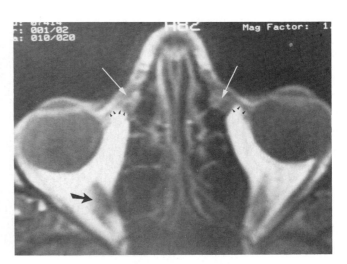

Fig. 10-86 Normal MRI anatomy. T₁W (800/20) MRI scan obtained 3 mm superior to view in Fig. 10-85 shows medial palpebral ligaments *(arrowheads);* lacrimal sacs *(white arrows);* and inferior rectus muscles *(black arrow).* The inferior portions of lenses are partially volumed in this section.

The bony orbits and their landmarks can be best visualized on CT scans with the aid of the bone extended scale and bone window technique (Fig. 10-80). The optic canals, the lateral and medial bony margins, the superior and inferior orbital fissures, the lacrimal fossa, lacrimal sac, nasolacrimal canal as well as the infraorbital canal and paraorbital sinuses are equally well seen on axial or coronal scans (Fig. 10-81). Coronal scans are best for assessing the floor and roof of the orbits. The lamina papyracea is a paper-thin plate that forms most of the medial orbital wall, separating it from the adjacent ethmoid air cells. This plate often appears to be dehiscent on CT scan; therefore, care should be taken not to make an erroneous suggestion of bone destruction or fracture.

Extraocular Muscles. The extraocular muscles are well visualized on CT scans and uniformly enhanced on postcontrast CT scans (Figs. 10-81 to 10-84). These muscles are seen with exquisite detail on MRI scans (Figs. 10-85 to 10-97). The extraocular muscles generally have a course parallel to the adjacent orbital wall. Consequently, only the horizontal recti (lateral and medial) may be seen in their entirety on an axial plane (Figs. 10-83 and 10-87). Likewise, vertical recti (inferior and superior) may be seen in the parasagittal (oblique) plane (Figs. 10-77, 10-78, and 10-98). The tapering of these muscles in their tendinous portions, as well as their origins at the annulus of Zinn, are well seen in parasagittal (vertical recti) and axial (horizontal recti) scans (Figs. 10-77 and 10-87). The superior and inferior recti are only partially visualized on any one axial section (Figs. 10-85, 10-86, 10-91, and 10-92). On coronal scans the recti muscles are seen cross-sectionally (Figs. 10-93 and 10-95). For accurate determination of the cross-sectional size of a muscle, reformatted images or direct oblique MRI scans would have to be done for each muscle separately. This is obviously not practical or necessary unless it is critical to determine whether a particular muscle is enlarged.[14] The levator palpebrae superioris is closely approximated with the superior rectus muscle, merges with it, and is only identified separately on anterior coronal images (Fig. 10-93) where it diverges and separates from the superior rectus. These two muscles can both be visualized at the same time or separately on sagittal and parasagittal (oblique) MR images (Fig. 10-98). The superior oblique muscle can be best visualized on coronal (its muscle portion) and axial (its tendinous portion) scans (Figs. 10-82, 10-84, and 10-94). The trochlear and reflected portions of its tendon are best seen on axial scans (Figs. 10-84 and 10-91). The trochlea is well seen on axial scans and is occasionally calcified. The inferior oblique muscle is best seen on coronal, sagittal, and parasagittal scans (Fig. 10-81). The muscle belly is poorly defined on axial scans. Only its insertion is seen well on axial scans.

Orbital Compartments. In descriptive terms the orbit has been divided into the extraperiosteal, subperiosteal, extraconal, conal, and intraconal spaces. The intraconal space is separated from the other spaces by the rectus muscles and their intermuscular septa, which are denser in the anterior orbit and best seen on coronal scans (Figs. 10-93 and 10-94). Certain lesions have a predilection to appear in a specific orbital space; and

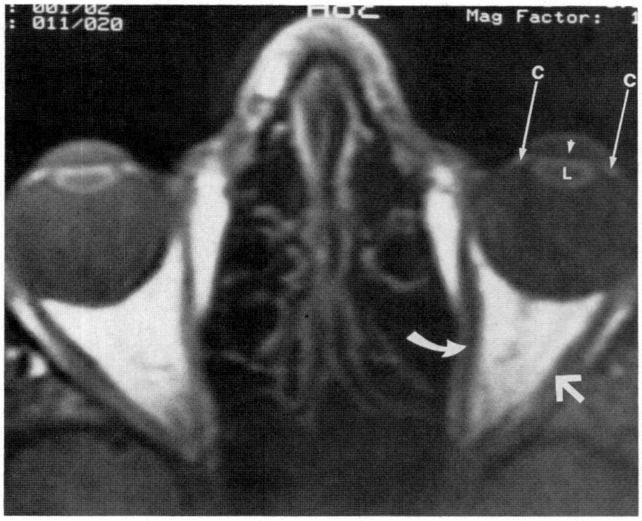

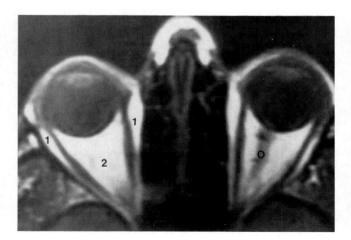

Fig. 10-87 Normal MRI anatomy. T_1W (800/20) MRI scan obtained 3 mm superior to view in Fig. 10-86 shows ciliary body *(C)*; anterior chamber *(arrowhead)*; lens *(L)*; medial rectus muscle *(curved arrow)*; and lateral rectus muscle *(straight arrow)*.

Fig. 10-88 Normal MRI anatomy. T_1W (800/20) MRI scan obtained 3 mm superior to view in Fig. 10-87 shows optic nerve *(o)*; extraconal orbital fat *(1)*; and intraconal orbital fat *(2)*.

the concept of various orbital spaces serves some practical value, which will be discussed later in this chapter.

Lacrimal Gland. The lacrimal glands are the only prominent structures that are readily identified in the lacrimal fossa in the superolateral extraconal space with the exception of a portion of the superior ophthalmic vein.[16] They are about the size and shape of an almond. They are adjacent to the tendons of the superior and lateral rectus muscles and separated from the globe by the lateral rectus muscles (Figs. 10-84, 10-90, and 10-91). The more anterior palpebral lobe is separated from the deeper orbital lobe by the lateral horn of the levator muscle aponeurosis.[19]

Vascular and Neuronal Structures. Vascular structures in the orbit can be seen frequently on noncontrast CT but are highlighted with contrast. They are seen on MRI as hypointense areas (signal voids). The ophthalmic artery can be seen in the apex of the orbit on the inferior aspect of the optic nerve as it swings laterally before looping around and over the optic nerve to its superior medial aspect (Fig. 10-95). Several of its branches, including the anterior and posterior ethmoidal and posterior ciliary branches, can usually be identified.[2,20,21]

The superior ophthalmic vein originates in the extraconal, anteromedial aspect of the orbit, and from here it courses near the trochlea to pass through the muscle cone medially to laterally beneath the superior rectus muscle and above the optic nerve, to exit the intraconal space through the superior orbital fissure (Figs. 10-90 and 10-91). This vein is routinely identified in axial, coronal, sagittal, and parasagittal images. The inferior ophthalmic and connecting veins are seen inconsistently.[2]

The intraconal and extraconal components of small nerves of the orbit, particularly the frontal, supraorbital, and inferior divisions of the third nerve, as well as the infraorbital nerve (a branch of the maxillary nerve) may be identified on CT and especially on MRI scans. The position of these nerves may be variable.[2] The frontal nerve can be seen between the levator palpebrae superioris muscle and the orbital roof (Figs. 10-93 and 10-94). Most of the small nerves can be seen on coronal scans of the orbital apex (Fig. 10-93).[21]

Optic Nerve. The optic nerve arises from the ganglionic layer of the retina and consists of coarse myelinated fibers, like the white matter of the central nervous system.[22] The orbital segment of the optic nerve is 3 to 4 mm in diameter and 20 to 30 mm long (Fig. 10-89). It has a serpentine course (with minimal inferior and lateral bowing in its midportion) in the orbit, which allows unrestricted movement of the globe. From its insertion on the posterior globe, it courses posteriorly, medially, and superiorly to exit the orbit at the optic

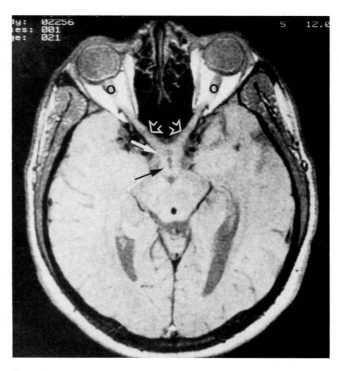

Fig. 10-89   Normal MRI anatomy. PW (2000/20) MRI scan shows intraorbital segment of optic nerves *(o);* intracanalicular segment of optic nerves *(hollow arrows);* chiasm *(white arrow);* and hypothalamus *(black arrow).*

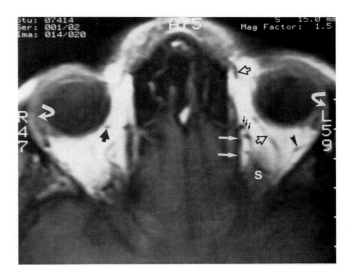

Fig. 10-90   Normal MRI anatomy. T_2W (800/20) MRI scan shows superior rectus muscle *(S);* lacrimal vein *(arrowhead);* lacrimal glands *(curved arrows);* superior ophthalmic vein *(hollow arrows);* medial ophthalmic vein *(three small arrows);* superior oblique muscle *(white arrows);* and presumed vorticose vein *(solid black arrow).*

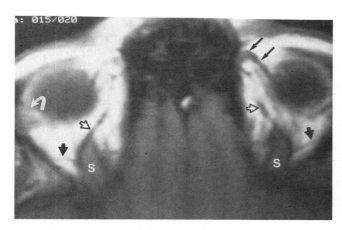

Fig. 10-91 Normal MRI anatomy. T₁W (800/20) MRI scan obtained 3 mm superior to view in Fig. 10-90 shows superior muscle complex *(S)*; superior ophthalmic vein *(hollow arrows)*; lacrimal glands *(curved arrow)*; reflected portion of superior oblique muscle tendon *(two black arrows)*; and lacrimal vein *(solid black arrow)*.

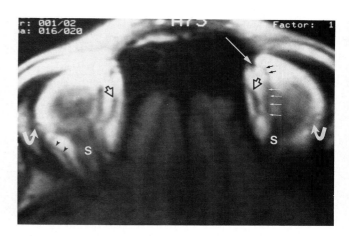

Fig. 10-92 Normal MRI anatomy. T₁W (800/20) MRI scan obtained 3 mm superior to view in Fig. 10-91 shows tendon of superior muscle complex *(S)*; superior ophthalmic veins *(hollow arrows)*; lacrimal glands *(curved arrows)*; presumed lacrimal nerve *(arrowheads)*; trochlea *(white solid arrow)*; presumed frontal nerve *(white arrows)*; and supratrochlear nerve *(small black arrows)*.

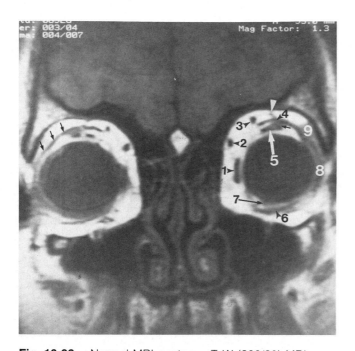

Fig. 10-93 Normal MRI anatomy. T₁W (800/20) MRI scan shows medial rectus muscle *(1)*; superior oblique muscle tendon *(2)*; superior ophthalmic/supratrochlear vein *(3)*; levator palpebrae superioris *(4)*; tendon of superior rectus *(single short arrow)*; tendon of superior oblique muscle *(5)*; inferior oblique muscle *(6)*; tendon of inferior rectus muscle *(7)*; tendon lateral rectus muscle *(8)*; palpebral portion of lacrimal gland *(9)*; supraorbital nerve *(white arrowhead)*; and intermuscular septum *(black arrows)*.

canal. The optic nerve is covered by layers of pia, subarachnoid membrane, and dura mater. All these layers fuse and become continuous with the sclera. At the superior aspect of the optic nerve, the three layers of covering are fused to each other and to the optic nerve and are fixed to the optic canal, protecting it from back-and-forth motion.[22] The intracranial segment of the optic nerve is located medially and then above the internal carotid artery in the suprasellar region (Fig. 10-89). The optic nerves join in the suprasellar cistern to form the optic chiasm (Fig. 10-89).[22] The subarachnoid space around the optic nerve sheath has a low density on CT scans and can be imaged during the course of iodinated contrast cisternography. The meningeal layers of the optic nerve show enhancement on postcontrast CT scans. On coronal scans immediately posterior to the globe, a small central density within the nerve represents the central retinal artery and vein.[2] The optic nerve/sheath measures between 3 to 5 mm in axial plane and 4 to 6 mm in the coronal plane.[16] The intracanalicular and prechiasmatic portions of the optic nerve are particularly well demonstrated by MRI (Fig. 10-89). Generally on T₁W, PW, and T₂W images, the optic nerve exhibits MRI characteristics similar to those of normal white matter.[22] A ring of T₁ hypointensity and T₂ hyperintensity representing cerebrospinal fluid (CSF) within the nerve sheath is frequently seen on coronal sections. This should not be confused with well-defined areas of hypointensity bordering the nerve, which are caused by chemical shift artifacts.

Globe. The three ocular coats (sclera, choroid, and retina) form a well-defined image on CT scans that enhance with IV contrast material. The lens is normally hyperdense on CT scans. The vitreous appears hypodense and shows no contrast enhancement. On MR images the ocular coats appear as a hypointense ring, and the vitreous has very similar characteristics as CSF. The lens is isointense to vitreous on T_1W and appears hypointense in T_2W images. The imaging of the globe is discussed in more detail in the ocular section of this chapter.

Bony Interorbital Distance. The distance between the orbits and their individual dimensions are important in the diagnosis of craniofacial anomalies. The eyes are often involved in craniofacial malformations, which include orbital clefts and orbital hypotelorism and hypertelorism. Measurement of the bony interorbital distance (BID) is useful in establishing the severity of the hypertelorism. This distance is commonly measured at the interdacryon level, the dacryon being the point of junction of the nasal bone, lacrimal bone, and nasal process of the maxilla.[17] Before CT most observers relied on standard radiographs for measuring the BID. Normal values for adults as well as younger age groups are available.[23-25] The BID was first defined by Cameron[26] in a small number of dried skulls as the maximum distance between the medial walls of the bony orbits measured at the juncture of the crista lacrimalis posterior with the frontolacrimal suture. Currarino and Silverman,[23] in their studies of arhinencephaly and trigonocephaly, measured the BID between the medial walls at what was described to be the junction between each medial angular process of the frontal bone with the maxillary and lacrimal bones.

To provide a statistically more reliable standard, Gerald and Silverman[24] repeated the original work of Currarino and Silverman[23] using the same technical factors and studied 100 patients in each year of age from birth to 12 years. Hansman[27] presented measurements of the interorbital distance and thickness of the skull based on radiographs of the skull and paranasal sinuses in a large group of healthy subjects. According to him, from "infancy to adulthood, the bony interorbital distance for girls is consistently narrower than for boys. Starting at 1 year 6 months, there is gradual increase in the size of the measurements for both sexes. At about 13 years of age the girl's growth began to level off. Since the boys continue to increase to the age of about 21 years, the measurements in girls fall more markedly below the boys as growth is completed." The average adult measurement in women is 25 mm and in men 28 mm.[27]

CT of the orbit provides an opportunity to evaluate the distance between the orbits and, if necessary, any other linear and angular measurements, as well as other information. The lacrimal bones and the orbital plates of the ethmoid (lamina papyracea) cast a thin line of increased density on the CT scan; therefore, the BID can

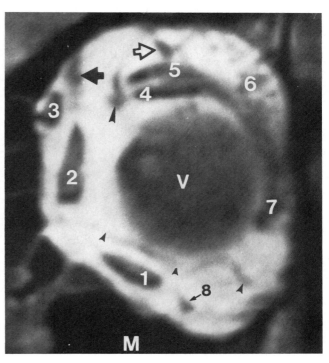

Fig. 10-94 Normal MRI anatomy. T_1W (800/20) MRI scan shows inferior rectus muscle *(1)*; medial rectus muscle *(2)*; superior oblique muscle *(3)*; superior rectus muscle *(4)*; levator palpebrae superioris *(5)*; partially volumed lacrimal gland *(6)*; lateral rectus *(7)*; presumed branch of oculomotor nerve *(8)*; collateral vein *(small arrowheads)*; medial ophthalmic vein *(solid black arrow)*; frontal nerve/supraorbital nerve *(hollow arrow)*; supraorbital/ophthalmic artery *(single arrowhead)*; vitreous *(V)*; and maxillary antrum *(M)*.

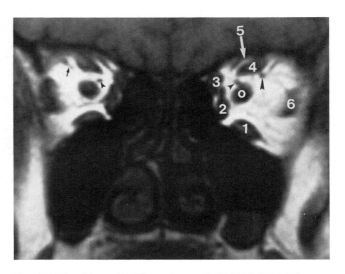

Fig. 10-95 Normal MRI anatomy. T_1W (800/20) MRI scan shows inferior rectus muscle *(1)*; medial rectus muscle *(2)*; superior oblique muscle *(3)*; superior rectus muscle *(4)*; levator palpebrae superioris *(5)*; lateral rectus muscle *(6)*; optic nerve *(o)*; superior ophthalmic vein *(large arrowhead)*; ophthalmic artery *(small arrowhead)*; and lacrimal nerve *(black arrow)*.

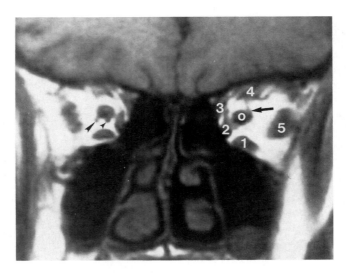

Fig. 10-96   Normal MRI anatomy. T₁W (800/20) MRI scan shows inferior rectus muscle *(1)*; medial rectus muscle *(2)*; superior oblique muscle *(3)*; superior rectus muscle *(4)*; lateral rectus muscle *(5)*; optic nerve *(o)*; long posterior ciliary arteries *(arrowheads)*; and presumed ciliary ganglion *(arrow)*.

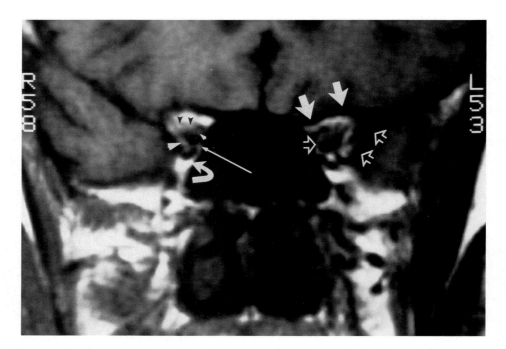

Fig. 10-97   Normal MRI anatomy. T₁W (800/20) MRI scan shows lesser *(double solid arrows)* and greater *(double hollow arrows)* wings of sphenoid bone; medial rectus muscle *(single hollow arrow)*; inferior rectus muscle *(long arrow)*; lateral rectus muscle *(large white arrowhead)*; superior muscle complex *(black arrowheads)*; optic nerve *(short white arrowhead)*; and fat in apex of orbit, along with inferior orbital fissure *(curved arrow)*. Common tendon of Zinn is seen as areas of hypointensity between rectus muscles. Relative position of nerves, veins, and ophthalmic artery entering orbital cavity through superior orbital fissure cannot be precisely resolved with current MRI technology.

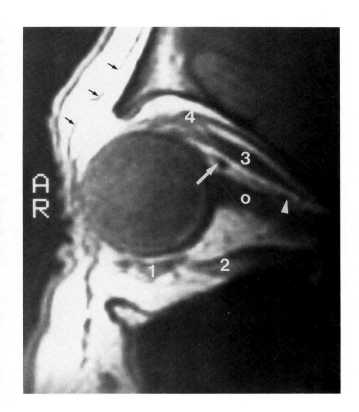

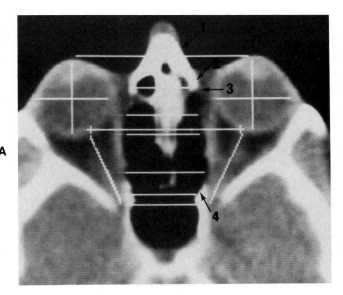

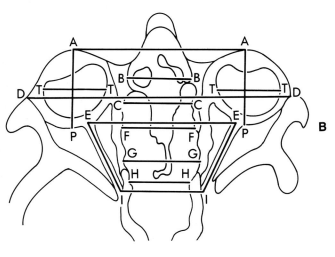

Fig. 10-98 Normal MRI anatomy. Sagittal PW (2000/20) MRI scan shows inferior oblique muscle *(1);* inferior rectus muscle *(2);* superior rectus muscle *(3);* levator palpebrae superioris *(4);* optic nerve *(o);* ophthalmic artery *(arrowhead);* superior ophthalmic vein *(white arrow);* and orbicularis muscle *(black arrows).*

Fig. 10-99 **A,** Axial CT scan of orbits at level of plane of optic nerves shows outline of globes, lenses, vitreous bodies; level of medial check ligament *(3);* medial and lateral rectus muscles; optic nerves; and retroorbital fat compartments. Note nasal bone *(1)* and frontal process of maxilla *(2)* on each side. Lamina papyracea is seen as very thin density hardly distinguishable from medial aspect of medial rectus muscle. Posterior to that is most posterior part of medial wall of bony orbit *(4),* which is related to anterior part of sphenoid sinus. **B,** Diagram shows different points selected for various measurements presented in Table 10-1. (From Mafee MF et al: CT in the evaluation of the orbit and the bony interorbital distance, AJNR 7:265, 1986.)

Table 10-1 CT orbital measurements in 400 adults

Line, Description	Minimum		Maximum		Mean	
	Male	Female	Male	Female	Male	Female
AA, Approximates interpupillary distance	6.26	6.21	7.51	7.50	6.78	6.63
BB, BIOD measured at posterior border of frontal processes of maxillae	2.29	2.29	3.21	3.20	2.67	2.56
CC, BIOD measured posterior or at level of orbital equator (useful orbits)	2.63	2.56	3.50	3.30	2.80	2.83
DD, Distance between anterior margin of frontal processes of zygomatic bones at level of plane of optic nerves	9.18	9.29	10.13	11.00	9.73	9.97
EE, Distance between optic nerves where they enter eyeballs	5.16	4.78	6.40	6.00	5.43	5.27
FF, BIOD measured at level of posterior poles of eyeballs	2.87	2.56	3.7	3.51	3.10	2.97
GG, BIOD measured at its widest part (usually posterior to FF line)	3.16	2.93	4.10	3.67	3.37	3.20
HH, BIOD measured at its most posterior part (apex of bony orbit)	2.16	2.43	3.37	3.23	2.73	2.80
II, Distance between superior orbital fissures at apex of bony orbit	2.90	2.70	3.83	3.63	3.10	3.00
JJ, Distance between central portion of cranial opening of optic canals	2.20	2.01	2.73	2.70	2.30	2.20
KK, Distance between tips of anterior clinoid processes	2.31	2.43	3.21	3.16	2.80	2.83
EI, Length of intraorbital part of optic nerve:						
Right	2.70	2.40	3.80	3.23	3.10	2.90
Left	2.60	2.40	3.80	3.21	3.20	2.80
AP, Anteroposterior diameter of eyeball:						
Right	2.50	2.39	2.90	2.70	2.80	2.50
Left	2.40	2.40	2.80	2.80	2.70	2.63
TT, Transverse diameter of eyeball:						
Right	2.50	2.40	2.80	2.90	2.70	2.71
Left	2.50	2.50	2.90	2.90	2.80	2.83
Angle between optic nerve axes (in degrees)	35°	36.5°	50°	51.5°	41°	42.3°

Note: BIOD = bony interorbital distance.

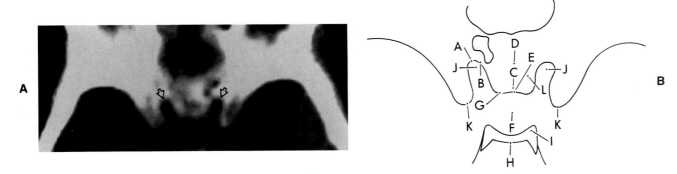

Fig. 10-100 **A,** Axial CT scan of head at level of planum sphenoidale and anterior roots of lesser wings of sphenoid bone shows cranial openings *(arrows)* of optic canals. **B,** Diagram shows structures in **A:** *A,* Cranial opening of optic canal; *B,* anterior root of lesser wing of sphenoid; *C,* posterior border of chiasmatic groove; *D,* planum sphenoidale; *E,* tuberculum sellae; *F,* pituitary fossa; *G,* middle clinoid; *H,* dorsum sellae; *I,* posterior clinoid; *J,* midportion of cranial opening of optic canal; *K,* anterior clinoid; *L,* anterior border of chiasmatic groove. (From Mafee MF et al: CT in the evaluation of the orbit and bony interorbital distance, AJNR 7:265, 1986.)

be measured at any desired point.[17] Mafee et al[17] presented the linear and angular measurements of the orbit in CT studies of 400 adults (200 men age 18 to 82, average age 52; 200 females age 17 to 88, average age 54) (Table 10-1). The data were collected from patients with normal orbits who were studied for suspicion of brain infarction, hearing loss, and brain tumors. None had any underlying craniofacial anomaly or congenital malformations. The patients were Caucasion except for a few who were Oriental. Their study data were collected only from nonrotated axial sections in the plane of the optic nerve (Fig. 10-99). A horizontal CT section through the orbits at this level generally shows two patterns: (1) a parallel separation of the medial orbital walls and (2) a fusiform or lateral spread of the ethmoidal air cells with the widest separation of the orbital walls occurring posterior to the posterior pole of globe.[17] The distance between the medial walls of the bony orbits at various points and other linear and angular measurements are illustrated in Fig. 10-99, *A* and *B*. Several reference points have been used. Anterior pole (A) is applied to the central point of the anterior curvature of the eyeball and posterior pole (P) to the central point of its posterior curvature. A line joining the two poles forms the optic axis (AP); the primary axes of the two globes are nearly parallel. The cranial opening of the optic canal is well demonstrated in Fig. 10-100. The optic canal lies between the roots of the lesser wing and is bounded medially by the body of the sphenoid bone (Fig. 10-100). The anterior root is broad and flat and is continuous with the planum sphenoidale (Figs. 10-97, *A* and 10-100, *A*). The posterior root is shorter and thicker (optic strut) and connected to the body of the sphenoid opposite the posterior border of the sulcus chiasmatis.[17] As seen in Table 10-1 the normal BID, measured at the posterior border of the frontal processes of

the maxilla on nonrotated CT scans in the plane of the optic nerve, ranges from 2.29 to 3.21 cm (average 2.67 cm) in men and 2.29 to 3.20 cm (average 2.56 cm) in women. The widest interorbital distance lies behind the posterior poles of the globes. This ranges from 3.16 to 4.10 cm (average 3.37 cm) in men and 2.93 to 3.67 cm (average 3.20 cm) in women. A line joining the lateral orbital margins in the axial plane (DD, line Table 10-1, Figs. 10-97, *A* and 10-99, *B*) will normally intersect the globe near its midportion with at least one third of the globe posterior to this line.

PATHOLOGY
Hypertelorism, Hypotelorism, Exophthalmus, and Exorbitism Defined

The terminology used to describe abnormalities of the orbit is complicated and may be confusing[28] to those unfamiliar with it; therefore, it will be briefly reviewed.

Hypertelorism literally translates from the Greek as "increased distance" ("hyper" meaning over and "tele" meaning distant). Orbital hypertelorism describes the anatomic situation in which the medial walls of the orbits are farther apart than normal.[28-30]

Patients with orbital hypertelorism almost always have eyes spaced more widely apart than normal. Telecanthus is a condition that may clinically mimic orbital hypertelorism. In this condition the distance between the apices of the medial canthal ligaments is increased and the eyes are spaced more widely apart than normal; however, the BID is not increased. These patients do not have orbital hypertelorism. They do have medial canthal hypertelorism. Telecanthus may be congenital or acquired; when acquired, it is often a consequence of trauma.[28]

Orbital hypotelorism refers to a decrease in the BID.

Patients with this condition may appear clinically to have either narrowly spaced or normally spaced eyes; surprisingly they may even appear to have widely spaced eyes. For example, patients with Down's syndrome and trisomy 13 were classically described as having hypertelorism on the basis of clinical evaluation, but in fact these patients have orbital hypotelorism.[28,30]

Exophthalmos describes abnormal prominence of the globe, while proptosis emphasizes abnormal protrusion of the globe. Exophthalmos and proptosis, however, commonly are used as synonyms. Exorbitism, on the other hand, refers to a decrease in the volume of the orbit. The orbital contents are greater in volume than the orbital capacity and generally protrude anteriorly (proptosis), causing the globe to be unusually prominent (exophthalmos).

Congenital and Developmental Abnormalities

There are many hereditary, as well as sporadic, abnormalities that involve the orbits, globe, and adjacent orbital tissues, and other craniofacial and skeletal structures. The study of these conditions is complicated by the variety of names used for the same syndrome and by the overlapping criteria utilized to establish the diagnosis of a syndrome.[31] To list all of the congenital malformations or syndromes is beyond the scope of this chapter. Many excellent books have detailed descriptions of these disorders.[31-34]

The eyes are often involved in craniofacial malformations, which include orbital clefts and orbital hypotelorism and hypertelorism. CT and MRI are very useful in the preoperative evaluation of such patients. Surgical treatment of hypertelorism involves translocation of the globes toward the midline by lateral wall osteotomy at a point posterior to the equator of the eye.[17] The CT and MRI may show an encephalocele or a porencephalic cyst as an additional feature of the malformation.[17]

Many congenital disorders involve the orbits, globe, and adjacent tissues.[31] A brief review of the embryonic development of the orbital and ocular structures is important in understanding the various congenital disorders that affect the orbit. By the third week of gestation, two indentations appear, one on each side of the neural groove or unclosed brain. These are the optic pits; and they deepen to form optic vesicles, which can be viewed externally in the 4 mm embryo (less than 4 weeks of gestation) as two lateral diverticula, on each side of the forebrain[35,36] (Figs. 10-98 and 10-101, A and B). The distal parts of the optic vesicles expand, whereas the proximal parts of the optic vesicles become the tubular optic stalks (Figs. 10-98 and 10-101, C). At the 5 mm embryonic stage (4 weeks of gestation), the external surface of each optic vesicle invaginates.[36] The concavity created by the invagination is known as the *optic cup.* The inner wall of the optic cup (the former

outer wall of the optic vesicles) gives rise to the sensory retina, and the outer wall of the cup is the forerunner of the retinal pigment epithelium (Fig. 10-101, C). The optic vesicle is covered by surface ectoderm (Figs. 10-98 and 10-101, C), which forms the lens.[35] Toward the fifth week, the lens vesicle has completely separated from the surface ectoderm to form the lens.[31] The mesenchyme around the developing eye gradually condenses to form sclera and choroid (Fig. 10-101). During the sixth week of gestation, pigment appears in the optic vesicles.[31] During the invagination of the optic vesicle, a groove remains open for some distance along the optic stalk at the inferior and slightly nasal aspect of the optic cup. This groove is known as the embryonic fissure, or cleft, through which mesenchyme extends into the optic stalk and cup, carrying the hyaloid artery with it (Fig. 10-101, C). As growth proceeds, the edges of the fissure become approximated and they close during the fifth week (15 mm). Failure of the tissues to fuse properly results in some of the congenital colobomatous defects to be discussed later. At the 7.5 mm stage the area in the optic cup where the optic nerve head will develop can be identified.[37] It is referred to as the primitive epithelial papilla and is located in the superior end of the embryonic fissure.[37] Once the axons pass through the primitive epithelial papilla, it is referred to as the *optic nerve head.*[37,38]

The orbit is formed from a combination of membranous and cartilaginous anlage, while the base of the skull, the cranial bone, and the ethmoid and sphenoid bones arise from the cartilage of the more primitive chondrocranium. The ethmoid and sphenoid bones contribute to a large portion of the orbit. The superior portions of the orbit and calvarium develop from a membranous anlage.[1,31]

During the sixth week the embryonic development of the face has progressed with the forward extension of the maxillary process beneath the corresponding optic vesicles. This results in the fusion of the paired maxillary processes with the lateral borders of the lateral nasal processes.[31] During the seventh week there is obvious development of the nose, lips, and chin. The facial clefts are almost completely closed.[31] The eyes continue their forward and medial development and become more prominent. The eyelids begin to form as archlike folds. The eyelids remain fused until the seventh fetal month. By the eighth week the face has assumed features that make it recognizable as human.[31,39-41]

Anatomic and Developmental Considerations. Congenital abnormalities of the orbit and eyes result from faulty development of the embryo and fetus. The eighth week of gestation is the last week of true embryonic development.[31,39-41] By the third week of gestation, the optic pits appear one on each side of the fore-

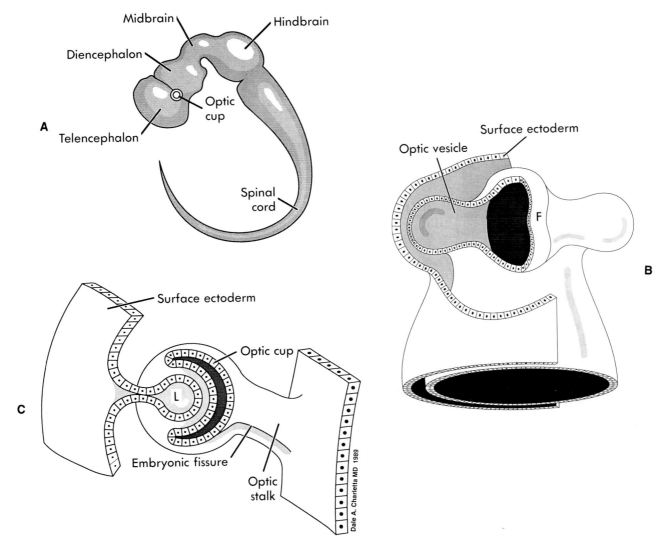

Fig. 10-101   A, 5 mm developing human embryo (4 weeks of gestation). By 3 weeks of gestation two indentations appear, one on each side of the neural groove. These are optic pits, which deepen to form the optic vesicles, one on each side of the forebrain. The optic vesicles give rise to an optic stalk and optic cup on each side. **B,** Development of the posterior ocular structures. In the 4 mm embryo, lateral diverticula on each side of the forebrain *(F)* have given rise to two optic vesicles. The distal portions of the optic vesicles expand, and the proximal portions become the tubular optic stalks. **C,** At the 5 mm stage, the external surface of each optic vesicle invaginates to form the optic cup. The inner wall of the optic cup (formerly the outer wall of the optic vesicle) gives rise to the retina, and the outer wall of the cup becomes the retinal pigment epithelium. The optic vesicle is covered by a layer of surface ectoderm, which forms the lens *(L)*. Note the embryonic fissure, through which mesenchyme extends into the optic stalk and cup. Failure of the embryonic fissure to close causes typical ocular colobomas. (From Mafee MF et al: CT of optic nerve colobomas, morning glory anomaly, and colobomatous cyst, Radiol Clin North Am 25:693, 1987.)

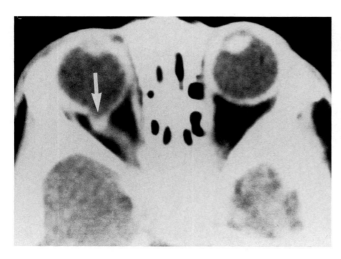

Fig. 10-102 Typical coloboma of optic disc. Axial CT scan shows large posterior global defect with optic disc excavation *(arrow)*.

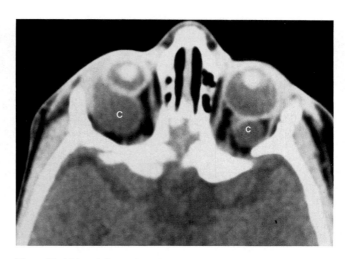

Fig. 10-103 Microphthalmos and colobomatous cysts. CT scan shows microphthalmos, right eyeball being greater than left eyeball with colobomatous cysts *(c)*.

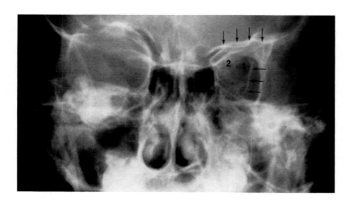

Fig. 10-104 Microphthalmia. Posteroanterior view of skull. Lesser wing of sphenoid *(2)* and left maxillary sinus are hypoplastic, superior orbital fissures are asymmetric *(1)*. Note difference between oblique lines *(horizontal arrows)*, which represent cortices of temporal surface of great wings of sphenoid bone. Notice hypoplasia of the roof of the left orbit *(vertical arrows)*. (From Mafee MF et al: CT in the evaluation of the orbit and the bony interorbital distance, AJNR 7:265, 1986.)

brain. Disturbance of the prosencephalic organizing center (prechordal mesoblast) can cause cyclopia, synophthalmia, or arhinencephaly. Anophthalmia occurs as a result of failure of the neuroectoderm of the optic pit to develop from the anterior portion of the neural plate. A variety of ocular and systemic abnormalities may be seen with an optic nerve coloboma (Figs. 10-97, 10-102, and 10-103). Craniosynotosis is caused from abnormal development of the blastemic stage of the skull bone, including the basicranium. Mandibulofacial dysostosis and otocephaly probably result from inhibition of mesodermal differentiation of the facial structures derived from the first and second branchial (visceral) arches.[31]

Under normal conditions the eye directs orbital growth. During the first year of life, the eye practically doubles in volume and attains more than 50% of its adult volume.[42] By the end of the third year, 75% of the adult volume is achieved (similar to neural growth).[42] The shape of the orbital cranial junction is also influenced by development of the brain and skull.[43] When the brain is underdeveloped but the eye is normal, the orbital plate of the frontal bone is usually elevated into the anterior fossa of the skull.[17] In microcephaly, the orbits are usually circular and the roofs are highly arched.[43] When the eye is underdeveloped but the brain is normal, the orbital plate of the frontal bone appears hypoplastic and the vertical or cranial portion is usually normal (Fig. 10-104). Enucleation of the globe in infancy and early childhood, if untreated with a prosthesis, leads to arrested development of the orbit.[31]

In coronal suture synostosis the orbit on the side of the fusion is elongated superiorly and laterally, imparting a harlequin appearance (Fig. 10-105). Correction of the cranial deformity can lead to spontaneous correction of the orbital deformity in some instances.[17,32] In mandibulofacial dysostosis the orbits may be defective inferolaterally because of malar bone hypoplasia. In cases of severe malar hypoplasia, the lateral wall of the orbit is formed by the greater wing of the sphenoid and the zygomatic process of the frontal bone.

Bony Abnormalities. Minor degrees of facial and or-

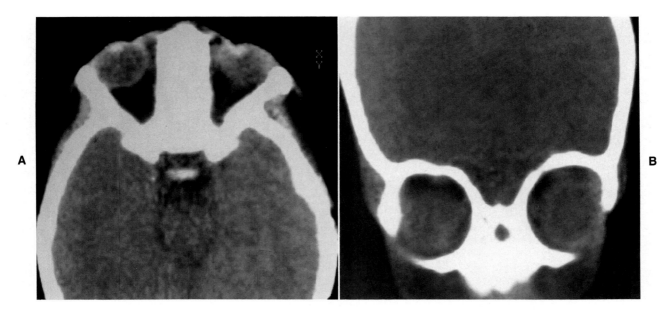

Fig. 10-105   Microphthalmia. Four-year-old boy born without nose and with left microphthalmos and apparent hypertelorism. **A,** Left globe is slightly smaller than right. Increased soft tissue between medial wall of orbit and globe anteriorly has clinical appearance of hypertelorism. In fact, interorbital bony distance is normal. **B,** Coronal scan shows irregular, thick compact bone in anterior midface with absent nasal structures and maxillary sinuses. (From Mafee MF et al: CT in the evaluation of the orbit and the bony interorbital distance, AJNR 7:265, 1986.)

bital asymmetry are the most common causes of pseudoproptosis.[2] For the most part these patients have minor degrees of asymmetry involving all of the hemifacial structures.[2] However, in a few instances, the asymmetry may be related to maxillary hypoplasia resulting in a relatively retroplaced orbit on the affected side. In many cases familial asymmetry may be evident when examining the siblings or parents. These minor developmental abnormalities of the orbit are considered to be anatomic variations. Anomalies of ossification may result in accessory sutures and supernumerary ossicles in the orbital walls.[31] On rare occasions congenital absence of bone in the frontal, maxillary, and orbital region may result in deformity of the bony orbit. Asymmetric enlargement of one bony orbit may result from eccentrically located lesions, such as neurofibroma, hemangioma, lymphangioma, dermoid, or other slow growing processes. A small orbit is seen in anophthalmia, microphthalmia, and postenucleation of the globe in infancy, if not followed by prompt prosthetic treatment.

Bony Orbit in Craniofacial Dysostosis. Craniofacial dysostosis and developmental anomalies may result in profound orbital abnormalities. Orbital malformations in craniofacial dysostosis result chiefly from coronal synostosis. Premature closure of one or more cranial sutures, termed *craniosynostosis* or *craniostenosis*, is the common denominator of many patients with craniofacial anomaly.

Primary Congenital Isolated Craniosynostosis. Any cranial suture may undergo premature closure, but several patterns are recognized more commonly than others. The incidence of congenital suture synostosis reported by Harwood-Nash[44,45] derived from a composite of his experience and from two large series reported by Anderson and Geiger[46] and Shillito and Matson[47] is as follows: Sagittal, 56%, single coronal, 11%; bilateral coronal, 11%; metopic suture, 7%; lambdoid, 1%; and three or more sutures, 14%. Depending on the suture that is prematurely closed, the skull and orbit, including the interorbital distance, have a characteristic shape. These can be grouped as follows:

1. Metopic; trigonocephaly (triangular head); hypotelorism is a constant feature of the trigonocephaly.[43]
2. Sagittal, scaphocephaly (dolicocephaly), in which the anteroposterior diameter of the bony orbit is usually increased and the vertical and transverse diameters of the bony orbit are usually decreased.
3. Unilateral coronal or lambdoid; plagiocephaly, in this condition, if the coronal suture is involved, there is characteristic deformity of the bony orbit (discussed later).
4. Bilateral coronal or lambdoid results in brachycephaly.
5. Coronal and sagittal; oxycephaly or acrocephaly (turricephaly).
6. Coronal, lambdoid, and sagittal; cloverleaf skull (Kleeblattschadel).

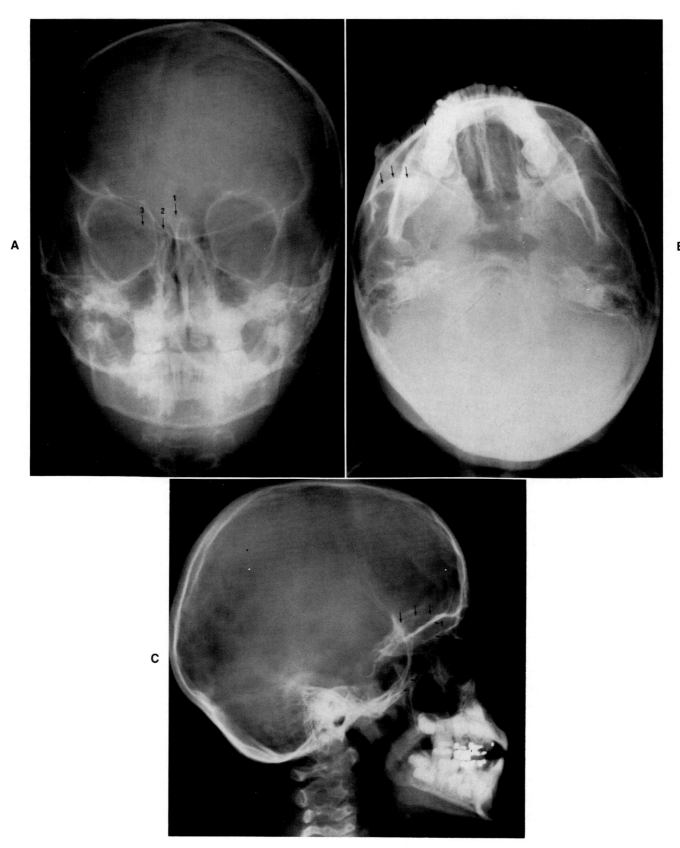

Fig. 10-106 For legend see opposite page.

Fig. 10-106   Plagiocephaly. Premature fusion of right coronal suture. Note elevation of right roof of orbit, giving harlequin appearance to right eye. Right lesser wing of sphenoid *(3)* and right ethmoidal plate (fovea ethmoidal [roof]) *(2)* are elevated. Right lateral margin of orbit is flattened, particularly in superior portion. Digital markings are somewhat increased on right side. Note shift of cristal galli *(1)*, ethmoid complex, and nasal septum to right. Volume of right anterior cranial fossa is decreased, usually a characteristic of premature coronal synostosis. **B,** Submentovertical view of same patient as in **A.** Note flattening of right frontal bone *(upper arrows)*, expansion of right greater wing of sphenoid *(lower arrows)*, and tilting of ethmoid complex to involved side. Note anterior displacement of right petrous bone and right temporomandibular joint and flattening of right side of occipital bone. **C,** Lateral view of same patient as in **A** and **B.** Note anterior displacement of right greater wing of sphenoid *(lower arrows)*, elevation of orbital surface of right anterior cranial fossa *(upper arrows)*, bony ridge along right *(1)* and left *(2)* medial border of orbital roof.

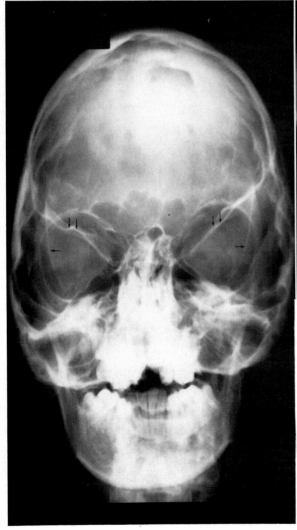

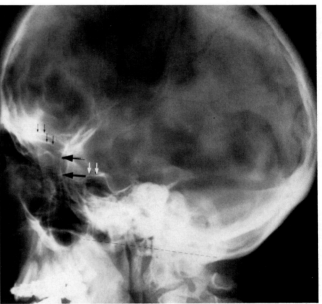

Fig. 10-107   Craniosynostosis caused by bilateral, premature fusion of coronal sutures. **A,** Posteroanterior view of skull shows hyperteloric orbits and marked increased digital markings. Note elevation of lesser wings of sphenoid *(vertical arrows)* and harlequin appearance of both orbits. Note stretched and laterally placed oblique lines *(horizontal arrows)* and flattening of lateral wall of orbits with recessed lateral orbital rim. **B,** Lateral skull view of same patient as in **A** shows absence of sutural lines, increased digital markings, downward and forward displacement of greater wings of sphenoid bone *(large black arrows)*, elevation of roof of orbits *(small black arrows)* and low position of planum sphenoidale *(white arrows)*.

Primary craniosynostosis may be associated with congenital syndromes. These conditions include the following: Crouzon's disease (craniofacial dysostosis), Apert's disease (acrocephalosyndactyly, type I), Saethre-Chotzen syndrome (acrocephalosyndactyly, type II),[44] Carpenter's syndrome (acrocephalopolysyndactyly), chondrodystrophia calcificans congenita (Conradi syndrome or punctate epiphyseal dysplasia), Brachmann-de Lange syndrome, Laurence-Moon-Biedl-Bardet syndrome, Treacher-Collins syndrome (mandibulofacial dysostosis), and craniotelencephalic dysplasia.[44,45]

Orbit in Plagiocephaly. Plagiocephaly results from unilateral closure of one of the paired sutures of the skull, frequently coronal or lambdoid, but rarely temporosquamous sutures. Each produces characteristic deformity of the skull. In practice, most of the time, plagiocephaly is seen in patients with hemicoronal premature synostosis.[44] Here an ipsilateral elevation of the lesser wing of the sphenoid is associated with upward extension of the superior lateral portion of the orbit, imparting a harlequin appearance to the orbit (Fig. 10-106, *A*). The flattening of the ipsilateral frontal bone is also characteristic of premature coronal synostosis (Fig. 10-107, *B*). The volume of the anterior cranial fossa on the side of fusion is decreased. The greater wing of the sphenoid is expanded, displaced forward and downward, and forms a relatively large, middle cranial fossa (Fig. 10-106, *B* and *C*). This occurs in addition to upward elevation of the roof of the orbit, which produces a shallow orbit. The ethmoidal plate (roof of the ethmoidal sinus) is elevated on the side of fusion (Fig. 10-106, *A*). The nasal septum, crista galli, and ethmoidal complex are tilted to the side of fusion (Fig. 10-106, *A*).

Premature fusion of both coronal sutures may occur with or without any other associated abnormality and may result in marked shortening of the anterior cranial fossa and orbital depth (Fig. 10-107). The brain impressions become more prominent on the inner table of the frontal bone (Fig. 10-107). Both a harlequin appearance of the orbit and the bony changes of the unilateral coronal synostosis are duplicated in the bilateral form (Fig. 10-107). Lombardi[48] noted a connection between sagittal or lambdoid synostosis or both in half the reported cases of coronal suture synostosis.

Orbit in Crouzon's and Apert's Diseases. Crouzon's disease, also known as craniofacial dysostosis, is an autosomal dominant disorder with considerable variability in expression.[44] Apert's disease, also known as acrocephalosyndactyly type I, is transmitted as an autosomal dominant disorder. The cranial and facial characteristics of Crouzon's disease are somewhat similar to Apert's syndrome, including brachycephaly, hypertelorism, bilateral exophthalmos, parrot beaked nose, maxillary hypoplasia, relative prognathism, and a drooping lower lip that produces a half-opened mouth. Bilateral exophthal-

mos is essentially a consequence of exorbitism, which in turn is a consequence of several factors that combine to produce a decrease in orbital volume. On the basis of the skull shape alone, Crouzon's and Apert's diseases cannot be distinguished.[44]

In any large series of patients with Crouzon's disease, no regular pattern of calvarial deformity exists. Oxycephaly, brachycephaly, scaphocephaly, and trigonocephaly may be present. In fact, there is too much heterogeneity to allow for a simplistic description. Generally, in Crouzon's disease, brachycephaly or oxycephaly is most often observed. Apert's disease is characterized by irregular craniostenosis with an acrobrachycephalic skull and syndactyly of the hands and feet. Associated skeletal abnormalities, such as ankylosis of the elbow, hip, or shoulder, as well as malformation of the cardiovascular, gastrointestinal, and genitourinary systems may be present.

The orbital malformation in Crouzon's and Apert's diseases is mainly caused by premature coronal synostosis. A striking harlequin appearance of the orbits is seen that results because of the elevation of the roofs and lateral walls of the orbits (Fig. 10-108). The su-

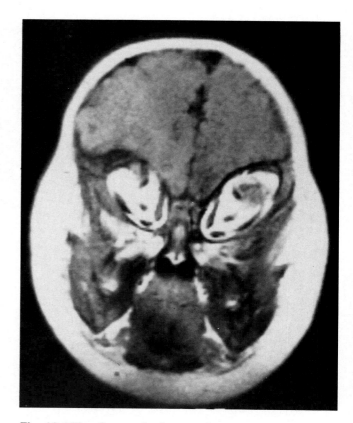

Fig. 10-108 Crouzon's disease. Coronal MRI scan shows striking harlequin appearance of orbits caused by elevation of roofs and lateral walls of orbits. Note deformity of extraocular muscles and hypoplasia of midface. One or more extraocular muscles may be absent in Crouzon's or Apert's disease.

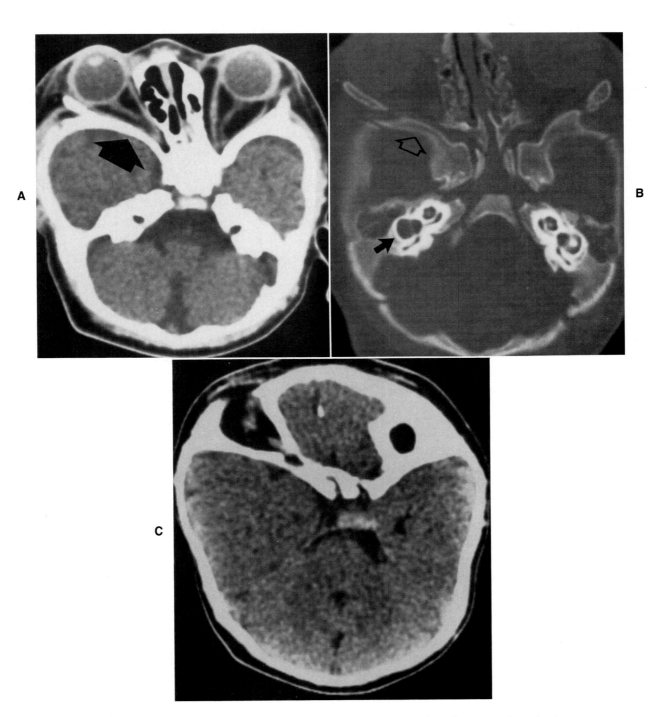

Fig. 10-109   Apert's syndrome. **A,** CT scan shows frontalization of greater wing of sphenoid *(arrow),* exorbitism, and lateral ballooning of ethmoid air cells, causing orbital hypertelorism. **B,** Slightly inferior section using bone algorithm; again, orbits are shallow, and greater wings have coronal orientation *(open arrow).* The lower portion of coronal sutures is open. Note also saccular dilation of lateral semicircular canal on right side *(black arrow).* **C,** Higher CT section shows near normal distance between intracranial opening of optic canals, which are narrow. Note brachycephalic contour of skull.

praorbital rim is recessed and the infraorbital rim is hypoplastic. The orbital depth is markedly reduced as the result of verticalization of the roof (upward tilt of the lesser wing and orbital plate of the frontal bone). Displacement of the greater wing of the sphenoid into a more coronal orientation, which is referred to as *frontalization of the greater wing of the sphenoid,* as well as ballooning of the ethmoid are other factors contributing to exotropia. Hypoplasia of the maxilla and the intermaxillary component contributes in part to the exophthalmos and relative prognathism (Figs. 10-108 and 10-109). Hypoplasia of the maxilla causes recession of the infraorbital rim and foreshortening of the orbital floor.[44] The optic canal in Crouzon's and Apert's diseases is usually narrow. This may lead to optic atrophy.[2] The distance between the intracranial openings of the optic canals is usually normal,[44] and this finding forms the basis for surgical procedures designed to correct or itbl hypertelorism by moving the bony orbits closer together without damaging the optic or oculomotor nerves. Of particular importance to the surgeon contemplating surgical correction of orbital hypertelorism is the orientation and degree of foreshortening of the lateral wall of the orbit. The type of lateral wall osteotomy performed (sagittal split or total mobilization) often depends on these anatomic factors.[28,29] Patients with craniosynostosis syndromes may have marked extraocular muscle anomalies ranging from an apparent absence of ocular muscles to abnormally inserted or very small extraocular muscles (Figs. 10-108 and 10-110).

Saethre-Chotzen Disease (Acrocephalosyndactyly Type II). Saethre-Chotzen disease was described by Saethre in 1931[44,49] and in 1932 by Chotzen.[50] The first family reported in the United States was described in 1970 by Bartsocas et al.[51] The Saethre-Chotzen disease is characterized by synostotic malformation of multiple sutures, facial asymmetry, mild midface hypoplasia, ptosis of the eyelids, an antimongoloid slant of the palpebral fissures, a beaked nose, a low set frontal hairline, variable brachycephaly, and variable cutaneous syndactyly, particularly of the second and third fingers. Other associated abnormalities include a high-arched palate, cleft palate, and deformity of the external ear. The orbital abnormalities in these patients are similar to Crouzon's and Apert's diseases.

Neurofibromatosis. The classic description of neurofibromatosis was published by Friedrich Daniel von Recklinghausen in 1882. Clinical criteria for diagnosing neurofibromatosis[52] include: (1) six or more cafe-au-lait spots, each greater than 1.5 cm in diameter; (2) axillary or other intertriginous freckles; (3) cutaneous neurofibromata, and (4) one or more unequivocally affected parents or siblings. The disease itself is characterized by abnormalities of both ectodermal and mesodermal origin. It is transmitted as an autosomal dominant dis-

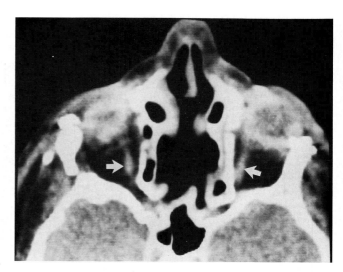

Fig. 10-110 Crouzon's syndrome. CT scan shows small inferior rectus muscles *(arrows).* Note hypertelorism and postsurgical changes of lateral orbital walls.

order of variable penetrance.[28] The incidence of neurofibromatosis is approximately 1 in 3000 live births.[53] About 50% of these patients have a positive family history of the disease, whereas the other 50% are the result of a spontaneous mutation; the mutation rate is about 10:4.[54]

The incidence of central nervous system tumors, including acoustic neuromas, gliomas, meningiomas, and ependymomas, is six times that of the general population.[55] Often multiple central nervous system tumors are present. Although 25% to 35% of neurofibromas occur in the head and neck region,[53] orbital abnormalities are relatively uncommon. Orbital abnormalities are often associated with exophtha¹mos, which may be pulsatile and can generally be classified into one of four categories[53]: (1) orbital neoplasms; (2) plexiform neurofibromatosis; (3) orbital osseous dysplasia (Fig. 10-111); and (4) congenital glaucoma. The most common orbital neoplasm seen in association with neurofibromatosis is optic glioma (Fig. 10-111, *A*). Meningioma is not unusual. Both optic gliomas and meningiomas may occur bilaterally. Bilateral optic gliomas are almost pathognomonic of neurofibromatosis (Fig. 10-112), whereas bilateral meningiomas are only suggestive of neurofibromatosis. Schwannoma, neurofibroma, and neurofibrosarcoma in the orbit also can be seen in these patients.

Orbital (Mesodermal) Defects. Osseous dysplasia of the cranial bones, in particular the bony orbit, may be part of the abnormality associated with von Recklinghausen's disease. The orbital defect is a consequence of partial or complete absence of the greater or the lesser wing of the sphenoid bone or both; the body of the sphenoid bone may also be involved, producing an ab-

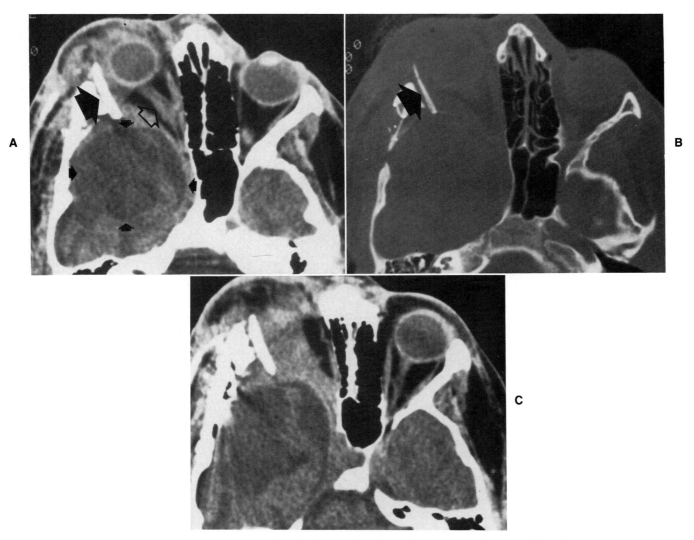

Fig. 10-111   Neurofibromatosis. Patient has had previous surgery for correction of orbital deformity. **A,** Note bone graft along lateral margin of right orbit *(large black arrow).* Note normal left and dysplastic right greater wing of sphenoid bone, with anterior herniation of porencephalic cyst of temporal lobe *(small arrows)* covered by dura. Right optic nerve is enlarged *(open arrow),* and right globe is proptotic. Enlargement of the optic nerve is thought to be caused by optic nerve glioma. **B,** Osseous abnormalities are better seen on this bone detail image. **C,** Sphenoid dysplasia and porencephalic cyst are again seen on this higher section. Note normal left optic nerve.

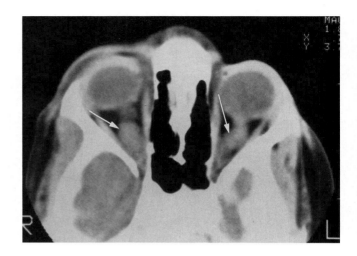

Fig. 10-112 Neurofibromatosis with bilateral optic nerve gliomas *(arrows).*

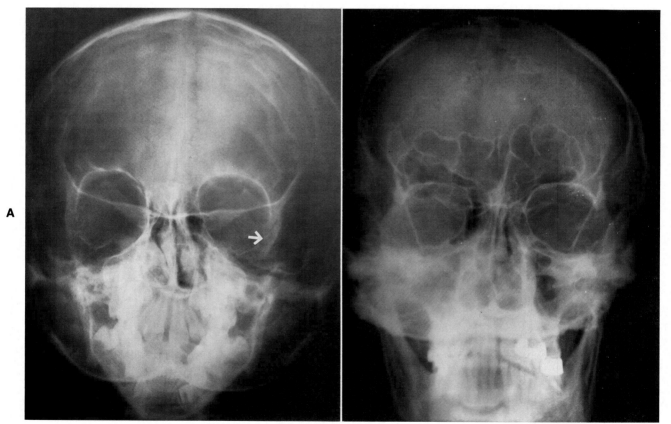

Fig. 10-113 **A,** Mandibulofacial dysostosis. Posteranterior (PA) view of skull shows hypoplastic mandible, hypoplastic malar bones, hypoplastic maxillary antra, and hypoplastic lateral wall of orbits *(arrow).* Oblique (innominate) lines are not visible because of hypoplasia of greater wing of sphenoid. **B,** Normal PA view of skull for comparison.

normal and dysplastic sella turcica[28,53] (Fig. 10-111). These osseous abnormalities allow the adjacent temporal lobe of the brain and its overlying, often thickened dural membrane to herniate anteriorly into the posterior aspect of the orbit, which causes anterior displacement of the globe (Fig. 10-111). The normal CSF fluid pulsations are transmitted to the globe, resulting in pulsatile exophthalmos. Associated findings include hypoplasia of the ipsilateral frontal and maxillary sinuses, as well as hypoplasia of the adjacent ethmoid air cells.[28,53]

Mandibulofacial Dysostosis

Orbital Defects. The malformation known as mandibulofacial dysostosis (MFD) was first reported in 1889 by ophthalmologist G.A. Berry.[56] Treacher-Collins,[57] whose name is attached to the disease of mandibulofacial dysostosis, described the disease and noted the characteristic malar hypoplasia and the associated flattening of the cheeks. In 1923 Pires deLima and Monteior[58] stated that MFD is probably caused by a developmental defect affecting the branchial arches (the hallmark of MFD is its varied expressivity). Franceschetti and Klein,[59] who coined the name MFD, classified the syndrome into five separate categories: complete, incomplete, abortive, unilateral, and atypical. Gorlin and Pindborg[32] stated that there is no unilateral form of the syndrome and that such cases are better classified as hemifacial microsomia. Poswillow[60] in his experimental study of a teratogenically induced phenocopy of MFD in an animal model showed that the disorder results from disorganization of the preotic neural crest about the time of migration of cells to the first and second branchial arches. There are now several recognized malformations in which abnormalities of the eye and associated abnormalities of structures derived from the first and second branchial arches are found.

Bony Orbital Defects. In MFD the maxillas and malar bones are usually poorly developed with small antra and shallow or incomplete orbital floors[44] (Fig. 10-113, A). The malar bones are hypoplastic, and the zygomatic arches are usually incomplete. The development of the zygomatic process of the maxilla varies among the cases described, and it may be aplastic. The radiographic orbital characteristics in MFD are the downward sloping floors of the orbits in line medially with a beaklike bony nasal contour. The lateral and lower rim of the orbit is often defective (Fig. 10-113, A). CT shows the deficiency of the lateral orbital floor as an orbital cleft that has considerable variability in degree. The greater wings of the sphenoid may be hypoplastic; therefore, the lateral orbital wall may be defective (Fig. 10-113, A). Herring[61] reported a patient with MFD with hypoplasia of the greater wing of the sphenoid with the temporal squamous bone extended anteriorly beyond its usual boundaries to replace the very hypoplastic

greater wing of the sphenoid. The squamous bone articulated directly with the frontal bone at the anterior end of the temporal fossa and formed a section of the lateral orbital wall. In MFD the infraorbital foramen may be absent. The fossa of the lacrimal sac may be larger than normal. The nasolacrimal canal is usually short.[61] The lacrimal bones are normal.

Bony Orbit in Craniofacial Microsomia. Craniofacial microsomia is known by many names, including first and second branchial syndrome, otomandibular dysostosis, and oculoauriculovertebral dysplasia.[32,44,62] In general, among the congenital oculoauriculocephalic syndromes, the term *first* and *second branchial arch syndrome* designates a characteristic congenital malformation that is usually unilateral but occasionally bilateral. The term *hemifacial microsomia* was advocated by Gorlin et al[32] to refer to patients with unilateral microtia, macrostomia, and failure of formation of the mandibular ramus and condyle. They included such malformations as the Goldenhar syndrome and oculoauriculovertebral dysplasia, which were previously described as separate entities but which are variants of this complex.[32] About 10% of the patients have bilateral involvement, but the disorder is nearly always more severe on one side.[32] The associated eye findings considered to be variable features of this syndrome include epibulbar dermoids or lipodermoids, microphthalmia, coloboma of the choroid and iris, and deformity of the bony orbit similar to MFD as a result of hypoplasia of the maxillary and malar bones.

Developmental Orbital Cysts. The most frequent developmental cysts involving the orbit and periorbital structures are the dermoid and epidermoid cysts and teratomas.[2,6,63,64] Both cysts result from the inclusion of ectodermal elements during closure of the neural tube. The dermal elements are pinched off along the suture lines, diploe, or within the meninges or scalp in

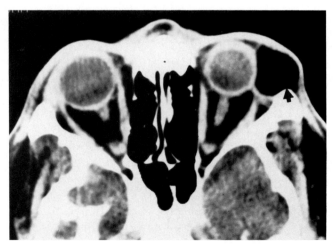

Fig. 10-114 Dermoid. CT scan shows a fat containing lesion *(arrow)* compatible with an orbital dermoid.

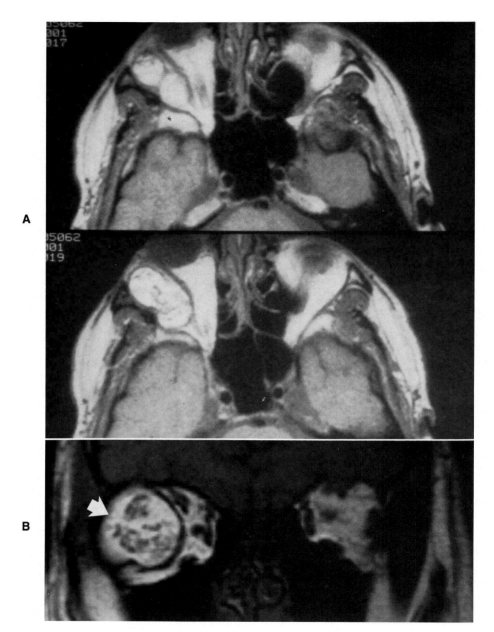

Fig. 10-115 Dermoid. **A,** PW axial MRI scans and **B,** PW coronal MRI scan show giant dermoid *(arrow).* Lesion is inhomogeneous and contains hyperintense areas caused by fat. Lesion appeared isointense to fat in T$_2$W MRI scans.

the course of embryonic development.[64] Both cysts have a fibrous capsule of varying degrees of thickness. The epidermoid has a lining of keratinizing, stratified epithelium. The dermoid contains one or more dermal adnexal structures such as sebaceous glands and hair follicles. Teratomas are choristomatous tumors that contain tissue representing two or more germ layers. Endodermal derivatives such as gut or respiratory epithelium, ectodermal tissues such as skin and its appendages, and neural and mesodermal tissues such as con-

nective tissues, smooth muscles, cartilage and bone, and vessels may be present. Teratomas are evident at birth as grossly visible cystic orbital masses.[6,64] The dermoid and epidermoid cysts favor the upper portion rather than the lower quadrants of the orbit for their growth (Figs. 10-114 and 10-115). They grow slowly; however, at times these cysts can grow rapidly, particularly in adults.[65] They are most frequently located at the superior temporal quadrant of the orbit, where they are fixed to the periosteum near the frontozygomatic suture line.[63-65] These cysts may be entirely confined to orbital adnexal tissues. Most of these cysts clinically appear during childhood as subcutaneous nodules near the orbital rim. In adults, the cysts most commonly arise behind the orbital rim, often near the lacrimal gland, and they may be difficult to distinguish from lacrimal gland tumors.[64,65] The cysts may contain cystic or solid components.

Other Less Common Congenital Anomalies of Orbit and Optic System. The orbit develops from mesodermal tissues, and the globe and optic pathway develop primarily from ectodermal tissues. Developmental defects of the eyeball result in a small orbit. The majority of orbital changes are found in association with deformities of the skull (Fig. 10-105) and skeleton.[31] Cyclopia, synophthalmia, clinical anophthalmia, and microphthalmia (Figs. 10-104 and 10-105) are developmental anomalies of the globe (Fig. 10-104) that are seen in fetal central nervous system anomalies associated with problems in forebrain differentiation (holoporosencephaly). MRI is particularly helpful in the detection of these anomalies.

Inflammatory Diseases

Orbital infections account for about 60% of primary orbital disease.[2] The process may be acute, subacute, or chronic. The majority of acute inflammatory disorders are of sinus origin. However, they may develop from an infectious process of the face or pharynx, trauma, foreign bodies or may be secondary to septicemia. The bacteria most commonly involved are staphylococcus, streptococcus, pneumococcus, pseudomonas, neisseriaceae, hemophillus, and mycobacteria.[66] Herpes simplex and herpes zoster are the major virus infections of the orbit. In immune-suppressed patients and poorly controlled diabetic patients, opportunistic infections such as fungal and parasitic pathogens may be responsible for severe sinonaso-orbital infections. Acute inflammation is characterized by a rapid development associated with soft tissue swelling, infiltration, destruction, and abscess formation. The location of the process is important. A preseptal infection (Fig. 10-116) rarely affects orbital functions. On the other hand, a retroseptal infection (Fig. 10-116) may have a profound and sudden effect on the optic nerve and orbital motility function. Pathologically in acute bacterial inflammation, polymorphonuclear leukocytes are usually the dominant cells, which along with their pharmacologic intermediates, lead to necrosis, rapid involvement, and destruction of the orbital tissue planes.

Orbital Cellulitis and Sinusitis. Sinusitis is the most common cause of orbital cellulitis. Even though antibiotics have decreased the incidence of complicated sinusitis with orbital involvement, it still occurs. The orbital manifestations may be the first sign of sinus infec-

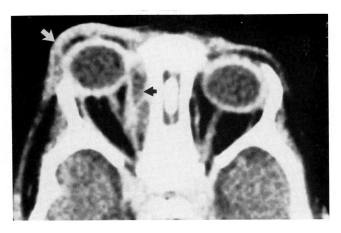

Fig. 10-116   Preseptal and retroseptal orbital inflammation. CT scan shows periorbital soft tissue infiltration and edema *(white arrow)* and retroseptal subperiosteal inflammation and edema *(black arrow)*.

tion in children.[64-67] Pathophysiologically, infection originating within the sinuses can spread readily to the orbit via the thin and often dehiscent bony walls and their many foramina, or by means of the interconnecting valveless venous system of the face, sinus, and orbit.[2] The classification of orbital cellulitis includes five categories or stages of orbital involvement from sinusitis: (1) inflammatory edema; (2) subperiosteal phlegmon and abscess; (3) orbital cellulitis; (4) orbital abscess; and (5) ophthalmic vein and cavernous sinus thrombosis.[2,64,67] Limiting a particular inflammatory lesion to one of these categories is difficult because they tend to overlap.[64,67]

Inflammatory Edema or Preseptal Cellulitis. Preseptal cellulitis is the first stage; it often is misdiagnosed as orbital or periorbital cellulitis. The infection in this early stage actually is still confined to the paranasal sinus.[67] This condition is characterized by swelling of the eyelids with mild orbital edema, usually involving the upper eyelid, especially medially. This reflects congestion of the venous outflow. In a slightly more advanced disease chemosis occurs. CT or MRI at this stage will demonstrate the edema of the eyelids and inflammatory changes of the infected sinus or sinuses.[6]

Subperiosteal Phlegmon and Abscess, Orbital Cellulitis, Orbital Abscess, and Ophthalmic Vein and Cavernous Sinus Thrombosis. As the reaction of the orbital periosteum begins and gradually advances, the edema of the eyelids and conjunctivae becomes more generalized and the eye begins to protrude. Inflammatory tissue and edema collects beneath the periosteum to form a subperiosteal phlegmon (Fig. 10-117). Subsequently, pus may form to represent a subperiosteal abscess (Fig. 10-118). As the disease progresses, the inflammatory pro-

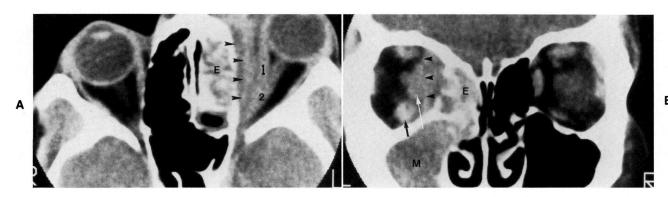

Fig. 10-117 Orbital subperiosteal phlegmon. **A,** CT scan shows proptosis of left eye with mucoperiosteal thickening of left ethmoid sinus *(E),* with soft tissue induration in medial subperiosteal space *(arrowheads).* Note lateral displacement of inflamed left medial rectus muscle *(1).* Optic nerve *(2).* **B,** Coronal CT scan, same patient as in **A,** shows clouding of right ethmoid *(E)* and maxillary *(M)* sinuses with subperiosteal soft tissue induration *(arrowheads)* and swelling of right medial rectus muscle *(white arrow)* and right inferior rectus muscle *(black arrow).* (From Mafee MF et al: CT assessment of periorbital pathology. In Gozalez CA, Beeker MH, and Flanagan JC, editors: Diagnostic imaging in ophthalmology, New York, 1985, Springer-Verlag New York, Inc, pp 281-302.)

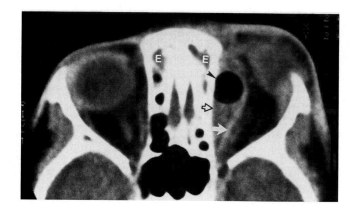

Fig. 10-118 Orbital subperiosteal abscess. CT scan shows proptosis of left eye with mucosal thickening of ethmoid air cells *(E),* with subperiosteal abscess *(hollow arrow).* Note air bubble *(arrowhead)* within abscess and swollen left medial rectus muscle *(arrow).*

Fig. 10-119 Orbital cellulitis and abscesses. CT scan shows right periorbital cellulitis and three abscesses. *A,* Right retroseptal abscess; *B,* left retrobulbar abscess; *C,* left eyelid abscess. Note slightly engorged left superior ophthalmic vein *(hollow arrow).*

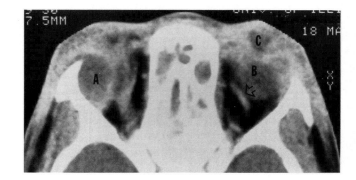

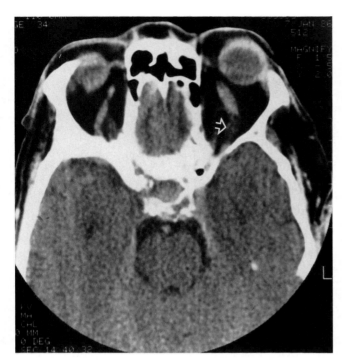

Fig. 10-120   Thrombosis of superior ophthalmic vein. CT scan shows engorged left superior ophthalmic vein with filling defect *(arrow),* which was caused by sphenoid sinus infection (moniliasis).

cess may infiltrate the periorbital and retroorbital fat to give rise to a true orbital cellulitis (Fig. 10-119). The subperiosteal abscess and orbital cellulitis frequently coexist.[64,67] At this stage, extraocular motility is progressively impaired. With severe involvement, visual disturbances can result from optic neuritis and/or ischemia (Fig. 10-117, A). Progression of intraorbital cellulitis or spread from the subperiosteal space leads to intraconal or extraconal loculation and abscess formation (Fig. 10-119).[2,64,67]

Ophthalmic vein thrombosis (Fig. 10-120) and cavernous sinus thrombosis are very serious complications of orbital and sinonasal infections. Cavernous sinus thrombosis is heralded by profound central nervous system deficit and orbital functional impairment.

Mycotic Infections. Another important and more complicated orbital inflammatory process is the extension of mycotic infection of both the nasal and paranasal sinuses into the orbit. Mycotic infection of the sinonasal cavities and craniofacial structures is a serious disease that requires prompt surgery and medical therapy to decrease its high morbidity rate.[64] Rhinocerebral mycotic infection may be caused by the members of the family Mucoraceae (mucormycosis)[64] and *Aspergillus* (aspergillosis) and other fungi. The fungi responsible for mucormycosis are ubiquitous and normally saprophytic in humans; they rarely produce severe disease, except in those patients with predisposing conditions.[64,66,68]

There are four major types of mucormycosis: rhinocerebral, pulmonary, gastrointestinal, and disseminated.[68] The most common form is the rhinocerebral form. The infection usually begins in the nose and spreads to the paranasal sinuses; then it extends into the orbit and cavernous sinuses.[64,68] Orbital involvement results in such orbital signs as ophthalmoplegia, proptosis, ptosis, loss of vision, and orbital cellulitis.[64] The inflammatory process soon extends along the infraorbital fissure and into the infratemporal fossa (Fig. 10-121).

Black necrosis of a turbinate is a diagnostic clinical sign, but it may not be present until late in the course of the disease.[64,68] The pathologic hallmark of mucormycosis is invasion of the walls of the vessels. Because of the invasion of the arterial and venous structures of the cavernous sinus, patients with sinonaso-orbitocerebral mycosis, particularly mucormycosis and aspergillosis, may rapidly develop brain infarction.[69]

Aspergillus is a ubiquitous mold found primarily in agricultural dust. It may produce rhinocerebral disease and orbital involvement similar to mucormycosis, although hematogenous spread from the lungs to the brain is more common.[68] This fungus also has a well-known propensity for invading blood vessels, including the internal carotid artery.[64] The combination of orbital and sinus involvement is not pathognomanic of rhinocerebral mucormycosis or aspergillosis; however, awareness of its possibility, particularly when any of the predisposing factors are present, helps in establishing an early diagnosis and the initiation of treatment of this aggressive and often fatal disease. The main contribution of CT and MRI to the diagnosis of sinonaso-orbital mycotic infections is its clear demonstration of the relationship between nasal, sinus, orbital, and cranial disease (Fig. 10-122).

Acute, Subacute, and Chronic Idiopathic Orbital Inflammatory Disorders (Pseudotumors). Idiopathic inflammatory syndromes are usually referred to as orbital "pseudotumors," a clinically and histologically confusing category of lesions.[2] In general, orbital pseudotumor comprises a broad category of orbital inflammatory diseases. It is defined as a nonspecific, idiopathic inflammatory condition for which no local identifiable cause or systemic disease can be found.[70,71] By definition this excludes orbital inflammatory disease caused by entities such as Wegener's granulomatosis, retained foreign bodies, sclerosing hemangioma, trauma, and sinusitis.

The condition was first described in 1905 by Birch-Hirschfield[72] and has remained somewhat of an enigma in the ophthalmology, radiology, and pathology literature.[71] In addition to the variety of classification systems and diagnostic criteria that have been offered over the years, this disease can include a wide range of clinical presentations, and many of the symptoms are nonspecific.

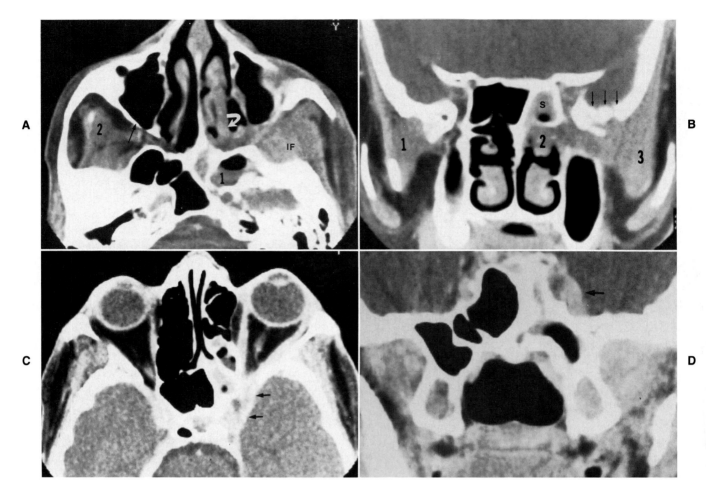

Fig. 10-121 Mucormycosis. **A,** CT scan shows soft tissue induration in left nasal cavity *(curved arrow)* and left infratemporal fossa *(IF)*. Note air fluid level in left sphenoid sinus *(1)*. Fascial planes in left infratemporal fossa *(IF)* region, compared with the right side *(2)*, are obliterated. Note rarefaction of posterior wall of left maxillary sinus compared to normal right side *(black arrow)*. **B,** Coronal CT scan, same patient as in **A,** shows soft tissue induration in left nasal cavity *(2)* and mucosal thickening of left sphenoid sinus *(S)*. Note soft tissue infiltration along inferior orbital fissure extending into infratemporal fossa *(3)*, as compared with normal right side *(1)*. Note irregularity of greater wing of sphenoid *(arrows)*, indicating osteomyelitis. Note normal fat planes along right superior and inferior orbital fissures and their effacement on the left side. **C,** CT scan, same patient as in **A** and **B,** shows involvement of left cavernous sinus *(arrows)* with enlargement (engorgement) of left lateral and medial rectus muscles. **D,** Coronal CT scan, same patient as in **A,** **B,** and **C,** shows involvement of left cavernous sinus *(arrow)*.

Fig. 10-122 Aspergillosis. **A,** PW MRI scan and **B,** T₂W MRI scan show soft tissue induration in left sphenoid sinus *(white arrow)*. Note internal carotid *(C)* and early soft tissue infiltration of left cavernous sinus *(hollow arrow)*. **C,** PW MRI follow-up scan and **D,** T₂W MRI follow-up scan show progression of pathological process, with marked infiltration of left cavernous sinus *(C)* and formation of left temporal lobe abscess *(arrowhead)* with marked peripheral edema. Note apical infiltration into left orbit *(black arrow in* **C***)* and inflammatory mycotic tissue in left sphenoid sinus *(white arrow)*. Mycotic process appears rather hypointense in T₂W MRI scan, a not uncommon finding with fungal infections. Note nonvisualization of left internal carotid artery (compare with **A** and **B**); this results from invasion of mycotic process, a finding confirmed by angiography and surgery. **E,** Postcontrast (Gd-DTPA) coronal MRI scan shows enhancement of mucosal thickening of left sphenoid sinus *(S)* and infiltrative process of left cavernous sinus *(C)* and temporal lobe abscess *(arrowhead)*.

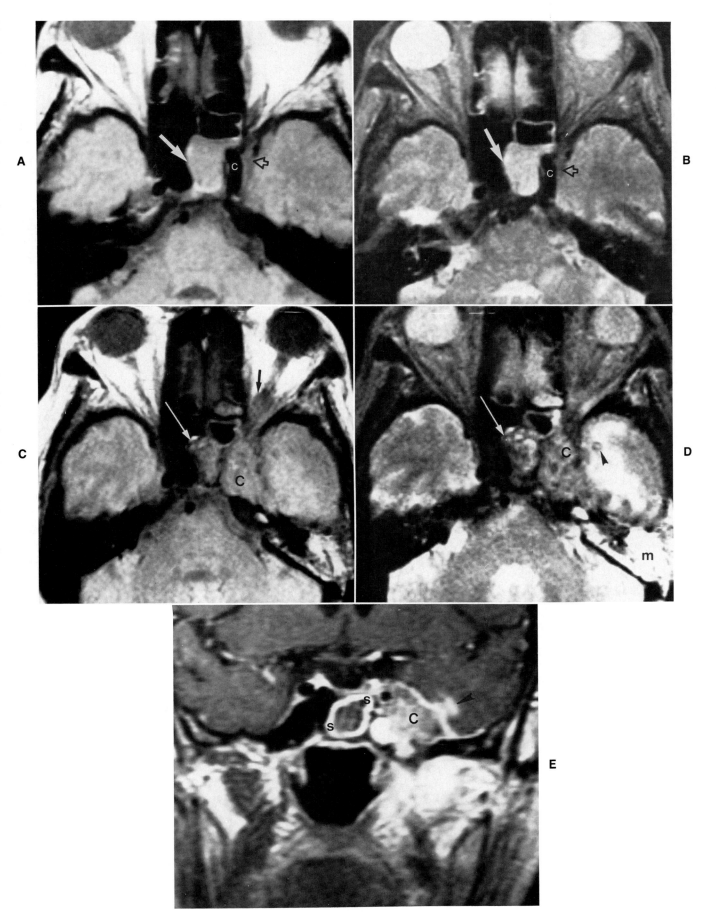

Fig. 10-122 For legend see opposite page.

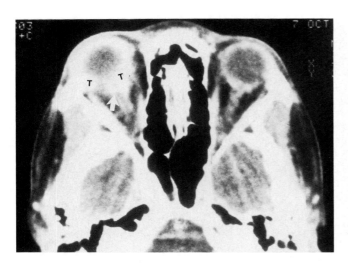

Fig. 10-123 Pseudotumor: periscleritis/perineuritis. Post-contrast CT scan shows diffuse thickening of scleral coat with inflammatory infiltration into Tenon's space *(T)* and perineuritis *(arrow)*.

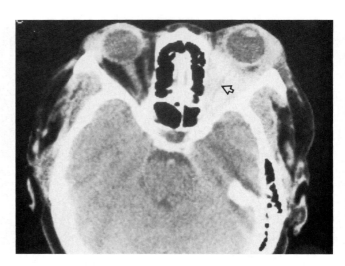

Fig. 10-124 Pseudotumor. CT scan shows diffuse infiltration of entire retrobulbar space. Optic nerve appears as lucent band *(arrow)* embedded within lesion.

The histopathology can vary from polymorphous inflammatory cells and fibrosis, with a matrix of granulation tissue, eosinophils, plasma cells, histiocytes, germinal follicles, and lymphocytes to a predominantly lymphocytic form. It is the chronic lymphocytic variety that is related to lymphoma.[71] Many cases of lymphocytic pseudotumor have been reported that, over a period of time, are found to harbor a malignant lymphoma without any evidence of systemic lymphoma. The presence of germinal follicles and increased vascularity is indicative of a reactive lesion, often associated with a favorable prognosis and responsiveness to steroids. An association has been noted between diffusely distributed lymphoblasts, steroid unresponsiveness and a probable neoplastic lymphoid lesion.[71] Not all steroid-resistant pseudotumors are destined to become lymphomatous. The peculiar behavior of pseudotumor has led some authors to speculate that some forms of pseudotumor are the result of an autoimmune process.[71,73] Pseudotumors may be classified as (1) acute and subacute idiopathic anterior orbital inflammation; (2) acute and subacute idiopathic diffuse orbital inflammation; (3) acute and subacute idiopathic myositic orbital inflammation; (4) acute and subacute idiopathic apical orbital inflammation; (5) idiopathic lacrimal adenitis; and (6) perineuritis.

Anterior Orbital Inflammation. In the anterior orbital pseudotumor group, the main focus of inflammation involves the anterior orbit and adjacent globe.[2] The major features of presentation are pain, proptosis, lid swelling, and decreased vision. Other findings may be ocular and include uveitis, sclerotenonitis (Tenon's capsule),

papillitis, and exudative retinal detachment (Fig. 10-123). The extraocular muscle (EOM) motility is usually unaffected. CT and MRI show thickening of the uveal-scleral rim with obscuration of the optic nerve junction, which enhances with contrast medium infusion on CT.[71,74] These findings result from leakage of proteinaceous edema fluid into the interstitium of the uvea and Tenon's capsule secondary to the inflammatory reaction.[71] Fluid in Tenon's capsule has been well documented with ultrasound (the T sign). Patients with posterior scleritis can develop retinal detachment and fundal masses, which simulate intraocular tumors.[71] The differential clinical diagnosis of anterior orbital pseudotumor includes orbital cellulitis, ruptured dermoid cyst or hemorrhage within a vascular lesion (hemangioma, lymphangioma), collagen vascular disease, rhabdomyosarcoma, and leukemic infiltration.

Diffuse Orbital Pseudotumor. Diffuse orbital pseudotumor is similar in many respects to acute and subacute anterior inflammation but with a greater severity.[2] The diffuse, tumefactive, or infiltrative type of pseudotumor may fill the entire retrobulbar space and mold itself around the globe while respecting the eye's natural shape. Even the largest of masses usually does not invade or distort the shape of the globe or erode bone (Figs. 10-124 and 10-125). This type of disease can be very difficult to differentiate from lymphoma. These large, bulky masses can be both intraconal or extraconal and must be differentiated from true tumors of the orbit, i.e., cavernous hemangioma, hemangiopericytoma, optic nerve sheath meningioma, optic nerve glioma, orbital schwannoma, and metastasis.[71] True tumors do

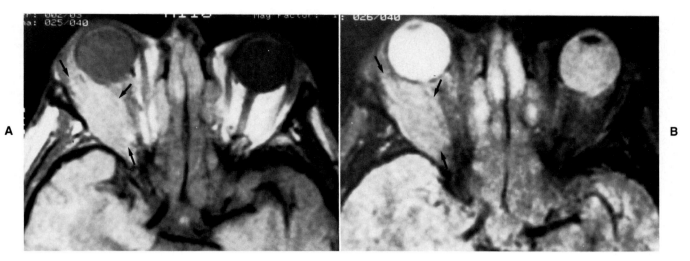

Fig. 10-125 Pseudotumor. **A,** PW MRI scan and **B,** T$_2$W MRI scan show infiltrative process *(arrows)* compatible with pseudotumor. Lesion is isointense to brain in PW and T$_2$W MRI scans.

not respect the boundaries of the globe; they push or indent its surface. Also, bone erosion and extraorbital extension are more typical of true tumors than pseudotumors.

Orbital Myositis. Idiopathic orbital myositis is a condition in which one or more of the EOMs are primarily infiltrated by an inflammatory process (Fig. 10-126). Myositis can be acute, subacute, or recurrent. The patient usually has painful extraocular movements, diplopia, proptosis, swelling of the lid, conjunctival chemosis, and inflammation over the involved EOM.[2,71] This disorder may be bilateral. The most frequently affected muscles are the superior complex and the medial rectus (Fig. 10-126). The major differential diagnosis is Grave's disease. However, dysthyroid myopathy is usually painless in onset, symmetric, slowly progressive, and associated with a systemic diathesis.[2] Trokel and Hilal[75] state that the typical CT finding in orbital myositis is enlargement of the EOMs, which extends anteriorly to involve the inserting tendon (Figs. 10-126 and 10-127). Other helpful indicators of inflammatory orbital myositis include a ragged, fluffy border of the involved muscle with infiltration and obliteration of the fat in the peripheral surgical space between the periosteum of the orbital wall and the muscle cone. Also observed is an inward bowing of the medial contour of the muscle belly, forming a shoulder as it passes behind the globe (Fig. 10-126). All these findings can be attributed to local tendinitis, fasciitis, and myositis of the involved muscle. In contrast, the fusiform appearance of an enlarged muscle in thyroid myopathy is produced by a myositis along only the belly of the muscle. The muscle

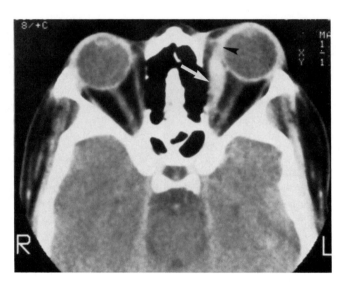

Fig. 10-126 Myositic pseudotumor. Postcontrast CT scan shows marked thickening and enhancement of left medial rectus muscle *(arrow).* Note extension of process into its tendinous insertion on globe *(arrowhead).*

borders are sharply defined, the fat in the peripheral surgical space is preserved, and usually there is no medial bowing or tendinous infiltration observed. Less common causes of EOM enlargement include arteriovenous fistula (e.g., carotid-cavernous fistula) and neoplasm (primary or metastatic).[71]

Apical Orbital Inflammation. Pseudotumor may present with infiltration of the orbital apex. Patients' presenting symptoms include a typical orbital apical syndrome of pain, minimal proptosis, and restricted EOM move-

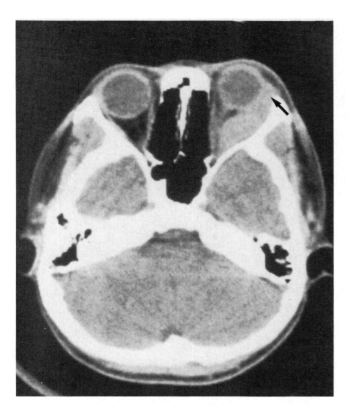

Fig. 10-127 Myositic pseudotumor (pseudorheumatoid nodule). CT scan shows enlargement of left lateral rectus muscle, including tendinous insertion on globe *(arrow)*. Soft tissue infiltration is present between left lateral rectus muscle and periosteum. Biopsy showed pseudorheumatoid nodule.

ments. The CT and MRI findings include an irregular infiltrative process of the apex of the orbit with extension along the posterior portion of the EOMs or the optic nerve (Fig. 10-75).

Lacrimal Adenitis. Acute idiopathic lacrimal adenitis presents with tenderness in the upper outer quadrant of the orbit in the region of the lacrimal gland.[71] Viral dacryoadenitis may present in a similar fashion, although it is commonly associated with an etiology such as mumps, mononucleosis, or herpes zoster. There can be adenopathy and lymphocytosis present in these cases. The differential diagnosis of nonspecific lacrimal adenitis includes viral and bacterial dacryoadenitis, rupture of a dermoid cyst in the lacrimal gland region, specific lacrimal gland inflammations such as sarcoidosis and Sjögren's disease, lymphoproliferative disorders, cysts, and neoplasia in this region. Because of the wide variety of pathology that involves the lacrimal gland, biopsy of this accessible site is necessary to define the correct diagnosis.[2]

Perineuritis. Idiopathic perineuritis can simulate optic neuritis by presenting with orbital pain, pain with extraocular motility, decreased visual acuity, and disk edema. In contrast to optic neuritis, pain is exacerbated with retrodisplacement of the globe and there is mild proptosis.[71] CT and MRI show a ragged, edematous enlargement of the optic nerve (Fig. 10-128).

CT Findings. Of the various CT characteristics associated with different features of pseudotumors, the most common CT findings include enhancement with IV contrast medium (95%), infiltration of the retrobulbar fat (76%), proptosis (71%), EOM enlargement (57%), apical fat infiltration and edema (48%), muscle tendon/ sheath enlargement (43%), and optic nerve thickening (38%).[71] Pseudotumor's enhancement with IV contrast medium is one of the distinguishing characteristics between it and similar appearing tumors, (i.e., lymphomas), which do not demonstrate significant enhancement. Thickening or edema of the eyelids, a feature of preseptal inflammatory conditions, is not usually present in pseudotumors and is another useful differentiating characteristic.[71] A key finding with pseudotumors is the virtual absence of bony erosion or distortion of the orbital contents. This finding is commonly present with both benign and malignant tumors.[71]

We have found no specific imaging findings nor are there any specific clinical signs to establish the diagnosis of pseudotumors with absolute certainty.[71] Classically the rapid development of unilateral, painful ophthalmoplegia, protosis and chemosis, with a rapid and lasting response to steroid therapy in an otherwise healthy patient, is highly suggestive of the diagnoses of pseudotumor. The majority of pseudotumors encountered in our practice were of the diffuse tumefactive and myositic varieties. These forms need to be differentiated primarily from a true orbital neoplasm and thyroid myopathy. A well-defined tumefactive pseudotumor with sharp borders cannot be reliably distinguished from a tumor and lymphoma using only CT and MRI criteria. Orbital manifestations of adjacent or systemic disease such as thyroid disease, lymphoma, leukemia, or metastases, are often diagnoses of exclusion. In the absence of a characteristic clinical presentation of pseudotumor or a poor response to steroids, biopsy is necessary. Myositic pseudotumor with its unilateral and usually single muscle enlargement that extends into the tendinous insertion has the most reliable CT and MRI findings to correlate with this diagnosis (Fig. 10-128, B-D).

Thyroid Orbitopathy. Thyroid myopathy occurs most commonly in middle-aged women. It is ophthalmologically characterized by exophthalmos and in some patients by the gradual onset of diplopia, which is usually of the vertical type. Initially in the acute congestive phase, the retrobulbar orbital contents are markedly swollen and congested. Later, a more chronic, noncongestive phase follows, in which a restrictive type of limited eye movement often develops, secondary to infil-

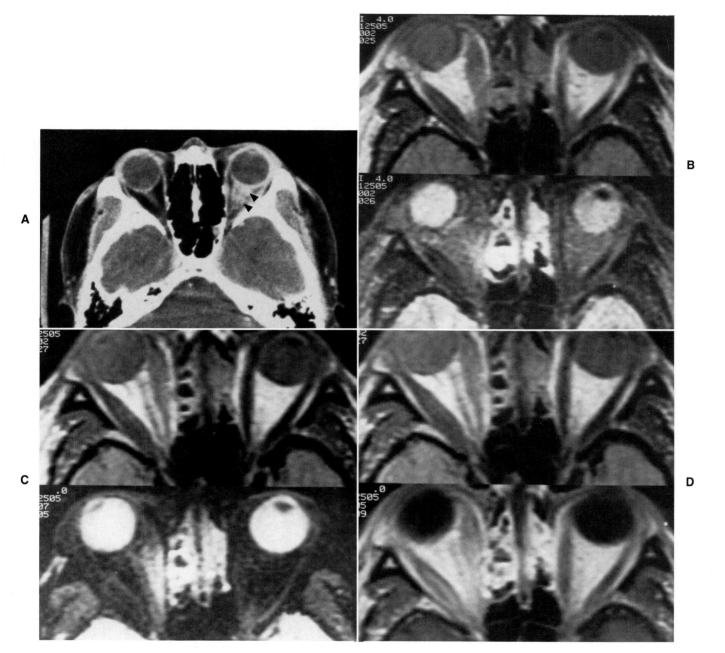

Fig. 10-128   A, Pseudotumor (perineuritis type). CT scan shows intraconal region of infiltration *(arrowheads)* surrounding left optic nerve. Slight thickening of posterior sclera indicates posterior scleritis and fluid (exudate) in Tenon's space. **B,** Pseudotumor (myositic type), PW *(top)* and T$_2$PW *(bottom)* MRI scans in another patient showing enlargement of the right lateral and medial rectus muscles. **C,** PW *(top)* and fat suppression; STIR *(bottom)* MRI scans showing enlargement of the right lateral and medial rectus muscles. Note hyperintensity of the right medial rectus in STIR image indicative of edema. The process appears to be more acute in right medial rectus than the right lateral rectus. **D,** PW *(top)* and T$_1$W post Gd-DTPA *(bottom)* MRI scans showing mild to moderate enhancement of the involved muscles.

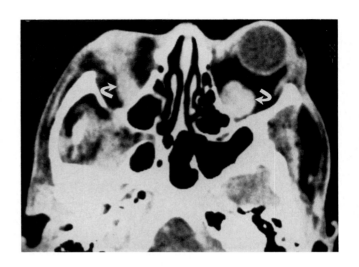

Fig. 10-129 Thyroid myopathy. CT scan shows enlargement of inferior rectus muscles *(arrows)*.

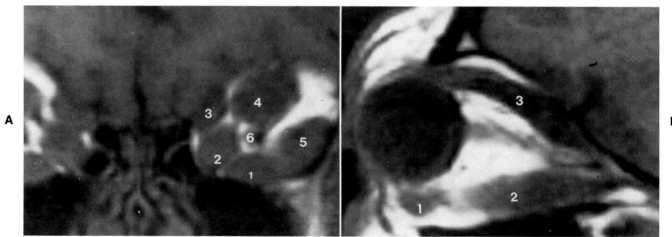

Fig. 10-130 Thyroid myopathy. **A,** Coronal T₁W MRI scan and **B,** saggital T₁W MRI scan show enlargement of extraocular muscles. In **A,** *1,* Inferior rectus muscle; *2,* medial rectus muscle; *3,* superior oblique muscle; *4,* superior rectus muscle; *5,* lateral rectus muscle; and *6,* optic nerve. In **B,** *1,* inferior oblique muscle; *2,* inferior rectus muscle; and *3,* superior rectus muscle.

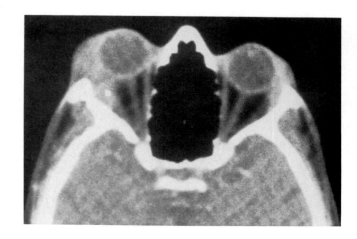

Fig. 10-131 Sarcoidosis chronic dacryoadenitis. CT scan shows enlargement of right lacrimal gland. Note mild enlargement of left lacrimal gland.

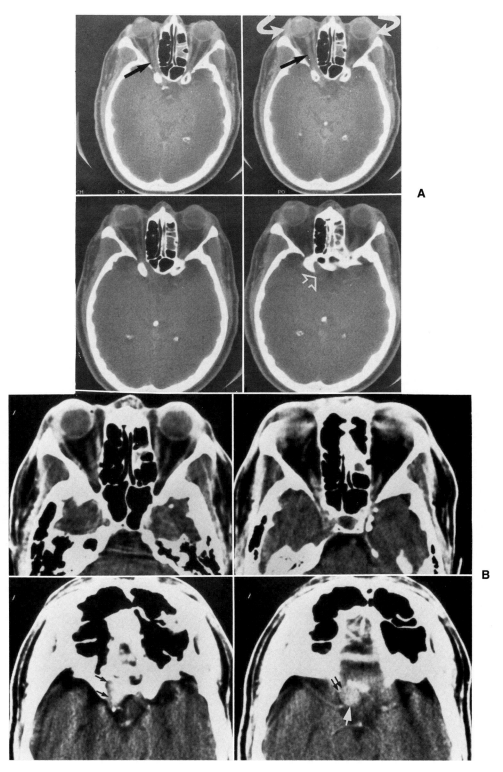

Fig. 10-132   Sarcoidosis with optic nerve involvement. **A,** Serial CT scans show enlargement of right optic nerve *(arrows),* including its intracranial segment. Note soft tissue mass in right side of chiasmatic cisterns *(hollow arrow)* and slight bilateral enlargement of lacrimal glands *(curved arrows).* **B,** Serial CT scans obtained for soft tissue detail, same patient as in **A,** show enhancing granulomas *(arrows).*

tration of the extraocular muscles and to subsequent loss of elasticity.[10] The involvement can be unilateral or bilateral; when it is bilateral, it is often fairly symmetric. The inferior rectus muscle is most commonly involved, leading to a limitation of elevation of the involved eye. The medial and superior rectus muscles are also frequently involved, and the lateral rectus and superior oblique muscles are less commonly affected. The forced duction test result is almost always abnormal.[10] Limitation of elevation is the most common disturbance of ocular motility in patients with Grave's disease.[13] The myopathy may occur at any time in the course of Grave's disease; laboratory evaluation may reveal hyperthyroidism, hypothyroidism, or euthyroidism.[10] In fact, the disease occasionally is found in patients who have been successfully treated for an overactive thyroid and who are euthyroid when first seen. Thyroid orbitopathy is considered to be an immunological response of an autoimmune disorder in which antithyroglobulin immune complexes bind to extraocular muscle membrane. EOM enlargement in Grave's disease and associated compressive neuropathy, if any, can be visualized by CT and MRI scanning (Figs. 10-129 and 10-130). About 90% of patients with thyroid orbitopathy will have bilateral CT abnormalities, even if the clinical involvement is unilateral.[2] Typically enlargement involves the muscle belly, sparing its tendinous portion. However, rare patients show thickening of the tendinous portion.[2] Another helpful finding in thyroid myopathy is the presence of low density areas within the muscle bellies. These are probably the result of focal accumulation of lymphocytes and mucopolysaccharide deposition.[2] Other CT and MRI findings in thyroid orbitopathy are increased orbital fat, enlargement (engorgement) of the lacrimal glands, edema (fullness) of the eyelids, proptosis, and stretching of the optic nerve with or without associated "tenting" of the posterior globe.

Sarcoidosis. Sarcoidosis is a granulomatous systemic disease of unknown etiology characterized by subacute or chronic inflammation involving multiple systems, including orbital and ocular structures.[2,76] It is an immunologically mediated disease affecting delayed hypersensitivity.[2] It is 10 to 20 times more common in black people than it is in whites. Virtually any part of the globe or orbit may be involved in sarcoidosis; Uveitis, chorioretinitis, kerato conjunctivitis, and conjunctival inflammatory nodules may be seen.[2] The most common form of orbital involvement in sarcoidosis is chronic lacrimal adenitis. This is often unilateral and may easily mimic a lacrimal tumor (Fig. 10-131). When it occurs bilaterally in the lacrimal and salivary glands, it is one of the causes of Mikulicz's syndrome.[76] Another type of orbital involvement with sarcoidosis is optic nerve involvement which may closely resemble a primary neoplasm of the optic nerve (Fig. 10-132).[22]

Sjögren's Syndrome. Sjögren's syndrome is an autoimmune disorder characterized by keratoconjunctivitis sicca and xerostomia. Patients may have an associated autoimmune disease such as rheumatoid arthritis, systemic lupus erythematosus, polymyositis, or scleroderma. The lacrimal and salivary glands are infiltrated by periductal lymphocytes. Eventually atrophy of the acini with hyalinization and fibrosis will occur. The early disappearance of lysozymes from the tears may help in differentiating Sjögren's syndrome from sarcoidosis, in which the lysozymes in the tears are increased.

Vasculitides (Angiitides)

The vasculitides (vasculitis) are an immunologic–complex-mediated group of diseases which include a variety of inflammatory angiodestructive processes. Clinically the vasculitides may show features of acute, subacute, and chronic inflammatory and vasoobstructive signs and symptoms.[2] The entire group includes a wide variety of disorders that are usually classified on the basis of the symptoms related to the organs affected as well as their histopathologic features.[2] The major ophthalmic or orbital diseases include polyarteritis nodosa, Wegener's granulomatosis, idiopathic midline destructive disease, giant cell arteritis (temporal arteritis), hypersensitivity (leukocytoclastic) angiitis, and connective tissue disease, including systemic lupus erythematosus, rheumatoid arthritis, scleroderma, and polymyositis.

Wegener's Granulomatosis. Wegener's granulomatosis is a multisystem disease characterized by a triad of necrotizing granulomas in the upper and lower respiratory tract; necrotizing vasculitis of the lung and upper respiratory tract, and other sites; and glomerulonephritis.[2,76] If left untreated, the disease is often fatal. The treatment of choice is combined corticosteroid-cyclophosphamide therapy.[2] Ocular manifestations of Wegener's granulomatosis may include scleritis, episcleritis, uveitis, retinal vasculitis, and rare conjunctival involvement. Orbital disease is seen in 18% to 22% of the patients with Wegener's granulomatosis. The condition is characterized by pain, proptosis, motility disturbance, chemosis, papilledema, and erythematous edema of the eyelids.[2,76] Characteristically ocular and orbital involvement is bilateral and either nonresponsive or temporarily responsive to corticosteroids, providing a clue to the diagnosis.[2] Involvement of the ocular adnexa includes lacrimal enlargement, nasolacrimal obstruction, or eyelid fistula formation.[2]

Orbital involvement with Wegener's granulomatosis should be differentiated from idiopathic pseudotumors, lymphoreticular proliferative disorders and metastatic carcinoma.[76] The CT and MRI appearances of Wegener's granulomatosis are similar to those of pseudotumors and lymphoma (Fig. 10-95).

Nasal and paranasal sinus involvement may be present in the majority of the cases. The definitive way to differentiate these lesions is by means of a biopsy.

Idiopathic Midline Destructive Granuloma. Idiopathic midline destructive disease, formerly called *lethal midline granuloma*, is a clinical entity characterized by extensive destructive lesions of the nose, sinuses, and pharynx, often with associated involvement of the orbit and central facial bones. It has some similarity to Wegener's granulomatosis, but pulmonary disease is rare and renal involvement is absent.[76] Although the pathogenesis is unknown, some cases may be caused by a central facial lymphomatoid process. The terms *lymphomatoid granulomatosis* and *polymorphic reticulosis* have been applied to this type of disease. If the biopsy indicates a granulomatous vasculitis, the preferred treatment is cyclophosphamide and corticosteroids as used for Wegener's granulomatosis. If the biopsy specimen shows a lymphomatous process, radiotherapy is considered the best treatment.[76]

Angiolymphoid Hyperplasia With Eosinophilia (Kimura's Disease). Kimura's disease is an idiopathic inflammation of the skin that characteristically involves the head and neck region.[76] It can affect the orbit. The lesion pathologically shows a central area of proliferation of fine blood vessels surrounded by benign lymphocytes. Numerous eosinophils and sometimes plasma cell and lymphocytes are scattered within the central vascular area.[76] In some cases marked fibrosis may occur after several years.[76] The CT and MRI appearance of Kimura's disease is nonspecific and resembles the pseudotumor group of orbital diseases. The best management of Kimura's disease of the orbit is complete excision when possible.[76]

Periarteritis Nodosa (Polyarteritis Nodosa). Periarteritis nodosa is a vasculitis of the medium and small arteries, adjacent veins, and occasionally arterioles and venules. The disease is segmental and leads to nodular aneurysms. The major ophthalmologic manifestations are retinal and choroidal infarcts leading to exudative retinal detachment. Orbital inflammation has been described. Proptosis may occur secondary to severe inflammation of the orbital arteries,[76] with secondary necrosis of the orbital connective tissues.[2,76]

Hypersensitivity (Leukocytoclastic) Angiitis. Hypersensitivity angiitis resembles periarteritis nodosa microscopically but affects smaller vessels. Pathologically the arterioles, venules, and capillaries are usually, but not necessarily, necrotic or they may simply have perivascular infiltration with neutrophils undergoing karyolysis (leukocytoclasis).[2] The spectrum of clinical disease varies from widespread multisystem involvement to primary dermatologic lesions.[2]

Lupus Erythematosus. Any of the connective tissue disorders may be associated with systemic vasculitis. The most common include systemic lupus erythematosus, rheumatoid arthritis, and dermatomyositis. Systemic lupus erythematosus is an autoimmune disease that affects many organs. It has a female:male ratio of 9:1 and occurs in second and third decades.[2] Histologically, the vasculitides in the connective tissue diseases resemble hypersensitivity angiitis.[2]

Evidence of antinuclear antibodies (ANA) is universally present in this syndrome. Twenty percent of patients have ocular involvement,[2] primarily affecting the retinal vessels. Orbital involvement is rare and is believed to be secondary to severe orbital vasculitis.[76] The CT and MR appearance of orbital lupoid disease may resemble that of pseudotumor and the lymphoreticular proliferative disorders.

Painful External Ophthalmoplegia (Tolosa-Hunt Syndrome). In 1954 Tolosa described a patient with unilateral recurrent painful ophthalmoplegia involving the third, fourth, and sixth cranial nerves and first division of cranial nerve V.[77] Carotid arteriography in this case showed segmental narrowing in the carotid siphon. The patient died after surgical exploration. Postmortem study showed adventitial thickening in the cavernous carotid artery surrounded by a cuff of nonspecific granulation tissue that also involved the adjoining cranial nerve trunks. In 1961 Hunt and co-workers[78] reported six patients with similar clinical symptoms and signs. After reviewing Tolosa's slides, these authors proposed a low-grade, nonspecific inflammation of the cavernous sinus and its walls as the cause of the syndrome. They also emphasized that angiography was essential to rule out an aneurysm or neoplasm.[78] In 1966 Smith and Taxdal[79] applied the term *Tolosa-Hunt syndrome* to this entity. They described five additional cases and stressed the diagnostic usefulness of the dramatically rapid therapeutic response to corticosteroid administration in this syndrome. In 1973 Sondheimer and Knapp[80] reported three patients with Tolosa-Hunt syndrome on whom orbital venography was performed. These investigators observed that the superior ophthalmic vein on the affected side was occluded in the posterior portion of the muscle cone in each case and that the ipsilateral cavernous sinus was partially or completely obliterated.

Painful external ophthalmoplegia, or Tolosa-Hunt syndrome, is now considered as an idiopathic inflammatory process and a regional variant of idiopathic orbital pseudotumors that, because of its anatomic location, produces typical clinical manifestations.[77] Pathologically there is an infiltration of lymphocytes and plasma cells along with thickening of the dura mater. The condition generally responds to systemic corticosteroid therapy. It is important to exclude the possibility of a neoplastic, inflammatory (particularly mycotic) or vasculogenic lesion (Figs. 10-121 and 10-122). Carotid angiography and MRI are most useful in excluding an aneurysm as the cause of the clinical signs and symptoms.[81] Certain parasellar lesions such as pituitary adenomas, meningiomas, craniopharyngiomas, neurogenic tumors, dermoid cysts, lymphomas, leukemic infiltrations, sinonasal and nasopharyngeal carcinomas, and metastatic lesions (i.e., melanoma, lung, breast, kidney, thyroid, and prostate) may produce similar symptoms.[81]

Amyloidosis. Amyloidosis is caused by deposition of an amorphous hyaline material (amyloid) in various tissues such as muscle, skin, nerve, adrenal gland, orbit, and other organs including the submucosal regions. Involvement of the orbit and ocular adnexa may occur as part of primary hereditary systemic amyloidosis, as part of secondary amyloidosis, or as a localized isolated process.[77,82] Clinical features of orbital and adnexal amyloidosis include blepharoptosis resulting from infiltration of the levator muscle of the upper eyelid and oculomotor palsies resulting from involvement of multiple extraocular muscles. When the lacrimal gland is involved, it resembles a lacrimal gland tumor. On CT amyloid deposits simulate pseudotumors as well as mass lesions, and amyloidosis can occasionally calcify.[82]

Miscellaneous Granulomatous and Histiocytic Lesions. A number of pathologic entities are recognized that rarely involve the orbit. This section briefly mentions some that could have been included with specific or nonspecific granulomatous inflammations, histiocytic disorders, or xanthomatous lesions including histiocytosis X (Langerhan's histiocytosis), Erdheim-Chester disease, juvenile xanthogranuloma, pseudorheumatoid nodules (Fig. 10-127), necrobiotic xanthogranuloma, and fibrous histiocytoma.[2] All of these lesions bear common features based on local or systemic infiltration by histiocytes.[2]

Langerhans Cell Histiocytosis. Langerhan's cell histiocytosis, formerly called *histiocytosis X,* includes three disorders (Hand-Schüller-Christian disease, Letterer-Siwe disease, and eosinophilic granuloma). These lesions do not behave as true neoplasia, and it has been suggested that the pathogenesis may be related to abnormal immune regulation.[2] Orbital involvement may vary, but the most common orbital manifestation is a solitary osseous destructive lesion. The differential diagnosis of orbital Langerhan's cell histiocytosis from the CT and MRI viewpoint includes nondestructive and destructive lesions usually in the superior temporal portion of the orbit simulating lacrimal gland tumors, rhabdomyosarcoma, metastatic neuroblastoma, and lymphoreticular proliferative disorders.

Erdheim-Chester Disease. Erdheim-Chester disease is a peculiar form of systemic xanthogranulomatosis that occurs in adults.[2,77] This condition is characterized by the infiltration of many organ systems, including the lung, kidney, heart, bones, orbit, and the retroperitoneal tissues. Orbital involvement tends to be bilateral. CT and MRI may show extensive soft tissue infiltration of the orbital fatty reticulum.[77,83] There may be no orbital enhancement following the administration of Gd-DTPA contrast material.[83] However, persistent delayed enhancement of the brain may be seen in these patients following IV injection of Gd-DTPA contrast material.[83]

Juvenile Xanthogranuloma. Juvenile xanthogranuloma develops in infants and consists of idiopathic multifocal cutaneous papules that are characterized histologically by a granulomatous inflammatory response frequently showing aggregation of histiocytes to form Touton giant cells.[76] The disease may involve the anterior uveal tract and orbital soft tissues.[76]

Pseudorheumatoid Nodules. Pseudorheumatoid nodules usually occurs as focal masses in the dermis of children. This disease may involve the anterior orbit and periorbital region (Fig. 10-127). The subcutaneous nodules consist of zonular granulomas surrounding necrobiotic collagen. These nodules are thought to be more common in sites of previous trauma, and they are easily managed by simple excision.[2]

Necrobiotic Xanthogranuloma. Necrobiotic xanthogranuloma is a histocystic disease characterized by the occurrence of multiple indurated xanthomatous subcutaneous nodules in patients with paraproteinemia and proliferative disorders such as multiple myeloma and leukemia.[2,76] Pathologically a zonular granulomatous inflammatory infiltrate, with Touton giant cells and xanthoma cells, surrounds an area of necrobiosis. Ophthalmic manifestations are common and include xanthogranulomas that involve the eyelid, orbit, conjunctiva, and orbital fatty reticulum.[2,76]

Tumors

Orbital Lymphoma. Lymphomas are solid tumors of the immune system. Most are composed of (monoclonal) B cells. The extranodal presentation of non-Hodgkin's lymphomas is common, with an incidence ranging from 21% to 64%.[84] Roughly 10% of non-Hodgkin's lymphomas appear in the head and neck region and lymphoid tumors account for 10% to 15% of orbital masses.[85]

Lymphoid neoplasms of the orbit span a large continuum of various classifications from the malignant lymphomas to the benign pseudolymphomas or pseudotumors to the reactive and atypical lymphoid hyperplasias.[84] There are no absolute imaging, clinical, or even laboratory tests that delineate all types of benign orbital lymphoid lesions from orbital lymphomas or lesions, which can simulate them.[84,86] A pleomorphic cellular infiltrate correlates with a more benign biologic activity. The more uniform the cellular appearance, the greater the likelihood that malignancy is present.[84] Of all patients with orbital lymphoma, 75% have or will have systemic lymphoma.[84] There is extensive overlap histologically from one type to another, and some forms of the benign process can transform over time into a more aggressive variety of lymphoma. The radiologist can be of most use in distinguishing the primary and secondary malignancies from the intermediate and benign lymphomas. True lymphoid tissue in the eye is found in the subconjunctiva and lacrimal gland.[84] These two areas account for most of the lymphoreticuloses developing at these sites.[87] The most common cytologic forms of malignant lymphoma involving the orbit are histiocystic and lymphocystic in various degrees of differentiation.

Diagnostic Imaging. Ultrasound, CT, and MRI can be used to evaluate orbital lymphomas. CT and MRI have made it possible to make a strong presumptive diagnosis of orbital lymphoma, especially when CT and MRI features are examined in conjunction with the clinical characteristics.[88] The CT and MRI features are usually nonspecific and at times are impossible to differentiate from orbital pseudotumors (Figs. 10-133 and 10-134), lacrimal gland tumors (Fig. 10-135), optic nerve tumors, Grave's orbitopathy, primary orbital tumors, or orbital cellulitis.[84,85,88,89] Orbital lymphomas are homogeneous masses of relatively high density and sharp margins, which are more often seen in the anterior portion of the orbit, retrobulbar areas (Fig. 10-136), or the superior orbital compartment (Fig. 10-137). Generally the lesions mold themselves to preexisting structures without eroding the bone or enlarging the orbit.[84,85] Mild enhancement is present[84,88] (Figs. 10-134 and 10-136).

The shared feature of all orbital lymphoid tumors is their tendency to mold themselves around the orbital structures without evidence of bony erosion (Figs. 10-135 to 10-137). In particular, a bulky lesion in the region of the lacrimal fossa not producing any bony erosion is most likely to be inflammatory or lymphoid[88] (Fig. 10-138). However, the aggressive malignant lymphomas can produce frank destruction of bone.[88]

Lacrimal gland lymphoma displaces the globe medially and forward and appears as a moderately enhancing mass in the lacrimal gland[84] (Fig. 10-138). Lacrimal gland lymphoma must be differentiated from other benign and malignant tumors of the lacrimal gland.

MRI has proved to be as sensitive as CT for the diagnosis of orbital lymphoma and pseudotumors. Both pseudotumors and lymphoma may have an intermediate or hypointense signal in T_1W[84] and PW MR images

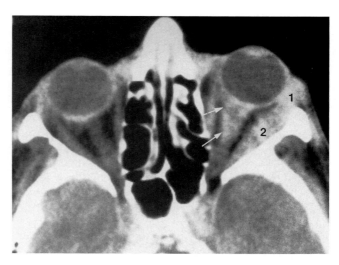

Fig. 10-133   Lymphoma. Postcontrast CT scan shows infiltrative process involving left lacrimal gland *(1)*, lateral orbital compartment *(2)*, and perioptic nerve region *(arrows)*.

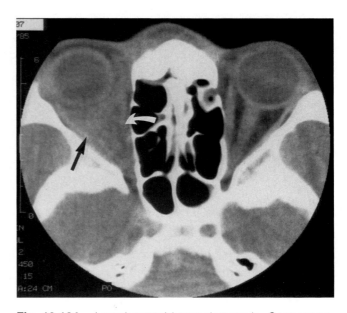

Fig. 10-134   Lymphomatoid granulomatosis. Contrast-enhanced CT scan shows diffuse infiltration of intraconal space of right orbit *(arrows)* with puttylike molding of process around posterior globe. CT features of this T-cell lymphoma precursor are virtually identical to those of true lymphoma, pseudotumor, lupoid infiltration, and metastatic carcinoma associated with marked proliferation of dense connective tissue surrounding malignant cells, such as in scirrhous carcinoma (breast, stomach).

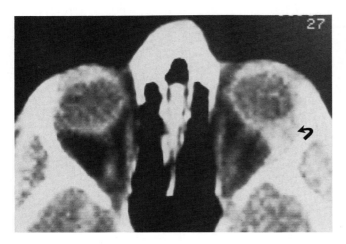

Fig. 10-135 Lymphoma (reticulum cell sarcoma). CT scan shows diffuse enlargement of left lacrimal gland (arrow).

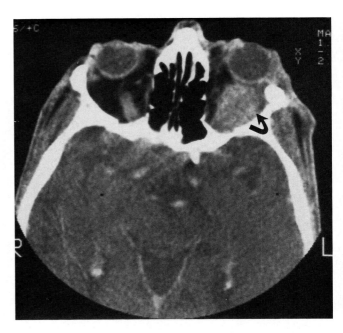

Fig. 10-136 Lymphoma. Postcontrast CT scan shows soft tissue mass (arrow) in left retrobulbar region.

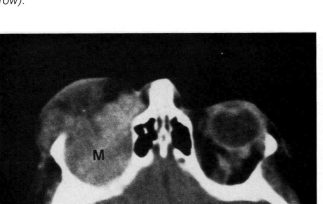

Fig. 10-137 Lymphoma. Postcontrast CT scan shows large mass (M) that molds itself around orbital structures.

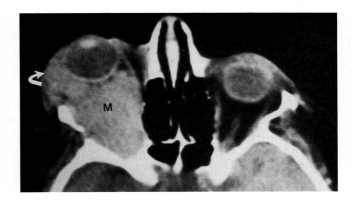

Fig. 10-138 Lymphoma. Postcontrast CT scan shows large mass (M) involving right lacrimal gland (arrow) and retrobulbar region.

and appear isointense to fat in T_2W MR images (Fig. 10-139). Lymphomas may be more hypointense in T_1W images than pseudotumors (Figs. 10-125 and 10-139). Lymphomatous lesions may be hyperintense in T_2W images (Fig. 10-140), and leukemic infiltrations can have similar MRI appearances to those of lymphomatous lesions (Fig. 10-141). Orbital lymphoma and psuedotumor demonstrate mild to moderate enhancement following IV injection of Gd-DTPA contrast material (see Fig. 10-128, B-D). All of the CT criteria used in the diagnosis of orbital pseudotumors and lymphomas should be used for MRI in the diagnosis of these conditions.[6]

Lymphoplasmacytic Tumors (Plasma Cell Tumor). Tumors composed of pure plasma cells (plasmacytomas) and those composed of B lymphocytes and plasma cells (lymphoplasmacytoid tumors) are closely related to the various lymphomas.[2,76] The plasma cell is actually a B lymphocyte modified to produce large quantities of immunoglobulin.[76] These so-called plasmacytoid lymphomas may secrete IgM paraprotein in sufficient quantities to cause a monoclonal peak in the serum; this is classically seen in Waldenstrom's macroglobulinemia.[2] An important tumor of plasma cells is multiple myeloma (Fig. 10-142). There are solitary forms of extramedullary plasmacytomas, which are not associated

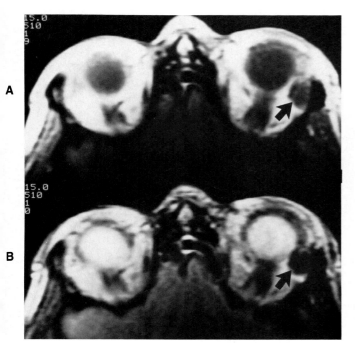

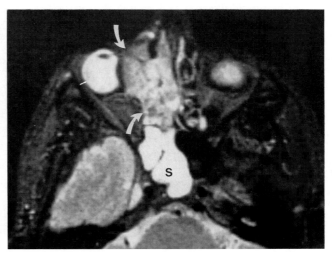

Fig. 10-139   Small cell lymphoma. **A,** Proton-weighted and **B,** T$_2$-weighted MRI scan showing lymphoma of the left lacrimal gland *(arrows)*.

Fig. 10-140   Lymphoma. T$_2$W MRI scan shows large mass *(arrows)* involving right ethmoid and orbit. Note retained secretion in right sphenoid sinus *(S)*.

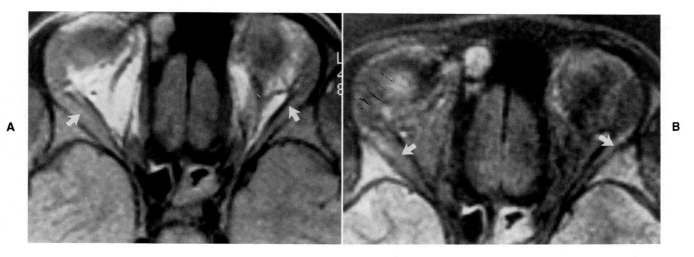

Fig. 10-141   Leukemic infiltration. **A,** PW MRI scan and **B,** T$_2$W MRI scan show bilateral subperiosteal leukemic infiltration *(arrows)*.

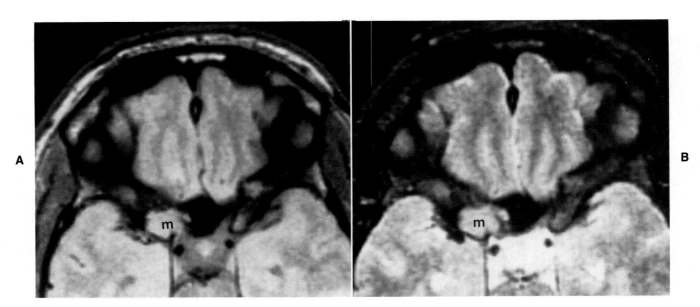

Fig. 10-142   Multiple myeloma. **A,** PW MRI scan and **B,** T₂W MRI scan show mass *(m)* involving right lesser wing and optic canal.

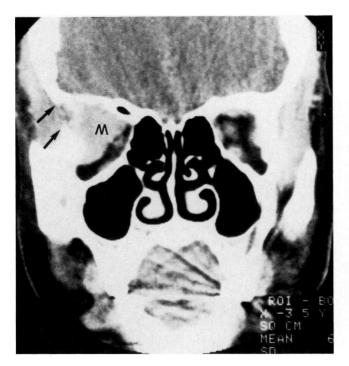

Fig. 10-143   Orbital myeloma. Postcontrast CT scan shows bone destruction of superolateral aspect of right orbit *(arrows)*, with large orbital mass *(M)*. This patient initially showed symptoms of proptosis. Biopsy of this mass revealed features compatible with lymphoplasmacytic tumor.

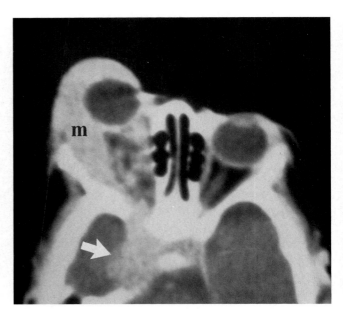

Fig. 10-144   Capillary hemangioma. Postcontrast CT scan shows enhancing mass *(m)* with involvement of eyelid and extension into right cavernous sinus *(arrow)*.

year, 35% are leukemia.[76] Leukemic disorders in children fall mainly into the lymphoid and myeloid groups. About 75% of cases are acute lymphoblastic leukemia, 20% are acute myelogenous leukemia, and 5% are chronic myelogenous leukemia.[76] Chronic lymphocytic leukemia is a disease of adulthood and almost never affects children.[76] The eye and adnexa are frequently involved (Fig. 10-141). Orbital involvement with leukemia is the result of direct infiltration of orbital bone or soft tissue by leukemic cells (Fig. 10-141). Such infiltration most often occurs in the form of a granulocytic sarcoma in patients with acute myelogenous leukemia. A granulocytic sarcoma is commonly called a *chloroma* because the myeloperoxidase within the tumor imparts a green hue as seen on gross examination.[76]

Vascular Conditions

Capillary Hemangioma (Benign Hemangioendothelioma). Capillary hemangiomas are tumors that occur primarily in infants during the first year of life. The tumor often increases in size for 6 to 10 months and then gradually involutes.[6,90] The tumor most commonly occurs in the superior nasal quadrant. Involution generally commences by the tenth month of life.[6,90] Microscopically the tumor is composed of endothelial and capillary vessel proliferation with benign endothelial cells surrounding small, capillary-sized vascular spaces.[6] Capillary hemangiomas in and around the orbit usually have an arterial supply from the external and/or the internal carotid arteries[6,90] and the tumors are capable of bleeding profusely.[6,90] These angiomas may extend intracranially through the superior orbital fissure (Fig. 10-144), optic canal, and orbital roof. On CT scans these lesions are seen as fairly well marginated (Fig. 10-144) to poorly marginated, irregular, enhancing lesions. In our series most of them were extraconal, although some of these lesions may be seen in the intraconal space. On dynamic CT study these capillary hemangiomas characteristically show an intense, homogeneous enhancement. The MRI of a capillary hemangioma is shown in Fig. 10-145.

Cavernous Hemangiomas. Cavernous hemangiomas of the orbit, the most common orbital vascular tumor in adults, have distinctive clinical and histopathologic features.[6,76] They tend to occur in the second to fourth decades of life. These tumors show a slowly progressive enlargement, which distinguishes them from capillary hemangiomas, which tend to gradually diminish in size. A prominent arterial supply is usually absent, in contrast to that of the capillary hemangiomas.[6] Cavernous hemangiomas possess a distinct fibrous pseudocapsule and therefore appear as well-defined masses (Figs. 10-146 and 10-147). This observation, in addition to the fact that they are usually independent of the general circulation, enables excision of the entire lesion without

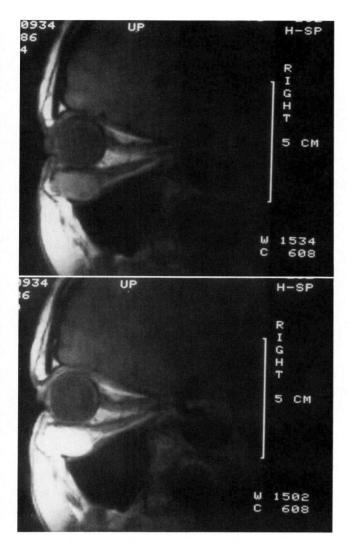

Fig. 10-145 Orbital hemangioma. Sagittal MR images (600/40) obtained without *(top)* and with *(bottom)* intravenous Gd-DTPA show hemangioma *(arrows)*. (Courtesy August F. Markl, MD.)

with systemic multiple myeloma.[76] Plasma cell tumors, particularly as they affect the orbit and ocular structures, display the same spectrum of clinical involvement as that seen in the lymphoproliferative disorders (Fig. 10-142).[2] Isolated plasmacytoma and Waldenstrom's macroglobulinemia produce a mass that can be visualized by both CT and MRI. The mass may be lobulated, densely enhancing, well defined with or without bony erosion (Fig. 10-143).[2] In cases of systemic myelomatosis, a permeative or moth-eaten pattern of bone destruction or obvious lytic destruction may be present.[64]

Orbital Leukemia. Leukemia is one of the most common childhood cancers. It is estimated that of approximately 7100 cancers in childhood in United States each

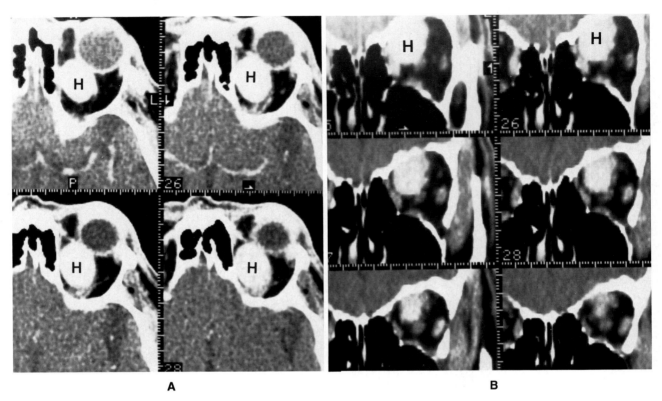

A   **B**

Fig. 10-146   Cavernous hemangioma. **A,** Serial axial CT scan and **B,** reformatted coronal CT scan show well-defined, intraconal, markedly enhancing hemangioma *(H).*

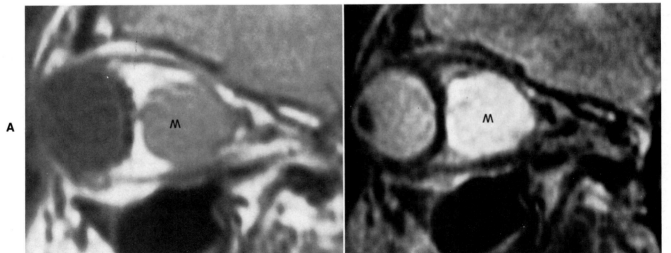

Fig. 10-147   Cavernous hemangioma. **A,** PW MRI scan and **B,** T$_2$W MRI scan show intraconal mass *(M),* which was presumed to be cavernous hemangioma.

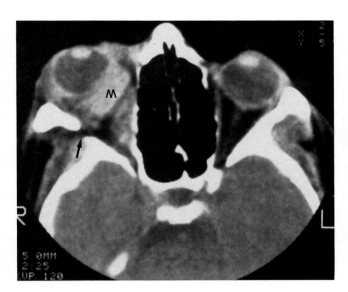

Fig. 10-148 Cavernous hemangioma. Postcontrast CT scan shows inhomogeneous enhancing mass *(M)* indenting nasal aspect of right globe. Note surgical defect *(arrow)*.

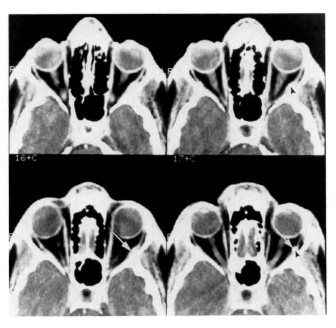

Fig. 10-149 Hemangioma. Serial contrast-enhanced CT scans show intramuscular hemangioma *(arrows)*.

fragmentation.[6] These hemangiomas may be located anywhere in the orbit[6] but frequently (83%) occur within the retrobulbar muscle cone (Figs. 10-146 and 10-147). On the CT scans cavernous hemangiomas appear as well-defined, smoothly marginated, homogeneous, rounded, ovoid, or lobulated soft tissue masses of increased density with variable degrees of contrast enhancement (Fig. 10-146). Cavernous hemangiomas always respect the contour of the globe, unless the tumor has been ruptured or surgically violated (Fig. 10-148). Orbital bone expansion is not uncommon in cavernous hemangiomas. At times calcification may be seen in these lesions. The MRI characteristics of these hemangiomas are shown in Fig. 10-147, *A* and *B*. Histologically cavernous hemangiomas are composed of large dilated vascular channels (sinusoid spaces) lined by thin, attenuated endothelial cells.[6] At times intraconal cavernous hemangiomas may be difficult to differentiate from other intraconal lesions such as meningiomas, hemangiopericytomas and schwannomas.[6] Occasionally hemangiomas may be intramuscular (Fig. 10-149). Sclerosing hemangiomas of the orbit may appear as an irregular mass with or without foci of calcification (Fig. 10-150).

Lymphangiomas. Orbital lymphangiomas occur in children and young adults. In contrast to the rapid, self-limited growth of infantile capillary hemangiomas, lymphangiomas gradually and progressively enlarge during the growing years.[6] Cavernous lymphangiomas are composed of delicate, endothelium-lined, lymph-

filled sinuses (filled with clear fluid or chocolate-colored unclotted fluid), which invade the surrounding connective tissue stroma.[6] The interstitial tissue often shows lymphoid follicles and lymphocytic infiltration.[6] Spontaneous hemorrhage within the lesion is common.[6] Lymphangiomas may have distinct borders but are typically diffuse and not well capsulated (Figs. 10-150 and 10-151), with portions of the lesion infiltrating the normal tissues of the lid and orbit.[6] They are usually multilobular (Fig. 10-151), complete surgical excision is seldom accomplished, and recurrence is common.[6] They are more common in the extraconal space.[6] On CT scans these lymphangiomas appear as poorly circumscribed, often heterogeneous masses of increased density in the extraconal or intraconal space (Fig. 10-150). Bony expansion may be present, calcification is rare, and minimal to marked contrast enhancement may be present (Fig. 10-150). On MRI scans lymphangiomas are seen as relatively hyperintense on T_1W and usually very hyperintense on T_2W images (Fig. 10-151). Their MRI characteristics should help to differentiate them from pseudotumors, hemangiomas, and many other lesions.[6]

Hemangiopericytomas. Hemangiopericytomas are rare, slow-growing vascular neoplasms that arise from the pericytes of Zimmermann,[6,91] which normally envelop the capillaries and postcapillary venules of practically all types of tissues.[92,93] Histologically these tumors are composed of scattered, capillary-like spaces surrounded by proliferating pericytes.[6] Hemangiopericytomas may be divided into lobules by fibrovascular sep-

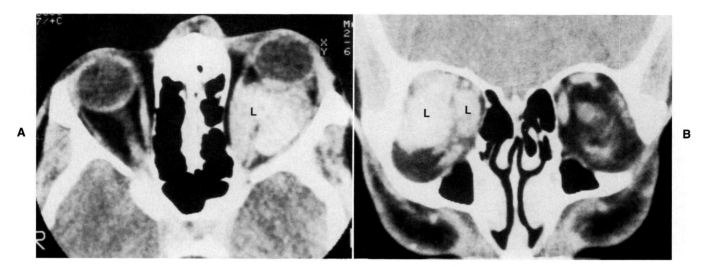

Fig. 10-150 Lymphangioma. **A,** Contrast-enhanced axial CT scan and **B,** coronal CT scan show large lobulated lymphangioma *(L)*.

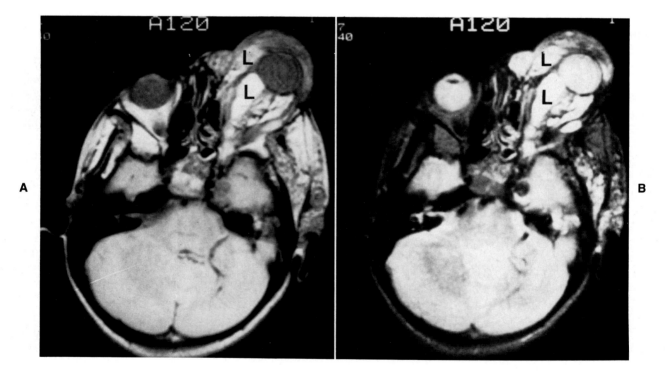

Fig. 10-151 Lymphangioma. **A,** PW MRI scan and **B,** T₂W MRI scan show large lymphangioma *(L)*.

ta.[6,91] About 50% of the cases are malignant[6,94]; and distant metastases, although uncommon, occur via the vascular and lymphatic routes, with the lungs as the most common sites for metastases.[6,91,93] These lesions tend to recur if not excised completely, and wide surgical excision is the treatment of choice.

On CT the margins of orbital hemangiopericytoma, in contrast to cavernous hemangioma, may be slightly less distinct because of their tendency to invade the adjacent tissues. Erosion of the underlying bone may be present (Fig. 10-152). Marked contrast enhancement is in favor of a hemangiopericytoma. MRI scans may not differentiate these tumors from cavernous hemangiomas, neurogenic tumors, meningiomas, and other lesions (Fig. 10-153). However, angiography may be very helpful in differentiating these lesions.[6] Hemangiopericytomas usually have an early florid blush,[6,81,95] and cavernous hemangiomas show late minor pooling of the contrast or often behave as avascular masses.[6,95,96] Meningiomas may show multiple tumor vessels and a late blush,[6,22,94] and schwannomas may show no tumor blush.[6,94] Hemangiopericytomas may be difficult to differentiate from other vasculogenic tumors such as angioleiomyomas or malignant hemangioendotheliomas (angiosarcomas) and from fibrous histiocytomas.[6]

Orbital Varix. Primary orbital varices are congenital venous malformations that are characterized by a proliferation of venous elements and massive dilation of one or more orbital veins, presumably associated with a congenital weakness in the venous wall.[6,81,96] Orbital varices are the most common cause of spontaneous orbital hemorrhage.[97] The CT appearance of an orbital varix may be normal in axial sections but quite abnormal in coronal sections, particularly when the scans are obtained with the patient in a prone position (Fig. 10-154). This varix prominence reflects the increased venous pressure in this position. Any time an orbital varix is suspected, additional CT sections should be made during a valsalva maneuver. Similarly, MRI should be obtained with the patient in the prone position. MRI of an orbital varix in one of our patients with bilateral varices showed hyperintense lesions in T_1W, PDW, and T_2W images (Fig. 10-155). An orbital varix may be seen as several round or tubular masses, occasionally with associated calcifications.[6]

Carotid Cavernous Fistulas. Carotid cavernous fistulas produce proptosis, chemosis, venous engorgement, pulsating exophthalmos, and an auscultable bruit. Ischemic ocular necrosis resulting from carotid-cavernous fistula has also been reported.[81] A carotid cavernous fistula may result from trauma or surgery or may occur spontaneously. Spontaneous carotid-cavernous fistulas have been reported in patients with osteogenesis imperfecta, Ehlers-Danlos syndrome, and pseudoxanthoma elasticum, probably caused by weakness of the vessel walls related to the connective tissue disease.[81] CT and MRI scanning will demonstrate proptosis with engorgement of the superior ophthalmic vein and frequent enlargement of the ipsilateral extraocular muscles. There may be CT or MRI evidence of venous

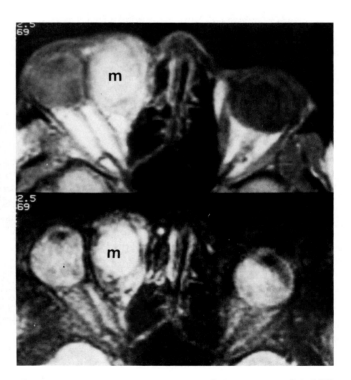

Fig. 10-153 Hemangiopericytoma/Schwannoma. PW MRI scan *(top)* and T_2W MRI scan *(bottom)* show mass *(m)* compatible with hemangiopericytoma/schwannoma. The initial diagnosis in this case on histologic examination of the surgical specimen was hemangiopericytoma. Further pathologic examination in another institution, however, revealed features compatible with schwannoma.

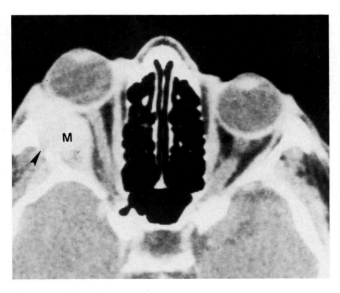

Fig. 10-152 Hemangiopericytoma. Contrast-enhanced CT scan shows enhancing mass *(M)* compatible with hemangiopericytoma. Note erosion of lateral orbital wall *(arrowhead)*.

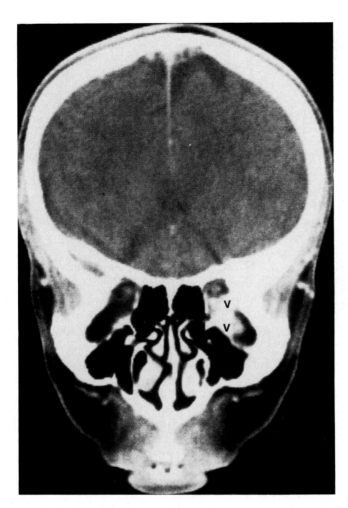

Fig. 10-154 Orbital varix. Coronal contrast-enhanced CT scan shows several round, enhancing masses compatible with orbital varix *(V)*.

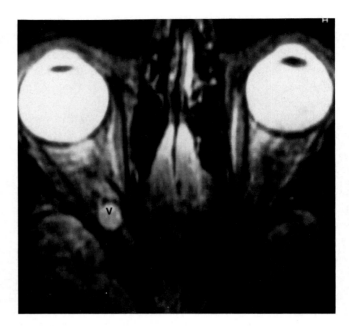

Fig. 10-155 Orbital varix. T$_2$W MRI scan shows round, hyperintense mass compatible with surgically proved orbital varix *(V)*.

thrombosis in the lumen of the superior ophthalmic vein or cavernous sinus. Angiographic demonstration of the exact location of the carotid-cavernous fistula is essential and aids in planning definitive therapy.[81]

Neural Lesions

Optic nerve meningiomas and gliomas are discussed in Chapter 11.

Orbital Schwannomas. Schwannomas are benign, slow-growing nerve sheath tumors, which account for 1% to 6% of all orbital tumors.[6,98-100] They may arise anywhere within the orbit, although they are most common in the intraconal space.[6] The malignant counterpart, the malignant schwannoma (neurogenic sarcoma and fibrosarcoma of the nerve sheath) is exceedingly rare in the orbit.[6,99,101] In general, neurofibromas and schwannomas are two benign tumors that originate from Schwann's cells. These tumors occur in the orbit either as isolated lesions or in association with neurofi-

bromatosis. The optic nerve has no Schwann's cells; therefore, orbital schwannomas must arise from the peripheral nerve fibers of the III, IV, V, VI, and VII cranial nerves. Schwannomas are well-capsulated neoplasms composed of Schwann's cells (Antoni types A and B). Histologically, schwannomas are sharply surrounded by a thin, fibrous capsule that is formed by compression of perineural tissue. The tumor is composed of compactly arranged, spindle-shaped cells that interlace in cords and whorls, which frequently are oriented with their long axes parallel to one another. This cellular pattern is referred to as Antoni type A.[6,98,99] Commonly the Antoni type B part of the tumor has a less cellular pattern, which is characterized by haphazardly distributed cells[6,98] in a collagenous matrix.[6,94,102] In contrast, neurofibromas are poorly encapsulated and less cellular. When most of the fascicles in a segment of peripheral nerve are involved, cylindrical enlargement of the entire nerve segment is observed. This clinical and gross pathologic configuration is referred to as *plexiform neurofibroma*.[6,102] Plexiform and diffuse infiltrating neurofibromas are highly vascular, poorly circumscribed tumors that are impossible to excise completely.[6,102] On CT scans the orbital schwannomas appear as sharply marginated, oval, fusiform often intraconal masses of increased density that show moderate to marked enhancement (Fig. 10-156). The optic nerve is always displaced or may be engulfed by the tumor (Fig. 10-156). The differential diagnoses are cavernous hemangioma, meningioma (Fig. 10-157), hemangiopericytoma, and metastasis.

Nontumoral Enlargement of the Optic Nerve Sheath.

Primary or secondary involvement of the optic nerve in cases of lymphoma (Fig. 10-128), sarcoid (Fig. 10-158), leukemia, tuberculosis, toxoplasmosis, and syphilis has been reported.[15,22]

Optic Neuritis. Optic neuritis is an acute inflammatory process that involves the optic nerve and that may appear as optic nerve enlargement.[15] Optic neuritis is sometimes an early manifestation of multiple sclerosis. In optic neuritis CT may show an enlarged optic nerve with some degree of contrast enhancement. On MRI the optic neuritis may appear hyperintense on T_2W MRI scans.[15] However, in some cases of optic neuritis the nerve can appear normal on CT and MRI. MRI visualization of MS plaques in cases of optic neuritis may be accentuated by fat suppression techniques (Fig. 10-159).[15]

Lacrimal Gland and Fossa Lesions

The lacrimal gland is about the size and shape of an almond and is located in the superolateral extraconal orbital fat in the lacrimal fossa, adjacent to the tendons of the superior and lateral rectus muscles. The more anterior palpebral lobe is separated from the deeper orbital lobe by the lateral horn of the levator muscle aponeurosis. The lacrimal gland region can be involved by a wide spectrum of orbital pathology. The excellent prognosis for benign mixed tumor, provided it is completely removed at first surgery, is now widely accepted. Proper management of this tumor requires preoperative recognition of the possibility that a benign mixed lacrimal gland tumor may be present. This preoperative diagnosis is imperative because in cases of a benign mixed tumor, no incisional biopsy should be performed but rather an en bloc excision including the adjacent tissues should be accomplished through a lateral orbitotomy to ensure complete tumor excision and to prevent late recurrences. Incisional biopsy of a benign mixed lacrimal gland tumor is associated with the spillage of tumor cells, leading to late recurrences and incomplete tumor resection. In general, epithelial tumors represent 50% of masses involving the lacrimal gland. The remaining 50% of lacrimal gland masses are of the lymphoid-inflammatory type. Metastases to the parenchyma of the lacrimal gland are rare. Dermoid cysts are not true lacrimal gland tumors but rather arise from epithelial rests located in the orbit, primarily in the superolateral quadrant. Epithelial cysts, on the other hand, are intrinsic lacrimal gland lesions that result from dilation of the lacrimal ducts.

Inflammatory diseases of the lacrimal gland can be divided into two categories, acute and chronic. Acute lacrimal adenitis (bacterial or viral) is more commonly seen in children and in younger persons and may be related to trauma. Such acute disease is associated with

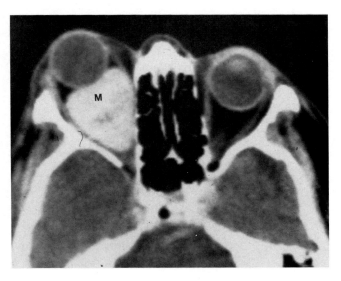

Fig. 10-156 Orbital schwannoma. Contrast-enhanced CT scan shows large enhancing mass (M).

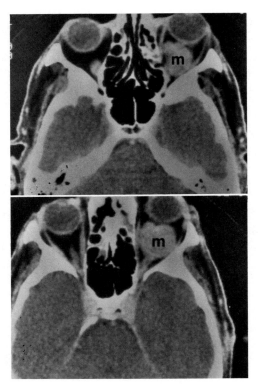

Fig. 10-157 Optic nerve sheath meningioma. Contrast-enhanced CT scans show large optic nerve sheath meningioma (m).

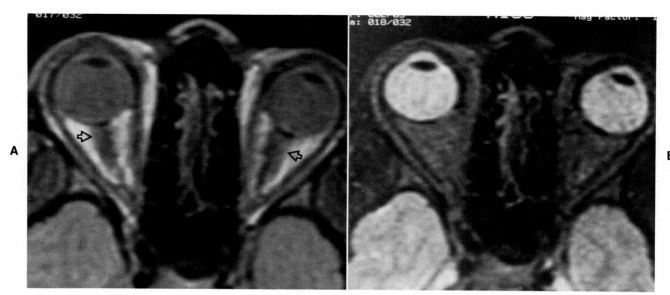

Fig. 10-158   Optic nerve sarcoidosis. **A,** PW MRI scan and **B,** T$_2$W MRI scan show irregular enlargement of optic nerves *(arrows)*. Lesion is isointense to fat in T$_2$W MRI scan.

local tenderness, erythema, lid swelling, conjunctival chemosis, discharge or suppuration, enlarged preauricular and cervical nodes, and systemic findings. Acute lacrimal adenitis is usually unilateral and tends to respond to therapy very rapidly. Acute lacrimal adenitis may be related to the broad spectrum of idiopathic inflammatory orbital pseudotumors. This diagnosis is often made on the basis of the clinical presentation, CT findings, and the prompt and favorable response to the administration of systemic corticosteroids.

Chronic lacrimal adenitis may follow acute infection or be caused by sarcoidosis (Fig. 10-160), thyroid ophthalmopathy, Mikulicz syndrome, "sclerosing pseudotumors" (Fig. 10-161) and Wegener's granulomatosis. In sarcoidosis, there is usually bilateral symmetric or asymmetric lacrimal gland enlargement (Fig. 10-160). Mikulicz's syndrome is a nonspecific swelling of the lacrimal and salivary glands, associated with conditions such as leukemia, lymphoma, tuberculosis, syphilis, and sarcoidosis. In Sjögren's syndrome the lacrimal glands are enlarged, with a lymphocytic infiltration of the glandular tissue. Half of these patients have connective tissue disease, such as rheumatoid arthritis, systemic lupus erythematosus, scleroderma, or polymyositis. Inflammatory pseudotumor in the region of the lacrimal gland accounts for about 15% of orbital pseudotumors. Although they are rare in the very young, the age range is very wide. The most common symptoms include proptosis, swollen lids, pain and dyplopia, with a duration of symptoms of less than 6 months in the majority of cases.

Ocular involvement in Wegener's granuloma is common, affecting 40% of patients with generalized disease. Involvement of the lacrimal gland is not uncommon. Histologic examination of involved lacrimal gland shows infiltration with histocytes, plasma cells, lymphocytes, polymorphs, and eosinophils, with giant cell formation. Massive enlargement of lacrimal glands may be present and has been demonstrated by CT scan.

Lymphomatous lesions of the lacrimal glands includes a broad spectrum from reactive lymphoid hyperplasia to malignant lymphomas of various types (Fig. 10-162). It can be very difficult to differentiate pathologically benign lymphocytic infiltration from lymphoma. Lymphomatous lesions usually occur in older patients. Shields and associates, in a review of 645 space-occupying orbital lesions that underwent biopsy, found 71 cases of lymphocytic and plasmacytic lesions. Of these, 12 were located in the lacrimal gland.

Benign mixed lacrimal gland tumors tend to occur in patients in the third to sixth decades of life. The tumors present with slowly progressive, painless upper lid swelling, proptosis, or both, without inflammatory symptoms or signs (Fig. 10-163).

Computed Tomography and MRI. Inflammatory lesions of the lacrimal gland show diffuse enlargement of the gland. Contrast enhancement may be marked and there may be associated acute lateral rectus muscle myositis. There may be an associated scleritis with fluid in Tenon's space and a ring of uveoscleral enhancement. In chronic lacrimal adenitis, the gland also shows diffuse oblong enlargement (Figs. 10-160 and 10-161). The

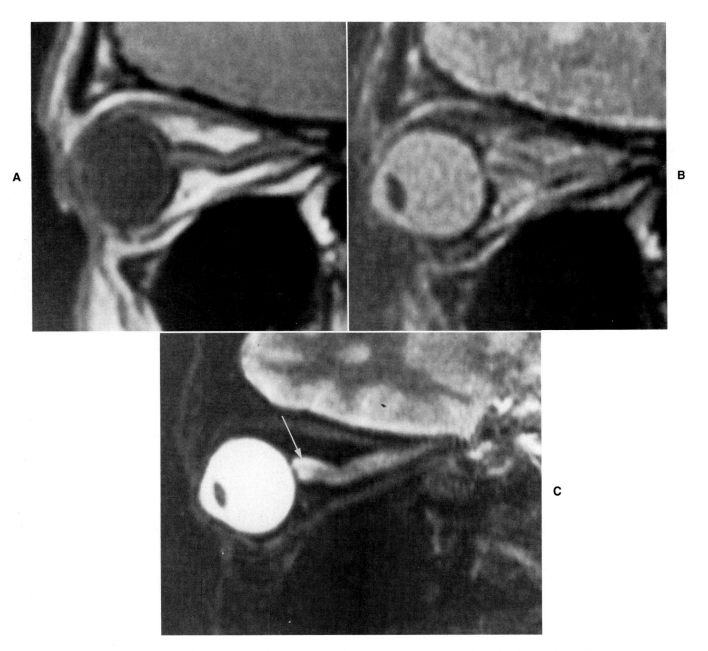

Fig. 10-159   Presumed optic nerve neuritis caused by multiple sclerosis. **A,** Sagittal PW MRI scan and **B,** sagittal T₂W MRI scan show no detectable abnormality of optic nerve. **C,** Fat-suppression (STIR) MRI scan shows apparent area of hyperintensity *(arrow)*. Part of hyperintensity is related to cerebrospinal fluid around optic nerve, which is irregular in this region.

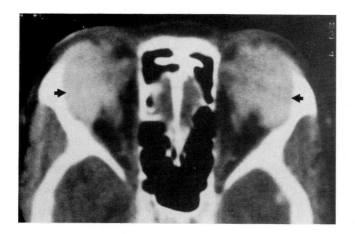

Fig. 10-160 Sarcoidosis. Axial CT scan shows bilateral, diffuse enlargement of entire lacrimal glands *(arrows)*.

Fig. 10-161 Lacrimal gland pseudotumor. Eighty-year-old patient with swelling of both eyes. Axial postcontrast CT scan shows bilateral, lobular enlargement of lacrimal glands *(arrows)*.

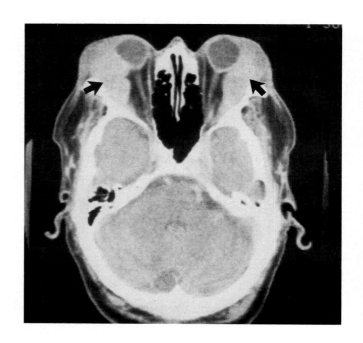

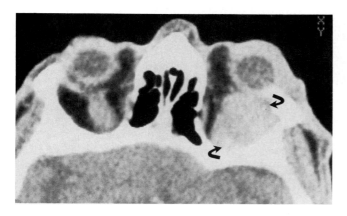

Fig. 10-162 Lymphoma. Axial postcontrast CT scan shows large mass in superior temporal quadrant extending posteriorly to orbital apex *(arrows)*; lacrimal gland is totally involved. Note postsurgical changes in lateral wall of left orbit.

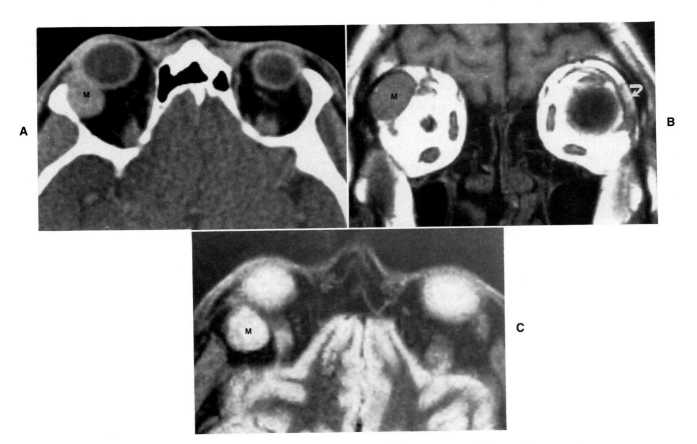

Fig. 10-163   Benign adenoma of lacrimal gland. **A,** Postcontrast CT scan shows well-defined mass *(M)*. **B,** T₁W MRI scan shows extraconal mass *(M)* involving right lacrimal gland. Note normal left lacrimal gland *(arrow)*. **C,** T₂W MRI scan shows hyperintense lacrimal mass *(M)*. Notice intact capsule around the mass, which is delineated by hypointensity of surrounding orbital fat and lateral orbital bone.

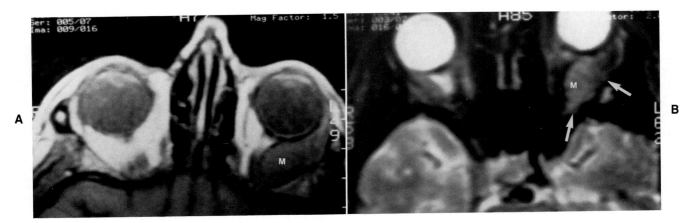

Fig. 10-164   Adenocarcinoma of lacrimal gland. **A,** T₁W MRI scan and **B,** T₂W MRI scan show large mass *(M)*. Lateral orbital wall is irregular *(arrows)*. CT scans showed erosion of bone.

glands may be massively enlarged in cases of sarcoidosis (Figs. 10-131 and 10-160) or other conditions such as Mikulicz's syndrome, pseudotumors (Fig. 10-161), and Wegener's granulomatosis.[6,76] However scleral enhancement is not an associated feature in these patients as it is in those patients with acute inflammations.

Benign and malignant lymphoid tumors situated in the lacrimal gland also display diffuse glandular enlargement with oblong contouring (Fig. 10-133). However, these lesions are very bulky (Fig. 10-162), have more frequent evidence of anterior and posterior glandular extension, with molding and draping of the gland upon the globe. In general, inflammatory processes and lymphomas tend to involve all aspects of the lacrimal gland, often including its palpebral lobe (Figs. 10-133 and 10-162). However, neoplastic lesions of the gland rarely originate in the palpebral lobe and therefore often have a tendency for posterior extension rather than anterior growth beyond the orbital rim (Fig. 10-163).

Since the lacrimal gland is histologically similar to the salivary gland, it is involved by similar disease processes. Epithelial tumors represent 50% of masses involving the lacrimal gland. Half of these are pleomorphic (benign mixed) adenomas; the other half are malignant tumors. Of the malignancies, adenoid cystic carcinoma is the most common lesion followed by malignant mixed tumor, mucoepidermoid carcinoma adenocarcinoma (Fig. 10-164), squamous cell carcinoma, and undifferentiated (anaplastic) carcinoma. A significant number of these tumors arise within pleomorphic adenomas. A benign mixed tumor is increasingly likely to undergo malignant degeneration the longer the patient has the tumor and experiences recurrences. In such a malignant mixed tumor, the malignant cell clone develops from the preexisting benign mixed tumor and often is poorly differentiated adenocarcinoma or an adenoid cystic carcinoma. In general, patients with these carcinomas have a poor prognosis.

In 1979 Stewart, Krohel, and Wright described a scheme for the clinical diagnosis and management of lacrimal fossa lesions that employed any distinguishing clinical features and plain radiographic studies for classifying lacrimal gland masses. Jakobiec et al performed a study on the clinical and CT findings for 39 patients with four different kinds of lacrimal gland swelling, sixteen of whom had parenchymal benign or malignant tumors. This study added a new diagnostic dimension of the shape of the soft tissue mass, "contour analysis," as another factor that can be combined with the clinical history.

Stewart et al reviewed 31 cases of benign and malignant lacrimal gland masses. Fourteen had benign mixed lacrimal gland tumors, and 13 had "pressure" changes characterized by enlargement of the lacrimal fossa without destruction of the bone. Sclerosis of bone was present in one patient. Malignant neoplasms accounted for 17 of the 31 tumors. Twelve had "pressure" changes, 2 had no bone changes, and 3 showed destructive changes. Three patients with "pressure" changes and malignant tumors had calcification in the lacrimal gland fossa. Two patients had sclerosis of the bone adjacent to the lacrimal fossa.

Jakobiec et al reviewed by CT 39 patients with solid masses in the lacrimal gland, 16 of which were parenchymal benign and malignant tumors (six benign mixed tumors, one schwannoma, and nine malignant epithelial tumors) and all of which exhibited rounded or globular soft tissue outlines. These were frequently associated with contiguous bone changes. Benign tumors had smooth encapsulated outlines, whereas the malignant tumors displayed microserrations indicative of infiltration. Inflammatory conditions in their series demonstrated diffuse, compressed, and molded enlargement of the lacrimal gland in an oblong fashion; and there were no associated bone defects. This study concluded that well-capsulated, rounded masses of long duration were likely to be benign mixed tumors. The epithelial neoplasms probably began unicentrically within the lacrimal gland and grew in a centrifugal fashion in all directions, sometimes indenting the globe, distorting its muscle cone, and creating fossa or bone destruction in the orbital walls. In contrast, inflammatory and lymphoid lesions of the lacrimal gland were seen as diffuse expansion of the lacrimal gland and the lesions molded themselves to preexisting orbital structures without eroding bone or enlarging the orbit.[88] The study found that the stroma of the epithelial tumors was often hyalinized or even cartilaginous, and that this type of tissue was more likely than the inflammatory or lymphoid lesions to mold itself in a putty-like fashion to the isthmus between the globe and the orbital bone.[88]

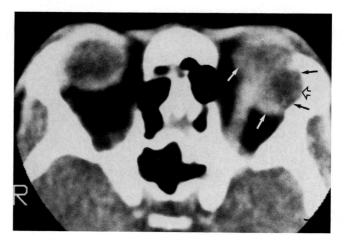

Fig. 10-165 Chronic hematic cyst ("cholesterol granuloma"). CT scan shows inhomogeneous mass *(arrows)*. Note compression deformity of orbital wall *(hollow arrow)*.

Bony changes in the lacrimal gland fossa may be produced by benign or malignant epithelial tumors, other parenchymal lacrimal gland tumors such as schwannomas, and lesions originating within the subperiosteal space or bone, including benign orbital cysts, hematic cysts (Fig. 10-165), eosinophilic granulomas, dermoid cysts, and metastatic carcinomas. Lymphoid and inflammatory processes rarely produce bony changes.

REFERENCES

1. Warwick R and Williams PL, editor: Gray's anatomy, ed 35 (British), Philadelphia, 1973, WB Saunders Co.
2. Rootman J, editor: Diseases of the orbit, Philadelphia, 1988, JB Lippincott Co.
3. Daniels DL, Yu S, Pech P et al: Computed tomography and magnetic resonance imaging of the orbital apex, Radiol Clin North Am 25:803-817, 1987.
4. Canalis RF and Burstein FD: Osteogenesis in vascularized periosteum, Arch Otolaryngol Head Neck Surg 3:511-518, 1985.
5. Duhamel HL: Sur le development et la crue des os des animax, Mem Acad R Sci 55:354-370, 1742.
6. Mafee MF, Putterman A, Valvassori GE et al: Orbital space-occupying lesions: role of CT and MRI; an analysis of 145 cases, Radiol Clin North Am 25:529-559, 1987.
7. Reeh MJ, Wobij JL, and Wirtschafter JD: Ophthalmic anatomy: a manual with some clinical applications, San Francisco, 1981, American Academy of Ophthalmology, pp 11-54.
8. Pansky B and House EL: Review of gross anatomy: a dynamic approach, New York, 1986, Macmillan Publishing Co, pp 11-54.
9. Gosling JA et al, editor: Atlas of human anatomy with integrated text, Philadelphia, 1985, JB Lippincott Co.
10. Mafee MF and Miller MT: Computed tomography scanning in the evaluation of ocular motility disorders. In Gonzalez CF, Becker MH, and Flanagan JC, editors: Diagnostic imaging in ophthalmology, 1985, Springer-Verlag New York, Inc, pp 39-54.
11. Dale RT, editor: Fundamentals of ocular motility and strabismus, New York, 1982, Grune & Stratton, Inc.
12. Helveston EM et al: The trochlea: a study of the anatomy and pathology. Ophthalmology 89:124-133, 1982.
13. Fink WH: The anatomy of the extrinsic muscles of the eye. In Allen JH, editor: Strabismus ophthalmic symposium, St Louis, 1950, The CV Mosby Co, pp 17-62.
14. Miller TM and Mafee MF: Computed tomography scanning in the evaluation of ocular motility disorders, Radiol Clin North Am 25:733-752, 1987.
15. Azar-Kia B et al: CT and MRI of optic nerve and sheath, Seminars in ultrasound, CT and MRI 9:443-454, 1988.
16. Peyster RG: Computed tomography of the orbit. In Gonzalez CF, Becker MH, and Flanagan JC, editors: Diagnostic imaging in ophthalmology, 1985, Springer-Verlag New York, Inc, pp 20-37.
17. Mafee MF et al: CT in the evaluation of the orbit and the bony interorbital distance, AJNR 7:265-269, 1986.
18. Mafee MF et al: Direct sagittal CT in the evaluation of temporal bone disease, AJNR 9:371-378, March/April 1988.
19. Mafee MF and Haik BG: Lacrimal gland and fossa lesions: role of computed tomography, Radiol Clin North Am 25:767-779, 1987.
20. Langer BG et al: MRI of the normal orbit and optic pathway, Radiol Clin North Am 25:429-446, 1987.
21. Zonneveld FW et al: Normal direct multiplanar CT anatomy of the orbit with correlative anatomic cryosections, Radiol Clin North Am 25:381-407, 1987.
22. Azar-Kia B et al: Optic nerve tumors: role of MRI and CT, Radiol Clin North Am 25:561-581, 1987.
23. Currarino G and Silverman FN: Orbital hypotelorism, arhinencephaly, and trigoncephaly, Radiology 74:206-216, 1960.
24. Gerald BE and Silverman FN: Normal and abnormal interorbital distances with special reference to mongolism, AJR 95:154-161, 1956.
25. Morin J et al: A study of growth in the interorbital region, Am J Ophthalmol 56:895, 1936.
26. Cameron J: Interorbital width: new cranial dimension; its significance in modern and fossil man and in lower mammals, Am J Phys Anthropol 15:509-515, 1931.
27. Hansman CF: Growth of interorbital distance and skull thickness as observed in roentgenographic measurements, Radiology 86:87-96, 1966.
28. Linder B, Campos M, and Schafer M: CT and MRI of orbital abnormalities in neurofibromatosis and selected craniofacial anomalies, Radiol Clin North Am 25:787-802, 1987.
29. Converse JM and McCarthy JG: Orbital hypertelorism, Scand J Plast Reconstr Surg 15:265-276, 1985.
30. DeMyer WM: Neurologic evaluation associated forebrain maldevelopment and orbital hypotelorism. In symposium on diagnosis and treatment of craniofacial anomalies, vol 20, St Louis, 1979, The CV Mosby Co, pp 153-163.
31. Becker MH and McCarthy JG: Congenital abnormalities. In Gonzalez CF, Becker MH, and Flanagan JC, editors: Diagnostic imaging in ophthalmology, 1985, Springer-Verlag New York, Inc, pp 115-187.
32. Gorlin RJ, Pindberg JJ, and Cohen MM Jr: Syndromes of the head and neck, ed 2, New York, 1976, McGraw-Hill Inc.
33. Smith DW: Recognizable patterns of human malformation, Philadelphia, 1970, WB Saunders Co.
34. Taybi H: Radiology of syndromes and metabolic disorders, ed 2, 1983, Chicago Year Book Medical Publishers.
35. Mafee MF et al: Computed tomography of optic nerve colobomas, morning glory anomaly, and colobomatous cyst, Radiol Clin North Am 25:693-699, 1987.
36. Mann I: Developmental abnormalities of the eye, ed 2, Philadelphia, 1957, JB Lippincott Co, pp 74-78.
37. Mann I: The development of the human eye, New York, 1969, Grune & Stratton, Inc.
38. Brown G and Tasman W, editors: Congenital anomalies of the optic disc, New York, 1983, Grune & Stratton, Inc, pp 97-191.
39. Arey LB: Developmental anatomy, ed 6, Philadelphia, 1970, WB Saunders Co.
40. Duke-Elder S and Wybar KC: System of ophthalmology: the anatomy of the visual system, vol 2, St Louis, 1961, The CV Mosby Co.
41. Hamilton WJ, Boyd JD, and Mossman HW, editors: Human embryology: development of form and function, ed 3, Baltimore, 1962, Williams & Wilkins.
42. Tessier P: The definitive plastic surgical treatment of the severe facial deformities of craniofacial dysostosis: Crouzon's and Apert's diseases, Plast Reconstr Surg 48:419-442, 1971.
43. Campbell JA: Craniofacial anomalies. In Newton TH and Potts DG, editors: Radiology of the skull and brain, book 2, vol 1, St. Louis, 1971, The CV Mosby Co, pp 571-633.
44. Mafee MF and Valvassori GE: Radiology of the craniofacial anomalies, Otolaryngol Clin North Am 14:939-988, 1981.
45. Harwood-Nash DC: Coronal sysostosis. In Rogers LF, editor: Disorders of the head and neck syllabus, second series, Chicago, 1977, American College of Radiology.
46. Anderson FM and Geiger L: Craniosynostosis: a survey of 204 cases, J Neurosurg 22:229-240, 1965.
47. Shillito J Jr and Matson DD: Craniosynostosis: a review of 519 surgical patients, Pediatrics 41:829-853, 1968.
48. Lombardi G: Radiology in neuro-ophthalmology, Baltimore, 1967, Williams & Wilkins.

49. Saethre H: Ein beitrag zum turnschädel problem (pathogenese, erblichkeit und symptomatologie), Deutsch Z Nervenh 119:533-555, 1931.

50. Chotzen F: Eine eigenartige familiare entwicklungsstorung (akrocephalosyndaktylie), dysostosis craniofacialis and hypertelorisms), Mschr Kinderb 55:97-122, 1932.

51. Bartsocas CS, Weber AL, and Crawford JD: Acrocephalosyndactyly type 2: Chotzen's syndrome, J Pediatr 77:267-272, 1970.

52. Lewis A et al: Von Recklinghausen neurofibromatosis II: incidence of optic glioma, Ophthalmology 91:929-935, 1984.

53. Zimmerman RA et al: Computed tomography of orbitofacial neurofibromatosis, Radiology 146:113-116, 1983.

54. Kobrin JL, Block FC, and Wiengiest TA: Ocular and orbital manifestations of neurofibromatosis, Surv Ophthalmol 24:45-51, 1979.

55. Jacoby CG, Go RT, and Beren RA: Cranial CT of neurofibromatosis, AJR 135:553-557, 1980.

56. Berry GA: Note on a congenital defect (? Coloboma) of the lower lid, Roy, London, Ophthal Hosp Rep 12:225, 1889.

57. Treacher-Collins E: Case with symmetrical congenital notches in the outer part of each lower lid and defective development of the malar bone, Trans Ophthal Soc 20:190, 1900.

58. Pires deLima JA, and Monteior HB: Aparello branquiale suas perturbacoes evolutivas, Arch Anat Anthrop (Lisboa) 8:185, 1923.

59. Francheschetti A and Klein D: The mandibulo-facial dysostosis, a new hereditary syndrome, Acta Ophthalmol 27:141-224, 1949.

60. Poswillo D: The pathogenesis of the Treacher-Collins syndrome (mandibulofacial dysostosis), Br J Oral Surg 13:1-26, 1975.

61. Herring SW, Rowlatt UF, and Pruzansky S: Anatomical abnormalities in mandibulofacial dysostosis, Am J Med Genet 3:225-259, 1979.

62. Pruzansky S, Miller M, and Krammer JF: Ocular defects in craniofacial syndromes. In Goldberg MF, editor: Genetic and metabolic eye disease, Boston, 1974, Little, Brown & Co, Inc, pp 487, 498.

63. Henderson JW: Orbital tumors, Philadelphia, 1973, WB Saunders Co, pp 116-123.

64. Mafee MF, Dobben GD, and Valvassori GE: Computed tomography assessment of paraorbital pathology. In Gonzalez CA, Becker MH, and Flanagan JC, editors: Diagnostic imaging in ophthalmology, 1985, Springer-Verlag New York, Inc, pp 281-302.

65. Grove AS: Giant dermoid cysts of the orbit, Ophthalmol 86:1513-1520, 1979.

66. Momose KJ: Infection of the orbit. In Gonzalez CA, Becker MH, and Flanagan JC, editors: Diagnostic imaging in ophthalmology, 1985, Springer-Verlag New York, Inc, pp 307-322.

67. Hawkins DD and Clark RW: Orbital involvement in acute sinusitis, Clin Pediatr 16(5):464-471, 1977.

68. Centeno RS, Bentson RJ, and Mancuso AA: CT scanning in rhinocerebral macor mycosis and aspergillosis, Radiology 140:383-389, 1981.

69. Courey WR, New PFJ, and Price DL: Angiographic manifestations of craniofacial phycomyeosis: report of three cases, Radiology 103:329-334, 1972.

70. Blodi FC and Gass JDM: Inflammatory pseudotumor of the orbit, Br J Ophthalmolo 52:79-93, 1968.

71. Flanders AE et al: CT characteristics of orbital pseudotumors and other orbital inflammatory processes, J Compu Assist Tomogr 13(1):40-47, 1989.

72. Birch-Hirschfield A: Zur diagnostik and pathologie der orbitaltumoren, Deutsche Ophth Ges 32:127-135, 1905.

73. Motto-Lippa L, Jakobiec FA, and Smith M: Idiopathic inflammatory orbital pseudotumor in childhood. II. Results of diagnostic tests and biopsies, Ophthalmology 88:565-574, 1981.

74. Mafee MF and Peyman GA: Choroidal detachment and ocular hypotony: CT evaluation, Radiology 153:697-703, 1984.

75. Trokel SL and Hilal SK: Recognition and differential diagnosis of enlarged extraocular muscles in computed tomography, Am J Ophthalmol 87:503-512, 1979.

76. Shields JA, editor: Diagnosis and management of orbital tumors, 1989, Philadelphia, WB Saunders Co.

77. Tolosa E: Periarteritic lesions of the carotid siphon with the clinical features of a carotid infraclinoid aneurysm, J Neurol Neurosurg Psychiatry 17:300, 1954.

78. Hunt WE et al: Painful ophthalmoplegia, Neurology 11 (suppl):56, 1961.

79. Smith JL and Taxdal DSR: Painful ophthalmoplegia: the Tolosa-Hunt syndrome, Am J Ophthalmol 61:1466, 1966.

80. Sondheimer FK and Knapp J: Angiographic findings in the Tolosa-Hunt syndrome: painful ophthalmoplagia, Radiology 106:105, 1973.

81. Tan WS, Wilbur AC, and Mafee MF: The role of the neuroradiologist in vascular disorders involving the orbit, Radiol Clin North Am 25:849-861, 1987.

82. Weber AL and Mikulis DK: Inflammatory disorders of the paraorbital sinuses and their complications, Radiol Clin North Am 25:615-630, 1987.

83. Tien RD et al: Cerebral Erdheim-Chester disease: persistent enhancement with Gd-DTPA on MR images, Radiology 172:791-792, 1989.

84. Flanders AE et al: Orbital lymphoma, Radiol Clin North Am 25:601-612, 1987.

85. Peyster RG and Hoover ED: Computerized tomography in orbital disease and neuro-ophthalmology, 1984, Chicago Year Book Medical Publishers, pp 21-56.

86. Char DM and Norman D: The use of computed tomography and ultrasonography in the evaluation of orbital masses, Surv Ophthalmol 27:49-63, 1982.

87. Fitzpatrick PJ and Macko S: Lymphoreticular tumors of the orbit, Int J Radiat Oncol Biol Phys 10:333-340, 1984.

88. Yeo JH et al: Combined clinical and computed tomographic diagnosis of orbital lymphoid tumors, Am J Ophthalmol 94:235-245, 1982.

89. Weber AL, Dallow R, and Oat R: CT evaluation of lymphoproliferative disease of the orbit in 48 patients. Abstract presented at the 13th Symposium on Neuroradiologicum, Stockholm, June 23-28, 1986.

90. Mafee MF et al: Dynamic computed tomography and its application to ophthalmology, Radiol Clin North Am 25:715-731, 1987.

91. Panda A et al: Hemangiopericytoma, Br J Ophthalmol 68:124-127, 1984.

92. Stout AP: Tumors featuring pericytes, glomus tumor and hemangioperibytoma, Lab Invest 5:217-223, 1956.

93. Stout AP and Murray MR: Hemangiopericytoma, Ann Surg 116:26-32, 1972.

94. Bockwinkel KD and Diddams JA: Haemangiopericytoma: report of care and comprehensive review of literature, Cancer 25:896-901, 1970.

95. Rootman J, Goldberg C, and Robertson W: Primary orbital schwannomas, Br J Ophthal 66:194-204, 1982.

96. Ruchman MC et al: Orbital tumors. In Gonzalez CA, Becker MH, and Flanagan JC, editors: Diagnostic imaging in ophthalmology, 1985, Springer-Verlag New York, Inc, pp 201-238.

97. Krohel GB and Wright JE: Orbital hemorrhage, Am J Ophthalmol 88:254, 1979.
98. Chisholm LA and Polyzoidus K: Recurrence of benign orbital neurilemmoma (schwannoma) after 22 years, Can J Ophthalmol 17:271-273, 1982.
99. Konrad EA and Thiel HJ: Schwannoma of the orbit, Ophthalmologica Basel 188:118-127, 1984.
100. Schatz H: Benign orbital neurilemmoma, Arch Ophthalmol 86:268-273, 1971.
101. Vidyakachole DL, Khalique MA, and Solanki BR: Malignant schwannoma of the orbit, Ind J Ophthalmol 1:35-43, 1979.
102. Harley RD, editor: Pediatric ophthalmology, Philadelphia, 1983, WB Saunders Co.
103. Jakobiec FA et al: Combined clinical and computed tomographic diagnosis of primary lacrimal fossa lesions, Am J Ophthalmol 94:785-807, 1982.
104. Stewart WB, Krohel GB, and Wright JE: Lacrimal gland and fossa leisons: an approach to diagnosis and management, Ophthalmol 86:886-895, 1979.

SECTION THREE
TEAR DUCT SYSTEM

CHARLES J. SCHATZ

DACRYOCYSTOGRAPHY

The radiographic evaluation of the lacrimal drainage system was first described by Ewing[1] and is of great value in the evaluation of patients with tearing (epiphora). Epiphora is commonly encountered by general ophthalmologists, and surgery is often indicated to relieve the symptom. Dacryocystography is capable of determining patency of the canaliculi, lacrimal sac, and nasolacrimal duct. When disease is present, the site and degree of obstruction and the presence of fistulae, diverticula, and concretions are evaluated with a dacryocystogram.

This section details the use of dacryocystography, including equipment, contrast materials, radiographic methods, and normal and pathologic conditions of the nasolacrimal apparatus.

Equipment

The equipment used is shown in Fig. 10-166. The dacryocystogram needle can be made by grinding off the sharp point of a 27-gauge lymphangiogram needle on a grinding stone. The tip of the modified needle should be rounded and polished so that no metallic burrs remain. An alternative to this needle is a tapered catheter as described by Iba and Hanafee[2] made from no. 18 Teflon tubing.

Contrast Materials

Ewing[1] used bismuth subnitrate in liquid petrolatum as the contrast material. Since then, many different opaque media have been described. Ethiodized oil (Ethiodol) was used by Campbell, Carter, and Doub.[3] Iodized oil (Lipiodol) was used by Hourn.[4] Iophendylate (Pantopaque) was used by Milder and Demorest.[5] Neohydriol was used by Agarwal.[6]

Oily materials, however, have disadvantages in the nasolacrimal system. First, if they are extravasated, they can remain in the soft tissues for many years. Sargent and Ebersole[7] reported such a case that revealed a considerable amount of residual contrast material more than 3 years after oily contrast material was extravasated into the periorbital tissues. Second, oily opaque material is not completely miscible with tears and can fail to fill the entire nasolacrimal system, causing diagnostic limitations. Third, it is more viscous than tears and often requires heating to reduce the viscosity before injecting, especially with iodized oil as described by Law.[8] When not heated, oily material requires a greater injection pressure than aqueous contrast material. "Physiologic" aqueous solution in the form of methylglucamine diatrizoate 40% (methylglucamine iodipamide 20%, Sinografin) has been used by Sargent and Ebersole[7] for dacryocystography. This material is nonirritating, water soluble, miscible with tears, and similar in viscosity and pH to tears. Sinografin is an excellent contrast material for dacryocystography. It can be used with all of the techniques used in this procedure.

Radiographic Techniques

Since the original description of Ewing[1] many radiographic techniques for dacryocystography have been described. The commonly used techniques are mentioned here.

Macrodacryocystography, first described by Campbell,[9] uses a magnification technique after van der Plaat's description[10] of radiographic magnification technique.

Kinetic dacryocystography, used by Epstein[11] and Trokel and Potter,[12] uses a cinematography format for evaluating the anatomy and function of the nasolacrimal apparatus.

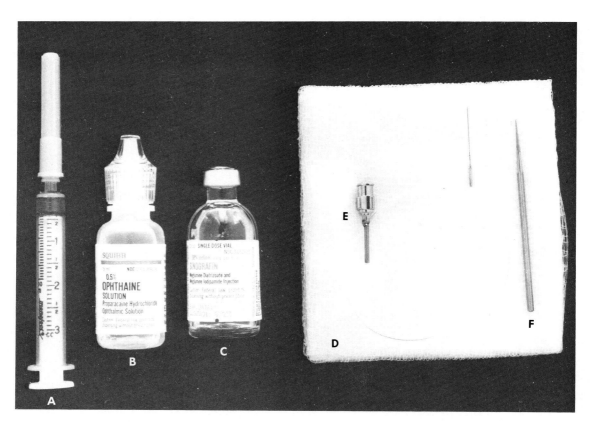

Fig. 10-166 Equipment used in dacryocystography: *A,* 3 ml syringe with 20-gauge needle. *B,* Topical ophthalmic anesthetic. *C,* Aqueous contrast material. *D,* Gauze pads. *E,* Blunt-tipped 27-gauge needle with approximately 25 cm of polyethylene tubing. *F,* Lacrimal dilator.

Distention dacryocystography, described by Iba and Hanafee,[2] involves plain radiographs that are obtained during injection of the contrast material.

Intubation macrodacryocystography, described by Lloyd, Jones, and Welham,[13] combines distention dacryocystography and macrodacryocystography.

Subtraction dacryocystography, described by Lloyd and Welham,[14] combines intubation macrodacryocystography with a standard photographic subtraction technique.

Tomographic dacryocystography, which uses complex-motion tomography, is the technique used by the author. This technique gives excellent detail of the nasolacrimal apparatus, and both the frontal and lateral planes are obtained. The technique demonstrates filling defects, obstruction, fistulae, and diverticula with improved detail over all other techniques because of the thin sections that complex-motion tomography can produce. Most of the illustrations in this section were obtained from examinations using this technique.

Injection Techniques

The injection procedure for dacryocystography requires local ophthalmic anesthesia. This is done after placing the patient on the examination table in the supine position. After scout films are taken, a few drops of the anesthetic agent are instilled into the conjunctival sac. Approximately 2 ml of the radiopaque material is drawn into the syringe and the lacrimal cannula and tubing are connected. The syringe, tubing, and cannula should be freed of all air bubbles. The lower lid is then slightly everted and the lower punctum is dilated with the lacrimal dilator. The region of the lacrimal sac is palpated; any fluid present in the sac should be expressed through the punctum or into the nose. The lacrimal cannula is then placed into the inferior punctum, where it should remain for the remainder of the procedure. The tubing is taped to the patient's face. The injection is then made and films are taken immediately. If distention dacryocystography or intubation dacryocystography is used, the films are obtained during the injection.

Indications for Dacryocystography

Dacryocystography is indicated in patients with epiphora when a mechanical obstruction, lacrimal apparatus fistula or diverticulum, lacrimal concretion, lacrimal sac operative failure, or recurrent inflammatory disease of uncertain cause is suspected after the clinical exami-

Fig. 10-167 Anatomy of normal lacrimal system. (From Campbell W: The radiology of the lacrimal system, Br J Radiol 37:1, 1964.)

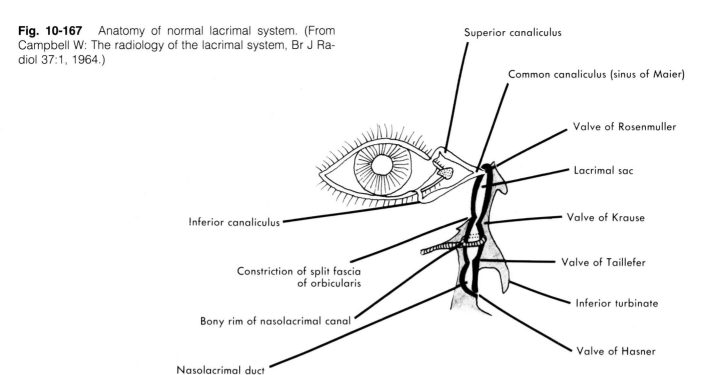

nation. When there is a definite chronic obstruction on the clinical examination, the only treatment is surgery. The dacryocystogram is used to determine the site of obstruction and the presence of fistulae or diverticula so that the appropriate surgical procedure can be performed. This procedure is usually a dacryocystorhinostomy.

The Normal Dacryocystogram

The lacrimal system consists of the inferior canaliculus, superior canaliculus, common canaliculus, lacrimal sac, and nasolacrimal duct (Fig. 10-167). Tears from the conjunctival sac enter the inferior or superior canaliculi through their respective puncta in the eyelids immediately lateral to the medial canthus. After a short vertical segment there is a horizontal segment of each canaliculus. The superior and inferior canaliculi merge medially to form the common canaliculus (sinus of Maier).

The common canaliculus is from 1 to 3 mm in length and enters the lateral aspect of the nasolacrimal sac near the junction of the upper and middle thirds. Radiographic measurements of the nasolacrimal apparatus were reported by Malik et al[15] (Table 10-2). Any distention of the sac greater than 4 mm on the frontal radiograph is considered pathologic. The lacrimal sac ends in a slight taper caused by a mucosal fold (valve of Krause) just above the rim of the orbit. At this level the nasolacrimal duct begins. There is a central mucosal constriction called the valve of Taillefer and a distal constriction called the valve of Hasner. The duct ends at the infe-

Table 10-2 Normal lacrimal passage dimensions*

Area	Dimension	Mean (in mm)	Range (in mm)
Lacrimal sac	Vertical diameter	11.10	6-14
	Lateral diameter	2.43	1-4
	Anteroposterior diameter	4.00	1-6
Nasolacrimal duct	Vertical diameter	20.97	13-26
	Lateral diameter	2.30	1-4
	Anteroposterior diameter	2.84	1-4

*From Malik SRK et al: Br J Ophthalmol 53:174, 1964.

rior meatus of the nose, beneath the inferior turbinate.

In the normal dacryocystogram the canaliculi, lacrimal sac, and nasolacrimal duct are not dilated, and contrast material is identified in the nose (Figs. 10-168 and 10-169). The lacrimal sac and nasolacrimal duct have a linear configuration. Frequently the patient will taste the contrast material within a few seconds of the injection because it drains from the nose into the pharynx and onto the base of the tongue in an unobstructed system.

Pathology of the Nasolacrimal System

Tears are secreted by the lacrimal gland situated laterally and superiorly to the globe. Under normal circumstances the tears either evaporate from the surface of the globe or drain into the lacrimal passages, where they pass into the inferior meatus of the nose. Epiphora has two causes, as described by Campbell.[9] The first is excessive lacrimation, which results in inadequate evaporation and drainage for the greater volume of tears. Dacryocystography in this entity is normal. The second cause is obstructive epiphora, which results from complete or incomplete obstruction of the lacrimal system. A normal flow of tears cannot be adequately handled by the diseased drainage system. Dacryocystography of these lesions is abnormal.

Obstruction. Complete or incomplete obstruction can occur and approximately 90% of obstructions are complete and 10% are incomplete. The most common site of obstruction is the junction of the lacrimal sac and nasolacrimal duct (Figs. 10-170 and 10-171). The second most common site of obstruction is the common canaliculus (Fig. 10-171). These statistics agree with Campbell[9] and Malik et al.[15] Less frequently the obstruction occurs within the lacrimal sac (Fig. 10-172).

Radiographically the lacrimal sac above the obstruction will usually be dilated and will have an ovoid or rounded configuration (Figs. 10-170 to 10-172), rather than the normal linear configuration. Because the dilated sac is palpable below the medial canthus, the lesion has been called a "mucocele of the lacrimal sac" by Campbell.[9] Rarely the sac will be constricted above the obstruction (Fig. 10-172).

When there is obstruction, there is usually reflux of the contrast material into the conjunctival sac through the uncannulated punctum and if the conjunctival sac is observed, (Figs. 10-171 to 10-173) this will be seen during the injection of a small volume of contrast material.

The obstruction may be incomplete (Fig. 10-174). In these cases, the dacryocystogram usually demonstrates a dilated lacrimal sac above the incomplete obstruction, and contrast material must be visualized in the nose to confirm the incomplete nature of the obstruction.

Various factors cause obstruction and include congenital stenosis, inflammatory processes, trauma including foreign bodies (Fig. 10-175), and tumors (Fig. 10-176). Occasionally with an inflammatory obstruction, a filling defect is seen in the canaliculi or obstructed nasolacrimal sac. This filling defect frequently represents a mycotic concretion of *Actinomyces israelii* (Fig. 10-177). A frequent artifact simulating a concretion is an air bubble injected into the nasolacrimal system during the dacryocystogram (Fig. 10-178). A crosstable lateral view will demonstrate the air bubble floating in the lacrimal sac (Fig. 10-178, *B*), whereas one concretion usually does not float in the contrast material.

Fistulae and Diverticula. Fistulae and diverticula of the canaliculi or lacrimal sac are usually the result of longstanding obstruction (Fig. 10-174). An obstruction

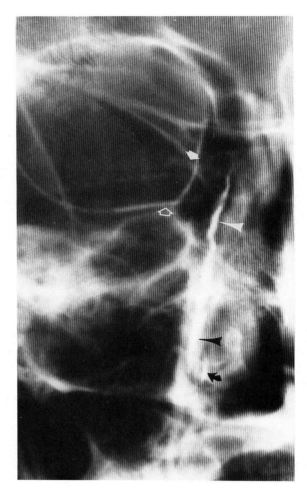

Fig. 10-168 Normal plain film dacryocystogram on right side. Superior canaliculus *(white arrow)*, inferior canaliculus with cannula in place *(open arrow)*, lacrimal sac *(white arrowheads)*, nasolacrimal duct *(black arrowhead)*, contrast material in nose *(curved arrow)*.

following trauma and facial fractures may result in a lacrimal sac−cutaneous fistula (Fig. 10-179).

Fistulae and diverticula are seen only in obstructed or partially obstructed nasolacrimal systems and will remain present until adequate drainage is restored. In addition, it is not possible to diagnose a diverticulum preoperatively without a dacryocystogram.

Surgical Devices. Occasionally surgery for epiphora is unsuccessful or the obstruction is too high in the nasolacrimal apparatus to allow for a dacryocystorhinostomy. In many of these cases a drainage tube is placed between the medial canthus and the nasal cavity, allowing relief of the epiphora. These tubes are radiopaque and should be recognized as iatrogenic foreign bodies (Fig. 10-180).

Text continued on p. 825.

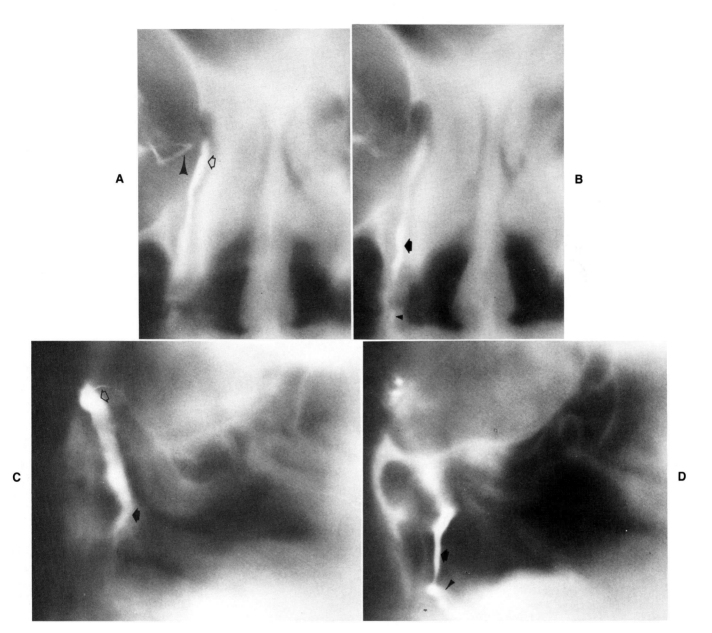

Fig. 10-169   Normal right tomographic dacryocystogram. **A,** AP view, anterior section shows canaliculi *(arrowhead)* and lacrimal sac *(open arrow).* **B,** AP view, posterior section shows nasolacrimal duct *(arrow)* and contrast material in nose *(arrowhead).* **C** and **D,** Lateral views show lacrimal sac *(open arrows),* nasolacrimal duct *(closed arrow),* and contrast material in nose *(arrowhead).*

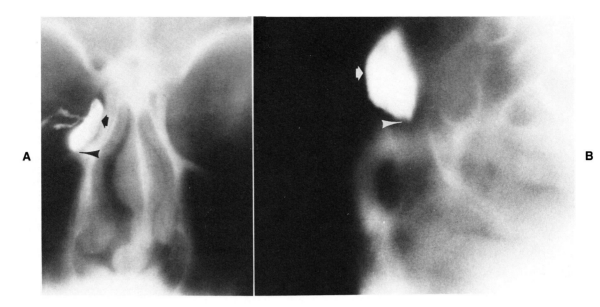

Fig. 10-170 Right tomographic dacryocystogram shows typical configuration of lacrimal drainage system in patient with history of chronic dacryocystitis and radiographic findings of obstruction at junction of lacrimal sac and nasolacrimal duct. **A,** Frontal tomogram. **B,** Lateral tomogram. *Arrowhead*, obstruction; *arrow*, dilated lacrimal sac.

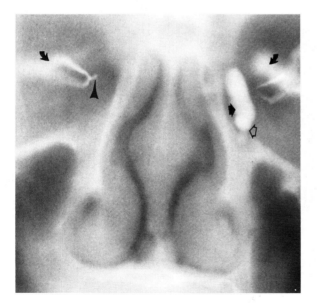

Fig. 10-171 Bilateral tomographic dacryocystogram reveals obstruction of common canaliculus *(arrowhead)* on right and obstruction at junction of lacrimal sac and nasolacrimal duct on left *(open arrow)*. Dilated lacrimal sac is seen on left *(arrow)*. Contrast material is seen in conjuctival sacs *(curved arrows)* from reflux through superior canaliculi.

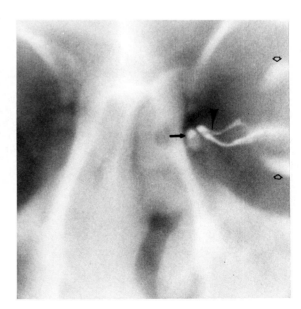

Fig. 10-172 Left tomographic dacryocystogram reveals obstruction in lacrimal sac *(arrow)*. *Arrowhead*, canaliculi; *open arrows*, contrast material in conjunctival sac.

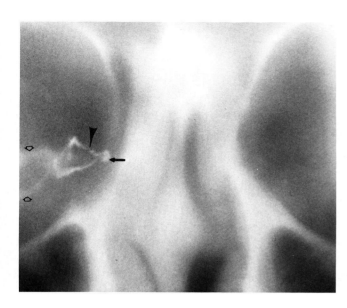

Fig. 10-173   Right tomographic dacryocystogram reveals high obstruction of lacrimal sac *(arrow)*. Note that lacrimal sac is not dilated above obstruction. *Arrowhead,* canaliculi; *open arrows,* contrast material in conjunctival sac.

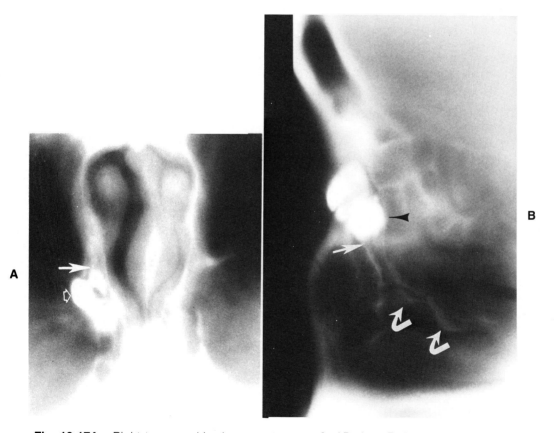

Fig. 10-174   Right tomographic dacryocystogram. **A,** AP view. **B,** Lateral view. Partial obstruction *(arrow)* is seen at junction of lacrimal sac and nasolacrimal duct. Note dilated lacrimal sac *(arrowhead)* proximal to obstruction. Also note diverticulum *(open arrow)* on AP view. Contrast material in nose *(curved arrows)* is seen on lateral view.

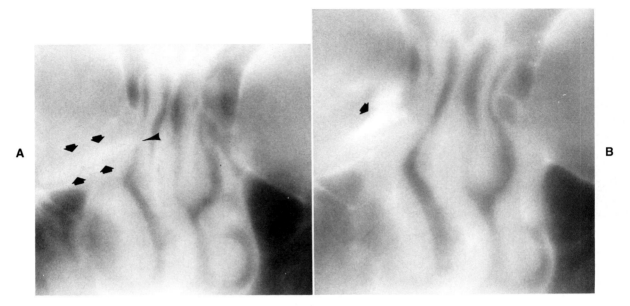

Fig. 10-175 Right tomographic dacryocystogram in patient with epiphora after operative repair of inferior "blow-out" fracture. **A,** Scout film shows silastic implant *(arrows)* with its medial end over nasolacrimal area *(arrowhead).* **B,** Contrast in obstructed and distorted lacrimal sac *(arrow)* at medial end of silastic implant.

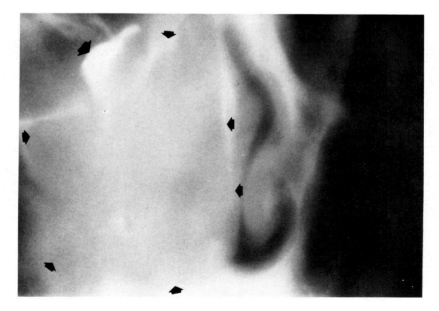

Fig. 10-176 Right tomographic dacryocystogram in 68-year-old woman with squamous cell carcinoma of right maxillary sinus and nasal airway. Patient had epiphora caused by tumor's invasion into lacrimal bone and lacrimal sac. *Small arrows,* tumor; *large arrow,* dilated lacrimal sac.

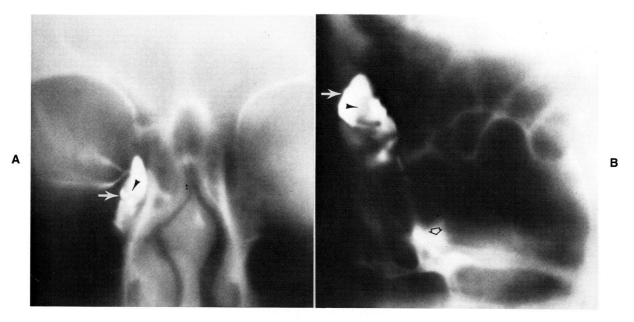

Fig. 10-177   Right tomographic dacryocystogram in patient with 10-year history of epiphora. **A,** AP view. **B,** Lateral view. Filling defect *(arrowhead)* in dilated lacrimal sac *(arrow)* represents concretion of *Actinomyces israelii* revealed by surgery. Obstruction was seen to be incomplete, because contrast material is seen in inferior meatus on lateral view *(open arrow).*

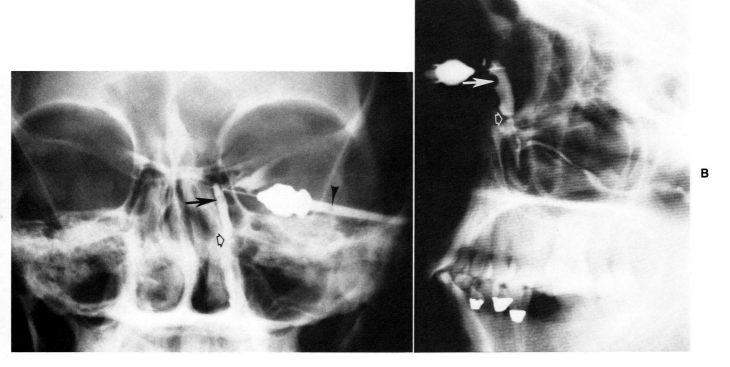

Fig. 10-178   Plain left dacryocystogram. **A,** Frontal view. **B,** Cross-table lateral view. Filling defects are air bubbles in dilated lacrimal sac *(arrow)* and in plastic tubing *(arrowhead).* Note appearance of air bubble on cross-table lateral view. Partial obstruction is present *(open arrow).*

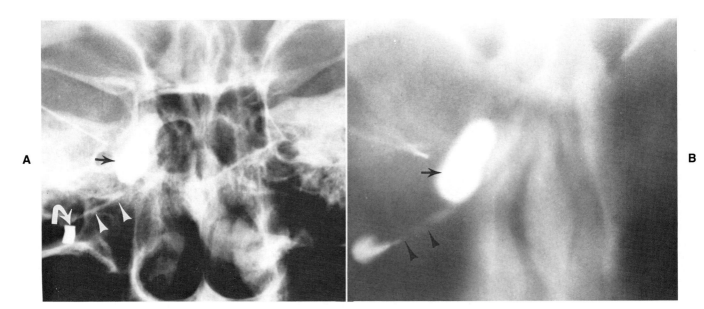

Fig. 10-179 Right dacryocystogram of 19-year-old patient with epiphora and dacryo-cystocutaneous fistula draining below inferior orbital rim. **A,** Frontal plain film view. **B,** Frontal tomographic view; *arrow,* dilated lacrimal sac; *arrowheads,* fistula; *curved arrow,* metallic marker on skin's surface at cutaneous end of fistula.

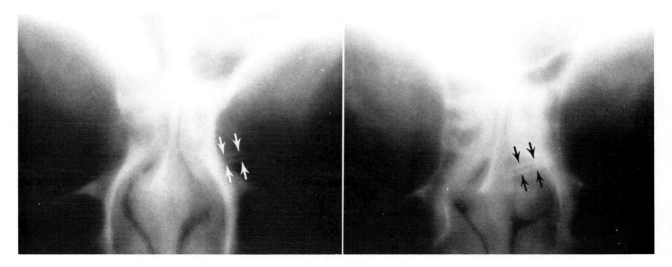

Fig. 10-180 AP tomograms demonstrate lacrimal drainage tube *(arrows)* between me-dial canthus and nose on left side. Patient had history of epiphora with unsuccessful dacryocystorhinostomy, requiring placement of drainage tube.

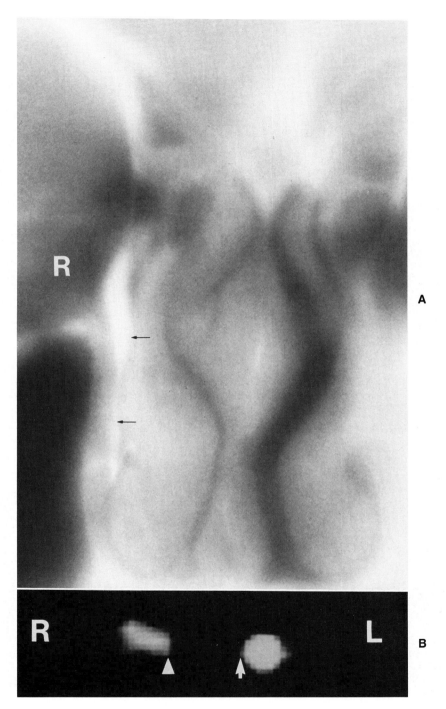

Fig. 10-181   A, Normal right dacryocystogram *(arrows)* in patient with epiphora on right side. **B,** Bilateral dacryoscintigram at 12 minutes. There is complete obstruction at the canaliculi bilaterally (right *[arrowhead]*, left *[arrow])*. Dacryocystogram **(A)** was normal on right because pressure of injection overcame functional obstruction at canaliculi. Patient did not complain of epiphora on left side.

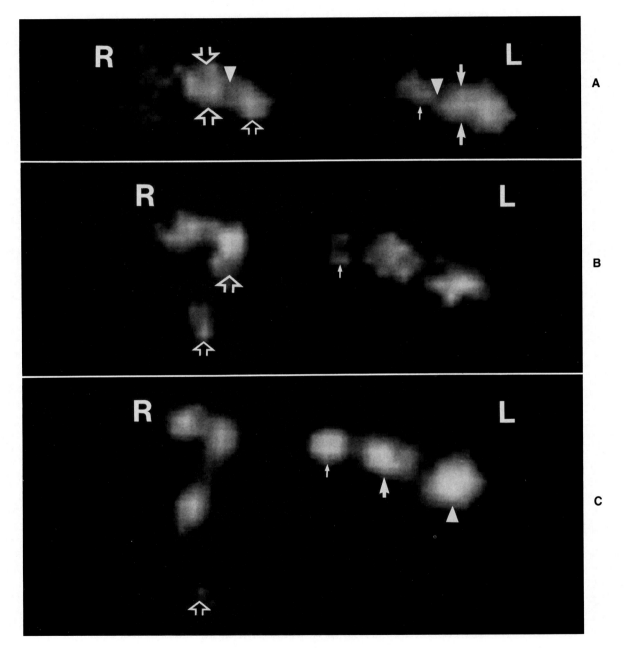

Fig. 10-182   For legend see opposite page.

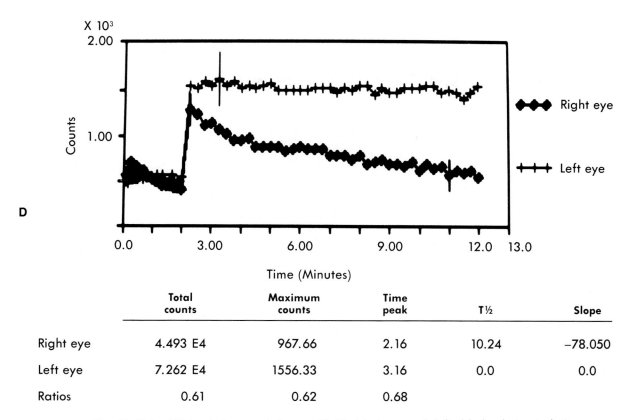

	Total counts	Maximum counts	Time peak	T½	Slope
Right eye	4.493 E4	967.66	2.16	10.24	−78.050
Left eye	7.262 E4	1556.33	3.16	0.0	0.0
Ratios	0.61	0.62	0.68		

Fig. 10-182   Bilateral dacryoscintigram. Right side is normal; left side is obstructed at lacrimal sac. **A,** Scan at 1 minute. Right: Tracer between upper and lower eyelid margins *(large open arrows),* canaliculi *(arrowhead),* and upper portion of lacrimal sac *(small open arrow).* Left: Tracer between upper and lower eyelid margins *(large arrows),* canaliculi *(arrowhead),* and upper portion of lacrimal sac *(small arrow).* **B,** Scan at 3 minutes. Right: Lacrimal sac *(large open arrow)* and nasolacrimal duct *(small open arrow).* Left: Upper lacrimal sac obstruction *(arrow).* **C,** Scan at 10 minutes. Right: Normal. Tracer in nose *(open arrow).* Left: Lower lid margin/conjunctival sac *(large arrow),* obstructed upper lacrimal sac *(small arrow),* tracer spilling over lower lid margin *(arrowhead).* **D,** Time activity curve. Right eye: Normal slope indicating normal drainage. T½ on right (normal range is 6 to 12 minutes) is 10.24 minutes. Left eye: No slope, indicating no drainage of tracer. T½ is beyond limits of scan time. Ratio indicates ratio of tracer in right eye/left eye.

DACRYOSCINTIGRAPHY

Although dacryocystography is the most commonly used imaging technique for evaluating the anatomy and pathology of the lacrimal drainage system, it does not provide adequate information about the physiology of this system. For example, in a patient with epiphora a normal dacryocystogram gives no information relating to a functional stenosis or site of obstruction of the lacrimal drainage system because the pressure of the injection overcomes the functional occlusion of the system (Fig. 10-181). Rossomondo et al[16] described dacryoscintigraphy as the imaging technique of choice since it provides a more physiologic, dynamic evaluation of lacrimal drainage than dacryocystography.

Moreover, when evaluating the physiology of tear drainage, dacryoscintigraphy can provide a quantitative analysis (Fig. 10-182, *D*).

Technique

99m Tc-pertechnetate in normal saline or 99m Tc-sulfur colloid are both useful tracers. The usual dose is 50 or 100 μCi. One drop of the solution (about 10 μl) is placed on the temporal portion of the conjunctiva. With a computer set up for two-phase dynamic acquisition, the following protocol is used:

Phase I: 5-second scans for 24 frames

Phase II: 15-second scans for 40 frames

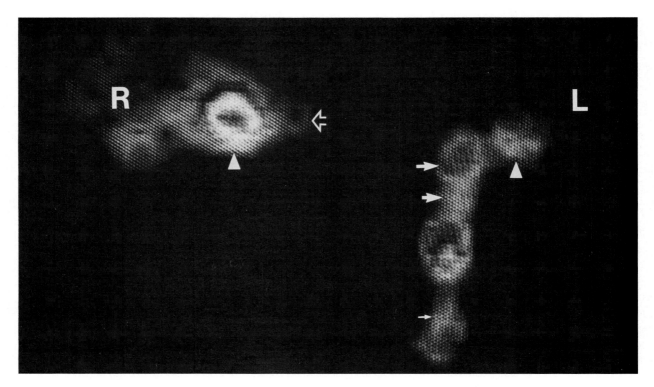

Fig. 10-183 Scan at 8 minutes. Right: Complete obstruction at canaliculi *(open arrow)* and lower lid margin *(arrowhead)*. Left: Normal. Lower lid margin *(arrowhead)*, lacrimal sac *(large arrows)*, and nasolacrimal duct *(small arrow)*.

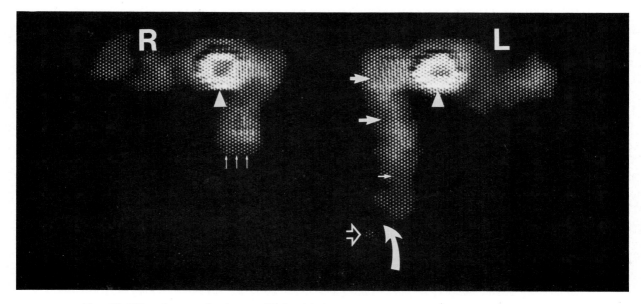

Fig. 10-184 Scan at 9 minutes. Right side has complete obstruction at junction of lacrimal sac and nasolacrimal duct *(triple arrows)*. Lower lid margin *(arrowhead)*. Left side is normal. Lower lid margin *(arrowhead)*, lacrimal sac *(large arrows)*, nasolacrimal duct *(small arrow)*, Hasner's valve *(curved arrow)*, and tracer in nose *(open arrow)*.

Bilateral studies are usually performed. A micropinhole collimator (1 mm) is placed anterior to the face between the two orbits, approximately 9 mm from the skin surface.

Normal Dacryoscintigraphy

See Figs. 10-182 to 10-184. Both lid margins are visualized. The canaliculi are visualized at approximately 10 seconds. Then the tracer can be seen in the lacrimal sac, the nasolacrimal duct, and finally in the nose. The valve of Hasner (Fig. 10-167) is usually seen as a reduction of scintillations at the lower end of the tracer column (Fig. 10-184).

Complete Obstruction

See Figs. 10-181 to 10-184. Total obstruction, if present, is always identified on dacryoscintigraphy. Even though the lacrimal sac may be filled with lacrimal secretions, debris, and even concretions, there is physiologic reflux[17,18] of the secretions into the conjunctival sac. Therefore, fresh secretions or tracer material from the dacryoscintigraphy will enter the lacrimal sac. The study is sensitive to the site of obstruction so that the appropriateness of surgery, such as a dacryocystorhinostomy, or placement of drainage tubes can be determined. The study of White et al[19] shows that the superior and inferior canaliculi are of equal importance in lacrimal drainage and that no statistical difference exists between the amount of tears that drains into either canaliculus. Therefore, if the dacryoscintigram shows an obstruction proximal to the lacrimal sac, it is most likely that the common canaliculus, or both the inferior superior canaliculi or puncta, are obstructed (Fig. 10-183).

Incomplete Obstruction

See Fig. 10-181. Patients with epiphora who have a normal dacryocystogram or normal lacrimal irrigation by the ophthalmologist usually have physiologic obstruction to the drainage of tears. In these patients bilateral, simultaneous dacryoscintigraphy studies are performed to evaluate the delay in transit of the tracer on the involved side. Comparing the two sides can reveal the amount of abnormal delay. Frequently the clinically normal side will also reveal abnormal flow. Amanant, Hilditch, and Kwok[20] reported that when there was a clinical unilateral abnormality, 42% of the patients had abnormal flow pattern by dacryoscintigraphy on the contralateral side. These authors believed that the "involved" side was so bothersome to the patient that the abnormality on the contralateral side went unnoticed or was felt to be an acceptable situation by the patient.

Summary

Dacryoscintigraphy reveals the dynamics of the lacrimal drainage system and can determine any functional obstruction or delay in transit. It is the best method of evaluating the dynamics of drainage of the canaliculi.[21] The time-activity curve provides a quantitative picture of lacrimal drainage (Fig. 10-182, *D*). To lessen the chance of surgical failure, the study is essential in the preoperative evaluation of the patient with epiphora so that the precise site of obstruction can be found and the appropriate surgical pathway can be established. However, to evaluate morphologic abnormalities such as a fistula (Fig. 10-179), diverticulum (Fig. 10-174), or concretion (Fig. 10-177), a contrast dacryocystogram is necessary.

REFERENCES

1. Ewing AE: Roentgen ray demonstration of the lacrimal abscess cavity, Am J Ophthalmol 26:1, 1909.
2. Iba GB and Hanafee WN: Distention dacryocystography, Radiology 90:1020, 1968.
3. Campbell DM, Carter JM, and Doub HP: Roentgen ray studies of the nasolacrimal passageways, Arch Ophthalmol 51:462, 1922.
4. Hourn GE: X-ray visualization of the naso-lacrimal duct, Ann Otol Rhinol Laryngol 46:962, 1937.
5. Milder B and Demorest BH: Dacryocystography. I. The normal lacrimal apparatus, Arch Ophthalmol 51:180, 1954.
6. Agarwal ML: Dacryocystography in chronic dacryocystitis, Am J Ophthalmol 52:215, 1961.
7. Sargent EN and Ebersole C: Dacryocystography: the use of Sinografin for visualization of the nasolacrimal passages, AJR 102:831, 1968.
8. Law FW: Dacryocystography, Trans Ophthalmol Soc UK 87:395, 1967.
9. Campbell W: The radiology of the lacrimal system, Br J Radiol 31:1, 1964.
10. van der Plaats GF: X-ray enlargement technique, J Belg Radiol 33:89, 1950.
11. Epstein E: Cine dacryocystography, Trans Ophthalmol Soc UK 81:284, 1961.
12. Trokel SL and Potter GD: Kinetic dacryocystography, Am J Ophthalmol 70:1010, 1970.
13. Lloyd GAS, Jones BR, and Wellman RAN: Intubation macrodacryocystography, Br J Ophthalmol 56:600, 1972.
14. Lloyd GAS and Wellman RAN: Subtraction macrodacryocystography, Br J Radiol 47:379, 1971.
15. Malik SRK et al: Dacryocystography of normal and pathological lacrimal passages, Br J Ophthalmol 53:174, 1969.
16. Rossomondo RM et al: A new method of evaluating lacrimal drainage, Arch Ophthal 88:523, 1972.
17. Amanat LA, Hilditch TE, and Kwok CS: Lacrimal scintigraphy. I. Compartmental analysis of data, Br J Ophthalmol 67:713, 1983.
18. Amanat LA, Hilditch TE, and Kwok CS: Lacrimal scintigraphy. III. Physiological aspects of lacrimal drainage, Br J Ophthalmol 67:729, 1983.
19. White WL et al: Relative canalicular tear flow as assessed by dacryoscintigraphy, Ophthalmology 96:167, 1989.
20. Amanat LA, Hilditch TE, and Kwok CS: Lacrimal scintigraphy. II. Its role in the diagnosis of epiphora, Br J Ophthalmol 67:20, 1983.
21. Denffer HW, Dressler J, and Pabst HW: Lacrimal dacryoscintigraphy, Semin Nucl Med 14:8, 1984.

CREDITS

Figs. 10-5, 10-19, and **10-25** from Mafee MF et al: Retinal and choroidal detachments: Role of MRI and CT, Radiol Clin North Am 25:487-507, 1977.

Figs. 10-7 and **10-140** from Mafee MF et al: Orbital space occupying lesions: Role of CT and MRI. An analysis of 145 cases, Radiol Clin North Am 25:529-559, 1987.

Figs. 10-9 and **10-56** from Mafee MF et al: Malignant uveal melanoma and similar lesions studied by CT, Radiology 156:403-408, 1985.

Fig. 10-11 from Mafee MF et al: CT in the evaluation of patients with persisitent hyperplastic primary vitreous (PHPV), Radiology 145:713-717, 1982.

Figs. 10-12 and **10-44 A-C** from Mafee MF et al: Persistent hyperplastic primary vitreous (PHPV): Role of CT and MRI, Radiol Clin North Am 25:683-692, 1987.

Figs. 10-22 and **10-66** from Mafee MF et al: Malignant uveal melanoma and simulating lesions: MRI evaluation, Radiology 160:773-780, 1986.

Fig. 10-31 from Mafee MF et al: Choroidal hematoma and effusion: Evaluation with MRI, Radiology 168:781-786, 1988.

Fig. 10-36 from Mafee MF et al: MRI versus CT of leukokoric eyes and use of in vitro proton magnetic resonance spectroscopy of retinoblastoma, Ophthalmology 96:965-976, 1989.

Figs. 10-37, 10-40, 10-49, 10-51, 10-58, and **10-70** from Mafee MF et al: Retinoblastoma and simulating lesions: Role of CT and MRI, Radiol Clin North Am 25:667-682, 1987.

Figs. 10-52, 10-53, and **10-54** from Mafee MF et al: CT of optic nerve colobomas, morning glory anomaly, and colobomatous cyst, Radiol Clin North Am 25:693-699, 1987.

Fig. 10-84 from Mafee MF et al: CT in the evaluation of Brown's superior oblique tendon sheath syndrome, Radiology 154:691-695, 1985.

Fig. 10-106 from Mafee MF et al: Radiology of the craniofacial anomalies, Radiol Clin North Am 14:939-988, 1982.

Figs. 10-109 and **10-111** from Linder B et al: CT and MRI of orbital abnormalities in neurofibromatosis and selected craniofacial anomalies, Radiol Clin North Am 25:787-802, 1987.

Fig. 10-126 from Flanders AE et al: CT characteristics of orbital pseudotumors and other orbital inflammatory processes, J Comput Assist Tomogr 13:40-47, 1989.

Fig. 10-161 from Mafee MF et al: Lacrimal gland and folla lesions: Role of CT, Radiol Clin North Am 25:707-779, 1987.

11 Imaging of the Visual Pathways

WILLIAM G. ARMINGTON
ROBERT A. ZIMMERMAN
LARISSA T. BILANIUK

The retrobulbar visual pathway (Fig. 11-1) includes all neural pathways involved in visual function from the point where the optic nerve originates from the posterior aspect of the globe through to the primary visual cortex lying within the medial aspects of the occipital lobes. The elements of the pathway can be affected by a variety of pathologic conditions, which, depending on their location, give rise to characteristic clusters of clinical symptomatology. The apparent symptoms, therefore, enable the pathologic condition to be located along the visual pathway with a high degree of certainty. Because of this, imaging techniques may be tailored to display optimally the expected condition. In the past, imaging techniques used to investigate the visual optic pathway included plain radiographs, orbital venography, pneumoencephalography, and complex motion tomography. In recent years computed tomography (CT) and magnetic resonance imaging (MRI) have

829

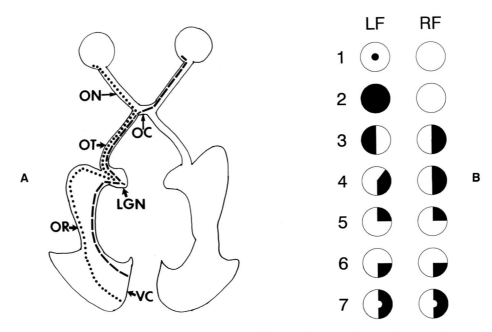

Fig. 11-1 A, Diagram of left visual pathway. (Dots indicate pathway that starts in temporal portion of retinae of left eye and ends in left occipital cortex; dashes indicate pathway from nasal portion of retinae of right eye that crosses to left in optic chiasm and ends in left occipital cortex; *ON,* optic nerve; *OC,* optic chiasm; *OT,* optic tract; *LGN,* lateral geniculate nucleus; *OR,* optic radiations; *VC,* visual cortex.) **B,** Visual field defects that can occur with abnormalities involving left visual pathway. Each visual field is represented separately; figure on reader's left represents patient's left visual field. (*LF,* left field; *RF,* right field.)

Site of lesion:
ON - 1. Left central scotoma
ON - 2. Complete blindness left visual field
OC - 3. Bitemporal hemianopia
OT, LGN - 4. Right incongruous homonymous hemianopia
OR - 5. Right congruous upper quadrantic hemianopia
OR - 6. Right congruous inferior quadrantic hemianopia
VC - 7. Right congruous homonymous hemianopia with macular sparing

become the mainstays of visual pathway imaging, because they allow direct visualization of the elements of the pathway and the pathologic processes contained therein.

This chapter defines the anatomy of the visual pathway, discusses the relevant embryology, delineates the role of CT and MRI, discusses the various pathologic entities that can affect the visual pathway and their clinical symptomatology, and illustrates the appearance of these pathologic conditions on the various imaging modalities.

EMBRYOLOGY OF THE RETROCHIASMATIC VISUAL PATHWAY

Embryologic development of the retrochiasmatic visual pathway is a complex process that occurs in a sequential, stepwise fashion. It involves the growth and development of both neural and vascular structures and is affected by influences stemming from developing osseous structures as well.[1,2] Development of the structures of the globe and optic nerve is described in general terms to place the development of the retrochiasmatic structures in perspective.

Within the embryonic period of fetal life,[1,2] specifically at 4 weeks of gestation, early vesicularization of the developing brain occurs. The optic pits appear on the surface of the rostral end of the developing embryo. Shortly thereafter the optic vesicles evaginate from the prosencephalon. The lens placode then begins developing within the optic vesicle. By the end of 5 weeks of gestation the optic vesicle has invaginated, forming the optic cup and the fetal fissure, a crease in the surface of the optic stalk in which the hyaloid artery travels to vascularize the lens vesicle. Subsequently, early development of the various layers of the retina occurs. Within the developing retina the ganglion cells begin to project their axons into the optic stalk, giving rise to the first discernible structure of the optic nerve. By the end of 6 weeks of gestation the lens capsule has formed about the lens vesicle, and progressive closure of the fetal fissure has begun. The anlagen of the extraocular muscles begin to develop, arising from mesodermal tissues of the orbit. The fetal fissure has closed completely by the end of 7 weeks of gestation. At this time the axons of the ganglion cells forming the optic nerve fibers reach the most proximal end of the optic stalk, with some crossing to form the chiasm. The lateral geniculate bodies begin to appear. The meningeal sheath surrounding the optic nerve forms and is contiguous with the dura covering the brain surfaces, as well as with the sclera enclosing the globe. Rods and cones begin to develop as a result of further retinal differentiation. By the end of 8 weeks of gestation retinal differentiation has progressed rapidly, and the bony orbit has begun to develop. The optic stalk is entirely filled with nerve fibers, and as a result the cavity of the optic vesicle no longer communicates with that of the forebrain. The optic chiasm is fully formed and separated from the floor of the third ventricle with only the optic recess remaining as a remnant at the proximal end of the optic vesicle.

In the fetal period of intrauterine development[1,2] the optic pathway develops further, particularly within the more central portions. By the end of 9 weeks of gestation early differentiation of the occipital cortex is noted. At this point the retina demonstrates a more mature layered appearance, and by the end of 10 weeks of gestation the optic tract has fully formed. The axons forming the optic nerve and tract reach the lateral geniculate bodies in the dorsolateral part of the mantle layer of the thalamus. Differentiation of the occipital cortex into marginal and mantle layers is completed by the end of 11 weeks of gestation with full elaboration of the peripheral cortical layer. By the end of 16 weeks of gestation the adult form of retinal vascularization is seen with entry of the central retinal artery via the optic nerve head, resulting from progressive atrophy of the hyaloid system. Myelination of the optic tracts begins at the lateral geniculate nuclei at 20 weeks of gestation and proceeds peripherally in a direction opposite that of axonal growth. The choroid now demonstrates three distinct layers. Myelination of the optic tract and chiasm continues from 24 through 28 weeks of gestation. Progressive enfolding of the calcarine cortex forming the calcarian fissure is noted. By the end of 32 weeks of gestation all layers of the retina have been entirely formed, and the eyelids, which previously were fused, are now unfused. By the end of 36 weeks of gestation the optic nerve has completed its myelination to the lamina cribrosa. Myelination of the optic radiations does not begin until approximately the time of birth. It then proceeds centrifugally over a 4-month period, beginning from the calcarine cortex toward the lateral geniculate bodies.

ANATOMY OF THE VISUAL PATHWAYS

Light enters the globe via the cornea and passes through the aqueous humor, lens, and vitreous humor and then strikes the retina, impinging upon photoreceptor cells in the most posterior layer of its laminated structure. Depolarizations occur within the rods and cones, which transmit impulses to the bipolar cells in the intermediate layer of the retina. These bipolar cells are the primary afferent neurons of the visual system. Impulses are then transmitted to the ganglion cells, which lie in the more superficial anterior layer of the retina. The axons of the ganglion cells course upon the most anterior surface of the retina, converging on the posterior pole of the eye, where they initiate a 90-degree turn and pierce the sclera at the lamina cribrosa, coalescing to form the optic nerve. Myelination of the axons of the optic nerve occurs after the axon exit the globe.[1]

The optic nerves pass dorsomedially to the orbital apex, entering the skull via the optic canal.[3] They then combine at the optic chiasm, which is superior to the sella turcica in the suprasellar cistern at the base of the brain. Axons from the nasal half of the retina decussate to contribute to the contralateral optic tract, whereas axons from the temporal half of the retina remain uncrossed. Central to the optic chiasm the fibers of the ganglion cells form the optic tracts.

Each visual field projects on parts of both retinae. The right visual field is projected on the nasal half of the right retina and the temporal half of the left retina. A monocular crescent of the most peripheral area of the right visual field is projected only onto the nasal half of the right retina because the nasal bridge precludes projection onto the left retina. Fibers from both retinae, which carry information about the right visual field, combine at the optic chiasm, forming the left optic tract. Therefore the whole right visual field projects to the left hemisphere.[1]

The optic tract courses dorsolaterally around the hypothalamus and the rostral part of the cerebral peduncle within the perimesencephalic cistern, synapsing with cells of the lateral geniculate bodies (see Fig. 11-1). A small number of fibers project in a medial caudal direction, forming the brachium of the superior colliculus, a projection to the superior colliculus and pretectal areas. The lateral geniculate nucleus lies in the dorsolateral aspect of the thalamus, ventral to the pulvinar and lateral to the medial geniculate body and cerebral peduncle. It is a precisely ordered six-layered structure. The contralateral half of the binocular visual field is represented in all layers of the lateral geniculate body. However, crossed and uncrossed fibers end in different layers. Crossed fibers project to layers 1, 4, and 6, whereas uncrossed fibers project to layers 2, 3, and 5.

Cell bodies of the lateral geniculate nucleus give rise to the optic radiations (geniculocalcarian tract), which pass to the ipsilateral primary visual cortex lying on the medial aspect of the occipital lobes surrounding the calcarian sulcus (see Fig. 11-1). Fibers of the optic radiations first pass through the retrolenticular part of the internal capsule (the most posterior part of the posterior limb of the internal capsule). They then arch laterally around the lateral ventricles and sweep posteromedially to synapse with cell bodies in the calcarine cortex. Fibers originating in the ventrolateral aspect of the lateral geniculate nucleus carry impulses from the inferior quadrant of the retina (superior visual field). They first sweep ventrally into the temporal lobe and then pass laterally over the inferior horn of the lateral ventricle before turning posterior to proceed to the calcarine cortex, inferior to the calcarine sulcus. Fibers from the dorsomedial aspect of the lateral geniculate nucleus, carrying information from the superior quadrant of the retina (inferior visual field), follow a more direct posterior course to the calcarian cortex, superior to the calcarian sulcus.

The calcarine cortex is topographically ordered in an anterior to posterior direction, as well as a superior to inferior one.[1] The most posterior area receives information from the central (macular) visual field. The middle third receives binocular information from the contralateral visual field. The most anterior third receives monocular information from the contralateral visual field. From the cell bodies lying within the calcarine cortex, axons project to visual association cortex in surrounding areas.

As a result of precise topographic localization of the visual fields at each part of the visual pathway, discrete lesions can be clinically localized with a high degree of accuracy. Lesions causing interruption of the optic nerve result in monocular blindness (Figs. 11-2 to 11-4). Lesions interrupting the decussating fibers at the optic chiasm cause bitemporal hemianopsia (Fig. 11-5). Interruption of the pathway at the optic tract causes contralateral homonymous hemianopsia. If the optic radiations are interrupted within the temporal lobe, a contralateral superior quadrantanopsia results (Fig. 11-6). Cortical lesions (Fig. 11-7) superior to the calcarine sulcus result in an inferior quadrantanopsia, whereas lesions inferior to the calcarian sulcus (Fig. 11-8) cause a superior quadrantanopsia. Lesions of the occipital pole result in central (macular) deficits.

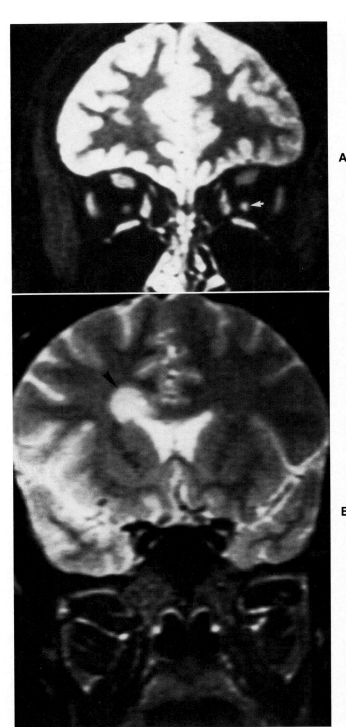

Fig. 11-2 Acute multiple sclerosis (MS) involving left optic nerve and periventricular white matter. **A,** Coronal STIR image of orbit shows high signal intensity within left optic nerve (arrow) at site of demyelinating disease. **B,** Same patient, coronal T$_2$WI, shows hyperintense right periventricular MS plaque (arrowhead).

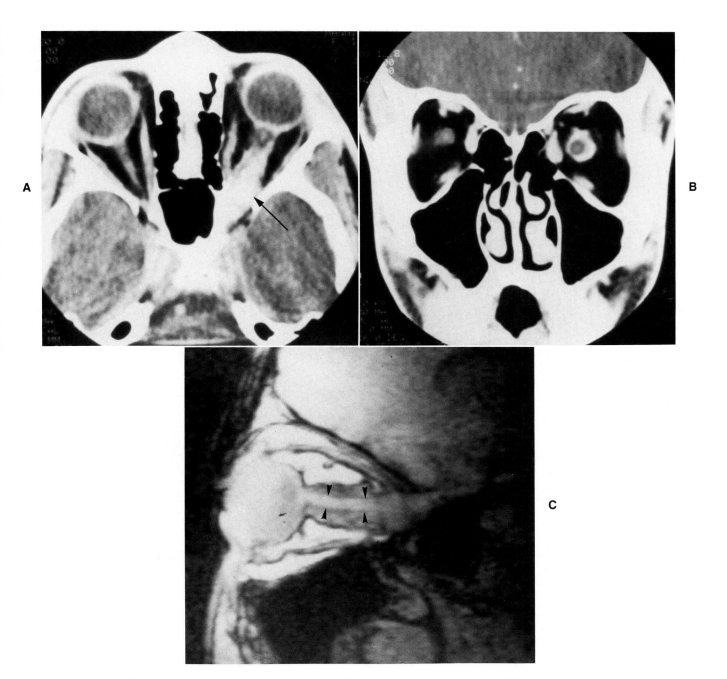

Fig. 11-3   Left perioptic meningioma. **A,** Axial contrast–enhanced CT shows hyperdense mass *(arrow)* enlarging optic nerve complex on left. Note that optic nerve appears less dense and surrounding mass more dense. **B,** Coronal CT after injection of contrast medium shows mass encasing optic nerve. Mass is thicker on lateral aspect than on medial aspect. Patient is a 16-year-old male with neurofibromatosis. **C,** Sagittal T_1WI shows optic nerve centrally *(arrowheads)* surrounded by irregular tumor mass that extends back toward optic foramen.

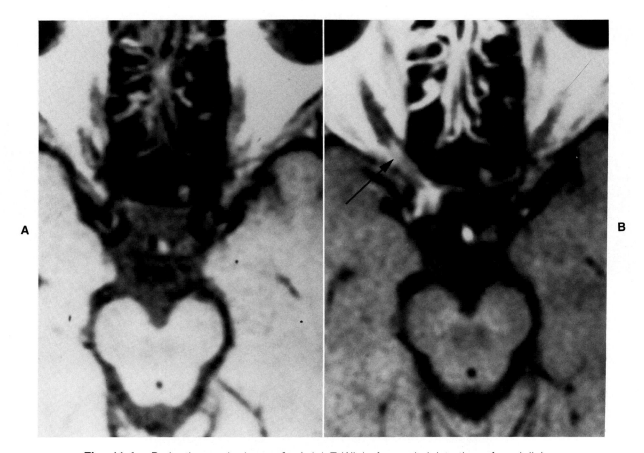

Fig. 11-4   Perioptic meningioma. **A,** Axial T$_1$WI before administration of gadolinium shows no specific abnormality. **B,** Axial T$_1$WI after intravenous administration of gadolinium shows enhancement of tumor *(arrow)* that extends from region of anterior clinoid process on right, through optic canal, along optic nerve. Surgery revealed perioptic meningioma.

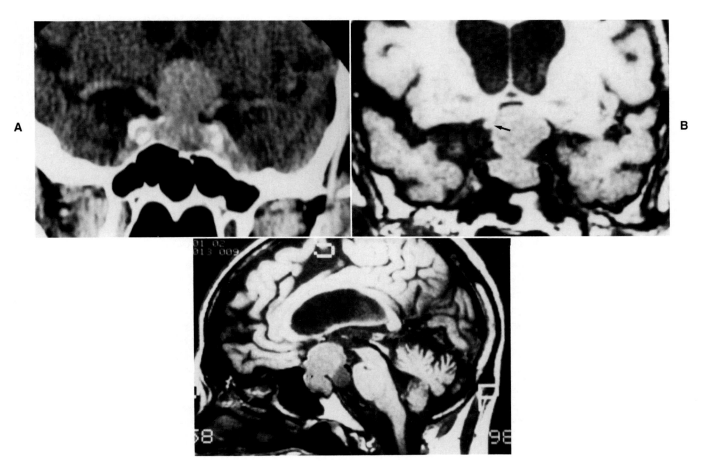

Fig. 11-5 Pituitary adenoma with chiasmal compression. Seventy-year-old male with bitemporal hemianopsia. **A,** Coronal CT after contrast enhancement shows intrasellar mass extending into suprasellar cistern. The pituitary fossa is enlarged. **B,** Coronal T₁WI shows isointense mass within sella, expanding it to left and extending through the diaphragma sella (site of the waist) into suprasellar cistern. Note compression of right optic nerve *(arrow).* **C,** Sagittal T₁WI shows intrasellar and suprasellar tumor mass. Optic chiasm is not distinguishable in this view.

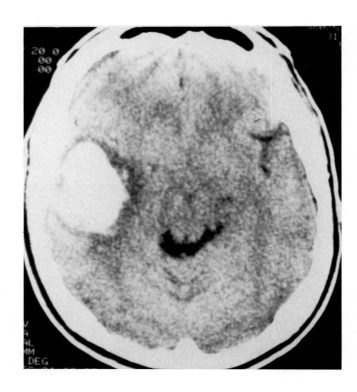

Fig. 11-6 Temporal lobe hematoma. Axial CT shows hyperdense mass in anterior aspect of right temporal lobe.

IMAGING TECHNIQUES

The indications for imaging of the optic pathways are based on clinical findings and symptomatology, which include some form of visual loss. The rapidity of onset of visual loss suggests the type of pathologic condition responsible, whereas the specific visual field deficit suggests the location of the pathologic process within the visual pathway. Sudden onset of monocular blindness when associated with pain suggests an optic nerve neuritis (see Fig. 11-2). Gradually progressive monocular blindness, especially if associated with proptosis, suggests a mass lesion such as perioptic meningioma involving the optic nerve sheath (see Figs. 11-3 and 11-4) as one of the likely causes. The ophthalmoscopic findings of papilledema or optic atrophy are frequently associated with neoplasia and mass effect or an inflammatory process. If the finding is unilateral, the optic nerve is the likely site of involvement. However, if bilateral papilledema or optic atrophy is present, an intracranial cause is more likely. Bitemporal hemianopsia is most commonly caused by a disease involving the optic chiasm; the most common such disease is a pituitary adenoma (see Fig. 11-5) causing compression of the decussating fibers of the optic pathway. Other conditions causing similar clinical findings include lesions that cause extrinsic compression of the chiasm (e.g., craniopharyngioma, meningioma, or carotid artery aneurysms) or intrinsic lesions of the chiasm, such as a chiasmatic glioma. Inflammatory conditions such as sarcoidosis, histiocytosis X, or tuberculosis may also involve the optic chiasm. Homonymous hemianopsia

suggests a disease process involving the retrochiasmatic portion of the visual pathway. Sudden onset of this visual field deficit suggests a vascular cause, whereas more gradual development suggests a mass lesion as the cause. If the deficit is incomplete and congruent (equally involving the superior and inferior quadrants of the contralateral visual field), the lesion is likely to lie within the calcarine cortex of the occipital lobe (see Fig. 11-7). If the deficit is incomplete and incongruous, then the lesion is likely to lie either in the temporal lobe involving Mayer's loop (superior quadrantinopsia) (see Fig. 11-6) or in the parietal lobe (inferior quadrantinopsia) (Fig. 11-9).

CT evaluation of the visual pathway should be obtained with intravenous contrast enhancement unless the patient has experienced trauma or has a history of severe contrast reaction, or unless a foreign body, hemorrhage, or infarction is suspected along the course of the optic pathway. Intravenous administration of a contrast medium in an adult should include a 50 ml bolus of 60% iodinated contrast, followed by 300 ml of 30% iodinated contrast solution administered as a continuous drip. Axially oriented contiguous CT scan sections 5 mm thick should be obtained from the foramen magnum to the orbital floor, then sections 3 mm thick should be obtained from the orbital floor to the orbital roof.[4] The remainder of the head can be imaged with contiguous cuts 10 mm thick. Coronal contiguous images 3 to 5 mm thick should be obtained with the patient's neck in maximally tolerated extension. This view should extend from the dorsum of the sella to the ante-

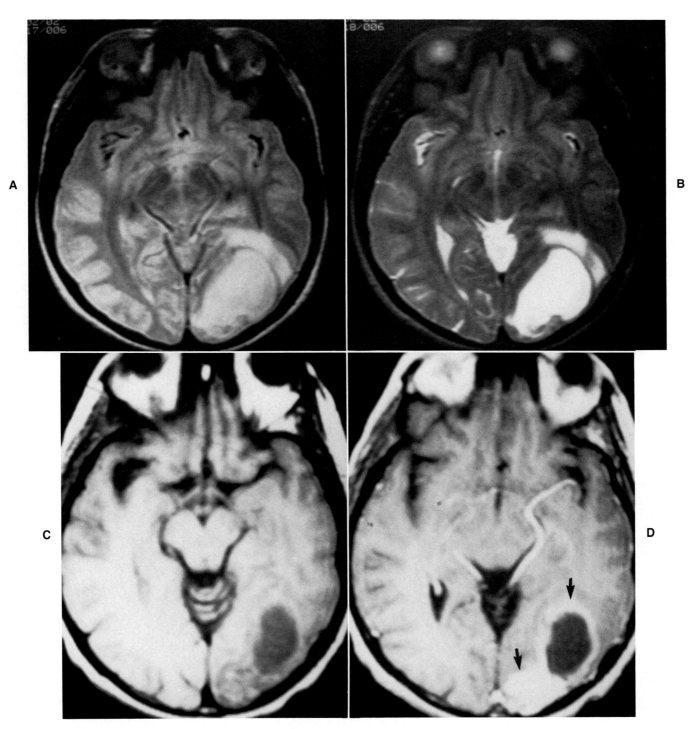

Fig. 11-7 Occipital lobe metastasis from carcinoma of the lung. **A,** Axial PDWI shows hyperintense mass in left temporal occipital region. **B,** Axial T₂WI shows same mass; point of separation exists between most posterior portion of mass and anterior segment of high-signal-intensity edema in adjacent white matter. **C,** Axial T₁WI without contrast medium shows hypointense cystic cavity and less hypointense solid soft tissue mass in occipital pole. **D,** Axial T₁WI after injection of contrast medium shows tumor enhancement *(arrows).*

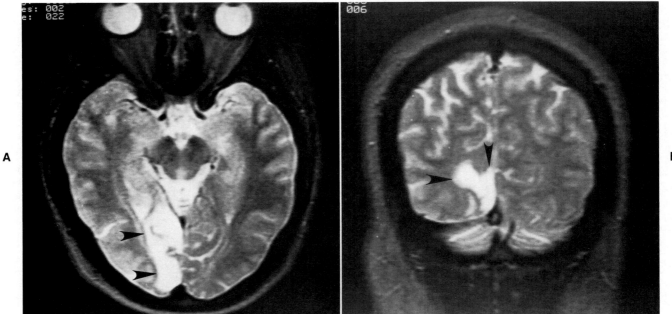

Fig. 11-8 **A,** Axial T$_2$WI shows a high signal intensity occipital infarct *(arrowheads)*. **B,** Coronal T$_2$WI. The infarct *(arrowheads)* lies below the calcarine fissure.

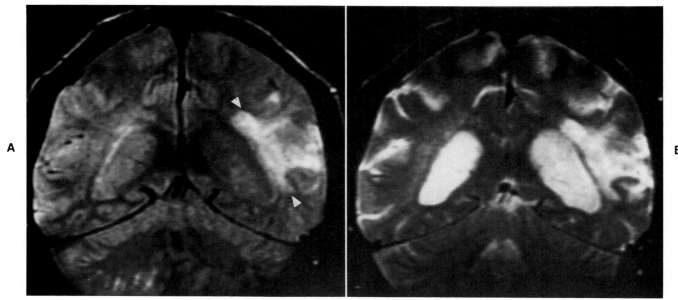

Fig. 11-9 Infarct posterior temporoparietal lobe. **A,** Coronal PDWI shows hyperintense area of high signal intensity *(arrowheads)* extending from cortex down to lateral margin of ventricle. **B,** Coronal T$_2$WI shows same area of abnormality.

rior aspect of the globe.[5] If MRI is unavailable, intrathecal water-soluble contrast medium administered by a lumbar puncture may be necessary to visualize the optic chiasm. A 20 cm field of view should be used for the axial images with subsequent magnification of the orbital region to display maximally the pathologic condition in this area. The coronal images should be obtained with a 12 to 15 cm field of view.

In general, MRI is the imaging modality of choice for visualization of the elements of the optic pathway except in patients with a history of trauma or when a fracture or foreign body with unknown ferromagnetic properties is suspected.[6] Once a modality for imaging has been chosen, the imaging protocol may be specifically altered to visualize optimally the region of the optic pathway most likely to contain the pathologic condition.

Magnetic resonance imaging of the elements of the optic pathway uses both a head coil and an orbit surface coil. Using the orbit surface coil, axial and coronal images with a TR of 500 to 800 msec and a TE of 20 msec should be obtained. Slices 3 mm thick with an interscan space either 0.5 or 1 mm thick, with 1 excitation, a 256 × 256 matrix and a 14 cm field of view optimally display the structures of the orbit.[6,7] The remainder of the intracranial optic pathway may be imaged using a sagittal TR 600, TE 20 spin echo sequence with 5 mm thick scan slices and a 1 mm thick interscan space using a 22 cm field of view with 2 excitations and a 192 × 256 matrix. This should be followed by an axial 2 echo study using a TR of 3000 and TE of 20 to 40 and 70 to 90, 5 mm thick slices, a 2.5 mm thick interscan space, 1 to 2 excitations, a 256 × 256 matrix, and a 20 cm field of view. The slices should be obtained from the low posterior fossa through the vertex of the skull, being certain to include the orbital structures within the scanning volume. If a pathologic condition involving the optic chiasm is suspected, high-resolution coronal and sagittal images of the area should be obtained using a TR of 600, a TE of 20, 3 mm thick scan slices, no interscan space, 2 to 4 excitations, a 256 × 256 matrix and a 20 cm field of view.[8,9] Techniques designed to suppress the signal from the orbital fat make pathologic conditions involving the optic nerve more visible and may be useful when subtle lesions are suspected. One such sequence involves the use of inversion recovery techniques (STIR). Such a technique uses a TR of 2500, a TE of between 30 and 60, a TI of 150, 2 excitations, a 128 × 256 matrix, 5 mm thick slices, and a 1 mm interscan space (see Fig. 11-2, A). Intravenous administration of gadolinium DTPA in a dose of 1 mmol/kg has demonstrated clinical utility in diagnosing both intraorbital and intracranial pathologic conditions, including neoplasms and inflammatory or infectious conditions. If intravenous gadolinium is used, the standard imaging protocol should be used, followed by spin echo images using a TR of 500 to 600, a TE of 20 with a scan thickness and spatial orientation chosen to display optimally the pathologic condition (see Figs. 11-4, A and B; 11-7, C and D).

NORMAL CT AND MRI ANATOMY

The normal intraorbital optic nerve/sheath complex is well visualized on axial and coronal CT because of the natural contrast between it and the surrounding retrobulbar adipose tissue.[4] The normal optic nerves are symmetrical and homogeneous in appearance. The normal diameter of the nerve is 3 to 5 mm (average 4.5 mm) on axial scans and 4 to 6 mm (average 5 mm) on coronal scans.[4] The intracanalicular portion of the optic nerve is poorly visualized with CT because of beam-hardening artifact from the surrounding bony canal. Unless intrathecal contrast material is used,[5] the intracranial portion of the nerve, as well as the optic chiasm and optic tract, are poorly visualized on CT because of inadequate contrast between the cerebrospinal fluid (CSF) and the neural tissues. Without contrast material in the CSF, the location of the intracranial portion nerve, the optic chiasm, and the optic tract is inferred on the basis of knowledge of their anatomic location relative to adjacent structures such as the suprasellar cistern, hypothalamus, medial aspect of the temporal lobes, and lateral aspect of the midbrain. The position of the lateral geniculate nucleus (LGN) is inferred by localizing the pulvinar of the thalamus, since the LGN is not directly visualized on CT. The optic radiations also are not directly seen, but their expected location may be inferred by observing the appropriate area of the temporal lobe adjacent to the temporal horn of the lateral ventricle and the parietal lobe adjacent to the atrium of the lateral ventricle. The most distal portion of the optic radiation can also be inferred by its position relative to the occipital horns of the lateral ventricles. The calcarine cortex is directly visualized along the medial aspect of the occipital lobes.

On MRI using short TR/TE (600/20) and long TR / short TE (3000/30) sequences, the intraorbital optic nerve demonstrates signal intensity similar to that of cerebral white matter.[5] It appears to be of lower intensity relative to the high signal intensity of the retrobulbar adipose tissue. On long TR / long TE (3000/90) images, the optic nerve has a signal intensity similar to that of orbital fat; however, occasionally a small amount of high-signal-intensity CSF can be visualized in the subarachnoid space between the nerve sheath and the optic nerve. The intracanalicular portion of the optic nerve is well visualized on MRI because of the absence of signal from the cortical bone forming the optic canal.[6] Short TR / short TE imaging sequences, particularly in the coronal projection, display the intracranial portion of the optic nerve as a relatively higher-signal-intensity structure within the lower-signal-intensity CSF of the suprasellar cistern. The optic chiasm and optic tracts demonstrate similar characteristics and are best visualized in either the coronal or sagittal planes.[9] Long TR with either short or long TE sequences tends to minimize the contrast between the intracranial optic nerves, chiasm, and optic tracts and the surrounding CSF, thereby inhibiting adequate display. The LGN occasionally may be seen on long TR / long TE images as a high-signal-intensity nuclear aggregation. More commonly the LGN is seen as a contour arising from the diencephalon and protruding into the ambiens cistern adjacent to the thalamus. The optic radiation may be seen as cerebral white matter intensity structures within the temporoparietal and occipital lobes; their course is inferred by knowledge of the anatomic location of this portion of the optic pathway. The calcarine cortex may be directly observed on either coronal, axial, or sagittal short or long TR images. The two gyri making up the primary visual cortex may be positively identified, since they are easily seen flanking the calcarine sulcus.

PATHOLOGIC CONDITIONS
Optic Nerve Visual Pathway Glioma

Gliomas of the optic nerve or visual pathway are relatively uncommon low-grade neoplasms that can involve various portions of the retrobulbar visual pathway, including the optic nerve, chiasm, optic tracts, and radiation. These tumors appear most frequently during the first decade of life, and there is a slight female preponderance. There is also an association between optic nerve gliomas and their visual pathway extension and neurofibromatosis.

Clinical Findings. Optic nerve gliomas constitute approximately 3% of all orbital tumors[10]; they outnumber perioptic meningiomas by approximately 4 to 1. Optic nerve gliomas occur most frequently in the first decade of life (median age is 5 years); however, they may be present at birth and have been reported in patients as old as 60 years of age.[10,11] They may occur at any point in the retrobulbar visual pathway, including the optic nerve, chiasm, or optic tract lateral geniculate bodies, and optic radiations.[10-12] Involvement of the optic chiasm with extension to involve both optic nerves is more common than involvement of a single optic nerve.[10] Invasion of the globe by the tumor, although extremely rare, has been observed.[11]

Approximately 15% of patients with optic nerve glioma demonstrate the findings of neurofibromatosis at the time of diagnosis (range is 12% to 38%).[10,11] Visual pathway gliomas appear early in life, often before the clinical stigmata of neurofibromatosis become evident.

The clinical picture of patients with optic nerve gliomas depends on whether the primary involvement is orbital or intracranial. Intraorbital gliomas usually appear early with painless proptosis. Globe motility usually is not restricted. Optic atrophy is the most frequent ophthalmoscopic finding, with occasional disc edema.[10] Loss or decreased vision with transient visual obscuration commonly occurs and may progress to total loss of vision. Occasionally peripheral visual constriction may be observed. Clinically, intraorbital optic nerve glioma and meningioma are difficult to differentiate.[11]

Intracranial optic nerve gliomas generally appear with symptoms related to the portion of the brain that is involved. These symptoms include seizures, nystagmus, hydrocephalus, and changes in mental status. Loss of vision is the most common initial symptom.[10] The presence of nystagmus is highly suspicious for chiasmal involvement.

Pathologic Findings. The cell of origin for optic nerve

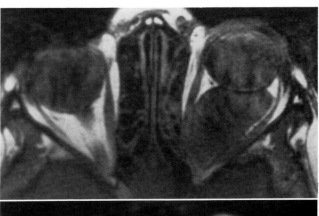

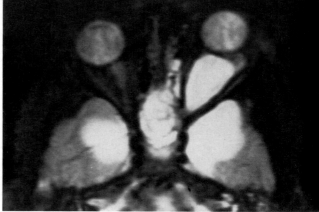

Fig. 11-10 Visual pathway glioma. **A,** Axial T_1WI shows fusiform expansion of left optic nerve, flattening of back of globe, and axial proptosis. **B,** Axial T_2WI shows high signal intensity involving optic nerve glioma and inferior extent of chiasmal tumor; high signal intensity also stems from associated arachnoid cysts compressing medial aspect of both temporal lobes.

gliomas has not been definitively elucidated, and thus these disorders are referred to in the general classification as gliomas. Specifically they are classified as grade I astrocytomas (juvenile pilocytic astrocytoma).[10,12] The tumors are slow growing with no tendency to metastasize. Malignant transformation does not occur in childhood gliomas. Development of optic nerve gliomas is observed to occur in stages from generalized hyperplasia of the glial cells within the nerve to complete disorganization with loss of landmarks within the nerve and the nerve sheath. The tumor usually causes smooth fusiform enlargement of the optic nerve (Fig. 11-10), although it may be somewhat asymmetric with respect to the nerve (Fig. 11-11). A reactive meningeal hyperplasia may be incited, which extends beyond the position of the tumor itself, making it difficult to differentiate from a perioptic meningioma.[12]

Microscopically, the tumor is composed of round, spindle-shaped cells similar in appearance to those of the normal optic nerve. Because no mitoses are present, the tumors do not enlarge by cell division but rather by hyperplasia of adjacent glial connective tissue and meninges with production of intracellular and extracellular mucopolysaccharides. Cystic changes may occur within the tumor as a result of mucinous substance production, infarction, or both.

CT Appearance. Optic nerve gliomas may be unilateral or bilateral. Unenhanced CT scan of these tumors typically demonstrates a marked diffuse enlargement of an optic nerve, often with a characteristic kinking or buckling (Fig. 11-12).[11,13] Fusiform enlargement of the nerve is common. Within the tumor, areas of lucency caused by mucinous or cystic changes may be observed, but calcification is not found in unradiated optic nerve gliomas. Following administration of a contrast medium, a moderate to intense enhancement of the tumor is often observed, frequently containing irregular parenchymal lucencies.[11,13] Bilateral optic nerve gliomas are thought be characteristic of neurofibromatosis (Fig. 11-13).[13] Extension of the tumor through the optic

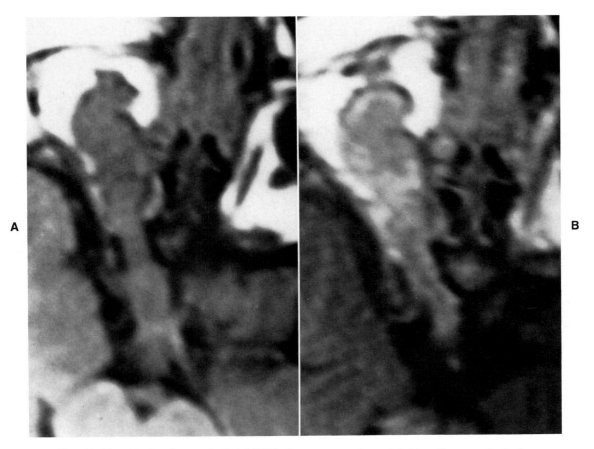

Fig. 11-11 Optic glioma. **A,** Axial T$_1$WI shows expansion of right optic nerve in its intraorbital, intracanalicular, and intracranial portions. **B,** Axial T$_1$WI after injection of gadolinium shows increased signal intensity of optic glioma. This tumor did not involve optic chiasm.

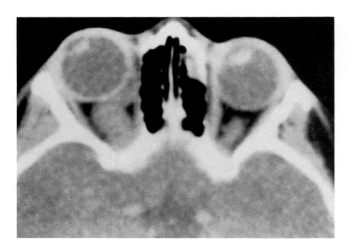

Fig. 11-12 Unilateral optic glioma. Axial CT shows fusiform enlargement of right optic nerve.

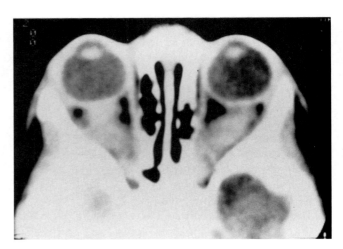

Fig. 11-13 Bilateral optic gliomas with neurofibromatosis. Axial contrast CT shows bilateral enlargement and enhancement of optic nerve gliomas.

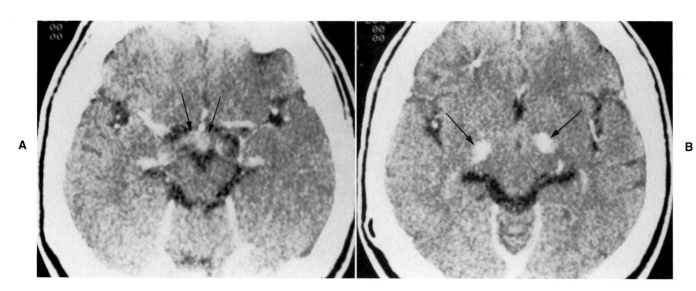

Fig. 11-14 Visual pathway glioma. **A,** Axial CT after injection of contrast medium shows enhancement of slightly enlarged optic chiasm *(arrows)*. **B,** Next higher CT section shows enhanced tumor extending along optic tracts *(arrows)* around cerebral peduncles.

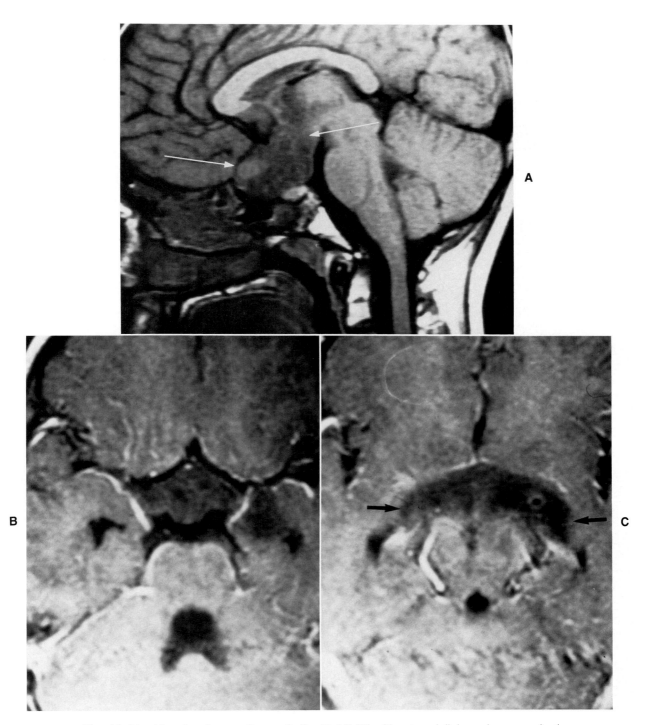

Fig. 11-15 Visual pathway glioma. **A,** Sagittal T₁WI without gadolinium shows marked hypointense tumor enlargement of optic chiasm *(arrows)* extending superiorly into hypothalamus. **B,** Axial T₁WI after injection of gadolinium shows hypointense mass expanding optic chiasm. **C,** Next higher MRI section shows visual pathway tumor extending into optic tracts *(arrows)* around cerebral peduncles of midbrain. Tumor does not enhance. Enhanced linear structures in **A** and **B** are veins.

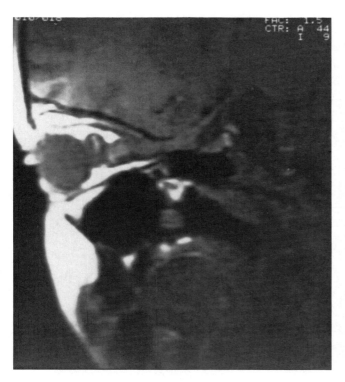

Fig. 11-16 Optic nerve glioma. Oblique sagittal T₁WI shows fusiform enlargement of optic nerve. Tumor extends through optic canal but does not reach optic chiasm.

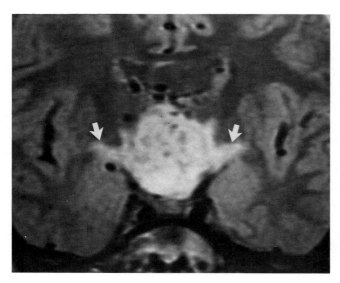

Fig. 11-17 Visual pathway glioma. Coronal PDWI shows marked expansion of optic chiasm by high-signal-intensity tumor, with tumor extending into both optic tracts (arrows).

foramen commonly results in enlargement of the optic canal. When the epicenter of the tumor involves the optic chiasm, both anterior and posterior extension of optic nerve glioma is seen (Figs. 11-14 and 11-15). Such involvement is a helpful feature in differentiating among lesions of the chiasm. Whatever imaging study is done, it must be adequate to evaluate the entire visual pathway, since frequently not only the optic nerve and chiasm but also the retrochiasmatic visual pathways are involved.[6]

MRI Appearance. When evaluating the visual pathways (specifically the optic nerves) for optic nerve glioma, thin sections (3 mm or less) should be obtained, since excessive slice thickness may make lesions inapparent as a result of volume averaging.[14] Precise anatomic definition of optic nerve gliomas is generally superior on MRI when compared with CT, especially where the lesion passes through the optic canal (Fig. 11-16).[15] Sagittal MRI give information not available with standard axial or coronal CT scanning techniques. In addition, the sensitivity of MRI to extension of optic nerve gliomas into the optic tracts, lateral geniculate bodies, and optic radiations appears to be much greater than that with CT (Figs. 11-17 and 11-18).[15] On MRI the lesion involving the optic nerve is generally well defined, revealing enlargement of the nerve with characteristic kinking and buckling (see Fig. 11-11). On short TR/TE images optic nerve gliomas are usually isointense to cortex and hypointense to white matter (see Fig. 11-10, *A*). Invariably they are hypointense to orbital fat. On long TR/TE images the lesions demonstrate a mixed to homogeneous appearance that is hyperintense to white matter cortex and orbital fat (see Fig. 11-10, *B*). Following administration of gadolinium contrast material, increased signal intensity on short TR/TE images is often seen (see Fig. 11-11).

Perioptic Meningioma

Perioptic meningiomas are benign tumors arising from the meningoendothelial cells of the arachnoid. The rests from which these arise occur in a variety of locations within both the orbit and cranial vault. Intraorbital meningiomas occur at the orbital apex, along the course of the optic nerve sheath or unrelated to the optic nerve, usually in the extraconal space from the periosteum of the orbital wall.[11] Meningiomas make up approximately 5% to 7% of all primary orbital tumors. They are more common in females than males (4 to 1) and appear most frequently in the fourth and fifth decades of life (median age is 38 years).[16] A significant portion of the tumors, however, occur in children (25% in the first decade), and then they are more frequent in patients with neurofibromatosis than is expected in the general population.

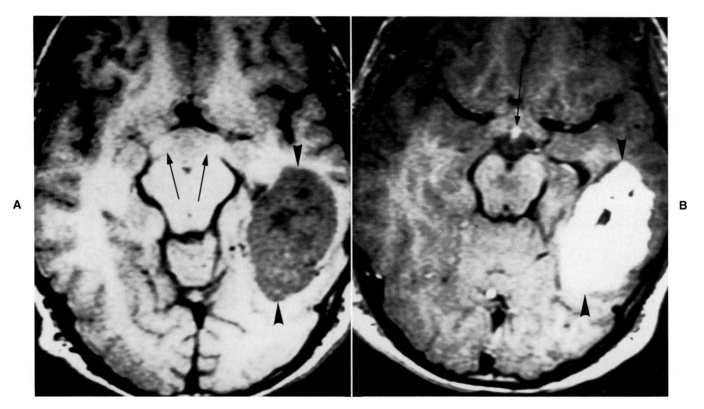

Fig. 11-18   Visual pathway glioma. **A,** Axial T₁WI shows enlarged optic chiasm *(arrows)* and hypointense mass *(arrowhead)* in optic radiations of left temporoparietal lobes. **B,** Axial T₁WI after intravenous injection of gadolinium shows marked enhancement of optic radiation portion of tumor *(arrowheads)* but no enhancement of chiasmal portion. Infundibular stalk of pituitary gland enhances *(arrow)*.

Clinical Findings. The symptoms the patient displays depend on the size of the tumor and its location within the orbit. Small intracanalicular perioptic meningiomas may be difficult to detect and yet cause significant symptomatology. Proptosis and visual loss are the usual symptoms in patients with perioptic meningiomas located close to the globe.[17] Papilledema, optic atrophy with central or peripheral scotomata, or both are commonly seen because of the tumor's proximity to the optic nerve. Diminished extraocular muscle motility is also common, since the tumor is unencapsulated, grows through the dura, and directly involves the extraocular muscles. Tumors that occur within the optic canal frequently appear with central scotomata, often without other symptoms.[16]

Pathologic Findings. Of the various histologic types of meningioma, the meningothelial variety is the most common within the orbit. Microscopically, the tumor consists of solid sheets of distinctively central vacuolated cells. Mitoses are rare. Within the orbit other histologic types of meningioma such as fibroblastic, transitional, syncytial, psammomatous, and angioblastic varieties are much less common. The rare orbital angioblastic meningioma may be differentiated with difficulty from hemangioblastoma and hemangiopericytoma only by an extensive capillary tumor network.[16] Regardless of the histology, pediatric perioptic meningiomas tend to be more aggressive than those in adults. These childhood tumors are often only partially encapsulated and have a propensity to grow by infiltration, breaking through the dura and involving other orbital structures. Orbital meningiomas, when adjacent to the bony wall, may induce a reactive hyperostosis. At or near the orbital apex a demineralization with enlargement of the optic canal can sometimes be seen.[16] Optic atrophy with a decrease in the number of axons within the nerve results from compression of the nerve by the tumor. The tumor grows as either an eccentric mass along one side of the optic nerve or as a circumferential lesion. Intratumoral psammomatous calcifications may be present, particularly within highly cellular areas of the tumor.

CT Appearance. On CT, perioptic meningiomas (see Fig. 11-3) appear as either a localized eccentric mass at the orbital apex[13] or as a well-defined tubular thickening (64%) or fusiform enlargement (23%) of the optic nerve.[11] Stippled calcification is common within the tumor (see Fig. 11-3), helping to differentiate it from the optic nerve glioma. Secondary enlargement of the optic canal, with bony hyperostosis, may be seen if the tumor is located in the appropriate position.[11,13] Because the detection of calcification and bony change is helpful in making the diagnosis of perioptic meningioma, a noncontrast enhanced CT scan may be considered superior to a nonenhanced MRI in evaluating small perioptic lesions.[15] After administration of a contrast medium with CT, moderate to marked enhancement of the tumor is seen. The so-called tram-track sign of perioptic meningioma is caused by uniform enhancement of a circumferential meningioma (see Fig. 11-3). This may simulate dural inflammation, a finding that may be present in cases of optic neuritis and idiopathic inflammatory pseudotumor.

MRI Appearance. Magnetic resonance imaging displays the tumor as an abnormally enlarged optic nerve silhouette (see Fig. 11-4). Signal characteristics depend on the pulsing sequence. On short TR/TE scans, as well as on long TR/TE scans, perioptic meningiomas show diminished signal intensity relative to normal brain tissue.[11] Relative to orbital fat, on short TR/TE images the lesions are hypointense, whereas on long TR/TE images, they are isointense. The calcifications within the tumor may be visualized as regions of signal void on MRI; however, most frequently intratumoral calcification is not seen. MRI may show bone involvement by meningioma as a region of absence of the expected signal void within an area of cortical bone.[18] Chemical shift artifact, resulting in a dark line on one side of the optic nerve, may mimic calcification, and similarly the subarachnoid space within the optic nerve sheath may appear dark on appropriate pulsing sequences, thereby mimicking circumferential calcification. This may be ruled out by using an appropriate pulsing sequence designed to increase the signal intensity of CSF.[6] The usefulness of gadolinium in the evaluation of perioptic meningiomas has been recently proved (see Fig. 11-4, B).[18]

Sarcoid

Sarcoidosis is a granulomatous disease of unknown cause that involves several organ systems, most commonly mediastinal and peripheral lymph nodes, lungs, liver, spleen, skin, eyes, and lacrimal glands.[16,19] Pathologically, it is characterized by noncaseating granulomas, which may occur in any tissue or organ of the body. Ophthalmic changes caused by involvement by sarcoid occur in up to 60% of cases.[19] The most frequently involved area within the orbit is the lacrimal gland; however, infiltration may be seen in any structure of the orbit.[18,20]

Clinical Findings. Two clinical presentations of sarcoidosis are noted. The subacute form generally occurs in patients under 30 years of age, particularly in women of Swedish, Puerto Rican, or Irish descent, and is characterized by rapid appearance of erythema nodosum, possibly with accompanying polyarthritis in association with bilateral hilar adenopathy. The second form is that of a chronic disease that affects patients over 30 years of age; the pulmonary parenchyma are involved, and the disease spreads beyond the thorax.[16] In general, the disease is seen predominantly in blacks 20 to 40 years of age.[19] Patients with subacute sarcoidosis tend to exhibit peripheral and cranial nerve involvement, most commonly of the seventh cranial nerve. The optic nerve is next most frequently involved. Involvement of the third, fourth, or sixth cranial nerves may produce extraocular muscle palsies. In the chronic form of sarcoidosis, CNS involvement is more common than peripheral nerve involvement. Optic nerve involvement is much more frequently seen in the chronic form of sarcoidosis than in the subacute form. (Recall that the optic nerve is an extension of a central brain tract and not a peripheral nerve.) Optic nerve involvement may occur at the chiasm or the intracanalicular or intraorbital portion. Optic nerve involvement in this form of the disease may lead to optic atrophy.

Anterior uveitis is characteristic of the subacute form of sarcoidosis, whereas a nonspecific granulomatous uveitis occasionally accompanied by cataract or secondary glaucoma is more indicative of the chronic form. Intracranial sarcoidosis is clinically evident in 5% of the cases, whereas 15% of autopsy cases demonstrate CNS involvement.[2] These patients may exhibit papilledema secondary to increased intracranial pressure. Optic atrophy may be present as a result of inflammation of the optic nerve, compression, or glaucoma caused by intraocular inflammation.

Pathologic Findings. The basic lesion of sarcoidosis is a noncaseating epithelioid cell tubercle. Langhans' giant cells are seen interspersed within the epithelioid cells centrally, and a thin rim of lymphocytes rings the individual tubercles. Inclusion bodies are characteristically seen within the giant cells in the tubercle. Although, as part of their natural course, the sarcoid granulomas may disappear without any evidence of scarring, they usually heal with sclerosis at the margins of the tubercles, and calcification does not occur during the healing process.[16]

Intracranial involvement by sarcoid generally occurs in one of two patterns. The most common one is granulomatous leptomeningitis with involvement of the leptomeninges, including those investing the optic nerves.

The second pattern is that of coalescence of sarcoid nodules into distinct parenchymal brain masses. In the leptomeninges, the cranial nerves, pituitary gland, third ventricle, hypothalamus, and (in rare cases) the pineal gland are involved.[19,21] Hydrocephalus may result from sarcoid lesions of the aqueduct, fourth ventricular outlet foramina, or the basal meninges.[22] The pathway of spread of sarcoidosis appears to be along the perivascular spaces, and noncaseating granulomas may be seen in the adventitia of small and medium-sized arteries and veins. True vasculitis with inflammation in and around the vessels is rare,[22] occasionally resulting in vessel obstruction with subsequent infarction.

CT Appearance. Diffuse infiltration of the leptomeninges is the most common CT finding. On the unenhanced study, areas of diffuse, irregularly increased attenuation along the leptomeninges may be seen; however, a normal study is the most frequent finding.[19] With orbital involvement the lacrimal gland may be enlarged and irregular thickening of the meninges of the optic nerve may be present. Brain parenchymal involvement produces discrete nodules that, on unenhanced CT, may be isodense or slightly hyperdense to the surrounding normal parenchyma. The nodules may be multiple or singular or may even form large, discrete masses upon coalescence (Fig. 11-19, A). Surrounding edema is usually not present. Following administration of a contrast medium, diffuse, irregular enhancement along the basal cisterns can be seen. The borders of the cortical sulci may enhance similarly as a result of leptomeningeal spread within the perivascular spaces of Virchow-Robin.[19] Homogeneous enhancement of parenchymal nodules also occurs after administration of the contrast medium (Fig. 11-19, A).[19,22,23] Obstructive hydrocephalus may be seen when structures adjacent to the third ventricle or the aqueduct or the outlet foramina of the fourth ventricle is involved. Cranial nerve involvement generally produces fusiform or irregular enlargement of the nerve with homogeneous enhancement after administration of a contrast medium.[19] Compression or direct invasion of the cranial nerves may occur as a consequence of infiltration of the basal meninges. Calcification is not a feature of sarcoidosis.[21]

MRI Appearance. Orbital sarcoid is well evaluated with MRI, which demonstrates a high degree of anatomic detail not seen with CT, particularly in areas where image degradation caused by beam-hardening artifact occurs (i.e., in the intracanalicular and intracranial portions of optic nerve). MRI demonstrates sarcoid involvement of the optic nerve as diffuse enlargement of the optic nerve sheath complex of a variable signal intensity that is usually isointense to extraocular muscle on short TR/TE images and minimally hyperintense to

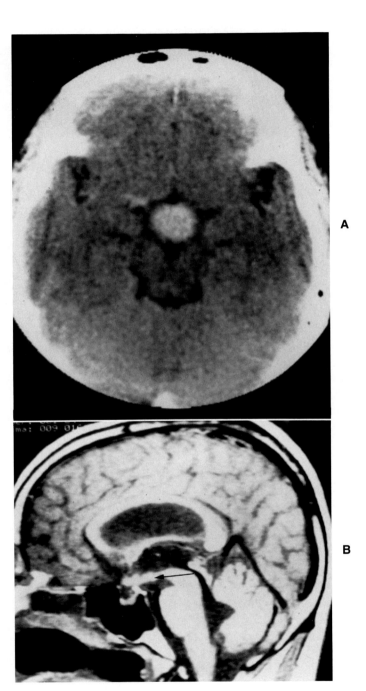

Fig. 11-19 Sarcoidosis involving optic chiasm. **A,** Axial CT shows contrast enhancement of thickened optic chiasm. **B,** Sagittal T$_1$WI shows irregular thickening of optic chiasm *(arrow)*.

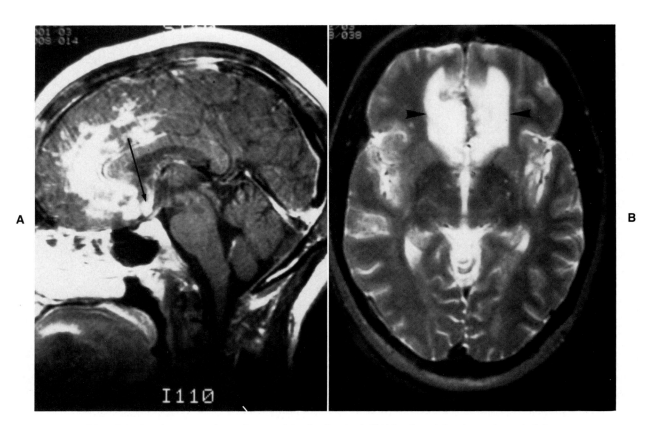

Fig. 11-20 Leptomeningeal sarcoid. **A,** Sagittal T_1WI after injection of gadolinium shows marked enhancement of leptomeninges between frontal lobes, extending along corpus callosum, and down onto surface of optic chiasm *(arrow).* **B,** Axial T_2WI shows bifrontal edema *(arrowheads)* within cortex and white matter of frontal lobes at site of leptomeningeal involvement by sarcoid.

orbital fat on long TR/TE images (Fig. 11-19, B).[18,20,24] Lacrimal gland involvement by sarcoid is generally seen as diffuse enlargement of the gland with a signal intensity pattern that may be either low or high on long TR/TE images.[18,20] The two major pathologic changes of intracranial sarcoid are well demonstrated by MRI. They consist of abnormal tissue involving the meninges (Figs. 11-20 and 11-21) and the brain parenchyma in addition to hydrocephalus and small areas of infarction.[25] Meningeal involvement by sarcoid tissue is most commonly seen in the region of the basal cisterns with focal areas of high-signal-intensity tissue on long TR/TE images (see Fig. 11-20, B). However, the signal intensity characteristics may vary, and the tissue occasionally may be hypointense to normal brain parenchyma on long TR/TE images. Periventricular involvement demonstrates similar signal intensity and is also a common location for visualization of abnormal sarcoid tissue. The parenchymal regions of sarcoid also have similar signal characteristics. MRI appears to have a greater sensitivity for detecting regions of sarcoidosis than does CT.[26] The hydrocephalus associated with sarcoid involvement of CSF is clearly identified with MRI. The site of obstruction responsible for the hydrocephalus may also be

determined through MRI techniques. Specifically, the absence of a flow void sign within the aqueduct or within the foramina of Magendie or Luschka may indicate these to be the primary sites of obstruction.[27] The use of gadolinium in evaluating sarcoid has proved helpful in demonstrating the extent of meningeal involvement (see Figs. 11-20, A, and 11-21, B).

Craniopharyngioma

Craniopharyngioma is a benign tumor that arises from remnants of Rathke's pouch. Craniopharyngiomas most commonly occur in a suprasellar location, as well as within the sella turcica. They make up between 1% and 3% of intracranial tumors. They are found most frequently in children but have two other age peaks, one in young adulthood and one in the fifth decade.[28]

Clinical Findings. Patients with craniopharyngioma most frequently complain of a headache. Visual disturbances also frequently occur, related to impingement of the tumor on the optic pathway at the level of the chiasm or optic tracts. Hypothalamic and pituitary dysfunction may be seen. When the tumor occurs in a child, growth failure may result.[29]

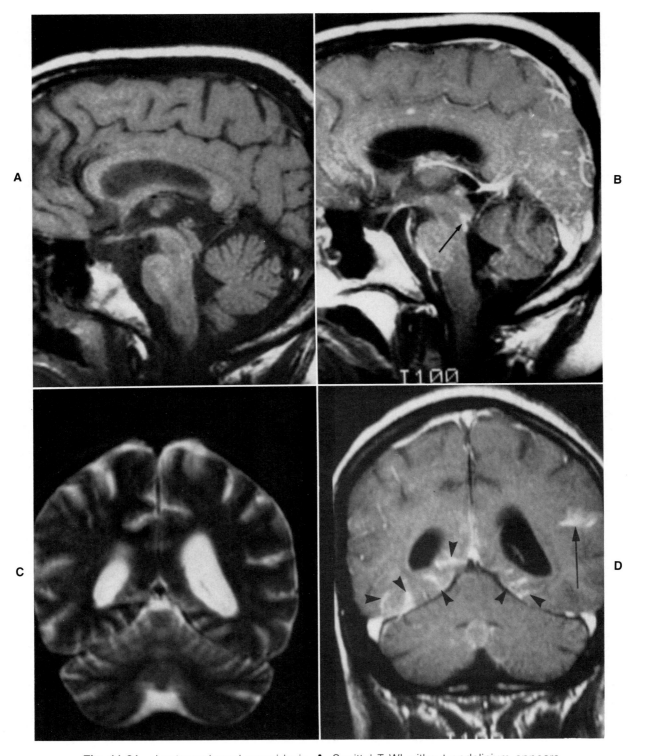

Fig. 11-21   Leptomeningeal sarcoidosis. **A,** Sagittal T₁WI without gadolinium appears normal. **B,** Sagittal T₁WI after gadolinium enhancement shows leptomeningeal enhancement in interhemispheric fissure and medial aspect of occipital lobe. Focus is present in sylvian aqueduct *(arrow).* **C,** Coronal T₂WI appears normal. **D,** Coronal T₁WI after injection of gadolinium shows enhancement of depths of sulci in occipital temporal region *(arrowheads),* enhancement of distal most portion of sylvian fissure on left *(arrow),* and thickening of leptomeninges over right parietal lobe.

Pathologic Findings. Craniopharyngiomas originate from squamous cell epithelial rests arising from Rathke's pouch. They are benign, slow-growing tumors. Grossly, the tumor is well encapsulated and adherent to surrounding tissues. As the tumor enlarges, the adjacent structures are compressed, including the optic chiasm anteriorly, the pituitary gland inferiorly, the hypothalamus superiorly, and the elements of the circle of Willis peripherally.[28] The tumor is usually cystic with interspersed solid areas. The cystic region contains either a liquid or semisolid dark brown, greasy material composed of cholesterol crystals, keratin, and calcified debris. Microscopically, the solid portions of the tumor consist of nests of stratified squamous or columnar epithelium in a fibrous stroma that is similar to that of the enamel organ of the tooth. Because of this, these tumors are considered to have an adamantinomatous histologic pattern.[29] Approximately 75% of craniopharyngiomas are found to contain significant amounts of calcium.

CT Appearance. With CT scan imaging, craniopharyngiomas usually appear as rounded, lobulated, or irregularly marginated masses occupying the suprasellar cistern (85% of the time) and occasionally involving the sella turcica (20% of the time). Cystic components are noted in 85% of the lesions. These cystic regions demonstrate a variable attenuation from either markedly hypodense to isodense relative to CSF (Figs. 11-22 and 11-23, A and B). The attenuation probably depends on the cholesterol content. Calcification is present in approximately 75% of the cases, varying from 70% to 90% in craniopharyngiomas occurring in children to 35% to 50% in craniopharyngiomas occurring in adults. The character of the calcification is generally conglomerate (see Fig. 11-23, A and B), although rimlike calcifications may occur about the cystic portions of the lesion (see Fig. 11-22). After administration of a contrast medium, the solid portions of the tumor usually are markedly enhanced.

MRI Appearance. Because of its multiplanar imaging capabilities, MRI well displays the anatomic configuration of the lesion relative to adjacent brain structures. On short TR/TE images the tumor generally displays increased to intermediate signal intensity as a result of T_1 shortening (Fig. 11-24, A). In rare cases the signal intensity is diminished, particularly if the lesion is predominantly cystic (see Fig. 11-23, C). Intermediate signal intensity on short TR/TE images is generally seen in tumors without elevated cholesterol content.[29] Focal areas of diminished signal intensity on short TR/TE and long TR/TE images may be secondary either to elevated carotin content within the cystic portions of the tumor or to calcification within solid portions. As a rule, hyperintense signal is seen on long TR/TE images as a

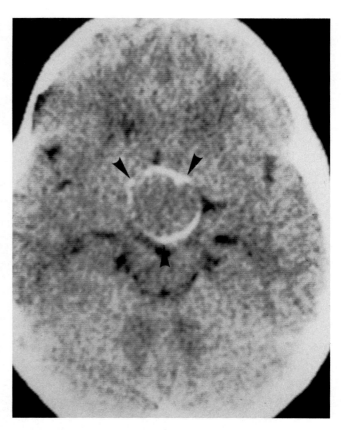

Fig. 11-22   Craniopharyngioma. Axial plain CT shows suprasellar tumor with peripheral rim of calcification *(arrowheads)* and central region that is isodense to brain.

result of T_2 prolongation (see Figs. 11-23, D, and 11-24, B).[29,30]

Comparison of CT and MRI reveals CT's greater sensitivity at displaying calcification; this makes it a more specific radiologic procedure for tumor identification, particularly when taken in conjunction with the clinical history. MRI, on the other hand, is more sensitive to the presence of a tumor and gives a more accurate preoperative demonstration of the extent and location of the tumor, which is important in planning the surgical approach.[29,30]

The role of gadolinium administration in evaluation of craniopharyngiomas by MRI has not yet been fully investigated; however, it has been shown that the tumor wall and solid portions are enhanced after administration of gadolinium (Fig. 11-25, B). Thus gadolinium may increase the sensitivity of MRI in evaluation of craniopharyngiomas, particularly in regard to tumor residual and recurrence after surgical excision.

Rathke's Cleft Cyst

Rathke's cleft cyst is a benign lesion consisting of a cystic remnant of Rathke's pouch that occurs within the

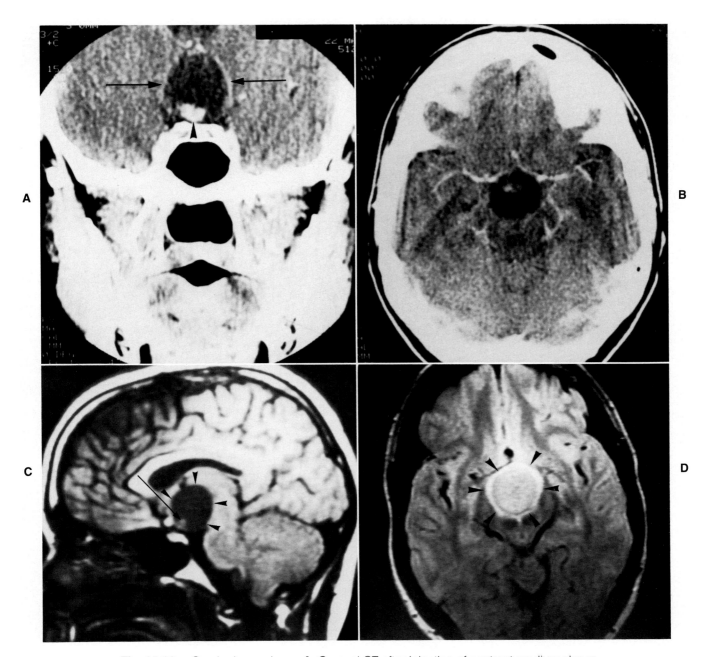

Fig. 11-23 Craniopharyngioma. **A,** Coronal CT after injection of contrast medium shows enhancement of cyst wall *(arrows)* and focus of calcification *(arrowhead).* **B,** Axial enhanced CT shows hypodense cystic mass with focus of calcification. **C,** Sagittal T_1WI shows cystic mass *(arrowheads)* in hypothalamus with inferior soft tissue density *(arrow)* at site of calcification seen on CT. Pituitary fossa is normal. **D,** Axial PDWI shows hyperintense wall to cyst *(arrowheads)* and slightly less intense contents. Cystic mass invaginates into midbrain, displacing cerebral peduncles to either side.

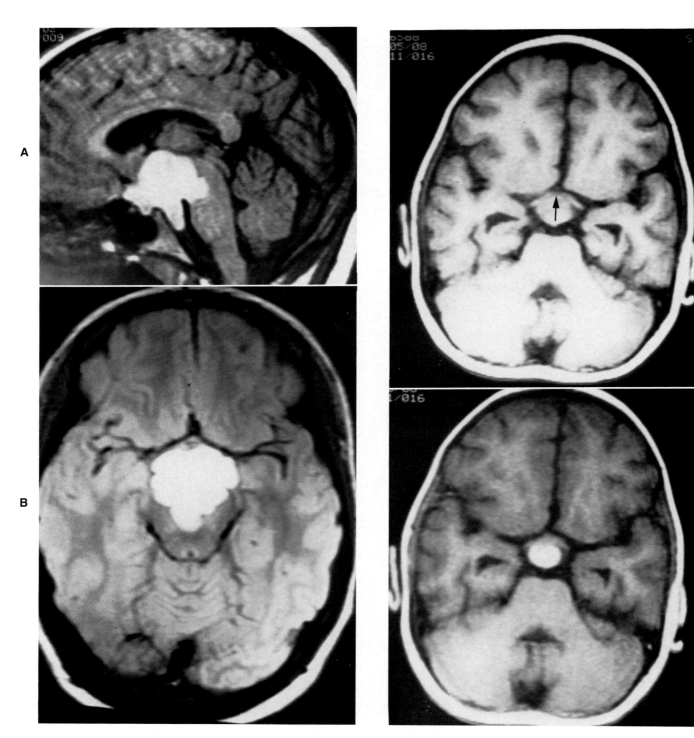

Fig. 11-24 Craniopharyngioma. **A,** Sagittal T₁WI shows hyperintense intrasellar, suprasellar, and retrosellar multilobulated mass involving hypothalamus and interpeduncular cistern and extending into prepontine space. **B,** Axial PDWI shows hyperintense, irregular mass displacing chiasm forward and separating cerebral peduncles.

Fig. 11-25 Craniopharyngioma. **A,** Axial T₁WI before gadolinium enhancement shows solid soft tissue mass in suprasellar cistern displacing optic chiasm *(arrow)* forward. **B,** Axial T₁WI after intravenous injection of gadolinium shows contrast enhancement of solid soft tissue mass in suprasellar cistern.

anterior portion of the sella turcica or the anterior aspect of the suprasellar cistern.

Clinical Findings. Rathke's cleft cysts usually are small and without discernible clinical symptoms. If they are symptomatic, they may appear with hypopituitarianism, diabetes insipidus, headache, or visual disturbances related to impingement on the visual pathway at the level of the optic chiasm or the optic tracts; however, only 60 symptomatic cases have been reported in the world literature.[31]

Pathologic Findings. Rathke's pouch, from which the anterior lobe of the pituitary, the pars tuberalis, and the pars intermedia are derived, is the organ of origin for the Rathke's cleft cyst. It is generally a simple cystic structure lying primarily within the anterior portion of the sella turcica, occasionally with protrusions into the suprasellar cistern region, forming a dumbbell-shaped lesion. Microscopically, the wall of the cyst in the intrasellar portion is lined by a simple cuboidal epithelium, which may be ciliated, whereas the suprasellar portion may be lined by stratified squamous epithelium.[28] The single cell layer forming the wall of the cyst often contains goblet cells. The cystic contents usually are of a serous or mucoid consistency with varying amounts of cellular debris. This variable protein content probably

accounts for the variable appearances of the cystic portion of the lesion on CT and MRI.

CT Appearance. Rathke's cleft cyst usually appears as a well-circumscribed cystic structure that has a mass effect, that lies within the sella turcica, and that occasionally has suprasellar extension. The wall of the cyst is generally thin, and the cyst contents usually are similar to CSF, although they may appear hypodense. The rim of tissue may enhance after administration of a contrast medium, and it occasionally contains small amounts of calcium. More complex cysts display a slightly increased density with septae partitioning the cystic portion.[31] Differential considerations for the simple form of the Rathke's cleft cyst include arachnoid cyst or cystic pituitary adenoma, whereas the more complex cysts may be impossible to differentiate from craniopharyngioma.

MRI Appearance. Simple cysts generally have signal intensity characteristics similar to CSF; that is, they usually appear hypointense to brain parenchyma on short TR/TE images and hyperintense to brain parenchyma on long TR/TE pulsing sequences. If the cyst fluid contains significant amounts of cholesterol, increased signal intensity is noted on short TR/TE images with diminishing intensity on progressively longer TR/

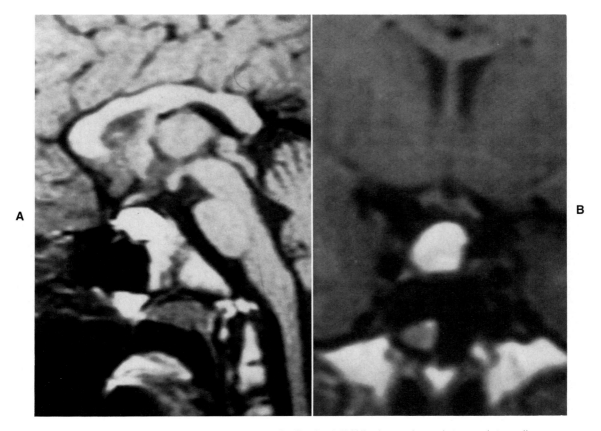

Fig. 11-26   Cyst of Rathke's pouch. **A,** Sagittal T$_1$WI shows hyperintense intrasellar mass bowing up into chiasmatic cistern, lying just below optic chiasm. **B,** Coronal T$_1$WI shows intrasellar mass with suprasellar extension; note that chiasm is not compressed.

TE images. Complex cysts, which represent a transitional form between a simple Rathke's cleft cyst and a craniopharyngioma, demonstrate signal heterogeneity on long TR/TE images with an isointense to hyperintense signal on short TR/TE images (Fig. 11-26). MRI better displays the relationship of the Rathke's cleft cyst to adjacent structures, particularly the optic chiasm and hypothalamus.

Pituitary Adenoma

Pituitary adenomas are benign neoplasms arising within the substance of the pituitary gland. They occur with equivalent frequency in males and females between 20 and 50 years of age. CT and more recently MRI have become the procedures of choice for evaluating tumors of the pituitary gland.

Clinical Findings. Adenomas of the pituitary gland can be separated into either microadenomas (less than 1 cm in diameter) or macroadenomas (greater than 1 cm in diameter). The microadenomas typically appear with endocrine abnormalities, the specific findings depending on which hormone is being elaborated by the adenoma. Macroadenomas, on the other hand, appear more often with symptoms caused by mass effect, such as those resulting from chiasmatic compression or pituitary insufficiency.

Pathologic Findings. Pituitary adenomas are usually unencapsulated solid tumors that may penetrate adjacent structures. The tumors can contain necrotic, cystic, or hemorrhagic regions and rarely contain calcification.[32] Of these adenomas, 25% to 30% are nonfunctional.[32] Prolactin-secreting tumors make up 25% of all secretory tumors, whereas growth hormone is elaborated in 20% and adrenocorticotropic hormone (ACTH) is elaborated in 10% of secreting tumors.[32] Microscopically, the adenomas are composed of sheets and cords of cells with a delicate stroma. The functional adenomas usually contain highly granulated cells indicative of their cytochemical activity. Ischemia with consequent necrosis and hemorrhage may occur secondary to compromise of the blood supply, which results from compression at the diaphragma sellae. This eventually may cause a rapidly expanding sellar mass, with consequent optic nerve compression, headache, and occasional meningeal irritation as the clinical findings. The incidence of malignant degeneration among pituitary adenomas is exceedingly small.

CT Appearance. The specific findings associated with pituitary adenoma vary, depending on the size of the lesion. Microadenomas typically are seen as focal hypodense areas within the surrounding pituitary gland, causing convexity of the upper surface of the gland and an increase in the height of the gland to a distance greater than 9 mm. Associated displacement of the infundibulum away from the side of the lesion may be seen, and thinning of the ipsilateral sellar floor may be

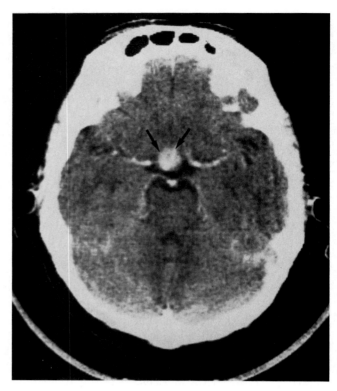

Fig. 11-27 Pituitary adenoma. Axial contrast CT shows homogeneous enhancement *(arrows)* of suprasellar extension of a pituitary adenoma.

present. These findings are more characteristically found in lesions elaborating prolactin. Lesions elaborating growth hormone or ACTH may be more difficult to visualize, since they tend to be less well encapsulated. After administration of a contrast medium, microadenomas tend to be hypodense relative to the surrounding (enhanced) pituitary gland.

Macroadenomas display findings that depend on the size of the lesion. They tend to enlarge the sella, causing sloping of the sellar floor (see Fig. 11-5, *A*) with possible extension into the sphenoid sinus. Depending on the degree of suprasellar extension, macroadenomas may displace the chiasm, temporal lobes, and even the third ventricle. After administration of a contrast medium, the macroadenomas generally appear isodense to slightly hypodense when compared with the cavernous sinuses (see Fig. 11-5, *A*). If the lesion is solid, homogeneous enhancement occurs (Fig. 11-27), whereas cystic or necrotic areas within a lesion tend to remain less dense relative to the remainder of the lesion. Macroadenomas may contain calcification either homogeneously distributed throughout the tumor or deposited in a rim. If infarction of the tumor occurs, a hypodense area secondary to edema may be seen or, alternatively, a hyperdense area may be seen secondary to hemorrhage (Fig. 11-28, *A*). However, these findings are often difficult to delineate on CT.[33]

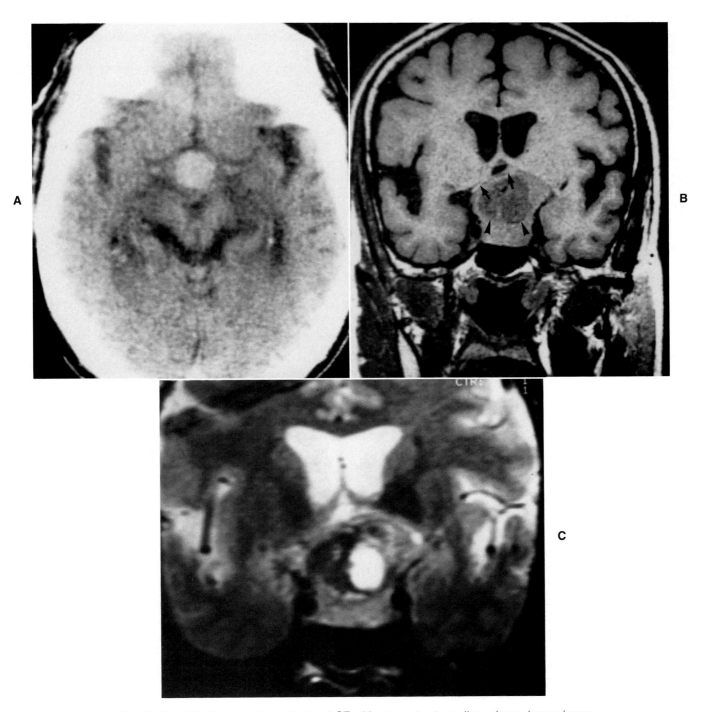

Fig. 11-28   Pituitary apoplexy. **A,** Axial CT without contrast medium shows hyperdense suprasellar mass consistent with either bleeding or calcification. **B,** Coronal T₁WI shows intrasellar and suprasellar mass extending slightly more to left. Chiasm is displaced and compressed from below *(arrows)*. Mass contains slightly less intense zone *(arrowheads)* consistent with deoxyhemoglobin. **C,** Coronal T₂WI shows same area of hypointensity within pituitary adenoma seen in **B** to be of both high and low signal intensity. High signal intensity more to left of midline is area of cystic necrosis, whereas low signal intensity represents deoxyhemoglobin.

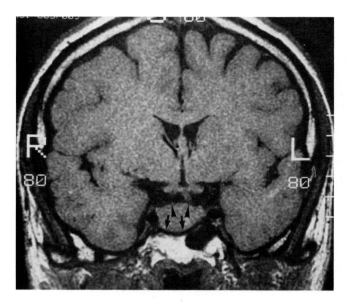

Fig. 11-29 Pituitary adenoma. Coronal T₁WI shows downward bowing of enlarged sellae *(arrows)*, upward convexity of gland *(arrowheads)*, and displacement of infundibular stalk to left.

MRI Appearance. MRI usually allows accurate delineation of pituitary adenomas greater than 3 mm in size.[31] In fact, smaller adenomas may be diagnosed but with less reliability.[34] A more specific diagnosis of a sellar mass may be achieved with MRI than with CT, and MRI is clearly better able to characterize subacute hemorrhage within the tumor.[31] Overall anatomic definition is more accurate with MRI than with CT.[33,35] Specifically, displacement of the optic chiasm, carotid artery, third ventricle, and infundibulum is more clearly seen with MRI than with CT (see Figs. 11-28, *B* and 11-29). Equivalent demonstration of dorsum sellar erosion is noted with the two imaging modalities.[35] CT is better able than MRI to demonstrate intratumoral calcification.

Findings of a pituitary adenoma on MRI are similar to those noted on CT. Specifically, the primary findings are an upward bulge at the top of the pituitary gland with contralateral deviation of the infundibulum and sloping of the ipsilateral sellar floor (Fig. 11-29).[31] On short TR/TE images the adenomas tend to be slightly hypointense to the surrounding normal pituitary gland and may or may not be associated with a mass effect.[31]

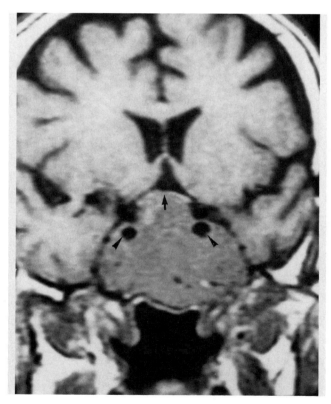

Fig. 11-30 Pituitary adenoma. Coronal T₁WI shows large pituitary adenoma elevating and compressing optic chiasm *(arrow)*. Both cavernous sinuses are invaded with tumor lateral to flow void of intracavernous internal carotid arteries *(arrowheads)*. Note outward convexity of lateral margin of cavernous sinuses.

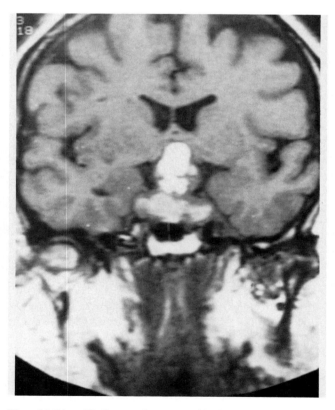

Fig. 11-31 Pituitary adenoma with intratumoral hemorrhage. Coronal T₁WI shows intrasellar and suprasellar mass of mixed signal intensity, which is caused by presence of methemoglobin. Note that mass extends laterally and compresses both cavernous sinus regions.

Occasionally pituitary adenomas may be isointense to the surrounding normal pituitary tissue.[35] On long TR/TE images the appearance of the adenomas varies[31] but may be moderately hyperintense relative to surrounding pituitary tissue.[35] Pituitary adenomas usually demonstrate homogeneous signal intensity; however, occasionally they are slightly inhomogeneous.[35]

Suprasellar extension with impingement on and displacement of the optic chiasm is best demonstrated on coronal and sagittal sections. Coronal sections are also better for demonstrating tumor extension into the cavernous sinuses (Fig. 11-30). Definitive display of extension into the cavernous sinuses is commonly difficult with MRI, since the medial wall of the cavernous sinus is very thin, and violation of this tissue plane may be difficult to see. There is no evidence of a difference in signal intensity between secretory and nonsecretory pituitary adenomas.[31] Cystic pituitary adenomas characteristically display high signal intensity on long TR/TE images and low signal intensity on short TR/TE images at the site of the cyst (see Fig. 11-28). Subacutely, hemorrhagic pituitary adenomas display high signal intensity on short TR/TE images because of the paramagnetic effect of methemoglobin (Fig. 11-31).

On short TR/TE images, after administration of a paramagnetic contrast agent such as gadolinium, a pituitary microadenoma is shown as a focal area of hypointensity relative to the surrounding enhancing normal pituitary tissue. This is true only if the images are acquired very early after administration of the contrast medium.[31] On images obtained late after administration of the medium, the adenoma enhances and may not be distinguished from the normal pituitary gland. Macroadenomas enhance with gadolinium.

Aneurysms

Aneurysms may be responsible for visual symptoms if they impinge directly on the visual pathway.[36,37] The most common aneurysms to do this arise from the internal carotid artery at the origin of the ophthalmic artery. Aneurysms occurring in this location compress either the optic chiasm, the intracranial portion of the optic nerve, or the proximal portion of the optic tract.

Clinical Findings. Aneurysms arising from the internal carotid artery at the origin of the ophthalmic artery most often appear in patients between 50 and 70 years of age. Most of these patients are female. Most aneurysms (75%) in this location are discovered at the time of angiographic evaluation for subarachnoid hemorrhage that has originated from another aneurysm. However, in approximately 25% of patients with these aneurysms, the presentation is solely because of visual symptoms. The aneurysms associated with visual symptoms are often found to be of large proportions (greater than 2.5 cm in diameter).[38] Also, more than half of the patients with these aneurysms have at least one other intracranial aneurysm. The most common site of the additional aneurysm is the same site on the contralateral side.[39]

A diverse range of visual abnormalities is encountered. Visual acuity is nearly always impaired. This usually begins on the side of the aneurysm and may be progressive over months or years, leading eventually to blindness. Visual field abnormalities are also diverse because of the variety of ways in which the optic nerves and chiasm can be displaced by the aneurysm. Most commonly, unilateral or bilateral temporal field defects are seen. The clinical presentation of aneurysms in this location can mimic that of pituitary tumors.

Pathologic Findings. Grossly, these aneurysms tend to be sacular ones arising from the upper surface of the internal carotid artery at the origin of the ophthalmic artery.[40] Microscopically, within the aneurysm dome there is fragmentation of the interna of the vessel with degeneration of the smooth muscle walls. Frequently the dome of the aneurysm contains layers of adherent thrombus of varying ages.

CT Appearance. Although aneurysms at the internal carotid–ophthalmic artery junction that cause visual pathway symptoms are usually intact, they are most frequently discovered when the patient seeks help for symptoms of a subarachnoid hemorrhage. Therefore the CT findings of an aneurysm in this location often coincide with the findings of subarachnoid hemorrhage. The CT appearance of subarachnoid hemorrhage is most commonly that of high-density material lying within the sulci and cysternal spaces. Depending on the location of the ruptured aneurysm, high-density material reflecting hemorrhage may be seen within the ventricular system or within the brain parenchyma itself.

The appearance of the aneurysm causing visual pathway symptoms depends on whether there is partial thrombosis within the aneurysmal dome. If no thrombus is present, the aneurysm usually appears as a rounded area of slightly increased density lying cephalad to the cavernous sinus adjacent to the optic chiasm. The structures in the region may be displaced. After injection of a contrast medium, there is homogeneous enhancement of the aneurysm by the iodinated contrast material (Fig. 11-32). Rim calcification may or may not be present (Fig. 11-33). A partially thrombosed aneurysm appears on unenhanced CT as a well-circumscribed mass with an isodense periphery and central hyperdensity. The hyperdense central patent lumen enhances upon administration of a contrast medium. A peripheral rim of enhancement may occur because of increased vascularity within the aneurysm wall. If the aneurysm is completely thrombosed, only isodense thrombotic material may be seen within its central por-

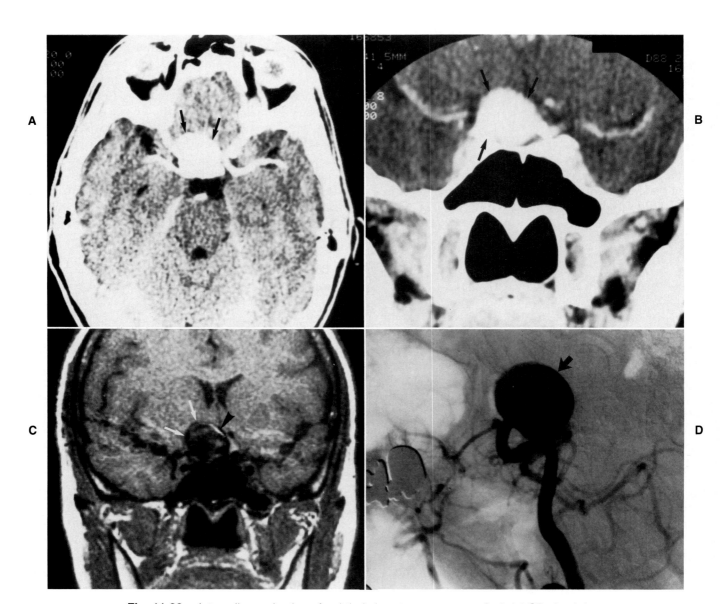

Fig. 11-32 Intrasellar projection of ophthalmic artery aneurysm. **A,** Axial CT after injection of contrast medium shows enhanced mass *(arrows)* in suprasellar space. **B,** Coronal CT after injection of contrast medium shows same mass *(arrows)* as in **A** lying partly within sella. **C,** Coronal T_1WI shows hypointense flow void of blood within lumen of intrasellar and suprasellar mass *(arrows)*. Small area of hyperintensity in superior margin may represent laminar clot *(arrowhead)*. Note irregular hyperintensity extending across sylvian fissures bilaterally at same level as aneurysm, representing flow artifacts in phase-encoding direction. **D,** Internal carotid arteriogram subtraction film shows ophthalmic artery aneurysm *(arrow)*.

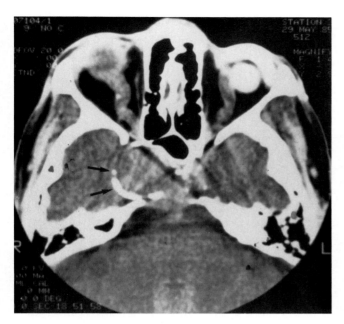

Fig. 11-33 Intracavernous aneurysm. Plain axial CT shows mass with peripheral calcification *(arrows)* that is eroding sphenoid bone and sellae.

tion.[41] Peripheral enhancement may still occur.

MRI Appearance. Compared to CT, MRI more precisely characterizes giant aneurysms and defines their location relative to adjacent anatomic structures. However, MRI is much less sensitive than CT for detecting acute subarachnoid hemorrhage. Therefore, in the setting of symptoms suggesting acute subarachnoid hemorrhage, CT scanning is the initial imaging modality of choice. MRI cannot definitely exclude the presence of an aneurysm. Angiography remains the most sensitive modality for detecting intracranial aneurysms. However, this modality is limited by its ability to demonstrate only the patent portions of the lumen of the aneurysm. Since many aneurysms contain thrombus partially or completely obliterating the lumen, the full extent of the lesion often cannot be defined by angiography.

The characteristic appearance of a partially thrombosed aneurysm on MRI has been well described.[42,43] On spin echo imaging, partially thrombosed aneurysms demonstrate a flow phenomenon, usually a flow void, within the patent portion of the lumen. The laminated thrombus along the margins of the aneurysm dome exhibits mixed signal intensities, reflecting the various stages of clot formation. A periluminal rim of hyperintensity is usually seen, reflecting methemoglobin surrounding the patent portion of the lumen (see Fig. 11-32, *C*). The parent vessel (i.e., the internal carotid artery) shows a signal void because of high velocity flow. Gradient echo acquisition images, which display high velocity flow as regions of high signal intensity, demonstrate blood flow within the lumen of the parent vessel and within the patent portion of the lumen of the aneurysm. In aneurysms with no thrombus formation, only the areas of signal void on spin echo images (Fig. 11-34) or high signal intensity on gradient echo acquisition images are seen in the region of the mass. If the aneurysm is completely thrombosed, mixed signal intensity caused by various stages of clot formation are seen on spin echo images within the aneurysmal mass (Fig. 11-35).

The relationship of the aneurysm to the elements of the visual pathway is delineated with MRI. The coronal plane is helpful for showing the relationship of the aneurysm to the optic chiasm, nerve, and tract, as well as the aneurysm's relationship to the structures of the sella turcica and the cavernous sinus.

Infarction

Cerebral infarction, a localized area of necrosis caused by circulatory insufficiency, is the most common pathologic disorder affecting the central nervous system. Cerebral infarctions may be further subdivided as either ischemic or hemorrhagic. They may occur in association with arteriosclerosis or with or without thrombosis, emboli, or venoocclusive disease.

Clinical Findings. Circulatory insufficiency may be caused by involvement of the anterior cerebral circulation (internal carotid arteries and their branches) or the posterior cerebral circulation (the vertebral basilar system). Amaurosis fugax, or transient loss of vision in one eye, is the most common ocular symptom of internal carotid artery ischemia. Specific findings vary from hemianopia to complete loss of light perception in the affected eye. Vision most commonly returns after a few minutes, and permanent visual loss is not a feature of the phenomenon. Cholesterol emboli may be found in association with episodes of amorosis fugax. Ophthalmoscopic evaluation reveals these emboli within the retinal arterials as characteristic bright yellowish orange plaques. Since the internal carotid artery and its branches supply the frontal and parietal lobes, portions of the temporal lobes, the corpus striatum, and the internal capsule, an occlusion may produce a variety of contralateral motor and sensory dysfunctions in addition to the visual findings.

Insufficiency of the circulation of the vertebral basilar system causes transient ischemic attack or infarction with complex and diverse neurologic symptoms. In addition to ocular symptoms, vertigo and nausea may be present if the cochlear vestibular system is involved. Involvement of the auditory system may produce tinnitus or partial deafness. Headache, dysphagia, dysarthria, and hiccupping may also occur. The ocular symptoms include transient homonymous hemianopsia, scin-

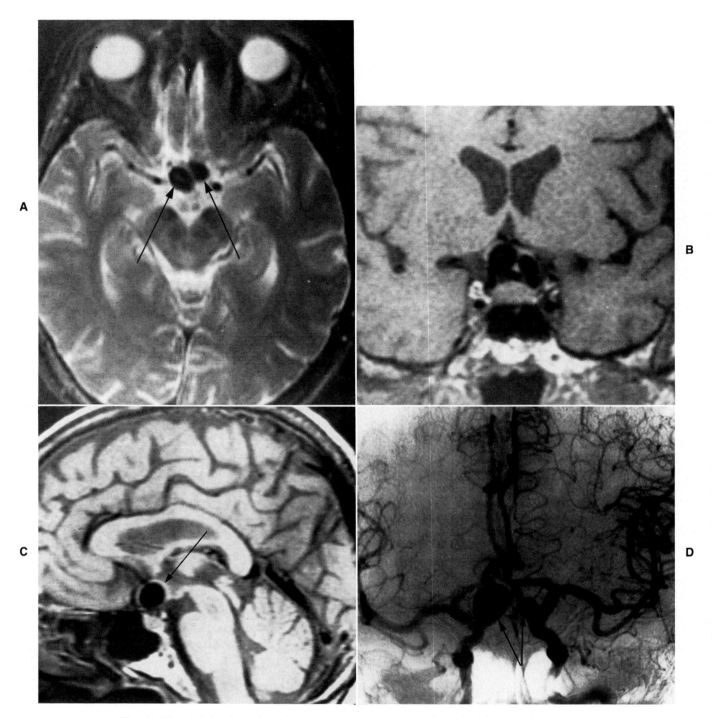

Fig. 11-34 Bilateral ophthalmic artery aneurysms appearing with bitemporal hemianopsia. **A,** Axial T$_2$WI shows two areas of hypointensity *(arrows)* in suprasellar cistern consistent with aneurysms. **B,** Coronal T$_1$WI shows two hypointense lumens of aneurysms projecting medially from region of internal carotid arteries and compressing optic chiasm bilaterally. **C,** Sagittal T$_1$WI shows larger aneurysm as hypointense flow void and depicts aneurysm's relationship to chiasm *(arrow)*, which is compressed from below. **D,** AP right and left carotid arteriogram subtraction films superimposed to show relationships of both ophthalmic artery aneurysms, which project medially *(arrows)*.

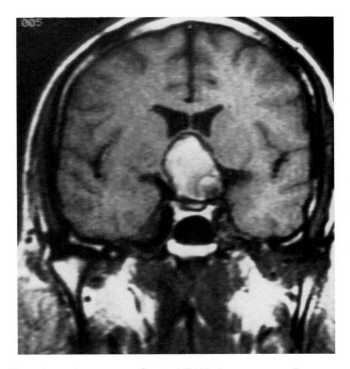

Fig. 11-35   Thrombosed aneurysm. Coronal T₁WI shows suprasellar mass composed of high-signal-intensity methemoglobin.

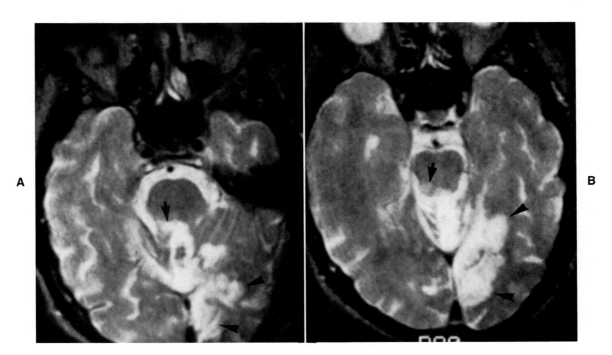

Fig. 11-36   Left occipital lobe and midbrain and upper brainstem infarction. **A,** Axial T₂WI shows hyperintense signal intensity at site of left occipital lobe infarct *(arrowheads)*. Note hyperintense focus of infarction in periaqueductal region of upper pons *(arrows)*. **B,** Next higher axial T₂WI shows further superior extent of hyperintense infarct involving left occipital and medial temporal lobes *(arrowheads)*. High-signal-intensity focus is present in dorsal aspect of right midbrain *(arrow)*.

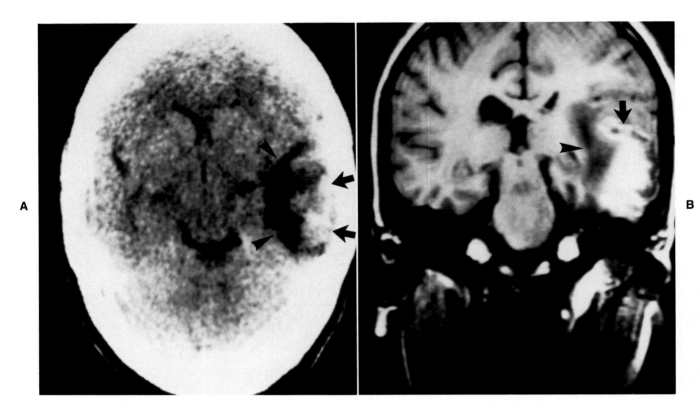

Fig. 11-37 Hemorrhagic infarct temporal lobe from cortical vein thrombosis. **A,** Axial CT without contrast injection shows zone of mixed hyperdensity *(arrows)* and hypodensity *(arrowheads)* with mass effect. **B,** Coronal T$_1$WI shows mass in left temporal lobe that is of both high signal intensity *(arrow)* and low signal intensity *(arrowhead).*

tillating scotomas, and possibly blurred vision with diplopia. The homonymous hemianopsia arises as a result of infarction of the occipital lobe's visual cortex, which is fed by branches of the posterior cerebral artery. Diplopia occurs because vascular insufficiency produces infarction in the brainstem nuclei of the third, fourth, and sixth cranial nerves. Internuclear ophthalmoplegia may occur as a result of interruption of the vascular supply to the medial longitudinal fasiculus (Fig. 11-36).

Pathologic Findings. Infarcts may be divided into two basic categories, depending on the amount of hemorrhage that occurs in the involved tissue. Infarction of thrombotic cause generally produces an anemic or nonhemorrhagic infarction, whereas infarctions of embolic cause often are associated with a variable degree of hemorrhage into the interstitial space.[28,32] Infarctions affecting the elements of the visual pathway are not dissimilar from infarctions in other regions of the brain, showing no discernible histologic differences. Their distinguishing factor is their position relative to the various portions of the visual pathway. The mechanism of infarction, whether hemorrhagic or anemic, is the same; that is, deprivation of blood supply to a given

area. In hemorrhagic infarctions, transitory occlusion of a vessel results in ischemic change of the brain tissue and the involved blood vessel's walls. When the blood supply is reestablished, blood elements penetrate the damaged vascular wall into the interstitial space, creating parenchymal hemorrhage.

The earliest grossly visible change in the evolution of an ischemic infarction is a slight discoloration and softening of the affected tissue, which occurs approximately 6 to 8 hours after occlusion of the vessel. Histologically, at this point there is diffuse swelling of the neurons with resultant cytotoxic edema. At 48 to 72 hours after occlusion of the vessel, tissue integrity is lost in the affected region and the surrounding tissue displays diffuse vasogenic edema. The combination of cytotoxic and vasogenic edema with the resultant mass effect may produce cerebral herniations that, depending on their site of occurrence, may damage neural transmission along the visual pathway (e.g., optic tract with temporal lobe herniation). Eventually, if the area of infarction is large enough, there is liquefaction and cyst formation surrounded by firm glial tissue. Histologically, in the final stages of evolution of an anemic infarction, gliosis both replaces and surrounds the necrotic region. Infarct

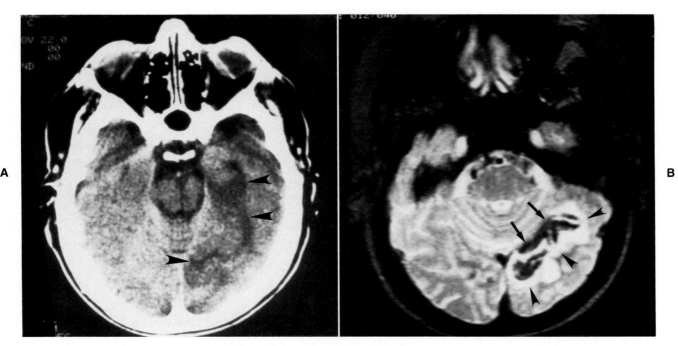

Fig. 11-38   Hemorrhagic infarct. **A,** Axial CT without contrast medium shows hypodensity *(arrowheads)* involving left occipital lobe and medial temporal lobe, a finding consistent with infarction. **B,** Axial T$_2$WI shows marked hypointensity of deoxyhemoglobin *(arrows)* in cortex of portions of hemorrhagic infarction. Surrounding hyperintensity is present *(arrowheads)*.

resolution may take weeks to many months.[32]

In addition to being associated with emboli, hemorrhagic infarctions may also be seen in association with hypertension and venous occlusion (Fig. 11-37) or bleeding dyscrasias. After extravasation of blood into the interstitial tissue, significant mass effect may occur, resulting in herniation. In fact, hemorrhagic infarction may result from a herniation that produced temporary compression of a trapped blood vessel. With reperfusion of the vessel on reduction of the herniation, blood suffuses through the damaged vascular wall into the infarcted brain.

CT Appearance. The effects of an ischemic infarction may be visible as early as 3 to 6 hours after the ictus. However, changes may be seen more reliably between 8 and 24 hours after the onset of ischemia. These changes are regions of hypointensity in the involved vascular distribution, including both white and gray matter (Fig. 11-38). The region of hypodensity, which represents intracellular (cytotoxic) edema, becomes more sharply defined over the next several days. Cytotoxic edema and tissue necrosis reach their maximum between the third and fifth day after the ictus, producing variable amounts of mass effect. In occipital lobe infarctions or infarctions involving the optic radiations, this may be perceived as effacement of the adjacent sulci and/or atrium and occipital horn of the lateral ven-

tricle. Larger infarctions may cause marked mass effect and result in descending transtentorial herniation with occlusion of the posterior cerebral artery when it is trapped on the tentorial edge. Occlusion of the posterior cerebral artery results in infarction of the posterior temporal and occipital lobes.

Vasogenic (interstitial) edema is seen more often with embolic infarction. This follows reperfusion of the affected area, usually occurs 2 to 14 days after the acute event, and is responsible for a significant degree of mass effect. Approximately 1 month after the ictus, cystic cavitation in the infarcted region occurs pathologically and is responsible for increasingly sharp definition of the region of the infarct. The infarcted region also becomes smaller because of progression of gliosis. The resultant increase in the depth of the adjacent sulci is also seen. Hemorrhagic infarctions, which result from embolic phenomena, overall are less frequent, representing only 20% of cases. The hemorrhage, when visible, is seen on unenhanced CT as a region of high density involving the cortex or the deep gray matter.

MRI Appearance. MRI is a valuable tool in the evaluation of cerebral infarction because of its high sensitivity both to increased tissue water content and to the absence of beam-hardening artifact. Thus the sensitivity of MRI in the early detection of infarction is much higher than that of CT. Experimentally, infarctions may

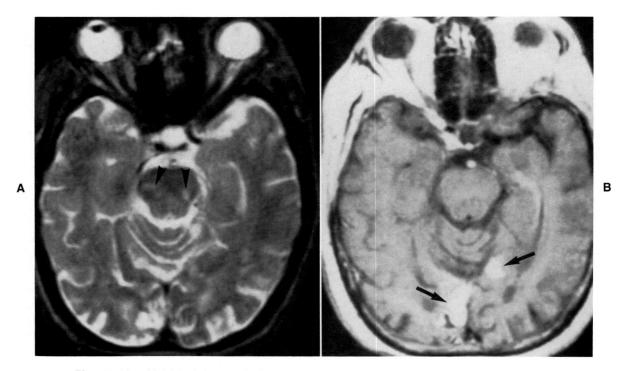

Fig. 11-39   Multiple infarcts. **A,** T$_2$WI shows several high-intensity foci in upper pons *(arrowheads)* that are consistent with small infarcts. **B,** T$_1$WI after injection of contrast medium shows enhancement of right occipital lobe and left medial temporal lobe infarcts *(arrows)* not seen on T$_2$WI.

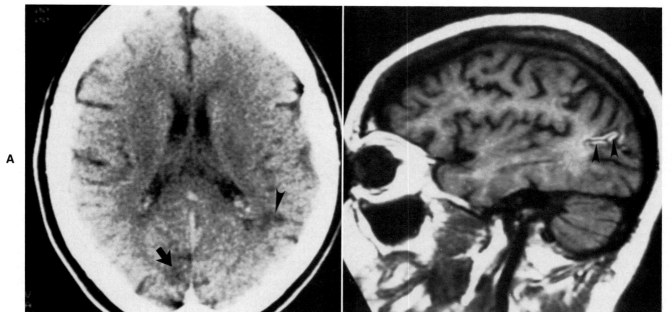

Fig. 11-40   Hemorrhagic infarcts of parietal and occipital lobes. **A,** Axial CT without contrast medium shows vague hypodensity in right occipital lobe *(arrow)* and another vague hypodensity *(arrowhead)* in left parietal lobe. **B,** Sagittal T$_1$WI shows hyperintense methemoglobin *(arrowheads)* in cortex.

be detected with MRI 2 to 4 hours after the onset of ischemia.[44] The earliest changes visible are caused by a prolongation of both T_1 and T_2 with resultant high signal intensity in the region of the infarction on long TR/ long TE images (see Fig. 11-9) and low signal intensity in the same region on short TR / short TE sequences. This is frequently visible 6 to 12 hours after the onset of symptoms and is attributable to the development of cytotoxic edema. With further evolution of the infarction, the absolute T_1 and T_2 prolongation becomes somewhat diminished and a slight alteration of signal intensity from the affected area results.[45] The mass effect produced by the region of infarction is clearly identified with MRI, with greater anatomic delineation of affected structures than is seen on CT. Contrast enhancement of the region of infarction after administration of gadolinium DTPA may be demonstrated as early as 16 to 18 hours after the ictus. Again, the region of enhancement correlates with areas of breakdown in the blood-brain barrier.[46] Interestingly, as edema and mass effect develop, the rapidity with which enhancement occurs declines, presumably as a result of compression of the microvasculature. The regions of enhancement following administration of gadolinium are seen as areas of increased signal intensity on short TR/TE images (Fig. 11-39).

Brain parenchymal change secondary to ischemia caused by vasculitis, as is seen in systemic lupus erythematosus, shows the same basic characteristics with regard to signal intensity as ischemia from either embolic or thrombotic phenomena. However, there is a difference in distribution in that the regions of ischemia are more diffuse throughout the brain, tending to occur in the regions of gray and white matter interface.

Hemorrhagic infarction may be demonstrated as areas of high signal intensity on short TR/TE images (Fig. 11-40, B) within the cortex or deep gray matter structures once deoxyhemoglobin (see Fig. 11-38, C) within the extravasated blood has been metabolized to methemoglobin. As evolution of the infarction proceeds and cystic encephalomalacia develops, the associated parenchymal volume loss is clearly delineated with MRI. Gliosis and demyelination within white matter tracks result in T_2 prolongation and consequently high signal intensity in the affected areas on long TR / long TE images.

Demyelinating Disease

The most common form of demyelinating disease to affect the optic pathway is multiple sclerosis. The characteristic changes seen in demyelination are caused by both plaque formation and gliosis, with resultant alteration in the appearance of the involved parenchyma. The neurophysiologic consequences of the loss of myelin are based on impaired transmission of neural impulses passing through the affected area.

Clinical Findings. Multiple sclerosis has a wide variety of signs and symptoms that are characteristically localized to at least two different anatomic areas within the central nervous system and that occur with a series of relapses and remissions separated in time by at least 1 month.[47] Initially the diagnosis may be difficult to confirm, since presentation may be caused by a single lesion or the course may be slowly progressive and not intermittent. Multiple sclerosis most characteristically affects patients between 10 and 50 years of age who reside in northern Europe or the northern United States. Females are affected more frequently than males in a ratio of 1.4 to 1.[48] Approximately half of patients with multiple sclerosis show clinical signs of optic nerve involvement. Visual evoked responses and electrophysiologic tests of optic nerve and pathway function are positive in approximately 90% of patients with multiple sclerosis. However, only 20% of patients show isolated optic neuritis as their initial clinical symptom.[12] Visual involvement, when present, is typically unilateral with dense regions of visual loss within the visual fields. Impaired color perception, ocular muscle palsies, and nystagmus are common, and internuclear ophthalmoplegia occasionally is present. Schilder's disease and Krabbe's disease are examples of other demyelinating diseases that may cause visual symptoms and involve the visual pathway. Schilder's disease usually appears during childhood, with progressive ataxia and loss of hearing and sight. Patients with Krabbe's disease may show symptoms of developmental delay, irritability, and spasticity, often beginning at 3 to 6 months of age.

Pathologic Findings. In multiple sclerosis the areas of demyelination are seen as focal lesions with well-circumscribed margins. Successive histologic changes occur consisting of demyelination followed by microglial reaction, followed by astrocytic proliferation.[12] In the initial stages oligodendrocytes and the myelin sheaths degenerate without change in the axon. At this time an associated vascular congestion with perivascular lymphocytic and plasma cell infiltrates is present. As a result, in the acute stage of the disease inflammation with swelling is present. Later the microglia phagocytize the myelin debris. This debris stimulates an intense gliosis that forms a firm glial scar in the late stage. Schilder's disease is characterized by large symmetrical zones of demyelination with degeneration of neural fibers and gliosis. These zones occur throughout the central nervous system, including the optic nerve and optic radiation.[12] Histopathologically, the lesions are identical to those seen in multiple sclerosis.[49]

CT Appearance. The plaques of multiple sclerosis are sometimes detectable by nonenhanced CT as hypo-

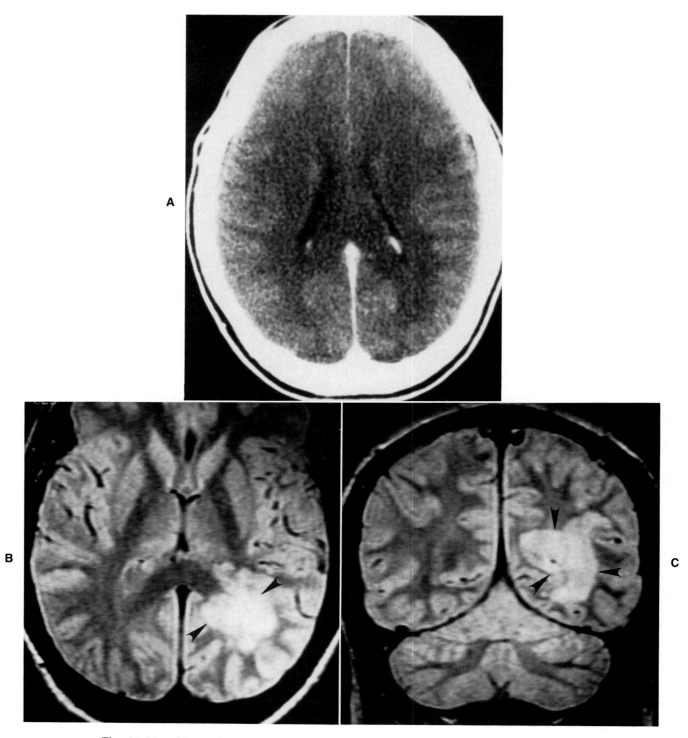

Fig. 11-41 Giant MS plaque producing acute homonymous hemianopsia. **A,** Axial CT after injection of contrast medium shows white matter in left parietal occipital region to be slightly fuller than white matter on right. This study was not labeled abnormal when read. **B,** Axial PDWI shows high–signal-intensity mass *(arrowheads)* in white matter of left temporoparietal occipital region (optic radiations). **C,** Coronal PDWI shows same high–signal-intensity mass *(arrowheads).*

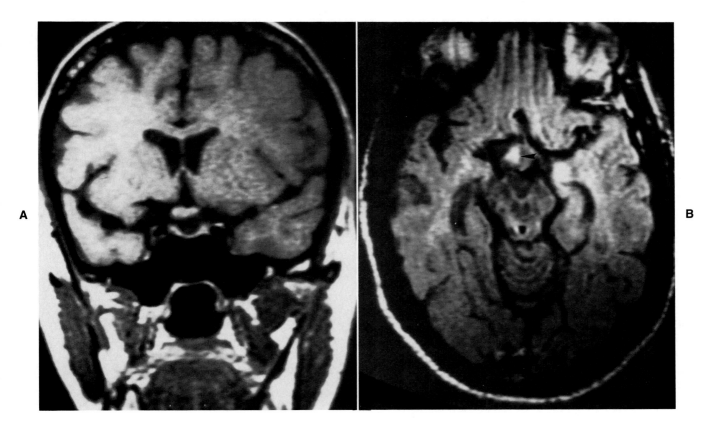

Fig. 11-42 Multiple sclerosis involving the optic chiasm. **A,** Coronal T$_1$WI shows focal enlargement of right side of optic chiasm. **B,** Axial PDWI shows high-signal-intensity change in right side of optic chiasm *(arrowhead).*

dense lesions within the periventricular white matter. Occasionally the plaques are large and demonstrate mass effect. However, they usually are less than 1.5 cm in greatest dimension. In approximately 5% of cases multiple sclerosis plaques may be seen within the cortical gray matter or deep gray matter of the cerebral hemispheres. After administration of a contrast medium, plaques in the acute phase may demonstrate enhancement. Enhancement patterns vary, with none being characteristic of multiple sclerosis. High-dose contrast media have been used to increase the sensitivity of CT in the detection of multiple sclerosis plaques.[50] Steroid administration, however, suppresses the enhancement of acute multiple sclerosis plaques because of stabilization of the blood-brain barrier. With chronic multiple sclerosis, generalized cerebral atrophy may be seen as a result of extensive gliosis.

The appearance of Schilder's disease on CT scanning has been described as large confluent areas of hypodensity within the deep cerebral hemispheric white matter, particularly the centrum semiovale. These areas may show peripheral contrast enhancement.

MRI Appearance. Because MRI is the most sensitive method of evaluation for patients with multiple sclero-

sis,[48,51] it has replaced CT in the diagnosis and follow-up of patients with that disease.[47]

Multiple sclerosis lesions characteristically demonstrate T$_2$ prolongation with consequent high signal intensity of the affected areas on long TR/TE scanning sequences (Figs. 11-41 and 11-42). The plaques usually are located within the periventricular white matter (see Fig. 11-2, *B*); however, an increased number of plaques have been detected within the white matter of the cerebellum, brainstem, and spinal cord. The activity of the plaques is difficult to ascertain. With intravenous administration of gadolinium, enhancement may be seen at the site of acute demyelination with breakdown of the blood-brain barrier. Use of short inversion time (inversion recovery sequences [STIR] for evaluating the optic nerve) in patients with clinically diagnosed optic neuritis has been helpful in demonstrating the plaque responsible for the observed clinical findings (see Fig. 11-2, *A*).[52] However, visual potentials remain more sensitive than MRI for detection of optic nerve lesions.

Cerebral Neoplastic Disease

Intracranial tumors affect the visual pathway either by disruption of the neural connections or by exertion of a mass effect, which causes distortion and subsequently impairs the functioning of the visual pathway. An extensive variety of neoplasms may involve the supratentorial brain and consequently the visual pathway.

Clinical Findings. The location of a particular neoplasm within the brain often can be determined by clinical signs and symptoms. Large tumors that involve the frontal lobes and those that raise intracranial pressure result in papilledema. Hemiplegia is present if the tumor involves the primary motor cortex. Neoplasms within the parietal lobe often result in visual field defects, particularly those involving the inferior quadrant of the contralateral visual field. If the neoplasm involves the angular gyri of the dominant hemisphere, there may be an inability to recognize printed words (alexia) and an inability to write (agraphia). Within the temporal lobe, neoplasms can produce visual field defects involving the superior quadrant of the contralateral visual field. If the tumor occurs at the confluence of the dominant frontal, temporal, and parietal lobes, an expressive aphasia frequently is present. Tumors occupying the occipital lobe often cause a congruous contralateral homonymous hemianopsia. If the tumor occupies the association areas of the occipital lobe, the patient may be unable to recognize familiar people (visual agnosia). A tumor that involves the most posterior aspect of the calcarine cortex may cause a visual field defect at the point of fixation. Other clinical findings with intracranial neoplasms include morning headache, nausea, lethargy, and impaired consciousness, depending on the size and location of the tumor. Papilledema may be observed in patients with tumors anywhere in the supratentorial brain.

Pathologic Findings. A wide variety of different tumor types[53] may involve the supratentorial brain and thus the visual pathway. In general terms the tissue types may be derived from the neural glia, which includes the astrocytes and oligodendrocytes, or from the ependyma and its homologues, neurons, primitive undifferentiated cells, and meninges. The tumors may also be metastatic from other regions of the body. Tumors derived from astrocytes include astrocytomas, juvenile pilocytic astrocytomas, and oligodendrogliomas. Astrocytomas range from well-differentiated, histologically benign lesions to highly aggressive anaplastic forms such as glioblastoma multiforme. Intracranial meningiomas arise from the dura, impairing the visual pathway by exertion of mass effect. Metastatic deposits to the brain from distant primary tumors are responsible for 20% to 25% of all intracranial tumors. The most frequent cell types are bronchogenic and breast carcinomas. Metastatic foci usually are multiple and are found

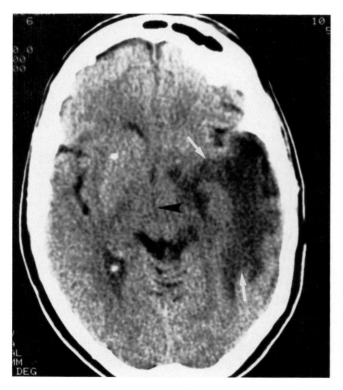

Fig. 11-43 Malignant astrocytoma and vasogenic edema. Axial plain CT shows hypodense mass *(arrows)* within left temporal lobe. Mass effect is exerted on third ventricle *(arrowhead)*.

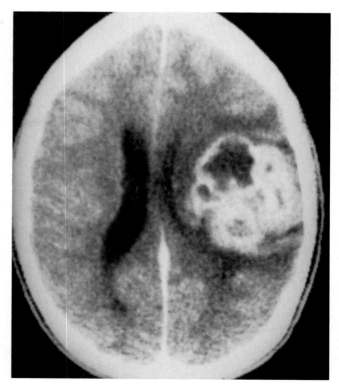

Fig. 11-44 Glioblastoma multiforme. Axial CT after injection of contrast medium shows marked enhancement of irregular mass in left frontal and parietal lobes. Body of left lateral ventricle is compressed.

most frequently at the junction of the gray and white matter. The brain tissue surrounding the metastatic focus may show a high degree of vasogenic edema. Microscopically, the metastatic foci are usually identical to the primary neoplasm.

CT Appearance. On CT, intracranial neoplasms are most often identified as mass lesions with or without contrast enhancement and with or without varying degrees of peritumoral edema. Depending on the tumor's location, there may be associated hydrocephalus or other physical distortion of the neuroaxis. Astrocytomas are usually isodense to hypodense to normal brain parenchyma on an unenhanced CT scan (Fig. 11-43). The amount of peritumoral edema frequently reflects the grade of the tumor, as does the degree of enhancement after administration of a contrast medium. More aggressive tumor types, in general, demonstrate a greater degree of enhancement and more peritumoral vasogenic edema. The glioblastoma multiforme often demon-

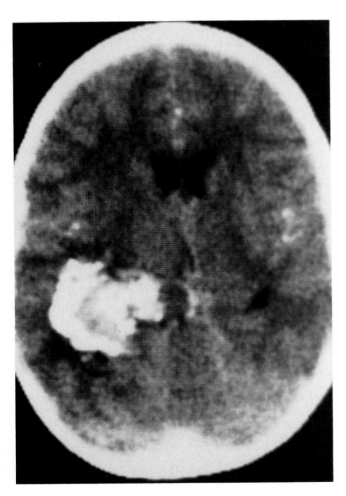

Fig. 11-45 Oligodendroglioma. Axial CT after enhancement shows dense (calcified) right temporal lobe—thalamic mass.

strates intense enhancement in a mixed or ring enhancing pattern and may have a markedly irregular margin (Fig. 11-44). Oligodendrogliomas tend to be of high density before administration of a contrast medium and to contain calcification in more than 90% of cases (Fig. 11-45). On plain CT, meningiomas are usually hyperdense relative to normal brain parenchyma. Calcification is found in approximately 20% of cases. Peritumoral edema may be present, and enhancement is usually homogeneous and intense. Metastatic lesions may be either single or multiple and vary in size.[54] From 3% to 14% of metastatic deposits contain intratumoral hemorrhage.[55] The metastatic lesions that are most prone to hemorrhage are (in descending order of likelihood) melanoma, choriocarcinoma, renal cell carcinoma, bronchogenic carcinoma, and thyroid carcinoma. Generally, metastatic lesions on an unenhanced scan are hypodense to surrounding brain unless they contain intratumoral hemorrhage. Edema is almost always present to some degree. Enhancement characteristics vary but enhancement is almost always present (97%).[54]

MRI Appearance. In general, MRI demonstrates greater sensitivity in tumor detection than does CT.[56] With the exception of the detection of calcification and bone abnormalities associated with intracranial tumors, MRI better characterizes a tumor once it is detected. With the lack of beam-hardening artifacts, direct multiplanar imaging and greater contrast sensitivity, MRI better depicts the anatomic extent of a tumor than does CT.

The appearance of the various tumor types on MRI is a function of many factors, including variations in water content, the presence or absence of hemorrhage, fat, calcification, or paramagnetic material such as melanin, and the degree of vascularity of the tumor.

Astrocytomas appear as mass lesions of high signal intensity on long TR/TE images (Fig. 11-46). Peritumoral edema may be seen as areas of high signal intensity spreading through the adjacent white matter on long TR/TE images. It is difficult to differentiate edema from a tumor solely on the basis of spin echo images (Fig. 11-46).[30] With increasing grade of the tumor, the tumor margins tend to be more irregular. Glioblastoma multiforme, which is the most anaplastic form of astrocytoma, appears as a markedly hyperintense, irregularly bordered mass lesion on long TR/TE images. Also, with increasing tumor grade there is a progressive disruption of the blood-brain barrier, which, after intravenous administration of gadolinium, results in a progressively intense T_1 shortening that is seen as an increased signal intensity on short TR/TE images (Fig. 11-47). Meningiomas demonstrate signal characteristics that reflect the amount of calcification, vascularity, and interstitial fluid present within the mass. In general, on short TR/TE images and long TR/TE images, meningiomas are isoin-

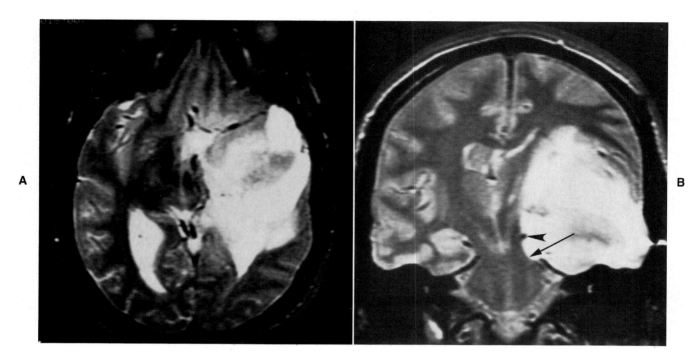

Fig. 11-46 Forty-three year-old male with malignant degeneration of low-grade astrocytoma of temporal lobe. **A,** Axial T$_2$WI shows hyperintense mass involving left temporal lobe. Edema and tumor are not separable. **B,** Coronal PDWI shows mass involving temporal lobe on left to have high signal intensity. Mass extends superiorly and medially. Tumor mass herniates *(arrow)* over free edge of tentorium and displaces medially basilar vein of Rosenthal *(arrowhead)* against mesencephalon. Optic tract is compressed.

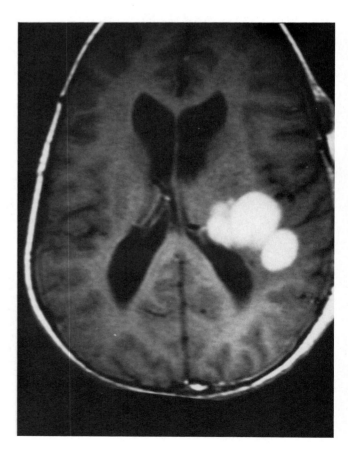

Fig. 11-47 Anaplastic astrocytoma of optic radiations. Axial T$_1$WI after administration of gadolinium shows enhancing tumor mass involving left optic radiations.

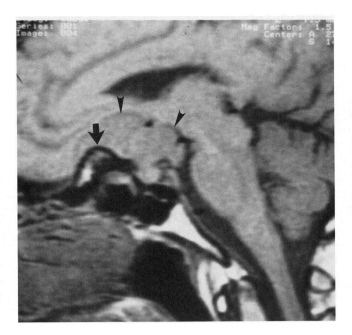

Fig. 11-48   Suprasellar planum sphenoidal meningioma. Sagittal T$_1$WI shows slightly hypointense suprasellar mass *(arrowheads)*. Hyperostosis of planum is present *(arrow)*.

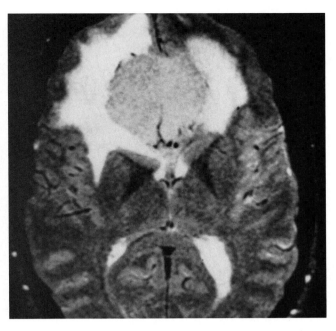

Fig. 11-49   Olfactory groove meningioma. Axial T$_2$WI shows isointense mass between frontal lobes surrounded by high-signal-intensity edema.

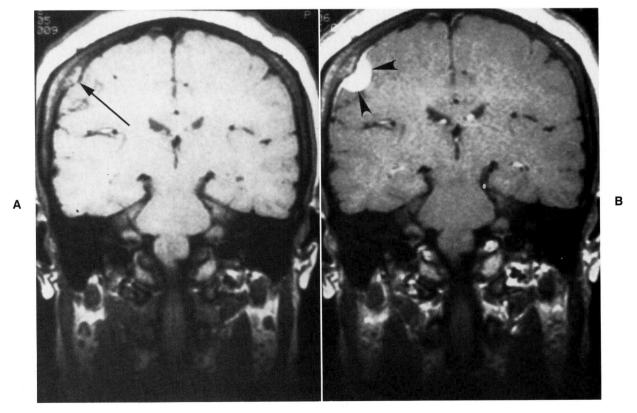

Fig. 11-50   Meningioma. **A,** Coronal T$_1$WI without gadolinium shows slight bony thickening *(arrow)* of right parietal bone. **B,** Coronal T$_1$WI with gadolinium shows intense enhancement of dural based mass *(arrowheads)* at site of bony hyperostosis.

tense to hypointense to surrounding normal brain parenchyma (Fig. 11-48). As a result of the decreased conspicuity of meningiomas on MRI, detection is based on the displacement of normal structures of the neuroaxis, including the white matter and vascular structures. On long TR / long TE images, surrounding edema helps to demarcate isointense meningiomas (Fig. 11-49). Intravenous administration of gadolinium much more clearly delineates meningiomas, since there is usually a moderate to marked homogeneous enhancement (Fig. 11-50).

Intracranial metastases display a variety of appearances on MRI. Characteristically, they appear as foci of increased signal intensity on long TR/TE images with their mass effect lying at the gray and white matter interface. Peritumoral edema is often present and may be difficult to distinguish from the tumor itself. Subtle differences in T_1 and T_2 relaxation times between the edema and the tumors may help in the differentiation; however, intravenous administration of gadolinium produces a clearer delineation. The sensitivity for detection of multiple metastatic foci is increased with the use of gadolinium, thereby increasing the certainty of the diagnosis of a metastatic cause.[57]

REFERENCES

1. Duke-Elder: System of ophthalmology, London, 1963, Henry Kimpton.
2. Newell FW: Ophthalmology: principles and concepts, St Louis, 1986, The CV Mosby Co.
3. Gray H: Anatomy of the human body, ed 29, Philadelphia, 1985, Lea & Febiger.
4. Unsold R, DeGroot J, and Newton TH: Images of the optic nerve: anatomic-CT correlation, AJNR 1:317, 1980.
5. Daniels DL et al: Computed tomography of the optic chiasm, Radiology 137:123, 1980.
6. Bilaniuk LT, Atlas SW, and Zimmerman RA: Magnetic resonance imaging of the orbit, Radiol Clin North Am 25:509, 1987.
7. Hershey BL and Peyster RG: Imaging of cranial nerve. II, Seminars in Ultrasound, CT and MR 8(3):164, 1987.
8. Albert A et al: MRI of optic chiasm and optic pathways, AJNR 7:255, 1986.
9. Daniels DL et al: Magnetic resonance imaging of the optic nerves and chiasm, Radiology 152:79, 1984.
10. Eggers H, Jakobiec FA, and Jones IS: Optic nerve gliomas. In Diseases of the orbit, New York, 1979, Harper & Row, Publishers, Inc, pp 417-433.
11. Azar-Kia B et al: Optic nerve tumors: role of magnetic resonance imaging and computed tomography, Radiol Clin North Am 25:561, 1987.
12. Naumann GOH and Atle DJ: Optic nerve. In Naumann GOH and Atle DJ, editors: Pathology of the eye, New York, 1986, Springer-Verlag New York, Inc, pp 723-770.
13. Mafee MF et al: Orbital space occupying lesion: role of computed tomography and magnetic resonance imaging, Radiol Clin North Am 25:529, 1987.
14. Sobel DF et al: MR imaging of orbital and ocular disease, AJNR 6:259, 1985.
15. Atlas SW et al: Orbit: initial experience with surface coil spin-echo MR imaging at 1.5T, Radiology 164:501, 1987.
16. Jones IS and Jacobiec FA, editors: Diseases of the orbit, New York, 1979, Harper & Row Publishers, Inc.
17. Sivony PA et al: Optic nerve sheath meningiomas: clinical manifestations, Ophthalmology 11:1313, 1984.
18. Atlas SW: Magnetic resonance imaging of the orbit: current status, Magn Reson Q 5:39, 1989.
19. Ey EH et al: Neurosarcoidosis involving optic nerves and leptomeninges: computed tomography findings, CT: J Comput Tomog 10:129, 1986.
20. Atlas SW et al: Surface coil MR of orbital pseudotumor, AJNR 8:141, 1987.
21. Wall MJ et al: A unique case of neural sarcoidosis with pineal and suprasellar involvement: CT and pathological demonstration, J Comput Assist Tomogr 9:381, 1985.
22. Mirfakhraee M et al: Virchow-Robin space: a path of spread in neurosarcoidosis, Radiology 158:715, 1986.
23. Clark WC, Acker JD, and Dohan FC: Presentation of central nervous system sarcoidosis as intracranial tumors, J Neurosurg 63:851, 1985.
24. Cooper SD et al: Neurosarcoidosis: evaluation using computed tomography and magnetic resonance imaging, CT: J Comput Tomogr 12:96, 1988.
25. Miller DH et al: Magnetic resonance imaging in central nervous system sarcoidosis, Neuroradiology 38:378, 1988.
26. Ketonen L, Oksanen V, and Kuuliaha I: Preliminary experience of magnetic resonance imaging in neurosarcoidosis, Neuroradiology 29:127, 1987.
27. Hayes WS et al: MR and CT evaluation of intracranial sarcoidosis, AJNR 8:841, 1987.
28. Kissane JM and Anderson WAD: Anderson's pathology, ed 9, St Louis, 1989, The CV Mosby Co.
29. Pusey E et al: MR of craniopharyngiomas: tumor delineation and characterization, AJNR 8:439, 1987.
30. Lee BCP and Deck MDF: Sellar and juxtasellar lesion: detection with MR, Radiology 157:143, 1985.
31. Kucharczyk W et al: Rathke cleft cysts: CT, MR imaging and pathologic features, Radiology 165:491, 1987.
32. Robbins SL, Cotran RS, and Kumar L: Pathologic basis of disease, ed 3, Philadelphia, 1984, WB Saunders Co.
33. Davis BC et al: CT surgical correlation in pituitary adenomas: evaluation in 113 patients, AJNR 6:711, 1985.
34. Davis PC et al: MR imaging of pituitary adenoma: CT, clinical, and surgical correlation, AJNR 8:107, 1987.
35. Karnaze MG et al: Suprasellar lesions: evaluation with MR imaging, Radiology 161:77, 1986.
36. Bull J: Massive aneurysms at the base of the brain, Brain 92:535, 1969.
37. Vinuela F et al: Clinico-radiological spectrum of giant super clinoid internal carotid artery aneurysms, Neuroradiology 26:93, 1984.
38. Ferguson GG: Carotid ophthalmic artery aneurysms. In Wilkins RH and Rengarchary SS, editors: Neurosurgery, New York, 1986, McGraw-Hill, Inc.
39. Deeb ZL et al: Diagnosis of bilateral intracavernous carotid artery aneurysms by computed tomography, CT: J Comput Tomogr 10:121, 1986.
40. Rhoton AL: Microsurgical anatomy of saccular aneurysms. In Wilkins RH and Rengarchary SS, editors: Neurosurgery, New York, 1986, McGraw-Hill, Inc.

41. Pinto RS et al: Correlation of computed tomographic, angiographic and neuropathological changes in giant cerebral aneurysms, Radiology 132:85, 1979.
42. Atlas SW et al: Partially thrombosed giant intracranial aneurysms: correlation of MR and pathologic findings, Radiology 162:111, 1987.
43. Olsen WL et al: Giant intracranial aneurysms: MR imaging, Radiology 163:431, 1987.
44. Unger EC et al: Acute cerebral infarction in monkeys: an experimental study using MR imaging, Radiology 162:789, 1987; AJNR 8:39, 1987.
45. Brant-Zawadzki M et al: MRI of acute experimental ischemia in cats, Am J Neuroradiol 7:7, 1985.
46. Virasponge C, Mancuso H, and Quisling R: Human brain infarcts: Gd-DTPA-enhanced MR imaging, Radiology 161:785, 1986.
47. Sheldon JJ et al: MR imaging of multiple sclerosis: comparison with clinical and CT examinations in 74 patients, AJNR 6:683, 1985.
48. Uhlenbrock D et al: MR imaging in multiple sclerosis: comparison with clinical CSF and visually evoked potential findings, AJNR 9:59, 1988.
49. Poser CM et al: Schilder's myelinoclastic diffuse sclerosis, Pediatrics 77:107, 1986.
50. Spiegel SM et al: CT of multiple sclerosis: reassessment of delayed scanning with high doses of contrast material, AJNR 6:533, 1985.
51. Paty DW et al: MRI in the diagnosis of MS: a prospective study with comparison of clinical evaluation, evoked potentials, oligoclonal banding and CT, Neurology 38:180, 1988.
52. Miller DH et al: Magnetic resonance imaging of the optic nerve in optic neuritis, Neurology 38:175, 1988.
53. Hart MN and Earle KM: Primitive neuroectodermal tumors of the brain in children, Cancer 32:890, 1973.
54. Pechova-Peterova V and Kalvach P: CT findings in cerebral metastases, Neuroradiology 28:254, 1986.
55. Atlas SW et al: Hemorrhagic intracranial malignant neoplasms: spin-echo MR imaging, Radiology 164:71, 1987.
56. Lee BCP et al: MR recognition of supratentorial tumors, AJNR 6:871, 1985.
57. Healy ME et al: Increased detection of intracranial metastases with intravenous Gd-DTPA, Radiology 165:619, 1987.

12 The Central Skull Base

IRA FRANKLIN BRAUN
LYN NADEL

SECTION ONE
INTRODUCTION TO THE CENTRAL SKULL BASE

NORMAL ANATOMY
The Sphenoid Bone

The sphenoid bone is the osseous foundation of the central skull base. This anatomically complex bone contains vital foramina that transmit important neurovascular structures, constitutes the floor of the middle cranial fossa, forms the floor of the parasellar cavernous sinuses, and contains the pituitary gland within the sella turcica. This strategically located bone and its foramina are involved by primary bone lesions, extracranial disease that extends intracranially, and intracranial disease that extends caudally through the skull base. A thorough understanding of this bony structure is essential before imaging the various disease processes that involve this region.

The shape of the sphenoid bone resembles that of a bird with outstretched wings. It consists of a central

The authors gratefully acknowledge the expert assistance provided by Mrs. Patricia Dimowski in the preparation of this chapter.

body, two sets of laterally directed wings (the greater and lesser), and two pterygoid processes, which are directed inferiorly (Fig. 12-1, *A* and *B*).

The body is cuboid and contains two air cells (the sphenoid sinuses) separated by a bony septum (Fig. 12-2). The superior surface of the body articulates anteriorly with the cribriform plate of the ethmoid, and contains a smooth central surface, the planum sphenoidale (Fig. 12-1, *B*). This portion of the sphenoid bone supports the overlying gyri recti and olfactory tracts of the base of the frontal lobes. Immediately posterior to the planum is a small bony ridge, the limbus, and behind this is the chiasmatic sulcus, which is a groovelike depression in one bone that leads laterally to the optic canals. The tuberculum sellae, another elevation of bone, is found just posterior to this sulcus. The sella turcica is situated immediately behind the tuberculum, and the thin dense bone of its anterior wall and floor is often called the lamina dura (Fig. 12-1, *B*). The middle clinoid processes, two small eminences, form the ante-

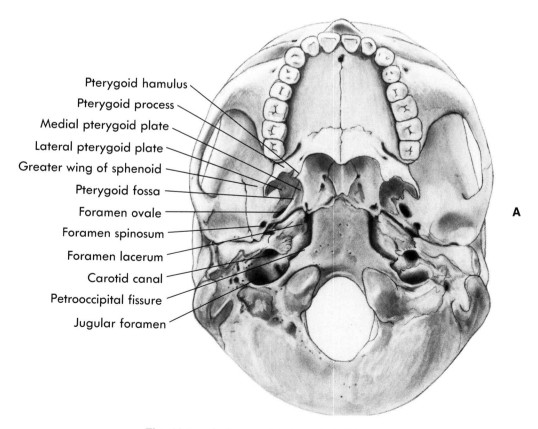

Pterygoid hamulus
Pterygoid process
Medial pterygoid plate
Lateral pterygoid plate
Greater wing of sphenoid
Pterygoid fossa
Foramen ovale
Foramen spinosum
Foramen lacerum
Carotid canal
Petrooccipital fissure
Jugular foramen

A

Fig. 12-1 **A,** Exocranial view of skull base.

rolateral boundaries of the sella; the dorsum sellae marks its posterior extent. The dorsum terminates superolaterally in the posterior clinoid processes, which provide attachment for the tentorium. The sphenoid body merges laterally with the greater wings and inferiorly with the pterygoid plates.[1]

Anteriorly, the body articulates with the perpendicular plate of the ethmoid bone. The sphenoid sinuses are contained within the body, usually divided into two separate air cells by a bony septum that is typically off center, thereby rendering the individual cells asymmetric (Fig. 12-2). The cells may extend laterally into the greater and lesser wings and into the base of the pterygoid plates. Anteriorly, each cell communicates with the nasal fossa via an opening in its upper anterior wall that leads into the sphenoethmoidal recess.

The greater wings course upwards and laterally from each side of the body (Fig. 12-1, B). Each upper or cerebral surface reflects the convolutions of the overlying brain and forms the main portion of the floor of the middle cranial fossa. The foramen rotundum, transmitting the maxillary nerve and the artery of the foramen rotundum, is found medially in the anterior portion of the greater wing. The foramen ovale is situated on the floor of the middle cranial fossa, lying posterolaterally to the foramen rotundum, and transmits the mandibular nerve, the accessory meningeal artery, and occasionally the lesser petrosal nerve. The foramen spinosum, transmitting the middle meningeal artery and meningeal branch of the mandibular nerve, is situated posterolateral to the foramen ovale (Fig. 12-1, B).[1]

A ridge is found on the lateral or exocranial surface of the greater wing; this ridge separates the wing into a superior temporal surface, which provides attachment for the temporalis muscle, and an inferior infratemporal surface, from which a portion of the lateral pterygoid muscle originates.

The orbital or anterior surface of the greater wing forms the posterior part of the lateral wall of the orbit (Fig. 12-1, B). It articulates superiorly with the orbital plate of the frontal bone and laterally with the zygomatic bone. Its inferior border forms the posterolateral margin of the inferior orbital fissure. Its medial margin forms the lateral border of the superior orbital fissure and near this margin a small tubercle arises, which provides attachment for the common tendinous ring from which the rectus muscles originate. The foramen rotundum is located below the medial end of the superior orbital fissure, and this portion of the greater wing also forms the posterior boundary of the pterygopalatine fossa.

The posteromedial edge of the greater wing extends from the body of the sphenoid laterally to the sphenoid spine, and its medial aspect forms the anterior edge of

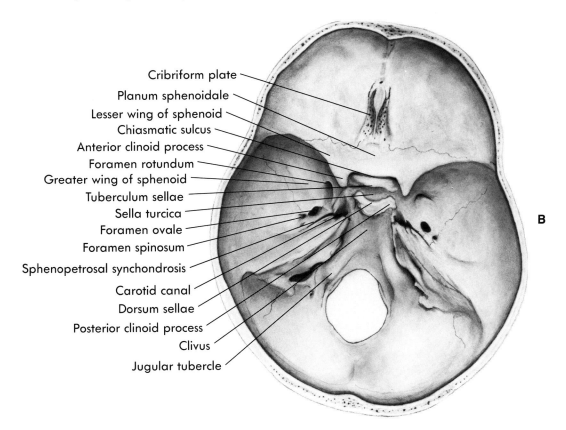

Cribriform plate
Planum sphenoidale
Lesser wing of sphenoid
Chiasmatic sulcus
Anterior clinoid process
Foramen rotundum
Greater wing of sphenoid
Tuberculum sellae
Sella turcica
Foramen ovale
Foramen spinosum
Sphenopetrosal synchondrosis
Carotid canal
Dorsum sellae
Posterior clinoid process
Clivus
Jugular tubercle

B

Fig. 12-1, cont'd   **B,** Endocranial view of skull base.

the foramen lacerum. The medial portion of the greater wing where it extends from the sphenoid spine to the body of the sphenoid forms the anterior edge of the foramen lacerum and contains the pterygoid (vidian) canal in the base of the pterygoid plates. The vidian canal transmits the corresponding vidian nerve and artery. The more lateral portion of the posterior edge of the greater sphenoid wing articulates with the petrous portion of the temporal bone via the sphenopetrosal synchondrosis (Fig. 12-1, *B*).[1]

The lesser wings are paired triangular bones that project laterally from the upper anterior parts of the body and end laterally in sharp points. Each lesser wing articulates anteriorly with the posterior edge of the orbital plate (roof) of the frontal bone. The lesser wing has a smooth superior surface, which is situated beneath a small portion of the frontal lobe, and an inferior surface, which forms not only the posterior roof of the orbit, but also the upper boundary of the superior orbital fissure. On the medial posterior aspect of the lesser wings are the anterior clinoid processes, which together form the anterior attachment of the tentorium (Fig. 12-1, *B*). The anterior and middle clinoid processes on each side are bridged by a fold of dura that occasionally ossifies forming the caroticoclinoid foramen, through which the carotid artery runs. The optic canal, transmitting the optic nerve and ophthalmic artery, traverses the medial attachment of the lesser wing to the body of the sphenoid.[1]

The triangular superior orbital fissure is bounded medially by the body of the sphenoid, above, by the lesser wing and below by the medial margin of the orbital surface of the greater wing. This fissure narrows laterally as the greater and lesser sphenoid wings converge. Through the fissure courses the oculomotor (III), trochlear (IV), and abducens (VI) nerves; the orbital branch of the middle meningeal artery; various sympathetic filaments of the internal carotid plexus; the recurrent meningeal branches of the lacrimal artery; and the ophthalmic veins.

The pterygoid processes descend from the undersurface of the medial aspects of the greater sphenoid wings, one on each side. Each pterygoid process is composed of a medial and lateral pterygoid plate, the upper parts of which are fused anteriorly (Fig. 12-1, *A*). The pterygoid fossa lies between these plates and is formed as the plates diverge posteriorly (Fig. 12-1, *A*). From the fossa arises the medial pterygoid muscle. The anterior surface of the pterygoid process forms the posterior boundary of the pterygopalatine fossa.

The lateral pterygoid plate forms a portion of the medial wall of the infratemporal fossa and provides attachment for the lateral pterygoid muscle; its medial surface forms the lateral wall of the pterygoid fossa, providing attachment for the medial pterygoid muscle (Fig. 12-1, *A*). The superior aspect of its anterior border forms the posterior boundary of the pterygomaxillary fissure.

The medial pterygoid plate terminates inferiorly in a hooklike process, the pterygoid hamulus, around which the tendon of the tensor veli palatini is slung. The lateral surface of the medial plate forms the medial wall of the pterygoid fossa (Fig. 12-1, *A*). The pharyngobasilar fascia is attached to the posterior margin of the medial plate; the superior pharyngeal constrictor takes origin more inferiorly.

Basal Foramina

Foramen Rotundum. The foramen rotundum, which is actually a canal in the base of the greater sphenoid wing, is situated just inferiorly and laterally to the superior orbital fissure (Fig. 12-1, *B*). The medial rim of the foramen may share a common wall with the lateral aspect of the sphenoid sinus, or occasionally the entire foramen may be situated within the sphenoid sinus itself. The canal extends obliquely forward away from the midline and slightly downward, connecting the middle cranial fossa to the pterygopalatine fossa.[2] It transmits the maxillary nerve (V2), the artery of the foramen rotundum, and emissary veins. This foramen is best visualized using coronal CT.

The maxillary nerve supplies sensation to the skin of the midface, lower eyelid, upper lip, mucosa of the nasopharynx, maxillary sinus, upper gums, and teeth. The artery of the foramen rotundum arises as a terminal branch of the internal maxillary artery within the pterygopalatine fossa, coursing alongside the maxillary nerve. It is an important anastamotic pathway between the cavernous branches of the internal carotid artery and the internal maxillary artery.[3]

Foramen Ovale. The foramen ovale, situated in the medial aspect of the greater wing of the sphenoid, transmits the mandibular nerve (V3), emissary veins, and the accessory meningeal artery from the middle cranial fossa to the infratemporal fossa. Endocranially it is situated posterolaterally to the posterior aspect of foramen rotundum (Fig. 12-1, *B*); exocranially it is found at the base of the lateral pterygoid plate (Fig. 12-1, *A*). The normal size of this foramen varies considerably, not only from patient to patient, but also from side to side in the same individual.[2] This foramen can be visualized on both axial and coronal CT, whereas the soft tissue lesions traversing it are best imaged using coronal MRI.

The mandibular nerve is both motor and sensory; it gives motor supply to the muscles of mastication and gives sensation to the skin over the temporal region, lower face, lips, gums, mandible, temporomandibular joints, and a portion of the dura. The motor root exits the skull base medially to the larger sensory root, both uniting exocranially in the region of the otic ganglion.

The accessory meningeal artery, supplying the pharynx, eustacian tube, and meninges, arises either from the middle meningeal artery directly, or from the internal maxillary artery, just distal to the middle meningeal. It courses anterior to the mandibular nerve as it extends through the foramen to supply the trigeminal ganglion, the lateral walls of the cavernous sinus, and the anterosuperior surface of the petrous temporal bone.[3]

Foramen Spinosum. The foramen spinosum connects the middle cranial fossa to the infratemporal fossa and is found on the posteromedial aspect of the greater sphenoid wing. Situated just posterolaterally to the foramen ovale on the endocranial aspect of the skull base (Fig. 12-1, B) and just anteriorly and laterally to the eustacian tube exocranially (Fig. 12-1, A). It transmits the middle meningeal artery, vein, and the recurrent branch of the mandibular nerve. The sphenoid spine is situated on the posterolateral border of the foramen (Fig. 12-1, A).[2] This foramen is best visualized radiographically using axial CT.

The middle meningeal artery arises from the proximal portion of the internal maxillary artery and ascends to enter the skull base through the foramen. It supplies the dura of the convexity, falx, and orbital roof and a variable portion of the infratentorial dura.[3] The foramen spinosum may be tiny or absent when the middle meningeal artery originates from the ophthalmic artery.

Foramen of Vesalius. This inconstant opening, connecting the middle cranial fossa to the scaphoid fossa (near the origin of the tensor veli palatini muscle), is situated anteromedially to the foramen ovale. The foramen of Vesalius is present in up to 22% of skulls,[2] transmits an emissary vein, and can be visualized with axial CT.

Foramen Lacerum. The exocranial aspect of this aperture (Fig. 12-1, A), which is not in reality a foramen, is covered with fibrocartilage. It is located at the base of the medial pterygoid plate, bounded anterolaterally by the greater wing of the sphenoid, posteriorly by the petrous apex, and medially by the sphenoid body and basiocciput. The pterygoid (vidian) canal opens posteriorly at the anterior aspect of the foramen lacerum; the rostral end of the carotid canal is found posteriorly.

The carotid artery is not transmitted through the canal as was formerly believed but rests on the endocranial aspect of the fibrocartilage that forms its floor.[2] An inconstant meningeal branch of the ascending pharyngeal artery[3] and the nerve of the pterygoid canal (vidian) actually pierce the cartilage and are therefore the only structures contained in the foramen.[2] The foramen lacerum may be visualized on axial and coronal CT and MRI.

Pterygoid (Vidian) Canal. The pterygoid (vidian) canal, which transmits the vidian artery and nerve, is situated in the base of the pterygoid plates below and me-

dial to the foramen rotundum in the body of the sphenoid bone. It may be located in the floor of the sphenoid sinus. It connects the pterygopalatine fossa anteriorly to the foramen lacerum posteriorly. This canal is best visualized on axial and coronal CT.

The nerve of the pterygoid (vidian) canal is the continuation of the greater superficial petrosal nerve after its union with the deep petrosal nerve. The greater superficial petrosal nerve is a preganglionic parasympathetic branch of the facial nerve, emanating from the genu. The deep petrosal nerve is a sympathetic branch from the carotid plexus. Following its exit from the canal the vidian nerve enters the sphenopalatine ganglion and provides autonomic supply to the lacrimal gland and mucous membranes of the nose, pharynx, and palate.[2]

The vidian artery, a branch of the terminal portion of the internal maxillary artery, arises in the pterygopalatine fossa, curves around the sphenopalatine foramen, and passes through the vidian canal posteriorly along the nerve of the same name. It supplies the mucosa of the nasopharynx, the sphenopalatine ganglion, and a portion of the auditory tube, where it terminates at its pharyngeal end.[3] Because of its proximity to the foramen lacerum, this vidian artery often provides important collateral supply to the internal carotid artery.

Pituitary Gland

The pituitary gland, continuous with the apex of the infundibulum, lies in the hypophyseal fossa and is covered by a circular fold of dura, the diaphragma sellae. The cavernous sinus borders the gland on each side (Fig. 12-2). The gland is divided into two main regions based on different embryological, morphological, and functional characteristics. The anteriorly located adenohypophysis is subdivided into a pars anterior and a pars intermedia, which are separated by the hypophyseal cleft, a vestige of a diverticulum of ectodermal tissue (Rathke's pouch) from which the adenohypophysis develops.[4] This cleft usually disappears during childhood, but remnants may persist as small cystic cavities in the center of the gland. The posterior neurohypophysis includes the median eminence, the infundibular stem, and the main posterior lobe. Both the adenohypophysis and the neurohypophysis include a portion of the infundibulum.

The diaphragma sellae is a sheetlike extension of the tentorium that extends from the posterior clinoid processes to the anterior clinoid processes. In this diaphragm is a hole through which the pituitary infundibulum extends down into the sella turcica.

Cavernous Sinuses

The cavernous sinuses (Fig. 12-2) are situated on each side of the body of the sphenoid bone, extend

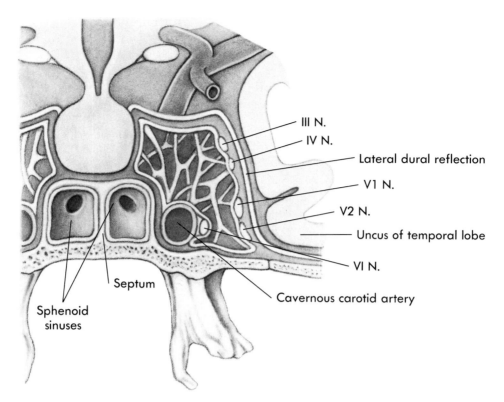

Fig. 12-2 Coronal view of the region of cavernous sinus.

from the superior orbital fissure anteriorly to the petrous apex posteriorly, and have an average length of 2 cm and width of 1 cm.[5] The internal carotid artery, suspended by fibrous trabeculae and surrounded by a sympathetic plexus, courses through the sinuses; abducens nerve is inferolateral to the artery. Proceeding superiorly to inferiorly, the oculomotor nerve, the trochlear nerve, and the ophthalmic and maxillary divisions of the trigeminal nerve are each contained within separate fibrous sheaths within the lateral wall of the cavernous sinuses. Endothelium separates these structures from the venous blood contained in the sinuses. The pituitary fossa above and sphenoid sinuses below are both medial to the cavernous sinuses. Meckel's cave, enclosing the trigeminal ganglion, is situated at the posteroinferior aspect of the sinuses.[5] The uncus of the temporal lobe is also related to the lateral sinus wall.

The superior ophthalmic veins, the superficial, middle, and inferior cerebral veins, and the sphenoparietal sinus are all tributaries of the cavernous sinuses. These drain into the transverse sinus via the superior petrosal sinus and into the internal jugular vein via the inferior petrosal sinus. Additional inferior drainage is into the pterygoid venous plexus via veins that pass through the emissary sphenoidal foramen, via the foramen ovale and foramen lacerum, and into the facial vein via the superior ophthalmic vein. Communication between the two cavernous sinuses is maintained by means of ante-

rior and posterior intercavernous sinuses and the basilar venous plexus situated on the clivus. Blood flow through the cavernous sinuses is attributed to the pulsatile arterial flow through the carotid artery and to the gravitational effects secondary to varying head position.[5]

Clivus

The clivus is that part of the skull base situated between the foramen magnum and the dorsum sellae. Most authors consider it to include both the basioccipital portion of the occipital bone and the body of the sphenoid bone.[6] Anterolaterally the clivus is bounded by the petrooccipital fissure, whereas more posteriorly there is the synchondrosis between the basioccipital and exoccipital portions of the occipital bone. The upper anterior margin of the clivus blends into the body of the sphenoid and the sphenoid sinus; below it slopes gently posteroinferiorly to merge with the anterior foramen magnum (Fig. 12-1, *A* and *B*). Inferiorly it is bounded by the nasopharynx. Two ridges, the jugular tubercles, are found along the lower lateral margins of the clivus, overlying the hypoglossal canals.

The inferior petrosal sinuses are found along the lateral border of the clivus, and a clival plexus of veins, frequently seen during angiography, lies on its endocranial aspect. The belly of the pons and medulla are also closely related to this clival surface.

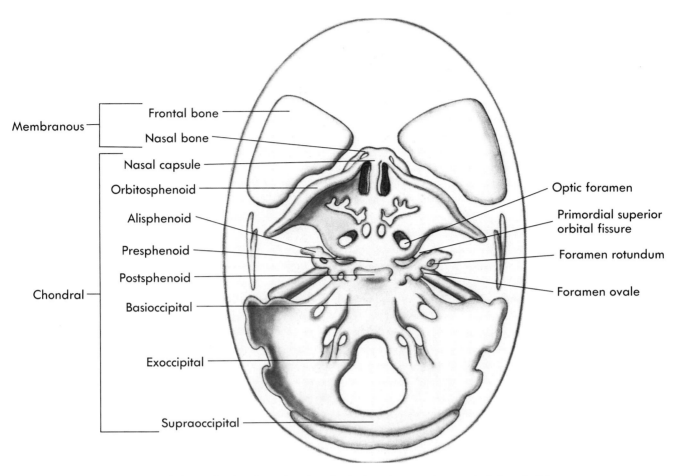

Fig. 12-3   Schematic drawing of embryological endocranial aspect of the skull base. (From Warwick R and Williams PL, editors: Gray's anatomy, ed 35 (Br), Philadelphia, 1973, WB Saunders Co.)

EMBRYOLOGY

The bones of the skull base are derived from cartilaginous precursors, known as the chondrocranium, whereas the phylogenetically newer calvarial bones, covering the newly expanded cerebral hemispheres, are formed from membrane (Fig. 12-3).[7] The chondrocranium also gives rise to the special sensory organs of hearing and olfaction. The growth and development of the skull base is closely coordinated with that of the face and cranial vault.

During the fourth week of gestation the formation of the ectomere capsule heralds the development of the skull. Mesenchymal condensation occurs between the developing forebrain and gut. By this time, initial development of the brain, cranial nerves, eyes, and blood vessels has already occurred.[7] The development of the cartilaginous skull base begins at around the 40th day of gestation by the conversion of mesenchyme into cartilage. This mesenchyme surrounds the developing notochord to form a floor for the base of the brain.

The notochordal plate develops cranial to the primi-

tive streak early in the third week of intrauterine life. During the fifth week of intrauterine life the notochord becomes enclosed by the bodies of the upper cervical vertebra and the basiocciput. It then lies directly in contact with the endoderm of the embryonic pharynx and finally terminates in the body of the sphenoid, just caudally to the pituitary fossa (Fig. 12-4). As development proceeds, the notochord becomes divided into segments and its only normal representation in the adult is the nucleus pulposus.

The cartilaginous masses that envelop the notochord are called the parachordal cartilages. The rostral termination of the notochord is situated immediately adjacent to the oropharyngeal membrane that closes off the stomadeum. Just rostral to this, the hypophyseal (Rathke's) pouch gives rise to the anterior pituitary or adenohypophysis, which therefore lies immediately rostral to the termination of the notochord (Fig. 12-4).[7]

The initially separate centers of cranial base chondrification fuse into a single, irregular, and greatly perforated *basal plate*.

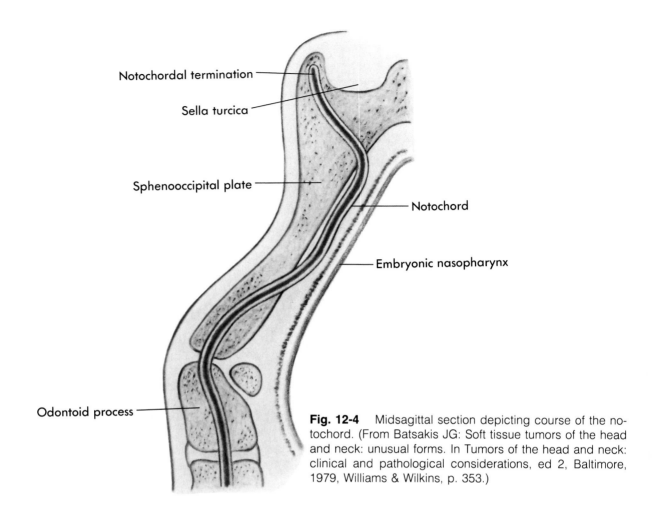

Notochordal termination

Sella turcica

Sphenooccipital plate

Notochord

Embryonic nasopharynx

Odontoid process

Fig. 12-4 Midsagittal section depicting course of the notochord. (From Batsakis JG: Soft tissue tumors of the head and neck: unusual forms. In Tumors of the head and neck: clinical and pathological considerations, ed 2, Baltimore, 1979, Williams & Wilkins, p. 353.)

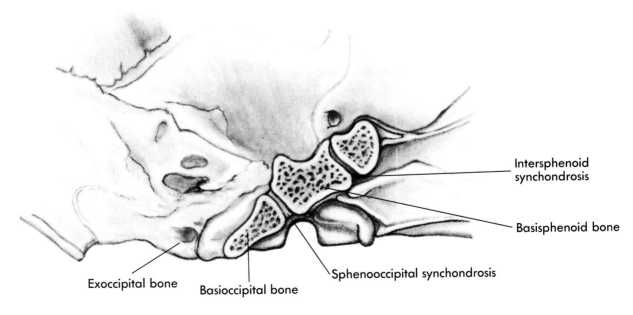

Intersphenoid synchondrosis

Basisphenoid bone

Exoccipital bone

Basioccipital bone

Sphenooccipital synchondrosis

Fig. 12-5 Midsagittal section of skull base in a newborn.

The basisphenoid (Fig. 12-5), the central cartilaginous precursor of the body of the sphenoid bone, is formed via fusion of the two lateral hypophyseal cartilages containing and surrounding the developing pituitary gland. Just rostral to this, two cartilages fuse to form the presphenoid (Fig. 12-3), which develops into the anterior part of the sphenoid bone. At the same time, laterally, there is fusion of the precursors of the lesser (orbitosphenoid) and the greater (alisphenoid) wings of the sphenoid bone. Preexisting blood vessels and cranial nerves determine the position and existence of the basal foramina both in the cartilaginous precursor and in the final bony skull base.

The optic foramen is formed as the orbitosphenoid cartilage joins the rostral part of the basal plate to surround the preexisting optic nerve and ophthalmic artery. The space between the orbitosphenoid and alisphenoid becomes the superior orbital fissure as the oculomotor and trochlear nerves, the ophthalmic division of the trigeminal nerve, and the ophthalmic veins course through it (Fig. 12-3).[7] The junction of the alisphenoid and the basal plate is perforated by the maxillary division of the trigeminal nerve to form the foramen rotundum, and by the mandibular division to form the foramen ovale. The middle meningeal artery perforates this region and forms the foramen spinosum. The foramen lacerum is formed by the persistence of cartilage between the ossification centers of the alisphenoid and the petrous apex; the carotid canal is formed by ossification around the artery at the junction of the alisphenoid, basal plate, and petrous apex.[7]

Centers of ossification within the basal plate, commencing with the basioccipital in the tenth intrauterine week, lay the basis for the enchondral bone portions of the occipital, sphenoid, and temporal bones and for the wholly endochondral ethmoid and inferior nasal conchae.[7]

Up to 15 separate endochrondral and intramembranous ossification centers compose the sphenoid bone. The greater wing of the sphenoid and the lateral pterygoid plate are derived from intramembranous ossification, whereas the medial plate, in the region of the foramen rotundum, originates from cartilage. The lesser wing (orbitosphenoid), a portion of the greater wing (alisphenoid), and the anterior (presphenoid) and the posterior (postsphenoid) parts of the body of the sphenoid bone are formed from cartilage. The presphenoid, with which the lesser wings are continuous, forms the body of the sphenoid anterior to the tuberculum; the postsphenoid, which is associated with the greater wings and pterygoid plates, forms the sella, dorsum, and basisphenoid.[7] The pharyngohypophyseal track (of Rathke's pouch), which gives rise to the anterior lobe of the pituitary, is obliterated by the postsphenoid ossification centers. In 0.4% of postnatal skulls, a persistent craniopharyngeal canal exists, which forms the basis of congenital craniopharyngeal tumors.[7] The synchondrosis (intersphenoid) between the presphenoid and the postsphenoid (Fig. 12-5) fuses shortly before birth, whereas the base of the pterygoid plates surround the vidian canal and fuse with the postsphenoid in the immediate postnatal period.

The skull base expands via growth of endochrondral remnants and because of forces applied to the growing sutures by the expanding brain. Growth takes place via appositional addition to sutural edges and separation at synchondroses. The sphenooccipital synchondrosis (Fig. 12-5), the last one to fuse, is primarily responsible for the growth of the skull base in the postnatal period. In summary, the entirety of the skull base, except for the orbital plates of the frontal bones and the most lateral parts of the greater wing of the sphenoid, is preformed in cartilage, whereas the remainder of the cranial vault undergoes membranous ossification.[7]

Portions of the chondrocranium (unossified cartilage) exist at birth, including, in the body of the sphenoid, the sphenooccipital and sphenopetrous junctions and the foramen lacerum at the petrous apex.[8] At birth the sphenoid is composed of three parts: the central part, consisting of the body and lesser wings, and two lateral parts, each made up of a greater wing and pterygoid process. Subsequently, in the first postnatal year, the greater wings and body fuse around the vidian canal, and the lesser wings fuse medially above the anterior part of the body to form an elevated smooth surface, the planum sphenoidale. The sphenoid and occipital bones are completely fused by the twenty-fifth year of life.[9]

The following illustrations (Figs. 12-6 to 12-12) are MRI and CT scans that demonstrate radiographic anatomy of the skull base.

Text continued on p. 895.

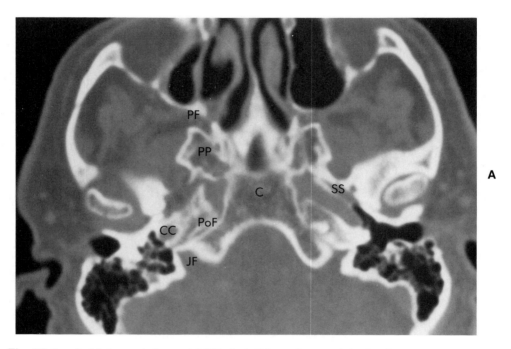

Fig. 12-6   A, High resolution axial CT of skull base in an adult. Sections are arranged from caudal, **A,** to rostral, **E.** *PF,* Pterygopalatine fossa; *PP,* pterygoid process; *SS,* sphenopetrosal synchondrosis; *C,* clivus; *PoF,* petrooccipital fissure; *CC,* carotid canal; *JF,* jugular fossa.

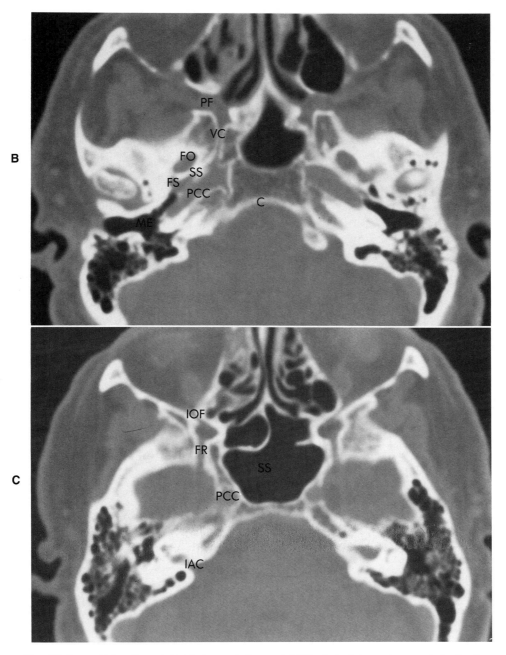

Fig. 12-6, cont'd   B and **C,** High resolution axial CT of skull base in an adult. Sections are arranged from caudal, **A,** to rostral, **E. B,** *PF,* Pterygopalatine fossa; *VC,* vidian canal; *FO,* foramen ovale; *SS,* sphenopetrosal synchondrosis; *FS,* foramen spinosum; *PCC,* petrous portion carotid canal; *ME,* middle ear; *C,* clivus. **C,** *IOF,* Inferior orbital fissure; *FR,* foramen rotundum; *SS,* sphenoid sinus; *PCC,* precavernous portion carotid canal; *IAC,* internal auditory canal.   *Continued.*

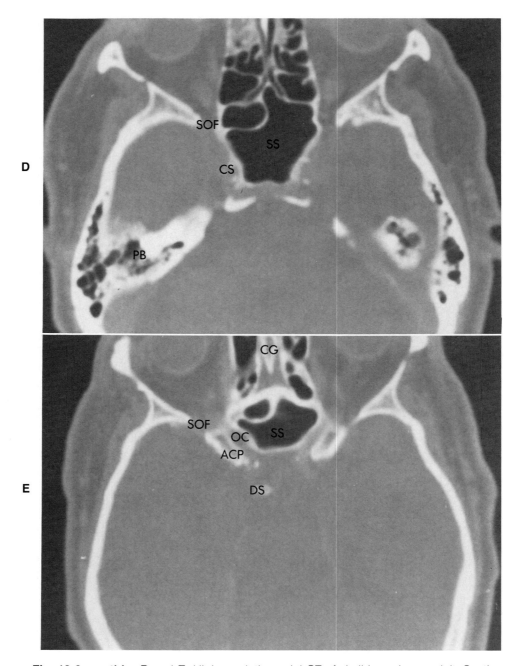

Fig. 12-6, cont'd **D** and **E,** High resolution axial CT of skull base in an adult. Sections are arranged from caudal, **A,** to rostral. **E. D,** *SOF,* Superior orbital fissure; *SS,* sphenoid sinus; *CS,* cavernous sinus; *PB,* petrous bone. **E,** *CG,* Crista galli; *SOF,* superior orbital fissure; *OC,* optic canal; *ACP,* anterior clinoid process; *SS,* sphenoid sinus; *DS,* dorsum sellae.

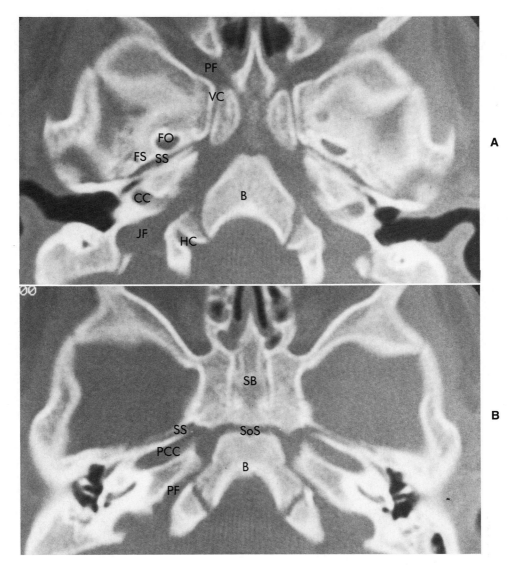

Fig. 12-7   **A** and **B,** Axial CT of the skull base in a 2-year-old child. **A,** *PF,* Pterygopalatine fossa; *VC,* vidian canal; *FO,* foramen ovale; *SS,* sphenopetrosal synchondrosis; *FS,* foramen spinosum; *CC,* carotid canal; *B,* basiocciput; *JF,* jugular fossa; *HC,* hypoglossal canal. **B,** *SB,* Body of sphenoid bone (basisphenoid); *SoS,* sphenooccipital synchondrosis; *SS,* sphenopetrosal synchondrosis; *PCC,* petrous portion carotid canal; *B,* basiocciput; *PF,* petrooccipital fissure.

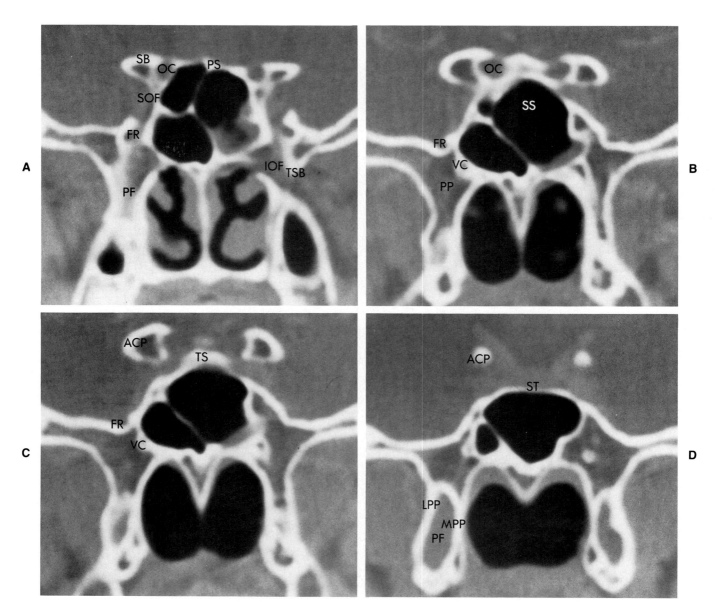

Fig. 12-8 **A** to **D,** High resolution coronal CT through skull base. Sections are arranged from anterior, **A,** to posterior, **G. A,** *PS,* Planum sphenoidale; *OC,* optic canal; *SB,* lesser wing of sphenoid bone; *SOF,* superior orbital fissure; *FR,* foramen rotundum; *IOF,* inferior orbital fissure; *TSB,* tubercle of sphenoid bone; *PF,* pterygopalatine fossa. **B,** *OC,* Optic canal; *SS,* sphenoid sinus; *FR,* foramen rotundum; *VC,* vidian canal; *PP,* pterygoid process. **C,** *ACP,* Anterior clinoid process; *TS,* tuberculum sellae; *FR,* foramen rotundum; *VC,* vidian canal. **D,** *ACP,* Anterior clinoid process; *ST,* floor to sella turcica; *LPP,* lateral pterygoid plate; *MPP,* medial pterygoid plate; *PF,* pterygoid fossa.

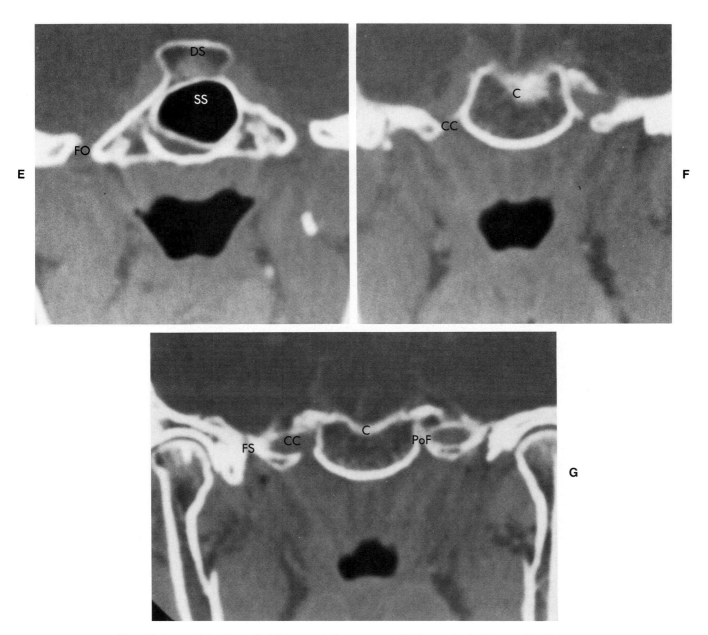

Fig. 12-8, cont'd   E to **G,** High resolution coronal CT through skull base. Sections are arranged from anterior, **A,** to posterior, **G. E,** *DS,* Dorsum sellae; *SS,* sphenoid sinus; *FO,* foramen ovale. **F,** *C,* Clivus; *CC,* carotid canal. **G,** *C,* Clivus; *CC,* horizontal petrous portion carotid canal; *FS,* foramen spinosum; *PoF,* petrooccipital fissure.

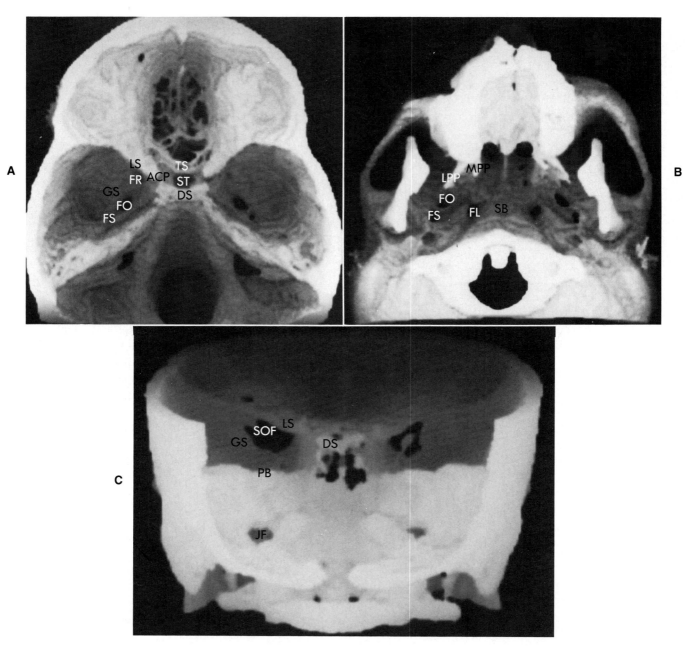

Fig. 12-9   A, Endocranial view of three-dimensional CT of the skull base. *TS,* Tuberculum sellae; *ACP,* anterior clinoid process; *LS,* lesser wing of sphenoid; *FR,* foramen rotundum; *ST,* sella turcica; *GS,* greater wing of sphenoid; *FO,* foramen ovale; *FS,* foramen spinosum; *DS,* dorsum sellae. **B,** Exocranial view of three-dimensional CT of the skull base. *MPP,* Medial pterygoid plate; *LPP,* lateral pterygoid plate; *FO,* foramen ovale; *FS,* foramen spinosum; *FL,* foramen lacerum; *SB,* body of sphenoid bone. **C,** View of three-dimensional CT of the skull base from behind. *LS,* Lesser wing of sphenoid bone; *SOF,* superior orbital fissure; *GS,* greater wing of sphenoid bone; *DS,* dorsum sellae; *PB,* petrous bone; *JF,* jugular foramen.

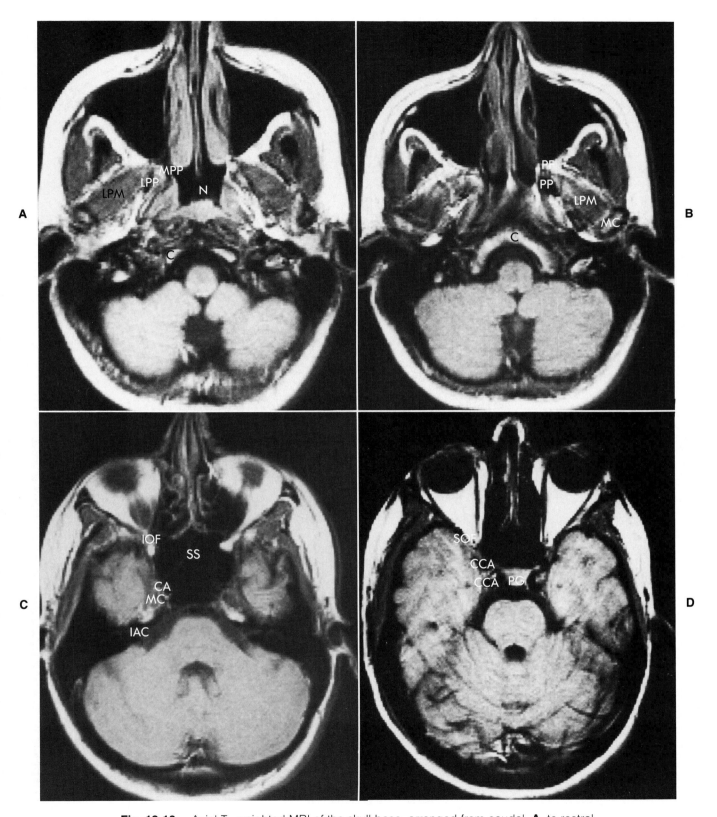

Fig. 12-10 Axial T₁-weighted MRI of the skull base, arranged from caudal, **A,** to rostral, **D. A,** *MPP,* Medial pterygoid plate; *LPP,* lateral pterygoid plate; *LPM,* lateral pterygoid muscle; *N,* nasopharynx; *C,* clivus. **B,** *PF,* Pterygopalatine fossa; *PP,* pterygoid process; *LPM,* lateral pterygoid muscle; *MC,* mandibular condyle; *C,* clivus. **C,** *IOF,* Inferior orbital fissure; *SS,* sphenoid sinus; *CA,* carotid artery; *MC,* Meckel's cave; *IAC,* internal auditory canal. **D,** *SOF,* Superior orbital fissure; *CCA,* cavernous carotid artery; *PG,* pituitary gland.

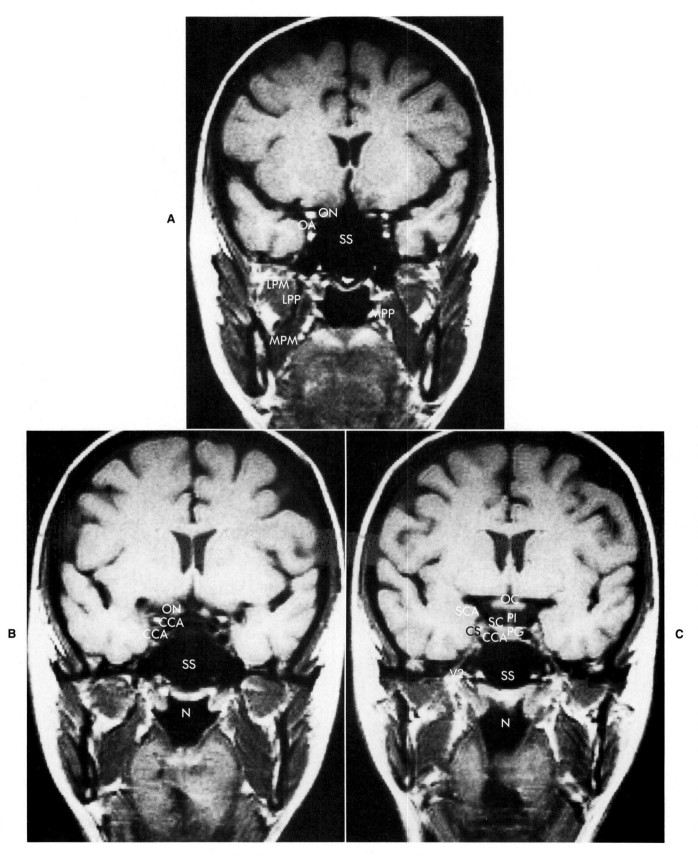

Fig. 12-11 For legend see opposite page.

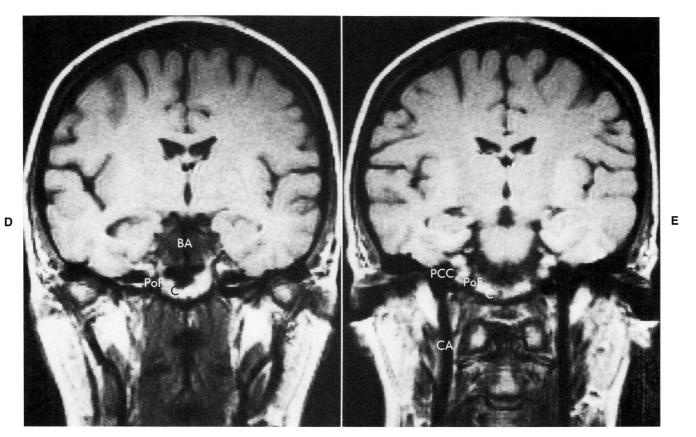

Fig. 12-11 Coronal T$_1$-weighted MRI of the skull base arranged from anterior, **A,** to posterior, **E. A,** *ON,* Optic nerve; *OA,* orbital apex; *SS,* sphenoid sinus; *LPM,* lateral ptery-goid muscle; *LPP,* lateral pterygoid process; *MPP,* medial pterygoid process; *MPM,* me-dial pterygoid muscle. **B,** *ON,* Optic nerve; *CCA,* cavernous carotid artery; *SS,* sphenoid sinus; *N,* nasopharynx. **C,** *OC,* Optic chiasm; *PI,* pituitary infundibulum; *SCA,* supracli-noid carotid artery; *SC,* suprasellar cistern; *CS,* lateral dural reflection of cavernous sinus; *CCA,* cavernous carotid artery; *PG,* pituitary gland; *V2,* V2 in foramen ovale; *SS,* sphe-noid sinus; *N,* nasopharynx. **D,** Coronal T$_1$-weighted MRI of the skull base arranged from anterior, **A,** to posterior, **E. D,** *BA,* Basilar artery; *PoF,* petrooccipital fissure; *C,* clivus. **E,** *PCC,* Petrous portion carotid canal; *C,* clivus; *CA,* carotid artery.

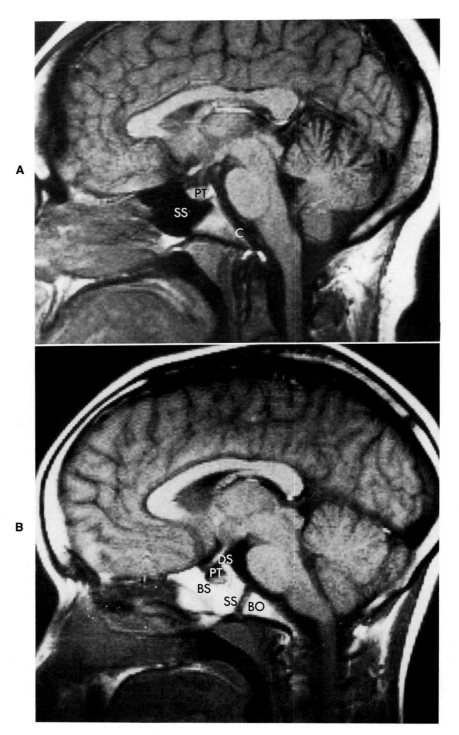

Fig. 12-12 **A,** Midline sagittal T₁-weighted MRI of skull base in an adult. *PT,* Pituitary within sella turcica; *SS,* sphenoid sinus; *C,* clivus. **B,** Midline sagittal T₁-weighted MRI of skull base in a child. *DS,* Dorsum sellae; *PT,* pituitary within sella turcica; *BS,* basisphenoid; *SS,* sphenooccipital synchondrosis; *BO,* basiocciput.

REFERENCES

1. Warwick R and Williams PL, editors: Gray's anatomy, ed 35 (Br), Philadelphia, 1973, WB Saunders Co, pp 288-291.
2. Sondheimer FK: Basal foramina and canals. In Newton TH and Potts DG, editors: Radiology of the skull and brain, New York, 1971, The CV Mosby Co, pp 287-347.
3. Djindjian R and Merland JJ: Super-selective arteriography of the external carotid artery, Berlin, 1978, Springer-Verlag, pp 24-25.
4. See reference 1, pp 1367-1371.
5. See reference 1, pp 695-696.
6. Coin CG and Malkasian DR: Clivus. In Newton TH and Potts DG, editors: Radiology of the skull and brain, New York, 1971, The CV Mosby Co, pp 348-356.
7. Sperber GH: Craniofacial embryology, Boston, 1981, Wright, pp 87-101.
8. See reference 1, p 115.
9. See reference 1, p 291.

SECTION TWO
IMAGING

IMAGING TECHNIQUES
CT Technique

The skull base is evaluated in both the axial and coronal planes. A slice thickness of 1.5 to 3 mm is used. For bone detail only, a high resolution bone algorithm is employed with a wide window setting (4000 HU). If soft tissue contrast is needed in addition to bone information, IV contrast is necessary. The axial study is performed in the plane of Reid's baseline, parallel to a line drawn from the infraorbital rim to the external auditory canal. Scans are obtained from the level of the foramen magnum to that of the suprasellar cistern. Direct coronal images are obtained perpendicular to Reid's baseline. If dental amalgam causes significant artifact in the direct coronal plane or if the patient cannot tolerate the coronal head position, reconstructed images can be obtained from thin (1.5 to 2 mm) axial scans.

Alternately, semicoronal scans can be obtained at an angle between 60 to 80 degrees of Reid's baseline. These scans can be angled either in front of or behind the amalgams and, although not completely coronal in orientation, they usually offer complementary information to the axial study.

MRI Technique

The skull base is imaged using a standard head coil. The routine examination consists of imaging in the midsagittal, axial, and coronal planes. T_1-weighted images are obtained with a TR of 600 to 1000 ms and TE of 17 to 20 ms for anatomic definition. A slice thickness of 3 to 5 mm is used. A midsagittal image is first obtained, which serves both as a "scout" view and to show the midline superior and inferior extent of disease. Because of the confusing aspects of anatomy, most often little use is made of parasagittal sections. Axial images are obtained from the suprasellar cistern to the nasopharynx. The axial study is usually repeated after the intravenous administration of gadolinium-DTPA (0.1 mM/ kg). Coronal images are then obtained from the anterior aspect of the sphenoid sinus to the foramen magnum.

T_2/proton density weighted sequences are usually of less value in examining the skull base because they add significant time to the total examination and the additional soft tissue contrast obtained can be achieved in most cases with the shorter gadolinium-DTPA–enhanced T_1-weighted sequence. If a T_2/proton density weighted spin echo sequence is desired, a TR of 2000 to 3000 ms is employed with echoes of TE 20 to 45/80 to 100 ms.

SECTION THREE
NONNEOPLASTIC DISORDERS

CONGENITAL AND DEVELOPMENTAL ANOMALIES
Arachnoid Cyst

Primary or congenital arachnoid cysts are developmentally abnormal arachnoid and collagen-lined cavities that are filled with CSF and that characteristically do not communicate with the ventricular system. They account for 1% of intracranial space–occupying lesions,[1] and usually appear in the first five decades of life.[2] Males are affected more commonly than females.

These lesions are developmental abnormalities of the subarachnoid space. During initial development there are no subarachnoid spaces, only loose mesenchyme, and all of the CSF is contained within the ventricular system.[3] It is hypothesized that as pulsations of the CSF force fluid into the subarachnoid space during normal development, the CSF becomes entrapped between the developing pia and arachnoid.[4]

These cysts may expand progressively during antenatal development and their most common location is in the middle cranial fossa. The exact mechanism of this enlargement is unknown, although many theories have been proposed.[4]

The CSF within the cyst has sectional imaging characteristics similar to those of intraventricular CSF on both CT and MRI. Bony changes of the skull base are better appreciated with CT and include thinning of the temporal bone, elevation of the lesser wing of the sphenoid, and anterior displacement of the greater sphenoid wing (Fig. 12-13).[2] These changes are more easily perceived with larger lesions.

Cephaloceles

Cephaloceles can occur anywhere in the cranial vault but are most commonly found in the midline, at the vertex, or in the skull base. The term describes a pro-

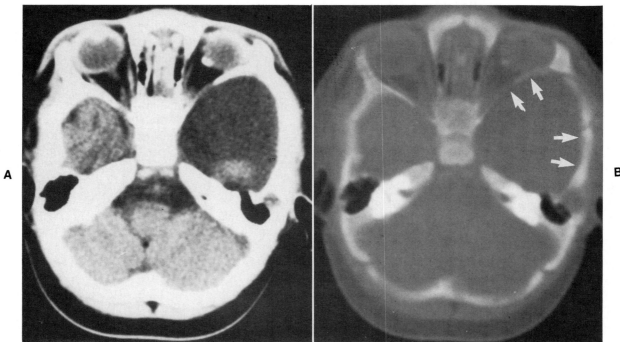

Fig. 12-13 7-year-old female with left-sided retinoblastoma with incidental arachnoid cyst. Axial CT slices through skull base obtained using **A,** soft tissue technique and **B,** bone technique reveal the presence of expanded middle cranial fossa on the left. This is associated with outward bowing of the squamous portion of the temporal bone and anterior displacement of the greater wing of the sphenoid *(arrows)*. The attenuation of the cyst material is similar to that of CSF.

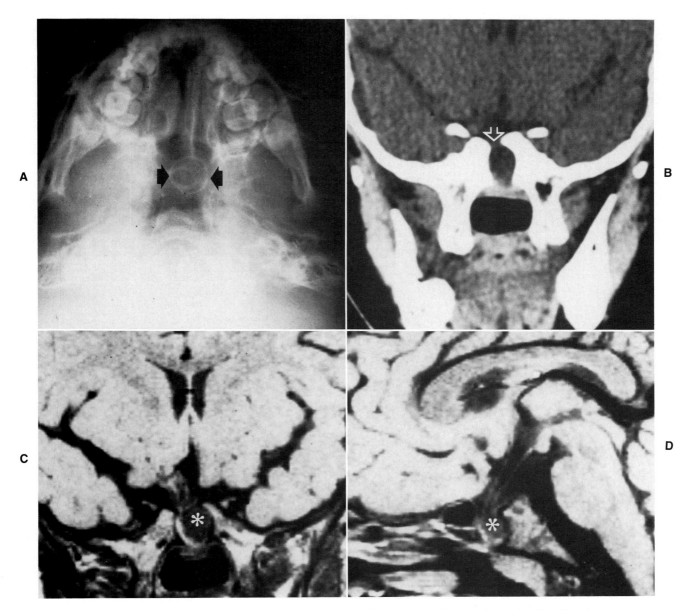

Fig. 12-14   8-year-old child who presents with recurrent bouts of meningitis. Basal cephalocele with persistent craniopharyngeal canal. **A,** Plain film of the skull, submento-vertex view. A well defined lucency surrounded by a thin rim of cortical bone is projected over the skull base *(arrows).* **B,** Coronal noncontrast CT scan through central skull base reveals presence of a persistent craniopharyngeal canal *(arrow)* in the sphenoid bone. **C,** Coronal and **D,** midsagittal T_1-weighted images through central skull base demonstrate herniation of the pituitary gland *(asterisk)* into the craniopharyngeal canal through the sphenoidal defect. Note the proximity of the pituitary gland to the roof of the nasopharynx. (Case courtesy of Dr. Das Narla.)

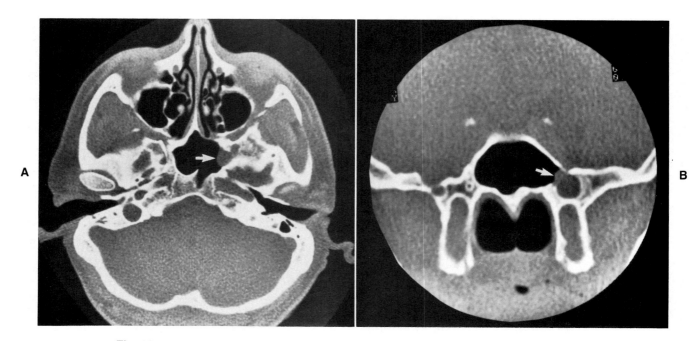

Fig. 12-15 35-year-old male who was found to have an incidental mass within his sphenoid sinus on a computed tomographic study performed for headache. Biopsy proven encephalocele. **A,** Axial and **B,** coronal computed tomography through central skull base and sphenoid sinus reveals the presence of a soft tissue mass within the left sphenoid sinus. The mass involves the base of the pterygoid plates on the left in the region of the vidian canal. A smooth, well-circumscribed defect in the bone is appreciated consistent with a benign process.

trusion of intracranial contents through a congenital, usually midsagittal defect in the calvarium and dura. If the cephalocele involves only meninges and subarachnoid space, it is called a meningocele. If, however, the defect contains brain as well, it is called an encephalocele. Cephaloceles, most of which occur sporadically, are estimated to be present in one in every 4000 births.[5] They comprise 10% to 20% of all craniospinal malformations, and most are thought to represent a failure of neural tube fusion at the level of the anterior neuropore on approximately the twenty-fifth day of gestation.[6] Extension of cephaloceles through the sphenoid bone, however, has been attributed to the persistence of the craniopharyngeal canal,[7] which is thought to be secondary to blood vessels that course through the sphenoid bone during development (Fig. 12-14).[8] A second cause is a developmental failure of the multiple and complex sphenoid ossification centers allowing herniation to occur through the resultant defect (Fig. 12-15).[7]

The dura usually is continuous with the periosteum of the external opening of the defect.[9] The external aspect of the cephalocele may be covered by various tissues depending on the origin and location of the specific calvarial defect. The covering can be derived from skin or mucous membrane from the nose, paranasal sinuses, or nasopharynx.[9] The area of bony dehiscence usually occurs at a suture or in an area where several bones coalesce. The aperture is smooth and defined by a rim of cortical bone. The defect may also arise in an area where ossification centers of a single bone, such as the sphenoid, unite (Fig. 12-15).

Of all encephaloceles, 10% occur in the region of the skull base (basal), 75% develop in the occipital region, and 15% arise around the nose and orbit. Basal cephaloceles can be grouped into five major categories[7]: (1) Sphenopharyngeal, in which the defect exists in the sphenoid bone and the cephalocele extends into the pharynx. If the herniated tissue only extends into the sphenoid sinus, then this subtype is termed transsphenoidal. (2) Sphenoorbital, which extends through the superior orbital fissure resulting in unilateral exophthalmos. This type is most commonly associated with neurofibromatosis. (3) Sphenoethmoidal, which extends through the sphenoid and ethmoid bones, appearing as a posterior nasal cavity mass. (4) Transethmoidal, which occurs in the cribriform plate, resulting in an anterior nasal fossa mass. (5) Sphenomaxillary, a theoretical type never documented clinically. Patients with basal cephaloceles may also have midface anomalies such as

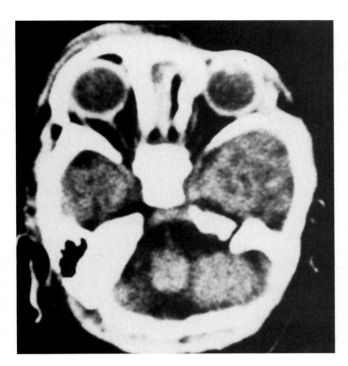

Fig. 12-16 Left unilateral coronal synostosis. Axial CT scan through skull base in an 18-month-old child with unilateral left coronal synostosis revealing the typical bulging calvarium in the region of the sphenozygomatic suture associated with a fullness of the middle cranial fossa on the left. Also note the resultant orbital deformity with associated decrease in the transverse dimension of the orbit.

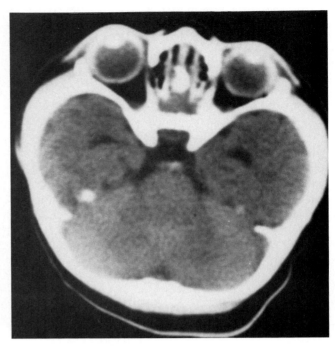

Fig. 12-17 Bilateral coronal synostosis. Axial CT scan through skull base in a 2-year-old child revealing changes typical of coronal synostosis, including bilateral calvarial bulging of the region of the sphenozygomatic suture and fullness of the both middle cranial fossae.

hypertelorism, broad nasal root, and cleft palate and lip. Various other congenital anomalies, including agenesis of the corpus callosum, have also been reported.[10]

A cephalocele may appear as a mass in the nose, nasopharynx, mouth, or posterior orbit. The most common type of basal cephalocele is the sphenopharyngeal, presenting as a pharyngeal mass, which may cause airway obstruction and act as a pathway for the development of CSF rhinorrhea and meningitis. Indeed, recurrent bacterial meningitis in a child with a normal immune system should occasion the search for a cephalocele.[9] Various cephaloceles may also appear with symptoms referable to the central nervous system. Sphenopharyngeal (also known as sincipital) cephaloceles may include frontal lobe involvement, whereas herniation of the hypothalamus and optic pathways may accompany the transethmoidal, sphenoethmoidal, and sphenonasopharyngeal varieties.[6]

Before the availability of CT imaging, the diagnosis of cephaloceles depended on the plain film recognition of a defect in the skull base, associated with a soft tissue mass. The defects usually were quite large in order to be so recognized. Base views of the skull, along with soft tissue studies of the nasopharynx, perhaps followed by tomography, were the modalities available for the

noninvasive diagnosis; angiography and pneumoencephalography were reserved for outlining the neural component of the lesion.

CT of the skull base now clearly shows the bony margins of the defect, as well as the soft tissue component of the lesion. Although cerebral angiography may be required to further define the contents of a cephalocele, the instillation of a low dose of intrathecal contrast before CT may aid in distinguishing a simple meningocele from an encephalocele. In the instance of an encephalocele, cortical sulci bathed in contrast material would be evident. The intrathecal instillation of a low dose of non-ionic contrast agent, in conjunction with a CT study, is the method of choice in the evaluation of the patient with a CSF leak.

MRI is obviating the necessity for the more invasive procedures needed in the evaluation of the soft tissue component of the lesion. In fact, MRI presently is the best modality for identifying the presence of brain tissue in a cephalocele (Fig. 12-14).

Craniosynostosis

The cranial sutures, which, when unfused, permit expansion of the cranial vault to accommodate the growing brain, normally begin to fuse by the age of 3 years, and usually completely fuse by the age of 6 years.[11] Premature fusion, or craniosynostosis, prevents normal growth and development of the brain and can cause permanent neurologic damage. Skull base deformities may be seen in addition to the usual calvarial abnormalities that accompany this condition.[12]

Unilateral coronal synostosis produces marked changes in the skull base, including anterior ipsilateral displacement of the sphenoid wing and petrous ridge, pterional thickening, and forward displacement and foreshortening of the bony orbit (Fig. 12-16). The resultant intracranial abnormalities include a smaller ipsilateral anterior cranial fossa and a bulging calvarium in the region of the sphenozygomatic suture associated with a full middle cranial fossa. In instances of bilateral coronal synostosis, these changes are seen bilaterally (Fig. 12-17). These findings are clearly evident on axial CT studies obtained through the skull base.

REFERENCES

1. Meche FGA and van der Braakman R: Arachnoid cysts in the middle cranial fossa: cause and treatment of progressive and nonprogressive symptoms, J Neurol Neurosurg Psychiatry 46:1102, 1983.
2. Sato K et al: Middle fossa arachnoid cyst: clinical, neuroradiological, and surgical features, Child's Brain 10:301, 1983.
3. James HE: Encephalocele, dermoid sinus, and arachnoid cyst. In McLaurin RL et al, editors: Pediatric neurosurgery, ed 2, Philadelphia, 1989, WB Saunders Co, pp 97-105.
4. Naidich TP, McLone DG, and Radkowski MA: Intracranial arachnoid cysts, Pediatr Neurosci 12:112, 1985-86.
5. Batsakis JG: Other neuroectodermal tumors and related lesions of the head and neck. In Tumors of the head and neck: clinical and pathological considerations, ed 2, Baltimore, 1979, Williams & Wilkins, p 334.
6. See reference 3, pp 97-106.
7. Pollock JA, Newton TH, and Hoyt WF: Transphenoidal and transethmoidal encephaloceles: a review of clinical and roentgen features in eight cases, Radiology 90:442, 1968.
8. Lowman RM, Robinson F, and McAllister WB: The craniopharyngeal canal, Acta Radiol (Diagn) 5:41, 1966.
9. Nager GT: Cephaloceles, Laryngoscope 97:77, 1987.
10. Sadeh M et al: Basal encephalocele associated with suprasellar epidermoid cyst, Arch Neurol 39:250, 1982.
11. Laurent JP and Cheek WR: Craniosynostosis. In McLaurin RL et al, editors: Pediatric neurosurgery, ed 2, Philadelphia, 1989, WB Saunders Co, pp 107-119.
12. Carmel PW, Luken MG III, and Ascherl GF Jr: Craniosynostosis: computed tomographic evaluation of skull base and calvarial deformities and associated intracranial changes, Neurosurg 9:366, 1981.

SECTION FOUR
TRAUMA

FRACTURES

Skull base fractures most commonly occur as extensions of cranial vault fractures.[1] These fractures may occur in a direct and isolated fashion or more commonly are the result of stress forces occurring on the basal foramina. Indirect forces transmitted from the mandible or vertebral column can also play contributing roles. The most common locations affected include the petrous temporal bone, the orbital surface of the frontal bone, and the basiocciput.[2] These fractures are typically difficult to recognize on plain film radiography and are usually suspected clinically when one or more of the following signs are present: CSF otorrhea or rhinorrhea, hemotympanum, mastoid region ecchymosis (Battle's sign), periorbital ecchymoses (raccoon eyes), or cranial nerve deficits. Anosmia and cavernous carotid fistula can also occur (Fig. 12-18).[3]

Fractures of the sphenoid bone are usually associated with other craniofacial injuries most commonly occurring with maxillary and zygomatic fractures. The sphenoid bone is involved in approximately 15% of patients with skull base fractures.[4]

Although the sphenoid bone appears to be relatively well protected by its position in the central skull base, it is actually quite vulnerable to fracture, for the lines of force can extend through its multiple osseous attachments.[4] Additionally, many muscles either insert into or take origin from the sphenoid, making muscular dysfunction an important sequela of trauma. Problems with ocular motility, mastication, speech, swallowing, and eustachian tube function may be seen.[4] The many neurovascular structures that either traverse the sphenoid or lie adjacent to it are also particularly vulnerable to injury.

The traumatic forces applied to the skull are presumably transmitted centrally to the sphenoid bone. An anterior impact causes maxillary, sphenoid, and pterygoid plate fractures. Lateral trauma results in zygomatic and sphenoid wing fractures.[4]

Trauma to the body of the sphenoid may result in a CSF leak with or without optic nerve damage associated with an optic canal fracture. Optic nerve injury may result from mechanical crush, concussion, hemorrhage, or frank tear.[5] This diagnosis should be sug-

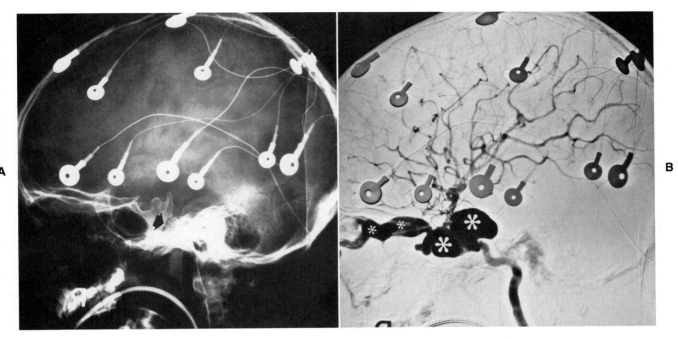

Fig. 12-18 23-year-old male who presents with pulsatile exophthalmos and decreased visual acuity following a motorcycle accident. Skull base fracture with resultant cavernous carotid fistula. **A,** Lateral plain film revealing the presence of a fracture *(arrow)* involving the sphenoid bone and clivus. **B,** Lateral subtraction view of an internal carotid artery angiogram revealing findings typical of a cavernous carotid fistula. Contrast from the arterial system has extravasated into the cavernous sinus *(large asterisks)* and subsequently into the superior ophthalmic vein *(small asterisks)*. Transmitted arterial pressure to the venous system in the superior ophthalmic vein causes the pulsatile exophthalmos.

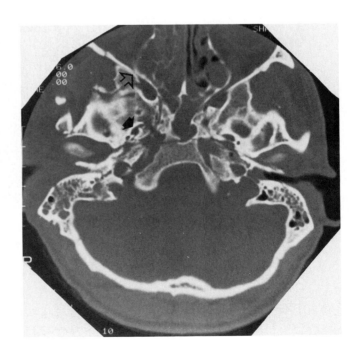

Fig. 12-19 23-year-old male following automobile accident presents with superior orbital fissure syndrome and multiple cranial nerve deficits. Multiple skull base fractures. Axial CT scan through the skull base revealing the presence of multiple fractures associated with fluid in the ethmoid and sphenoid sinuses. Multiple fractures causing narrowing of the orbital apex and superior orbital fissure *(open arrow)* are appreciated as well as a fracture involving the foramen ovale *(black arrow)*.

gested when the patient experiences sudden or progressive visual loss following trauma. Visual loss associated with an identifiable fracture in the region of the optic canal is strongly suggestive of optic nerve injury.[5]

In instances of sphenoid wing fracture, patients usually have various combinations of motor and sensory disturbances referable to the regional cranial nerves. Foramen ovale involvement could result in sensory disturbances in the course of V3, along with loss of motor function in the muscles of mastication (Fig. 12-19). Superior orbital fissure trauma could result in the superior orbital fissure syndrome, which in more extreme cases could consist of a dilated pupil, ptosis, and extraocular muscle dysfunction.[4]

Abnormalities of mastication should be expected with fractures of the pterygoid plates and associated injury to the regional musculature. Dysphagia, caused by compromise of the superior constrictor and tensor veli palatini, can also be seen. Additionally, eustachian tube dysfunction can result in a middle ear effusion (serous otitis).

Axial, thin slice, high resolution CT is the obvious method of choice for the initial evaluation of patients with skull base fractures. In instances of suspected CSF leak, a study using water soluble intrathecal contrast to define the leak is indicated (see following discussion of CSF fistula).

CSF FISTULA

The most common cause of CSF fistula is skull base trauma, occurring in 2% of unselected head injuries.[6] Nontraumatic CSF leaks are much less common and may persist for years, whereas the traumatic variety usually resolves within 1 week. The onset of a CSF leak usually occurs within 48 hours of trauma; the leak is usually unilateral, and anosmia is a concomitant symptom in 78% of cases. The risk of infection is high, with infection occurring in 25% to 50% of untreated cases.[6]

Fractures that pass through the frontoethmoidal complex and middle cranial fossa are those most commonly associated with CSF leaks. A temporal bone fracture passing parallel to the long axis of the petrous bone commonly results in CSF otorrhea. CSF flow is usually scanty, with profuse leakage being unusual. This contrasts with the spontaneous nontraumatic variety of CSF leakage, in which CSF flow is usually profuse. Tumors, especially those arising in the pituitary gland, are the most common causes of nontraumatic CSF leakage,

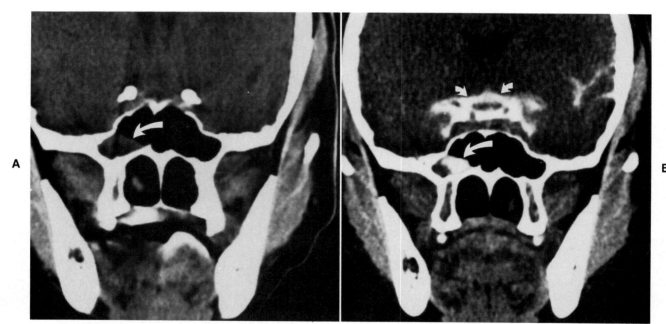

Fig. 12-20 25-year-old male status post head trauma with persistent CSF rhinorrhea and recurrent meningitis. Traumatic cerebrospinal fluid fistula demonstrated by water soluble contrast cisternography. Coronal CT through the sphenoid sinus obtained **A,** prior to and **B,** following the intrathecal instillation of water soluble contrast material. A soft tissue density is appreciated involving the right lateral floor of the sphenoid sinus (curved arrow) as seen on the study prior to the instillation of contrast material. Following the instillation of contrast, increased density is appreciated in this region consistent with the accumulation of contrast, documenting the presence of a CSF fistula. Also noted is the presence of contrast material within the suprasellar cistern (small curved arrows) outlining the chiasm and vascular structures. The fracture site was not identified.

with congenital anomalies, such as encephaloceles, being the next most common causes.[6]

Precise localization of the site of CSF leakage is mandatory before any surgical intervention. Because CT cisternography can more accurately demonstrate the site of injury, it has replaced radioisotopic studies as the modality of choice when evaluating a patient with a CSF leak.[7] These procedures are usually successful in demonstrating the fistula only if the patient is actively leaking at the time of the study. In the CT examination, a precontrast study is obtained using a high resolution, thin section technique in the coronal plane. The study is centered either through the cribriform plate or through the sphenoid sinus, depending on the area of clinical interest. The study is scrutinized for area(s) of bony dehiscence. A small volume of intrathecal contrast is then instilled into the lumbar subarachnoid space, and the patient is restudied in a similar fashion. The precontrast and postcontrast examinations are compared to determine if there are any density differences that could be due to the contrast leakage (Fig. 12-20).

REFERENCES

1. Gurdjian ES and Webster JE: Head injuries: mechanisms, diagnosis, and management, Boston, 1958, Little, Brown & Co, p 76.
2. McLaurin RL and McLennan JE: Diagnosis and treatment of head injury in children. In Youmans JR, editor: Neurological surgery, ed 2, Philadelphia, 1982, WB Saunders Co, pp 2084-2136.
3. Thomas LM: Skull fractures. In Wilkins RH and Rengachary SS, editors: Neurosurgery, New York, 1985, McGraw-Hill Book Co, pp 1623-1626.
4. Ghobrial W, Amstutz S, and Mathog RH: Fractures of the sphenoid bone, Head Neck Surg 8:447, 1986.
5. Manfredi SJ et al: Computerized tomographic scan findings in facial fractures associated with blindness, Plast Reconstr Surg 68:479, 1981.
6. Ommaya AK: Cerebrospinal fluid fistula. In Wilkins RH and Rengachary SS, editors: Neurosurgery, New York, 1985, McGraw-Hill Book Co, pp 1637-1647.
7. Drayer BP et al: Cerebrospinal fluid rhinorrhea demonstrated by metrizamide CT cisternography, AJR 129:149, 1977.

SECTION FIVE
TUMORS AND TUMORLIKE CONDITIONS

BENIGN TUMORS
Juvenile Angiofibroma

The angiofibroma is a highly vascular, locally invasive lesion that originates either in the nasopharynx or posterior nares of adolescent males. This lesion commonly spreads through the central skull base to involve the middle cranial fossa. It accounts for approximately 0.5% of all head and neck neoplasms[1] and is the most common benign tumor of the nasopharynx.[2] Patients usually have nasal obstruction, recurrent and severe epistaxis, and less commonly facial deformity. The site of origin is usually broad based and can involve the adjacent posterolateral wall of the nasal cavity. The lesion, on presentation, may be unilateral or may entirely fill the nasopharynx.

Extranasopharyngeal spread at the time of presentation is common. These lesions usually extend into the infratemporal fossa via the pterygopalatine fossa and in so doing anteriorly displace the posterior wall of the maxillary antrum. Once the tumor gains access to the pterygopalatine fossa it may spread to the orbit via the inferior orbital fissure and thence into the middle cranial fossa via the superior orbital fissure, considered to be the major route of intracranial spread. Sphenoid sinus invasion is present in nearly two thirds of the cases as the lesion erodes the floor of this sinus (Figs. 12-21 and 12-22). Angiofibromas may spread through the natural ostia of the regional paranasal sinuses to involve them as well. Extension through the skull base into the cavernous sinus can be perceived angiographically as this tumor parasitizes blood supply from the dural branches of the cavernous carotid artery (Fig. 12-22). Although histologically benign, the lesion can be highly aggressive and locally invasive.

This neoplasm has an intermediate signal intensity on T_1-weighted images, compared to the relatively hyperintense fat and the relatively low signal intensity of muscle (Fig. 12-23). Discreet punctate or serpentine areas of hypointensity, representing the vascular flow voids of the larger tumor vessels, can be seen. This MRI appearance is similar to that observed with paragangliomas and other highly vascular neoplasms.[3] Although small areas of bony destruction are difficult to recognize on MRI, the soft tissue mass itself and the extent of its anatomic involvement are most easily assessed using MRI (Fig. 12-23).[4]

Meningioma

Meningiomas, typically benign tumors that arise from arachnoidal cells of the meninges, usually occur in adults between the ages of 20 to 60 years and account

Text continued on p. 908

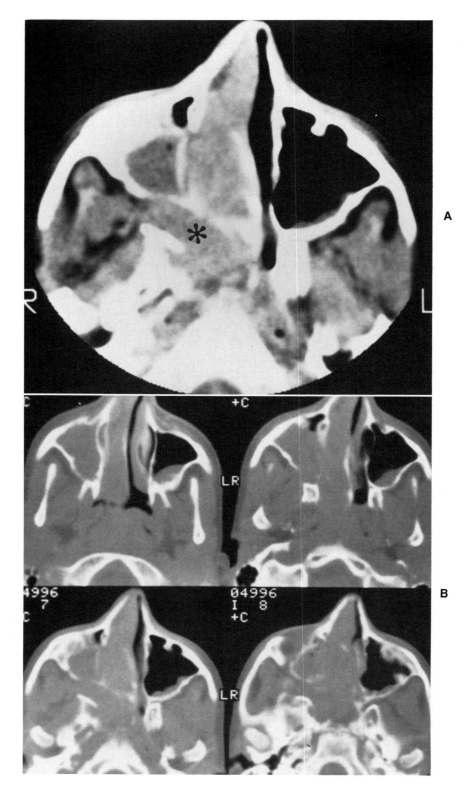

Fig. 12-21 For legend see opposite page.

C

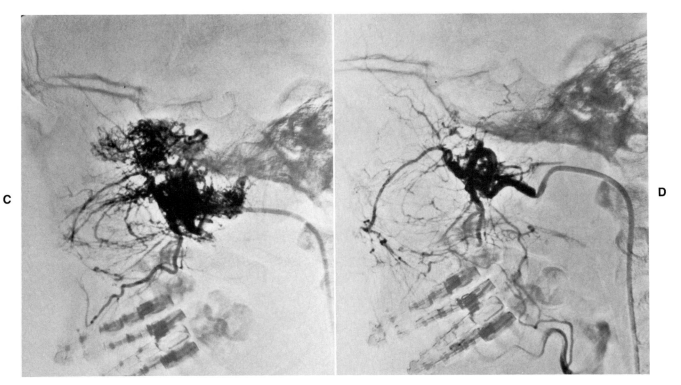

D

Fig. 12-21   17-year-old male who presented with nasal stuffiness and epistaxis. Juvenile nasopharyngeal angiofibroma. **A,** Axial contrast enhanced CT scan revealing the presence of hyperdense tumor causing expansion of the pterygopalatine fossa *(asterisk)* and involving the base of the pterygoid plates. Tumor extends anteriorly into the nasal fossa. **B,** Axial images through the skull base revealing bony destruction of the base of the sphenoid bone. Lateral, subtraction angiography of the internal maxillary artery. **C,** Preembolization angiogram reveals the typical hypervascularity of this neoplasm demonstrated in the subselective internal maxillary artery angiogram. **D,** Following embolization normal vascularity is appreciated. The lesion was removed with minimal blood loss.

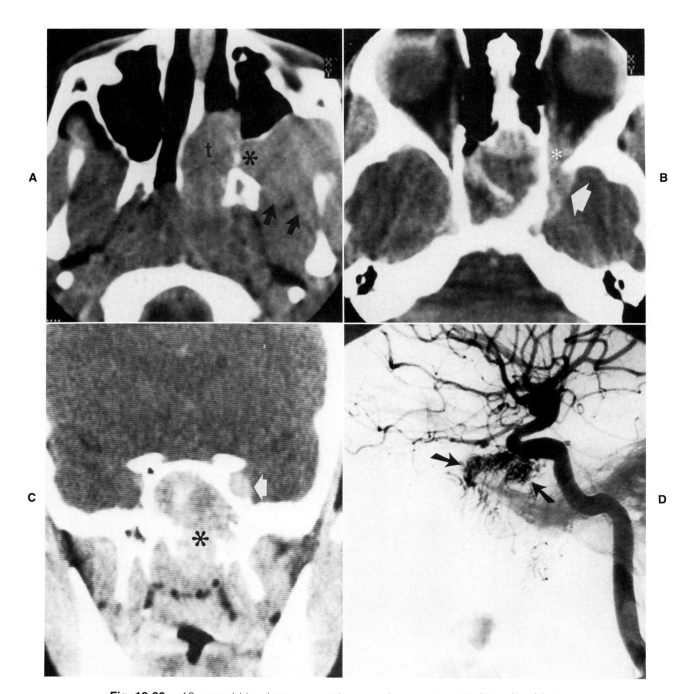

Fig. 12-22 12-year-old in whom a nasopharyngeal mass was noted at adenoidectomy. Juvenile nasopharyngeal angiofibroma. **A,** Axial CT scan demonstrating the presence of a tumor within the left nasal fossa *(t)* with extension through the widened pterygopalatine fossa *(asterisk)* into the infratemporal fossa laterally *(arrows)*. Note the characteristic anterior displacement of the posterior wall of the maxillary antrum. **B,** Axial contrast enhanced CT scan obtained through the skull base demonstrates enhancing tumor within the orbital apex *(asterisk)* and left cavernous sinus *(arrow)*. Destruction of the central skull base is also appreciated. **C,** Coronal contrast enhanced study reveals the presence of tumor extending through the skull base *(asterisk)* into the sphenoid sinus with extension into the cavernous sinus *(arrow)*. **D,** Lateral subtraction view of an internal carotid artery angiogram reveals the presence of supply to this juvenile angiofibroma via dural branches of the cavernous carotid artery *(arrows)*, consistent with tumor invasion of the cavernous sinus.

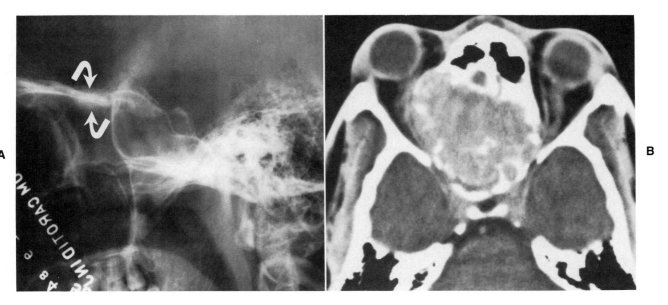

Fig. 12-23   14-year-old male presenting with recurrent epistaxis. Juvenile nasopharyngeal angiofibroma. **A,** Midsagittal and **B,** parasagittal T₁-weighted MRIs demonstrating the presence of a large mass in the nasal fossa and nasopharynx *(af)* with growth posteriorly and destruction of the base of the sphenoid bone *(asterisk)* with involvement of the sphenoid sinus. The parasagittal image reveals the mass coursing up to the region of the cavernous carotid artery *(arrows)* within the cavernous sinus. The signal intensity is intermediate compared to fat and muscle. (Used with permission from Braun IF: MRI of the nasopharynx, Radiol Clin North Am 27(2): 315, 1989.)

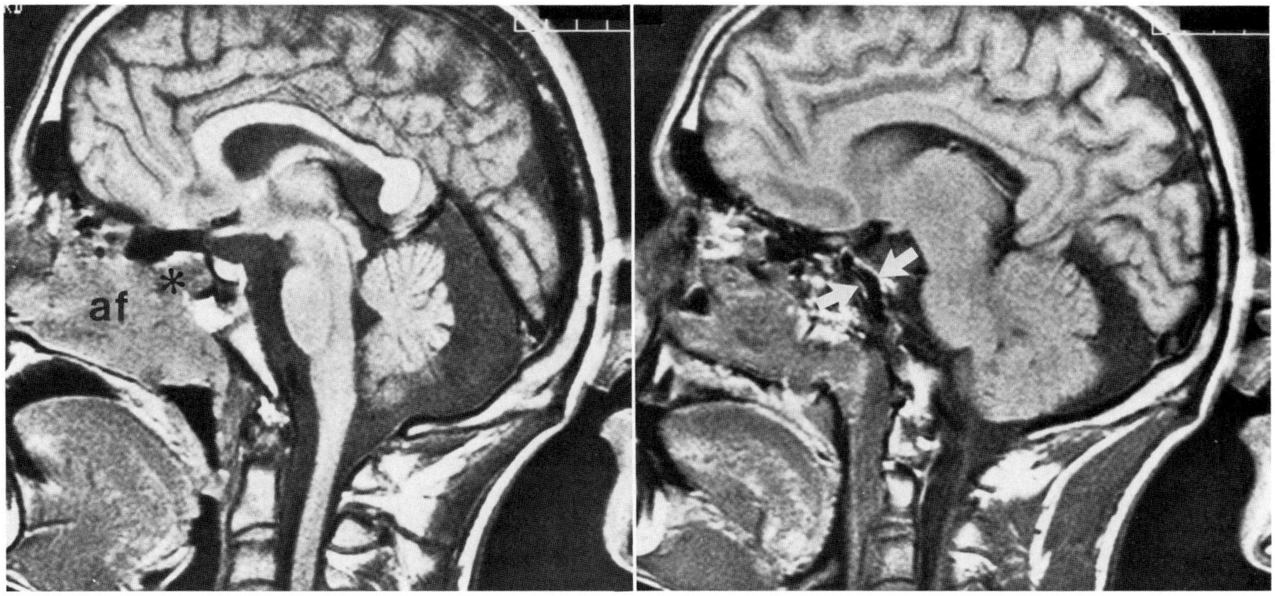

Fig. 12-24   52-year-old female presents with headache and altered mental status. Meningioma. **A,** Lateral plain film of the skull demonstrating hyperostosis in the region of the planum sphenoidale *(curved arrows).* **B,** Axial contrast enhanced CT slice through the region of the planum demonstrating a large expansile mass occupying the floor of the anterior cranial fossa emanating from the planum sphenoidale. Irregular enhancement and bony destruction is apparent.

for about 15% of all primary brain tumors. These tumors are often located parasagittally or along the cerebral convexities. Involvement of the skull base is less common. In a surgical series on 200 consecutive patients with meningiomas, 65 tumors (33%) emanated from the skull base and most arose from the sphenoid wing.[5] Other locations included the olfactory groove, tuberculum sellae, and floor of the anterior and middle cranial fossae.

Olfactory groove meningiomas arise between the crista galli and tuberculum, along the floor of the anterior cranial fossa. Patients most commonly experience altered mental status and headache. Seizures, anosmia, and visual disturbances are less commonly noted (Fig. 12-24).[5]

Patients with tuberculum meningiomas usually experience asymmetrical visual loss and headache. Optic atrophy is commonly found on ophthalmological examination.

Sphenoid wing meningiomas can be categorized into hyperostosing meningioma en plaque, meningiomas arising from the middle third of the sphenoid ridge, and those arising from the clinoid. The en plaque variety (Fig. 12-25) usually is associated with slowly progressive, unilateral painless exophthalmos. Headache, numbness in the distribution of V1 or V2, and seizures occasionally may be present.[5] Meningiomas arising from the middle third of the sphenoid wing (Fig. 12-26) compress the regional frontal and temporal lobes, and headache and seizure are the usual presenting complaints. Those tumors arising more medially usually involve either the medial sphenoid wing or the clinoid. Those principally involving the medial wing tend to encase both the carotid and middle cerebral arteries and compress the optic nerve, the chiasm, and the regional parenchyma. Those involving the clinoid may also involve the cavernous sinus. These patients may have decreased vision, third cranial nerve palsy, and sensory loss in the V1 distribution.

Since arachnoid cells accompany the cranial nerves,[6] it is not surprising that meningiomas can be found adjacent to and traversing the various skull base foramina. This relationship is presumed to account for the association of meningiomas with these cranial nerves.[7] These meningiomas can cause erosion of the foramina, simulating neuromas (Fig. 12-27). Grossly destructive changes in the skull base can also be seen as these tumors extend exocranially (Fig. 12-28). Indeed, in these instances, it may be difficult to distinguish these lesions from malignant processes.

Smaller meningiomas are usually best imaged using CT. Focal areas of hyperostosis (which may be the

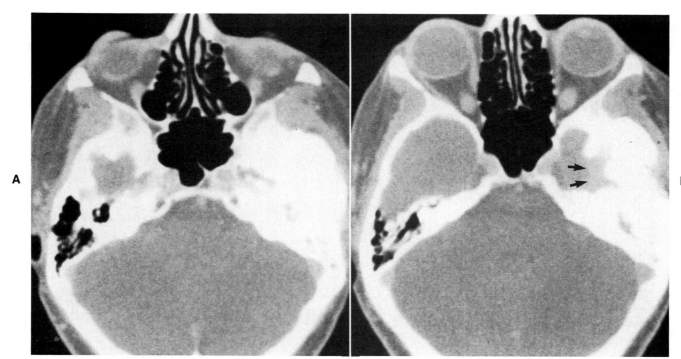

Fig. 12-25 54-year-old female who presents with temporal lobe seizures. Meningioma. Axial contrast enhanced CT scans obtained through the floor of the **A,** middle cranial fossa and **B,** orbital apex demonstrates a predominantly hyperostotic en plaque variety meningioma with a minimal soft tissue component (**B,** *arrows*).

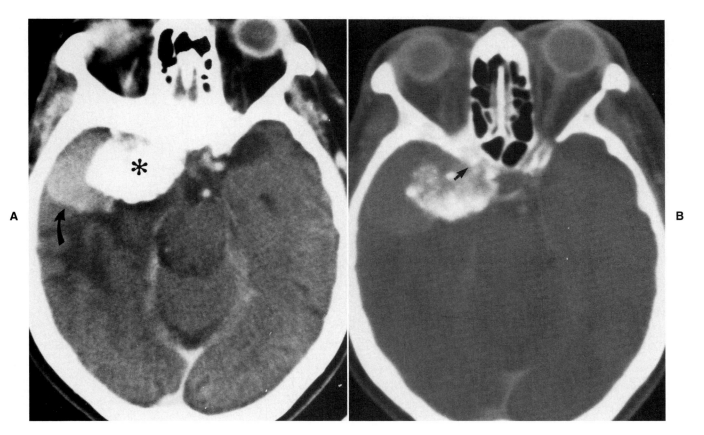

Fig. 12-26   40-year-old female presenting with decreased visual acuity in the right eye. Meningioma. Axial contrast enhanced CT study obtained through the middle cranial fossa using **A,** soft tissue technique and **B,** bone technique. **A,** A large calcified lesion is noted emanating from the medial sphenoid wing on the right *(asterisk).* The enhancing soft tissue component *(curved arrow)* is seen peripherally. **B,** Bone window reveals that the calcified portion of the meningioma is adjacent to the anterior clinoid process *(arrow).* The proximity of this lesion to the optic canal is evident.

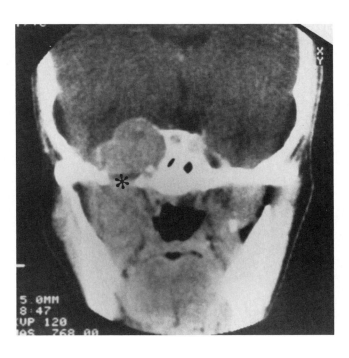

Fig. 12-27   21-year-old female who presents with sensory disturbances along the course of the fifth cranial nerve. Meningioma. Coronal contrast enhanced CT scan reveals the presence of an enhancing lobular mass in the floor of the left middle cranial fossa extending exocranially through the skull base via a widened foramen ovale *(asterisk)* into the region of the parapharyngeal space.

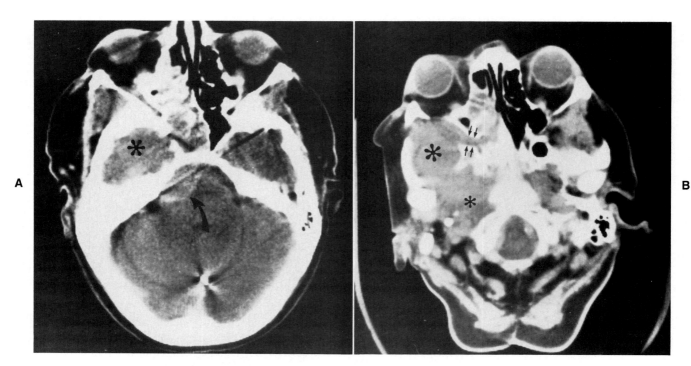

Fig. 12-28 55-year-old female who presents with decreased visual acuity and facial pain. Meningioma. Axial contrast enhanced CT studies through the **A,** middle cranial fossa and **B,** lower skull base demonstrate the presence of a large enhancing lesion occupying the middle cranial fossa *(asterisk)*. The lesion extends posteriorly into the infratentorial region causing brainstem distortion *(arrow)*. Involvement of the body of the sphenoid bone is also apparent. **B,** Extension of the neoplasm inferiorly through the skull base into the pterygopalatine fossa *(arrows)*, the infratemporal fossa *(large asterisk)* and posteriorly into the region of the carotid sheath and upper reaches of the parapharyngeal space *(smaller asterisk)* is apparent. The differential diagnosis of this lesion would have to include a malignant process.

only abnormality seen) can easily be identified using wide bone window settings. The soft tissue component, when present, usually enhances intensely following the administration of intravenous contrast material.

On MRI, meningiomas often have relaxation times similar to those of brain parenchyma; therefore MRI can be relatively insensitive to their presence (Fig. 12-29). The T_1-weighted images should be carefully scrutinized for any distortion of anatomy, and areas of parenchymal hyperintensity (caused by brain edema) should be sought on the T_2-weighted images. The administration of paramagnetic contrast causes dramatic enhancement (T_1 relaxation time shortening) of these lesions and therefore its usage is mandatory when investigating meningiomas of the skull base (Fig. 12-30).

Pituitary Tumors

Approximately 15% of all intracranial neoplasms are pituitary tumors, the majority of which are benign adenomas that arise in adenohypophyseal cells. Incidental adenomas found at unselected routine autopsies occur in 8% to 23% of cases.[8] These lesions are usually slow growing, histologically benign, and confined to the sella. Some lesions may, however, grow more rapidly and display invasive tendencies. The most common symptoms are headaches and visual disturbances. Pituitary adenomas can be classified according to size, with microadenomas being less than 1 cm and macroadenomas being greater than 1 cm in diameter.

Pituitary adenomas are also classified according to their endocrine features. They can secrete abnormal amounts of growth hormone, prolactin, ACTH, TSH, follicle stimulating hormone (FSH)/luteinizing hormone (LH), or multiple hormones or secrete none at all. Most are prolactinomas.

Superior extension into the suprasellar cistern, lateral extension into the cavernous sinuses, and inferior extension through the skull base into the sphenoid sinus and nasopharynx can be seen (Fig. 12-31). Indeed, differentiation of such a lesion from a nasopharyngeal carcinoma may at times be impossible.[9]

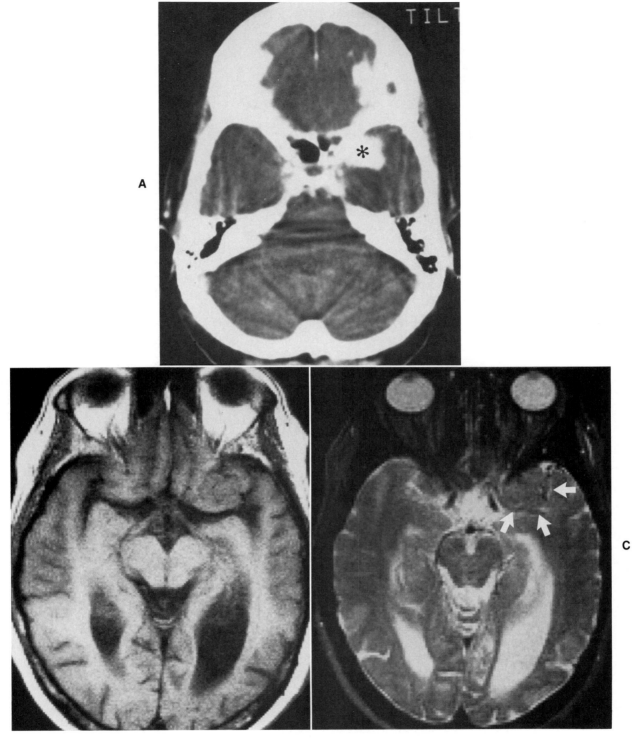

Fig. 12-29 38-year-old male presents with seizures. Meningioma. **A,** Contrast enhanced axial CT image reveals the presence of an enhancing mass adjacent to the left anterior clinoid *(asterisk).* The noncontrast study (not shown) revealed that this mass is not calcified. **B,** Axial T_1- and **C,** T_2-weighted images reveal the relative insensitivity of MRI to the presence of this meningioma. The relaxation characteristics of the tumor and brain are sufficiently similar that they are isointense to one another. The mass is somewhat better seen on the T_2-weighted image (**C,** *arrows*). No parenchymal edema is apparent.

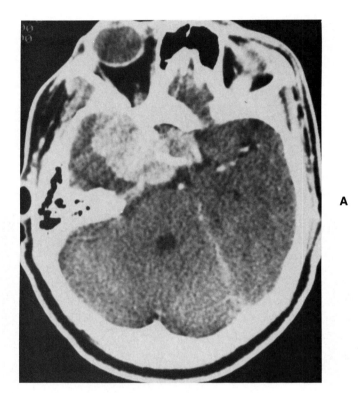

A

Fig. 12-30   42-year-old female with decreased visual acuity and seizures. Meningioma. **A,** Axial contrast enhanced CT reveals the presence of a right sphenoid wing meningioma extending to the cavernous sinus, middle cranial fossa and prepontine cistern infratentorially. **B,** Axial proton density (left) and T_2-weighted image (right) obtained in this same patient reveal the presence of this mass, which has a slightly increased signal intensity compared to the regional brain parenchyma. The conspicuity of this lesion is much less on MRI than when compared to CT. **C,** Axial T_1-weighted image obtained pre- (left) and post- (right) administration of gadolinium-DTPA. The mass on the noncontrast T_1-weighted image is inconspicuous, but enhances intensely following the administration of gadolinium.

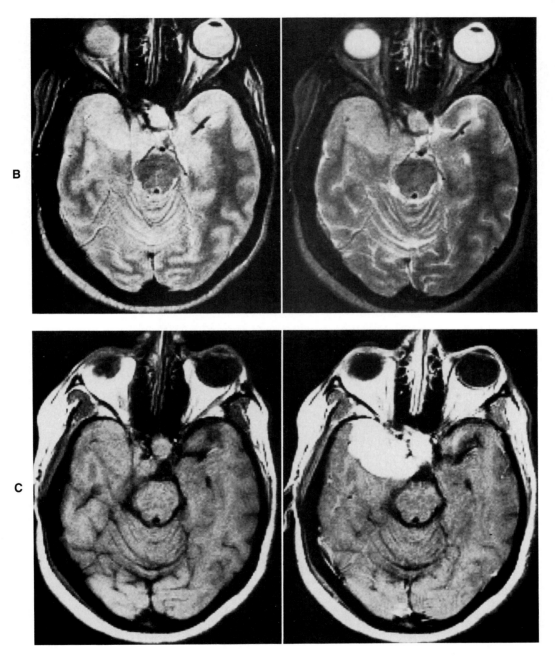

Fig. 12-30   For legend see opposite page.

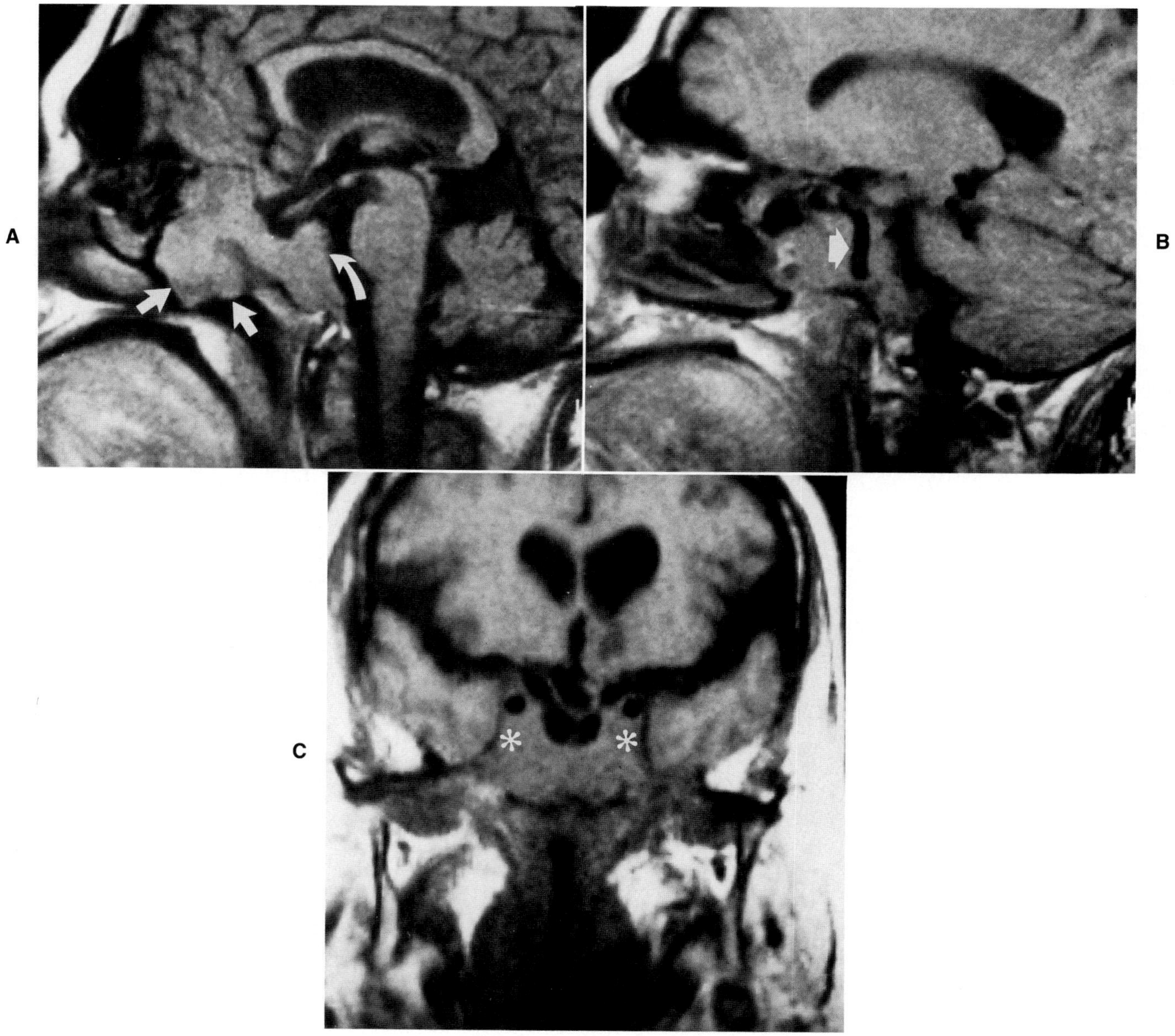

Fig. 12-31 38 year-old female presenting with amenorrhea, galactorrhea, and hyperprolactinemia. Invasive benign pituitary adenoma. **A,** Midsagittal, **B,** parasagittal, and **C,** coronal T$_1$-weighted images reveal the presence of a mass involving the body of the sphenoid bone which is relatively isointense to brain. The mass extends inferiorly to the nasal fossa and nasopharynx (**A,** *straight arrows*), posteriorly to involve the clivus (**A,** *curved arrow*), laterally to envelope the cavernous carotid artery (**B,** *arrow*) and it invades both cavernous sinuses (**C,** *asterisk*). A sphenoid sinus malignancy or chordoma would also be in the differential diagnosis.

MALIGNANT TUMORS
Chondrosarcoma

Chondrosarcomas of the head and neck constitute 6.7% of all reported sites of occurrence.[10] These lesions may arise directly from cartilage, endochondral bone, or tissue without a cartilaginous component,[11] such as in the brain or in the meninges. Lesions occurring in areas not normally associated with cartilage are thought to arise from differentiation of primitive mesenchymal cells. Since the bone of the skull base is cartilaginous in nature, the occurrence of this neoplasm in this region is embryologically predictable.

These lesions typically spread by local invasion and when removed surgically, recurrence is common. Systemic metastases are infrequent, but when they occur they usually have a more aggressive nature.[12] Intracranially, the most common locations for these lesions are the parasellar region, the cerebellopontine angles, and along the convexities.[13] The parasellar lesions commonly extend through the skull base.

Lee and Van Tassel,[14] in a study of 15 cases of craniofacial chondrosarcomas, described 3 cases that arose from the undersurface of the skull base, in the pterygoid plate region. An additional 6 cases arose in the region of the vomer and sphenoethmoidal area, with extension into the infratemporal fossa and parapharyngeal space. They found that the most common bony changes were a combination of erosion and destruction, usually with a narrow zone of transition. Calcification of the tumor matrix was a hallmark of these lesions, being similar to that seen in the more common extracranial chondrosarcomas. The differential diagnosis of skull base chondrosarcomas includes chondroma, meningioma, plasmacytoma, chordoma, carcinoma of the sphenoid sinus, and metastases. It may be impossible to establish a precise histological diagnosis based solely upon the imaging findings of these tumors.

As with all skull base lesions, the newer, more agressive surgical approaches to the skull base mandate that the radiologist be very accurate in defining the extent of these lesions. This is best accomplished with MRI because of its greater soft tissue contrast resolution and its ability to easily obtain multiplanar imaging. CT still retains an important complementary role because of its ability to evaluate calcifications, which may be helpful in the differential diagnosis. In addition, subtle bone erosions can only be seen on CT (Fig. 12-32).

Chordoma

Chordomas are malignant neoplasms that arise in residual remnants of embryonic notochord. More than one third of these tumors occur in the region of the skull base, usually in the clivus and around the sphenooccipital synchondrosis.[15] These lesions typically extend inferiorly into the nasopharynx, and occasionally may reach the nasal cavity and maxillary antrum.[16] The relationship of these neoplasms to this particular region of the skull base is easily understood when one considers the embryology of the notochord in this region (Fig. 12-4). Various common points of origin of this neoplasm in the skull base include the dorsum sellae, the clivus, and the retropharyngeal region.

During the eighth intrauterine week, reorganization of the myotomes, sclerotomes, and dermatomes ensues. Some researchers believe that it is during this time of rapid developmental upheaval that notochordal tissue can separate from the true notochord and form ectopic rests.[17] Since this same degree of developmental activity does not take place in the cervical and thoracolumbar regions of the spine, notochordal ectopia rarely is found in these areas.

Chordomas constitute less than 1% of all intracranial tumors and 3% to 4% of all primary bone tumors.[18] Chordomas can occur at any age, although in the cranioverterbral region the greatest number are diagnosed between the ages of 20 and 40 years. This contrasts to sacrococcygeal chordomas, which have a peak occurrence between the ages of 40 and 60 years. Males are more commonly affected than females.

Common presenting symptoms of craniovertebral chordomas include orbitofrontal headache, visual disturbances, ophthalmoplegia, ptosis and symptoms referable to cranial nerves V, VII, and VIII. Pituitary or brainstem abnormalities may develop as a result of intracranial tumor spread.

Although these lesions grow slowly and metastases are rare, the ultimate outlook is considered poor. Their infiltrative growth pattern accounts for an almost 100% recurrence rate despite radical surgery,[19] and their central skull base location makes complete removal almost impossible. In addition, chordomas are radioresistant.

Chordomas appear radiographically with bone destruction usually associated with a soft tissue mass. They commonly contain areas of calcification and bony fragments.[20] The degree of bone destruction present depends on the site of the lesion's origin and the direction of tumor spread. Chordomas are avascular on angiography and may act as an extraaxial mass, displacing the basilar artery and brainstem posteriorly. The extent of bony destruction, best demonstrated with the use of CT, typically involves the clivus, but may extend into the petrous apices and sphenoid bone. The soft tissue component usually enhances when intravenous contrast material is given. MRI, however, should provide the most accurate assessment of the true tumor margins. Sze et al,[21] in a study comparing CT and MRI in the evaluation of 20 intracranial and upper cervical chordomas, found that although MRI and CT were equivalent

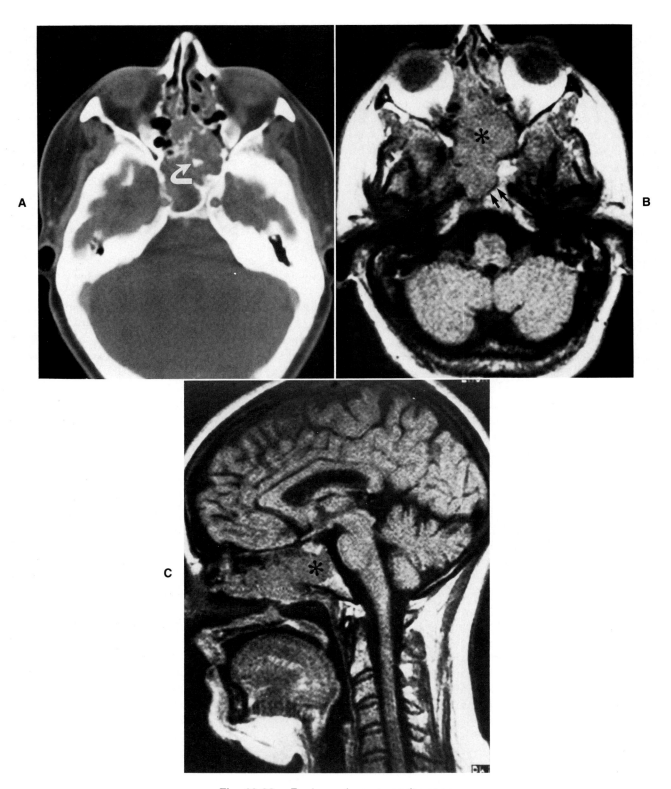

Fig. 12-32 For legend see opposite page.

Fig. 12-32 65-year-old male presenting with epistaxis and facial pain. Chondrosarcoma. **A,** Axial CT scan performed using a wide window to accentuate bony detail reveals the presence of a midline destructive lesion involving the body of the sphenoid bone extending anteriorly to the ethmoids and nasal fossa. An area of increased density *(arrow)* is appreciated within the mass which may represent tumoral calcification. The presence of this calcification may lead one to suggest the diagnosis of chondrosarcoma. **B,** Axial T_1-weighted MRI obtained through the same level as the CT depicted in **A.** Note the presence of the relatively homogeneous midline mass *(asterisk)* slightly less intense than brain. Associated destruction of the clivus *(arrows)* is appreciated. Note that the previously noted area of increased density, felt to represent tumoral calcification in **A** is inconspicuous on MRI. **C,** Midsagittal T_1-weighted MRI demonstrates the presence of a midline destructive mass that is in the ethmoid sinuses and nasal fossa and that courses posteriorly into the body of sphenoid and clivus *(asterisk)*. The midsagittal image is ideal for demonstrating the extent of disease. While the MRI studies in this patient may be somewhat less specific than the CT owing to the inconspicuousness of the calcification, the MRI better illustrate the true disease extent.

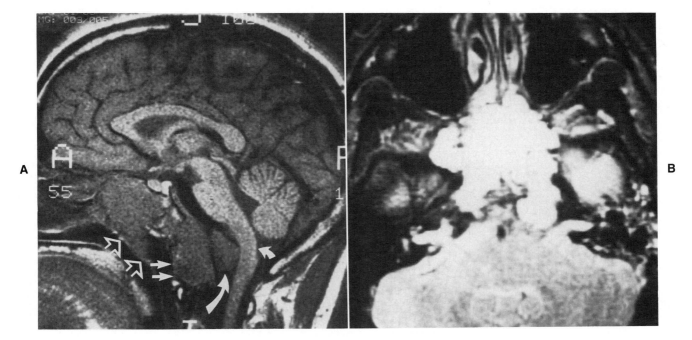

Fig. 12-33 Middle-aged female presenting with brainstem symptoms. Chordoma. **A,** Midsagittal T_1-weighted image demonstrates the presence of a destructive lesion involving the central skull base, which is relatively isointense to brain. The mass extends anteroinferiorly to involve the roof of the nasopharynx *(open arrows)*, inferiorly to involve C1 *(closed straight arrows)* and extends posteriorly to involve the medullary cistern *(large curved arrow)* causing kinking of the medulla around the mass *(small curved arrow)*. **B,** Axial T_2-weighted image demonstrates prolongation of the T_2 relaxation time of this mass. (Case courtesy of Dr. Gordon Sze.)

in detecting the lesion, MRI was considerably better in delineating the true extent of tumor. Fifteen of the neoplasms appeared isointense on T_1-weighted images, with the remaining five tumors being hypointense on T_1-weighted images. High signal intensity was seen in all 20 lesions on T_2-weighted sequences (Fig. 12-33). Oot et al, in another study, evaluated MRI and CT in the detection of both clival chordomas and chondrosarcomas. Their conclusions were the same as those of Sze et al.[22] The diagnosis of a chordoma should be considered when there is a destructive lesion in the clivus or basiocciput occurring in a middle-aged adult.

Nasopharyngeal Carcinoma

The incidence of nasopharyngeal carcinoma in white populations is between 0.25% to 0.5% of all malignant tumors.[23,24] There is, however, a distinctly high racial incidence in the Chinese population. This predisposition exists not only for native Chinese, but also for those members of this racial group who have been transplanted to other countries. In Hong Kong, for instance, nasopharyngeal carcinoma accounts for 18% of all malignant neoplasms.[25] Males are afflicted more often than females, and the mean age of presentation is 40 years, somewhat earlier than for other forms of adult malignancies. Because of their nasopharyngeal location, these lesions often remain asymptomatic for a long time, which often results in a delay in diagnosis.

Nasopharyngeal carcinomas spread primarily by infiltrating neighboring regions such as the cranium, orbit, or parapharyngeal space.[26] Extension to and invasion of the skull base is commonly encountered with this malignancy. Once tumor has spread laterally from the nasopharyngeal wall, it easily can gain access to the prestyloid portion of the parapharyngeal and then to the masseteric space. From these areas, spread to the skull base in the region of the foramen ovale, the foramen spinosum, and the floor of the middle cranial fossa is facilitated.

The common intracranial spread of carcinoma of the nasopharynx to involve the caverous sinus and cranial nerves III, IV, (V1 and V2), and VI is thought to be secondary to the close proximity of the fossa of Rosenmuller to the foramen lacerum. Neoplasm is thought to spread along the canal of the foramen lacerum, along the carotid artery, and thence into the cavernous sinus to involve the aforementioned cranial nerves.[26] The fifth cranial nerve is the earliest and most commonly affected nerve, and involvement produces numbness or pain along the distribution of the various branches. The next most commonly involved cranial nerve is the abducens, and involvement causes a lateral rectus palsy and diplopia.

On MRI, nasopharyngeal carcinomas have a homogeneous signal intensity similar to that of the adjacent mucosa. This signal intensity is intermediate between

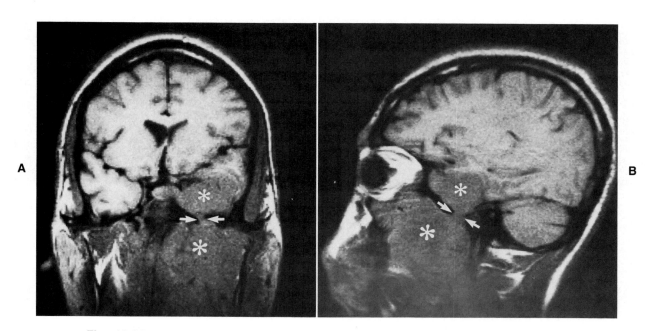

Fig. 12-34 17-year-old male presents with nasal stuffiness. Nasopharyngeal carcinoma. **A,** T_1-weighted coronal and **B,** parasagittal images reveal the presence of a large nasopharyngeal carcinoma which has spread to the parapharyngeal space (large asterisk), coursed superiorly through a widened foramen ovale (arrows) to involve the middle cranial fossa (small asterisk). These imaging planes are especially advantageous when imaging transcranial spread of tumor. (Used with permission from Braun IF: MRI of the nasopharynx, Radiologic Clinics NA 27[2]:315, 1989.)

that of fat and that of muscle on T_1-weighted images. The distinction between tumor and musculature is further increased with the use of proton-density or T_2-weighted images. These lesions, especially the smaller ones, are much more easily identified on MRI than on CT. The superior soft tissue contrast resolution of MRI allows more accurate localization of the lesion and better definition of its extent, especially with regard to involvement of the adjacent musculature. Although axial images are used for the initial localization, imaging in the coronal plane is necessary to rule out transcranial spread of tumor (Fig. 12-34).[4] Enhancement with paramagnetic contrast material may prove useful in evaluating any intracranial spread of neoplasm.

Rhabdomyosarcoma

Rhabdomyosarcoma, the most common soft tissue sarcoma in children, represents between 5% and 15%[27] of all malignant solid tumors and between 4% and 8% of all cases of malignant disease in children under 15 years of age.[28] Seventy percent of patients are under 10 years of age at clinical presentation, and the peak incidence is in children between 2 and 5 years of age. The head and neck is the most common site of origin.[29]

Approximately 29% of all head and neck rhabdomyosarcomas involve the pharynx,[30] the majority of which involve the nasopharynx and are the embryonal type. The mean age of 49 subjects studied by Dito and Batsakis[30] was 6 years. Local recurrences and distant spread are the hallmarks of this disease. Skull base invasion, seen in as many as 35% of patients, usually involves the cavernous sinus, is associated with cranial nerve palsies, and is a grave prognostic sign.[29] Lymph node involvement occurs in one half of the patients; the lungs and bones are the common sites of metastases. Although surgery and irradiation were the treatments of choice, more recently chemotherapy has become a primary treatment approach because of the associated improved survival rate compared with the dismal survival statistics of earlier treatment plans.

These lesions appear as bulky nasopharyngeal masses on MRI, commonly extending through the skull base to involve the cavernous sinus. The signal intensity is homogeneous and intermediate between that of muscle and that of fat on T_1-weighted images. Although small areas of bony destruction are more difficult to perceive on MRI than on CT, intracranial tumor extension is most easily seen on coronal MRI (Fig. 12-35).

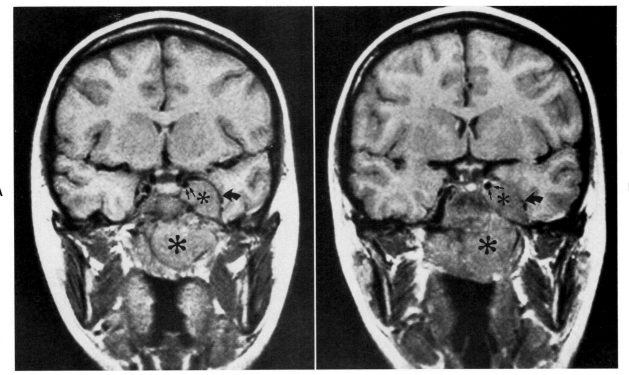

Fig. 12-35   12-year-old male presents with restriction of ocular motion and nasal stuffiness. Rhabdomyosarcoma of the nasopharynx with extension through the skull base. **A** and **B,** Coronal T_1-weighted images revealing the presence of a mass within the nasopharynx *(large asterisk)* with skull base destruction and invasion of the left cavernous sinus *(small asterisk)*. Note the lateral deviation of the lateral dural reflection of the cavernous sinus *(curved arrow)*. The mass abuts the cavernous internal carotid artery *(small arrows)*. (Used with permission from Braun IF: MRI of the nasopharynx, Radiologic Clinics NA 27[2]:315, 1989.)

Perineural Tumor Spread

Perineural and transcranial spread of head and neck malignancies via the cranial nerves is an important, yet underemphasized, mode of disease transmission. Neural invasion by tumor was first described in 1842, and has been noted to occur in malignancies of a number of organs.[31] Ballantyne, in 1963, determined that neural invasion was relatively common in carcinomas of the head and neck, and more importantly, frequently influenced prognosis.[32] Although epithelial tumors in general show a propensity for this mode of spread, such tumor extension occurs most commonly with squamous cell carcinoma and adenoid cystic carcinoma.

Perineural tumor involvement usually indicates a poor, although not hopeless, prognosis. The prognosis becomes bleaker with intracranial tumor spread. Most of these patients have advanced disease; some may be candidates for surgical resection, and a preoperative knowledge of such neural infiltration will alter the surgical approach.

Although in theory any cranial nerve may be involved, most cases described in the imaging literature are confined to the fifth and seventh nerves. Before MRI, the radiographic signature of this manner of spread was bony erosion of basal foramin, this was best evaluated by CT. However, extensive neural involvement could be present before any foraminal expansion and thus before radiographic detection. This was especially true of the larger apertures such as the superior orbital fissure and the jugular foramen. With the advent of MRI this form of metastasis can be detected at an earlier stage, perhaps affecting patient treatment and improving prognosis. T_1-weighted MRI has the ability to demonstrate such intracranial and extracranial perineural tumor extension. Nerve involvement is seen as a smooth, isointense thickening of the nerve. This finding, in association with concentric enlargement of the basal foramen, is direct evidence of perineural and transcranial tumor spread (Fig. 12-36).[33] Gadolinium-DTPA T_1-weighted images can also identify neural invasion by showing high signal intensity enhancement of the involved nerve.

Metastatic Disease

Metastatic lesions of the central skull base are infrequent but more common than primary bone lesions.

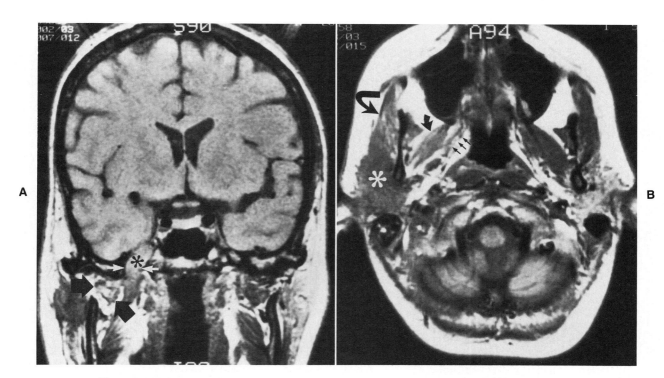

Fig. 12-36 Adenoid cystic carcinoma of the parotid gland with perineural spread involving V3. **A,** Coronal T_1-weighted image demonstrates infiltration of V3 by tumor *(asterisk)*. There is an isointense enlargement of the nerve as it enters the skull base through a widened foramen ovale *(small arrows)*. Denervation atrophy and fatty infiltration of the lateral pterygoid muscle *(large arrows)*, due to involvement of the motor portion of V3, which supplies the muscles of mastication, is easily appreciated. **B,** Axial T_1-weighted image through the parotid region reveals the primary location of the adenoid cystic carcinoma within the right parotid gland *(asterisk)*. Also seen is the presence of denervation atrophy of the muscles of mastication: masseter *(large curved arrow)*, lateral pterygoid muscle *(small curved arrow)*, and medial pterygoid muscle *(small arrows)*.

They most commonly occur from carcinoma of the prostate, lung, or breast. Prostate metastases typically produce hyperostosis with an associated soft tissue mass, which may be mistaken for a meningioma. Lung and breast metastasis are generally lytic and may also have a soft tissue component. Lytic and blastic metastatic lesions will generally demonstrate enhancement. The bony destruction as well as the soft tissue components are best evaluated with CT scanning. Differentiation between primary and metastatic neoplasm based on imaging characteristics alone may be difficult.

MISCELLANEOUS CONDITIONS
Paget's Disease

Paget's disease, a condition of unknown etiology, is seen primarily in older adults, and, depending on the series, from 29% to 65% of patients are reported to have skull involvement.[34] Paget's disease can be seen radiographically as a continuum that ranges from osteoporosis circumscripta, which represents the active phase of the disease, to dense sclerosis, which represents the healing phase. When the base of the skull is involved, sclerosis and bone thickening are the most common findings, at times simulating the appearance of fibrous dysplasia (Fig. 12-37). Basilar invagination and platybasia are frequent occurrences with skull base disease and are the result of bony softening and the mechanical stresses of muscular attachments.

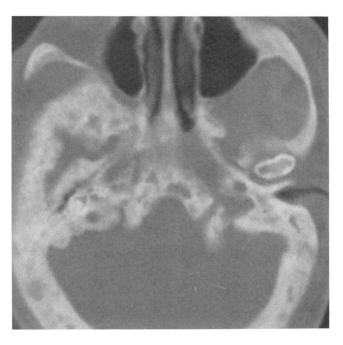

Fig. 12-37 Paget's disease. Axial CT study through the skull base in an elderly male showing the bony thickening and fluffy sclerosis that are typical of this disorder.

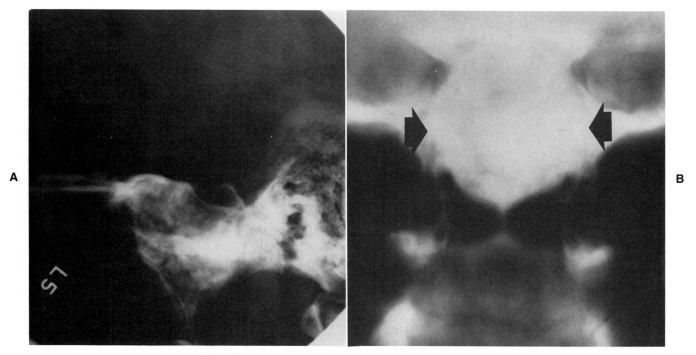

Fig. 12-38 20-year-old patient presents with headache. Monostotic fibrous dysplasia. **A,** Lateral film and **B,** anteroposterior tomogram reveal a sclerotic, hazy, bony lesion that causes widening of the sphenoid bone (**B,** *arrows*).

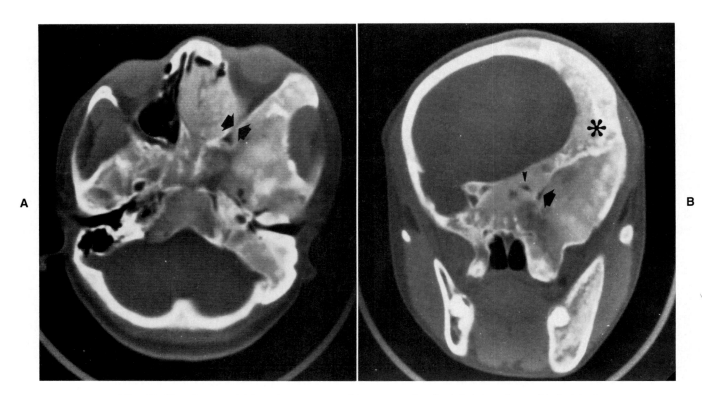

Fig. 12-39 9-year-old female presents with progressive facial deformity and left-sided blindness. Polyostotic fibrous dysplasia. **A,** Axial and **B,** coronal computed tomography demonstrates the sclerotic type of fibrous dysplasia with involvement of the central skull base, calvarium, mandible, and other facial bones. The widened diploic spaces (*asterisk,* **B**), osseous expansion and hazy sclerosis are typical of this lesion. **A,** Encroachment of the orbital apex *(arrows)* is easily appreciated. **B,** Narrowing and encroachment of the superior orbital fissure on the left *(arrow)* is appreciated. Involved bone is seen surrounding the optic canal *(arrowhead).*

Fibrous Dysplasia

Fibrous dysplasia, a developmental anomaly of the mesenchymal precursor of bone, manifests itself as a defect in osteoblastic differentiation and maturation. The etiology is unknown and it is not hereditary.[35] In 70% to 80% of cases, a single bone is involved; in the remainder of cases there is polyostotic disease. Any bone can be affected. Calvarial involvement is usually monostotic, whereas the skull base and facial bones are commonly involved in the polyostotic form. The polyostotic variety is usually associated with a younger age group and has more severe bony involvement than does the monostotic form.

Up to 50% of patients with polyostotic fibrous dysplasia have skull and facial bone involvement, whereas these bones are affected in only 10% to 25% of patients with the monostotic form.[35] The most commonly involved bones are the sphenoid, frontal, maxillary, and ethmoid, followed in frequency by the occipital and temporal bones.[36]

Patients may have facial asymmetry and deformity. Symptoms and signs referable to the orbit include exophthalmos, visual impairment, and blindness; these are caused by bony encroachment on the optic nerve secondary to involvement of the optic canal and sphenoid lesser wing.

Three radiologic appearances of fibrous dysplasia of the skull have been described by Fries[37]: Pagetoid, sclerotic, and cystic. The sclerotic type most commonly involves the skull base and sphenoid bone.[38] This sclerosis, which may be extensive, can be seen on plain radiography (Fig. 12-38) and may mimic Paget's disease, neurofibromatosis, and meningioma. Concomitant facial bone involvement should, however, lead to the diagnosis of fibrous dysplasia. The presence of widened diploic spaces, osseous expansion, and hazy, poorly defined sclerotic lesions are common findings. The foraminal encroachment of the skull base caused by the disease is readily imaged with CT (Fig. 12-39).

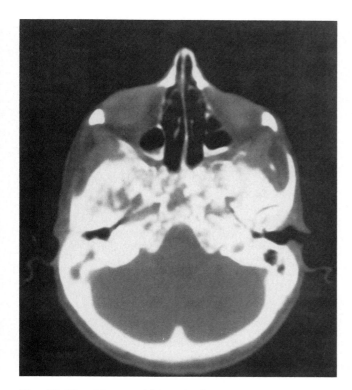

Fig. 12-40   62-year-old female 5 years status post skull base irradiation for nasopharyngeal carcinoma. Axial CT image shows a pattern of mixed sclerosis with slight bony thickening. This appearance is consistent with radiation necrosis or osteitis. Differentiation from a chronic osteitis, such as that seen with chronic osteomyelitis, is difficult.

Radiation Necrosis

The osseous changes of radiation necrosis are believed to be secondary to an osteoblastic destruction, which is often followed by vascular compromise and further bony damange.[39] These changes are dependent on a variety of factors, including radiation dosage, the specific type of therapy employed, the time since treatment, the specific bone involved, and the presence of concurrent trauma and infection.[40] The bones of children are more sensitive to the effects of radiation than are the bone of adults, and the bony growth centers in children are easily damaged by irradiation.[39] The changes of radiation necroses are slowly progressive and are first noted about 1 year after treatment.

Recent studies have indicated that this entity is not as uncommon as previously thought. In a study of 92 patients irradiated for pituitary lesions, 17% to 18.5% had radiation injury of the skull base.[41] The radiographic findings included areas of lysis and mixed scle-

rosis, which were most prevalent in the central region of the beam and diminished towards the beam's periphery (Fig. 12-40). The entity is best investigated with axial CT.

REFERENCES

1. Batsakis JG: Vasoformative tumors. In Tumors of the head and neck: clinical and pathological considerations, ed 2, Baltimore, 1979, Williams & Wilkins, p 297.
2. Lingeman RE and Shellhamer RH: Benign neoplasms of the nasopharynx. In Cummings CW et al, editors: Otolaryngology-head and neck surgery, St. Louis, 1986, The CV Mosby Co, p 1269.
3. Som PM et al: Tumors of the parapharyngeal space and upper neck: MR imaging characteristics, Radiology 164:823, 1987.
4. Braun IF: MRI of the nasopharynx, Radiol Clin North Am 27(2):315, 1989.
5. Ojemann RG: Meningiomas: clinical features and surgical management. In Wilkins RH and Rengachary SS, editors: Neurosurgery, New York, 1985, McGraw-Hill Book Co, pp 635-654.
6. Cushing H: The meningiomas (dural endothelioma): their source and favoured seats of origin, Brain 45:282, 1922.
7. Batsakis JG: Other neuroectodermal tumors and related lesions of the head and neck. In Tumors of the head and neck: clinical and pathological considerations, ed 2, Baltimore, 1979, Williams & Wilkins, p 348.
8. Kovacs K, Horvath E, and Asa SL: Classification and pathology of pituitary tumors. In Wilkins RH and Rengachary SS, editors: Neurosurgery, New York, 1985, McGraw-Hill Book Co, pp 834-842.
9. Hoffman JC Jr: Radiology of sellar and parasellar lesions. In Wilkins RH and Rengachary SS, editors: Neurosurgery, New York, 1985, McGraw-Hill Book Co, pp 822-834.
10. Pritchard DJ et al: Chondrosarcoma: a clinicopathologic and statistical analysis, Cancer 45:149, 1980.
11. Jones HM: Cartilaginous tumors of the head and neck, J Laryngol Otol 87:135, 1973.
12. Guccion JC et al: Extraskeletal mesenchymal chondrosarcoma, Arch Pathol 95:336, 1973.
13. Bahr AL and Gayler BW: Cranial chondrosarcoma, Radiology 124:151, 1977.
14. Lee YY and Van Tassel P: Craniofacial chondrosarcomas: imaging findings in 15 untreated cases, AJNR 10:165, 1989.
15. Mabrey RE: Chordoma: a study of 150 cases, Am J Cancer 25:501, 1935.
16. Batsakis JG and Kittleson AC: Chordomas: otorhinolaryngologic presentation and diagnosis, Arch Otolaryngol 78:168, 1963.
17. Wright D: Nasopharyngeal and cervical chordoma: some aspects of their development and treatment, J Laryngol Otol 82:1337, 1968.
18. Krol G, Sundaresan N, and Deck M: Computed tomography of axial chordomas, J Comput Assist Tomogr 7:286, 1983.
19. Batsakis JG: Soft tissue tumors of the head and neck: unusual forms. In Tumors of the head and neck: clinical and pathological considerations, ed 2, Baltimore, 1979, Williams & Wilkins, p 353.
20. Firooznia J et al: Chordoma: radiologic evaluation of 20 cases, AJR 127:797, 1976.
21. Sze G et al: Chordomas: MR imaging, Radiology 166:187, 1988.
22. Oot RF, Melville GE, and New PFJ: The role of MR and CT in evaluating clival chordomas and chondrosarcomas, AJNR 9:715, 1988.
23. Godtfredsen E: Ophthalmologic and neurologic symptoms of ma-

lignant nasopharyngeal tumors: a clinical study comprising 454 cases, with special references to histopathology and the possibility of early recognition, Acta Psychiatr Neurol 34:1, 1944.

24. Schnohr P: Survival rates of nasopharyngeal cancer in California: a review of 516 cases from 1942 through 1965, Cancer 25:1099, 1970.

25. Digby KH, Fook WL, and Che TY: Nasopharyngeal malignancy, Br J Surg 28:517, 1941.

26. Lederman M: Cancer of the nasopharynx: its natural history and treatment, Springfield, Ill, 1961, Charles C Thomas, p 10.

27. Feldman BA: Rhabdomyosarcoma of the head and neck, Laryngoscope, 92(4):424, 1982.

28. Young JL and Miller RW: Incidence of malignant tumors in U.S. children, J Pediatr 86:254, 1975.

29. Malogolowkin MH and Ortega JA: Rhabdomyosarcoma of childhood, Pediatr Ann 17(4):251, 1988.

30. Dito WR and Batsakis JG: Intraoral, pharyngeal, and nasopharyngeal rhabdomyosarcoma, Arch Otolaryngol 77:123, 1963.

31. Dodd GD et al: The dissemination of tumors of the head and neck via the cranial nerves, Radiol Clin North Am 8(3):445, 1970.

32. Ballantyne AJ, McCarten AB, and Ibanez ML: The extension of cancer of the head and neck through peripheral nerves, Am J Surg 106:651, 1963.

33. Laine FJ et al: Perineural tumor extension through the foramen ovale: evaluation with MR imaging, Radiology 174:65, 1990.

34. Olmstead WM: Some skeletogenic lesions with common calvarial manifestations, Radiol Clin North Am 19(4):703, 1981.

35. Resnick D and Niwayama G: Diagnosis of bone and joint disorders, vol 6, Philadelphia, 1988, WB Saunders Co, p 4057.

36. Daffner RH et al: Computed tomography of fibrous dysplasia, AJR 139:943, 1982.

37. Fries JW: The roentgen features of fibrous dysplasia of the skull and facial bones, AJR 77:71, 1957.

38. Leeds NE and Seaman WB: Fibrous dysplasia of the skull and its differential diagnosis, Radiology 78:570, 1962.

39. Resnick D and Niwayama G: Diagnosis of bone and joint disorders, vol 5, Philadelphia, 1988, WB Saunders Co, p 3034.

40. Rubin P and Casarett GW: Mature cartilage and adult bone. In Clinical radiation pathology, vol 2, Philadelphia, 1968, WB Saunders Co, p 557.

41. Shimanovskaya K and Shiman A: Radiation injury of bone, New York, 1983, Pergamon Press.

13 The Temporal Bone

R. THOMAS BERGERON
WILLIAM W.M. LO
JOEL D. SWARTZ
ANTON N. HASSO
DAVID P.C. LIU
RONALD E. BROADWELL

SECTION ONE
INTRODUCTION TO THE TEMPORAL BONE

R. THOMAS BERGERON

EMBRYOLOGY AND DEVELOPMENTAL ANATOMY

Each of the organs of special sense has a fascinating phylogeny. None surpasses the ear, however, in demonstrating the resourcefulness and richness of invention of a biologic system in making adaptive modifications so as to deal successfully with a changing environment.

The ear began as an organ of balance. In the fish of 350 million years ago it existed as a fluid-filled pocket, sunken beneath the surface of the skin on either side of the head. The pocket communicated directly with the ocean water in which the ancient fish swam, providing a mechanism whereby the fish could sense its orientation in the sea. It is physically possible for such a structure to be sensitive to low-frequency vibrations transmitted through the water, and indeed such was likely the case. Hearing nonetheless was only incidental, if not accidental, to a structure primarily developed to provide balance.

By the time evolution had produced creatures that existed on land the vestibular system had become much more highly developed. But in so doing, it lost its continuity with the external environment, becoming deeply encased and sealed off within the base of the skull. To become successful land dwellers, however, perception of sound had become important to survival. The economy of nature prevailed. Connection between the external environment and the inner ear was reestablished and the middle and external ear were evolved. Concurrently, the hearing portion of the inner ear structure became much more highly specialized (Fig. 13-1).

The following is the story of the development of the ear as we know it. It bears great relevance to the understanding of congenital anomalies, malformations, anatomic variations, and the "normal" state.

Streeter[1,2] provides the definitive account of the embryologic development of the inner ear. Numerous others also have studied the development of the ear in this and previous centuries, but the most complete single source of information relating to development of all portions of the temporal bone remains in Bast and Anson,[4] *The Temporal Bone and Ear*. Shambaugh[5] presents the essence of their work in abbreviated form in *Surgery of the Ear*. Iurato[6] presents an even more concise precis in *Submicroscopic Structure of the Inner Ear*.

Inner Ear

Inner ear development may be considered in three stages: (1) endolymphatic (otic or membranous) labyrinth, (2) perilymphatic (periotic) labyrinth, and (3) bony labyrinth.

Inner ear formation commences about the third week of fetal life. A platelike thickening of neuroectoderm on either side of the head forms midway alongside the hind brain; this is called the *otic placode*. This invaginates in a few days and forms the *otic pit*. By the fourth week of embryonic life the pit has deepened and narrowed, its lips have fused to form the *otocyst* (otic ves-

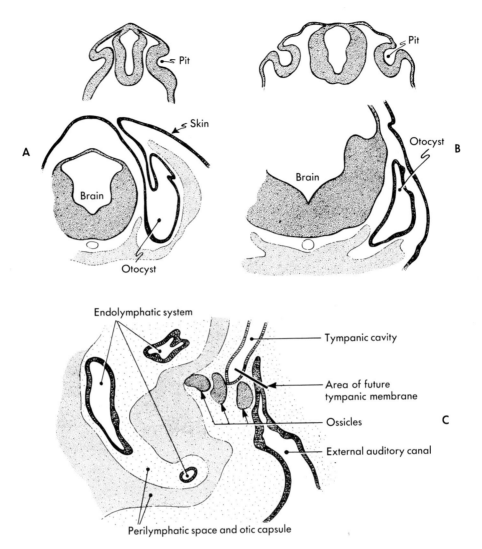

Fig. 13-1   Comparative embryology of ear. **A,** In shark, otocyst is in communication with circumambiant water. **B,** Human endolymph contained within membranous labyrinth is surrounded by another fluid, perilymph. Aqueous system of human progenitors is restored in this way and equilibratory function of inner ear is maintained. **C,** Auditory function, which is subserved by wave transmitting system, is brought about in humans by conversion of branchial arch apparatus of shark. (Modified from Anson B, Harper D, and Winch T: The vestibular and cochlear aqueducts: developmental and adult anatomy of their contents and parietes, Third Symposium on the Role of the Vestibular Organs in Space Exploration, NASA SP 152:125, 1967.)

sicle), and it has descended away from its surface ecto-dermal origin.

The otocyst is fluid filled and ectodermal lined and constitutes the primitive endolymphatic (otic), or membranous, labyrinth. The otocyst comes to lie opposite the fifth neuromere and is in contact rostrally with the facial-acoustic ganglionic mass. Accompanied by these neural cells, the cyst then migrates to the developing skull base.

By 4½ weeks, the otocyst has elongated and started to divide into two main sections, the longer utricular-

saccular portion and the smaller endolymphatic portion that arises at the point on the otocyst wall that originally joined the neuroectoderm. The *utricle* and *semicircular canals* differentiate from the posterolateral aspect of the otocyst, while the *saccule* and *cochlear duct* and the communication between the two, the *ductus reuniens*, arise anteromedially.

By the sixth week, two flattened pouches have developed on the otocyst. The superior and posterior semicircular ducts will eventually arise from the one pouch at the dorsal margin of the otocyst, while the lateral semicircular duct differentiates from the more lateral outpouching. By the seventh week, the central portions of the walls of these pouches flatten and fuse into epithelial plates. By this process, canals are left at the periphery of each pouch, and the region into which these canals join the otocyst becomes the utricle. The central epithelial plates eventually break down, leaving the semicircular canals.

The saccule originates from the anteromedial portion of the otocyst. At the sixth developmental week the future cochlea makes its first appearance in the form of the cochlear duct, which develops as an evagination of the saccule. By 8 weeks, the duct is elongated and beginning to coil; by 11 weeks, it has formed 2½ turns.

Later, the communication between the cochlear duct and the saccule becomes narrowed to form the ductus reuniens. Similarly, parts of the utricle and saccule become constricted to form the *utricular duct* and the shorter *saccular duct*, which eventually join together to form the common *endolymphatic duct*.

The membranous labyrinth is surrounded by mesenchyme, which differentiates into cartilage that envelops the entire labyrinth. The membranous labyrinth enlarges within its cartilaginous encasement until midterm, by which time it has reached its complicated adult form.

The surrounding cartilaginous otic capsule then ossifies. No further growth of these structures occurs for the lifetime of the individual, with the exception of the endolymphatic duct and sac. Interestingly, these structures are the earliest appendages of the otic vessicle to appear; but unlike the rest of the membranous labyrinth, which reaches adult shape and size by midterm, the endolymphatic duct and sac continue to change throughout infancy and childhood until after puberty. At full adulthood the endolymphatic sac is three times larger than at birth. Its function will be discussed later.

As the mature anatomic configuration of the labyrinth develops (by approximately 6 to 7 months of fetal age, when the membranous labyrinth is completely developed), its sensory end-organs emerge, appearing in the utricle and saccule between 7 and 8 weeks, within the semicircular ducts by 8 weeks, and within the cochlea at 12 weeks. Differentiation in the cochlear duct goes on at the slowest rate, not being completed until after midterm. It is noteworthy that the cochlea not only is the last of the labyrinth to differentiate but also is less stable and more subject to developmental malformations and acquired disease than are the phylogenetically older vestibular end-organs.

Perilymphatic (Periotic) Labyrinth

The development of the mesenchyme immediately around the membranous labyrinth is complex.[1,2] By 7 weeks of fetal age it has become precartilage. At 8 weeks the precartilage changes to an outer zone of true cartilage that forms the *otic capsule*, while the inner zone begins to loosen and vacuolize and forms the *perilymphatic space*. Fluid-filled cavities appear around the vestibule and cochlear duct and finally surround the semicircular ducts. These spaces all eventually fuse and become confluent, forming a continuous perilymphatic labyrinth containing a delicate matrix composed of arachnoid-like connective tissue. The perilymph circulates within the interstices of the filaments as they traverse the distance between the membranous labyrinth and the endosteum of the otic capsule. This filamentous matrix is present to some degree in all portions of the perilymphatic space, except around the cochlear duct in the spaces known as the *scala tympani* and *scala vestibuli*. The absence of filaments within the scalae permits undampened pulsatile movement of the perilymph between the oval and round windows in the adult cochlea. The kinetic energy of the sound waves is absorbed by the membranes of the cochlear duct and the "secondary tympanic membrane" of the round window.

The perilymphatic space has three prolongations into the surrounding osseous otic capsule: the *cochlear aqueduct* (perilymphatic duct), the small *fissula ante fenestram*, and the *fossula post fenestram*. These latter two structures are of only remote radiologic interest; however, either or both of them may be involved as a focus of diseased bone in otosclerosis.

The cochlear aqueduct extends from the scala tympani near the round window to the subarachnoid space near the emergence of the glossopharyngeal nerve on the inferior surface of the petrous pyramid. It will be described in further detail in the section on anatomy.

Bony Labyrinth

Ossification of the otic capsule commences only when the cartilage has attained maximum growth and maturity. Once the membranous labyrinth has become encased by enchondral bone all growth of the inner ear structures ceases and there is no possibility for future expansion of this rigid structure. The enchondral bone formed in the cartilage of the otic capsule is never removed and replaced by haversion bone; i.e., there is no remodeling. Along with the ossicles, the otic capsule is unique within the human body. They remain as a primitive, relatively avascular type of bone that is exceptionally hard and poor in osteogenic response.[7]

Ossification occurs between the sixteenth and twenty-third weeks of fetal life, with 14 separate centers identifiable. No suture lines are visible because ossification begins only after all growth has ceased. The bony otic capsule is complete except for an area over the lateral semicircular canal, a narrow rim of cartilage that remains around the oval window, and the fissula ante fenestram.

The otic capsule is made up of concentric layers of dense enchondral bone with a thin uniform layer of endosteal bone being laid down against the endosteal membrane that lines the labyrinth. Outside the enchondral layer, periosteal bone is laid down in parallel lamellae.

The endosteal layer and the thick middle enchondral layer of the capsule remain relatively inert and unchanged through life. In response to infection or trauma the endosteal membrane lining the labyrinth may proliferate, obliterating the lumen of the labyrinth (see section on infections of the temporal bone: obliterative labyrinthitis).

The enchondral layer participates very feebly in osteogenic repair, so fractures of the labyrinth may remain completely unhealed except by fibrous union. However, there are also advantages to this poor bone repair. The poor osteogenic response made possible the construction of a labyrinthine fenestra that remained permanently open in early operations for stapedial otosclerosis. One of the conditions that prompted the development of stapes prosthesis implantation surgery following stapes mobilization procedures in early otosclerosis surgery was the failure of fractured stapedial crura or footplates to heal.

The periosteal bone of the labyrinthine capsule (i.e., the bone that lies peripheral to the dense middle endochondral bone) continues to be added to by apposition during infancy and up until early adult life. In due course this periosteal bone is removed and replaced by haversion bone. Eventually pneumatic cells invade most of the periosteal layer of the capsule along with much of the remainder of the temporal bone. As with other periosteal bone, that of the otic capsule reacts readily to infection or trauma with osteogenesis. Rarely, there may be a profound response such as that occurring with a meningioma.

As has been noted, ossification about the entire otic capsule is relatively uniform and complete with the exception of three areas: the area around the oval window, the area of the fissula ante fenestram, and an area over the lateralmost bulge of the lateral semicircular canal. Ossification in this latter region is unique because in early stages it is the same as in the remainder of the otic capsule, with the production of three layers of bone; however, at approximately midterm the portion covering the lateralmost sweep of the lateral semicircular canal undergoes dissolution. By the thirteenth week, the periosteal layer and varying amounts of the middle enchondral layer have been removed. Eventually there is reconstitution with a varying thickness of the periosteal bone. In some circumstances this reconstitution is (normally) very thin and for that reason it

can appear radiographically as a site of bony dehiscence; this can be misinterpreted as a sign of labyrinthine fistula when occurring in the presence of cholesteatoma. One should therefore be circumspect and not overinterpret this finding on imaging.

Outer and Middle Ear

Although it is apparent that the sound-perceiving neurosensory apparatus of the inner ear comes from the neuroectodermal otocyst, the sound-conducting mechanism arises from totally different and widely separated anlages. The sound-conducting mechanisms of the outer and middle ear are derived from the branchial or gill apparatus of the embryo.

At 4 weeks of fetal age three branchial arches separated by two external branchial grooves have developed on either side of the head. The first branchial groove deepens to become the primitive external auditory meatus, while the corresponding evagination from the pharynx, the first pharyngeal pouch, grows outward and upward toward it, forming the primitive eustachian tube. For a brief moment in embryologic time the epithelium of the first branchial groove touches the endoderm of the first pharyngeal pouch at the site of the future tympanic membrane. However, soon mesoderm grows between and separates these two layers so that the mature tympanic membrane is formed by all three germinal layers.

Over the next 5 fetal months the first branchial groove contributes to the development of the mature configuration of the *external acoustic meatus*, the outer, cuticular layer of the *tympanic membrane*, and the *tympanic ring*.

The auricle develops from around the first branchial groove from six knoblike outgrowths or hillocks arising from the first and second branchial arches, appearing at the sixth week of embryonic life and fusing by the third month.

The first pharyngeal pouch becomes the *eustachian tube* and *middle ear cavity*; the cartilages of the first and second branchial arches form the ossicles. The first branchial arch forms the bodies of the malleus and incus; the second branchial arch forms the crura of the stapes, the lenticular process and long crus of the incus, and the manubrium of malleus. The footplate of the stapes comes from the otic capsule. With further development the ossicles separate from their parent cartilages and fuse. These separate processes then develop independent growth.

The ossicles, similar to the otic capsule and labyrinth, grow only through the first half of uterine life and then ossify. Each of these bones ossifies from a single center; the incus appears at 16 weeks, the malleus at 16½ weeks, and the stapes at 18 weeks. The ossicles are formed of enchondral bone that persists for the rest of the individual's life, as does the enchondral layer of the labyrinthine capsule. The malleus and incus remain solid and relatively constant in size and shape. The stapes, however, undergoes a process of erosion and thinning soon after it ossifies. The adult stapes is less bulky and considerably more delicate and fragile than it is in mid–fetal life. With this diminution in bulk and weight there develop exceptional variations in size, shape, and strength of the adult crura and footplate. A normal adult footplate varies from being thick and uniform to being thin and irregular. It even may be dehiscent in its central portion. One therefore should abstain from characterizing an irregular, thick, thin, or dehiscent footplate as abnormal based on its imaging appearance.

As the ossicles differentiate and ossify, the surrounding mesenchymal connective tissue becomes less dense and less cellular; by 18 to 21 weeks the tissue filling the space of what is to become the middle ear is very loose, somewhat vacuolated, and mucoid in character. By 22 weeks this vacuolated, mucoid connective tissue gives way to the upward expanding tympanic epithelium of the first pharyngeal pouch. The latter encroaches on and wraps around the ossicles and their tendons and ligaments, investing them with epithelial tissue derived from endoderm. Communication between the pharynx and middle ear is thus established. At maturity only the eustachian tube remains as an anatomic reminder of the upward migration of the first pharyngeal pouch in the formation of the tympanic cavity and communicating spaces.

By the thirtieth week "pneumatization" of the tympanum proper is almost complete. Pneumatization of the antrum soon follows and progresses rapidly from the thirty-fourth to the thirty-fifth week, but in the epitympanum it lags and is not completed until the last month of fetal life.

Pneumatization at this stage of development has nothing to do with the actual presence of air in the ear; used in this context it relates rather to the process of focal dissolution and displacement of mesenchymal connective tissue with eventual formation of the space that comes to be lined by an advancing layer of endodermal (respiratory) epithelium arising from the first pharyngeal pouch. This space will become the aerated cavities of the eustachian tube, the middle ear, antrum, etc., at term. Pneumatization thus comes to refer to the creation of an epithelial-lined space to be aerated later.

Pneumatic Cells of the Temporal Bone

The air cells of the temporal bone develop as outpouchings of the antrum, epitympanum, tympanic cavity, and eustachian tube. Despite tentative epithelial evaginations appearing from the antrum as early as 34 weeks, no significant pneumatic cellular expansion into the remainder of the temporal bone occurs until after birth, with the stimulation caused by the presence of air within the middle ear. The pneumatizing process then goes into a period of high activity, proceeding over several years. The petrous apex may demonstrate continued pneumatization into early adult life.

Pneumatization occurs as a result of epithelial-lined projections arising from the lining of the middle ear and its extensions. These evaginations probe the spaces between spicules of new bone that are forming and the spaces created by the degeneration of bone marrow into a loose connective tissue stroma. The air cells will invade bone only after the marrow has been converted into a loose mesenchymal tissue. It is averred by Wittmaack[8] that the presence of middle ear infections in infancy causes the embryonic subepithelial connective tissue to fibrose; this prevents its condensation and thinning and impedes the progress of the advancing fingers of evaginating pneumatic cells. This would explain pneumatization arrest following otitis media in infants and children.

The Neonatal Temporal Bone

At birth the anatomic portions of the hearing and vestibular system are virtually fully developed with the exception of the formation of the osseous portion of the external acoustic canal. Even the internal acoustic canal (which is not part of the bony labyrinth but is by common clinical practice considered to be part of the inner ear because of its juxtaposition and functional relationship to the labyrinth) is of nearly adult vertical dimension and will grow probably no more than 1 mm in height during the remainder of the individual's life. (The length of the internal acoustic canal, however, will increase substantially during childhood.)

Shambaugh[5] emphasizes that the remainder of the neonatal temporal bone, however, is small and differs from the adult both in shape and position, occupying the inferolateral surface of the skull rather than the lateral aspect as in mature individuals. He notes that, as viewed from the side, the infant temporal bone consists of a large squamous portion, a diminutive tympanic portion, and no mastoid. Whereas in the adult the mastoid lies posterior to the tympanic ring, in the child the petrous portion lies behind the tympanic ring and below the squamous portion.

Formation of the Mastoid Process

The mastoid process is a postnatal structure and begins to develop during the second year of life as a result of downward extension of the squamous portion and partially as a result of extensions of the petrous portion. These two parts of the mastoid process come together at the petrosquamous suture line. Within the mastoid process air cells grow down from the antrum vertically in the petrous portion to the mastoid tip and laterally and radially into the squamous portion. A dividing bridge of bone separating these two cell tracks is known as *Koerner's septum*. This is visible radiographically as a pointed bony spicule directed obliquely downward, originating from the antral roof.

With further maturation of the mastoid, the thin, incomplete infantile ring that constitutes the tympanic portion of the bone grows laterally and inferiorly to form the osseous extension of the (heretofore) cartilaginous auditory canal. Two suture lines are formed: the *tympanosquamous suture* arising in the anterosuperior meatal wall and the posteriorly positioned *tympanomastoid suture*.

NORMAL ANATOMY

The anatomy of the temporal bone is complex and in many circumstances confusing. Part of the complexity has to do with 350 million years of evolutionary modification of this organ and part has to do with unfortunate anatomic terminology, ambiguity, imprecision, and redundancy that has become fixed in scientific nomenclature. The following section is a compendium gathered from many anatomic sources.[3,4,6,7,9-13]

Temporal Bone

The temporal bones are situated at the sides and base of the skull. Each consists of five parts: squamous, mastoid, petrous, tympanic, and the styloid process.

Squamous Portion. The squamous portion forms the anterolateral and upper part of the bone; it is shell-like and thin. The external surface is smooth and convex, giving attachment to the temporalis muscle; it forms part of the wall of the temporal fossa. A gently arching *zygomatic process* arises from the lower portion of the squama and is directed anteriorly. Its lateral surface is convex and lies directly beneath the skin and subcutaneous tissue. The medial surface is concave and serves as the origin of the masseter muscle. The anterior end of the zygomatic process articulates with the zygomatic bone. The posterior portion of the zygomatic process is divided into an anterior and posterior root. The posterior root lies above the external auditory canal and becomes continuous with the temporal line posterior to the external auditory canal.

The anterior root becomes the articular tubercle of the condylar (glenoid or mandibular) fossa. The condylar fossa is bound posteriorly to the anterior surface of the tympanic bone.

The mandibular fossa is cleaved in the coronal plane by the tympanosquamous suture laterally and by that suture's inward extension, the petrotympanic (Glaserian) fissure, medially. The portion of the condylar fossa anterior to the fissure is the articular portion of the joint; that portion posterior to the Glaserian fissure is the nonarticular portion.

The internal surface of the squama is concave and irregular. Meningeal vessels groove the inner surface. The superior border articulates with the parietal bone, and the anteroinferior border articulates with the greater wing of the sphenoid.

Mastoid Portion. The mastoid portion has a rough outer surface and serves as origin to a portion of the occipital and the posterior auricular muscles. In the adult the mastoid portion is continued inferiorly into a conical projection, the mastoid process. This process gives attachment to the sternocleidomastoid, splenius capitis, and longissimus capitis muscles. On the medial side of the process is a deep groove, the mastoid notch or digastric groove, for the attachment of the digastric muscle. Medial to this is a shallow furrow, the occipital groove, which lodges the occipital artery.

The inner or intracranial surface of the mastoid presents a deeper groove, the sigmoid sulcus, which lodges part of the transverse sinus.

The superior border is broad and serrated and articulates with the parietal portion of the temporal bone. The posterior border, similarly serrated, articulates with the inferior border of the occipital bone. Anteriorly and above, the mastoid portion is fused with the descending process of the temporal squama; below, it enters into the formation of the external acoustic meatus and the tympanic cavity.

The mastoid process is hollowed to form a number of spaces, the mastoid cells, which exhibit great variety in size and number. In the upper and anterior part of the process, these cells are large and irregular, toward the middle part they diminish in size, and those in the apex of the process frequently are small. In addition to these cells there occurs a large irregular cavity, the tympanic antrum, that is situated at the upper and anterior part of the mastoid portion of the bone. The antrum communicates with the remainder of the mastoid cells and with the epitympanum (attic), which is situated anteroinferiorly and medially by way of the narrow channel, the *additus ad antrum*.

Petrous Portion. The petrous pyramid is wedged in at the base of the skull between the sphenoid bone anteriorly and the occipital bone posteriorly. Its apex is directed medially, forward, and slightly upward. It contains the inner ear.

The petrous portion resembles a toppled three-sided pyramid lying on the flat surface of one of its sides. Its base is laterally positioned and is fused with the internal surfaces of the squamous and mastoid portions. The apex points medially and forward and is inserted into the angular interval between the posterior border of the greater wing of the sphenoid bone and the basilar part of the occipital bone. The anterior (middle fossa) face of the petrous pyramid has a more horizontal orientation and is "longer" than the posterior surface, which is relatively vertical and "shorter."

The anterior face (surface) forms the posterior limit of the middle cranial fossa and is continuous laterally with the inner surface of the squamous portion; it is united at these edges by the petrosquamous suture. Its surfaces are somewhat irregular and marked by depressions for convolutions of the brain and by a shallow depression medially for the reception of the semilunar ganglion (Meckel's cave) of the fifth canial nerve. The arcuate eminence, which marks the site of the underlying superior semicircular canal, is near its midportion. In front of and slightly lateral to this eminence is a depression that marks the position of the tympanic cavity. The layer of bone that separates the tympanic and cranial cavities is usually very thin and is known as the *tegmen tympani.* A nearby groove leads laterally and posteriorly to an oblique opening, the hiatus of the facial canal, which transmits the greater superficial petrosal nerve and the petrosal branch of the middle meningeal artery.

The posterior face (surface) of the petrous pyramid forms the anterior bony limit of the posterior fossa and is continuous with the inner surface of the mastoid portion of the temporal bone at the petromastoid suture. To reiterate, this face has a more vertical orientation than the anterior surface. Near the center of this surface is the opening to the internal auditory (acoustic) canal (meatus), which transmits the seventh and eighth cranial nerves, the nervus intermedius, and the internal auditory artery. The opening of the internal auditory canal is known as the *porus acusticus.*

The lateral end of the internal auditory canal is closed by a vertical plate of bone, the *lamina spiralis,* which separates the fundus of the canal from the vestibule. The fundus is divided by a transverse crest of bone, the *crista falciformis,* into a smaller upper and a larger lower compartment. The crista, which arises anteriorly, usually extends medially no more than 2 to 3 mm. The upper compartment occupies about 40% and the lower about 60% of the vertical dimension of the canal. In the upper compartment the facial nerve (VII) lies anteriorly and the superior vestibular division of cranial nerve VIII lies posteriorly. The branches of the latter go to the utricle and superior and lateral semicircular canals. A thin crest of arachnoid tissue separates the lateral portion of this upper compartment into its anterior and posterior portions. This crest occasionally ossifies and is known as *Bill's bar.*

In the compartment beneath the crista falciformis there are three sets of foramina. Anteriorly, a set is arranged spirally about the central canal of the cochlea (the *modiolus*) to accommodate the cochlear division of the eighth cranial nerve. Posteriorly, branches of the inferior division of the vestibular nerve take their exit, one set of foramina leading to the saccule and the remainder leading to the posterior semicircular canal.

Posteroinferior to the internal acoustic meatus is a small slit that leads to the vestibular aqueduct. This transmits the endolymphatic duct along with the accompanying artery and vein.

The inferior face (surface) of the petrous pyramid is a rough and irregular surface and forms part of the exterior of the base of the skull. It furnishes partial attachment for the *levator veli palatini* and the cartilaginous portion of the eustachian tube. It is pierced anteriorly by the aperture of the carotid canal. The cochlear aqueduct opens on the inferior surface, lying almost vertically beneath the porus acousticus. Behind the opening of the cochlear aqueduct lies the jugular fossa.

There are two minute canals that perforate the inferior surface of the petrous portion within or near the jugular fossa.

- The *inferior tympanic canaliculus,* which accommodates the tympanic branch of the glossopharyngeal nerve (Jacobson's nerve), lies between the carotid canal and the jugular fossa.
- The *mastoid canaliculus,* which serves as entrance for the auricular branch of the vagus nerve (Arnold's nerve), is located within the lateral part of the jugular fossa.

The styloid process originates from the inferior face of the pyramid. The *stylomastoid foramen* is situated between the downward projections of the mastoid process and the styloid process. This foramen constitutes the terminus of the bony facial canal.

The superior angle (border) of the petrous portion of the temporal bone is grooved for the superior petrosal sinus and gives attachment to the tentorium cerebelli. This superior angle commonly is referred to as the "petrous ridge"; it represents the line of the intersection between the anterior and posterior surfaces of the pyramid. The anteromedial extremity of the ridge is notched for the reception of the roots of the trigeminal nerve.

The posterior angle of the pyramid is defined by the junction of the lower aspect of the posterior surface with the posterior limits of the inferior surface. From the perspective of the inner surface of the skull within the posterior fossa, the posterior angle is marked by a sulcus of the petrous portion that along with a corresponding sulcus on the occipital bone forms the channel for the inferior petrosal sinus. An excavation on the inferior and medial aspect of the posterior surface of the pyramid, in continuity with this sulcus, is known as the *jugular fossa.* The corresponding depression, in continuity with the sulcus arising from the anterolateral surface of the occipital bone, is known as the *jugular notch.* These semilunar cavities face one another and together form the *jugular foramen.* The dilated portion of the internal jugular vein that occupies the foramen is the *jugular bulb.*

The anterior angle of the pyramid marks the junction between the pyramid and the bones of the floor of the middle cranial fossa. The anterior border is divided into two parts: the medial part, which articulates with the greater wing of the sphenoid, and the lateral portion, which adjoins the squamous part at the petrosquamous suture.

At the angle of the junction of the petrous and squamous portions, there are two (semi) canals placed one above the other, which are separated by a thin plate of bone. This septum is known as the *septum canalis musculotubarii* (cochleariform process). The upper canal contains the tensor tympani muscle, and the lower canal is the bony portion of the eustachian tube.

Tympanic Portion. The tympanic portion of the temporal bone is a curved plate lying below the squamous part and in front of the mastoid process. Its *posterior* surface is somewhat C-shaped and forms the *anterior* wall, the floor, and the posteroinferior aspect of the bony external auditory canal. At the medial end of the canal there is a narrow furrow, the *tympanic sulcus*, for the attachment of the tympanic membrane. The lateral border of the tympanic portion of the temporal bone is roughened, forming a large part of the margin of the opening of the external auditory canal; this is continuous with the cartilaginous part of the canal. The lateral part of the upper border is fused with the back of the postglenoid tubercle. Its medial extension forms the posterior boundary of the petrotympanic fissure.

There is considerable ambiguity in anatomic descriptions regarding the terms *petrotympanic fissure*, *tympanosquamous fissure*, and *Glaserian fissure*. Many anatomic depictions point unassailably to a junction between the *squamous* and tympanic portions, labeling the area "petrotympanic fissure." This is more easily understood if one recognizes that the tympanosquamous fissure (squamotympanic) is merely the lateral extension of the petrotympanic fissure, while the Glaserian fissure is the medial extension of the petrotympanic fissure. This serves as a passageway for the anterior tympanic branch of the internal maxillary artery. In the medialmost extreme portion of the petrotympanic fissure is the small canal for the chorda tympani, the *iter chordae anterius (anterior tympanic aperture)*.

The lower border of the tympanic bone encloses the root of the *styloid process*. Posteriorly, the tympanic portion blends with the squamous and mastoid portions, forming the anterior boundary of the tympanomastoid fissure.

Styloid Process. The styloid process of the temporal bone averages about 2.5 cm in length and projects downward and forward from the undersurface immediately anterior to the stylomastoid foramen. It gives origin to muscles and ligaments of the hyoid, pharyngeal and glottic regions.

External Auditory Canal

The walls of the external auditory canal (meatus) are formed laterally of fibrocartilage and medially of bone, while both parts are lined by skin reflected inward. The osseous portion of the meatus, which comprises slightly more than half of the canal, is a tunnel through the temporal bone. The bony canal is about 16 mm long and directed inward, forward, and downward. On a sagittal scan section the canal is oval or elliptical in shape, with its long axis directed downward and slightly backward. The anterior wall, floor, and lower part of the posterior wall are formed by the tympanic component of the temporal bone; the remainder of the posterior wall and the roof arise from the squamousal portion.[11]

The tympanic membrane makes a compound angle with the external acoustic meatus. The inferior border of the tympanic membrane lies closer to the midsagittal plane than does the superior border. Additionally, the anterior border lies closer to the midsagittal plane than does the posterior border. This means that the tympanic membrane is sloping both downward and inward. The posterosuperior wall of the external auditory meatus measures about 25 mm in the adult, while the anteroinferior wall is over 30 mm.

Vessels and Nerves. The arteries of the external auditory meatus are derived from the external carotid artery through branches from the posterior auricular, superficial temporal, and internal maxillary arteries. The veins and lymphatics connect with those of the auricle. The veins ultimately empty into the internal and external jugular veins and occasionally into the sigmoid sinus by way of mastoid emissary veins.

The lymphatics of the external acoustic canal and auricle empty into all adjacent regional nodes, including the parotid, superficial cervical, and retroauricular groups.

Because the development of the external ear is embryologically complex, the cutaneous innervation is similarly complex and subject to considerable variation. Innervation is derived from the auriculotemporal branch of the mandibular division of the trigeminal nerve and from cutaneous branches of the cervical plexus, primarily the greater auricular nerve from C2 and C3. There are also contributions from sensory fibers originating in the eighth, ninth, and tenth cranial nerves.

The Middle Ear

The middle ear or tympanic cavity is an irregular, laterally compressed space within the temporal bone. It is filled with air that is conveyed to it from the nasopharynx through the eustachian tube. It is traversed by the ossicular chain, which connects the lateral and medial walls. The ossicles both transmit and amplify the vibrations incident on the tympanic membrane across the cavity to the inner ear.

The tympanic cavity consists of three parts: the *tympanic cavity proper* (or mesotympanum) opposite the tympanic membrane, the *attic* (or epitympanic recess or epitympanum) above the level of the membrane, and the *hypotympanum*, a variable inferior and medial extension occurring below the level of the tympanic membrane.

Shaped more like a cleft than a box, the vertical dimension (including the attic) and the anteroposterior dimension of the cavity are each about 15 mm. The transverse dimensions measure about 6 mm superiorly and 4 mm inferiorly. Opposite the center of the tympanic membrane it may measure only about 2 mm. The lateral extent of the cavity is defined by the tympanic membrane or *membranous wall* and the medial or *labyrinthine wall* by the otic capsule. The roof is known as the *tegmental wall* and the floor, which is separated from the jugular fossa by a thin plate of bone, is known as the *jugular wall*. Anteriorly the space is delimited by the *carotid wall* and posteriorly by the *mastoid wall*.

Roof or Tegmental Wall. The tegmen tympani is a plate of bone that arises from the petrous portion of the temporal bone. Its forward prolongation becomes the roof of the canal for the tensor tympani muscle and its backward continuation forms the roof of the mastoid antrum. The tegmen tympani separates the middle ear cavity from the middle cranial fossa. The lateral margin of the tegmen interdigitates with the squamous portion of the temporal bone at the petrosquamous suture. In children this may be unossified and may allow a direct passage of infection from the middle ear to the epidural space of the middle cranial fossa. In adults, veins from the middle ear perforate this suture to end in the petrosquamous sinus (present in about 50% of cases) and the superior petrosal sinus. They may transmit infection directly into the cranial venous sinuses.[10]

Floor or Jugular Wall. The floor or jugular wall of the middle ear cavity lies either at or slightly below the level of the floor of the external auditory meatus and is usually a very thin plate of bone that separates the cavity from the internal jugular vein. If the jugular bulb is particularly small, then the floor may be correspondingly thick—even as much as a centimeter—and it may contain air cells intervening between the middle ear cavity and the internal jugular vein. The inferior extent of the tympanic cavity below the level of the inferior attachment of the tympanic membrane, along with its medial extension, is known as the *hypotympanum*.

If the jugular bulb is very large it may bulge upward into the floor of the tympanic cavity, giving it a convex margin. This bulging reduces the potential size of the hypotympanum. Occasionally the bone may be dehiscent (see section on high jugular bulb), with the jugular bulb present within the hypotympanum. The importance of recognition of this anatomic variation is obvious in the differential diagnosis of glomus tumor, jugular diverticulum, and aberrant position of the carotid canal in the circumstance of pulsatile tinnitus.

A small aperture for the passage of the tympanic branch of the glossopharyngeal nerve (Jacobson's nerve) is present within the jugular wall near the labyrinthine wall.

Mastoid or Posterior Wall. The mastoid or posterior wall is wide above and below and presents the *additus ad antrum* (entrance to the tympanic antrum), the *pyramidal eminence*, and the *incudal fossa*. The additus ad antrum is a large, irregular aperture that leads posteriorly from the epitympanic recess to the mastoid antrum. The pyramidal eminence is situated immediately behind the oval window and in front of the vertical (mastoid) portion of the facial canal; it is hollow and contains the origin and belly of the stapedius muscle. Its summit projects forward toward the oval window, and it is pierced by a small aperture that transmits the tendon of the muscle. The cavity of the pyramidal eminence is prolonged downward and backward in front of the facial canal and communicates with it by a minute aperture that transmits a twig from the facial nerve to the stapedius muscle.

There are two important recesses in the posterior wall, the *sinus tympani* and the *facial recess* (Fig. 13-2). They may be the sites of occult extension of disease within the middle ear. They are demonstrated with ease by means of axial scans in CT.

The tympanic sinus is a space that is bounded by the labyrinthine wall medially and by the pyramidal eminence laterally.

The facial recess is bounded by the pyramidal eminence, styloid complex, and facial canal medially and by the bony tympanic annulus laterally. The facial recess is an important surgical landmark when the middle ear cavity is entered from the posterior aspect by means of a mastoid approach.

The incudal fossa is a small depression in the lower and posterior portion of the epitympanic recess; this is the site of attachment of the posterior ligament of the short process of the incus.

Just lateral and usually slightly inferior to the aperture transmitting the tendon of the stapedius muscle is the aperture for the chorda tympani nerve as it separates from the mastoid portion of the facial nerve.

Carotid or Anterior Wall. The carotid or anterior wall is wider above than below and corresponds with the carotid canal, from which it is separated by a thin plate of bone that is perforated by the tympanic branch of the

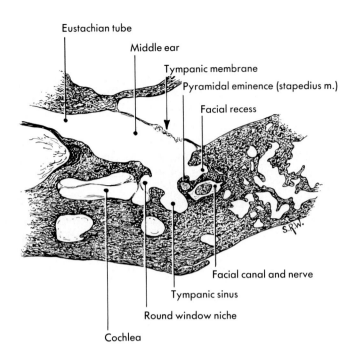

Eustachian tube
Middle ear
Tympanic membrane
Pyramidal eminence (stapedius m.)
Facial recess
Facial canal and nerve
Tympanic sinus
Round window niche
Cochlea

Fig. 13-2   Relationships of sinus tympani, facial recess, and facial canal within posterior wall of middle ear. Axial section through temporal bone at level of round window niche. These relationships are of paramount importance to operating surgeon because they affect surgeon's ability to gain access to diseased tissue. Tympanic sinus may be site of occult disease. Primary facial nerve pathologic processes may also obliterate these spaces. This minute anatomy is exquisitely defined on axial computed tomography.

internal carotid artery and also by the caroticotympanic nerve. At the upper part of the anterior wall are the orifice of the semicanal for the tensor tympani muscle and the tympanic orifice of the eustachian tube, separated from each other by the septum canalis musculotubarii. These semicanals run from the tympanic cavity forward and downward to the angle between the squamous and petrous portion of the temporal bone. These semicanals lie one above the other rather than side by side.

The semicanal for the tensor tympani is the superior and smaller of the two; it is cylindrical and lies beneath the tegmen tympani. It extends to the labyrinthine wall of the tympanic cavity and ends immediately above the oval window. In current usage the septum canalis musculotubarii is more commonly known as the *processus cochleariformis*. This bony structure forms the lateral wall and floor of the semicanal for the tensor tympani.

The Eustachian Tube. The eustachian tube is the lower of the two channels and the one through which the tympanic cavity communicates with the nasopharynx. Its length is about 3.5 cm, and its direction is downward, forward, and medially. It forms an angle of about 45 degrees with the sagittal plane and one of about 30 degrees to 40 degrees with the horizontal plane. Part of the eustachian tube is composed of bone, and part is composed of fibrous tissue and cartilage.

The osseous portion is a little over a centimeter in length. It begins in the carotid wall below the process cochleariformis and, tapering slowly, ends at the angle of junction of the squamous and petrous portions of the temporal bone. Its distalmost end has a serrated margin for the attachment of the cartilaginous portion.

The cartilaginous portion is around 2.5 cm in length. The cartilage lies in a groove between the petrous part of the temporal bone and the greater wing of the sphenoid. This groove ends opposite the upper posterior margin of the medial pterygoid plate.

The tube is not of uniform diameter; its narrowest portion (the isthmus) lies at the junction of the bony and cartilaginous portion. It is at its widest diameter at the pharyngeal orifice. The cartilaginous and bony portions of the tube are not in the same vertical plane, the cartilaginous portion being slightly more steeply inclined than the bony portion.

Lateral or Membranous Wall. The tympanic cavity extends above the level of the tympanic membrane as the epitympanic recess. The lateral boundary of the tympanic cavity proper, therefore, is the tympanic membrane together with the small rim of the temporal bone to which it is attached. The osseous tympanic ring is complete superiorly at the notch of Rivinus. Close to this notch are three small apertures: the petrotympanic (glaserian) fissure and the anterior and posterior tympanic apertures (iter chordae anterius and posterius).

The petrotympanic fissure transmits the tympanic branch of the internal maxillary artery and houses the anterior process of the malleus and its anterior ligament.

The chorda tympani nerve gains entrance and finds egress from the tympanic cavity by way of the posterior and anterior tympanic apertures, respectively. The chorda tympani traverses the tympanic cavity but gives off no branches to it.

The tympanic membrane is directed obliquely downward and inward, forming an angle of about 50 degrees with the floor of the external acoustic canal and about 15 degrees with the midsagittal plane. The manubrium of the malleus is attached to the medial surface of the tympanic membrane at its center and pulls the membrane inward; the lateral surface of the membrane therefore appears concave, and the central depression of this concavity is called the *umbo.*

Medial or Labyrinthine Wall. The medial wall of the tympanic cavity is that part of the petrous portion of the temporal bone that surrounds the internal ear and separates the cavities of the middle and internal ears.[10] Several bulges and depressions are apparent, reflecting the various contours of the inner ear structures.

Posteriorly and superiorly, in what would be considered the medial wall in the region of the additus, is the prominence produced by the anterior limb of the lateral semicircular canal. Below this and extending more anteriorly is the prominence of the facial canal produced by the bone overlying the intratympanic portion of the facial nerve. Anterior to the prominence of the facial canal is the curving terminus of the septum canalis musculotubarii; this also serves as a landmark for the position of the geniculum of the facial nerve (geniculate ganglion), which lies immediately anterior to the first knee of the facial nerve.

Immediately below the mesotympanic facial canal is the laterally directed oval window niche, which contains the oval window at its medial terminus. Below the oval window lies the promontory, a convexity that bulges into the tympanic cavity and represents a portion of the otic capsule over the basal turn of the cochlea. Below and behind the back part of the promontory is the round window niche, which leads to the round window. The round window has an orientation very close to the coronal plane and is directed downward. Posterior to the promontory is a smooth bony projection, the *subiculum promontorii,* which forms the inferior border of the deep depression known as the *tympanic sinus.* Inferior to the subiculum lies the round window niche.

The superior border of the sinus tympani is bounded by another smooth, bony bridge, the ponticulus. The oval window niche lies superior to the ponticulus.

To recapitulate, there are two bony bridges: the upper or ponticulus and the lower or subiculum. Between the two lies the sinus tympani. Above the ponticulus lies the oval window niche. Below the subiculum lies the round window niche.

Epitympanic Recess. That portion of the tympanic cavity that extends above the level of the tympanic membrane is known as the epitympanic recess, or attic. This is a chamber having a height about one third that of the entire tympanic cavity; the attic projects lateral to the plane of the tympanic membrane. This small portion of the tympanic cavity therefore has as its lateral wall a part of the squamous portion of the temporal bone; the inferior, medially directed pointed terminus of the lateral attic wall is known as the *scutum,* which is directly above the tympanic membrane.

The attic contains the head of the malleus and the body and short process of the incus. Superiorly the epitympanic recess is bounded by the tegmen tympani; medially by the prominence of the lateral semicircular canal and the prominence of the facial nerve; laterally by the scutum; and inferiorly by the incudal fossa and the bony surface just behind it. The boundary line between the tympanic cavity proper and the epitympanic recess is marked by the prominence of the facial canal medially, the inferior limit of the incudal fossa inferiorly, and the scutum laterally. The additus ad antrum originates from the posterosuperior aspect of the epitympanic recess.

Contents of Tympanic Cavity

Auditory Ossicles. Three small bones span the width of the tympanic cavity. The *malleus* consists of a head, a neck (manubrium), and two processes. The head lies within the epitympanum. The *manubrium* is attached to the tympanic membrane. The *lateral process* abuts the tympanic membrane immediately below the pars flaccida. The *anterior process* is a slender spicule of bone that passes forward and downward into the petrotympanic fissure.

The *incus* is shaped somewhat like a premolar tooth, with two widely diverging roots that differ in length. The *body* is somewhat cuboid but compressed transversely. On its anterior surface is a deeply concavoconvex facet that articulates with the head of the malleus. The body of the incus and the head of the malleus are bound to one another by a thin capsular ligament, forming a diarthroidial joint known as the *incudomalleolar articulation.*

The two crura of the incus diverge from one another narrowly at right angles. The *short crus* or short process projects almost horizontally backward and is attached to the incudal fossa in the lower and posterior portion of the epitympanic recess.

The *long crus* (long process) descends nearly vertically behind and parallel to the manubrium of the malleus and bends medially to end in a rounded projection, the *lenticular process,* which is tipped with cartilage and articulates with the head of the stapes. This is also a diarthroidal joint and is called the *incudostapedial articulation.*

From its articulation with the incus, the stapes passes almost horizontally across the tympanic cavity to meet the wall of the labyrinth at the oval window.

The *stapes* resembles a stirrup and consists of a head, a neck, two crura, and a base. The *head* has a depression that is covered by cartilage and articulates with the lenticular process of the incus. The *neck* is the constricted part of the bone succeeding the head, and its posterior aspect gives insertion to the tendon of the stapedius muscle.

The *anterior* and *posterior crura* diverge from the neck and are connected at their ends to the flattened oval plate known as the *base*, which forms the footplate of the stapes and is fixed to the margin of the oval window by the annular ligament. The anterior crus is shorter and less curved than the posterior. The edge of the stapedial base is covered with cartilage, as is the rim of the oval window; the junction thereof constitutes the *tympanostapedial syndesmosis*.

Ligaments. The ossicles are connected with the walls of the tympanic cavity by ligaments: three for the malleus, and one each for the incus and stapes.

The *anterior ligament* goes from the neck of the malleus just above the anterior process to the carotid wall near the petrotympanic fissure. The *superior ligament* descends from the roof of the epitympanic recess to the head of the malleus. The *lateral ligament* goes from the posterior part of the notch of Rivinus to the head of the malleus.

The *posterior ligament* of the incus is a short, thick band connecting the neck and end of the short crus to the posterior wall of the incudal fossa.

The *annular ligament* of the base of the stapes has been described previously. It represents the fibrous ring that encircles the base of the stapes and attaches to the margin of the oval window.

Muscles. The muscles of the tympanic cavity have already been alluded to; one each arises from the anterior and posterior walls.

The *tensor tympani*, the larger muscle, is contained in the bony canal above the osseous portion of the eustachian tube, from which it is separated by the processus cochleariformis. It passes backward through the canal and ends in a slender tendon that enters the tympanic cavity; it makes a sharp bend around the terminus of the process cochleariformis and is inserted into the neck of the malleus, which is at the upper end or root of the manubrium. It is supplied by a branch of the mandibular nerve that passes through the otic ganglion.

The *stapedius* muscle rises from the walls of the conical cavity hollowed out of the interior of the pyramidal eminence. Its tendon emerges from the orifice at the apex of the pyramidal eminence; as it moves forward, it is inserted into the posterior surface of the neck of the stapes. It is supplied by a branch of the facial nerve.

By their actions both the tensor tympani and stapedius muscles reduce the efficiency of the sound-conducting mechanism. The tensor tympani accomplishes this by tightening the drum of the tympanic membrane and thereby diminishing the amplitude of excursion of the malleus. The stapedius muscle exerts its action by pulling the head of the stapes backward, which causes the base of the bone to rotate on a vertical axis drawn through its own center. The posterior part of the base is pressed inward toward the vestibule and the forward portion is withdrawn from it. This reduces the amount of area effectively transmitting the vibration at the footplate and diminishes the mechanical advantage of the lever mechanism. Both of these muscles therefore serve to protect the inner ear from excessive amplitude oscillations of the footplate of the stapes when there is a very loud noise. This protective reflex is invoked with low-frequency vibration only and is most effective at frequencies under 5000 Hz.

Nerves and Vessels. The nerves of the middle ear cavity are represented by the tympanic plexus, which lies on the cochlear promontory under the mucosa, within grooves or canals in the bone. This plexus is formed chiefly by the tympanic branch (nerve of Jacobson) of the ninth cranial nerve but is reinforced by one or more caroticotympanic nerves derived from the internal carotid sympathetic plexus. The facial nerve also makes a minor contribution to the tympanic plexus. These fibers are mostly parasympathetic secretomotor fibers. The tympanic branch of cranial nerve IX supplies sensory innervation to the mucosa of the middle ear.

Glomus tympanicum tumors take their origin in cell groups associated with the tympanic branch of the ninth cranial nerve (the tympanic plexus).

The chorda tympani arising from cranial nerve VII traverses the middle ear cavity but is not a source of innervation to the cavity.

The tympanic cavity derives its arterial supply from a number of vessels, most of which are branches of the external carotid artery. These include the *anterior tympanic* artery arising from the internal maxillary artery; the *inferior tympanic* artery arising from the ascending pharyngeal artery; the *stylomastoid* artery arising from either the posterior auricular or the occipital artery, which gives off a *posterior tympanic* artery; a *superior tympanic* and *petrosal* artery arising from the middle meningeal artery; and *caroticotympanic* branches arising from the internal carotid artery.

The veins roughly parallel the arteries and empty into the superior petrosal sinus and pterygoid plexus. The lymphatics begin as a network in the mucous membrane and end chiefly in the retropharyngeal lymph nodes.

Route of the Facial Nerve (Cranial Nerve VII)

The facial or seventh cranial nerve emerges from the brainstem as two roots, *motor* and *sensory*. The motor root is the larger. It leaves the medulla oblongata at the inferior border of the pons, medial to the acoustic nerve. The smaller sensory root or *nervus intermedius* (of Wrisberg) contains efferent and visceral efferent fibers. It emerges from the medulla between the motor root of the facial nerve and the acoustic nerve.

Motor Root. As the motor root leaves the medulla it pierces the pia mater and receives its sheath. The bundle then continues forward and laterally in the posterior fossa to the internal auditory meatus, where it enters in conjunction with the nervus intermedius and acoustic nerve. As it spans the distance between the medulla and the porus acousticus the motor root aligns itself in a groove on the superior surface of the cochlear division of the acoustic nerve. This intracranial segment is 23 to 24 mm in length.

The internal auditory canal segment is 7 to 8 mm in length and lies in a superior relationship to the cochlear nerve, passing above the crista falciformis. While within the canal, the motor root is separated from the acoustic bundle by the nervus intermedius, but the three nerve bundles are all surrounded by one sheath or arachnoid and dura and by continuations of the subarachnoid and subdural spaces. While still within the canal, the motor root and the nervus intermedius unite to form the combined nerve trunk.

The labyrinthine segment of the nerve measures 3 to 4 mm in length and passes forward and laterally within its own bony channel, the *fallopian canal.* When it reaches a point just lateral and superior to the cochlea, it angles sharply forward, nearly at a right angle to the long axis of the petrous pyramid, to reach the geniculate ganglion. At the ganglion the direction of the nerve reverses itself, executing a hairpin turn so that it runs posteriorly. This is the so-called first knee or *first genu* of the facial nerve. At this point the facial nerve is lying just above the base of the cochlea, i.e., above and medial to the promontory.

The first genu of the facial nerve, in the limb distal to the geniculate ganglion, delineates the anteriormost extent of the tympanic segment of the nerve. This tympanic segment is around 12 mm in length and passes posteriorly and laterally, perpendicular to the long axis of the petrous bone on the medial wall of the tympanic cavity. It lies above the oval window and below the bulge of the lateral semicircular canal. At the level of the sinus tympani the nerve changes direction at the *second genu.* At this point the nerve assumes a vertical position, dropping downward in the posterior wall of the tympanic cavity and the anterior wall of the mastoid to exit at the base of the skull from the stylomastoid foramen. This mastoid segment is about 15 to 20 mm in length.[12]

There are three primary branches of the facial nerve: the greater superficial petrosal nerve, the nerve to the stapedius muscle, and the chorda tympani.

The greater superficial petrosal nerve arises from the geniculate ganglion and exits the petrous bone and facial canal just anterior to the geniculate ganglion by way of the facial hiatus along the anterior aspect of the petrous pyramid. The greater superficial petrosal nerve is a mixed nerve, containing both parasympathetic fibers (from the nervus intermedius) and motor fibers. This nerve will receive sympathetic fibers from the deep petrosal nerve, at which point it becomes the vidian nerve.

The nerve to the stapedius muscle is a small twig given off from the facial nerve as it descends in the posterior wall of the tympanic cavity behind the pyramidal eminence.

The chorda tympani takes its origin about 5 mm above the stylomastoid foramen and is composed mainly of sensory fibers, although it also contains a few motor fibers and is therefore a mixed nerve. As it leaves the trunk of the facial canal, it pursues a slightly recurrent course upward and forward in the canaliculis chorda tympani *(iter chordae posterius),* a minute canal in the posterior wall in the tympanic cavity. It enters the tympanic cavity close to the border of the tympanic membrane. It then crosses the cavity, running on the medial surface of the tympanic membrane at the junction of its upper and middle thirds. It is covered by mucous membrane lining of the tympanic cavity and passes to the medial side of the manubrium of the malleus above the tendon of the tensor tympani. It therefore passes *between* the malleus and the incus. It leaves the tympanic cavity by way of a canal in the petrotympanic fissure to pass to the base of the skull through a small foramen, the *iter chordae anterius* (anterior tympanic aperture). It eventually joins the lingual nerve in the parapharyngeal space to supply taste sensation to the anterior two thirds of the tongue.

Bony Dehiscences. It is customary to consider the facial canal to be a closed bony tube except where branches make their exit. Such is not invariably the case. Baxter[14] reported dehiscence in more than half of over 500 temporal bones studied microscopically. Dehiscences in the canal were most common in the tympanic portion near the oval window region and were occasionally present in the mastoid segment and near the region of the geniculate ganglion. The average dimension of these dehiscences was less than 1 mm. The radiologic demonstration of a substantial loss of bone in any region of the facial canal, therefore, should be considered abnormal.

Anomalous Course in Petrous Bone. Although the course of the facial nerve through the temporal bone is one of the most constant of anatomic relationships, anomalous courses do occur. Such a circumstance may be extremely treacherous for a surgeon, and everyone involved in the interpretation of temporal bone images must be alert to the possibility of such an anomaly.

An anomalous course of the mastoid portion is to be expected in the presence of atresia of the external acoustic canal (discussed later), but numerous such courses have been reported in the absence of any other significant developmental abnormality.

Most of the anomalous courses reported are involved in that part of the nerve peripheral to the geniculate ganglion. The interested reader is referred to the work of Basek,[15] Schucknecht,[12] Shambaugh,[7] Dunkin et al,[16] and Wright et al.[17]

The main trunk of the facial nerve in its tympanic portion may take an anomalous course along the medial wall of the tympanic cavity, the most common having a position anterior and inferior to the oval window rather than above it. More importantly, the nerve may divide into two or more branches at any position along its course, and these two branches may either parallel one another or diverge.

An anomalous course of the facial nerve within the tympanic cavity is a diagnosis unlikely to be made other than by direct inspection by the operating surgeon. On the other hand, an unusual course or absence of an identifiable canal in the mastoid portion of the facial nerve canal is an observation that should be made by use of CT scans. Otherwise, the surgeon may inadvertently injure the abnormally positioned nerve.

The Inner Ear (Fig. 13-3)

Bony Labyrinth. The bony labyrinth consists of the *vestibule, semicircular canals,* and *cochlea.*

Vestibule. The central portion of the cavity of the bony labyrinth is the vestibule. The vestibule is a relatively large ovoid perilymphatic space measuring approximately 4 mm in diameter, leading anteriorly into the cochlea and posteriorly into the semicircular canals. There are cribrose areas, minute openings for the entrance of the nerve branches from the vestibular nerve on the medial wall and floor of the vestibule, where it abuts on the lateral end of the internal acoustic canal. The vestibule has two other openings: the oval window for the footplate of the stapes and the vestibular aqueduct.

Semicircular Canals. The three semicircular canals are continuous with the vestibule. Each of the canals makes about two-thirds of a circle and measures about 1 mm in cross-section diameter. Each is enlarged anteriorly by an *ampulla.* The nonampulated ends of the superior and posterior semicircular canals join to form the bony *common crus.*

A portion of the superior semicircular canal usually forms a ridge (arcuate eminence) on the anterior surface of the petrous bone (the posterior delimitation of the middle cranial fossa). The lateral (horizontal) semicircular canal projects as a ridge on the medial wall of the attic.

The perilymphatic space of the semicircular canals opens and communicates freely with the vestibule at both their ends.

The superior and posterior semicircular canals are both arranged in a vertical orientation at approximately right angles to one another. The superior canal is directed anterolaterally at an angle about 45 degrees to the midsagittal plane, and the posterior canal is directed posterolaterally at a corresponding angle. It

should be noted therefore that the angles of the vertical canals are oriented within both temporal bones so that the superior semicircular canal of one side has the same sagittal orientation as the posterior canal of the opposite side, and vice versa.

The lateral semicircular canal does not occupy a horizontal plane and for this reason the older terminology ("horizontal") has been discarded. The anterior limb of the lateral semicircular canal lies in the plane higher than the posterior limb, making an angle of about 30 degrees with the horizon. In the erect position therefore the neck would have to be flexed about 30 degrees for the lateral semicircular canal to be "horizontal."

Cochlea. The perilymphatic cavity of the vestibule is also continuous with the cochlea anteriorly. The cochlea is a conical structure, its base lying on the internal auditory canal and its apex or *cupola* directed anteriorly, laterally, and slightly downward. The base measures around 9 mm, and its axis height is about 5 mm. The base is perforated by numerous apertures for the passage of the cochlear nerve.

The cochlea consists of a conical central axis, the modiolus; a bony canal wound spirally around the central axis for a little more than 2½ turns; and a delicate *osseous spiral lamina,* which projects from the modiolus into the canal and partially divides it. In the living state the division of the canal is completed by the *basilar membrane,* which stretches from the free border of the osseous spiral lamina to the outer wall of the bony cochlea. The two passages into which the cochlear canal is thus divided communicate with each other at the apex of the modiolus by a small opening, the *helicotrema.*

The modiolus is the conical central pillar of the cochlea. Its base is broad and appears at the lateral end of the internal acoustic canal, where it corresponds with the cochlear outflow of the eighth cranial nerve. It is perforated by numerous orifices for the transmission of the branches of the nerve.

The bony *cochlear canal* takes between 2½ and 2¾ turns around the modiolus. The first turn bulges toward the tympanic cavity, and this elevation on the medial wall of the tympanic cavity is known as the *promontory.* The bony cochlear canal is about 30 mm long and diminishes gradually in diameter from the base to the summit, where it ends in the cupola, which forms the apex of the cochlea. The cross-sectional diameter of the beginning of the canal is about 3 mm. The openings in or near the first portion of the cochlear canal include the round window, which is covered by the secondary tympanic membrane; the oval window (actually an opening of the vestibule), which is covered by the footplate of the stapes; and the aperture of the *cochlear canaliculus,* which leads to a small canal that communicates with the subarachnoid space by an opening on the inferior surface of the petrous portion of the temporal

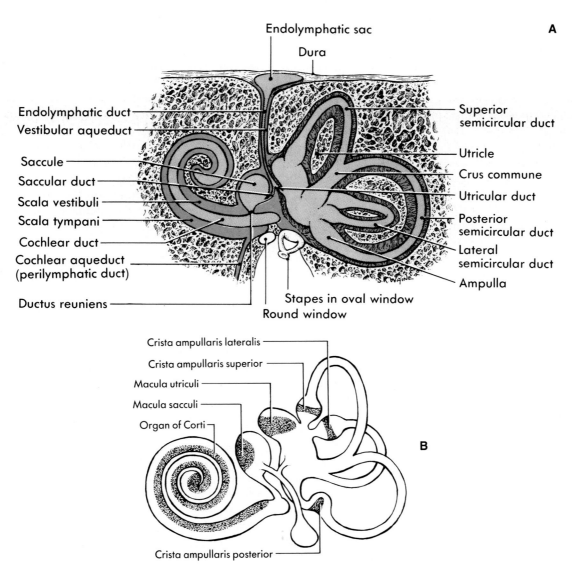

Endolymphatic sac

Dura

A

Endolymphatic duct

Vestibular aqueduct

Saccule

Saccular duct

Scala vestibuli

Scala tympani

Cochlear duct

Cochlear aqueduct
(perilymphatic duct)

Ductus reuniens

Superior
semicircular duct

Utricle

Crus commune

Utricular duct

Posterior
semicircular duct

Lateral
semicircular duct

Ampulla

Stapes in oval window
Round window

Crista ampullaris lateralis

Crista ampullaris superior

Macula utriculi

Macula sacculi

Organ of Corti

B

Crista ampullaris posterior

Fig. 13-3 **A,** Inner ear, schematic drawing. Membranous labyrinth is enclosed within bony labyrinth and separated from it by perilymphatic space. Cochlear and vestibular portions of membranous labyrinth are surrounded by perilymph. Vestibule and semicircular canals tend to be suspended from walls of bony labyrinth by myriad tiny arachnoid-like filaments. No such filaments exist around cochlear duct. Membranous labyrinth encloses endolymphatic space and is filled with endolymph. Endolymphatic sac and duct are in continuity with endolymphatic space. Cochlear aqueduct communicates with subarachnoid space and is in continuity with perilymphatic space. Oval window abuts against vestibule; round window is located at commencement of basilar turn of cochlea. Perilymphatic space is dark gray. **B,** Specialized sensory areas of membranous labyrinth. Sensory cells mediating hearing are located in organ of Corti within cochlear duct. Sensory organs of vestibular labyrinth are located in maculae of utricle and saccule and within ampullae of semicircular canals. Macula of utricle mediates most of sensations related to linear acceleration of head; ampullary cristae are sensitive to changes in angular acceleration of head.

bone. The cochlear canaliculus, also known as the *cochlear aqueduct* or *perilymphatic duct*, allows at least theoretical equilibration between the perilymphatic space and the subarachnoid space; however, it is usually completely filled with arachnoid and fibrous tissue.

Membranous Labyrinth (Fig. 13-3, *B*). The interconnecting spaces of the membranous labyrinth constitute the endolymphatic cavity. The labyrinth consists of the cochlear duct, the vestibular sense organs, the endolymphatic duct and sac, the round window membrane, and the vascular system.

Cochlear Duct. The *cochlear duct* is a spiral tube lying within the cochlea and attached to its outer wall. The cochlear duct is a blind pouch; it cleaves the perilymphatic space within the bony labyrinth and divides it into two portions, the scala vestibuli and the scala tympani. The cochlear duct is triangular, its roof being formed by Reisner's membrane, its outer wall by the endosteum lining the bony canal, and its floor by the basilar membrane and the outer part of the osseous spiral lamina. It contains the organ of Corti, which is the site of placement of the supporting and sensory (hair) cells that mediate hearing.

The Vestibular Sense Organs. The sensory organs of the vestibular labyrinth are located in the maculae of both the utricle and saccule and within the ampullae of the semicircular canals. The epithelium consists of supporting and hair cells (sensory cells) covered by a gelatinous layer into which the cilia project.

Vestibular physiology is complex. The maculae are referred to as organs of static balance because the otoliths, under the influence of gravity (they have a specific gravity of 2.71), exert traction on the cilia of the hair cells in varying positions of the head. The macula of the utricle mediates most of the sensations that have to do with linear acceleration of the head. The ampullary crests located within the semicircular canals are called organs of kinetic balance because they are stimulated by the movement of or pressure changes in the endolymph caused by the angular acceleration of the head; this produces deviation of the cupulae.

The utricle resides within the elliptical recess of the vestibule. The sensory cells of the utricle lie within the *macula*. The semicircular ducts all open into the utricle. From the anteromedial part of the utricle the *ductus utriculosaccularis* takes its origin and opens into the endolymphatic duct.

The saccule lies in the spherical recess near the opening of the scala vestibuli of the cochlea. The macula of the saccule is located along its anterior wall.

The saccule communicates with the sinus of the endolymphatic duct by way of the saccular duct and with the cochlear duct by way of the ductus reuniens. From the lower part of the saccule the ductus reuniens communicates with the basal end of the cochlear duct.

The semicircular ducts are about one quarter of the diameter of the semicircular canals. Each has an ampulla at one end that lies within the ampulla of the corresponding bony canal. The semicircular ducts open by five orifices into the utricle, the common crus being a single opening for the junction of the medial end of the superior and the upper end of the posterior semicircular ducts. A crestlike septum, the *ampullary crest*, crosses the base of each ampulla and is made up of sensory epithelium distributed on a mound of connective tissue and covered by a gelatinous cupula.

Endolymphatic Duct and Sac. The *endolymphatic duct* begins within the vestibule as a dilated portion, the *endolymphatic sinus*. It arises at the confluence of the utricular and saccular ducts. As it leaves the vestibule, it narrows into an isthmus and passes through the vestibular aqueduct. As the endolymphatic duct reaches the dural opening of the vestibular aqueduct, it widens again into the flat *endolymphatic sac*. The remainder of the sac lies between the periosteum of the petrous bone and the dura mater.

Round Window Membrane. The round window membrane (secondary tympanic membrane) measures about 3 mm in its horizontal axis and about 1.5 mm in its transverse axis. The round window membrane is of particular importance in acoustic energy transfer within the inner ear, where it performs as a yielding area of the bony labyrinth to permit movement of the perilymph in association with excursions of the stapedial footplate. Movements of these two diaphragms should be typically 180 degrees out of phase with one another.

Vascular System. The arterial blood supply to the membranous labyrinth originates within the cranial cavity and effectively is distinct from the vessels that supply the otic capsule in the tympanic cavity, although there are a few terminal branches that penetrate the endosteal layer. In a study of 100 human specimens Mazzoni[18] reported finding a consistent arterial loop in the region of the internal auditory canal. This loop is either the main trunk or a branch of the anterior inferior cerebellar artery in 80% of cases, of the accessory anterior cerebellar artery in 17%, or a branch of the posterior inferior cerebellar artery in 3%. The loop was found inside the internal auditory canal in 40%, at the porus in 37%, and within the cerebellopontine angle cistern in 33% of cases.

The anterior inferior cerebellar artery arterial loop gives rise to the *internal auditory artery* (labyrinthine artery) and also frequently to the *subarcuate artery*. It then takes a recurrent course to the cerebellum. The internal auditory artery distributes to the dura and nerves in the internal auditory canal to adjacent bone of the canal and to the medial aspect of the inner ear before dividing into the *common cochlear artery.*[18] The further ramifications of these arteries to the membranous labyrinth are discussed by Hawkins[19] and further elaborated on by Schuknecht.[12]

The main venous channels of the cochlea are the *posterior* and *anterior spiral veins*. These join together near the base of the cochlea to form the *common modiolar vein. The common modiolar vein is joined by the vestibulocochlear vein to become the vein of the cochlear aqueduct*. This main channel enters a bony canal near (but not within) the cochlear aqueduct to empty into the inferior petrosal sinus.

The semicircular canals are drained by vessels that pass toward the utricular end to form the *vein of the vestibular aqueduct*, which accompanies the endolymphatic duct and drains into the lateral venous sinus.

Bast and Anson[4] describe an *internal auditory vein* that traverses the internal auditory canal and drains into the inferior petrosal sinus, but this is an inconstant vessel.

Perilymphatic Spaces and Fluid Systems. The perilymphatic space (see Fig. 13-2) of each semicircular canal is continuous at both ends with the perilymphatic space of the vestibule, and this space is in turn continuous widely with that of the scala vestibuli. The scala vestibuli is continuous with the scala tympani at the helicotrema. All the perilymphatic spaces therefore open widely into each other.

The total volume of fluid contained within the developmentally mature periotic space is estimated to be approximately 0.2 ml—about three drops. Without those three drops of fluid, however, the transmission of sound waves from the oval window to Reissner's membrane in the cochlea could not be mediated.

There are several actual or potential dehiscences in the compact bone of the petrous portion of the temporal bone that could theoretically permit communication between the perilymphatic space and the middle and inner ears.[10] These include (1) the oval window, normally sealed off from the middle ear cavity by the footplate of the stapes and its annular ligament, (2) the round window, normally sealed off from the middle ear by the secondary tympanic membrane, (3) the *fissula ante fenestram* and the *fossula post fenestram*, two small extensions of the perilymphatic space extending from the vestibule toward the middle ear cavity that are usually obliterated by connective tissue, and (4) the vestibular aqueduct, a channel that extends through the otic capsule from the vestibule to the posterior cranial fossa and transmits the endolymphatic duct and accompanying vein. The duct, vein, and connective tissue surrounding them so fill the aqueduct that there is no perilymphatic *space* and, therefore, no actual communication between the perilymphatic space of the vestibule and the epidural space. (5) The fifth actual or potential dehiscence is the cochlear aqueduct (perilymphatic duct, cochlear canaliculus), a normally minute canal that opens on the inferior surface of the petrous part of the temporal bone and permits communication between the subarachnoid space and the scala tympani.

Occasionally the cochlear aqueduct is very patulous, although filled with arachnoid and fibrous tissue, and this provides at least a theoretical possibility of free communication of the perilymphatic space with the subarachnoid space. Whether this is physiologically important in the transport of potentially noxious substances to the inner ear from the violated subarachnoid space is yet unproved.

How the Ear Amplifies Sound

Once the inner ear becomes sequestered within the base of the skull it becomes necessary in the evolutionary sense to reestablish continuity with the external environment so as to provide a suitable apparatus for the reception of sound. Evolution elegantly fashioned a method based on the simplest of hydraulic principles, solving the problem of acoustical impedance mismatch between sound waves traveling in the fluid of the inner ear—the ossicular lever mechanism vibrating in an air chamber and attached to the large area diaphragm (tympanic membrane) on one side and the small area diaphragm (stapes footplate) on the fluid side.

Sound waves are amplified by three different mechanisms by the time the vibrations in the air of the external acoustic canal are changed to fluid pulsations of the perilymph within the membranous labyrinth.

The first mechanism is the "organ pipe" resonance of the external canal. The resonant frequency of the column of air enclosed within the external acoustic canal accounts for approximately doubling of the pressure at the tympanic membrane compared to that at the entrance to the canal for frequencies between 2000 and 5400 Hz.

Secondly, the area of the tympanic membrane varies between 15 and 30 times the area of the oval window. This concentration of force at the stapes footplate amplifies the incoming vibrations of sound approximately 15 to 30 times.

Finally, the lever mechanism of the ossicular chain reduces the amplitude of the excursion of the bone at the footplate of the stapes in comparison to the long handle of the malleus and thereby increases the force by a factor of two to three.

The sound waves therefore may be amplified by a factor of up to 180 by the time that they encounter the perilymph.[20]

REFERENCES

1. Streeter GL: The development of the scala tympani, scala vestibuli and perioticular system in the human embryo, Am J Anat 21:299, 1917.
2. Streeter GL: The histogenesis and growth of the otic capsule and its contained periotic tissue spaces in the human embryo, Contrib Embryol 20:5, 1918.
3. Anson BJ and Donaldson JA: Surgical anatomy of the temporal bone, ed 3, Philadelphia, 1981, WB Saunders Co.
4. Bast TH and Anson BJ: The temporal bone and ear, Springfield, Ill, 1949, Charles C Thomas, Publisher.

5. Shambaugh G Jr: Surgery of the ear, ed 2, Philadelphia, 1967, WB Saunders Co, pp 5-39.
6. Iurato S: Submicroscopic structure of the inner ear, New York, 1967, Pergamon Press, Inc.
7. Shambaugh G Jr: Surgery of the ear, ed 2, Philadelphia, 1967, WB Saunders Co, pp 565-599.
8. Wittmaack K: Uber die normale und die pathologische. Pneumatisation des Schlafenbeines, Jena, 1918, Fischer.
9. Goss CC, editor: Gray's anatomy, Philadelphia, 1959, Lea & Febiger.
10. Hollinshead WH: Anatomy for surgeons, vol 1, The head and neck, ed 2, New York, 1968, Harper & Row, Publishers, Inc.
11. Schaeffer and Parsons J, editors: Morris' human anatomy, Philadelphia, 1942, Blakiston.
12. Schuknecht HF: Pathology of the ear, Cambridge, Mass, 1974, Harvard University Press.
13. Warwick R and Williams PL editors: Gray's anatomy, ed 35 (Br), Philadelphia, 1973, WB Saunders Co.
14. Baxter A: Dehiscence of the fallopian canal, J Laryngol Otol 85:587, 1971.
15. Basek M: Anomalies of the facial nerve in normal temporal bones, Ann Otol Rhinol Laryngol 71:392, 1962.
16. Dunkin D et al: Bifurcation of the facial nerve, Arch Otolaryngol 86:619, 1967.
17. Wright J Jr, Taylor C, and McKay D: Variations in the course of the facial nerve as illustrated by tomography, Laryngoscope 77:717, 1967.
18. Mazzoni A: Internal auditory artery supply to the petrous bone, Ann Otol Rhinol Laryngol 81:13, 1972.
19. Hawkins J: Vascular patterns of the membranous labyrinth, Third symposium on the role of the vestibular organs in space exploration, NASA SP 152:241, 1967.
20. Stevens SS and Warshowsky F: Sound and hearing, New York, 1965, Time-Life Books, Inc.

SECTION TWO

IMAGING

DAVID P.C. LIU
WILLIAM W.M. LO

CT AND MR IMAGING OF THE NORMAL PETROUS TEMPORAL BONE (David P.C. Liu)

Rapid advances in medical technology have contributed greatly to improved imaging of the temporal bone in the past decade. High resolution computerized tomography (HRCT), magnetic resonance imaging (MRI), and digital subtraction angiography (DSA) have largely supplanted plain films, pluridirectional tomography, and selective angiography.[1-4] Indications for the use of these individual modalities remain in evolution primarily as a consequence of the fast-paced changes made in MRI.[5-11] Decrease in slice thickness, advances in surface coil design, and reduction of background noise have contributed to the betterment of both spatial and contrast resolution.

Needless to say, the foundation of diagnosis requires optimization of image quality as well as familiarity with local anatomy. This section provides (1) an overview of the technical details germane to the imaging of fine anatomic structures of the temporal bone using state of the art technology and (2) a discussion of relevant anatomic relationships. The idealized imaging workup provides a comprehensive, "definitive" examination coupled with economy of data acquisition and exposure. This is particularly true for HRCT, where radiation dose to the lens is a relevant consideration and must be minimized.

CT Anatomy

Familiarity with the local anatomy is critical when examining the petrous temporal bone. Although the structures within the middle and inner ear cavities are small, they can be clearly identified if well imaged. This is in part because of the presence of air within the middle ear cavity and mastoid air cells that provides a natural contrast with the surrounding bony and soft tissue structures.

The ability of high resolution computerized tomography (HRCT) to provide exquisite contrast and spatial resolution at a lower radiation dose is one of the clearest advantages over routine complex motion tomography. As a result, HRCT is the current method of choice for the delineation of fine structures of the temporal bone. These can be resolved easily with direct axial or direct coronal planar scanning, or both; other planes of interest, such as sagittal imaging, are available, but rarely necessary.[12-21]

Because fine bony detail is imperative, sections as thin as 1.5 mm should be obtained. Software algorithms selected to emphasize bony detail also should be employed. This accentuation usually is accomplished by processing the raw data in a retrospective fashion so that the right and left sides may be imaged separately.

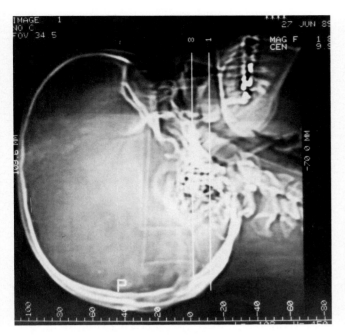

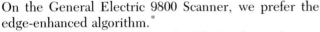

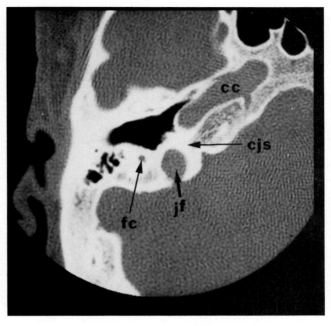

Fig. 13-4 Lateral scout film demonstrating slight degree of hyperextension needed to achieve plane of scanning without changing angle of the gantry. First and last slices are illustrated here as landmarks.

Fig. 13-5 Most inferior transverse section demonstrates jugular foramen *(jf)* and descending or vertical mastoid segment of facial canal *(fc).* Carotid canal *(cc).* Caroticojugular spine *(cjs).*

On the General Electric 9800 Scanner, we prefer the edge-enhanced algorithm.[*]

Thin-section axial images should be obtained commencing inferiorly from the lower margin of the external auditory meatus and extend upward to the level of the arcuate eminence of the superior semicircular canal. These landmarks are easily ascertained on a lateral scout view, with the chin slightly extended (Fig. 13-4). This slightly extended position precludes the necessity of angling the gantry and provides axial images that are effectively 10 degrees negative to the orbitomeatal line. It should be noted that this positioning avoids direct exposure to the lens of the eye. Of additional benefit is that 0-degree tilt ensures the shortest reformatting time possible.

The indications for intravenous contrast depend strictly on the history and the pertinent clinical information. In most cases a study without contrast is ade-

quate, especially if the suspected lesion is within the petrous temporal bone itself. Intravenous contrast is useful if the following conditions are suspected: (1) a hypervascular lesion, e.g., glomus tumor; (2) a cerebellopontine angle mass in a patient with sensorineual hearing loss; or (3) extension of disease intracranially or below the skull base.

The axial plane (Figs. 13-5 to 13-14) allows exquisite delineation of the tympanic cavity and its contents, the inner ear structures, and the entire course of the facial nerve. The anatomic relationships are demonstrated as sections are obtained from the lowest level of the hypotympanum inferiorly to the level of the tegmen tympani (the bony roof of the petrous portion of the temporal bone) superiorly (see Fig. 13-4).

Coronal images (Figs. 13-15 to 13-20) serve as an adjunctive plane (when lesions or congenital variants need to be clarified further). It is imperative, therefore, that temporal bone CT studies be monitored carefully. Coronal images should be obtained from the plane of the cochlea anteriorly to the plane of the posterior semicircular canal posteriorly (Fig. 13-21). This orientation is particularly useful in evaluating the bony crista falciformis within the internal auditory canal, the tegmen tympani forming the roof of the epitympanic cavity, and the individual superior, posterior, and lateral semicircular canals.

---

*Scans were performed with a General Electric 9800 QUICK CT Scanner. The raw data, acquired at 1.5 mm contiguous slice intervals, were geometrically enlarged to obtain a spatial resolution of 0.6 mm. The individual right and left sides were then enlarged to a 9.6 cm square field of view.

For display and hard copy imaging, a window level of 300H and a window width of 4,000H were selected. The scans were performed at 120KV and 300MAS.

Text continued on p. 950.

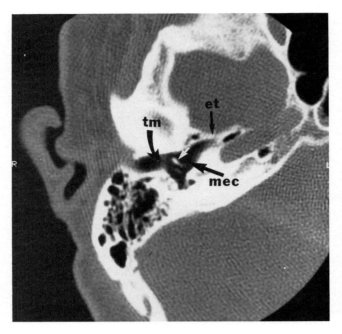

Fig. 13-6 Transverse section at level of middle ear cavity *(mec)*. Mesotympanum contains manubrium of the malleus *(white arrow)*, which is immediately medial to tympanic membrane *(tm)*. Eustachian tube *(et)*.

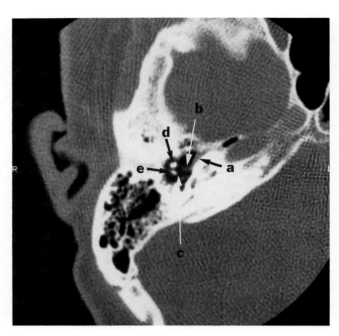

Fig. 13-7 Transverse section, slightly higher in the mesotympanum, demonstrates tensor tympani muscle *(a)*, with its attached tendon *(b)*. Incudo-stapedial articulation *(c)* is at same level as neck of the malleus *(d)* and long process of the incus *(e)*.

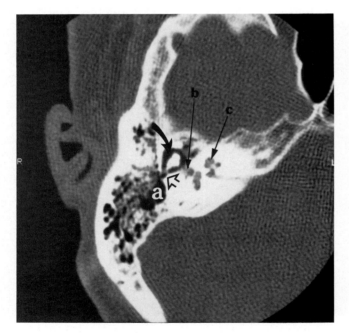

Fig. 13-8 Transverse section through the attic shows typical figure-of-eight appearance created by attic *(curved arrow)*, aditus ad antrum *(open arrow)* and mastoid antrum *(a)*. Oval window *(b)*. Second turn of cochlea *(c)*.

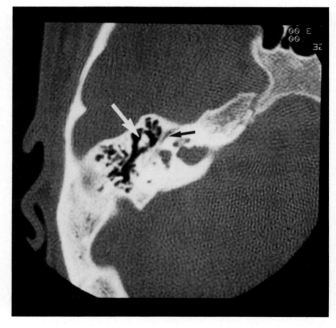

Fig. 13-9 Transverse section at level of the incudomalleal articulation *(white arrow)* often demonstrates horizontal or tympanic portion of the facial canal *(black arrow)* as a fine linear structure.

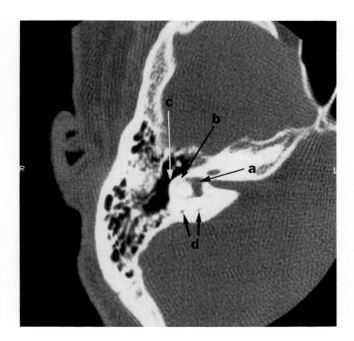

Fig. 13-10 Transverse section at level of the vestibule *(a)*, lateral semicircular canal *(b)*, bony covering of lateral semicircular canal *(c)*, and posterior semicircular canal *(d)*.

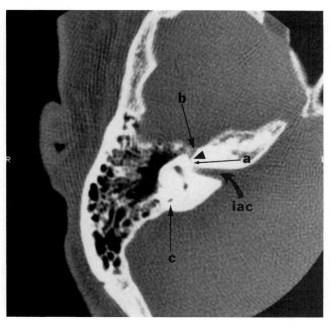

Fig. 13-11 Transverse section through internal auditory canal *(iac)* demonstrates first portion of the facial canal *(a)*, geniculate ganglion *(arrowhead)*, canal for the greater superficial petrosal nerve *(b)*, and posterior semicircular canal *(c)*.

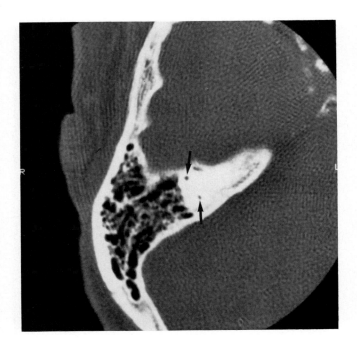

Fig. 13-12 Transverse section through level of the superior semicircular canal *(black arrows)*.

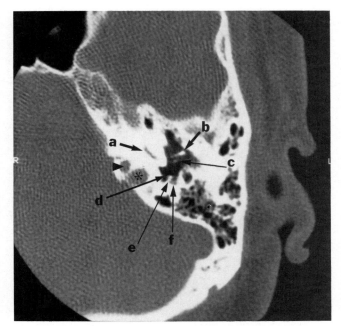

Fig. 13-13 Transverse section through basal turn of the cochlea *(a)* demonstrates pars nervosa *(arrowhead)* separate from the pars jugularis *(asterisk)*, neck of the malleus *(b)*, and long process of the incus *(c)*. Pyramidal eminence *(e)* separates the sinus tympani *(d)* from the facial recess *(f)*.

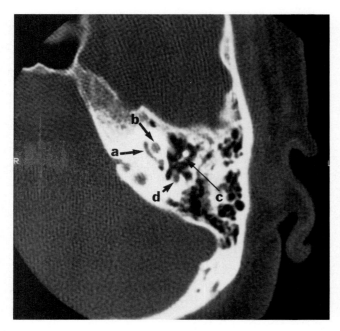

Fig. 13-14 Slightly higher transverse section through first turn *(a)* and second turn *(b)* of the cochlea includes a view of incudomalleolar articulation *(c)* and stapedius muscle *(d)*.

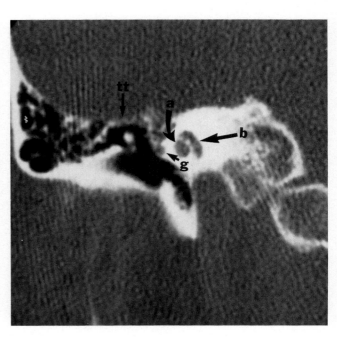

Fig. 13-15 Coronal image (most anterior, at level of the cochlea). First turn *(a)* and second turn *(b)* of cochlea. Genu of facial nerve *(g)*. Tegmen tympani *(tt)*.

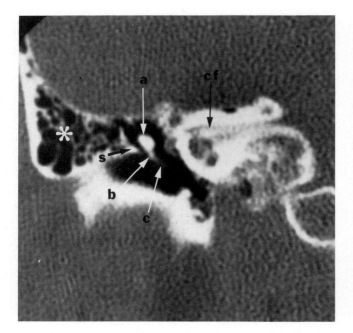

Fig. 13-16 Coronal image at head of malleus *(a)*. Neck *(b)* and manubrium *(c)* of malleus. Bony scutum *(s)* marks lateral border of Prussak space. Crista falciformis *(cf)* within internal auditory canal. Pneumatized mastoid air cells *(asterisk)*.

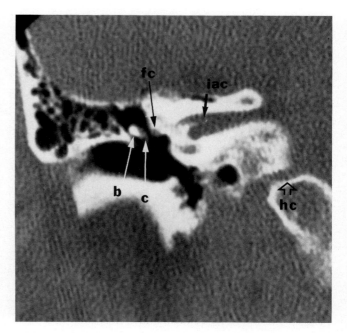

Fig. 13-17 Slightly posterior coronal section, through midportion of internal auditory canal *(iac)*. Body of incus *(b)* with its lenticular process *(c)*. Horizontal (tympanic) segment of facial nerve canal *(fc)*. Hypoglossal canal *(hc)*.

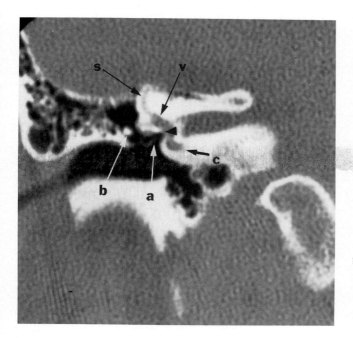

Fig. 13-18   Coronal section through vestibule *(v)* demonstrates adjacent oval window *(arrowhead)*. Anterior crus of stapes *(a)*. Short process of incus *(b)*. Superior semicircular canal *(s)*. First turn of the cochlea *(c)*.

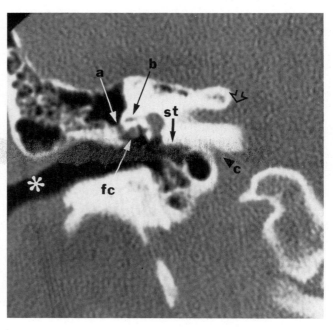

Fig. 13-19   Coronal section through aditus ad antrum *(a)*. Tympanic segment of facial nerve canal *(fc)* lies immediately inferior to lateral semicircular canal *(b)*. Sinus tympani *(st)*. Porus acusticus *(open arrow)*. Cochlear aqueduct *(c)*. External auditory canal *(asterisk)*.

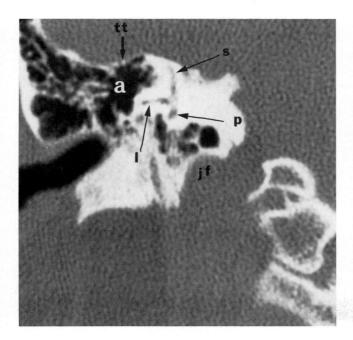

Fig. 13-20   Coronal image [most posterior, at level of mastoid antrum *(a)*]. Superior *(s)*, lateral *(l)*, and posterior *(p)* semicircular canals. Jugular foramen *(jf)*. Tegmen tympani *(tt)*.

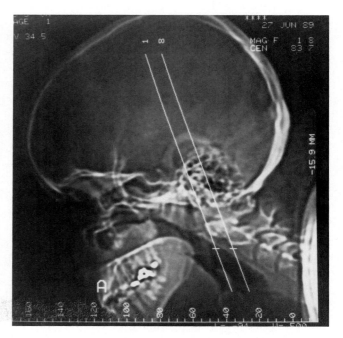

Fig. 13-21   Coronal scout film illustrating positions of the first and last slices, as well as the plane of scanning.

The contents of the middle ear cavity are easily identified on both axial and coronal images. The auditory ossicles and their articulations are well seen, and the suspensory ligaments may occasionally be demonstrated. In the attic (see Figs. 13-8 and 13-14), the head of the malleus and the more posterior body of the incus are connected by a small, diarthrodial joint lined with synovial tissue. More inferiorly (see Fig. 13-7), the neck of the malleus, the long process of the incus, and the incudostapedial articulation are visualized. The remainder of the ossicular chain, including the lenticular process of the incus and rarely the footplate of the stapes covering the oval window, is best seen on direct coronal projections (see Fig. 13-18). Anteriorly, the long process of the incus forms a right angle and bends medially to form the lenticular process. Since this process is parallel to the transverse (axial) plane, the right-angle bend is more easily resolved in the coronal plane (see Fig. 13-17). The relationship of the head of the malleus with its neck and manubrium is quite clearly seen on coronal scans (see Fig. 13-16).

In the axial plane the configuration of the ossicles can be used to help localize the vertical level of the scan in the middle ear cleft. In the attic the ossicles have an "ice cream cone" configuration, with the "ball of ice cream" being the head of the malleus and the "cone" being the body and short process of the uncus. In the mesotympanum, opposite the tympanic membrane, the ossicles have a "wishbone" appearance, with the anterior limb being the manubrium of the malleus and the posterior limb being the long process of the uncus. In between these scan levels is the neck of the manubrium, which is at the level of the scutum.

Two normal soft tissue structures in the middle ear cavity that are routinely visualized on HRCT are the tensor tympani and the stapedius muscles. The tensor tympani (see Fig. 13-7) is identified as it exits its bony canal, located superior to the eustachian tube. It travels posteriorly over the surface of the cochlea, executes nearly a right-angle turn at the process cochleariformis, and continues laterally as a tendon, finally inserting on the manubrium of the malleus.[22] The stapedius muscle (see Fig. 13-14) arises from a cavity within the pyramidal eminence posteriorly (see Fig. 13-13) and courses anteriorly through the middle ear to insert on the neck of the stapes.[22]

Two notable recesses are in the posterior region of the middle ear cavity, created by a bony projection on the posterior wall (the pyramidal eminence). The medial recess is the sinus tympani, the lateral is the facial recess (see Fig. 13-13). They are important sites of clinically occult inflammatory disease.

Examination of the inner ear structures is straightforward. The anteriorly located cochlea consists of 2½ spirals, of which only the basal and second turns are most constantly resolvable on HRCT (see Figs. 13-8, 13-13 to 13-15). The vestibule (with its communicating semicircular canals) is immediately lateral and posterior to the internal auditory canal (see Figs. 13-10 to 13-12).

As the facial nerve exits from the fundal portion of the internal auditory meatus (see Fig. 13-11), its labyrinthine segment projects anteriorly and laterally; executing a "U turn" just beneath the cortical bone that constitutes the middle fossa surface of the petrous temporal bone, the nerve widens briefly to form the geniculate ganglion. A small branch, the greater superficial petrosal nerve (see Fig. 13-11) then continues anteriorly and medially. The remaining (larger) portion of the facial nerve continues posteriorly, coursing under the lateral semicircular canal, as the tympanic (second) segment of the nerve. The relationship of this segment, as it travels inferiorly to the lateral semicircular canal, is best seen on the coronal projection (see Fig. 13-19). As the nerve reaches the posterior portion of the middle ear, at the level of the sinus tympani, it executes a right-angle turn downward (the second genu) and continues on a relatively vertical course through the mastoid to exit via the stylomastoid foramen. This mastoid (vertical) segment is identifiable in cross section on axial images (see Fig. 13-5) but is most recognizable on direct or reformatted sagittal images. It may be difficult to identify in a well-pneumatized and aerated mastoid. It is frequently difficult to see in its entirety on coronal sections as well, since the plane of section often is not totally parallel to the course of the entire segment.

The major vascular structures traveling through the petrous temporal bone have a predictable course, although a wide variety of congenital variations is possible.[18] The horizontal (petrous) portion of the carotid canal is separated from the jugular foramen at this level by a bony septum, the caroticojugular spine (see Fig. 13-5). The jugular foramen, in turn, comprises two compartments, the more medial *pars nervosa* and the laterally positioned *pars vascularis* (see Fig. 13-13). The pars nervosa contains the inferior petrosal sinus as well as the glossopharyngeal (IX) nerve; the larger pars vascularis contains the internal jugular vein and the vagus (X) and spinal accessory (XI) nerves. However, considerable variation in the position of these cranial nerves can occur. Delineation of the vascular structures separate from the adjacent cranial nerves within the jugular foramen is beyond the resolution of HRCT. The very small cochlear aqueduct is frequently identified as a well-corticated notch immediately medial to the pars nervosa and just inferior to the porus acousticus of the internal auditory canal (see Figs. 13-13 and 13-19). The cochlear aqueduct serves as a potential communication between the subarachnoid space and the inner ear perilymph.[15] The vestibular aqueduct is a less constantly identifiable structure, extending from the vestibule in a posteroinferior direction, finally opening onto the posterior margin of the petrous pyramid. Its primary function appears to be the resorption of endolymph, a process that is instrumental in maintaining equilibration between endolymph and the cerebrospinal fluid.[17] There is wide variation in size of these structures.

Correlative MRI Anatomy

Inasmuch as CT is excellent in depicting bony detail, MRI functions as an adjunctive modality in defining soft tissue structures as well as fluid-containing structures. Current technology allows a slice thickness as thin as 3 mm, with or without the use of surface coils. Surface coils increase the signal-to-noise ratio (SNR); however, their main disadvantages at this time are (1) inhomogeneous signal generated by the surface coil and (2) ability to image only one side at a time. At present, use of the standard head coil with thin sections provides comparable resolution to that obtained by using surface coils. However, this situation may change with further development of surface coil technology.

Despite all the imperfections of the technology, MRI is an excellent tool in visualizing soft tissue structures: the cochlear and vestibular apparati, the contents of the internal auditory canal, the facial nerve, and the greater superficial petrosal nerve (Figs. 13-22 to 13-28). On both T_1-weighted (T_1WI) and T_2-weighted images (T_2WI), signal is noted to arise from the endolymph and perilymph of the labyrinthine structures. More specifi-

cally, the liquid may be discriminated within the first and second cochlear turns (see Figs. 13-23, 13-24, and 13-29); the vestibule (see Figs. 13-23 and 13-24); and the individual superior, lateral, and posterior semicircular canals (see Figs. 13-26 to 13-28).

One of the primary differences between HRCT and MRI images is the inversion of contrast when imaging bone. On CT, both compact and spongy bone appear white; on MRI, cortical bone appears black because of the paucity of mobile protons. On conventional MRI, the middle ear cleft is not seen since it is normally filled with air and surrounded by the dense cortical bone of the temporal bone. The ossicular chain is also composed of dense cortical bone and produces no MR signal. The soft tissue structures, such as the suspensory ligaments of the ossicles, and the tensor tympani and stapedius muscles are too small to be resolved, even with the use of surface coils. Nevertheless, the air and ossicular filled middle ear cavity can be localized by its relationship to the cochlear and vestibular semicircular canal systems, which are filled with intermediate to high signal perilymph.[11]

On thin axial images, the anterior portion of the attic, or the epitympanum, lies directly lateral to the basal turn of the cochlea (see Fig. 13-23, A). The midportion of the attic, more specifically at the level of the incudomalleal articulation, lies immediately lateral to the tympanic portion of the facial nerve.

The entire course of the facial nerve within the petrous bone is resolvable on T_1WI.[5-7] The facial nerve is located within the anterior superior compartment of the internal auditory canal. The superior compartment is

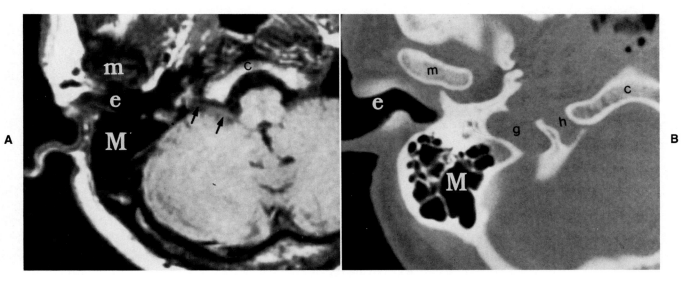

Fig. 13-22 Corresponding transverse **A** MRI and **B,** CT images illustrate hypoglossal nerve *(black arrows)* within hypoglossal canal *(h)*. Clivus *(c)*, mandibular condyle *(m)*, external auditory meatus *(e)*, and mastoid air cells *(M)*. Jugular foramen *(g)*.

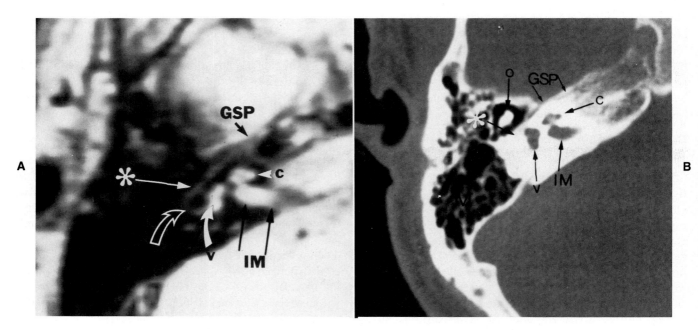

Fig. 13-23 **A,** This T$_2$-weighted MRI compared to **B,** a similar CT slice, demonstrates seventh and eighth cranial nerve complex within the internal auditory meatus *(IM)*. Horizontal portion of facial nerve *(asterisk)* is identified lateral to cochlea *(c)* and vestibular apparatus *(v)*. Greater superficial petrosal nerve *(GSP)* arises anterior to cochlea *(c)*. Lateral semicircular canal *(open, curved arrow)*.

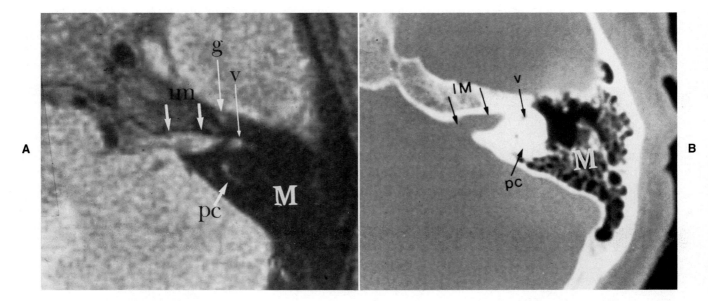

Fig. 13-24 **A,** Another T$_2$-weighted transverse MRI and **B,** a corresponding CT image through internal auditory meatus *(IM)* are able to identify vestibule *(v)*, posterior semicircular canal *(pc)*, and mastoid air cells *(M)*. Geniculate ganglion *(g)*.

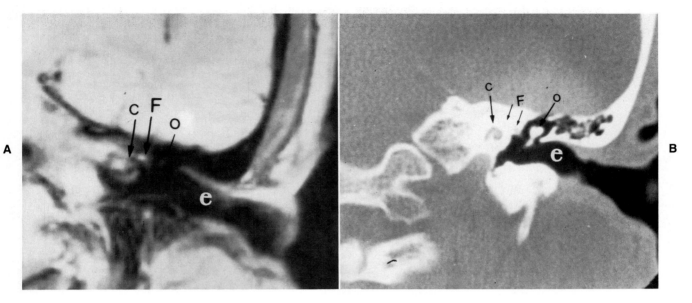

Fig. 13-25   A, Coronal T₁-weighted image through level of the cochlea *(c)* is compared to **B,** a similar coronal CT image. At this level, horizontal portion of facial canal *(F)* is seen in cross-section and is immediately lateral to the cochlea *(c)*. Head of malleus *(o)* may also be seen as a small focus of signal. External auditory meatus *(e)*.

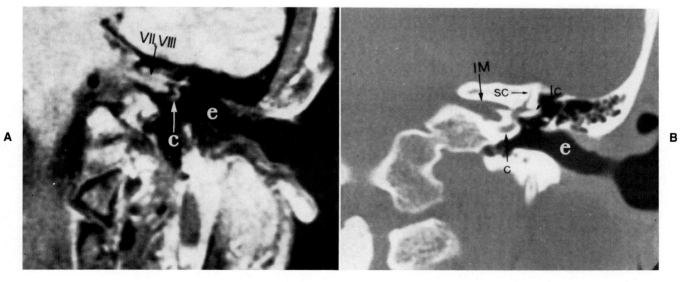

Fig. 13-26   A, Another T₁-weighted coronal MRI compared to **B,** a coronal CT image demonstrates separate seventh and eighth nerves (VII, VIII) coursing through internal auditory meatus *(IM)*. Superior semicircular canal *(sc)*, lateral semicircular canal *(lc)*, and cochlea *(c)* are also identified. External auditory meatus *(e)*.

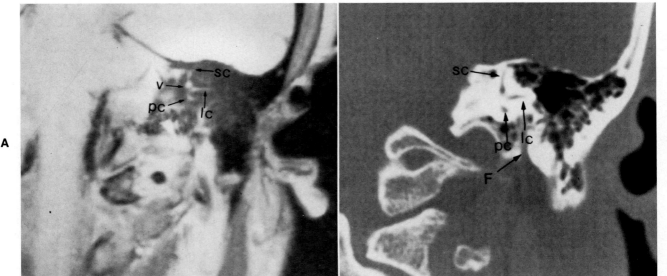

Fig. 13-27 **A,** A more posterior coronal T$_1$-weighted MRI demonstrates clearly the vestibule *(v)* and separate superior semicircular *(sc)*, lateral semicircular *(lc)*, and posterior semicircular *(pc)* canals. **B,** Corresponding CT section also shows mastoid (third or vertical) portion of facial canal *(F)*.

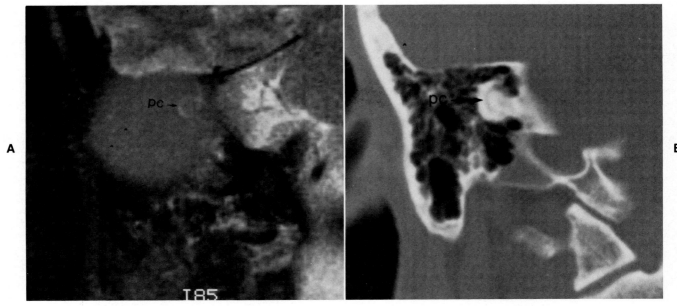

Fig. 13-28 **A,** Most posterior coronal T$_2$-weighted MRI demonstrates isolated posterior semicircular canal *(pc)* and **B,** its companion CT image.

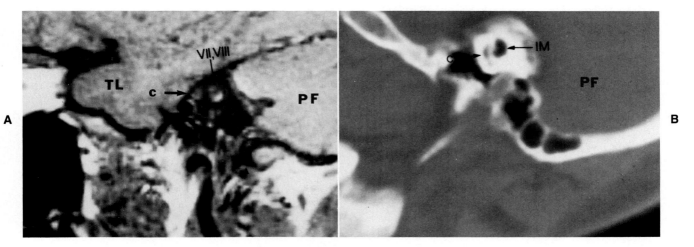

Fig. 13-29   Comparison of **A,** a T_1-weighted sagittal image with **B,** a comparable direct sagittal CT image demonstrates seventh and eighth cranial nerves *(VII, VIII)* within internal auditory meatus *(IM)*. Signal from the cochlea *(c)* arises slightly anterior to these nerves. Anterior is on left side of image. Posterior fossa *(PF)*. Temporal lobe *(TL)*.

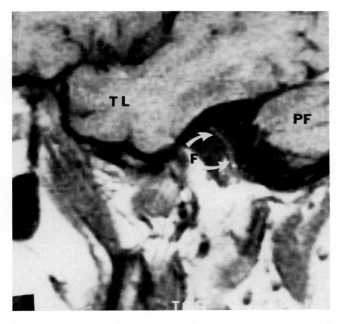

Fig. 13-30 T_1-weighted sagittal image depicts mastoid (vertical) portion of facial nerve *(F)*. Temporal lobe *(TL)*. Posterior fossa *(PF)*.

separated from the inferior compartment by the crista falciformis; because it is bony, it maintains low signal on both T_1W1 and T_2W1. The superior vestibular nerve is located posteriorly in the upper compartment. The inferior compartment confines the inferior vestibular nerve posteriorly and the cochlear nerve anteriorly. These compartments are best viewed on sagittal and coronal projections (see Figs. 13-26 and 13-29).

As the facial nerve exits the internal auditory canal,

its labyrinthine segment widens into the geniculate ganglion, which then serves as the origin of the greater superficial petrosal nerve; this structure courses anteriorly and medially as a thin, linear structure (see Fig. 13-23). The facial nerve proper then continues posteriorly as the tympanic segment, lateral to the cochlea and vestibule and semicircular canals, and is best seen on T_1W1 in the axial projection (see Fig. 13-23). At the second genu, within the mastoid portion, the nerve takes a more vertical course. This mastoid segment is best seen in the sagittal plane (Fig. 13-30).

The mastoid antral cavity is normally filled with air and is surrounded by dense cortical bone. Therefore, in the absence of disease, this area is devoid of MR signal. The individual septations that separate the air cells also are not seen; however, they can be localized because of their lateral position to the lateral semicircular canal, which has high signal perilymph (see Fig. 13-26).*

HIGH-RESOLUTION CT ANATOMY OF THE JUGULAR FORAMEN (William W.M. Lo)

The jugular foramen is bounded anterolaterally by the petrous portion of the temporal bone and posterolaterally by the occipital bone.[18,23] It is a complex canal that courses anteriorly, laterally, and then inferiorly as it exits through the base of the skull. Hence its appear-

---

*Fig. 13-26 MR images are courtesy of Dr. George Krol, Memorial Sloan Kettering Cancer Center. The images were created on a GE 1.5 Tesla signal system, without the use of surface coils, with 3 mm thick slices and with 1.5 mm interslice gaps. T_1-weighted images were obtained at a TR 800 msec, TE 25 msec; T_2-weighted images at TR 2000 msec with the first and second echo at TE 40 and TE 80 msec, respectively. Matrix size was 256 × 256, with a total of 6 excitations.

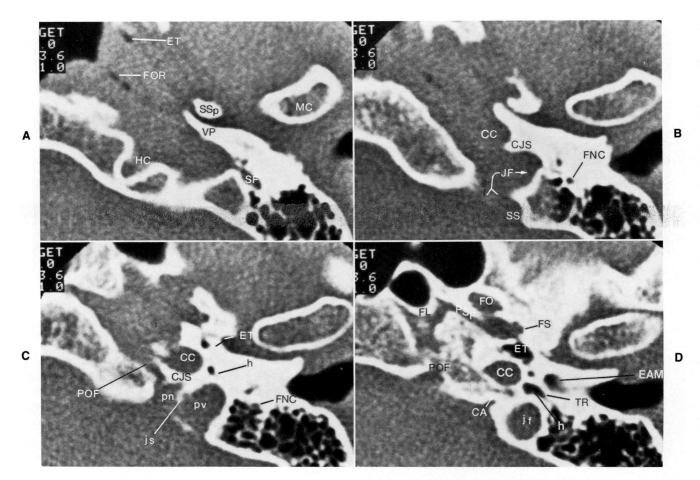

Fig. 13-31 A series of 1.5 mm high-resolution computed tomographic (HRCT) sections through left jugular foramen area with 0-degree angulation from anthropologic baseline (infraorbital rim to superior margin of external meatus) at 3 mm intervals rostrally. **A,** Level of floor of endocranial opening. Note medially the exocranial opening of hypoglossal canal *(HC),* and laterally stylomastoid foramen *(SF).* Other structures: vaginal process *(VP),* mandibular condyle *(MC),* spine of sphenoid *(SSp),* air in eustachian tube *(ET),* and fossa of Rosenmüller *(FOR).* **B,** Level of midendocranial opening. Note course of terminal portion of sigmoid sinus *(SS),* which drains anteriorly and then laterally to form jugular bulb before descending as the internal jugular vein. Jugular foramen (JF) is separated from ascending carotid canal *(CC)* by top of caroticojugular spine *(CJS).* Laterally facial nerve canal *(FNC)* descends toward the stylomastoid foramen. NOTE: The larger the jugular fossa, the closer it approaches the descending facial nerve canal. **C,** Level of top of endocranial opening. At this level pars nervosa *(pn)* is well demarcated from pars vascularis *(pv)* by jugular spine *(js).* Medially inferior petrosal sulcus overlies petrooccipital fissure *(POF).* Laterally is descending facial nerve canal *(FNC).* Anteriorly caroticojugular spine *(CJS)* separates ascending carotid canal *(CC)* from jugular foramen. Small amounts of air are in eustachian tube *(ET)* and inferior recess of hypotympanum *(h),* respectively. **D,** Level above endocranial opening. Notice close relationship of carotid and jugular canals to hypotympanum *(h).* In this subject jugular fossa *(jf)* domes above level of inferior tympanic ring *(TR).* Eustachian orifice *(ET)* along with peritubal cells is anterior to carotid canal *(CC).* Unlabeled small air-filled structure lateral to carotid canal can be traced to air cells on adjacent sections. Semicanal housing tensor tympani muscle lies above this section and is not seen. Other structures: external auditory meatus *(EAM),* foramen spinosum *(FS),* foramen ovale *(FO),* petrosphenoidal fissure *(PSF),* foramen lacerum *(FL),* petrooccipital fissure *(POF),* cochlear aqueduct *(CA).* (From Lo WWM and Solti-Bohman LG: High-resolution CT of the jugular foramen: anatomy and vascular variants and anomalies, Radiology 150:743, 1984.)

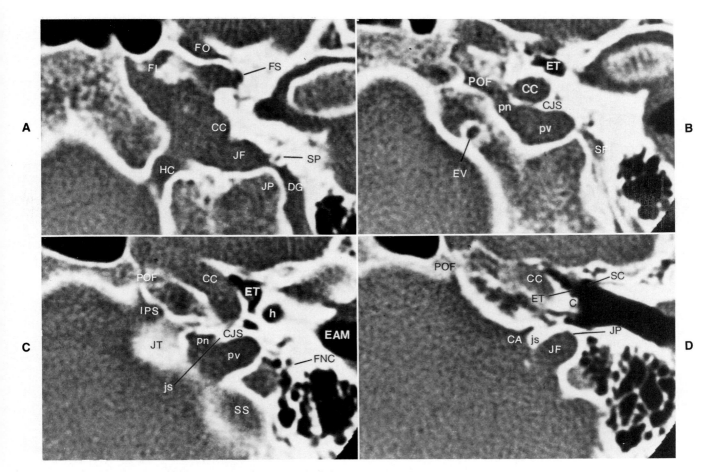

Fig. 13-32　A series of 1.5 mm HRCT sections through left jugular foramen area with 30-degree angulations from anthropologic baseline at 3 mm intervals rostrally. **A,** Level just below exocranial opening. Hypoglossal canal *(HC)* tunneling under jugular tubercle lies at this level. Jugular process *(JP)* of occipital bone forms posterior border of jugular foramen *(JF)*. Laterally lies base of styloid process *(SP)*, posterior to which is groove for digastric muscle *(DG)*. Other structures: foramen spinosum *(FS)*, foramen ovale *(FO)*, foramen lacerum *(FL)*. **B,** Level of exocranial opening of jugular foramen. Caroticojugular spine *(CJS)* separates ascending carotid canal *(CC)* and jugular fossa. "Alembic" configuration of jugular fossa, consisting of pars nervosa *(pn)* and pars vascularis *(pv)*, can be recognized. Other structures: stylomastoid foramen *(SF)*, eustachian tube *(ET)*, petrooccipital fissure *(POF)* underlying inferior petrosal sinus, and emissary vein *(EV)*. **C,** Level of inferior border of endocranial opening. Foramen approaches "bird" shape. Pars nervosa *(pn)* and pars vascularis *(pv)* are well marked by jugular spine *(js)*. Horizontal carotid canal *(CC)* is well seen. External auditory meatus *(EAM)*, inferior recess of hypotympanum *(h)*, and eustachian tube *(ET)* with adjacent air cells appear similar to Fig. 13-31, *D*. Other structures: petrooccipital fissure *(POF)*, jugular tubercle *(JT)*, sigmoid sulcus *(SS)*, facial nerve canal *(FNC)*, inferior petrosal sulcus *(IPS)*, caroticojugular spine *(CJS)*. **D,** Superior border of endocranial opening. Note proximity of jugular foramen *(JF)* to hypotympanum separated from each other by jugular plate *(JP)*. Inferior surface of promontory of cochlea *(C)* is visible. Eustachian tube *(ET)* joins protympanum. Semicanal *(SC)* is only partially seen in this subject. Other structures: jugular spine *(js)*, cochlear aqueduct *(CA)*, carotid canal *(CC)*, petrooccipital fissure *(POF)*. (From Lo WWM and Solti-Bohman LH: High-resolution CT of the jugular foramen: anatomy and vascular variants and anomalies, Radiology 150:743, 1984.)

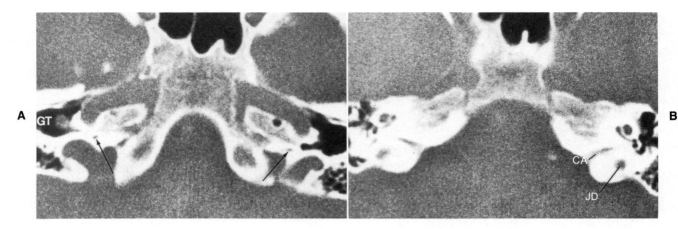

Fig. 13-33 **A,** Inferior tympanic canaliculus on caroticojugular spine *(arrows)*. A small glomus tympanicum tumor *(GT)* is present on the right. **B,** Trumpet-shaped cochlear aqueduct *(CA)* anterior to jugular dome *(JD)* should not be confused with higher and larger internal auditory canal (not shown). (From Lo WWM and Solti-Bohman LH: High-resolution CT of the jugular foramen: anatomy and vascular variants and anomalies, Radiology 150:743, 1984.)

ance on a scan section varies according to the level through the foramen and the inclination of the section (Figs. 13-31 and 13-32).

The jugular foramen is divided by a fibrous septum into a smaller anteromedial neural compartment (pars nervosa) and a larger posterolateral vascular compartment (pars vascularis) (see Figs. 13-31 and 13-32). The terminal portion of the sigmoid sinus flows anteriorly to enter the jugular foramen; turns laterally to expand into the jugular bulb in the jugular fossa; and then drains inferiorly as the internal jugular vein, which is posterolateral to the cervical segment of the internal carotid artery, in the carotid sheath.

Immediately medial to the internal jugular vein, in an anterior to posterior order, exit the ninth (glossopharangeal), tenth (vagus), and eleventh (spinal accessory) cranial nerves through the foramen. The ninth nerve passes alone through the neural compartment; and the tenth and eleventh together through the vascular compartment posterolateral to the jugular vein.[24] The inferior petrosal vein exits the posterior fossa through the pars nervosa medial to the ninth nerve, crossing laterally, in most cases, between the ninth nerve and the tenth and eleventh nerves, to join the internal jugular vein immediately outside the skull.[24] The neurovascular anatomy is better demonstrated on MR than on CT.[25,26]

Within the jugular foramen, the glossopharangeal nerve gives rise to its tympanic branch, which enters

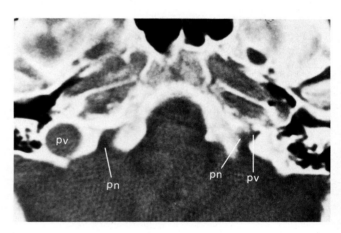

Fig. 13-34 Normal variation in size and symmetry between the two jugular fossae. Pars nervosas *(pn)* are nearly equal while the right pars vascularis *(pv)* is much larger and closer to hypotympanum than the left. (From Lo WWM and Solti-Bohman LH: High-resolution CT of the jugular foramen: anatomy and vascular variants and anomalies, Radiology 150:743, 1984.)

the tympanic cavity through the inferior tympanic canaliculus along the inferior tympanic artery (Fig. 13-33). Similarly, the vagus nerve gives rise to its auricular branch, which reaches the descending facial nerve canal through the mastoid canaliculus. These two glomus-bearing branches of nerves are also known, respectively, as the nerves of Jacobson and Arnold.[27]

The jugular foramen averages 15 mm in length and 10 mm in width.[28] The smaller pars nervosa, averaging about 5 mm in width, is relatively constant in size. The larger pars vascularis varies considerably in size depending on the size of the jugular vein it transmits (Fig. 13-34). Using the sum of the width of the two compartments and the total length of the foramen as an index, Di Chiro[28] found that the two sides may differ by as much as 18 mm. When the two sides are unequal, the dominant one is more often on the right than on the left.

The caroticojugular spine, a wedge-shaped bone, oriented essentially in a coronal plane and pointed inferiorly, separates the jugular foramen from the carotid canal. It is perforated by a number of tiny foramina, including the inferior tympanic canaliculus, which transmits the inferior tympanic nerve and artery into the tympanic cavity.[23] On rare occasions, this submillimeter canal can be identified on axial high resolution CT (see Fig. 13-34). The mastoid canaliculus is difficult to identify with certainty.

Other bony structures seen adjacent to the jugular foramen include the carotid canal, the eustachian tube, the facial nerve canal, the sigmoid sulcus, the hypoglossal canal, the petrooccipital fissure, and the cochlear aqueduct (see Figs. 13-31 and 13-32).

REFERENCES

1. Littleton JT et al: Temporal bone: comparison of pluridirectional tomography and high resolution computed tomography, AJR 137:835, 1981.
2. Shaffer KA, Haughton VM, and Wilson CR: High resolution computed tomography of the temporal bone, Radiology 134:409, 1980.
3. Mafee MF et al: Computed tomography of the middle ear in the evaluation of cholesteatomas and other soft tissue masses: comparison with pluridirectional tomography, Radiology 148:465, 1983.
4. Swartz JD: Current imaging approach to the temporal bone, Radiology 171:309, 1989.
5. Valvassori GE et al: MR of the normal and abnormal internal auditory canal, AJNR 9:115, 1988.
6. Press GA and Hesselink JR: MR imaging of the cerebellopontine angle and internal auditory canal at 1.5T, AJNR 9:241, 1988.
7. Teresi L et al: MR imaging of the intratemporal facial nerve using surface coils, AJNR 8:49, 1987.
8. Teresi LM et al: MR imaging of the intraparotid facial nerve, AJNR 8:253, 1987.
9. Lo WWM et al: Intratemporal vascular tumors: detection with CT and MR imaging, Radiology 171:443, 1989.
10. Daniels DL et al: Surface coil magnetic resonance imaging of the internal auditory canal, AJNR 6:487, 1985.
11. Koenig H, Lenz M, and Sauter R: Temporal bone region: high resolution MR imaging using surface coils, Radiology 159:191, 1986.
12. Swartz JD: High resolution computed tomography of the middle ear and mastoid. I. Normal radioanatomy including normal variations, Radiology 148:449, 1983.
13. Virapongse C et al: Computed tomography of temporal bone pneumatization. I. Normal pattern and morphology, AJNR 6:551, 1985.
14. Swartz JD: The facial nerve canal: CT analysis of the protruding tympanic segment, Radiology 153:443, 1984.
15. Bhimani S, Virapongse C, and Sarwar M: High resolution computed tomographic appearance of the normal cochlear aqueduct, AJNR 5:715, 1984.
16. Kapila A, Chakeres DW, and Blanco E: The Meckel cave: computed tomographic study, Radiology 152:425, 1984.
17. Valvassori GE: The large vestibular aqueduct and associated anomalies of the inner ear, Otolaryngol Clin North Am 16(1):95, 1983.
18. Lo WWM and Solti-Bohman LG: High resolution CT of the jugular foramen: anatomy and vascular variants and anomalies, Radiology 150:743, 1984.
19. Mafee MF et al: Direct sagittal CT in the evaluation of temporal bone disease AJNR 9:371, 1988.
20. Manzione JV, Rumbaugh CL, and Katzberg RW: Direct sagittal computed tomography of the temporal bone, J Comput Assist Tomogr 9:417, 1985.
21. Turski PA et al: High resolution CT of the petrous bone: direct vs. reformatted images, AJNR 3:391, 1982.
22. Schuknecht HF: Pathology of the ear, Boston, 1974, Harvard University Press, pp 25-26.
23. Warwick R and Williams PL, editors: Gray's anatomy, ed 35 (Br), Philadelphia, 1973, WB Saunders Co, pp 272, 294.
24. Rhoton AL Jr and Buza R: Microsurgical anatomy of the jugular foramen, J Neurosurg 42:541, 1975.
25. Daniels DL et al: Magnetic resonance imaging of the jugular foramen, AJNR 6:699, 1985.
26. Daniels DL et al: Gradient recalled echo MR imaging of the jugular foramen, AJNR 9:675, 1988.
27. Guild SR: The glomus jugulare, a non-chromaffin paraganglion, in man, Ann Otol Rhinol Laryngol 62:1045, 1953.
28. Di Chiro G, Fisher RL, and Nelson KB: The jugular foramen, J Neurosurg 21:447, 1964.

SECTION THREE
CONGENITAL ANOMALIES

ANTON N. HASSO
RONALD A. BROADWELL

The temporal bone develops from the pars branchialis and the pars otica. The pars branchialis radiates from the first and second branchial arches, the first branchial groove, and the adjacent mesenchyme. The pars otica develops from the auditory vesicle and adjacent mesenchyme. The development of the outer and middle ear is independent of the development of the inner ear. Anatomic variations, congenital anomalies, or both reflect the fact that one portion of the ear may be normal while another portion may be grossly malformed. Because outer and middle ear development is more closely linked, significant malformations of the external auditory canal are usually accompanied by middle ear deformities and vice versa. Inner ear anomalies usually occur independently. However, some inner ear anomalies are more frequently seen among patients who have concomitant anomalies of the other two compartments as compared to the normal population.

Since mesenchyme is involved in the development of all portions of the ear, there are certain situations where combined malformations can occur. The toxic embryopathy subsequent to maternal ingestion of thalidomide is an example of such a situation. Some of the otocraniofacial dysplasias show similar combined malformations (see Table 13-4).

The internal auditory canal, which is not part of the ear, may be normal in the presence of a grossly deformed inner ear. Cases of dysplasia or aplasia of the internal auditory canal may occur in the presence of a normal labyrinth, but extreme hypoplasia or aplasia of the internal auditory canal is more commonly associated with significant bony malformations of the inner ear. The development of the internal auditory canal is distinct from that of the labyrinth. The underlying mechanism explaining the coexistence of these congenital deformities is not apparent.

Anatomic variations comprise the range of dimensions, contours, and spatial orientation of the bony structures within the temporal bone region encountered in a normal population that demonstrates neither functional impairment nor anatomic substrate carrying the potential for imperiling the well-being of the individual. These two tests provide the crucial distinction between a "variation" and an anomaly.[1]

NORMAL VARIATIONS

The bony external auditory canal shows considerable variation in both size and configuration. It comprises the medial one half to two thirds of the complete external auditory canal, the lateral portion being cartilaginous. The bony portion is usually narrower than the cartilaginous portion and is directed medially, anteriorly, and slightly inferiorly, forming in its course a slight curve, the convexity of which is posterosuperior in position. There is a wide spectrum of shapes of the external auditory canal, varying from circular to oval to heart-shaped to triangular. The long axis of an oval canal may change its orientation, spiraling from medial to lateral. The bone that forms the anterior wall of the external auditory canal and separates it from the temporomandibular joint (TMJ) averages about 1.5 mm in thickness, with a range varying from about 0.2 mm to almost 4 mm in thickness.[1]

The middle ear, including its epitympanic recess, measures 15 mm in its anteroposterior and vertical diameters. The transverse diameter measures about 6 mm above and 4 mm below; opposite the center of the tympanic cavity, its transverse diameter is only about 2 mm. The hypotympanum is the pneumatized inferior extension of the middle ear cavity below the level of the tympanic ring. This is variable both in depth and in medial extension. The bone of the floor of the tympanic cavity, which separates it from the jugular bulb below, is thick when the hypotympanum is underdeveloped and small and thin when it is deep. Air cells of the mastoid group variably pneumatize this bony separation, particularly if the floor of the cleft is some distance removed from the jugular bulb.[1]

An important variation exists in the depth and angle of the sinus tympani, which forms a bony cavity lying between the bony labyrinth medially and the pyramidal eminence laterally. The sinus tympani is of surgical significance in that it may contain diseased tissue, most commonly an acquired cholesteatoma that is not visible by the usual surgical approach. The difficulty in approaching the sinus tympani depends on how deeply and in what direction the sinus extends. The retroauricular surgical approach to the sinus tympani requires an entry between the facial nerve and posterior or lateral semicircular canals or both. The distance between the sinus tympani and facial nerve is therefore important, as is the distance between the facial nerve and the posterior semicircular canal. The normal measurements for the sinus tympani are a depth of 3 mm (range 0.6 to 6.0 mm) and a width of 2 mm (range 1 to 3 mm). The deepest and widest portion of the sinus tympani is usually located at the level of the round window membrane. The distance between the sinus tympani and facial nerve is about 1 mm (range 0.1 to 1.6 mm). The distance between the facial nerve and posterior semicircular canal is about 3 mm (range 2.0 to 3.5 mm) at a distance between 2 and 3 mm below the inferior border of the footplate of the stapes. Although such minute differences may seem to be of interest only to the surgeon, they emphasize the need for precise diagnostics in this field of imaging.[1]

There is essentially no variation in size or shape of the osseous labyrinth.[1] People of all ages have virtually the same size and shape labyrinthine structures.[2]

The cochlea is conical, measuring about 5 mm from base to apex, and its breadth across the base is about 9 mm. It normally has 2½ to 2¾ coils, appearing as three "stories." Minor alterations in the size of the cochlea, minor variation in the number of coils, or both is not significant. Marked reduction of the lumen of the various coils is more important. The vestibule is ovoid but flattened transversely. It measures about 5 mm from the front backward; the same from above downward and about 3 mm across. No normal variants exist for the vestibule.

Each of the semicircular canals is about 0.8 mm in diameter, and each has a dilatation of one end, called the ampulla. The superior semicircular canal is oriented transversely to the long axis of the petrous temporal bone and measures about 15 to 20 mm in length. The posterior semicircular canal is also vertically placed and is directed backward, nearly parallel with the posterior surface of the petrous portion. It is the longest canal, measuring from 18 to 22 mm. The lateral semicircular canal is the shortest of the three, its arch being directed horizontally backward and laterally. It is inclined 30 degrees with the horizontal, the anterior limb of which lies in the superior plane. As with the vestibule, there are no normal variants, although an anatomically abnormal vestibule or semicircular canal may be present without clinical symptoms.[1]

Table 13-1   Classification of outer and middle ear anomalies

Entity	Extent of middle ear involvement*	Ear structures derived from entity	Specific malformations
Tympanic ring dysplasia	0 to ++	External auditory canal, tympanic membrane, short process of malleus	Varying degrees of external ear canal stenosis. May have ossicular deformity and/or small middle ear cavity.
Tympanic ring aplasia	+	External auditory canal, tympanic membrane, short process of malleus	Bony plate obliterating external canal, absent tympanic membrane, anterior process of malleus fused to atresia plate, facial canal immediately dorsal to a posteriorly displaced TMJ.† Tympanic cavity may be small.
First branchial arch dysplasia	++	Marjority of malleus, incus; mandible	Deformities of malleus and incus and/or fusion to attic/antrum or atretia plate (if present). Hypoplastic mastoid air spaces with obliteration of attic/antrum. If atretic plate present, terminal portion of facial nerve lies within plate. Tympanic cavity may be slitlike. Usually associated with mandibular anomalies.
Second branchial arch dysplasia	+++	Stapes superstructure, lateral lamina of footplate; facial nerve, styloid process, mastoid process, stylohyoid ligament, superior cornu of hyoid bone	Defects of the stapes superstructure and footplate. Abnormal positioning of the facial nerve with absent bony covering. Nerve is exposed across floor of middle ear, may have bipartite or tripartite forms.

*0 = No involvement
 + = Mild involvement
 ++ = Moderate involvement
 +++ = Severe involvement
†TMJ = Temporomandibular joint

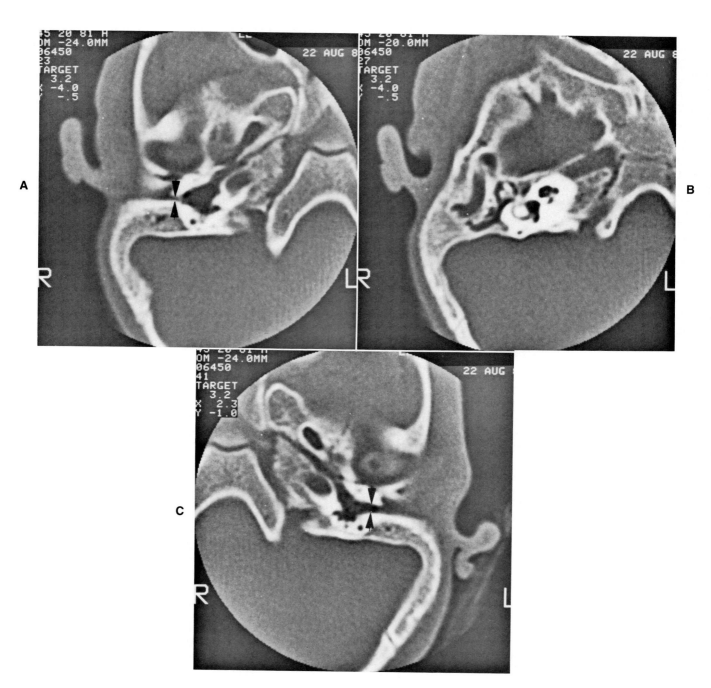

Fig. 13-35   Bilateral tympanic ring dysplasia. Axial CT scans. **A,** Bony stenosis of right external auditory canal is evident *(arrowheads)*. There is a soft tissue mass representing embryonic debris within tympanic cavity. **B,** Middle and inner ear structures appear normal. Ossicular chain is well developed and is not fused to walls of tympanic cavity. **C,** Similar, less severe stenosis of left external auditory canal *(arrowheads)*. There is opacification of tympanic cavity, which may be due to residual embryonic debris.

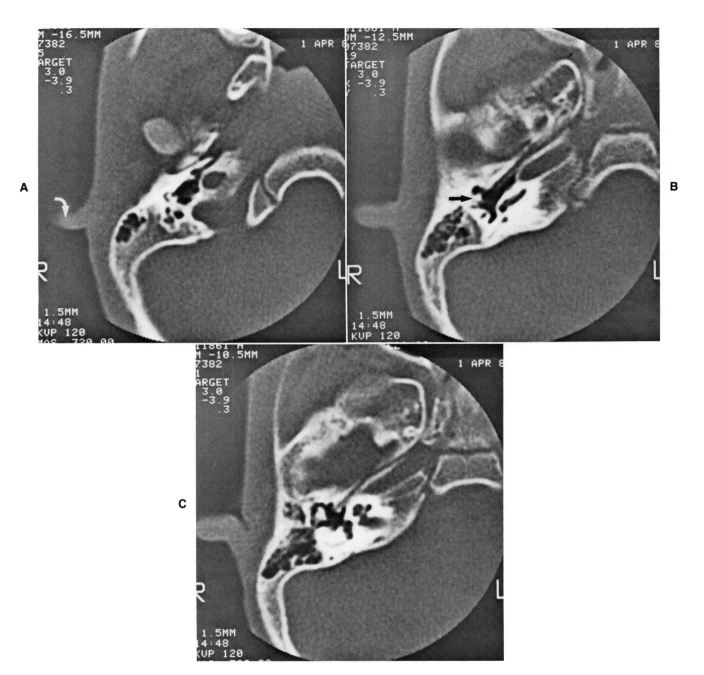

Fig. 13-36 Tympanic ring aplasia of right ear. Axial CT scans. **A,** Osseous atretic plate obliterates external auditory canal. There is severe microtia with a skin tag representing outer ear *(curved arrow)*. Lack of support from tympanic ring has allowed posterior migration of temporomandibular joint. **B,** Fusion of normal ossicles (neck of malleus and body of incus) to atresia plate *(arrow)*. Note well-developed tympanic cavity and mastoid air cells. **C,** Epitympanic cavity recess, mastoid air cells, facial nerve canal, and inner ear structures are normal.

ANOMALIES OF THE OUTER EAR

Malformations of the outer ear may involve the auricle or the external auditory canal. The auricle develops around the first branchial groove and contains tissues contributed by both the first (mandibular) and second (hyoid) branchial arches.[3] An anomaly of the auricle (microtia) may occur as an isolated event but is usually associated with other anomalies. Severe microtia is typically associated with atresia or stenosis of the external auditory canal[4] (Table 13-1).

The external auditory canal is a derivative of the first ectodermal branchial groove between the mandibular and hyoid arches. The first ectodermal branchial groove comes in contact with connective tissue from the adjacent mesoderm and forms the tympanic membrane and tympanic ring.[3] Ossification of the tympanic ring forms the tympanic portion of the temporal bone in adult life.

Stenosis of the External Auditory Canal

Dysplasia of the tympanic ring may lead to the development of stenosis of the external auditory canal (Fig. 13-35). The canal may be diffusely narrowed, or there may be variable focal stenosis. Severe stenosis may trap epithelial debris in the medial end of the canal (Fig. 13-35, A and C). This normal squamous epithelium may subsequently undergo metamorphosis to form an acquired cholesteatoma of the external canal. As the cholesteatoma enlarges, the medial end of the canal expands with concomitant pressure effects on the tympanic membrane and ossicles. In some cases perforation of the tympanic membrane leads to gross bone destruction, with the predictable consequences of an untreated cholesteatoma.[5]

Atresia of the External Auditory Canal

Atresia of the external auditory canal typically is caused by tympanic ring aplasia and may be complete or partial, unilateral or bilateral. Complete osseous atresia of the external auditory canal consists of a bony plate across the external auditory canal, where the tympanic membrane is usually located. This deformity is associated with fusion of the neck of the malleus to the atresia plate (Fig. 13-36).[6,7] The short or anterior process of the malleus originates from the tympanic ring[3] and may be the only absent portion of the ossicles when there is no concomitant involvement of the first or second branchial arches (see below). With isolated tympanic ring anomalies, the tympanic cavities are normal in size, and the mastoids are well developed (unless there is a history of infection).

In some cases there may be a fibrous atresia of the external auditory canal. Instead of the tympanic membrane, a "plug" of soft tissue is located at the site of the tympanic membrane. This relatively mild anomaly is caused by failure of recanalization[1] with or without fusion of a portion of the malleus to the lateral wall of the tympanic cavity (Fig. 13-37).[7]

Patients with atresia of the external auditory canal cannot be examined otoscopically. It is essential to examine these patients with high resolution computed tomography (HRCT) in order to rule out the presence of a concomitant dysplasia of the middle ear cleft or a congenital cholesteatoma of the middle ear.[7] In these cases CT will show either a dysplastic nonaerated middle ear or an opaque tympanic cavity with possible erosion of its walls. These patients may require early surgery to remove the cholesteatoma and preserve facial nerve function with or without reconstruction of the external auditory canal.

Temporomandibular Joint Anomalies

Since the tympanic ring is significantly involved in all anomalies of the outer ear, there may be alterations in the usual architecture of the temporomandibular joint (TMJ). Deformity of the mandibular condyle is frequently associated with tympanic ring anomalies, along with a shallow joint space.[8] The temporal squama may be pushed downward, and the glenoid fossa may be markedly flattened or even absent.[5] The position of the TMJ is frequently abnormal, being relatively higher and more posterior in relationship to the middle ear[8] (Fig. 13-36, A). Normally, the distance from the posterior aspect of the ramus of the mandible to the anterior surface of the tympanic bone is approximately 8 mm. In some congenital cases, depending on the degree of hypoplasia or agenesis of the tympanic bone, the distance may reach 40 mm.[5] The abnormal position of the TMJ may affect the ability of the surgeon to reconstruct the external auditory canal.[8] Furthermore, the facial nerve canal may exit in the narrow space between the glenoid fossa and mastoid process, directly in the surgical field.

ANOMALIES OF THE MIDDLE EAR

Anomalies of the middle ear form a continuum with varying degrees of involvement. Minimal middle ear involvement is represented by tympanic ring dysplasia or aplasia. Mild to moderate involvement occurs when there is anomalous development of the first branchial arch. Severe involvement represents additional involvement of the second branchial arch (Table 13-1).

Tympanic Ring Dysplasia

Tympanic ring dysplasia first appears with varying degrees of external auditory canal stenosis (Fig. 13-35, A and C). The size of the middle ear cavity may be completely normal. The ossicles may be normal or partially fused to each other or to the lateral wall of the at-

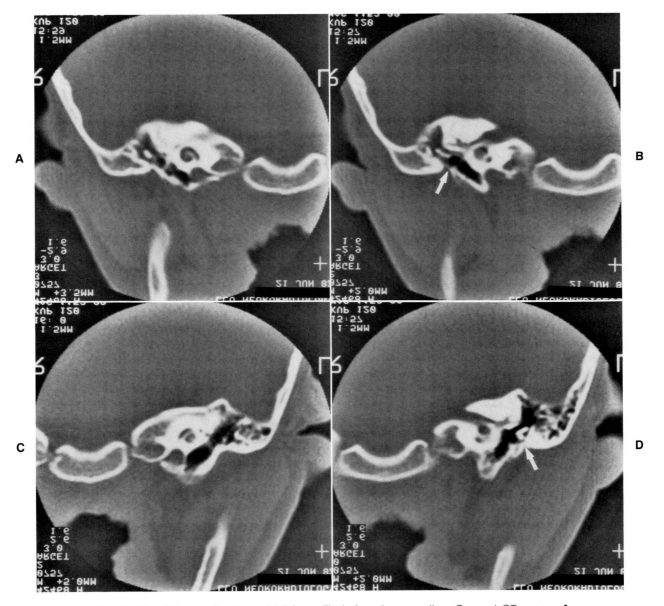

Fig. 13-37 Bilateral first branchial (mandibular) arch anomalies. Coronal CT scans. **A** and **B,** Membranous atresia of right external auditory canal. There is microtia with a rudimentary right auricle. Absent external auditory canal is replaced by soft tissue attached to tympanic membrane *(arrow)*. Ossicular chain is only partially developed. Epitympanic recess is opacified, which may be due to residual embryonic debris. Inner ear structures are normal. **C** and **D,** Osseous atresia of left external auditory canal. There is microtia and absence of external auditory canal. A thick bony septum or atresia plate substitutes for absent tympanic membrane *(arrow)*. Ossicles are malformed, and inner ear structures are normal.

tic or both. Obliteration, erosion of the middle ear and mastoid air cells, or both may result from the presence of embryonic debris in these spaces (congenital cholesteatoma)[9] or from an acquired cholesteatoma arising from a stenosed external auditory canal.[5]

Tympanic Ring Aplasia

Under certain conditions, especially common in the thalidomide malformations, complete aplasia of the tympanic ring may occur.[9] A bony plate forms in place of the tympanic ring and obliterates the external ear canal and tympanic membrane (Fig. 13-36). This atresia plate redirects the terminal portion of the facial nerve, causing it to course more anteriorly within the plate and to exit at the bottom of the plate near the TMJ (Figs. 13-38 and 13-39).[6,10] The lack of posterior support allows dorsal positioning of the TMJ with abutment of the glenoid fossa against the anterior aspect of the mastoid process (see Fig. 13-36, A).[4,7,9]

A constant finding is fusion of a portion of the malleus to the atretic plate.[6] Most of the malleus develops from Meckel's (first branchial arch) cartilage. The short or anterior process originally forms from the tympanic ring through intramembranous ossification. In later embryologic development the malleus annexes this small portion of the ring, creating the anterior process.[3] When no tympanic ring forms, the neck of the malleus is fused to the atretic plate (see Figs. 13-36, B, and 13-39, A, B, and E). The tympanic cavity may be of normal size but may be slightly reduced, depending on the size of the bony atresia plate (see Figs. 13-39, A to C).[1,4,8,9] The mastoids are usually well pneumatized.[4] Complete tympanic ring aplasia consists of absence of the external auditory canal and tympanic membrane, presence of a bony atretic plate including fusion of the neck of the malleus, anterior displacement of the facial nerve, and posterior positioning of the temporomandibular joint.

First (Mandibular) Branchial Arch Dysplasia

Maldevelopments of the first branchial arch result in various congenital malformations of the eyes, ears, mandible, and palate, which together constitute the first arch syndrome. The complete syndrome is believed to be caused by insufficient migration of cranial neural crest cells into the first branchial arch.[11] Dysplasias of the first branchial arch have characteristic otologic anomalies, the more obvious manifestations resulting from defects of Meckel's (first branchial arch) cartilage. This cartilage forms the incus and most of the malleus.[3] These ossicles are usually anomalous with varying maldevelopments of the external auditory canal, middle ear cavity, and mastoid air cells (see Fig. 13-39, A to C, E, and F). First arch dysplasias also show mandibular anomalies since the formation of the mandi-

ble is guided by the first arch cartilage template (Fig. 13-40 and see Fig. 13-39, D).

Second (Hyoid) Branchial Arch Dysplasia

Second branchial arch dysplasias include anomalies of the stapes superstructure, lateral lamina of the stapes footplate, and the facial nerve canal. Normally, the facial nerve migrates anteroinferiorly after exiting the stylomastoid foramen to extend directly to the facial musculature innervated by this nerve. As a result of defective formation of the stapes superstructure and a portion of the footplate, the facial nerve is unimpeded in its anterior migration, lying exposed directly across the floor of the middle ear (Fig. 13-39, F). The facial nerve may appear as a soft tissue mass within the floor of the tympanic cavity. An aberrant course of the facial nerve canal should be suspected whenever the structures originating from Reichert's (second branchial arch) cartilage (i.e., the superstructure and lateral lamina of the stapes footplate, styloid process, stylohyoid ligament, and superior cornu of the hyoid bone) are maldeveloped (see Fig. 13-39, D).

The anomalous facial nerve may have a bipartite or tripartite form. The most common bifid nerve is one that extends just beneath the lateral semicircular canal as one trunk, splits into two trunks through its vertical course downward in the temporal bone, and unites either at or just outside the stylomastoid foramen into a single trunk. The more lateral of these trunks is usually the larger one and is usually the one that receives the chorda tympani. A soft tissue mass may be seen on the promontory of the cochlea inferior to the oval window, which, when combined with absence of the bony facial canal superior to the oval window, suggests the anomalous course. In general, most congenitally aberrant facial nerves are short and relatively thick.[5] Occasionally, the facial nerve is in normal position but is exposed owing to failure of development of a complete bony wall. In other cases the nerve lies exposed in submucosal tissue and may cross an anomalous middle ear cavity in the region of the oval or round windows.[8]

ANOMALIES OF THE INNER EAR

Approximately 20% of patients with congenital sensorineural hearing loss have radiographic anomalies of the inner ear.[12] These anomalies represent a broad range of histopathologies. In the past, attempts at classifying these anomalies have relied heavily on certain restricted categorical types. Since many of the observed anomalies did not fit these defined types, there were many difficulties in classification. A description based on anatomic terms appears to be more accurate and practical. Some of the histologic types are described below because they represent classic descriptions that are widely used in the literature.

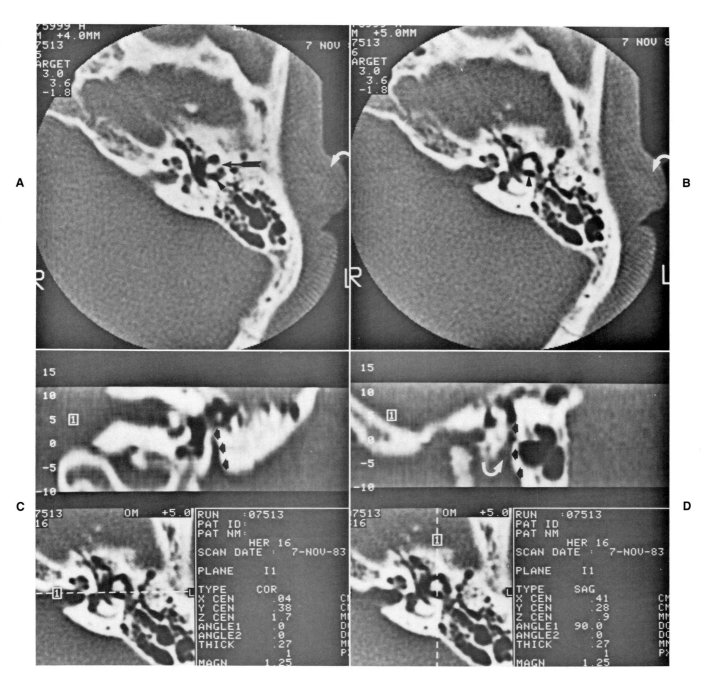

Fig. 13-38 Tympanic ring aplasia of left ear. **A** and **B,** Axial CT scans. Outer ear *curved arrow* consists of a nubbin of tissue. Note absence of external auditory canal. Ossicles are fused to bony atresia plate *(long arrow, **A**)*. Genu of facial nerve canal lies in center of tympanic cavity *(arrowheads **A, B**)*. **C,** Coronal reformatted image performed at site of arrowheads in **A** and **B.** Note third portion of facial nerve canal extending directly beneath ossicles in tympanic cavity *(arrowheads)*. **D,** Sagittal reformatted CT scan performed at site of arrowheads in **A** and **B.** Third portion of facial nerve canal extends directly into floor of tympanic cavity *(arrowheads)*. Condyle of mandible and temporomandibular joint lie in close proximity to stylomastoid foramen *(curved arrow)*.

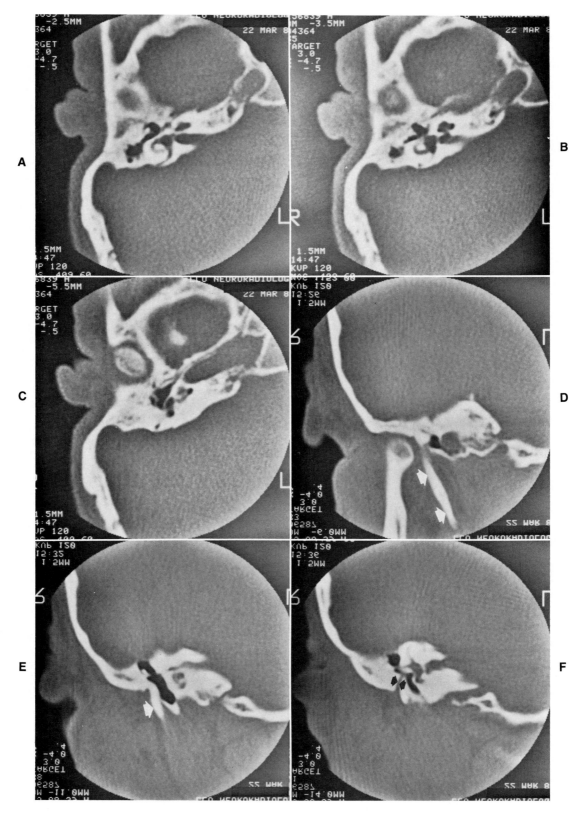

Fig. 13-39 For legend see opposite page.

Fig. 13-39 First (mandibular) and second (hyoid) branchial arch anomalies of right ear (Goldenhar's syndrome). **A, B,** and **C,** Axial CT scans. Stigmata of first branchial arch anomalies are clearly evident with atresia of external auditory canal, maldevelopment of middle ear, and osseous atresia plate obliterating external auditory canal. Ossicles are fused to the thick atresia plate. Size of middle ear cavity is reduced to a slitlike aperture. There is poor development of mastoid air cells. Outer ear consists of a skin tag. Temporomandibular joint has migrated posteriorly. **D, E,** and **F,** Coronal CT scans. A small slitlike middle ear cavity is evident. There is atresia of external auditory canal, fusion of ossicles and flattening of temporomandibular joint. Due to involvement of second branchial arch cartilage and its derivative, facial nerve is unimpeded in its anterior migration, exiting in a more anterior position close behind temporomandibular joint *(arrowheads,* **F**). Enlarged styloid process *(arrowheads,* **D, E**) is positioned directly adjacent to stylomastoid foramen.

Membranous Labyrinth

The membranous labyrinth is the fundamental part of the ear. It is the first to form prior to the development of other portions of the inner ear. As the acoustic nerve develops, its peripheral process reaches the membranous wall. The epithelium then becomes modified into the neural epithelium for the end organs of hearing and equilibrium.[3]

Many genetically determined anomalies, such as the Siebenmann-Bing and Scheibe types, involve portions of the membranous labyrinth, including the basilar membrane, organ of Corti, or spiral ganglia. Radiographic diagnosis is precluded in these anomalies since the osseous labyrinth is normal.[12]

Bony Labyrinth

Semicircular Canals. Malformation of the lateral semicircular canal is the most common inner ear anomaly.[4,9,10,12] Malformation of the superior and posterior semicircular canals without involvement of the lateral canal is unusual. The malformed canals are either narrow or short and wide (Fig. 13-41). In extensive malformation the vestibule is dilated and forms a common lumen with the lateral canal. In some cases it may not be possible to identify the canals because the lumen is obliterated or the canals are absent. When the canals are absent, there is typical flattening of the corresponding portion of the otic capsule.[10]

Vestibule. Anomalies of the vestibule rarely occur as an isolated event; more frequently they are present in association with other inner ear anomalies.[13] The vestibular anomalies consist of complete or partial assimilation of the semicircular canals (usually the lateral semicircular canal) into the vestibule.[10,12] Rarely, an enlarged, globular vestibule may be found (Fig. 13-42). This anomaly of the inner ear has been associated with thalidomide-induced deafness.[13]

Cochlea. Jackler[12] has advanced a classification of cochlear anomalies based on the hypothesis that the various morphologic patterns result from an arrest of maturation during stages of inner ear embryogenesis. The following represents the spectrum of cochlear abnormalities corresponding to the arrested stage of development (Fig. 13-43).

Complete Labyrinthine Aplasia (Michel's Deformity). There is no inner ear development. In place of the normal inner ear structures, a small, single cystic cavity is present. This description corresponds to the histopathology classically described by Michel and represents an early failure in development correlating to the third gestational week.

Common Cavity. During the fourth week, the otic placode invaginates to form a simple cavity called the otocyst. A lack of normal differentiation beyond this stage results in a common cavity with the cochlea and vestibule, forming a large cystic cavity with no internal architecture. The semicircular canals may be normal or malformed.

Cochlear Aplasia. Arrested development of the cochlea during the fifth week of embryogenesis produces this defect. The cochlea fails to form and appears as a single cavity. The other elements of the inner ear (i.e., the vestibule and semicircular canal) may be normal or malformed (Figs. 13-44 and 13-45, *C* and *D*).

Cochlear Hypoplasia. Cochlear hypoplasia displays a small rudimentary cochlear bud associated with a normal or malformed vestibule and semicircular canals. A cessation of cochlear development during the sixth week of intrauterine life is the probable cause of this lesion (Fig. 13-45, *A* and *B*).

Incomplete Partition (Classic Mondini's Malformation). This entity represents a small cochlea with incomplete or no intrascalar septa. Anomalies of the remaining in-

Text continued on p. 976.

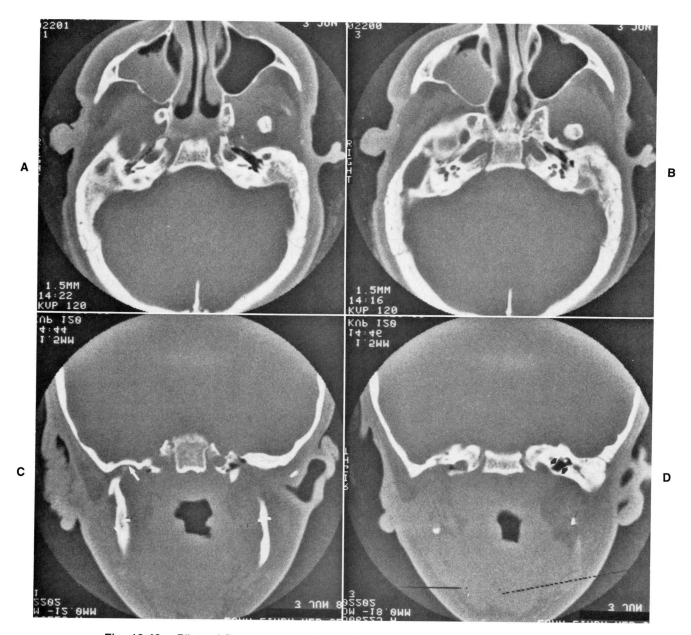

Fig. 13-40 Bilateral first and second branchial arch anomalies (Treacher-Collins syndrome). **A** and **B,** Axial CT scans. These images document stigmata of first arch dysplasia consisting of malformed ossicles with maldevelopment of external auditory canals, middle ear cavities, and mastoid air cells. Osseous atresia plates obliterate external auditory canals, fusing ossicles, and reducing size of middle ear cavities. Involvement of tympanic ring allows for posterior migration of temporomandibular joints. There is severe dysplasia of auricles bilaterally. **C** and **D,** Coronal CT scans. Small slitlike middle ear cavity on left side (*arrowheads,* **D**) and atretic external auditory canal are seen. Note deformed rami of mandible bilaterally and flattening of right temporomandibular joint (*arrow,* **C**). Auricles consist of deformed tissues with multiple irregular skin tags.

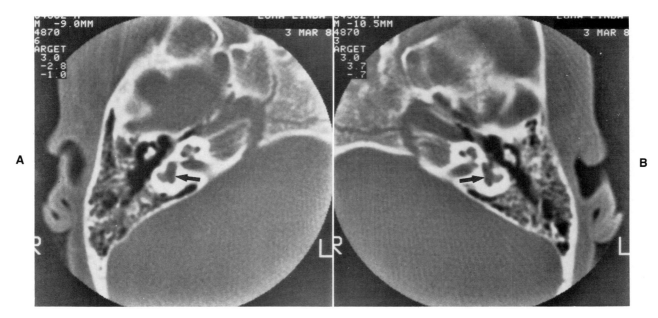

Fig. 13-41   Bilateral mild anomalies of posterior and lateral semicircular canals. **A,** Axial CT scan of right ear. Dilated bud represents lateral and posterior semicircular canals *(arrow)*. This is a common inner ear anomaly. **B,** Axial CT scan of left ear. A similar anomaly is documented *(arrow)*. Note that middle ear structures and mastoid air cells are well developed.

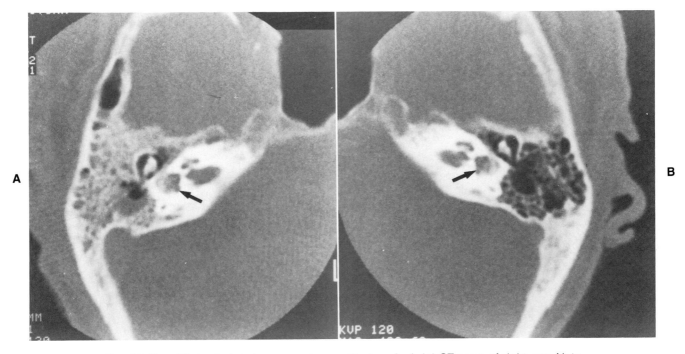

Fig. 13-42   Bilateral globular-appearing vestibules. **A,** Axial CT scan of right ear. Note that enlarged vestibule is partially assimilated with lateral semicircular canal *(arrow)*. Remainder of inner ear structures are normal. **B,** Axial CT scan of left ear. A similar anomaly is identified on left side *(arrow)*. Epitympanic recess, ossicles, and mastoid air cells are normal.

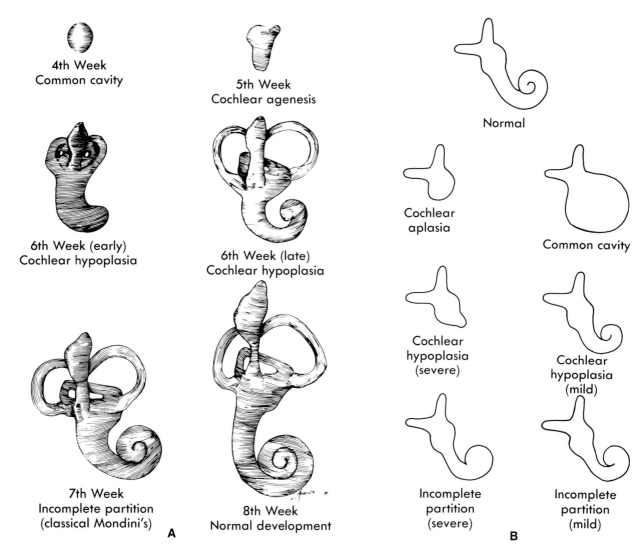

Fig. 13-43 **A,** Schematic representation of labyrinthine malformations. Anomalies are depicted as a result of arrests during various stages of embryrogenesis. **B,** Schematic representation of radiographic appearance of continuum of labyrinthine malformations. (Reproduced by permission from *The Laryngoscope,* "Congenital Malformations of the Inner Ear," suppl 40, vol 97, no 3, part II, March 1987, by Robert K. Jackler and William M. Luxford.)

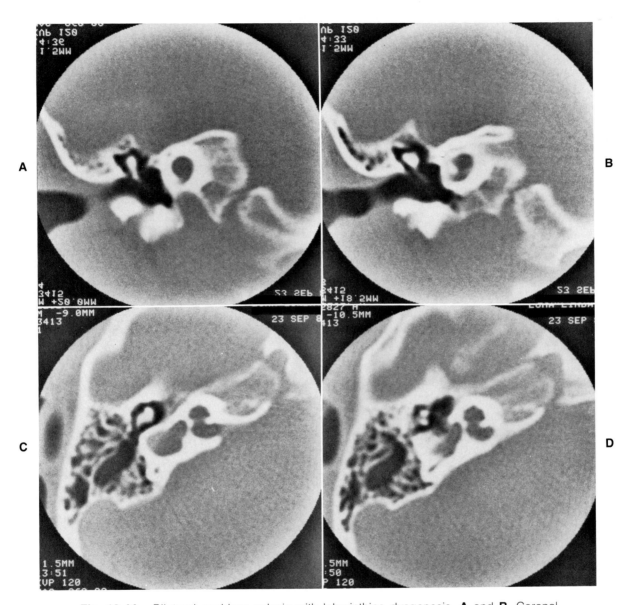

Fig. 13-44 Bilateral cochlear aplasia with labyrinthine dysgenesis. **A** and **B,** Coronal CT scans of right ear demonstrating hypoplastic cochlear cavity. **C** and **D,** Axial CT scans of right ear. Note poorly developed vestibule and semicircular canals. Anomalies of inner ear correspond to cochlear aplasia occurring at about fifth week of gestation.

Continued.

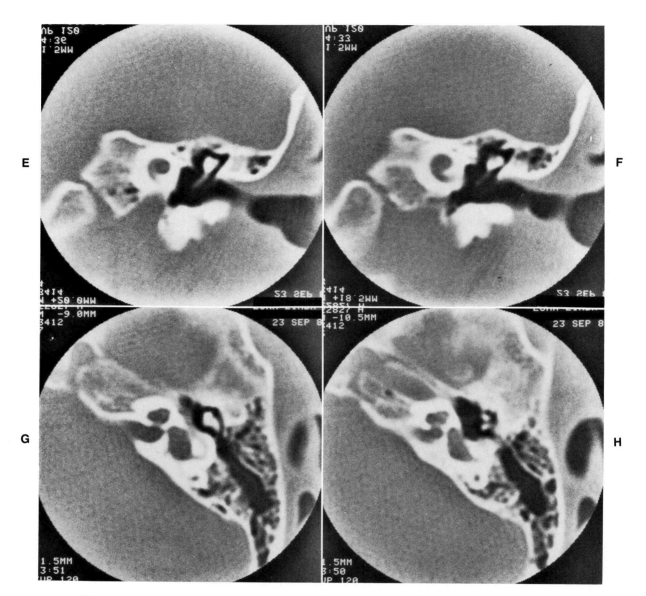

Fig. 13-44, cont'd **E** and **F,** Coronal CT scans of left ear. There are similar anomalies involving the left cochlea. **G** and **H,** Axial CT scans of left ear. There is a rudimentary lateral semicircular canal, but remainder of vestibule and semicircular canals form a single cavity.

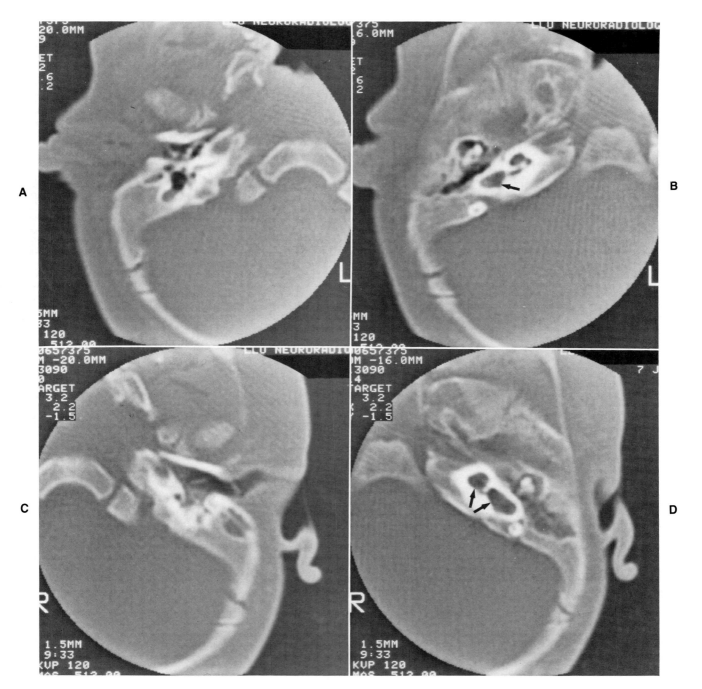

Fig. 13-45   Combined bilateral tympanic ring dysplasia and cochlear hypoplasia. **A** and **B,** Axial CT scans of right ear. There is severe microtia with auricular skin tags. Cartilaginous portion of external auditory canal is not visible. There is mild stenosis of external auditory canal. Cochlea is partially developed. Semicircular canals and vestibules are malformed *(arrow).* **C** and **D,** Axial CT scans of left ear. There is less severe microtia with less stenosis of cartilaginous portion of left external auditory canal. There is more severe involvement of inner ear with significant hypoplasia of cochlea, vestibule, and semicircular canals *(arrows).*

ner ear, such as dilatation of the vestibular aqueduct, may be present (Figs. 13-46 and 13-47). Arrest of maturation at the seventh week of intrauterine life may result in these findings. Incomplete partition of the cochlea characterizes a classic histologic malformation first described by Carlo Mondini in 1791. Mondini documented a flat cochlea, having 1½ turns instead of the normal 2½ to 2¾ turns. He also described a large vestibule with wide, small, or missing semicircular canals and immature sensorineural structures.[14] Aside from Scheibe's deafness, Mondini's malformation is probably the most common form of genetic deafness.[15]

Internal Auditory Canal. The internal auditory canal may be characterized by stenosis or even atresia. Isolated dilatation of the canal is of unknown pathologic significance.[2] A bony septum may be present, partitioning this structure into two or more separate canals.

Vestibular Aqueduct. The anomalies of the vestibular aqueduct have been described as ranging from total obliteration to a widely dilated form (see Fig. 13-46). Gradations between these two extremes have been documented, most notably a filiform aqueduct, which may or may not be associated with Ménière-like disturbances.[4]

Valvassori and Clemis[16] describe the dilated vestibular aqueduct in detail, including its incidence and presentation. According to their study of 3700 consecutive patients, 50, or 1.5% of cases, showed an enlarged vestibular aqueduct (greater than 1.5 mm diameter). Sixty percent of the patients had radiographically identifiable anomalies of the vestibule, semicircular canals, and cochlea. The hypoplastic cochleas were classified into the Mondini type of cochlear anomalies (see Fig. 13-47). The remaining 40% of patients showed no other identifiable anomalies of the inner ear and may have had associated pathology of the membranous labyrinth, which would not be visible by radiographic means. The clinical findings in these patients with enlargement of the vestibular aqueduct included 5 patients with vestibular symptoms. The remaining 45 patients first demonstrated a variety of pure sensorineural and mixed hearing loss.

The association of vestibular aqueductal dilatation and incomplete partition of the cochlea (classic Mondini's deformity) appears likely when the embryology of these structures is understood. The vestibular aqueduct and partitioning of the cochlea are the last developing entities within the inner ear. A teratogen exerting its effects in this late stage of development can easily involve both structures simultaneously.

VASCULAR ANOMALIES (Table 13-2)
Internal Carotid Artery

Aberrant (Lateral) Course. An aberrant course of the internal carotid artery through the middle ear is rare.[17]

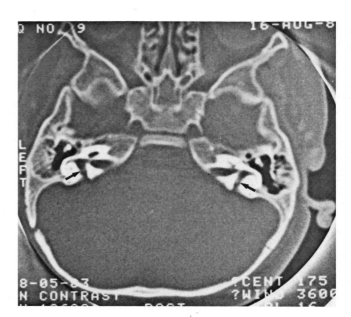

Fig. 13-46 Bilateral giant vestibular aqueducts. Axial CT scan of both ears. There is marked dilatation of vestibular aqueducts bilaterally (arrows). Cochleas (not shown) are also malformed.

More than 90% of the cases described in the literature occur in females, with the majority occurring on the right side.[18] No convincing explanation for this predominance in females or of the right side has been presented.[19]

There is no universally accepted etiology for this anomaly.[17] Among the proposed mechanisms is a congenital failure of ossification of the bony limiting wall of the petrous carotid canal. Some authors have reported that the bony plate is frequently less than 0.5 mm thick.[19] With age, as the vessel elongates and becomes tortuous, it may protrude through the defect into the tympanic cavity.[18,19] Persistence of embryonic vessels may produce sufficient traction to pull the artery into the middle ear (Fig. 13-48).[18]

Otalgia has been reported as one of the initial symptoms.[20] Other signs and symptoms include tinnitus, hearing loss (mostly conductive), a red-blue pulsatile mass behind the tympanic membrane, vertigo, and the presence of a fullness sensation in the ear.[18,19] The tinnitis may be caused either by the direct mechanical transmission of the vessel's pulsations to the tympanic membrane and ossicles or by the audible sound produced by arterial blood flow emanating from the abnormal vessel within the middle ear. The hearing loss may be the result of the mass effect of the vessel (e.g., the dampening of the tympanic membrane vibrations or encroachment or erosion of the ossicles).[18] Many patients are asymptomatic.

Not infrequently, the red-blue mass behind the tym-

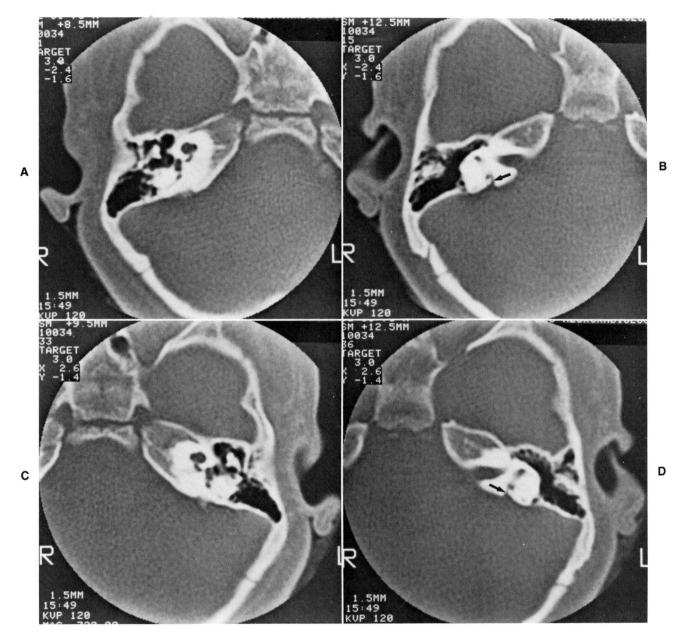

Fig. 13-47   Bilateral Mondini malformations with incomplete partition of cochlea and en-largement of vestibular aqueducts. **A** and **B,** Axial CT scans of right ear. Cochlea is small with incomplete partition. Vestibular aqueduct is slightly dilated *(arrow).* **C** and **D,** Axial CT scans of left ear. There is a similar anomaly of left cochlea. Left vestibular aqueduct is also enlarged *(arrow).*

Table 13-2 Vascular anomalies associated with malformations of the petrous bone

Anomaly	Proposed etiology	Clinical presentation	Diagnostic imaging
Internal carotid artery			
Aberrant (lateral)	Absence of the hypotympanic bony plate because of congenital failure of ossification (with age the artery elongates and becomes tortuous, protruding through the defect); abnormal persistence of embryonic vessels (e.g., stapedial artery, producing traction pulling artery through osseous defect into middle ear)	Tinnitus, hearing loss (usually conductive), red-blue pulsatile mass behind TM,* otalgia, vertigo, fullness in the ear. May be asymptomatic.	CT†—Soft tissue mass in the hypotympanum extending toward the oval window area, indenting promontory or displacing the TM laterally; may have associated grooving of the apical, middle, and basilar turns of the cochlea; lateral wall of the carotid canal not visualized on coronal views; bony posterolateral portion of the canal is absent on axial views. Angio‡—Lateral deviation of the internal carotid artery past the "vestibular line"; caliber of the artery usually increased; persistent stapedial artery a common finding
Partial absence	Alternate blood flow theory; blood flow preferentially courses through the inferior tympanic artery and the hyoid/caroticotympanic arteries, bypassing the vertical portion of the intrapetrous carotid	Can present as above	CT—Vertical part of carotid canal may be absent; soft tissue mass in hypotympanum. Angio—Internal carotid artery enters the middle ear with a reduced caliber, through Jacobson's canal (inferior tympanic artery course); then courses below and against the promontory inferior and anterior to the stapes; proceeds forward to join the horizontal portion of the carotid canal
Complete absence	Unilateral absence possibly resulting from mechanical causes in early development, such as amniotic adhesions, excessive bending of the cephalic end of embryo	Can present as an incidental finding during workup of neurologic symptoms	CT—Absence of the carotid canal. Angio—Unilateral or bilateral absence of the internal carotid arteries with varied associated anomalies of the remaining vasculature
Jugular vein			
High jugular bulb	Anatomic variation	Silent, unless inadvertently entered during attempted myringotomy, paracentesis, or turning of a tympanomeatal flap	CT/Veno§—High position of the jugular bulb with a thin hypotympanic plate
Protruding jugular bulb	Congenital dehiscence of the bony plate covering the jugular bulb, with protrusion of the bulb through the defect	Bluish mass behind TM on otologic exam. Pulsatile tinnitus, headaches, hearing loss (usually conductive) from loss of mobility of the ossicular chain and/or TM or impingement on the oval window	CT—Dehiscence of the bony floor of the hypotympanum. Soft tissue mass in the middle ear. Veno—Jugular bulb projecting through bony defect into middle ear cavity
Jugular diverticulum	Unknown	Hearing loss (sensorineural) tinnitis (nonpulsatile), vertigo, symptoms mimicking Ménière's disease	CT—Jugular diverticulum lying more medial and posterior in the petrous bone than a high jugular bulb; does not invade middle ear; at times erodes into IAC,‖ causing direct pressure on the acoustic nerve; can obliterate the vestibular aqueduct. Veno—Jugular diverticulum extending superiorly into the petrous bone (superiormost extension of the medial diverticulum lies in a plane higher than the level of a high jugular bulb)

*TM = Tympanic membrane
†CT = Computed tomography
‡Angio = Carotid angiography
§Veno = Jugular venography
‖IAC = Internal auditory canal

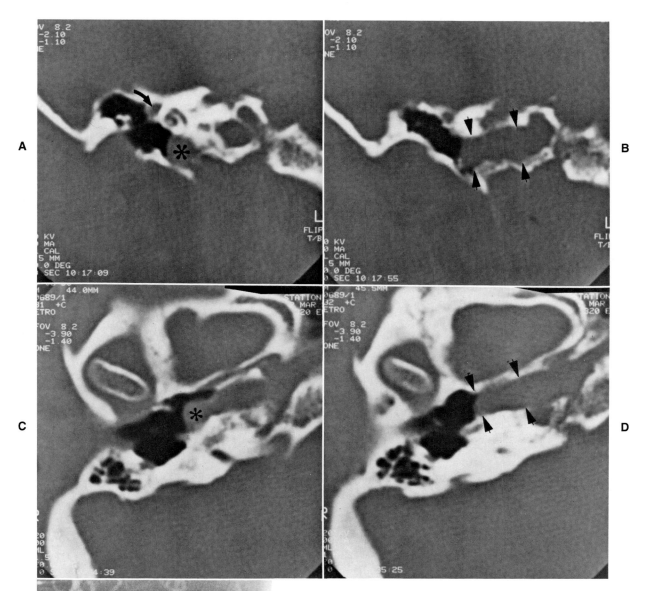

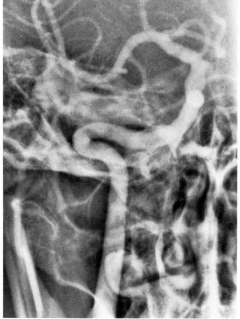

Fig. 13-48 Aberrant lateral course of right internal carotid artery. **A** and **B,** Coronal CT scans of right ear. There is a soft tissue mass in floor of tympanic cavity *(asterisk)* representing boneless portion of internal carotid artery. There is enlargement of facial nerve canal *(curved arrow)* due to presence of a stapedial artery that exits tympanic cavity with facial nerve. Horizontal carotid canal is enlarged *(arrowheads).* **C** and **D,** Axial CT scans. A round soft tissue mass *(asterisk),* continuous with carotid canal, bulges into anterior inferior floor of tympanic cavity. Horizontal portion of carotid canal is enlarged *(arrowheads).* **E,** Anteroposterior view of right internal carotid angiogram. Lateral course of internal carotid artery through middle ear is apparent. Note looping of this vessel laterally and its prominent intratympanic course. (Case courtesy of C. Roger Bird, M.D., Phoenix, AZ.)

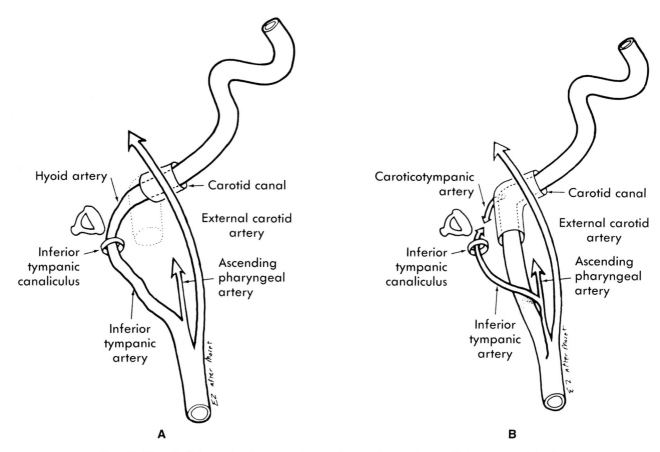

Fig. 13-49   A, Schematic diagram of normal vascular anatomy of internal carotid artery. Note bony vertical and horizontal segments of carotid canal. Small inferior tympanic artery extends through skull base via inferior tympanic canaliculus and anastomosis with caroticotympanic artery (vestige of embryologic hyoid artery). Anastomosis occurs on cochlear promontory medial to stapes. **B,** Schematic diagram of partial absence of internal carotid artery. Cervical portion of carotid artery has failed to develop, causing agenesis of vertical segment of carotid canal. As a result of compensatory hypertrophy of inferior tympanic artery, there is enlargement of inferior tympanic canaliculus. Inferior tympanic artery courses through tympanic cavity under cochlear promontory to anastomose with persistent hyoid artery and then enter horizontal carotid canal via a cleft in carotid plate. (Reproduced by permission from *Radiographics,* vol 5, no 6, November 1985, by William W.M. Lo, Livia G. Solti-Bohman, and John T. McElven, Jr.)

panic membrane has been inadvertently ruptured during therapeutic myringotomies, biopsy for suspected glomus tumors, or both. This has resulted in catastrophic hemorrhage from the middle ear, emergently treated by ear packing.

CT reveals an enhancing soft tissue mass in the hypotympanum extending toward the oval window area, indenting the promontory, and displacing the tympanic membrane laterally.[18] Grooving of the apical, middle, and basilar turns of the cochlea by the artery may also be seen.[17] A stapedial artery, which is depicted as a soft tissue mass in the middle ear enlarging the facial canal, is often present. On coronal views, the limiting lateral

wall of the carotid canal is absent.[1] The enlarged facial canal is visible above the cochlea (see Fig. 13-48, *A* and *B*). On axial views the bony posterolateral portion of the canal is absent (see Fig. 13-48, *C* and *D*).[17]

Internal carotid angiography documents a large carotid artery that is deviated laterally and buckled beyond the "vestibular line." The vestibular line represents a vertical line drawn tangential to the lateral margin of the vestibule on anteroposterior views (see Fig. 13-48, *E*).[17,18,20] In one examination of 100 normal patients, none of the normal arteries were found lateral to this line.[21] The caliber of the artery is normal or dilated at the site of the bony defect (see Fig. 13-48).

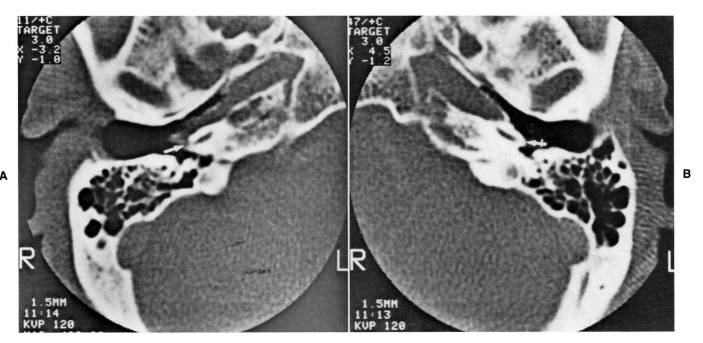

Fig. 13-50   Unilateral partial absence of internal carotid artery. **A,** Axial CT scan of abnormal right ear. Carotid artery lies medially and inferiorly in tympanic cavity. Carotid canal is small and irregular in appearance due to partial agenesis of internal carotid artery. Resultant hypertrophy of inferior tympanic branch of external carotid artery enters horizontal carotid canal through a cleft beneath eroded cochlear promontory *(arrow).* **B,** Axial CT scan of normal left ear. Note bony covering over internal carotid artery. This vessel lies along medial margin of cochlea. Cochlear promontory is unaffected *(crossed arrow).* (Case courtesy of William W.M. Lo, M.D., Los Angeles, CA.)

Asymptomatic aberrant arteries require no treatment. Therapy is usually reserved for patients with pulsatile tinnitus, hemorrhage, or cranial nerve palsies. Intervention ranges from the interposition of synthetic material between the artery and ossicles, disarticulation of the ossicular chain, or ligation of the internal carotid artery in cases of hemorrhage.[18]

Partial Absence. A small segment of the intrapetrous portion of the internal carotid artery may be absent, resulting in an aberrant arterial course through the middle ear. Embryologically, a variation in flow leads to regression of blood flow through the cervical internal carotid artery with preferential flow through the inferior tympanic artery and hyoid artery, which then joins the horizontal petrous portion of the normal internal carotid artery (Fig. 13-49).[4] Thus lack of flow results in atrophy of the internal carotid artery up to the horizontal petrous portion. Under such conditions the tympanic canaliculus transmits an unusually prominent inferior tympanic artery. This vessel appears as an aberrant internal carotid artery in the middle ear with the associated signs and symptoms described before (Fig. 13-50).

CT shows an enhancing soft tissue mass in the hypo-

tympanum and absence of the vertical portion of the bony carotid canal. Internal carotid angiography demonstrates the artery entering the middle ear with a reduced caliber as a result of the bony confines of the tympanic canaliculus. From that point it courses below and against the promontory inferior and anterior to the stapes and proceeds forward to join the horizontal petrous portion of the carotid canal.[4]

Agenesis. The etiology of congenital absence of the internal carotid artery is unknown. Keen[22] has suggested that unilateral absence of the internal carotid artery may be from mechanical causes in early development such as pressure effects, excessive bending of the cephalic end of the embryo from side to side, or the effects of amniotic adhesions. No explanation has been offered for bilateral absence, which is extremely rare.

Symptoms may or may not preclude the discovery of an absent internal carotid artery. The agenesis may be discovered as an incidental finding during the workup of an unrelated problem or, more commonly, may be discovered during the workup of neurologic symptoms. In 42 reported cases of congenital absence, 12 patients initially had subarachnoid hemorrhage caused by rup-

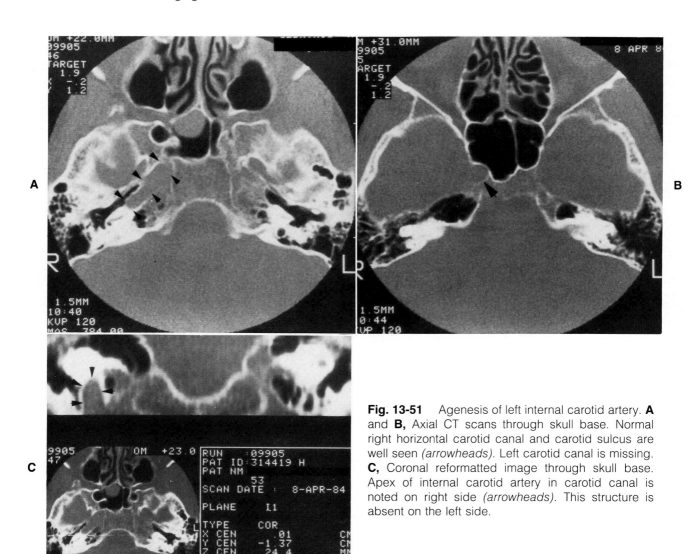

Fig. 13-51 Agenesis of left internal carotid artery. **A** and **B,** Axial CT scans through skull base. Normal right horizontal carotid canal and carotid sulcus are well seen *(arrowheads).* Left carotid canal is missing. **C,** Coronal reformatted image through skull base. Apex of internal carotid artery in carotid canal is noted on right side *(arrowheads).* This structure is absent on the left side.

tured intracranial aneurysm. Other clinical presentations include multiple cranial nerve palsies caused by compression of a dilated loop of the basilar artery, hemiparesis after minor head trauma, and various other neurologic signs and symptoms resulting from major head injuries.

CT shows no carotid canal in the petrous bone or a small vertical cleft, possibly representing an abortive carotid canal (Fig. 13-51). Internal carotid angiography demonstrates absence of the internal carotid artery. This examination reveals the frequent occurrence of associated anomalies of the remaining vasculature; i.e., dilated basilar artery collaterals, ipsilateral dilation of the posterior communicating artery filling the corresponding anterior or middle cerebral arteries or both,

and ipsilateral ophthalmic or anterior cerebral arteries arising from the middle cerebral artery.

Jugular Vein

High Jugular Bulb. A high jugular bulb is a jugular bulb located above the level of the bony annulus of the temporal bone.[23,24] Because of this high position, the bony covering of the jugular bulb may be thin, rendering the bulb vulnerable to trauma. In three separate studies, this anatomic variant was found to be present in 7%, 6%, and 3.5% of temporal bones examined histologically, making it the most common vascular anomaly of the petrous bone.[24]

This entity bears some relation to the degree of pneumatization of the mastoid air cells. In a poorly

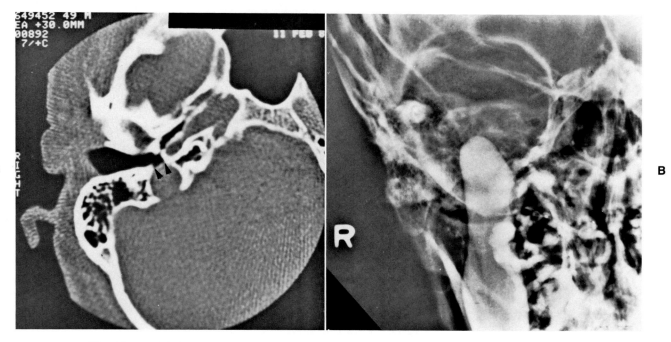

Fig. 13-52 High jugular bulb. **A,** Axial CT scan of right ear. High jugular bulb does not extend into right tympanic cavity *(arrowheads)*. **B,** Anteroposterior view of a right internal jugular venogram. High right jugular bulb is confirmed. There is no evidence of a diverticulum.

pneumatized mastoid, the sigmoid sinus is more anterior, the jugular fossa tends to be deep, and the jugular bulb has a correspondingly high dome.[24] The height of the bulb is significant because of the risk of inadvertently entering the vein during myringotomy or middle ear procedures. CT and jugular venography show the high position of the bulb and the thin hypotympanic limiting wall (Fig. 13-52).

Protruding Jugular Bulb. The second most common vascular anomaly is the jugular bulb initially seen as a vascular mass in the middle ear. This entity has two components, a dehiscence of the floor of the middle ear and a protrusion of a portion of the jugular bulb through the dehiscence (Fig. 13-53). A bony dehiscence overlying the jugular bulb in one cadaveric study was found to have a 7% incidence of occurrence.[19]

Patients may have pulsatile tinnitus, headaches, hearing loss (usually conductive, with the jugular bulb impinging on the ossicles, tympanic membrane, oval window, or a combination), a bluish mass behind the tympanic membrane, or hemorrhage after myringotomy.[19,23,25,26] CT shows an enhancing soft tissue mass in the middle ear as well as a bony defect above the jugular bulb in the floor of the hypotympanum (see Fig. 13-53). Jugular venography reveals the jugular bulb projecting through the defect into the middle ear.

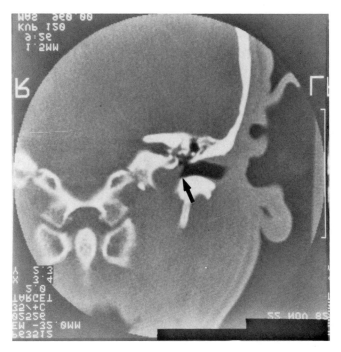

Fig. 13-53 Protruding left jugular bulb. Coronal CT scan of left ear. A small portion of left jugular bulb protrudes into middle ear cavity via a defect in floor of hypotympanum *(arrow)*.

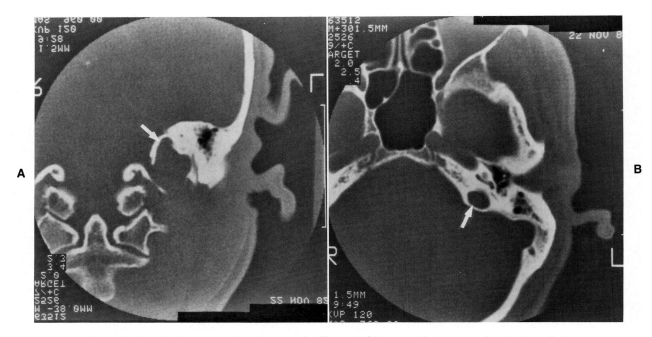

Fig. 13-54 Left jugular diverticulum. **A,** Coronal CT scan. There is a diverticulum that protrudes into roof of petrous bone behind internal auditory canal *(arrow).* **B,** Coronal CT scan of left ear. Smooth walled jugular diverticulum extends superiorly to level of osseous labyrinth. Note indentation on posterior wall of petrous bone *(long arrow).*

Jugular Diverticulum. A jugular diverticulum is an irregular outpouching of the jugular bulb that rises superiorly and medially in the petrous pyramid. The etiology of this venous anomaly is unknown.[24]

There are characteristic differences between a jugular diverticulum and a protruding jugular bulb. A jugular diverticulum is situated more medially and posteriorly in the petrous bone than is a protruding jugular bulb (Fig. 13-54). A jugular diverticulum does not invade the middle ear, is not visible on inspection, and is not exposed to surgical trauma from a myringotomy or tympanotomy. The diagnosis of a jugular diverticulum is only made radiographically. A protruding jugular bulb is diagnosed by both radiologic and otoscopic examinations.[24]

The hearing loss from a jugular diverticulum is sensorineural from encroachment on the endolymphatic duct or on the internal auditory canal. Tinnitis, if present, is continuous or intermittent in patients with a jugular diverticulum. Patients with a jugular diverticulum may be dizzy or vertiginous, symptoms that are commonly associated with a protruding jugular bulb. Sometimes, a jugular diverticulum may cause signs and symptoms that mimic classic Ménière's disease.[24]

CT demonstrates the irregular diverticulum extending superiorly into the petrous pyramid (see Fig. 13-54). The diverticulum may show encroachment on the internal auditory canal, vestibular aqueduct, or both. Jugular venography shows the irregular outpouching of the diverticulum extending superiorly into the petrous bone. The most superior extension of the diverticulum lies in a plane higher than the level of a protruding jugular bulb.[1]

Agenesis. Agenesis of the jugular bulb and sigmoid sinus is extremely rare. In these cases the absent sigmoid sinus redirects the flow from the transverse sinus into a canal posterior and superior to the petrous bone. This canal then drains directly through the transmastoidian venous channels into adjacent scalp veins. CT of the temporal bone and skull base will document the absent sigmoid sinus and jugular bulb along with the aberrant venous drainage system (Fig. 13-55).

MALFORMATIONS OF THE PETROUS BONE ASSOCIATED WITH MENINGITIS (Table 13-3)

Cerebrospinal fluid (CSF) leakage from the petrous bone structures is a rare and potentially life-threatening condition.[27] This cryptic condition typically develops as a result of trauma or following the destructive effects of infection. An associated congenital abnormality of the temporal bone should always be suspected in cases of recurrent meningitis, especially when there is hearing impairment. Most of these patients have a history of recurrent meningitis and persistent otorrhea, rhinorrhea,

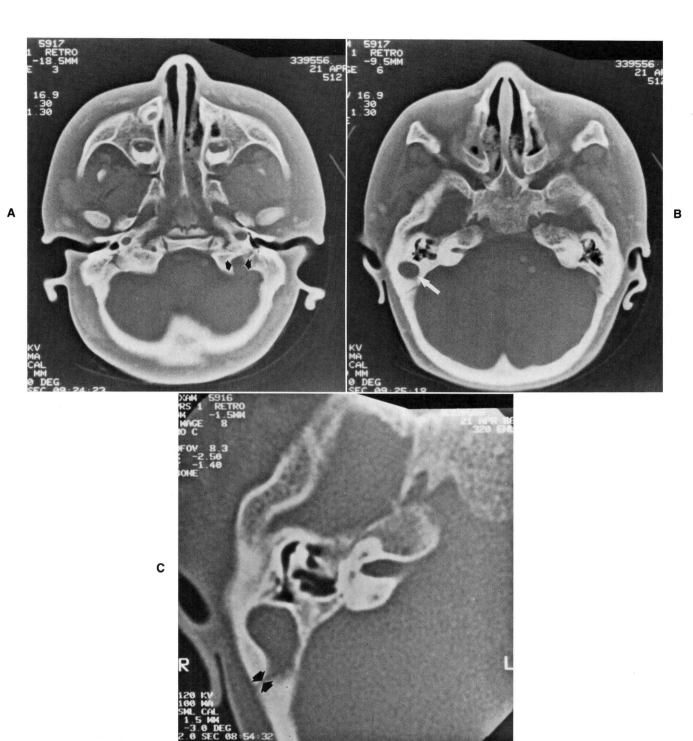

Fig. 13-55   Absent sigmoid sinus and jugular bulb. **A** and **B,** Axial CT scans of skull base. There is a normal left jugular foramen (*arrowheads,* **A**), but no evidence of a right jugular foramen. There is a dilated cavity in right mastoid portion of temporal bone representing alternate drainage pathway of transverse sinus through enlarged mastoid emissary vein (*arrow,* **B**). **C,** Enlarged axial CT scan of right temporal bone. Enlarged mastoid emissary vein shows a connection through calvarium into scalp *(arrowheads).* (Case courtesy of C. Roger Bird, M.D., Phoenix, AZ.)

Table 13-3 Malformations of the petrous bone associated with meningitis

Anatomic entrance	Mechanism of CSF leak	Clinical presentation	Diagnostic imaging
Internal auditory canal	Defect in lamina cribrosa separating the IAC* and vestibule. CSF† may follow perineural sheaths as they pierce this thin portion of bone. Perilymphatic hydrops develops with secondary displacement of the stapes footplate.	Recurrent meningitis, otorrhea (if TM‡ perforated), rhinorrhea, hearing loss, serous otitis media, lack of caloric responses, pseudo Ménière's disease.	Abnormal accumulation of subarachnoid injected tracer material behind the TM, in the external canal, eustachian tube, or middle ear of the involved side. CT§ scan may show abnormalities of the inner ear.
Dehiscence of the tegmen tympani	Dehiscence of the tegmen with an accompanying meningocele, allowing direct access to the middle ear.	Usually an adult patient with no otologic signs, but can present as above.	Similar to above. CT may show meningocele and/or dehiscence of the tegmen.
Wide cochlear aqueduct	Persistence of a wide fetal-type cochlear aqueduct, allowing perilymphatic hydrops with subsequent "gushing" of CSF via the round or oval windows.	Similar to first entity (above); hearing loss of a progressive, fluctuating, mixed type.	Positive radioactive tracer studies and a wide cochlear aqueduct on CT.

*IAC = Internal auditory canal
†CSF = Cerebrospinal fluid
‡TM = Tympanic membrane
§CT = Computed tomography

or both; but some may have no otologic symptoms. When suspected, it is essential to document subtle sites of bone-dura discontinuities.

Cerebrospinal fluid fistulas have conveniently been described as comprising various entrances and exits[28] occurring across the complex anatomy of the temporal bone (see Table 13-3). The following discussion classifies these lesions according to their entrances with identification of their corresponding exits.

Internal Auditory Canal

The internal auditory canal is one of the most frequently observed entrances of CSF into the middle ear.[9] The canal is normally filled with CSF to its most lateral extent, where it is separated from the vestibule by the thin lamina cribrosa. The vestibular and cochlear nerves penetrate this thin bony layer to enter the inner ear. It has been shown that defects in the development of the lamina cribrosa[9,13,29] or the existence of patent perineural pathways[27,30] accompanying the nerves piercing this plate can allow communication between the subarachnoid space and the perilymphatic fluid.

This abnormal communication between CSF and perilymph causes the hydrostatic pressure within the inner ear to increase. This state of "perilymphatic hydrops" has been postulated to cause displacement, perforation, or both of the stapes footplate.[2,28] (The round window is less frequently involved.) This defect allows communication to the middle ear, or communication may be established when the surgeon manipulates or removes the stapedial footplate ("stapes gusher").[9] Depending on the competency of the tympanic membrane, the patient may experience otorrhea, rhinorrhea, or both. Other symptoms may include hearing loss, serous otitis media, loss of caloric responses,[31] and pseudo Ménière's diseases.[28] At times, no clinical evidence of a fistula occurs.[4] Associated with the fistula may be a variety of inner ear malformations, the most common being an enlarged and confluent vestibule and lateral semicircular canal (see Figs. 13-41 and 13-42). The cochlea is often cystic and devoid of internal architecture (Figs. 13-44 and 13-45).[9,12]

Owing to the complex anatomy and at times the lack of obvious leakage, the diagnosis of a fistula may be difficult to elucidate. Various imaging materials have been injected into the subarachnoid space to document these fistulas. Nuclear tagged substances (i.e., technetium DTPA, radioactive iodinated serum albumin, or indium) may accumulate in and localize the affected ear.[14,27,31] Dyes, such as indigo carmine, may be injected and visualized either as leaking into the middle ear or as discoloration of the tympanic membrane, nose, and nasopharynx. An intrathecal injection of a nonionic radiographic contrast agent may be used to outline the defect. CT of the petrous bone has become an integral part of the workup. Not only may defects be directly visualized (i.e., intrathecally injected contrast material may be seen in the labyrinth), but any associated inner ear abnormalities can be demonstrated simultaneously.

Surgical closure of the fistula should be undertaken some time after complete recovery from meningitis.[30] The method of correction is dictated by the functional status of the ear, the size of the fistula, and the quantity of fluid issuing from the fistula. If hearing and vestibular function are to be preserved, a tissue graft of fat, venous wall, or fibrous tissue is placed to inhibit the leakage. If the leakage continues, the stapes can be removed and a graft placed to cover the oval window. A stapes prosthesis is then placed to preserve hearing and to hold the graft in place. If preservation of vestibular or auditory function, or both, is not an issue, the fistula may be closed by a tissue implant into the vestibule.[14]

Dehiscence of the Tegmen Tympani

A CSF fistula may arise from congenital absence of a portion of the tegmen tympani.[28] If there is an associated defect in the adjacent meninges, CSF can reach the middle ear.[4] In contradistinction to internal auditory canal defects, these patients tend to be adults. As a result of the lack of inner ear involvement, the patients usually have no otologic signs.[4,28]

Coronal CT scanning of the petrous bone typically demonstrates incomplete development of the tegmen tympani, which may have an associated meningocele protruding into the middle ear. Treatment consists of neurosurgical repair of the bone and meningeal defects.

Wide Cochlear Aqueduct

Many investigators have confirmed a communication of CSF and perilymph through the cochlear aqueduct.[27] Normally the flow is directed through the aqueduct to the cisternal spaces. Some authors believe that the narrow adult aqueduct is not patent at all and that the fluids intermingle by diffusion through the membrane of the aqueduct. In contrast to the adult state, the cochlear aqueduct in children is patulous and short and may communicate directly with the subarachnoid space. The persistence of this fetal-type wide aqueduct has been postulated as causing a retrograde flow of CSF into the vestibule.[28,30] This entity sets the stage for "perilymphatic hydrops" with its accompanying lesions in or near the stapes footplate ("stapes gusher"). Patients are seen with progressive, fluctuating mixed hearing loss that was not present earlier in life.[28]

CT demonstrates a short, widely patent cochlear aqueduct (Fig. 13-56). This anomaly may be associated with a variety of inner ear malformations as described with internal auditory canal fistulas. Treatment may include ablation of the cochlear aqueduct,[9] tight packing of the vestibule with tissue grafts, or a combination.

CONGENITAL SYNDROMES INVOLVING THE EAR
(Table 13-4)

Syndromes associated with congenital anomalies of the ear are usually the result of an inherited disorder, although substrate damage in utero as a result of an external teratogen may occur in some cases. Hearing loss associated with these syndromes tends to be severe and less responsive to correction since the onset is early and

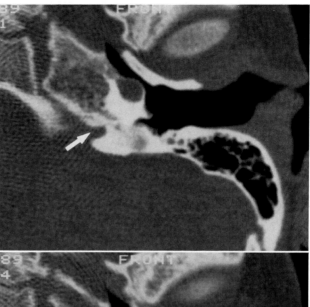

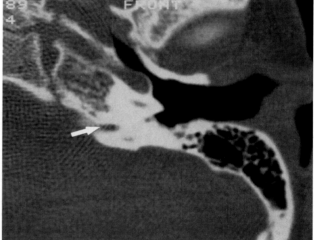

Fig. 13-56   Dilated cochlear aqueduct. **A** and **B,** Axial CT scans of left temporal bone. Enlarged aqueduct and its dilated orifice are well seen *(arrows).*

there are significant architectural anomalies present (see Fig. 13-39).

It is convenient to organize these syndromes into major classification groups according to their dominant morphologic features. The clinical and radiographic findings in these syndromes have been collected and categorized into various clinical groups. The groups consist of the otocraniofacial syndromes, otocervical syndromes, otoskeletal syndromes, and miscellaneous syndromes. These groups are described and classified in Table 13-4.

Otocraniofacial Syndromes

The otocraniofacial syndromes consist of anomalies of the ear, skull, and face. This group contains dominantly inherited syndromes involving the structures derived from the first and second branchial arches. These arch

Table 13-4 Syndromes with congenital abnormalities of the ear

Syndromes	Outer	Ear abnormalities Middle	Inner	Major associated anomalies
Otocraniofacial syndromes				
Treacher-Collins' syndrome (mandibulo-facial dyostosis)	+++ Deformed, low-set auricles; varying degrees of stenosis to atresia of external canal	+++ Deformed to absent ossicles, decreased size of middle ear cavity, underdeveloped mastoids, abnormal course of the facial nerve (usually anteriorly displaced)	0 to +* Occasionally abnormal vestibule with a short, wide LSCC†	Antimongoloid slant of palpebral fissures, coloboma of internal third of lower lid, malar/mandibular hypoplasia, scalp hair projecting onto side of face
Crouzon's disease (craniofacial dysostosis)	+++ Stenosis to atresia of external canal	+++ Narrow tympanic cavity, ossicle chain fixation via ankylosis of malleus to attic or of stapes to promontory	0	Ocular proptosis, hypertelorism, hypoplasia of the maxilla, parrotlike nose, craniosynostosis
Apert's syndrome (acrocephalosyndactyly)	0	+ Fixation of the stapes footplate	0	Craniosynostosis, midface hypoplasia, exophthalmos, high palatal arch, syndactyly of hands and feet, hypertelorism, antimongoloid slant, crowded teeth
Hemifacial microsomia	+++ Microtia, atresia/stenosis, vertically oriented external canal	+++ Descent of tegmen, ossicles deformed or absent	0	Unilateral mandibular/maxillary hypoplasia, macrostomia, hypoplastic TMJ,‡ hemivertebrae or hypoplasia, coloboma of upper lid
Otocervical syndromes				
Goldenhar's syndrome (oculoauriculovertebral dysplasia)	+++ Preauricular appendages; deformed auricle, atresia of canal	+++ Severe dysplasia with narrow cavity, absent ossicles	++* Hypoplastic cochlea and petrous ridge, short IAC§ with acute upward inclination	Epibulbar dermoids, hemi and/or block vertebrae, unilateral hypoplasia of maxilla/mandible, coloboma of upper lid, pharyngeal anomalies
Klippel-Feil syndrome	++ Microtia, atresia/vertical orientation of external canal	++ Thickening and fixation of stapes, bony obliteration of tympanic cavity	+++ Range from hypoplasia of cochlea and SCCs to a simple otocyst. Stenotic IAC	Short neck, fusion of two or more cervical vertebrae, low occipital hairline

*0 = No abnormalities
+ = Mild abnormalities
++ = Moderate abnormalities
+++ = Severe abnormalities
†LSCC = Lateral semicircular canal

‡TMJ = Temporomandibular joint
§IAC = Internal auditory canal
‖PSCC = Posterior semicircular canal
SCC = Semicircular canal

Table 13-4   Syndromes with congenital abnormalities of the ear—cont'd

Syndromes	Ear abnormalities Outer	Ear abnormalities Middle	Ear abnormalities Inner	Major associated anomalies
Otocervical syndromes—cont'd				
Wildervanck syndrome (cervico-occuloacoustic syndrome)	0	0	+++ Aplasia or hypoplasia of various structures	Manifestations of Klippel-Feil syndrome plus deafness, abducens palsy, and retraction of the orbits
Cleidocranial dyostosis	+ Narrowed canal	+ Marked sclerosis of mastoid	++ Marked sclerosis of petrous bone	Large brachycephalic head, large fontanelles with wide sutures, partial or total aplasia of clavicles, spinal abnormalities, and small, poorly developed facial bones
Otoskeletal syndromes				
Craniometaphyseal dysplasia (Pyle's syndrome)	+ Sclerosis of canal	++ Osseous proliferation within tympanic cavity, constriction of facial nerve canal, obliteration of the mastoids	++ Sclerosis of IAC	Flask-shaped enlargement of the metaphysis of the long bones, overgrowth of the craniofacial skeleton, obliteration of the sinuses
Frontometaphyseal dysplasia (Hart's syndrome)	0	+ Deformed ossicles	++ Osseous infiltration around cochlea	Large supraorbital ridge, absent pneumatization of the frontal sinuses, micrognathia, metaphyseal splaying of the tubular bones, wide nasal bridge, flaring of the iliac wings
Osteogenesis imperfecta (van der Hoeve's syndrome)	0	+ Stapes abnormalities	+++ Loss of otic capsule (changes identical to cochlear otosclerosis)	Deformity and bending of extremities, short stature, hyperextensibility of ligaments, dental defects, blue sclerae, fine hair, thin cornea
Osteopetrosis (Albers-Schönberg disease)	++ Narrowed canal	++ Sclerotic bone thickening that narrows facial canal and tympanic cavity, covering oval and round windows, obliterating mastoid sinuses	+++ IAC narrowed	Generalized increase in bone density with narrowed neural foramina, obliterated paranasal sinuses and mastoid cells, fractures, anemia, facial paralysis

Continued.

Table 13-4   Syndromes with congenital abnormalities of the ear—cont'd

Syndromes	Ear abnormalities			Major associated anomalies
	Outer	Middle	Inner	
Other syndromes				
Pendred's syndrome	0	0	++ Incompletely developed cochlea with hypoplasia, flattening of promontory	Triad of goiter, malformed inner ear, and pathologic perchlorate test
Waardenburg syndrome	0	0	++ PSCC absent,‖ LSCC slightly dilated, vestibule slightly irregular in shape	Hypertelorism, broad, high nasal root, white forelock, pigmentary disorders of the eye
Möebius' syndrome	+ Auricular malformation	++ Facial canal absent with no enlargement at geniculate ganglion	+++ SCC and vestibule dilated, hypoplastic cochlea, which may be a cystic cavity	Facial and abducens nerve palsy, possible additional cranial nerve involvement
Chromosome 18 deletion syndrome	++ Low-set auricles, stenosis to atresia of external canals	++ Ossicular abnormalities	0	Hypertelorism, hypoplasia of midface, epicanthic folds, carp-shaped mouth, foot anomalies, mental retardation, congenital heart disease
DiGeorge syndrome	0	+++ Ossicular deformities of small tympanic cavity	+++ Varying degrees of aplasia/dysplasia of cochlea	Congenital absence of parathyroid and thymus gland, heart and kidney abnormalities
Thalidomide embryopathy	+++ Complete absence of auricle, atresia of canal	+++ Forwardly displaced mastoid process, contracted tympanic cavity, absent, fixed, or abnormally situated ossicles	+++ Range from saccular dilation of LSCC to severe dysplasia of the otic cystic remnant	Varying degrees of limb reduction defects, cardiac anomalies, deafness, gastrointestinal malformations, hemangiomas, cranial nerve palsies

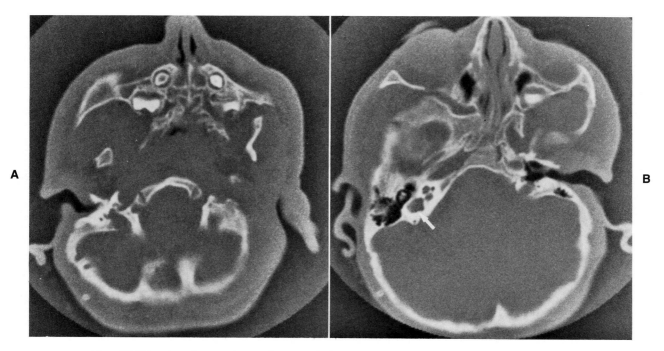

Fig. 13-57 Apert's syndrome (acrocephalosyndactyly). **A** and **B,** Axial CT scans of skull base. There is a deformity of skull base and facial bones causing an apparent plagiocephaly. Left middle and posterior cranial fossae are smaller than those on the right side. Right vestibule and semicircular canals form a single cavity *(arrow).*

anomalies invariably involve the external auditory canal with varying degrees of stenosis or atresia. The middle ear is typically involved with ossicular and facial canal abnormalities (see Fig. 13-40). Various facial asymmetries, as well as calvarial anomalies, are present in all cases. Occasionally, there may be inner ear anomalies (Fig. 13-57).

Otocervical Syndromes

Otocervical syndromes include anomalies of the ear, neck, and shoulder. The ear anomalies occur less frequently with the otocervical syndromes than with the otocraniofacial syndromes. The dominant features of this group are malformations of the cervical vertebrae. There may be fusion of one or more of the vertebral bodies. There typically tends to be more inner ear involvement, with occasional anomalies of the branchial arch systems.

Otoskeletal Syndromes

The otoskeletal syndromes consist of anomalies of the ear, face, and limbs. The common feature is abnormalities involving portions of the osseous skeleton. The otic manifestations of the otoskeletal syndromes portray a bony hyperactivity with osseous infiltration and narrow-

ing of the various bony fissures and foramina. The associated skeletal anomalies tend to repeat this common theme of bony overgrowth.

Other Syndromes

Several other syndromes have associated otic anomalies representing a broad range of morphologic types. The prominent features range from metabolic disorders to purely structural anomalies. The range of otic anomalies crosses over anatomic boundaries to engulf every aspect of the ear, representing a basic mesenchymal defect caused by a particular teratogen, for example, thalidomide.

REFERENCES

1. Bergeron RT, Osborn AG, and Som PM: Head and neck imaging: excluding the brain, St Louis, 1984, The CV Mosby Co, pp 778-791.
2. Jørgen J: Congenital anomalies of the inner ear, Radiol Clin North Am 12:473, 1974.
3. Anson BJ and Donaldson JA: Surgical anatomy of the temporal bone and ear, ed 2, Philadelphia, 1973, WB Saunders Co, pp 30-74.
4. Vignaud J, Jardin C, and Rosen L: The ear, diagnostic imaging, Paris, 1986, Masson Publishing USA, Inc, pp 104-145.
5. Wright JW Jr: Polytomography and congenital external and middle ear anomalies, Laryngoscope 91:1806, Nov 1981.

6. Jahrsdoerfer R: Congenital malformations of the ear: analysis of 94 operations, Ann Otol 89:348, 1980.

7. Swartz JD and Faerber EN: Congenital malformations of the external and middle ear, AJNR 6:71, Jan/Feb 1985.

8. Lapayowker MS: Congenital anomalies of the middle ear, Radiol Clin North Am 12:463, 1974.

9. Phelps PD and Lloyd GAS: Radiology of the ear, Oxford, 1983, Blackwell Scientific Publications, pp 22-48.

10. Petasnick JP: Congenital malformations of the ear, Otolaryngol Clin North Am 6:413-428, June 1973.

11. Moore KL: The developing human, ed 3, Philadelphia, 1982, WB Saunders Co, pp 179-215.

12. Jackler RK and Luxford WM: Congenital malformations of the inner ear, Laryngoscope 97:1, March 1987.

13. Lagundoye SB, Martinson FD, and Fajemisin AA: The syndrome of enlarged vestibule and dysplasia of the lateral semicircular canal in congenital deafness, Radiology 115:337, 1975.

14. Schuknecht HF: Mondini dysplasia: a clinical and pathological study, Ann Otol Rhinol Laryngol 89:1, Jan/Feb 1980.

15. Paparella MM: Mondini's deafness: a review of histopathology, Ann Otol Rhinol Laryngol 89:1, Mar/Apr 1980.

16. Valvassori GE and Clemis JD: The large vestibular aqueduct syndrome, Laryngoscope 88:723, May 1978.

17. Swartz JD et al: Aberrant internal carotid artery lying within the middle ear, Neuroradiology 27:322, 1985.

18. Sinnreich AI et al: Arterial malformations of the middle ear, Otolaryngol 92:194, 1984.

19. Glasscock ME III et al: Vascular anomalies of the middle ear, Laryngoscope 90:77, 1980.

20. Saito H, Chikamori Y, and Yanagihara N: Aberrant carotid artery in the middle ear, Arch Otorhinolaryngol 209:83, 1975.

21. Lapayowker MS et al: Presentation of the internal carotid artery as a tumor in the middle ear, Radiology 98:293, Feb 1971.

22. Keen JA: Absence of both internal carotid arteries, Clin Proc 4:588, 1946.

23. Overton SB and Ritter FN: A high placed jugular bulb in the middle ear: a clinical and temporal bone study, Laryngoscope 83:1986, Dec 1973.

24. Jahrsdoerfer RA, Cail WS, and Cantrell RW: Endolymphatic duct obstruction from a jugular bulb diverticulum, Ann Otol 90:619, 1981.

25. Lloyd TV, Van Aman M, and Johnson JC: Aberrant jugular bulb presenting as a middle ear mass, Radiology 131:139, 1979.

26. Lo WWM and Solti-Bohman LG: High-resolution CT of the jugular foramen: anatomy and vascular variants and anomalies, Radiology 150:743, 1984.

27. Clark, JL, DeSanto LW, and Facer GW: Congenital deafness and spontaneous CSF otorrhea, Arch Otolaryngol 104:163, 1978.

28. Pimontel-Appel B and Vignaud J: Liquorrhea in congenital malformation of the petrous bone, J Belge Radiol 63:283, 1980.

29. Sykora GF, Kaufman B, and Katz RL: Congenital defects of the inner ear in association with meningitis, Radiology 135:379, May 1980.

30. Curtin HD, Vignaud J, and Bar D: Anomaly of the facial canal in a Mondini malformation with recurrent meningitis, Radiology 144:335, July 1982.

31. Carter BL, Wolpert SM, and Karmody CS: Recurrent meningitis associated with an anomaly of the inner ear, Neuroradiology 9:55, 1975.

SECTION FOUR
INFLAMMATORY DISEASE

JOEL D. SWARTZ

Primary *pneumatization* of the middle ear is a complicated developmental process that depends on numerous factors, including nutrition, heredity, and environment.[1,2] Aeration of existing cells is, however, a dynamic process that depends on a normally functioning *eustachian tube*. Atticoantral aeration is further dependent on the patency of the *anterior* and *posterior tympanic isthmi*, which provide communication between the middle ear and attic.[3,4] Eustachian tube compromise (dysfunction or obstruction) with resultant decreased *intratympanic pressure* (ITP) has been widely accepted as the primary cause for most subsequently discussed varieties of inflammatory disease of the middle ear and mastoid.[1,5-8]

MIDDLE EAR EFFUSION

Middle ear effusions result from decreased ITP and may occur as an isolated phenomenon or in association with other manifestations of chronic otitis media.[6,8,9] Those occurring in infants and children are usually treated without the aid of radiologic intervention.[8] Imaging of middle ear effusions occurring spontaneously in an adult must include examination of the nasopharynx in order to exclude an obstructing neoplasm.

Such effusions may occur anywhere in the middle ear cleft (tympanic cavity proper), or within the attic, antrum, or mastoid air cell system. Diagnosis is made by demonstration of an air-fluid level, preferably in two orthogonal planes (Fig. 13-58).[9] Unfortunately, the diagnosis of an effusion in the completely opaque middle ear often is not possible. CT attenuation numbers are unreliable because of the diversity of the components of the collection. *Tympanostomy tubes* are used in these patients both for drainage and as a means of ITP normalization.[6,10,11] These tubes are made of various plastics and metals, including stainless steel (Fig. 13-59). They are of widely varying shapes and are consistently visible at CT except when obscured by adjacent soft tissue debris.[12-14]

MASTOIDITIS

The CT appearance of *acute mastoiditis* is nonspecific—patchy opacification of multiple mastoid air cells by mucopurulent secretions (Fig. 13-60). The mastoid will clear if the patient is treated properly. If treatment is inadequate, complications may develop. These are heralded by demineralization of trabeculae with eventual formation of a single large cavity (*coalescent mas-*

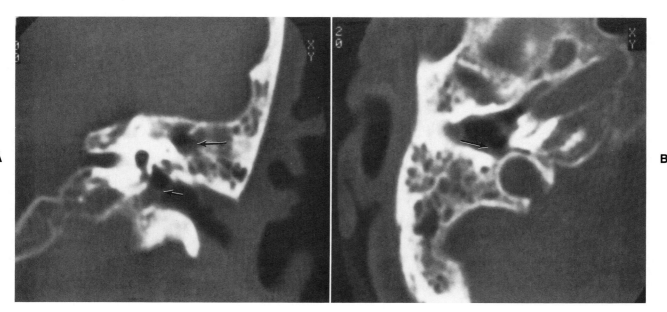

Fig. 13-58 Middle ear effusion. Multiple air/fluid levels *(arrows)* are demonstrated in both coronal **(A)** and axial **(B)** projections.

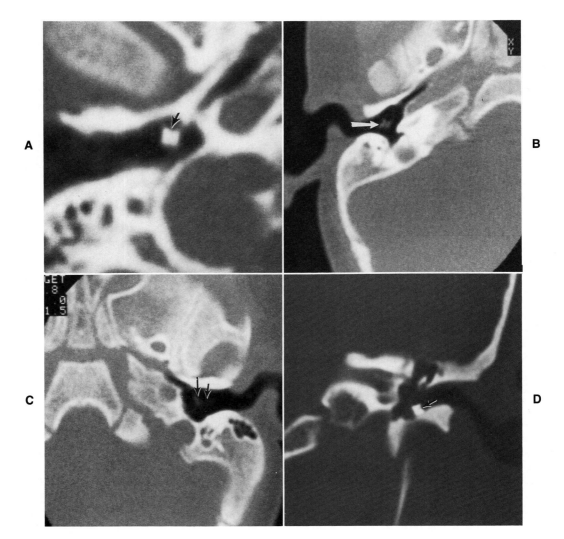

Fig. 13-59 Tympanostomy tubes *(arrows).* **A,** Axial view of metallic bobbin tube. **B,** Axial view of nonmetallic bobbin tube. **C,** Axial view of nonmetallic intratympanic phalange. **D,** Coronal view of extruded metallic bobbin type tube. (**A** through **C** from Swartz JD et al: High resolution computed tomography of the middle ear and mastoid, Part III, Surgically altered anatomy and pathology, Radiology 148:461, 1984.)

toiditis) (Fig. 13-61).[15] With continued progression, *thrombophlebitic complications* may result in destruction of the lateral mastoid cortex (palpable subperiosteal abscess), zygomatic root, external auditory canal (EAC), or the mastoid tip *(Bezold abscess).* Involvement of the *petrous apex* classically results in *Gradenigo's syndrome* (a triad of sixth nerve palsy, pain in the distribution of the fifth nerve, and chronic otitis media). If the internal or superior mastoid cortex is disrupted, grave complications such as *sigmoid sinus thrombosis, meningitis, epidural abscess,* or *brain abscess* may ensue. These intracranial findings are more easily evaluated with magnetic resonance imaging (MRI) than with CT.[15a,15b,15c]

GRANULATION TISSUE

The inexperienced observer rarely considers the common pathologic entity of granulation tissue in the differential diagnosis of middle ear debris.[14] Although pathologically manifested in several ways, the CT appearance may be identical both in distribution and CT density to most other manifestations of chronic otitis media. Importantly, granulation tissue, although often vascular, rarely causes bony erosion when it occurs as an isolated phenomenon and is often present concurrently with other middle ear maladies.[3,9,16,17]

Cholesterol granuloma (CG), a distinctive subtype of granulation, has received recent attention in the radiologic literature and is of considerable diagnostic impor-

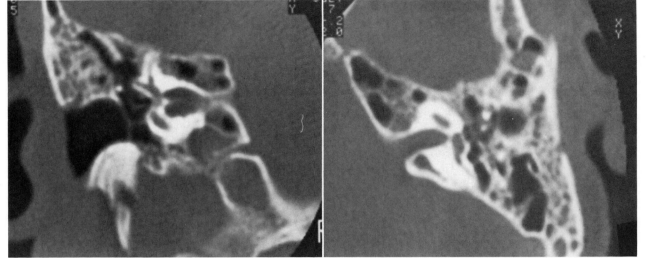

Fig. 13-60 Acute mastoiditis. Multiple nonspecific fluid levels are identified in coronal **(A)** and axial **(B)** projections.

tance for a number of reasons.[1,18-25] CG may be present anywhere in the middle ear cleft from the middle ear cavity proper to the petrous apex. When originating in the latter location, the mass has a smooth erosive quality that may be responsible for a variety of clinical symptoms (Fig. 13-62). The latter lesion may occur in the absence of a history of chronic otitis in patients with otherwise normal mastoid pneumatization. These are also referred to as giant cholesterol cysts.[25] Those occurring in the mastoidectomy cavity are variously referred to as chocolate cysts or blue-domed cysts. All of the aforementioned lesions are histopathologically identical.

Regardless of their location, CG consists of brownish hemorrhagic fluid, containing cholesterol crystals.[20] The crystals form as a result of hemorrhage, and the lesion may thus have a short T_1 relaxation time and appear bright (high signal intensity) on short TR / short TE MRI.[20a,20b] Equally bright signal is present on T_2-weighting indicating the predominance of methemoglobin. The pathologic nature of this lesion causes it to impart a bluish tint, which may appear quite ominous otoscopically when visualized in the middle ear cavity proper.[21,24] The clinical differential diagnosis can include *paraganglioma, dehiscent jugular bulb,* or *aberrant internal carotid artery,* so a vascular study may be needed. Even if no tint or other vascular abnormality is present, there may be little consolation for the surgeon since considerable bleeding may occur with CG. The absence of tympanic membrane bulging in the CG patient is helpful in differentiating this entity from a paraganglioma (glomus tympanicum).[14]

TYMPANIC MEMBRANE RETRACTIONS

The retracted tympanic membrane (TM) is obvious otoscopically and in and of itself is not an important CT diagnosis. The TM has a small wedge-shaped superior portion, the *pars flaccida,* and a larger inferior portion, the *pars tensa.* Retraction of the pars flaccida is particularly important to the clinician because of its association with the common acquired atticoantral cholesteatoma, which may not be visible otoscopically.[17] Retraction of the pars tensa, particularly when thickened, is more easily visible on CT and may extend to the promontory (Fig. 13-63).[9] These retractions may be associated with ossicular defects (long process of incus) and perhaps even in an ossicular discontinuity whereby the tympanic membrane is in direct apposition to the stapes capitulum ("nature's myringostapediopexy") (Fig. 13-64). These patients will often have normal conductive hearing.[2,9] Cholesteatomas arising from the pars tensa are much less common. When associated with middle ear opacification, TM retraction indicates the absence of mass lesion (cholesteatoma, paraganglioma, etc.), which is helpful in differential diagnosis.

ACQUIRED CHOLESTEATOMA

A cholesteatoma is a concentrically enlarging collection of exfoliated keratin within a sac of stratified squamous epithelium.[2,7,17] Cholesteatomas may be congenital or acquired. Congenital cholesteatomas occur in the suprasellar cistern, cerebellopontine angle, or many other intracranial locations.[26,27] Those occurring in the diploic space are in the differential diagnosis of the solitary lytic calvarial lesion. Congenital cho-

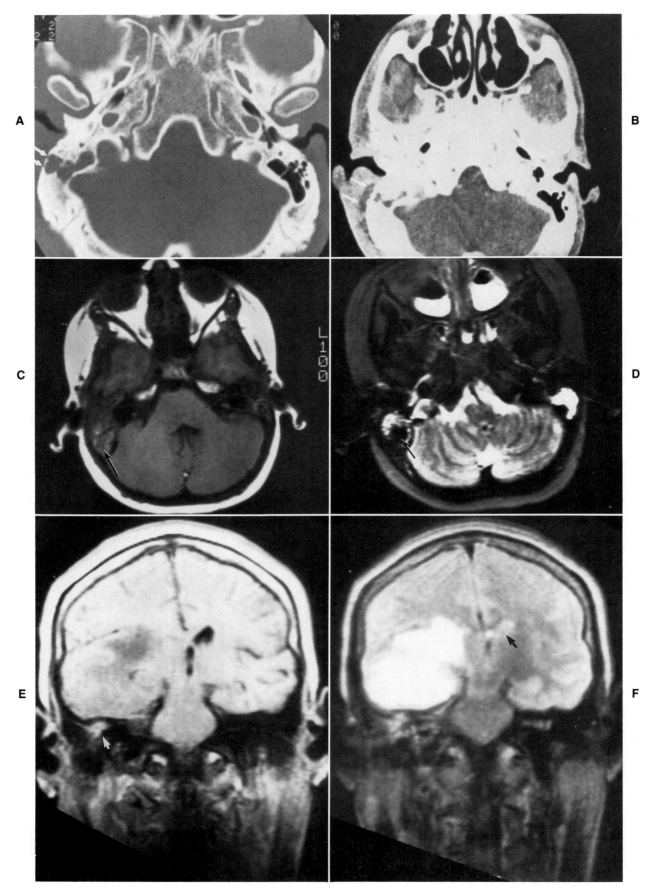

Fig. 13-61   For legend see opposite page.

Fig. 13-61 Coalescent mastoiditis. **A,** Axial view, bone window. A coalescent cavity has formed in right mastoid. There is a defect in lateral mastoid cortex *(white arrows).* **B** Axial view, soft tissue window. A subperiosteal abscess *(white arrows)* was drained. **C** and **D,** Sigmoid sinus thrombosis (different patient). **C,** Axial short TR, short TE (T₁-weighted) image. **D,** Axial long TR, long TE (T₂-weighted) image. Laminated region of low signal intensity *(arrow)* consistent with deoxyhemoglobin. **E** and **F,** Coalescent mastoiditis, cerebritis. **E,** Coronal T₁-weighted image reveals abnormal signal in the right mastoid *(arrow).* There is a mass effect in the right temporal lobe. **F,** Corresponding T₂-weighted image demonstrates extensive bright signal (edema) in the right temporal lobe. Signal (CSF) in mastoid is identical to that of the left frontal horn *(arrow).* (**C** and **D** from Swartz JD: Current imaging approach to the temporal bone, Radiology 171:309, 1989. **E** and **F** from Holliday RA: MRI of mastoid and middle ear disease, Radiol Clin North Am 27:283, 1989.)

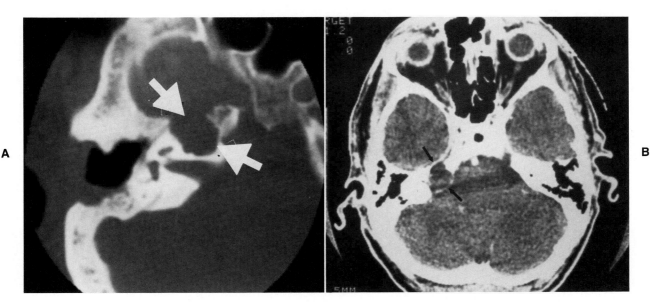

A   B

Fig. 13-62 Cholesterol granuloma, petrous apex. **A,** Axial image demonstrates a smoothly erosive lesion of petrous apex *(white arrows).* Patient has had previous mastoid surgery. (From Swartz JD: Imaging of the temporal bone, New York, 1986, Thieme Medical Publishers, Inc.) **B, C,** and **D,** Different patient. **B,** Axial CT. Smooth expansile lesion *(arrows).*

Continued.

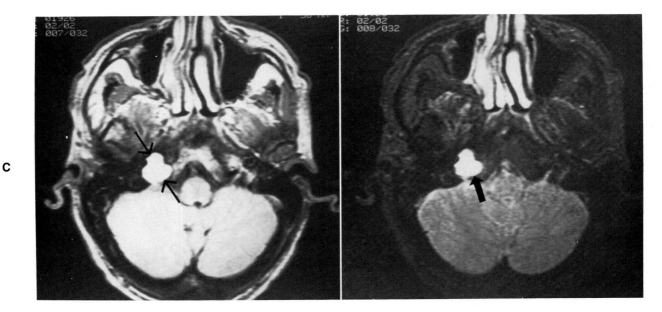

Fig. 13-62, cont'd   C, Axial MRI (short TR, short TE) bright signal (*arrow*). **D,** Axial MRI (long TR, long TE) identically bright signal (*arrow*). Signal suggests extracellular methemoglobin is the major constituent of the hemorrhagic byproducts of this mass. (Case courtesy Beverly Hershey, M.D.)

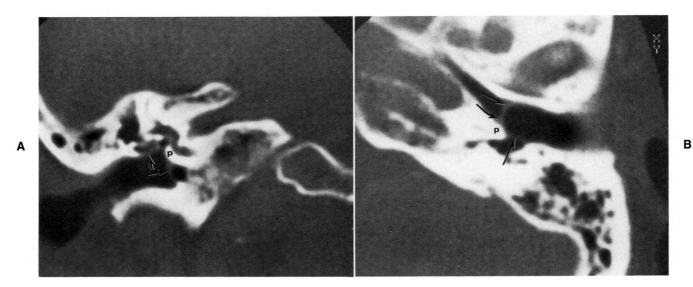

Fig. 13-63   Pars tensa retraction. **A,** Coronal and **B,** axial views reveal clearly definable retraction *(arrows)* extending to level of promontory *(P)*.

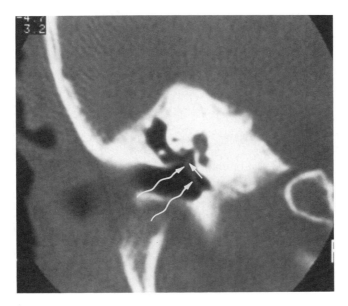

Fig. 13-64 Myringostapediopexy. Coronal image demonstrates retraction *(long white arrows)* articulating with head of stapes *(small arrow)*.

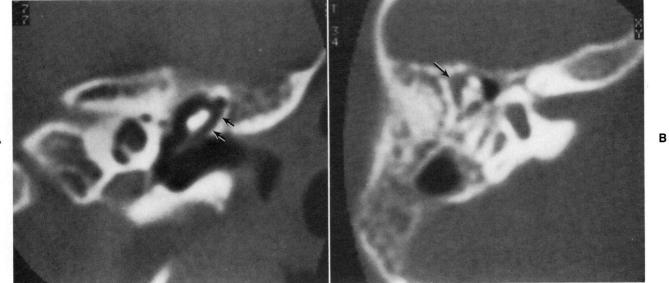

Fig. 13-65 Early Prussak cholesteatoma. Soft tissue mass is demonstrated *(arrows)*. **A,** Coronal view. **B,** Axial view.

lesteatoma also occurs in the temporal bone, particularly in the middle ear cleft; however, the vast majority occurring in the latter location (98%) are acquired.[27]

The acquired cholesteatoma is essentially unique to the middle ear.[7,28,29] The skin lining the tympanic membrane grows quite rapidly and normally migrates externally with the cerumen, which develops in the lateral cartilagenous third of the external auditory canal.[7,30] Although there are a number of suggested etiologies, perhaps the most compelling suggests that tympanic membrane retraction disrupts this normal physiology and epithelial ingrowth subsequently occurs in "pockets."[31-33] Such collections easily become trapped and may grow rapidly. Once a tympanic membrane retraction pocket has developed, it must be cleansed on a regular basis. Repeated bouts of otitis media in the absence of retraction may cause epithelial immigration into the middle ear, and this represents an additional proposed etiology.[31,33]

The majority of acquired middle ear cholesteatomas are therefore secondary to tympanic membrane defects. The tympanic membrane consists of a smaller, more superior, pars flaccida (Shrapnell's membrane) and a larger, more inferior, pars tensa.

Pars flaccida cholesteatoma is especially common since this portion of the TM lacks a fibrous layer and therefore retracts more easily.[34] As indicated in the previous section, decreased ITP resulting in pars flaccida retractions can occur not only in association with eustachian tube dysfunction but also in the presence of nonpatency of the tympanic isthmi (attic block).[4] Cholesteatomas arising in this locale originate in Prussak's space, which is bordered laterally by the attic wall, medially by the malleus head and incus body, and superiorly by the lateral mallear ligament (Fig. 13-65).[4,35] This type of cholesteatoma is the easiest to diagnose because the mode of extension is classic. Prussak's space opens posteriorly into the posterolateral attic; therefore the path of least resistance for these lesions is in this direction (Fig. 13-66). From here the mass easily extends to the antrum via the aditus ad antrum and subsequently inferiorly into the central mastoid tract and mastoid air cells. Note that the epithelium in the attic and antrum is much flatter (pavement epithelium), and the periosteum is predisposed to compromise by any expansile process. By virtue of their location, acquired Prussak cholesteatomas generally displace the malleus head (and incus body) medially (Fig. 13-67), and they erode the adjacent scutum.[28,35-37] Extension from the attic inferiorly into the posterior tympanic recesses is not rare with larger lesions.

Most pars tensa cholesteatomas arise from posterosuperior retractions and initially involve the recesses of the posterior tympanum, specifically the sinus tympani medially and facial recess laterally (Fig. 13-68).[29] Superior extension of these lesions into the attic will generally displace the ossicular mass (malleus head and incus body) laterally.

Cholesteatomas provide an excellent medium for bacterial growth, and there is always a potential for superinfection. This was responsible for most life-threatening intracranial complications such as meningitis, abscess, and venous sinus thrombosis, which were common in the preantibiotic era but are fortunately now rare.[17,38-41] Individuals with clinical evidence of one of these intracranial maladies should probably undergo MRI before CT.

The precise etiology of bony destruction secondary to

Fig. 13-66 Early Prussak cholesteatoma. Axial image demonstrates mass *(arrows)* extending from Prussak's space posteriorly through aditus *(arrowhead)* into mastoid antrum.

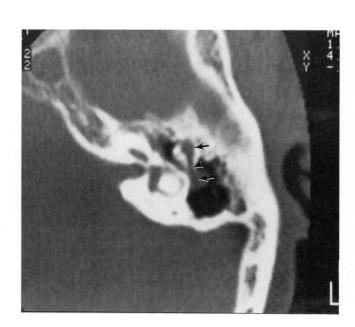

cholesteatoma has not been pinpointed; however, there has been excellent documentation that stratified squamous epithelium in the absence of associated granulation tissue does not erode bone.[7,40,42,43] Simple mechanical pressure also has been disputed as a cause. Some observers believe that a collagenase may be elaborated by abnormal fibroblasts. Others suggest that adjacent granulation tissue is the culprit. Regardless of the etiology, it is the capacity of the lesion to destroy bone that is responsible for all of the local complications of cholesteatoma. Ossicular destruction is the most prevalent of these. The otolaryngologic literature indicates that such ossicular compromise occurs in 75% of pars flaccida cholesteatomas and in as many as 90% of pars tensa cholesteatomas.[42-45] The long process of the incus, by virtue of its poor ligamentous support and blood supply, is the most common segment of the ossicular chain to be involved by both of these types of acquired cholesteatoma. The stapes must also be carefully evaluated when the lesion involves the oval window niche. Amputation of the malleus head and incus body occurs classically in far advanced lesions, particularly those arising in Prussak's space (Fig. 13-69).

Labyrinthine fistula is another potentially serious complication of the erosive properties of cholesteatoma.[17,46-49] By far the most commonly compromised re-

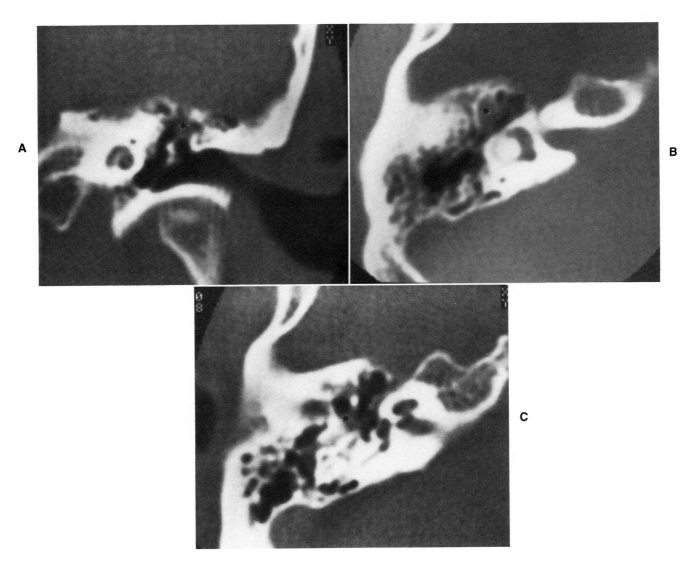

Fig. 13-67 Prussak cholesteatoma. **A,** Coronal image demonstrates mass *(asterisk)* displacing malleus head medially. **B,** Axial image demonstrates mass *(asterisk)* in attic. **C,** More inferior axial image demonstrates that mass is extended inferiorly into facial recess *(asterisk).*

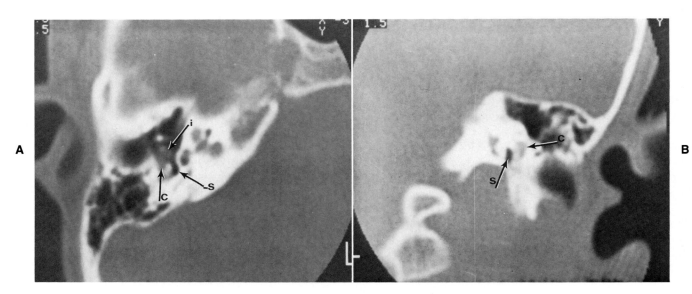

Fig. 13-68 Facial recess cholesteatoma. **A,** Axial image demonstrates soft tissue mass *(C, arrow)* within facial recess. Mass does not extend medially into clear sinus tympani *(S, arrow)*. Incudostapedial articulation *(i, arrow)* is intact. **B,** Coronal image demonstrates mass *(C, arrow)* in more laterally oriented facial recess. Again, more medial sinus tympani *(S, arrow)* is clear.

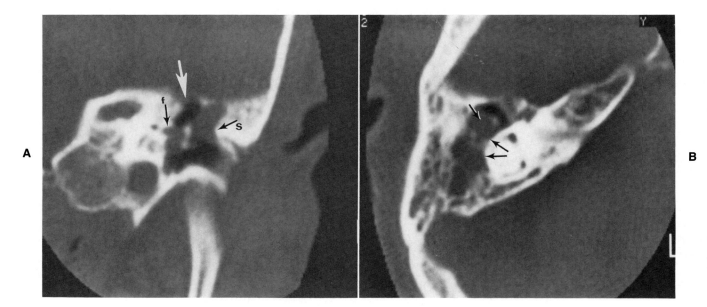

Fig. 13-69 Aggressive acquired cholesteatoma. **A,** Coronal image demonstrates mass displacing malleus head medially. There is striking erosion of scutum *(S, arrow)*. This image also demonstrates tegmen defect *(white arrow)*. Mass is extended medially and is in direct apposition to proximal tympanic segment of facial nerve canal *(f, arrow)*. **B,** Axial image demonstrates that ossicular mass in attic has been essentially destroyed *(single arrow)* (compare Fig. 13-65, *B*). Lateral semicircular canal *(double arrows)* is intact indicating absence of fistula.

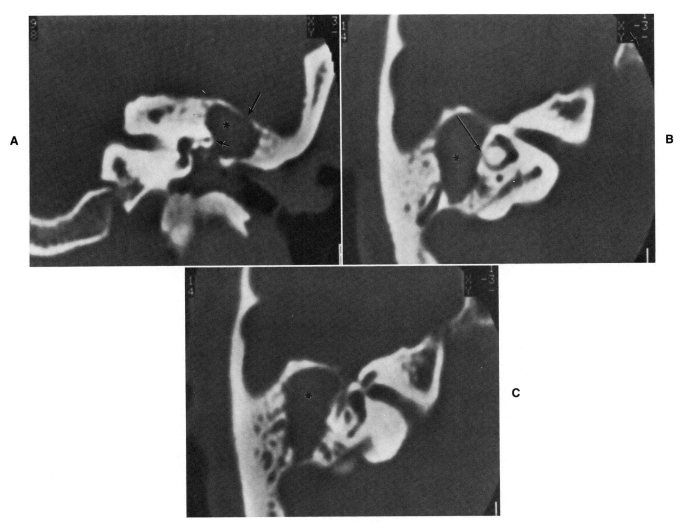

Fig. 13-70   Erosive cholestateoma. **A,** Coronal image demonstrates large smoothly erosive mass *(asterisk)* eroding tegmen *(long arrow)* and lateral semicircular canal *(short arrow)*. **B,** Axial image demonstrates mass *(asterisk)* clearly focally eroding lateral semicircular canal *(long arrow)*. **C,** Additional axial image demonstrates large mass *(asterisk)*.

gion is the lateral semicircular canal (Fig. 13-70). This area should be carefully evaluated on both coronal and axial images for evidence of cortical thinning in all patients with middle ear disease. The diagnosis of fistula can be made when the mass is in direct apposition to the membranous portion of the labyrinth. The patient will usually have presenting symptoms of vertigo intermittently complicating long-standing chronic otitis. Classically the patient may have an acute vertiginous episode during otoscopic manipulation of the lesion in the clinician's office. Identification of bony erosion in the absence of a gross fistula is also important to note since surgical removal of the adjacent mass may cause an acute fistula. Complications of fistula formation include the potential for total hearing loss and persistant

unremitting *vertigo*.[38] The latter complication may necessitate *labyrinthectomy*.

The facial nerve canal must be carefully evaluated for evidence of erosion or invasion.[49] Unfortunately, the most common areas involved (the first and second genu) may be covered by an ultra-thin layer of bone in normal circumstances, and subtle erosions are difficult if not impossible to demonstrate (Fig. 13-69, *B*).[14,17,50] Gross invasion of the facial nerve canal in these regions is quite demonstrable, however (Figs. 13-71 and 13-72). The midtympanic segment of the facial nerve canal along the undersurface of the lateral semicircular canal is another problematic area. The mass may commonly extend to this region, and involvement is quite difficult to discern. The observer should indicate if the mass is

Text continued on p. 1008.

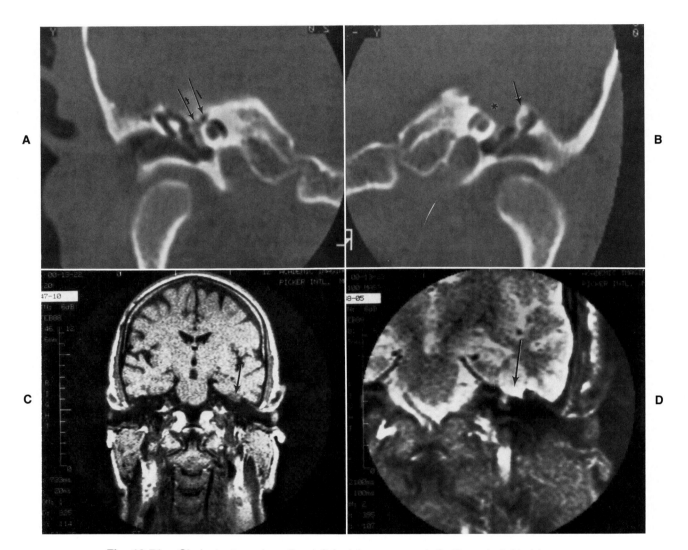

Fig. 13-71 Cholesteatoma invading left facial nerve canal. **A,** Normal, right side, coronal image: *l (arrow)*, labyrinthine segment; *t, arrow,* tympanic segment. **B,** Mass *(asterisk)* noted obliterating both segments. Note deformed malleus (tympanosclerosis). Tegmen is defective. **C,** Coronal T_1 WI. Mass noted *(arrow)*. **D,** Coronal (magnified) T_2 WI. Bright signal represents mass *(arrow l* cf. B).

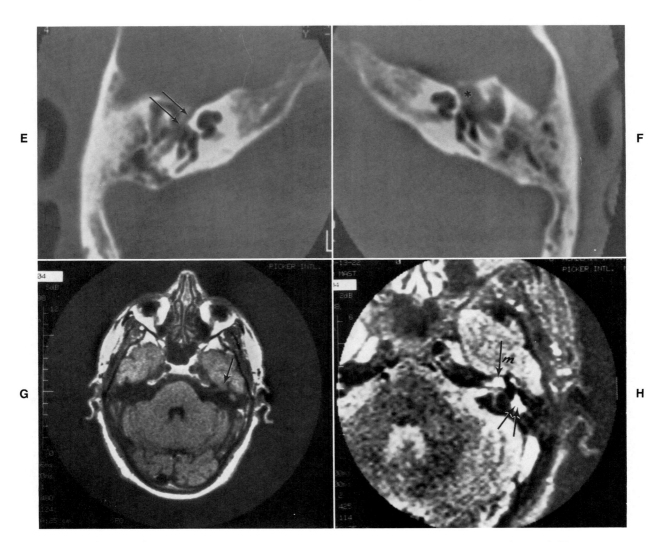

Fig. 13-71, cont'd   E, Normal axial image right side—tympanic segment *(arrows).* **F,** Mass (*) noted obliterating tympanic segment. **G,** Axial T₁ WI. Mass noted *(arrow).* **H,** Axial (magnified) T₂ WI. Mass of bright signal (M, *arrow*) other bright signal *(double arrows)* represents mastoid debris.

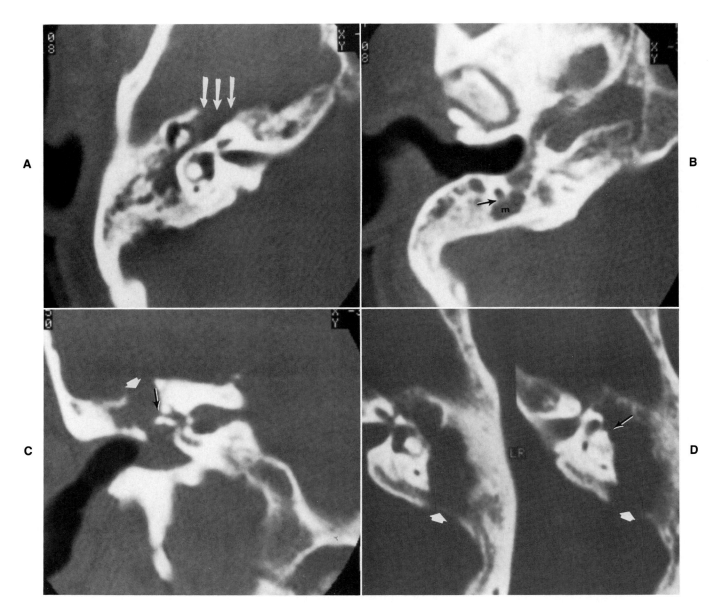

Fig. 13-72 Erosive cholesteatoma. **A,** Axial image demonstrates soft tissue mass throughout the attic and antrum. There is a large defect anteriorly indicating that the mass may be in direct apposition to the middle cranial fossa dura *(3 white arrows).* **B,** The mass (m) has eroded the sinus tympani and has extended posterolaterally to come in direct contact with the mastoid segment of the facial nerve canal. There is erosion in the posterior margin of this structure *(arrow).* **C,** Different patient. Coronal image demonstrates large mass throughout middle ear. There is a large tegmen defect *(white arrowhead)* and obvious labyrinthine fistula *(arrow).* **D,** Contiguous axial images demonstrate in addition to large fistula *(arrow)* the presence of defect in the sigmoid sinus plate *(white arrowhead).*

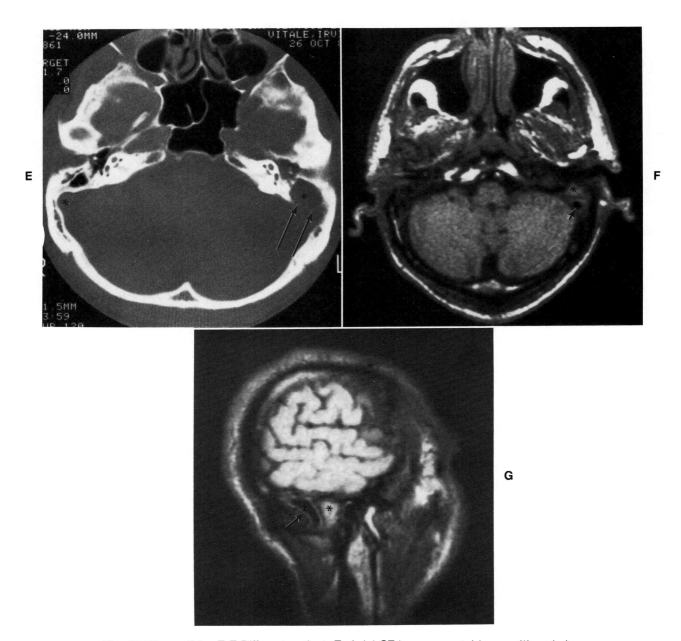

Fig. 13-72, cont'd   E-F Different patient. **E,** Axial CT image. mastoid mass (*) and sigmoid sinus plate defect *(arrows).* **F,** Axial T₁ Wᵢ MRI. Mastoid mass (*) patent sigmoid sinus, flow void *(arrow).* **G,** Sagittal T₁ Wᵢ MRI. Mastoid mass (*). Patent sigmoid sinus, flow void *(arrows).*

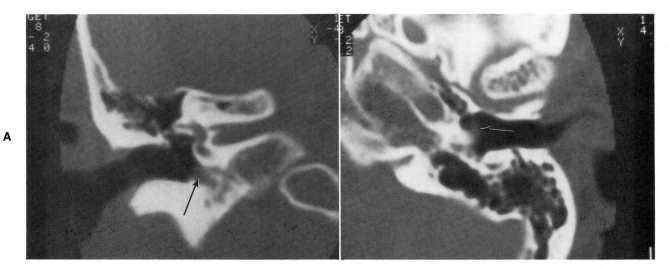

Fig. 13-73 Glomus tympanicum. **A,** (Coronal) and **B,** (axial) demonstrate a soft tissue mass *(arrows)* in the hypotympanum. This is quite unlikely to represent cholesteatoma as it is in an atypical location and the mastoid is normally aerated.

in direct apposition to one of these segments of the canal and suggest the possibility that such invasion could indeed have taken place.

Bony alteration occurs at several other locations. Especially ominous is involvement of the tegmen tympani and sigmoid sinus plate (Fig. 13-72). MRI is recommended when defects occur at these sites, as this could indicate epidural invasion by cholesteatoma or the potential for development of meningitis, cerebritis, or abcess should the lesion become superinfected. The CT density of middle ear debris is in no way histologically specific.[14] The observer must rely on secondary factors in order to arrive at an appropriate diagnosis. Such factors include age, location and distribution, calcification or ossification, tympanic membrane status (bulge or retraction), bony erosion, degree of mastoid pneumatization, and the amount of conductive hearing deficit (Fig. 13-73). Bony alteration is commonly associated with attic cholesteatoma, and this diagnosis should be questioned if such changes are not present. Findings include scutum blunting, attic expansion (lateral wall remodeling), and erosion of the anterior tympanic spine. The latter structure is best appreciated in the sagittal plane.[51]

Holotympanic debris in the absence of TM alteration or significant conductive hearing deficit quite likely represents granulation or fluid.[52] In the presence of tympanic membrane retraction and conductive deficit, the possibility of inflammatory ossicular fixation should be considered, especially when there is associated calcification or ossification. Such debris associated with tympanic membrane bulging may represent congenital cholesteatoma in a child or glomus tympanum in an adult.

CONDUCTIVE DEAFNESS IN NONCHOLESTEATOMATOUS CHRONIC OTITIS MEDIA

The high incidence of conductive hearing deficit (CHD) in individuals with congenital and acquired cholesteatoma is well known. Ossicular erosions are the predominant cause. Less well described is the commonplace occurrence of CHD in patients with noncholesteatomatous chronic otitis media. These patients could possibly have a healed tympanic membrane, and fenestral otosclerosis may be suspected clinically. CHD in these patients may be secondary to erosive changes in the ossicles or ossicular fixation.

Histochemical analysis of the middle ear in the presence of chronic otitis media (COM) has yielded a number of substances that may perpetuate bony lysis.[53,54] Collagenase, lipopolysaccharides, and prostaglandins have all been implicated. Some attention was given to a proposed osteoclast activating factor, which was believed to be discharged from white blood cells. Many researchers have demonstrated acid phosphatase, a well-known marker for lysosomal activity, within the diseased middle ear.[54] This substance is probably produced by histiocytes developing subsequent to foreign body reaction. Capillary proliferation and high oxygen tension may contribute to the activity of the enzyme.[43]

There is a distinct predisposition for erosive changes to develop in the distal incus, specifically the long and lenticular processes.[43] The stapes is also commonly involved. Attic changes (malleus head or incus body) are less common but do occur on occasion (Fig. 13-74). Both axial and coronal images must be carefully studied

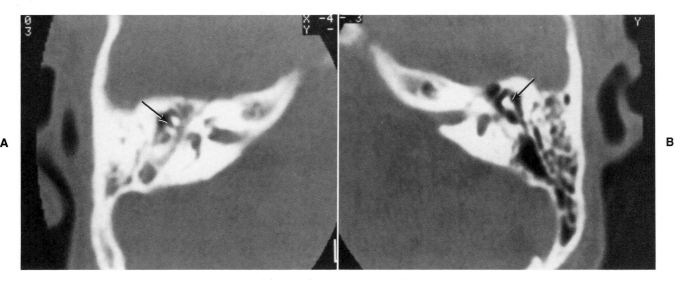

Fig. 13-74 Non-cholesteatomatous erosion. **A,** There is an erosion of the head of the malleus and body of the incus in the vicinity of the malleo-incudal articulation *(arrow)*. **B,** Normal axial section for comparison (malleoincudal articulation indicated with arrow).

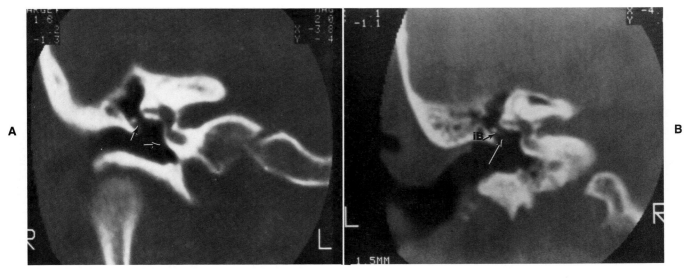

Fig. 13-75 Non-cholesteatomatous erosion. **A,** Coronal image. Incus body is intact *(upper arrow)*. Long process is absent. Lower arrow indicates the retracted tympanic membrane. **B,** Normal patient for comparison. Normal incus body (IB, *arrow*) and incus long process (L, *arrow*) are indicated.

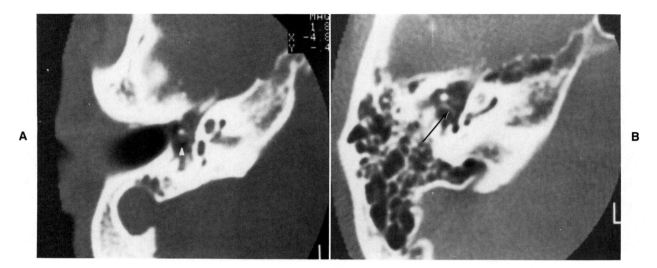

Fig. 13-76   Non-cholesteatomatous erosion. **A,** Axial image (right ear) indicates absent lenticular process *(white arrowhead)*. **B,** Normal patient for comparison (right ear). Normal lenticular process and stapes head are present. The incudostapedial articulation is indicated with an arrow. More anteriorly one can see the malleus head and the tensor tympani tendon.

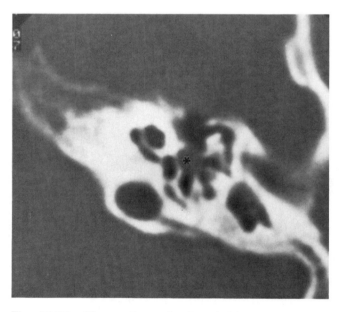

Fig. 13-77   Fibrous tissue fixation. Axial section reveals non-specific soft tissue (*) in oval window niche. Patient had maximal conductive deficit.

to make a specific anatomic diagnosis.[53] The coronal images yield the best information regarding the status of the vertically oriented long process (Fig. 13-75). The remainder of the chain is best visualized on axial CT sections. Images obtained in this projection just inferior to the oval window are particularly helpful in these individuals. One should visualize two parallel "lines."[14,53]

More anteriorly the tensor tympani tendon and malleus neck are seen. More posteriorly, and more importantly, the lenticular process of the incus and the stapes superstructure are identified with the intervening incudostapedial joint (ISJ) (Fig. 13-76). This region should be carefully scrutinized. A widened ISJ could be secondary to erosive changes associated with fibrous replacement.[53a] Ossicular defects are seen to best advantage in the nonopaque "dry ear."

Ossicular fixation may also be responsible for postinflammatory CHD.[55-58] Fibrous tissue, tympanosclerosis, and new bone formation may occur in these patients. At CT, fibrous tissue has a nonspecific appearance (Fig. 13-77). The observer should be alerted to this diagnosis in the presence of nonerosive and nonexpansile changes in the middle ear of a patient with a wide audiometric air-bone gap. Fibrous tissue may be generalized or focal. If focal, there is a propensity for involvement in the region of the oval window and in Prussak's space.

Tympanosclerosis refers to deposits of hyalinized collagen within the tympanic cavity.[55,59-61] Involvement of the tympanic membrane is common but often asymptomatic (Fig. 13-78, A). CHD results when the process involves or encases the ossicles or their suspensory ligaments and tendons.[62] The CT appearance consists of punctate or weblike calcific density(s) (Fig. 13-78). Peristapedial tympanosclerosis may be treated with prosthetic stapedectomy, a procedure with an increased incidence of poor results in this clinical setting.[63]

New bone formation (fibroosseous sclerosis) is the

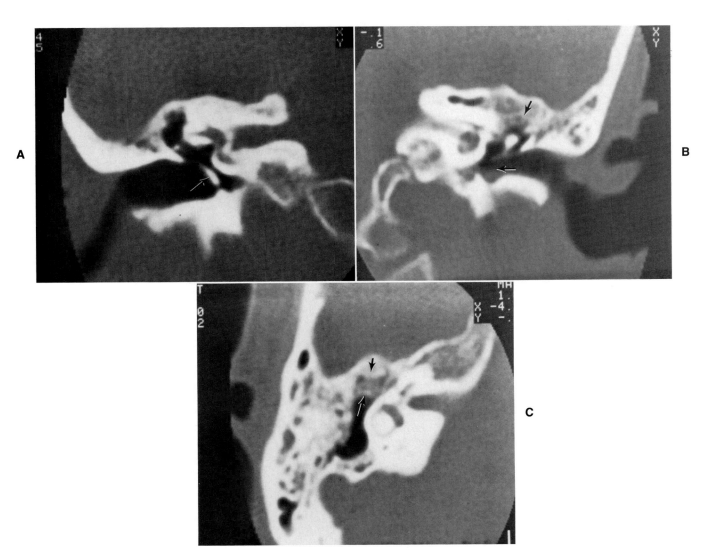

Fig. 13-78   Tympanosclerosis. **A,** Coronal image demonstrates tympanosclerosis *(arrow)* involving tympanic membrane. This was asymptomatic. **B, C,** Different patient. Note patchy calcification *(arrow)* in attic on coronal **(B)** and axial **(C)** images. The patient had substantial conductive deficit. Incidental note is made of fluid level on coronal image *(lower arrow, coronal image).*

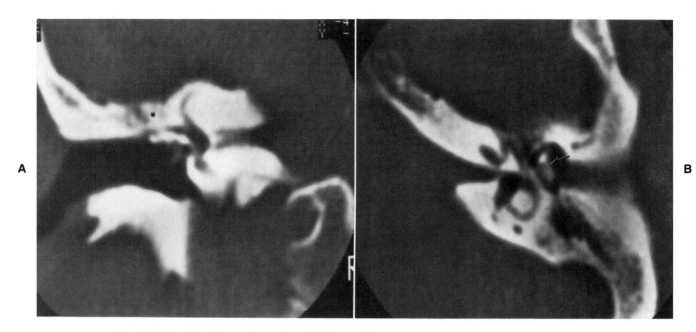

Fig. 13-79   New bone formation. **A,** Coronal image demonstrates homogeneous new bone (*) within attic. **B,** Axial image beneath level of new bone formation reveals anky-losed malleoincudal articulation *(arrow).*

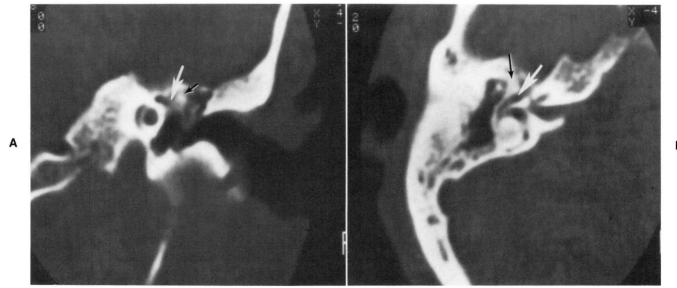

Fig. 13-80   New bone formation. Coronal **(A)** and axial **(B)** images demonstrate new formation *(outlined arrow)* in medial aspect of attic in direct apposition to proximal tym panic segment of facial nerve canal *(white arrow).*

least common histologic type of postinflammatory ossicular fixation.[55] This is most likely to occur in the attic and cause encasement of the ossicular chain (Figs. 13-79 and 13-80).[62]

POSTOPERATIVE MIDDLE EAR AND MASTOID

CT has become an indispensible tool for evaluation of the postoperative middle ear and mastoid.[13,14,46,64] This examination is especially helpful when the surgery was performed many years before or by an individual other than the physician referring the study. We routinely recommend CT in evaluation of the symptomatic postmastoidectomy patient as well as for the asymptomatic patient who was recently operated on, in which circumstance the study serves as an informative baseline examination should future problems arise. CT is also informative for evaluation of the prosthetic stapedectomy and other forms of ossiculoplasty.[14,63,65]

A structured CT evaluation of the postmastoidectomy patient should include (1) categorization of the surgical defect, (2) evaluation of the cavity for residual debris, (3) careful study of the margins of the cavity for bony defects, (4) observation of the status of the ossicular chain, (5) evaluation of the inner ear structures to exclude fistula formation, and (6) careful study of the margins of the facial nerve canal.

Regardless of the exact surgical approach (postauricular, endaural, transcanal), the object of surgery for chronic otitis media and cholesteatoma is the removal of all diseased tissue while sparing as many normal structures as possible.[66] Mastoidectomy defies categorization since no two procedures are identical; however, certain guidelines do exist.[67,68] Removal of limited mastoid air cells with maintenance of the external auditory canal (EAC) wall and ossicular chain (OC) constitutes simple (cortical) mastoidectomy (Fig. 13-81, A). This procedure, although still performed in the approach to the CP angle or endolymphatic sac, has been largely abandoned as treatment for COM because of the high recurrence rate. Removal of *all* mastoid air cells with sparing of the EAC wall and OC is termed intact canal wall mastoidectomy (ICWM) (Fig. 13-81, B).[67,69] This procedure avoids the tympanomastoid cavity; however, again, published recurrence rates are unacceptable by many standards. Both of these procedures are categorized as closed cavity mastoidectomy.

The open cavity procedures (radical mastoidectomy, modified radical mastoidectomy) are much more commonly encountered.[67,68,70] In modified radical mastoidectomy (Bondy procedure), which is performed primarily for atticoantral cholesteatoma, the ossicular chain is meticulously preserved (Fig. 13-81, C). With radical mastoidectomy the bulk of the ossicular chain is sacrificed, with preservation of the stapes superstructure, if possible (Fig. 13-81, D). Type III tympanoplasty (articulation of graft with stapes superstructure) is often performed in this circumstance. For this reason both preoperative and postoperative CT evaluation should include an investigation of the status of the stapes superstructure (Fig. 13-82, B).

It is virtually impossible to make a histologic diagnosis based on the CT appearance of debris in a tympanomastoid cavity (Figs. 13-83 and 13-84). Recurrent cholesteatoma, granulation tissue, and even simple redundant mucosa or surgical packing may appear identical on CT. Fortunately, such a specific diagnosis is not important, for the surgeon will be much more concerned about associated findings. Regardless of histopathology, most debris is identified in the posterosuperior aspect of the cavity. An attempt should be made to distinguish debris in the mastoid bowl from that in the middle ear or attic proper (deep or superficial to tympanoplasty, if present).

Prior to reoperation the surgeon will want to be assured that the margins of the cavity are intact. Our experience has been that focal bony defects, especially in the region of the tegmen or sigmoid sinus plate, can be especially significant (Fig. 13-83, B). Debris adjacent to such a defect can represent encephalocele or, conversely, may indicate that residual or recurrent debris is extending through the defect into the epidural compartment (Fig. 13-85). Individuals with defects adjacent to the sigmoid sinus plate are at risk for the development of sigmoid sinus thrombosis should complications arise. MRI is strongly recommended in the presence of unexplained bony defects.[70a]

The margins of the ossicular chain must be carefully studied, particularly if the surgeon plans a definitive procedure, which may include tympanoplasty and ossiculoplasty. The distal incus is especially vulnerable in the preoperative patient with a long history of chronic otitis media. The labyrinth, particularly the lateral semicircular canal, should be carefully evaluated for thinning, which would suggest fistula formation.

The facial nerve canal, particularly the mastoid segment, may be dangerously close to the surgical defect, and the referring physician should be cautioned.

Under unusual circumstances the contents of an acquired cholesteatoma may drain externally, leaving only the aggressive peripheral microscopic membrane that consists of keratinizing stratified squamous epithelium. The CT appearance in these patients is reminiscent of mastoidectomy as no soft tissue mass is seen (automastoidectomy [mural cholesteatoma]) (Fig. 13-85).[70b]

Prosthetic stapedectomy is performed most commonly in individuals with fenestral otosclerosis.[71] CT evaluation can be quite rewarding if the observer is

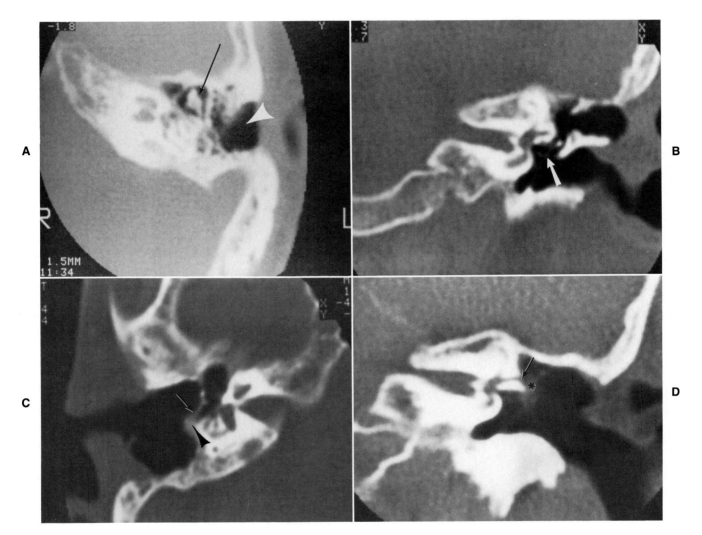

Fig. 13-81   Mastoidectomy. **A,** Cortical mastoidectomy. Several mastoid air cells have been removed *(white arrowhead).* Ossicular chain is entirely intact *(arrow).* **B,** Intact canal wall mastoidectomy. Mastoid air cells have been removed. External auditory canal is intact. Ossicular chain *(white arrow)* is preserved. **C,** Modified radical mastoidectomy. Mastoid air cells and external auditory canal have been removed. Ossicular chain is intact. In this patient the short process of incus *(arrow)* was fixed within residual fibrous tissue *(arrowhead)* adjacent to lateral semicircular canal. **D,** Radical mastoidectomy. Coronal image demonstrates absence of mastoid air cells, external auditory canal wall, and ossicular chain. There is labyrinthine fistula *(arrow)* with adjacent soft tissue debris representing residual cholesteatoma (*).

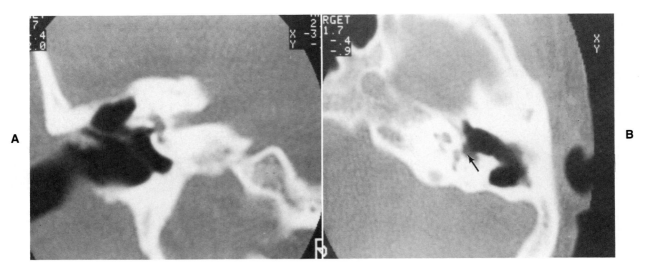

Fig. 13-82   Radical mastoidectomy, intact stapes. **A,** Coronal image. Tympanoplasty noted. **B,** Axial image. An intact stapes remnant *(arrow)* is demonstrated. This is an important observation if reoperation is planned.

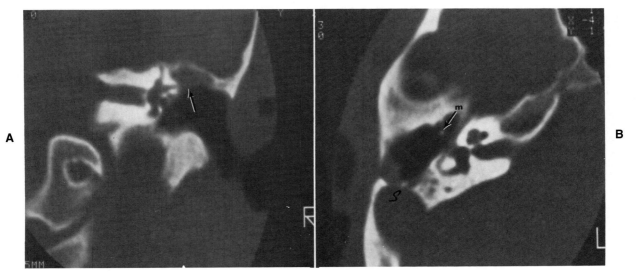

Fig. 13-83   Radical mastoidectomy, recurrent debris. **A,** Coronal section. There is residual soft tissue debris representing residual cholesteatoma *(arrow)* in the mastoid bowl. **B,** Axial image demonstrates a residuum of malleus neck *(m, arrow).* There is an anteriorly and laterally placed sigmoid sinus (S) with overlying focal bony defect. The surgeon should be cautioned if reoperation is planned.

aware of the normal appearance of the prosthesis.[63] Various materials are used, including Teflon, Silastic, stainless steel, and various plastics. Many surgeons use a 35-gauge stainless steel wire, which can be difficult to visualize on CT (Fig. 13-86). Usually the tip of the wire can be identified with overlapping, thin axial sections. The metallic piston is easily seen in all projections (Fig. 13-87). Identification of the Teflon and Silastic devices is intermediate in difficulty (Fig. 13-88). The normally functioning prosthesis may be located in the anterior, central, or posterior portion of the oval window (Fig. 13-89).

CT is often requested for evaluation of recurrent conductive deficit, vertigo, and sensorineural hearing loss in the poststapedectomy patient.[67,71-73] Vertigo and sensorineural hearing loss may have several etiologies, many of which are beyond CT resolution. These symptoms are common in the immediate postoperative period and are usually self-limited; however, persistent or recurrent and fluctuating symptoms of this type may have significant implications. Perilymph fistula, an abnormal communication between the inner ear and middle ear, can cause such symptomatology.[74] This diagnosis is crucial to the surgeon, since reoperation must be planned to prevent labyrinthitis and possible meningitis. CT diagnosis is difficult and depends on fluid dynamics within the vestibule (Fig. 13-90). Unexplained fluid collections emanating from the oval window or pooling in the middle ear or mastoid should be viewed with suspicion (Fig. 13-91). A pneumolabyrinth is obviously highly suggestive. Unfortunately CT findings in these cases may be nonexistent. It should be emphasized that perilymph fistula does occur spontaneously in individuals with no known preexistent conditions. The CT findings in these cases are even more sparse.

Sensorineural hearing loss and/or vertigo may also result from abnormal penetration of the prosthesis into the vestibule with compromise of the utriculosaccular organ. The CT diagnosis may be simple but depends on the type of prosthesis used.

Acute labyrinthitis, endolymphatic hydrops, and intravestibular fibrous adhesions are additional causes for poststapedectomy dizziness, vertigo, and sensorineural hearing loss.[75] There are no known CT manifestations.

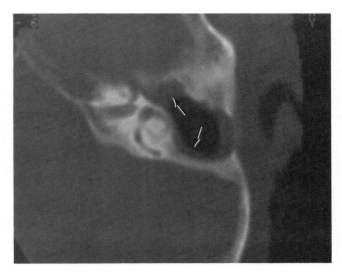

Fig. 13-84 Radical mastoidectomy, residual debris. Axial image demonstrates circumferential debris *(arrows)* in mastoid bowl. No reoperation was performed on this patient.

Ossification of the labyrinth may develop in long-standing chronic labyrinthitis.[14] In such a circumstance the CT findings are quite obvious (Fig. 13-92).

Recurrent conductive deficit, on the other hand, is commonly associated with specific CT findings.[76] Causes include prosthesis subluxation, incus necrosis, granuloma or fibrous tissue formation, or recurrent growth of otosclerosis and incus dislocation.[63]

The initial CT clue in cases of prosthesis subluxation is a "vacant" oval window. Careful evaluation of the posterior recesses and ridges in the axial projection usually yields evidence of the dislocated prosthesis itself (Fig. 13-93).

Incus necrosis occurs at the attachment of the wire to the long process.[73] CT diagnosis is difficult and depends on careful evaluation of high-quality overlapping coronal images (Fig. 13-94). Any defects in the long process should be viewed with intense scrutiny.

CT findings in granuloma or fibrous tissue formation are nonspecific and consist of abnormal soft tissue de-

Text continued on p. 1023.

Fig. 13-85 Encephalocele. **A,** Coronal image demonstrates thinned but seemingly intact tegmen *(arrow)*. The remains of the scutum (S) are demonstrated. **B,** Axial image, however, demonstrates absent bone *(arrows)* between mass (*) and middle cranial fossa. At surgery an encephalocele was present. **C, D,** and **E,** Automastoidectomy axial sections, left ear. This patient has had no surgery. Note the extensive remodeling caused by the aggressive cholesteatoma membrane *(arrows)*. *O,* residual ossicular chain; *S,* stapes superstructure.

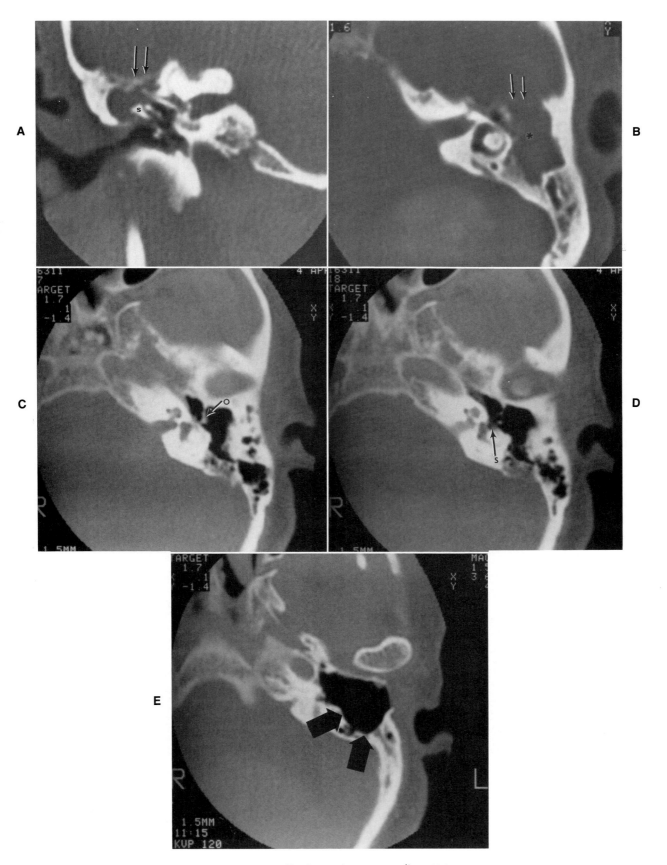

Fig. 13-85   For legend see opposite page.

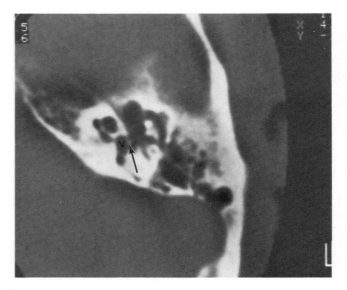

Fig. 13-86   Stapes prosthesis, wire. Axial image demonstrates tip of wire prosthesis *(arrow)* located centrally within oval window. Vestibule (v).

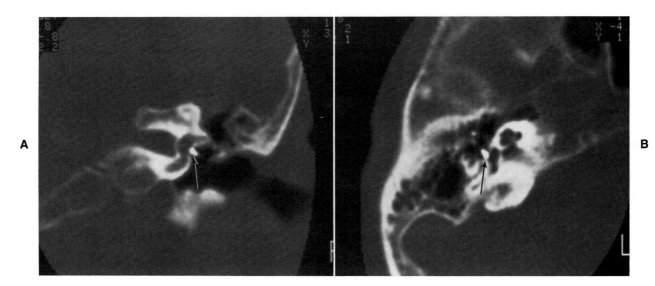

Fig. 13-87   Stapes prosthesis, metallic piston. **A,** Coronal image. **B,** Axial image. Prosthesis *(arrow)* is identified centrally within oval window.

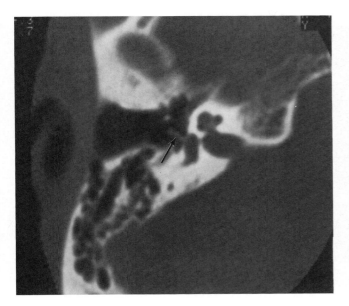

Fig. 13-88   Stapes prosthesis, teflon. Axial image demonstrates non-metallic prosthesis *(arrow)* seen in its entirety.

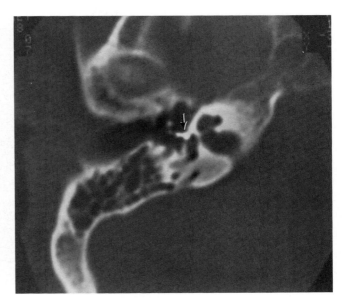

Fig. 13-89   Stapes prosthesis, metallic piston, anteriorly placed. Axial image demonstrates metallic prosthesis *(arrow)* within oval window anteriorly. This was a normally functioning device.

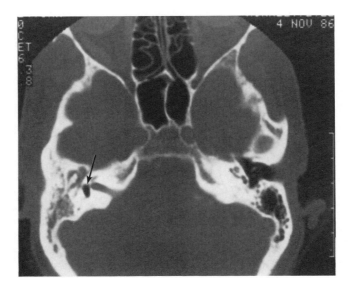

Fig. 13-90   Air in vestibule. Axial image demonstrates a collection of air within vestibule *(arrow)*. This is of profound significance as it indicates a direct communication between middle and inner ear.

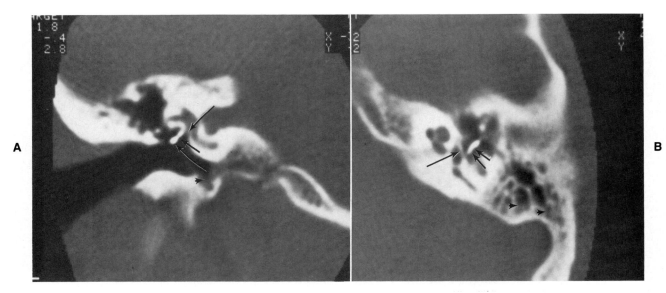

Fig. 13-91 Perilymph fistula. Prosthesis *(double arrows)* is located superficial and superior to otosclerotic oval window *(arrow)*. Several fluid levels *(arrowheads)* are identified on both the coronal **(A)** and axial **(B)** images.

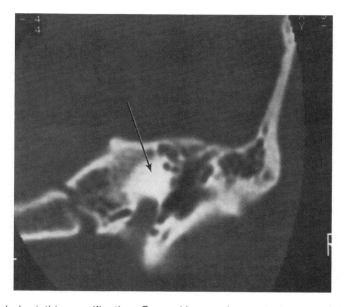

Fig. 13-92 Labyrinthine ossification. Coronal image demonstrates complete ossification of membranous labyrinth with resultant absence of delineation of cochlear turns.

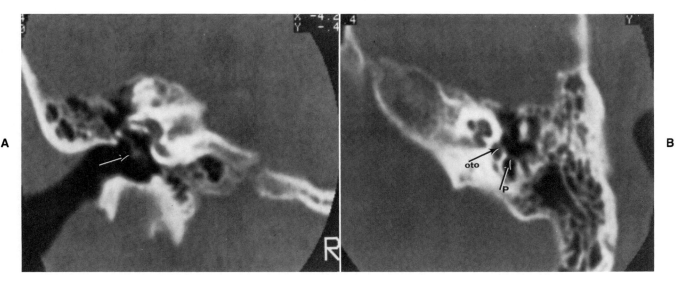

Fig. 13-93   Stapes prosthesis, dislocation. **A,** Coronal image demonstrates lateralization of graft *(arrow).* **B,** Axial image. Oval window niche is vacant. Stapes footplate is abnormally thickened by otosclerosis *(oto, arrow).* The dislocated prosthesis *(p, arrow)* is identified posteriorly.

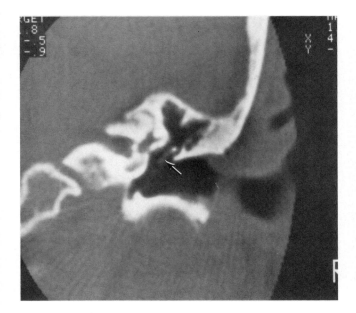

Fig. 13-94   Incus necrosis. Coronal image demonstates focal defect *(arrow)* in long process of incus. Patient had recurrent conductive deficit several months subsequent to prosthetic stapedectomy.

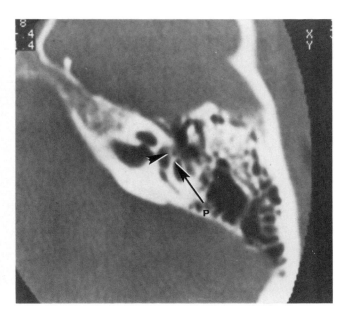

Fig. 13-95   Compromised prosthesis. Axial image demonstrates prosthesis *(P, arrow)* located posteriorly in oval window. Recurrent otosclerotic overgrowth of oval window *(arrowhead)* has compromised the function of prosthesis.

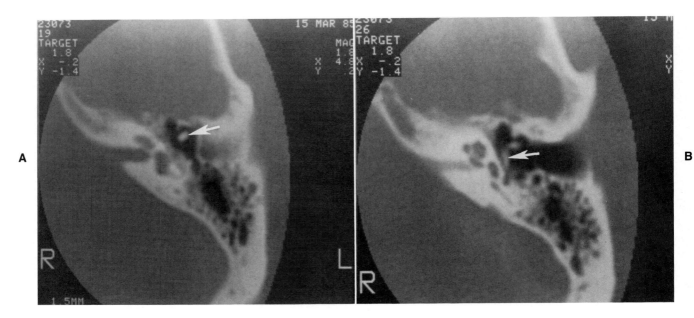

Fig. 13-96   Incus dislocation. **A,** Axial image demonstrates that malleus head *(arrow)* is in normal position. Incus is absent. **B,** A more inferior image demonstrates malpositioned incus *(arrow)* adjacent to oval window. The patient is status post-prosthetic stapedectomy.

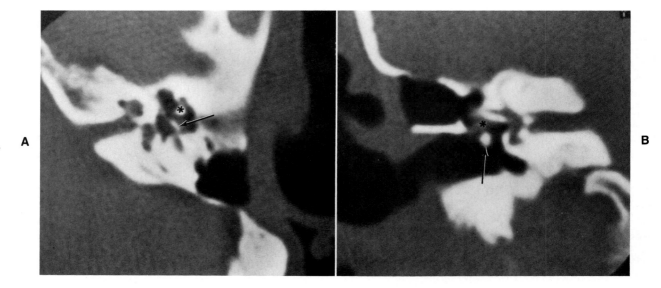

Fig. 13-97   Incus interposition. **A,** Axial image—malleus head (*) in normal position (note anterior mallear ligament). Incus interposition graft is transversely oriented *(arrow)*. Stapes superstructure cannot be visualized on this image (was present and visible on monitor screen). **B,** Coronal image demonstrates intact canal wall mastoidectomy. Incus interposition graft *(arrow)* is well demonstrated en face. There is residual soft tissue debris (*) between graft and undersurface of lateral semicircular canal. This represented postoperative fibrous tissue and limited the function of prosthesis somewhat.

bris in the oval window niche surrounding the prosthesis. Such tissue may also develop more laterally at the incus attachment and is especially likely to occur in the individual with preexistent chronic otitis. (Prosthetic stapedectomy in individuals with tympanosclerosis has a much higher incidence of poor surgical results.)

Although drilling is required when obliterative otosclerotic disease is present, these foci are usually not surgically removed. The prosthesis is instead placed in such a way as to bypass existing disease. Continued growth of otosclerotic plaques can, of course, further narrow the oval window and compromise function of the prosthesis. A specific diagnosis often can be inferred when this occurs, although it is quite difficult in the absence of preoperative images (Fig. 13-95).

We have encountered secondary incus dislocation on several occasions (Fig. 13-96).[77] The cause is not clear; however, all patients also had obliterative disease. Severe torsional stresses may contribute to this complication.

Ossiculoplasty is commonly performed in order to reestablish conductive hearing in individuals with a damaged ossicular chain.[78] Such damage is most likely caused by chronic otitis media with or without cholesteatoma but can result from trauma. Synthetic as well as homograft devices are used depending on the preference of the individual surgeon.

The most common homograft procedure is the incus interposition.[66,78,79] In short, this involves removal of the incus (or its remnants) with resculpting and drilling so that the redesigned incus can be interposed between the drum and intact stapes superstructure (Fig. 13-97). This is a highly successful procedure in experienced hands and remains in use today. Possible complications include dislocation or postinflammatory fixation, or both, by granuloma or fibrous tissue formation. CT is quite valuable in postoperative evaluation.[13,77]

The search for a synthetic material that would not incite foreign body reaction in the middle ear was rewarded with the development of *Proplast* (polytetrafluoroethelene-vitrous carbon) and *Plastopore* (high-density polyethelene sponge). Both are trademarks of Richard's Medical, Memphis, Tennessee.[80,81] The porous nature of these materials allows for infiltration by histiocytes and fibroblasts, which provide stabilization over time. These substances can be formed into countless shapes and are usually referred to as *TORP (total ossicular replacement prosthesis)* and *PORP (partial ossicular replacement prosthesis)*. The TORP is interposed between the drum and the oval window, while the PORP is interposed between the drum and an intact stapes superstructure (Fig. 13-98). CT examination is diagnostically challenging since the entire length of the prosthesis is usually not seen because of its oblique course.[65] The thickness and density of these substances

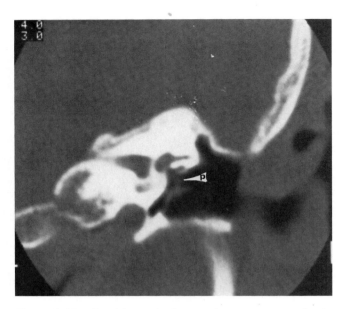

Fig. 13-98 Partial ossicular replacement prosthesis (PORP). Coronal image demonstrates prosthesis *(p, white arrowhead)* articulating with tympanoplasty and extending toward oval window. Often articulation with stapes is difficult to discern.

usually preclude confusion with a normal ossicular chain. Delineation of these devices is commonly simple in the well-pneumatized middle ear; however, if recurrent debris has developed adjacent to the device, it may not be perceptible because the CT density may be identical to that of its surroundings. The complications include subluxation and granuloma formation. Fortunately, the clinical and audiometric findings are most important, and the CT is not required for diagnosis of a poorly functioning device.

Simple tympanoplasty is performed in individuals with an unhealed perforation of the tympanic membrane. CT usually plays no role in the evaluation of this procedure. Both the homograft and synthetic replacements referred to in the previous paragraphs require tympanoplasty. In the absence of ossiculoplasty, five types of tympanoplasty are defined. These are classified on the basis of the degree of ossicular bypass. Most commonly encountered in our experience is the type III tympanoplasty in which the graft is articulated directly with the head of the stapes.

Cochlear implantation has become increasingly available as an alternative to the conventional hearing aid for individuals with severe to profound sensorineural deafness. Single channel and multichannel devices are in clinical use at several institutions.[82,83,84] They are inserted via the round window for a variable distance into the cochlea for the purpose of stimulating the cochlear nerve. Temporal bone imaging has been used for both

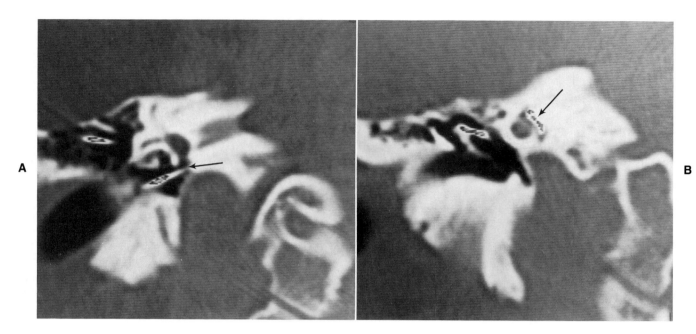

Fig. 13-99   Multichannel cochlear implant. Two coronal images demonstrate device entering round window *(single arrow, **A**)* and continuing into middle turn *(arrow, **B**)*. (From Harnsberger HR et al: Cochlear implant candidates: assessment with CT and MR imaging, Radiology 164:53, 1987.)

preoperative and postoperative evaluation. CT can be helpful in identification of the site of termination of the electrode in those cases in which placement was technically difficult. Preoperative evaluation is more critical, particularly for the multichannel device, which must be inserted 22 to 26mm into the middle cochlear turn (Fig. 13-99). Absolute contraindications to implantation include bilateral acoustic neuromas, severe fractures, and obliterative labyrinthine (cochlear) ossification. Relative contraindications include congenital cochlear malformation, cochlear otosclerosis (otospongiosis), and uncontrolled otitis media or mastoiditis.

THE EXTERNAL AUDITORY CANAL

CT identification of abnormal soft tissue debris in the external auditory canal (EAC) is not uncommon and is of variable clinical significance. In most cases the appearance is histologically nonspecific. Often, simple otoscopic manipulation will cause transient mucosal thickening within the canal, which may cause confusion unless such a history is available. Granulation tissue or fibrous tissue is often visualized otoscopically. CT can demonstrate contiguity with the middle ear, which is of great diagnostic significance to the physician because the medial extent of such debris is usually inapparent.

The majority of significant EAC pathology, both inflammatory and neoplastic, occurs in elderly patients, especially those with long-standing chronic otitis media.[85-90]

Inflammatory Disorders

Otitis externa is usually a benign self-limited process; however, it may become a life-threatening condition in the elderly diabetic or immunocompromised patient ("malignant" external otitis) (Fig. 13-100).[87,89,91] The exact etiology is obscure, although excess moisture, hyperglycemia, and ischemic perichondritis have all been postulated. This disease often begins in an insidious fashion at the osseous-cartilaginous junction, and the clinician must remain alert so that there is no failure to recognize potentially serious complications. The TM is resistant to the infectious process; middle ear and mastoid involvement is believed to arise secondary to propagation via tiny clefts in the cartilaginous portion of the canal, the fissures of Santorini. TMJ involvement is not uncommon. Facial palsy is a grave prognostic sign and may occur as a result of mastoid destruction or, more commonly, secondary to subtemporal spread of infection to the stylomastoid foramen. Intracranial involvement is a preterminal event and may be heralded by the development of meningitis, abscess formation, infarcts, or sinus thrombosis.

Pseudomonas aeroginosa, a gram-negative motile aerobic rod that tends to proliferate in moist devitalized tissue, particularly when host defenses are impaired, is classically the offending organism.[92] This organism produces a variety of endotoxins, exotoxins, neurotoxins, and destructive enzymes. Among the latter, elastase and collagenase are the most significant since they al-

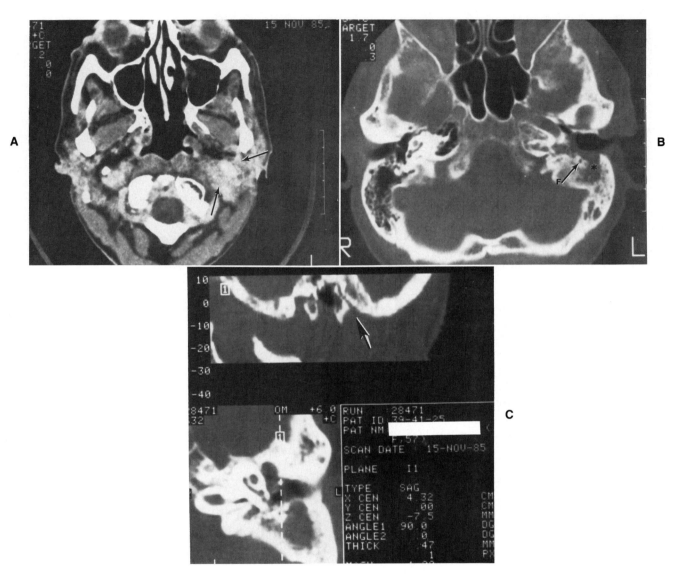

Fig. 13-100 Malignant external otitis. **A,** Contrast enhanced axial image demonstrates enhancing debris *(arrows)* in subtemporal regions surrounding styloid process. **B,** More superior axial image targeted for bone demonstrates debris eroding into mastoid (*). Mastoid segment of facial nerve canal (F, *arrow*) is intact. **C,** Sagittally reformatted image demonstrates some expansion in region of stylomastoid foramen *(arrow)* in this patient with early signs of facial palsy.

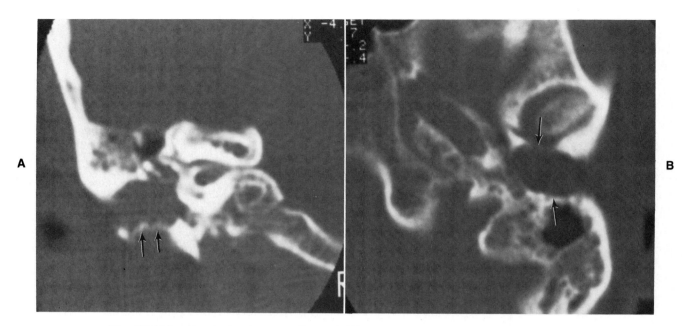

Fig. 13-101   Keratosis obturans. Coronal **(A)** and axial **(B)** reveals smooth expansion and erosion of the canal wall *(arrows)*. The mass clearly extends into middle ear and surrounds ossicular chain.

low invasion across fascial planes. The increased severity of this process in diabetic patients presumably results from their increased susceptibility to endarteritis and defective chemotaxis of leukocytes.

Both CT and MRI provide excellent delineation of soft tissue invasion in the subtemporal region as well as accurate information about the status of the stylomastoid foramen.[72,76,93] CT is needed for the evaluation of details regarding involvement of the middle ear, mastoid, and intratemporal bony facial nerve canal. Because of its high sensitivity, radionuclide evaluation probably still has a role in initial disease identification.[87] When intracranial pathology is suspected, MRI is most desirable.

Neoplastic Disorders*

Malignant neoplasia involving the external auditory canal (EAC) may be intrinsic or extrinsic and usually will have squamous cell, basal cell, or salivary gland origin.[28,94,95] *Melanomas, metastases,* and *gliomas* are extremely rare. *Squamous cell carcinoma,* a disease of the elderly, may originate in the canal or extend from the middle ear. In the latter circumstance there is usually a long-standing history of chronic otitis media. *Basal cell carcinoma* invading the external auditory canal often will originate in the postauricular sulcus. Neoplasms of

*Neoplasms of the temporal bone are addressed in detail in one of the following sections.

salivary origin (i.e., *mucoepidermoid carcinoma, adenoid cystic carcinoma*) may originate in the parotid gland or arise from minor salivary gland rests within the external canal or middle ear.

The imprecise term *ceruminoma* remains in use for describing all neoplasms of ceruminous gland origin. This term should be discarded in favor of *ceruminous adenoma* and adenocarcinoma, *pleomorphic adenoma,* and *adenoid cystic carcinoma,* which have all specifically been described as having ceruminous gland origin within the canal. This is more appropriate terminology since the malignant varieties (i.e., adenoid cystic carcinoma, ceruminous adenocarcinoma) are much more aggressive lesions.

The most common benign "neoplasm" of the external canal is the *exostosis.*[96] This lesion arises in the osseous portion of the canal, usually in patients with a prolonged exposure to cold sea water. Bilaterality is common, and the lesions are often broad based. They usually arise along the tympanomastoid or tympanosquamous suture lines. Although clinically similar, the exostosis is distinct from the *osteoma.*[97] The latter is much less common and usually unilateral, and temporal bone origin is not limited to the external canal.

Keratosis obturans (KO) and *external auditory canal cholesteatoma* (EACC) are entirely different clinical and pathologic processes.[85,90,98] Although they both represent accumulations of exfoliated keratin within the bony EAC, KO usually is diagnosed in patients under the

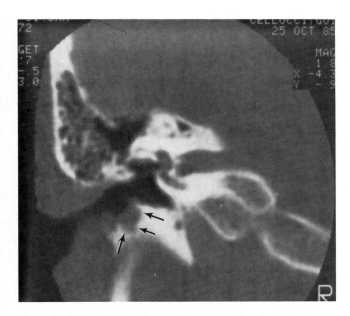

Fig. 13-102 External auditory canal cholesteatoma. There is soft tissue mass in external canal. There are punched out erosions in the floor of external auditory canal demonstrated on this coronal image *(arrows).*

age of 40 years who have a history of sinusitis or bronchiectasis. There is often severe pain and conductive deficit, but only rarely otorrhea. KO is often bilateral, associated with an abnormal tympanic membrane, and heralded by a keratin plug and smooth widening of the canal on otoscopic inspection.

EACC patients in contrast have a chronic dull ear pain and no hearing loss. These are often elderly patients with unilateral lesions, and otorrhea is common. There is no association with sinusitis or bronchiectasis, and there will be no evidence of a keratin plug on otoscopic inspection. The tympanic membrane will usually be normal. Rather than smooth widening as in KO, the bony changes with EACC are much more focal and consist of localized erosions and periostitis, possibly with sequestration.

The soft tissue components of the aforementioned benign and malignant neoplasms (excluding exostosis and osteoma) are virtually identical by CT criteria.[86] CT is of value primarily for determining the extent of disease and the presence of bony erosion or destruction (Figs. 13-101 and 13-102). Since the mastoid segment of the facial nerve canal is constantly located immediately adjacent to the posterior tympanic annulus, CT, particularly in the axial projection, is well suited for determination of the proximity of the disease process to this crucial structure.

REFERENCES

1. Plester D: Hereditary factors in chronic otitis media in general and cholesteatoma in particular. In McCabe BS, Sade J, and Abramson M, editors: Cholesteatoma, First international Conference, Birmingham, Ala, 1977, Aesculapius.
2. Schuknecht HF: Pathology of the ear, Boston, 1974, Harvard University Press.
3. Mafee MF et al: Chronic otomastoiditis: a conceptual understanding of CT findings, Radiology 160(1):193, 1986.
4. Proctor B: Chronic otitis media and mastoiditis. In Paparella MM and Shumrick DA, editors: Otolaryngology, vol 2, The ear, Philadelphia, 1980, WB Saunders Co, pp 1465-1489.
5. Beaumont GD: Radiology and the management of chronic suppurative otitis media, Australasian, Radiology 24:238, 1980.
6. Bluestone CD and Cantekin EI: Eustachian tube dysfunction. In English GM, editor: Otolaryngology, New York, 1979, Harper & Row, Publishers, Inc.
7. Moran WB Jr: Cholesteatoma. In English GM, editor: Otolaryngology, New York, 1980, Harper & Row, Publishers, Inc.
8. Paparella M: The middle ear effusions. In Paparella MM and Shumrick DA, editors: Otolaryngology, ed 2, vol 2, The ear, Philadelphia, 1980, WB Saunders Co, pp 1422-1444.
9. Swartz JD et al: High resolution computed tomography of the middle ear and mastoid. II. Tubotympanic disease, Radiology 148:455, 1983.
10. Buckingham RA: Cholesteatoma in chronic otitis media following middle ear intubation, Laryngoscope 91:1415, 1981.
11. Pratt LL and Murray J: The placement of middle ear ventilation tubes: some indications and complications, Laryngoscope 83:1022, 1973.
12. Klein MA, Kelly JK, and Eggleston D: Recognizing tympanostomy tubes on temporal bone CT: typical and atypical appearances, AJR 150:1411, 1988.
13. Swartz JD et al: High resolution computed tomography of the middle ear and mastoid. III. Surgically altered anatomy and pathology, Radiology 148:461, 1983.
14. Swartz JD: Imaging of the temporal bone: a text/atlas, New York, 1986, Thieme Medical Publishers, Inc.
15. Mafee MF et al: Acute otomastoiditis and its complications: role of CT, Radiology 155:391, 1985.
15a. Holliday RA: Inflammatory diseases of the temporal bone: evaluation with CT and MR, Seminars in Ultrasound, CT, and MR 10(3):213-235, 1989.
15b. Holliday RA: MRI of mastoid and middle ear disease, Radiol Clin North Am 27:283-299, 1989.
15c. Swartz JD: Current imaging approach to the temporal bone, Radiology 171:309-317, 1989.
16. Paparella MM and Meyerhoff WC: Clinical significance of granulation tissue of chronic otitis media. In Sade J, editor: Cholesteatoma and mastoid surgery, Amsterdam, 1982, Kugler, pp 387-395.
17. Swartz JD: Cholesteatomas of the middle ear: diagnosis, etiology and complications, Radiol Clin North Am 22(1):15, 1984.
18. Amedee RG, Marks HW, and Lyons GD: Cholesterol granuloma of the petrous apex, Am J Otol 8(1):48, 1987.
19. Beumont GD: Cholesterol granuloma, J Otolaryngol Soc Aust 2:28, 1967.
20. Lo WWM et al: Cholesterol granuloma of the petrous apex: CT diagnosis, Radiology 153:705, 1984.
20a. Martin N et al: Cholesterol granulomas of the middle ear cavities: MR imaging, Radiology 172:521-525, 1989.
20b. Greenberg JJ et al: Cholesterol granuloma of the petrous apex, AJNR 9:1205-1214, 1988.
21. Miglets AW and Booth JB: Cholesterol granuloma presenting as an isolated middle ear tumor, Laryngoscope 91:410, 1981.

22. Phelps PD and Lloyd GA: Vascular masses in middle ear, Clin Radiol 37(4):359, 1986.

23. Pickles JM, Tucker AG, and Cowie JW: Computerized tomography of vascular middle ear masses, J Laryngol Otol 100(4):405, 1986.

24. Plester D and Steinbach E: Cholesterol granuloma, Otolaryngol Clin North Am 15:655, 1982.

25. Latack JL et al: Giant cholesterol cysts of the petrous apex, AJNR 6(2):409, 1985.

25a. Gomori JM and Grossman RI: Mechanisms responsible for the MR appearance and evolution of intracranial hemorrhage, Radiographics 8:427, 1988.

26. Nager GT: Epidermoids (congenital cholesteatomas) involving the temporal bone. In Sade J, editor: Cholesteatoma and mastoid surgery, Amsterdam, 1982, Kugler, pp 41-60.

27. Swartz JD et al: Congenital middle ear deafness: CT study, Radiology 159:187, 1986.

28. Crabtree JA, Britton BH, and Pierce MK: Carcinoma of the external auditory canal, Laryngoscope 86:405, 1976.

29. Nager GT: Cholesteatoma of middle ear: pathogenesis and surgical indication. In McCabe BS, Sade J, and Abramson M, editors: cholesteatoma, First International Conference, Birmingham, Ala, 1977, Aesculapius, pp 191-203.

30. Sade J: Pathogenesis of attic cholesteatoma, J Royal Soc Med 71:716, 1978.

31. Cody DTR: The definition of cholesteatoma. In McCabe BF, Sade J, and Abramson M, editors: Cholesteatoma, First International Conference, Birmingham, Ala, 1977, Aesculapius, pp 6-9.

32. Ruedi L: Acquired cholesteatoma, Arch Otolaryngol 78:252, 1983.

33. Sade J: Pathogenesis of attic cholesteatoma: the metaplasia theory. In McCabe BS, Sade J, and Abramson M, editors: Cholesteatoma, First International Conference, Birmingham, Ala, 1977, Aesculapius, pp 212-232.

34. Swartz JD and Varghese S: Pars flaccida cholesteatoma as demonstrated by computed tomography, Arch Otolaryngol 110:515, 1984.

35. Buckingham RA and Valvassori GE: Tomographic evaluation of cholesteatomas of the middle ear and mastoid, Otolaryngol Clin North Am 6(2):363, 1973.

36. Mafee MF et al: CT of the middle ear in evaluation of cholesteatoma and other soft tissue masses, Radiology 148:465, 1983.

37. Phelps PD and Lloyd GAS: The radiology of cholesteatoma, Clin Radiol 31:501, 1980.

38. Fisch U: Intracranial complications of cholesteatoma. In Sade J, editor: Cholesteatoma and mastoid surgery, Amsterdam, 1982, Kugler, pp 369-382.

39. Mathews TJ and Marcus G: Otogenic intradural complications: a review of 37 patients, J Otolaryng Otol 102(2):121, 1988.

40. Ritter FN: Complications of cholesteatoma. In McCabe BF, Sade J, and Abramson M, editors: Cholesteatoma, First International Conference, Birmingham, Ala, 1977, Aesculapius, pp 430-437.

41. Sheehy JL, Brackman N, and Graham MN: Complications of cholesteatoma: a report of 1024 cases. In McCabe BF, Sade J, and Abramson M, editors: Cholesteatoma, First International Conference, Birmingham, Ala, 1977, Aesculapius, pp 420-429.

42. Sade J, Berco E, and Buyanover D: Ossicular damage in chronic middle ear inflammation. In Sade J, editor: Cholesteatoma and mastoid surgery, Amsterdam, 1982, Kugler, pp 347-358.

43. Sade J, Berco E, and Halevy A: Bone resorption in chronic otitis media with and without cholesteatoma. In McCabe BF, Sade J, and Abramson M, editors: Cholesteatoma, First International

Conference, Birmingham, Ala, 1977, Aesculapius, pp 128-135.

44. Nager GT: Theories on the origin of attic retraction cholesteatoma. In Proceedings of the Shambaugh Fifth International Workshop on Microsurgery and Fluctuant Hearing Loss, Huntsville, Ala, 1977, Strobe Publishers.

45. Tos M: Can cholesteatoma be prevented? In Sade J, editor: Cholesteatoma and mastoid surgery, Amsterdam, 1982, Kugler Publishing, pp 591-598.

46. Hasso AN, Vignaud J, and Bird CH: Pathology of the temporal bone and mastoid. In Newton TH, Hasso AH, and Dillon WP, editors: Computed tomography of the head and neck, vol 3, Modern neuroradiology, New York, 1988, Raven Press. Chapter 5.

47. Jackler RK, Dillon WP, and Schindler RA: A correlation of surgical and radiographic findings, Laryngoscope 94:746, 1984.

48. Johnson DW et al: Computed tomography of local complications of temporal bone cholesteatomas, J Comput Assist Tomogr 9:519, 1985.

49. Silver AJ et al: Complicated cholesteatomas: CT findings in inner ear complications of middle ear cholesteatomas, Radiology 164:47, 1987.

50. Swartz JD: Facial nerve canal: CT analysis of the protruding tympanic segment, Radiology 153:443, 1984.

51. Manzione JV, Rumbaugh GL, and Katzberg RW: Direct sagittal computed tomography of the temporal bone, J Comput Assist Tomogr 9:417, 1985.

52. O'Donoghue GM et al: The predictive value of high resolution computerized tomography in chronic suppurative ear disease, Clin Otolaryngol 12(2):89, 1987.

53. Swartz JD et al: Ossicular erosions of the dry ear: CT diagnosis, Radiology 163:763, 1987.

53a. Swartz JD et al: Acquired disruptions of the incudostapedial joint, Radiology 171:779-781, 1989.

54. Thomsen J, Balslev-Jorgensen M, and Bretlau P: Bone resorption in chronic otitis media: a histological and ultrastructural study. I. Ossicular necrosis, J Laryngol Otol 88:975, 1974.

55. Kenney SE: Post-inflammatory ossicular fixation in tympanoplasty, Laryngoscope 88:821, 1978.

56. Lumio JS: Contribution to the knowledge of chronic adhesive otitis: the diagnosis, Acta Otolaryngol 39:196, 1981.

57. Swartz JD et al: Post-inflammatory ossicular fixation: CT analysis with surgical correlation, Radiology 154:697, 1985.

58. VanBaarle PW, Huygen PL, and Brickman WF: Findings in surgery for chronic otitis media: a retrospective data analysis of 2225 cases followed for two years, Clin Otolaryngol 8:151, 1983.

59. Gibb AG: Tympanosclerosis, Ear Nose Throat J 60:565, 1981.

60. Goodhill WJ and Jesse RA: Malignant neoplasms of the external auditory canal and temporal bone, Arch Otolaryngol 106:675, 1980.

61. Zollner F: Tympanosclerosis, J Laryngol Otol 70:77, 1956.

62. Tos M: Bony fixation of the malleus and incus, Acta Otolaryngol 70:95, 1970.

63. Swartz JD et al: Stapes prosthesis: evaluation with CT, Radiology 158:179, 1986.

64. Johnson DW: CT of the postsurgical ear, Radiol Clin North Am 22:67, 1984.

65. Swartz JD et al: Synthetic ossicular replacements: normal and abnormal CT appearance, Radiology 163:766, 1987.

66. Shambaugh GE and Glasscock ME, editors: Surgery of the ear, ed 3, Philadelphia, 1980, WB Saunders Co, pp 251-287.

67. Cody DTR and Taylor WF: Mastoidectomy for acquired cholesteatoma: long term results. In McCabe BS, Sade J, and

Abramson M, editors: Cholesteatoma, First International Conference, Birmingham, Ala, 1977, Aesculapius, pp 337-351.

68. Paparella MM and Meyerhoff W: Mastoidectomy and tympanoplasty. In Paparella MM and Shumrick DA, editors: Otolaryngology, vol 2, The ear, ed 2, Philadelphia, 1980, WB Saunders Co, pp 1510-1547.

69. Sheehy JL: Intact canal wall tympanoplasy with mastoidectomy. In Snow JB, editor: Controversy in otolaryngology, Philadelphia, 1980, WB Saunders Co, pp 213-222.

70. Kohut RI: Cholesteatoma: the advantages of modified radical and radical mastoidectomy. In Snow JB, editor: Controversy in otolaryngology, Philadelphia, 1980, WB Saunders Co, pp 223, 227.

70a. Martin N et al: Brain herniation into the middle ear cavity: MR imaging, Neuroradiology 31:184, 1989.

70b. Nardis PF et al: Unusual cholesteatoma shell: CT findings, J Comp Asst Tomog 12:1084, 1988.

71. Sheehy JL, Nelson RA, and House HP: Revision stapedectomy: review of 258 cases, Laryngoscope 91:43, 1981.

72. Curtin HD, Wolfe P, and Snyderman N: Facial nerve between the stylomastoid foramen and the parotid, Radiology 149:165, 1983.

73. Gibbon KT: The histopathology of the incus after stapedectomy, Clin Otolaryngol 4:343, 1979.

74. Dawes JD and Watson RT: Perilymph fistula, Clin Otolaryngol 4:291, 1979.

75. Belal L and Yukoski J: Post stapedectomy dizziness: a histopathologic agent, J Otol 3:187, 1982.

76. Crabtree JA, Britton BH, and Powers WH: An evaluation of recent stapes surgery, Laryngoscope 90:224, 1980.

77. Swartz JD et al: Computed tomography of the disarticulated incus, Laryngoscope 96:1207, 1986.

78. Hilding DA et al: Reconstruction of the ossicular chain. In Snow JB, editor: Controversy in otolaryngology, Philadelphia, 1980, WB Saunders Co, pp 57-83.

79. Hough JVD: Ossicular malformations and their correction. In Shambaugh GE and Shea JJ, editors: Proceedings of the Shambaugh Fifth International Workshop in Middle Ear Microsurgery and Fluctuant Hearing Loss, Huntsville, Ala, 1977, Strobe Publishers, pp 186-194.

80. Brackman DE, Sheehy JL, and Luxford WM: TORPS and PORPS in tympanoplasty: a review of 1042 operations, Otolaryngol Head Neck Surg 92:337, 1984.

81. Glasscock ME et al: Ossicular chain reconstructions: the TORP and PORP in chronic ear disease, Laryngoscope 93:981, 1983.

82. Ball JB, Miller GW, and Hepfner ST: Computed tomography of single channel cochlear implants, AJNR 7:41, 1986.

83. Harnsberger HR et al: Cochlear implant candidates: assessment with CT and MR imaging, Radiology 164:53, 1987.

84. Mueller DT et al: Temporal bone computed tomography in the preoperative evaluation for cochlear implantation, Ann Otol Rhinol Laryngol 98:346, 1989.

85. Biber JJ: The so-called primary cholesteatoma of the external auditory meatus, Laryngol Otolaryngol 67:474, 1953.

86. Chakeres DW, Kapila A, and LaMasters D: Soft tissue abnormalities of the external auditory canal: a review of CT findings, Radiology 166:105, 1985.

87. Mendelson DS et al: Malignant external otitis: the role of computed tomography and radionuclides in evaluation, Radiology 149:745, 1983.

88. Naiberg J, Berger G, and Hawke M: The pathologic features of keratosis obturans and cholesteatomas of the external auditory canal, Arch Otolaryngol 110:69, 1984.

89. Ostfeld E, Aviel A, and Pelet D: Malignant external otitis: diagnostic value of bone scintigraphy, Laryngoscope 91:916, 1981.

90. Piepergerdes JC, Kramer BM, and Behnke EE: Keratosis obturans and external auditory canal cholesteatoma, Laryngoscope 90:388, 1980.

91. Bergeron RT, Osborn AG, and Som PM: Head and neck imaging: excluding the brain, St. Louis, 1984, The CV Mosby Co, pp 728-846.

92. Meyerhoff WL, Gates GA, and Montalbo RJ: Pseudomonas mastoiditis, Laryngoscope 87:483, 1977.

93. Gherini SG, Brackmann DE, and Bradley WG: Magnetic resonance imaging and computerized tomography in malignant external otitis, Laryngoscope 96(5):542, 1986.

94. Goodwin WJ and Jesse RA: Malignant neoplasms of the external auditory canal and temporal bone, Arch Otolaryngol 106:675, 1980.

95. Hicks GW: Tumors arising from glandular structures of the external auditory canal, Laryngoscope 93:326, 1983.

96. DiBartolomeo JR: Exostosis of the external auditory canal, Ann Otolaryngol 88(suppl 61):1, 1979.

97. Deni A et al: Extracanalicular osteomas of the temporal bone, Arch Otolaryngol 105:706, 1979.

98. Bunting WP: Ear canal cholesteatoma and bony resorption, Trans Am Acad Ophthalmol Otolaryngol 72:161, 1968.

SECTION FIVE
TRAUMA AND MISCELLANEOUS DISORDERS

JOEL D. SWARTZ

TRAUMA

Individuals with a history of trauma can be seen by the imaging specialist under a variety of clinical circumstances. Magnetic resonance imaging (MRI) is recommended for those in whom intracranial abnormalities are the greatest clinical concern because of its highly desirable ability to delineate parenchymal abnormality and extracerebral collections.[1] In those with the predominant complaint of hearing loss, vertigo, cerebrospinal fluid (CSF) leak or seventh nerve paralysis (often delayed phenomenon), CT eclipses all other imaging modalities because of its ability to demonstrate

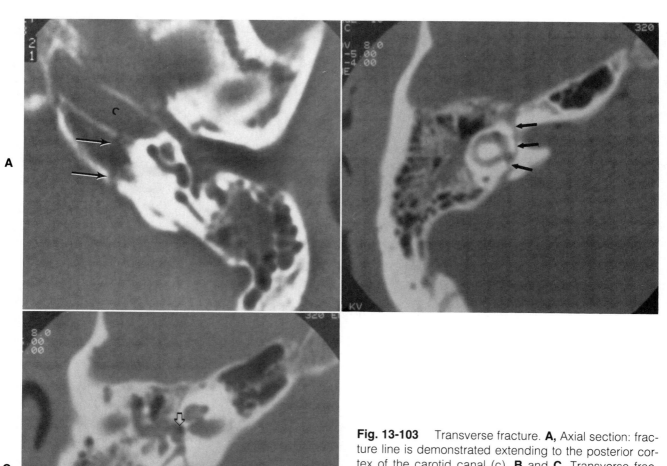

Fig. 13-103 Transverse fracture. **A,** Axial section: fracture line is demonstrated extending to the posterior cortex of the carotid canal (c). **B** and **C,** Transverse fracture, different patient. Axial sections, right ear. **B,** Fracture line *(arrows)* extends through the fundus of the internal auditory canal *(IAC).* **C,** Pneumovestibule *(arrow).*

bony detail, which allows characterization of fracture deformity and associated ossicular derangements.[2-9]

In the past most of the emphasis on imaging evaluation of the temporal bone concerned the evaluation of fracture deformity.[10] Temporal bone fractures are described as being longitudinal (occurring in the direction of the long axis of the temporal bone), transverse (perpendicular to the long axis), or mixed (Figs. 13-103 and 13-104).[11] Classically, most fractures are described as longitudinal, with estimates of occurrence of up to 86%. Our experience, as well as that of others, indicates that with the advent of CT the majority of fractures are now characterized as mixed (Fig. 13-105). Most temporal bone fractures are visualized on images obtained in the axial projection, since the long axis of the temporal bone is so exquisitely depicted in this manner. The observer should remember that these fractures may be of little significance in the absence of related clinical symptomatology.

Longitudinal fractures generally result from blows to the temporoparietal region. There is a high incidence of ossicular derangement with this type of fracture; however, the inner ear structures are usually spared.[11] Tympanic membrane perforations occur commonly. Facial paralysis is noted in 10% to 20%; however, it is usually delayed and incomplete.[12-14] If squamous epithelium debris invades the fracture line prior to callus development, the patient is at increased risk for formation of acquired cholesteatoma (see Fig. 13-105).[15] A cholesteatoma developing in this clinical context may be quite aggressive and dangerous.[16]

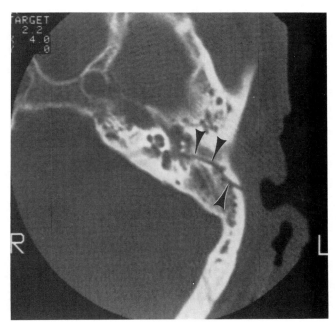

Fig. 13-104 Longitudinal fracture. Fracture line is demonstrated through the mastoid *(arrowheads)* extending to but not disrupting the ossicular chain. (From Swartz JD: Imaging of the temporal bone, New York, 1986, Thieme Medical Publishers, Inc.)

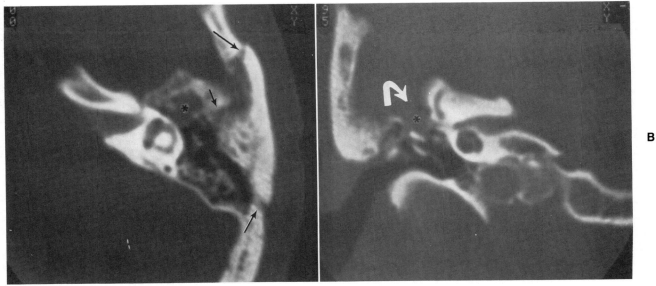

Fig. 13-105 Complicated mixed fracture. **A,** Axial section—fracture lines are demonstrated *(arrows)*. A soft tissue mass is identified in the attic (*). **B,** Coronal image—a large tegmen defect is present *(curved white arrow)*. There is a soft tissue mass identified in the attic *(asterisk)*. This mass could represent encephalocele or cholesteatoma invading fracture line. MRI was recommended in this case.

Transverse fractures usually result from a frontal or occipital impact.[10,11] Involvement of the labyrinth is relatively common. This can result in acute complete hearing loss or severe vertigo caused by involvement of the cochlear or vestibular apparatus. Such a fracture may also cause these symptoms by transsection of the internal auditory canal, usually at the fundus.

Detailed imaging is especially critical in those patients with facial nerve paralysis, since early operative intervention may be necessary to reverse or impede the nerve damage (Fig. 13-106).[17] As previously discussed, facial nerve impingement can result from either a transverse or longitudinal fracture, more commonly from the former.[18] If the observer fails to identify a fracture, then the entire course of the facial nerve must be studied in both coronal and axial projections, if possible, in search of fracture fragments or evidence of localized expansion that could result from intraneuronal hematoma or edema. The most common site of injury occurs in the distal labyrinthine segment, just proximal to the geniculate ganglion with transverse fracture, and in the proximal tympanic segment, just distal to the geniculate ganglion, with longitudinal fracture.[19]

Disruption of the tegmen tympani is the most common cause of CSF otorrhea (see Fig. 13-105).[20,21] This more commonly results from longitudinal than from transverse fractures. The entire border of the temporal bone must be studied when this history is present. Direct sagittal imaging or sagittal reformations are also highly desirable in this clinical circumstance.[6] Of course, in order to develop true CSF otorrhea, the tympanic membrane must be perforated. We have seen several cases of CSF rhinorrhea developing subsequent to retromastoid craniectomies that have breached the mastoid air cell system.[8] In these individuals the middle ear cleft is filled with CSF; and, as a result of the intact tympanic membrane, CSF will egress through the eustachian tube and subsequently into the nasopharynx and nasal cavity. Obviously, clinical correlation is needed in this circumstance.

Vertigo and hearing loss are the most common posttraumatic complaints. Although vertiginous complaints can be related to temporal bone fracture, the cause often defies imaging evaluation. Such vertigo, associated with fluctuating sensorineural or mixed hearing loss, may indicate perilymph fistula, believed by many to indicate a surgical emergency.[22] Unfortunately, there is a paucity of CT findings in this disorder, and the diagnosis usually will be the sole responsibility of the clinician (see Fig. 13-91).[23] The observer should keep in mind that vertiginous complaints following injury are relatively common and self-limited, requiring only symptomatic treatment.

Hearing loss is obviously a common sequela of temporal bone trauma. Sensorineural hearing loss (SNHL) may of course result from fracture involving the internal auditory canal or cochlea; however, as with the evaluation of vertigo, the cause of the SNHL may not be apparent even after thorough imaging. In the absence of demonstrable fracture, patients are often labeled with the diagnosis of labyrinthine concussion.[11,20,24] The length and degree of such a sensorineural loss is variable.

CT evaluation of posttraumatic conductive deafness provides the highest likelihood of making a pinpoint diagnosis.[7,8] Loss of conductive hearing occurring secondary to tympanic membrane damage occurs commonly. This may occur with or without a fracture of the tympanic ring. Shrinkage of the audiometric air-bone gap (hearing improvement) should occur after repair or spontaneous healing of the perforation. Hematotympanum is also a common sequela of trauma that can also result in disturbance of the conductive mechanism. Loss of conductive hearing that persists after tympanic membrane healing and resorption of middle ear debris usually results from ossicular derangement. Obviously, the observer must exclude a preexistent condition such as otosclerosis or chronic otitis media.

The ossicular chain can be disrupted at multiple sites. The malleus and stapes are well anchored by ligamentous and tendinous structures, which are described earlier in the chapter.[25,26] Fractures of the stapes do occur but may be difficult to characterize at CT. Overlapping axial images usually will demonstrate both the anterior and posterior crus of the stapes in the normal patient.[26] Lack of visualization of these structures should provoke suspicion. Fractures of the malleus are rare but have been reported (Fig. 13-107).

The incus, as a result of its relative lack of support, is the most vulnerable ossicle.[13,27] Malleoincudal subluxations are not uncommon, and this articulation should be carefully studied during evaluation of axial sections (Fig. 13-108).[8] Complete incus dislocations have been well described and are easy to diagnose (Fig. 13-109).[9] The residual incus may be identified within the middle ear cavity or external auditory canal or may not be visible. In the latter case the incus may indeed disintegrate. Occasionally, the ossicular chain is so fragmented as to defy description (Fig. 13-110). Disruptions of the incudostapedial joint are believed by many to be the most common cause of posttraumatic conductive deficit. This articulation is best appreciated in the axial projection because of its oblique orientation (Fig. 13-111, A).[28] A distance of 1 mm or less is normally present between the lenticular process of the incus and the capitulum of the stapes, and there should be neither an anterior nor a posterior offset between these two structures. Overlapping axial sections provide the greatest diagnostic latitude for adequate evaluation of this region (Fig. 13-111, B).

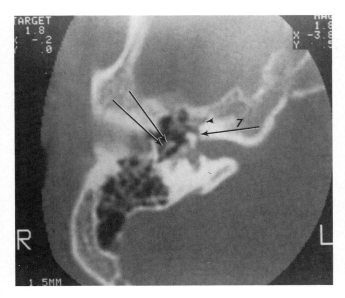

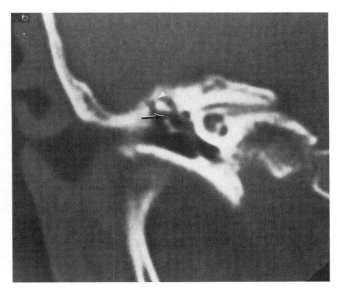

Fig. 13-106   Fracture, facial nerve paralysis. Axial section demonstrates a fracture *(arrow)* extending to labyrinthine segment of facial nerve canal (7, *arrow*). Malleus is absent. Incus body *(double arrows)* is noted. (From Swartz JD: Imaging of the temporal bone, New York, 1986, Thieme Medical Publishers, Inc.)

Fig. 13-107   Fractured malleus. Coronal image demonstrates this unusual fracture whereby malleus head is separated from malleus neck *(arrow)*. Notice that superior mallear ligament *(arrowhead)* is intact.

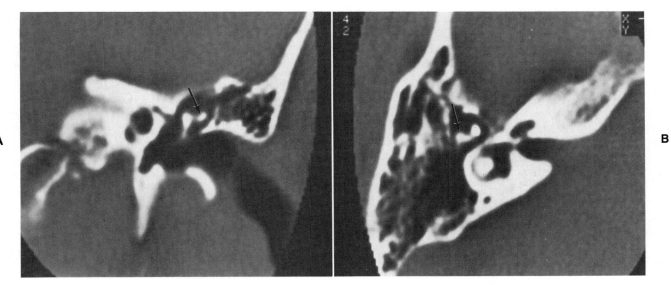

Fig. 13-108   Malleoincudal disruption. **A,** Coronal image demonstrates unusual vertical orientation of malleus head. An additional bony "fragment" is demonstrated laterally *(arrow)*. **B,** Axial image demonstrates disruption of the malleoincudal articulation with abnormal lateral and anterior position of incus body *(arrow)*.

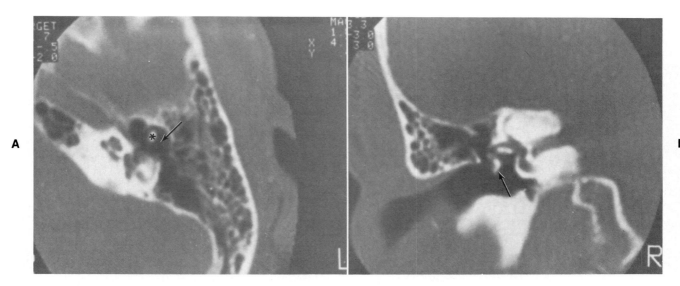

Fig. 13-109 Incus dislocation. **A,** Axial section—normally positioned malleus head is indicated (*). The incus body is absent (arrow). **B,** Coronal section—dislocated incus is identified in mesotympanum (arrow).

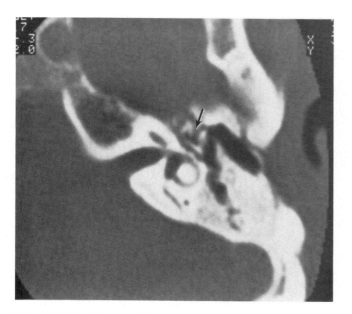

Fig. 13-110 Shattered ossicular chain. Multiple ossicular remnants are identified in the attic (arrow).

DISTURBANCES OF GROWTH, METABOLISM, AND AGING
Paget's Disease

Although primarily a disease of the axial skeleton and calvarium, involvement of the temporal bone in *Paget's disease (osteitis deformans)* occurs frequently.[29-32] Patients may have hearing loss, tinnitus, or dysequilibrium. The same pathologic changes occur here as elsewhere: osteoclastic resorption followed by osteoblastic proliferation. The disease begins at the *petrous apex* (site of greatest marrow deposition) and progresses inferolaterally. Demineralization of the otic capsule is a later manifestation. There is a well-known male predominance (80%). The aforementioned hearing loss may be conductive, sensorineural, or mixed. Conductive deficit is less common and may result from stapediovestibular encroachment or, very rarely, pagetoid involvement of the ossicular chain.[32] Sensorineural loss has been proved to be of cochlear etiology, refuting previous suggestions of compressive neuropathy caused by narrowing of the internal auditory canals.

The CT appearance is classic. There is generalized (not focal) demineralization that may involve the entire temporal bone (Figs. 13-112 and 13-113).[33-36] In our experience Paget's disease of the temporal bone has usually been an asymmetric, predominately unilateral process. Virtually all patients have obvious calvarial involvement, and a significant number also have basilar invagination.[37]

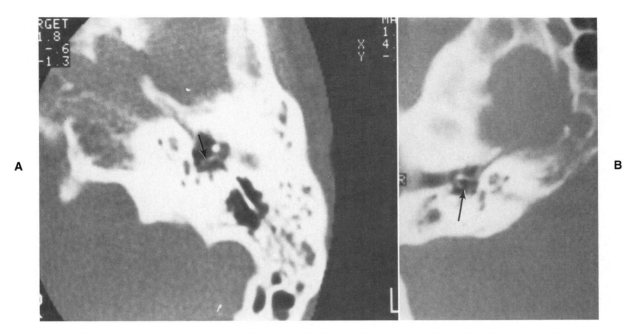

Fig. 13-111   Incudostapedial disruption. **A,** Normal incudostapedial articulation on axial section *(arrow).* **B,** Disrupted right incudostapedial articulation.

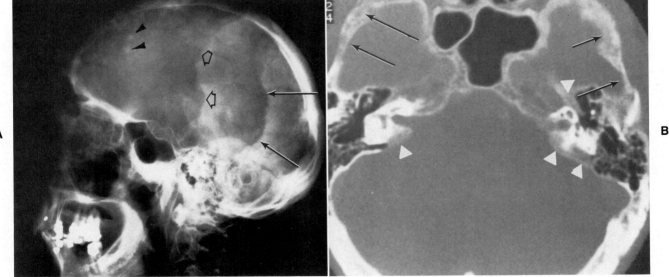

Fig. 13-112   Paget's disease—calvarium and temporal bone. **A,** Lateral skull film demonstrates classical changes of osteoporosis circumscripta. Posterior margins *on each side* ("advancing edge") are demonstrated *(outlined arrowheads and outlined arrows).* Countless dense foci *(black arrowheads)* are noted; these probably indicate subacute nature of process. **B,** CT scan; axial section demonstrates demineralization of squamous portion of temporal bone *(outlined arrows).* Asymmetric demineralization of petrous temporal bone and region of otic capsule is also appreciated *(white arrowheads).*

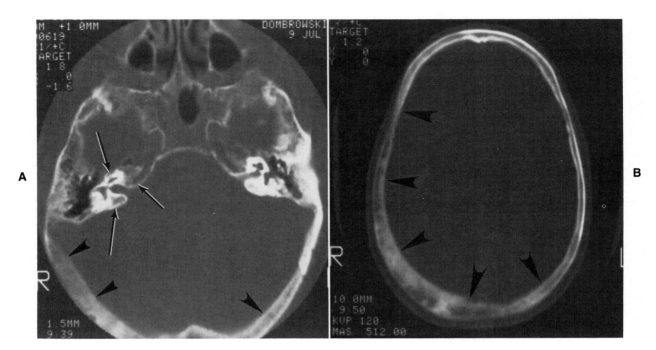

Fig. 13-113 Paget's disease—calvarium and temporal bone. **A,** CT scan; axial section—demineralization of right temporal bone is identified *(outlined arrows)*. Calvarial changes, which are bilateral, are also appreciated on this image *(black arrowheads)*. **B,** CT scan; axial section—pagetoid changes in calvarium are appreciated. There is obvious thickening with central inhomogeneous high density *(black arrowheads)*.

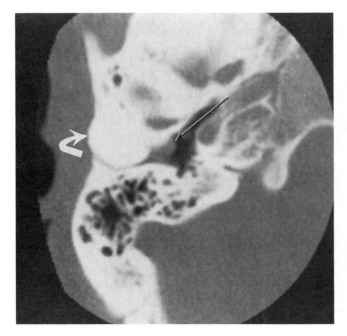

Fig. 13-114 Fibrous dysplasia. Axial section. There is bony occlusion of external auditory canal *(curved white arrow)*. Soft tissue density *(outlined arrow)* medial to occluding plug represented cholesteatoma. (From Swartz JD: Imaging of the temporal bone, New York, 1986, Thieme Medical Publishers, Inc.)

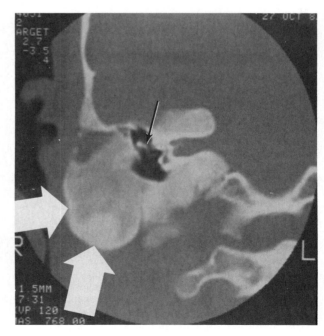

Fig. 13-115 Fibrous dysplasia. Coronal image demonstrates homogeneous bony overgrowth of entire temporal bone, particularly mastoid *(large white arrows)*. Ossicular chain *(outlined arrow)* is intact.

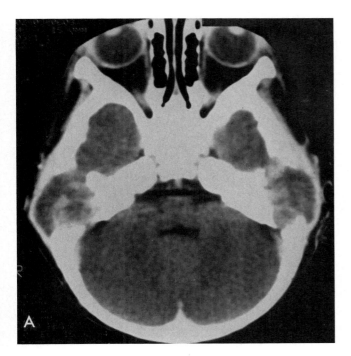

Fig. 13-116 Histiocytosis X. Bilateral temporal bone involvement by destructive soft tissue masses is demonstrated. (With permission from WB Saunders Co, Thieme Medical Publishers; case courtesy, HD Curtin, MD.)

Fibrous Dysplasia

The CT appearance of fibrous dysplasia of the temporal bone is completely different from that of Paget's disease. This mesenchymal disorder results in fibroosseous deposition without demineralization.[33-36,38] The inner ear is spared. The external auditory canal is commonly involved and may be occluded or severely stenotic.[39] An external canal cholesteatoma may be associated medial to the occluding plug (Fig. 13-114). Bony expansion of the mastoid and external auditory canal are the most common characteristics (Fig. 13-115). Impingement on the ossicular chain has been reported.[32,40]

Histiocytosis X

Involvement of the temporal bone in individuals with histiocytosis X form of reticuloendotheliosis is not rare, occurring in perhaps 30% of cases.[41] Thirty percent of those with temporal bone involvement have bilateral disease. Clinical symptomatology may masquerade as chronic otitis, and the diagnosis subsequently may be delayed. The granulomatous mass and associated bony erosion are well demonstrated by CT (Fig. 13-116).

Osteogenesis Imperfecta Tarda

Patients with osteogenesis imperfecta tarda often have hearing loss. The CT appearance is virtually identical to otosclerosis; indeed, some authors have suggested a common genetic abnormality (Fig. 13-117).[32]

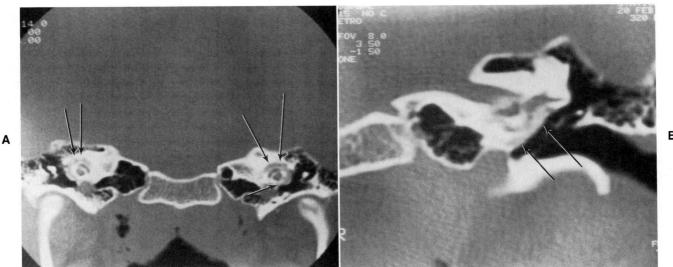

Fig. 13-117 Osteogenesis Imperfecta. **A,** Coronal image demonstrates demineralization in cochlea *(outlined arrows)* identical to that seen with cochlear otosclerosis (otospongiosis). **B,** Magnified coronal image demonstrates demineralization of basilar turn of cochlea extending to the oval window *(outlined arrows).* (From Swartz JD: Imaging of the temporal bone, New York, 1986, Thieme Medical Publishers, Inc.)

Osteopetrosis

Defective resorption of the primary spongiosa with persistence of calcified cartilage is believed to be the etiology for osteopetrosis, which results in thick, dense, and fragile bones.[32,37] Dense bony sclerosis is the end result. Identical findings may occur in pyknodysostosis, Englemann's disease (progressive diaphyseal dysplasia), and Pyle's disease (craniometaphyseal dysplasia) (Fig. 13-118). In the early phase of osteopetrosis increased bone density is not a prominent feature. Rather, more subtle findings prevail: prominent subarcuate fossae, trumpet-shaped internal auditory canals, and limited mastoid pneumatization.[41a] These findings suggest that delayed maturation is the primary abnormality with bone thickening and sclerosis being a secondary manifestation.

Otosclerosis

The temporal bone is unique because there normally is endochondral persistence within the otic capsule between the outer endosteum and inner periosteum.[37,42] Resorption of this endochondral layer, with deposition of spongy vascular new bone, is referred to as otosclerosis (otospongiosis). This is a slowly progressive disorder with a 65% female predominance and an 80% incidence of bilaterality. Otosclerosis usually manifests initially in the second or third decade.[29,43] The bilaterality is often asynchronous.[44]

Tinnitus may be the presenting symptom; however, hearing loss will always develop eventually. The deficit may be sensorineural, conductive, or mixed.[45]

Sensorineural hearing loss is associated with areas of demineralization at various locations within the otic capsule that can be appreciated with CT (Figs. 13-119 to 13-121).[35,36,46-48] When present in the cochlea, they represent a relative contraindication to cochlear implant surgery.[49-52] Cytotoxic enzymes are implicated as the cause of these foci.[53,54] Diffusion of these enzymes into the cochlear fluid is responsible for hyalinization of the spiral ligament and subsequent hearing loss.

The basilar membrane forms the boundary between the cochlear duct and the scala tympani. This membrane widens as it approaches the apical turn. High-frequency tones have maximum amplitude at the basilar turn, and low-frequency tones toward the apex. One can therefore predict the type of sensorineural hearing loss from the CT location of these foci (see Fig. 13-120).[48]

It has been suggested that areas of demineralization (otospongiosis) are associated only with the active phase of this disease. Cochlear otosclerosis in the chronic phase may have no CT manifestations other than subtle

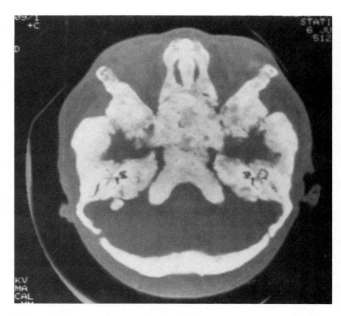

Fig. 13-118 Progressive diaphyseal dysplasia. Remarkable bony density involving entire cranial base including temporal bones is demonstrated. (From Swartz JD: Imaging of the temporal bone, New York, 1986, Thieme Medical Publishers, Inc.)

periosteal thickening. This may explain the relatively high incidence of otherwise asymptomatic sensorineural hearing loss occurring in young individuals with normal CT scans. The observer should be aware that diffuse labyrinthine ossification is not a consequence of otosclerosis.[55] In this situation a history of previous labyrinthectomy should be sought (Fig. 13-122). Otherwise this finding will likely represent a long-standing residuum of labyrinthitis (labyrinthitis ossificans). This entity may have a tympanogenic, meningogenic, hematogenic, or traumatic etiology. CT with densitometric measurements has been proposed as an objective approach to the study of the cochlear capsule.[56,57] Comparison of densitometries performed before and after medical treatment provides an opportunity to monitor the process.

Images obtained in both the axial and coronal position should be carefully evaluated for otospongiotic foci. This disease is often profoundly symmetric.

Conductive deficit is more common and virtually always secondary to stapediovestibular compromise (fenestral otosclerosis). The most common lesion of otosclerosis occurs in the anterior oval window region at the approximate location of the embryologic fissula ante fenestrum, which is an area of cartilage and connective tissue lying in the endochondral layer between the oval

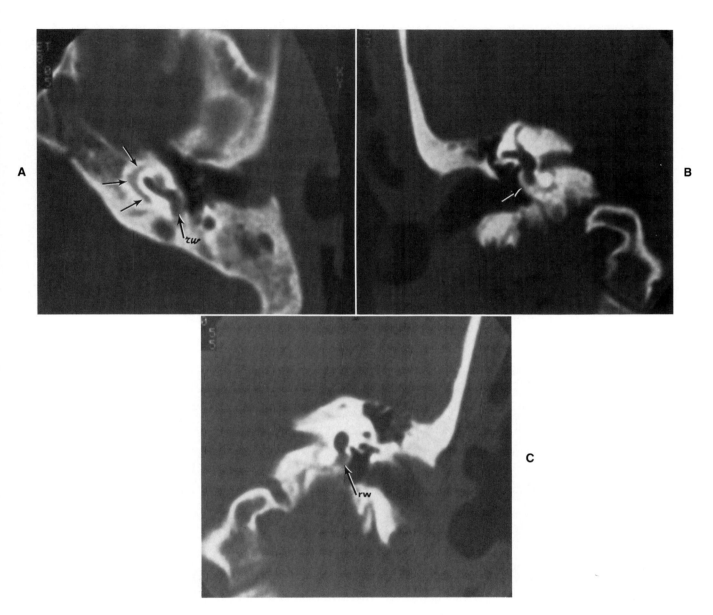

Fig. 13-119   Cochlear otosclerosis (otospongiosis). **A,** Axial section, left ear—there is clearly definable bony demineralization in middle and proximal basilar turn of cochlea *(unlabeled outline arrows)*. Abnormality extends to round window *(rw, arrow)*. **B,** Coronal image, left ear—demineralization of basilar turn is demonstrated *(outlined arrow)*. **C,** Coronal image, right ear—demineralization of basilar turn extending to and occluding round window is demonstrated *(rw, arrow)*.

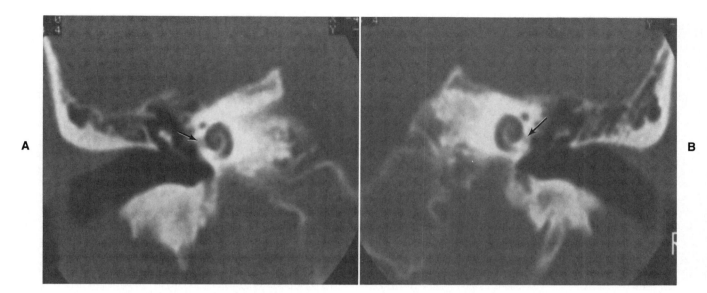

Fig. 13-120 Cochlear otosclerosis (otospongiosis)—apical turn. **A** and **B,** Coronal images. Foci of demineralization in apical turn *(arrows)* are demonstrated. Notice symmetry. Patient had bilateral low frequency sensorineural deficit.

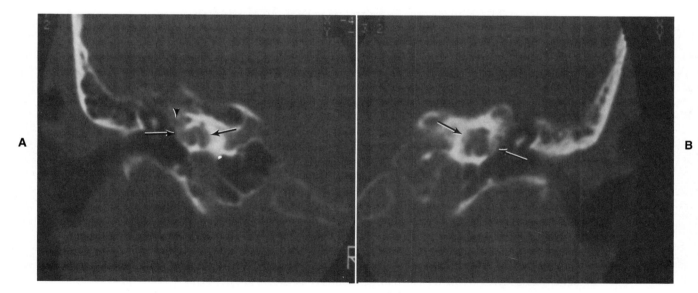

Fig. 13-121 Cochlear otosclerosis (otospongiosis). **A** and **B,** Coronal images demonstrate extensive demineralization throughout apical and middle turns of cochlea bilaterally. Again, notice symmetry.

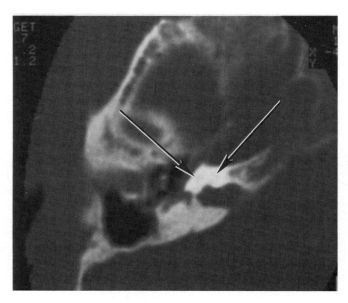

Fig. 13-122   Labyrinthitis ossificans. Axial image, right ear. There is diffuse bony sclerosis involving cochlea *(arrows)*. Patient is status post labyrinthectomy. This should not be confused with otosclerosis.

window and cochleariform process (origin of tensor tympani tendon) (Fig. 13-123, *A* to *E*).[42,45,58] Careful study of the oval window in the axial projection, using overlapping CT sections, is necessary to make this diagnosis. More extensive disease may also be appreciated in the coronal plane, particularly when the oval window is completely occluded (obliterative fenestral otosclerosis), which occurs in approximately 2% of cases (Fig. 13-124).

Fenestral otosclerosis has been treated surgically for a number of years. Many different procedures, including stapes mobilization and fenestration of the lateral semicircular canal, have been used in the past. Currently most surgeons perform stapedectomy followed by prosthesis insertion.

Preoperative evaluation of individuals with noninflammatory conductive deficit must always include careful evaluation of the oval window for subtle otosclerotic plaque formation.[60,61] Most patients have the typical anterior dense focus; however, others may have a posterior focus, or both (Fig. 13-123, *D* to *G*). The contralateral ear must also be studied, since the incidence of bilaterality is high. On occasion patients will have only a subtle thickening of the stapes footplate–annular ligament complex. The latter situation may also occur as a postinflammatory phenomenon (tympanosclerosis).[35] When oval window disease is not appreciated, the ossicular chain must be carefully studied for evidence of congenital anomaly. On occasion no abnormality will be evident despite intensive careful study, and congenital stapes fixation may be the ultimate surgical diagnosis. This entity may have no CT manifestations.[35]

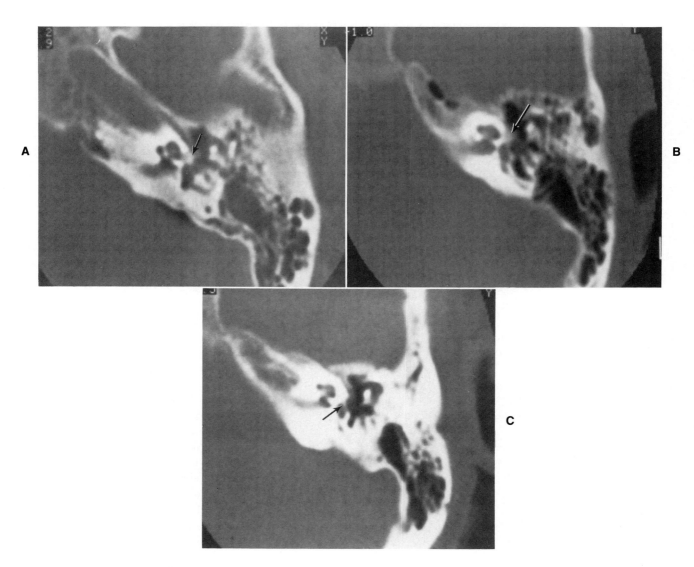

Fig. 13-123 Fenestral otosclerosis. **A-C,** Three different patients with typical anterior plaques of otosclerosis of varying sizes *(arrows).*

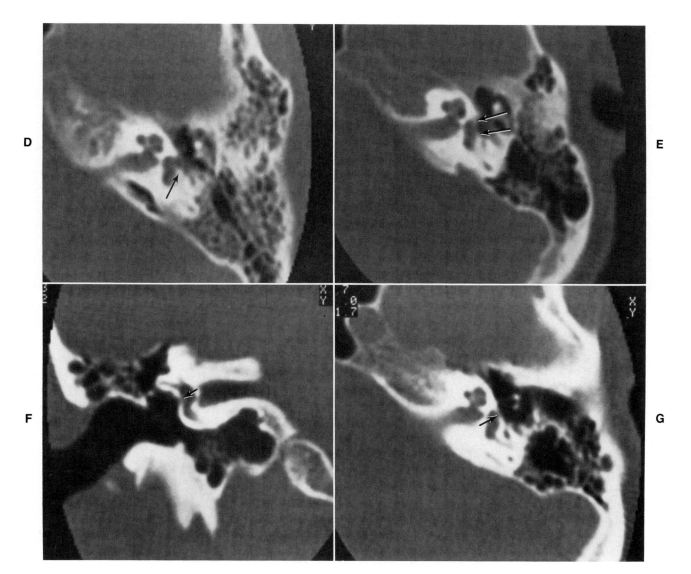

Fig. 13-123, cont'd   D, Unusual posterior plaque *(arrow).* **E,** Anterior and posterior plaques *(arrows).* **F,** Coronal and **G,** axial images demonstrate homogeneous thickening of stapes footplate/annular ligament *(arrows).* Note that this can also be seen with tympanosclerotic involvement of oval window in individuals with postinflammatory ossicular fixation.

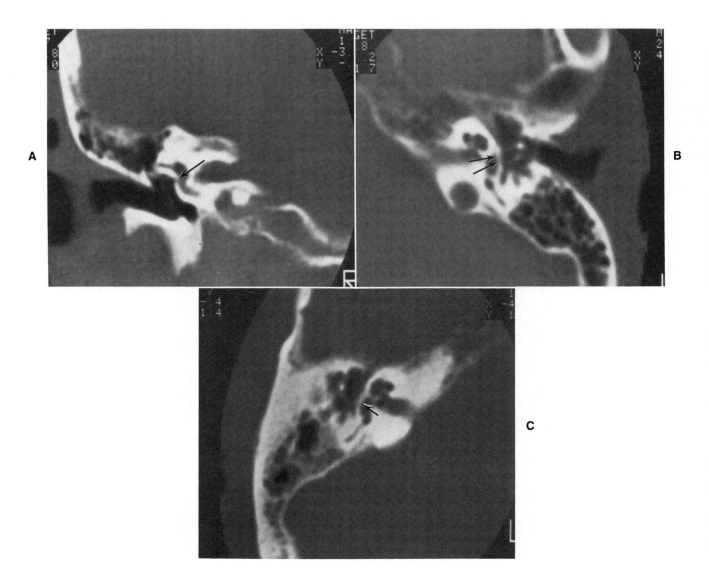

Fig. 13-124 Fenestral otosclerosis, obliterative. **A,** Coronal section and **B,** axial section demonstrates remarkable bony overgrowth in oval window niche. **C,** Axial image, right ear (different patient). Again, notice heaped up bone in right oval window *(arrow)*.

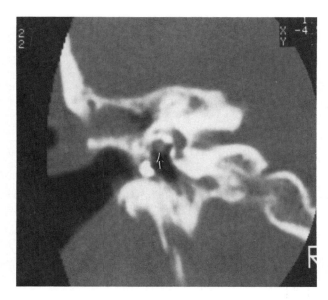

Fig. 13-125 Facial nerve dehiscence. Coronal image demonstrates soft tissue fullness *(arrow)* beneath lateral semicircular canal. This represents dehiscence of tympanic segment of facial nerve canal.

CT evaluation of the round window, facial nerve canal, jugular foramen, and cochlear aqueduct are always necessary for satisfactory preoperative examination.[61] Round window obliteration secondary to otosclerosis is unusual but does occur (see Fig. 13-119, *A* and *C*). Many surgeons will not operate in this circumstance since it will quite likely compromise the surgical results. Facial nerve dehiscence may be appreciated with CT, and preoperative demonstration of this anomaly is very desirable as well (Fig. 13-125).[62] Both of these circumstances are best appreciated in the coronal plane. Profuse flow of CSF following oval window manipulation (the *"stapes gusher"*) is said to occur in individuals with a large ipsilateral cochlear aqueduct. The surgical hazard of a dehiscent jugular vein is obvious.

REFERENCES

1. Zimmerman RA et al: Magnetic resonance imaging in temporal bone fracture, Neuroradiology 29(3):246, 1987.
2. Hasso AN, Vignaud J, and Bird CH: Pathology of the temporal bone and mastoid. In Newton TH, Hasso AH, and Dillon WP: Computed tomography of the head and neck, vol 3, Modern neuroradiology, New York, 1988, Raven Press. Chapter 5.
3. Holland BA and Brant-Zawadski M: High resolution CT of temporal bone trauma, AJNR 5:291, 1984.
4. Johnson DW et al: Temporal bone trauma high resolution computed tomographic evaluation, Radiology 151:411, 1984.
5. Lipkin AF, Bryan RN, and Jenkins HA: Pneumolabyrinth after temporal bone fracture: documentation by high resolution CT, AJNR 6(2):294, 1985.
6. Manzioni JV, Rumbaugh CL, and Katzberg RW: Direct sagittal computed tomography of the temporal bone, J Assis Tomogr 9:419, 1985.
7. Schubiger O et al: Temporal bone fractures and their complications: examination with high resolution CT, Neuroradiology 28(2):93, 1986.
8. Swartz JD et al: CT evaluation of the middle ear and mastoid for post-traumatic hearing loss, Ann Otol Rhinol Laryngol 94:263, 1985.
9. Swartz JD et al: Computer tomography of the disarticulated incus, Laryngoscope 96(11):1207, 1986.
10. Wright JW: Trauma of the ear, Radiol Clin North Am 12(3):527, 1974.
11. Lindeman RC: Temporal bone trauma and facial paralysis, Otolaryngol Clin North Am 12:403, 1979.
12. Fisch U: Facial paralysis and fractures of the petrous bone, Laryngoscope 84:2141, 1974.
13. Hough JVD: Otologic trauma. In Paparella MM and Shumrick DA, editors: Otolaryngology, vol 2, The ear, ed 2, Philadelphia, 1980, WB Saunders Co pp 1656-1679.
14. McCabe BF: Injuries to the facial nerve, Laryngoscope 82:1891, 1972.
15. Brooks BG and Graham MD: Post traumatic cholesteatoma of the external auditory canal, Laryngoscope 94:667-670, 1984.
16. Freeman J: Temporal bone fractures and cholesteatoma, Ann Otol Rhinol Laryngol 92(6):558, 1983.
17. Aquilar EA III et al: High resolution CT scan of temporal bone fractures: association of facial nerve paralysis with temporal bone fractures, Head Neck Surg 9(3):162, 1987.
18. Harker LA and McCabe BF: Temporal bone fractures and facial nerve injury, Otolaryngol Clin North Am 7:425, 1974.
19. Tos M: Course of and sequela to 248 petrosal fractures, Acta Otolaryngol 75:353, 1973.
20. Cannon CR and Jahrsdoerfer JA: Temporal bone fractures: review of 90 cases, Arch Otolaryngol 109:285, 1983.
21. Neely JG, Neblett CR, and Rose JE: Diagnosis and treatment of spontaneous cerebrospinal fluid otorrhea, Laryngoscope 92(6):608, 1982.
22. Althaus SR: Perilymph fistulae, Laryngoscope 91:531, 1982.
23. Swartz JD et al: Stapes prosthesis: evaluation with CT, Radiology 158:179, 1986.
24. Goodwin WJ: Temporal bone fractures, Radiol Clin North Am 16:651, 1983.
25. Schuknecht HF: Pathology of the ear, Boston, 1974, Harvard University Press, pp 291-318.
26. Swartz JD: High resolution CT of the middle ear and mastoid. I. Normal anatomy including normal variations, Radiology 148:449, 1983.
27. Bellucci RJ: Traumatic injuries of the middle ear, Otolaryngol Clin North Am 16:633, 1983.
28. Swartz JD: Imaging of the temporal bone: a text/atlas, New York, 1986, Thieme Medical Publishers, Inc.
29. Goodhill V: Ear: diseases, deafness and dizziness, New York, 1979, Harper & Row, Publishers, Inc, pp 388-457.
30. Gussen R: Early Paget's disease of the labyrinthine capsule, Arch Otolaryngol 91:341, 1970.
31. Najer GT: Paget's disesae of the temporal bone, Ann Otol Rhinol Laryngol 84 (suppl 22):1, 1975.
32. Schuknecht HF: Pathology of the ear, Boston, 1974, Harvard University Press, pp 351-414.
33. Hasso AN, Vignaud J, and Bird CH: Pathology of the temporal bone and mastoid. In Newton TH, Hasso AH, and Dillon WP, editors: Computed tomography of the head and neck, vol 3, Modern neuroradiology, New York, 1988, Raven Press. Chapter 5.
34. Swartz JD et al: High resolution computed tomography. 6. Craniofacial Paget's disease and fibrous dysplasia, Head Neck Surg 8(1):40, 1985.
35. Swartz JD: Imaging of the temporal bone: a text/atlas, New York, 1986, Thieme Medical Publishers, Inc.

36. Vignaud J, Jardin C, and Rosen L: The ear: diagnostic imaging, New York, 1986, Masson Publishing USA, Inc.

37. Valvassori GE: Otodystrophies. In Barrett A, Brunner S, and Valvassori GE, editors: Modern thin section tomography, Springfield, Ill, 1973, Charles C Thomas, Publisher, pp 109-117.

38. Barrionuevo CE et al: Fibrous dysplasia and the temporal bone, Arch Otolaryngol 106:298, 1980.

39. Cohen A and Rosenwasser H: Fibrous dysplasia of the temporal bone, Arch Otolaryngol 89:39, 1969.

40. Smouha EE, Edelstein DR, and Parisier SC: Fibrous dysplasia of the temporal bone: report of three new cases, Am J Otol 8(2):103, 1987.

41. Cunningham MJ, Curtin HD, and Butkiewicz BL: Histiocytosis X of the temporal bone: CT findings, J Comp Assist Tomogr 12(7):70, 1988.

41a. Bartynski WS, Barnes PD, and Wallman JK: Cranial CT of autosomal recessive osteopetrosis, AJNR 10:543, 1989.

42. Valvassori GE: Otosclerosis, Otolaryngol Clin North Am 6(2):379, 1973.

43. Lindsay JR: Otosclerosis. In Paparella MM and Shumrick DA, editors: Otolaryngology, vol 2, The ear, ed 2, Philadelphia, 1980, WB Saunders Co, pp 1617-1644.

44. Ruedi L: Pathognesis of otosclerosis, Arch Otolaryngol 78:469, 1963.

45. Rovsing H: Otosclerosis: fenestral and cochlear, Radiol Clin North Am 12:505, 1974.

46. Mafee MF et al: Use of CT in stapedial otosclerosis, Radiology 156:709, 1985.

47. Swartz JD et al: Cochlear otosclerosis (otospongiosis): CT analysis with audiometric correlation, Radiology 155:147, 1985.

48. Swartz JD et al: Fenestral and cochlear otosclerosis: CT evaluation, Am J Otol 6(6):476, 1985.

49. Balkany TJ, Dreisbach JN, and Seibert CE: Radiographic imaging of the cochlear implant candidate: preliminary results, Otolaryngol Head Neck Surg 95(5):592, 1986.

50. Ball JB Jr, Miller GW, and Hepfner ST: Computed tomography of single channel cochlear implants, AJNR 7:41, 1986.

51. Harnsberger HR et al: Cochlear implant candidates: assessment with CT and MR imaging, Radiology 164:53, 1987.

52. O'Donoghue GM et al: Cochlear implantation in children: the problem of head growth, Otolaryngol Head Neck Surg 94(1):78, 1986.

53. Antoli-Candela F Jr, McGill T, and Peron D: Histopathological observations on the cochlear changes in otosclerosis, Ann Otol Rhinol Laryngol 86:813, 1977.

54. Parahy C and Linthicum FH: Otosclerosis: relationship of spiral ligament hyalinization to sensorineural hearing loss, Laryngoscope 93:717, 1983.

55. Swartz JD et al: Labyrinthine ossification: CT appearance and possible etiology, Radiology 157:395, 1985.

56. Valvassori GE: CT densitometry in otosclerosis, Adv Otorhinolaryngol 37:47, 1987.

57. Valvassori GE and Dobben GD: CT densitometry of the cochlear capsule in otosclerosis, AJNR 6:661, 1985.

58. Bretlau P: Relationship of the otosclerotic focus to the fistula antefenestrum, J Otolaryngol Otol 83:1187, 1959.

59. Swartz JD et al: Stapes prosthesis: CT evaluation, Radiology 158:179, 1986.

60. Mafee MF et al: Use of CT in stapedial otosclerosis, Radiology 156:709, 1985.

61. Swartz JD et al: Fenestral otosclerosis: significance of preoperative CT evaluation, Radiology 151:703, 1984.

62. Swartz JD: The facial nerve canal: CT analysis of the protruding tympanic segment, Radiology 153:443, 1984.

SECTION SIX

TUMORS OF THE TEMPORAL BONE AND THE CEREBELLOPONTINE ANGLE

WILLIAM W.M. LO

CLINICAL OVERVIEW

A discussion of tumors of the temporal bone is not complete without including tumors of the cerebellopontine (CP) angle. The fifth through twelfth cranial nerves exit the posterior cranial fossa either through the temporal bone or immediately adjacent to it. Clinically, in most cases presentations of tumors of the temporal bone are similar to those of tumors of the CP angle. Radiologically, therefore, when searching for tumors of the temporal bone, lesions of the CP angle should also be considered.

The temporal bone and the CP angle form the junctional region where neurosurgery and otology overlap.[1,2] In neurotology, the most common clinical problems that warrant radiologic evaluation for a possible tumor include:

1. Investigation of the CP angle syndrome in search of an acoustic neuroma or one of the other tumors of this region.
2. Investigation of pulsatile tinnitus or the jugular foramen syndrome in search of a paraganglioma or one of the other tumors or vascular lesions of the region (see preceding discussion on imaging).
3. Investigation of peripheral facial nerve dysfunction in search of a tumor.
4. Investigation of other tumors of the temporal bone whether they are visible or invisible externally.

Each of these clinical settings points out different differential diagnostic possibilities. The following discussions will be organized with these settings in mind.

IMAGING OVERVIEW

Historically, the investigation of acoustic schwannomas (neuromas) and other tumors of the CP angle and temporal bone has progressed through plain films,[3] tomography,[4] pneumoencephalography,[5] positive contrast meatocisternography,[6] and angiography.[7] With all of these modalities, the diagnosis made was based on indirect signs such as erosion and displacement of either vessels or contrast material.

Modern imaging uses predominantly either magnetic resonance imaging (MRI) or computed tomography (CT), both of which image the lesions directly. They are supplemented in selected cases by angiography. These newer modalities have been indispensable allies to the recent advances in surgical management of temporal bone tumors,[8] and the imaging discussions in this section will be solely directed to them.

A retrospective study of 75 CP angle and petromastoid masses by Gentry et al compared the diagnosis made by MRI and CT and showed that *both* modalities were accurate and had similar abilities for detecting a wide variety of masses including those of neoplastic, nonneoplastic, or vascular origin.[9] MRI was often more helpful for characterization of neuromas, epidermoid cysts, exophytic gliomas, and vascular lesions, while CT was usually more informative for meningiomas, metastases, and tympanomastoid cholesteatomas.[9]

For the investigation of vestibulocochlear symptoms when a retrocochlear lesion is suspected, MRI is the imaging method of choice. When a labyrinthine or cochlear lesion is suspected, high-resolution CT with bone detail is appropriate.[10]

MRI is preferred over CT for the investigation of other cranial nerve dysfunctions; and if the MRI examination is normal, no other diagnostic studies are usually performed.

On the other hand, for the investigation of pulsatile tinnitus, conductive hearing loss, or a retrotympanic mass, which suggest the presence of a paraganglioma or a vascular anomaly, high-resolution CT is preferred over MRI. If a mass lesion is found localized within the tympanic cavity or if a vascular anomaly is recognized, no other imaging is usually needed.

Angiography is usually reserved for the detection of arterial stenotic lesions and arteriovenous fistulae, for the evaluation of tumor vascularity, and for preoperative embolization.

MRI and CT, however, must not be considered mutually exclusive. Each may be employed to supplement the other whenever indicated for problem-solving. For example, if the differentiation between a CP angle meningioma or epidermoid is not conclusive on MRI, one should not hesitate to use CT to determine the lesion's attenuation (density), degree of enhancement, and presence of calcification and/or hyperostosis.[9] Conversely, MRI may be used to supplement CT by better defining or to determine the extent of a paraganglioma.[11]

ACOUSTIC SCHWANNOMAS (NEUROMAS)
Incidence and Terms

Acoustic schwannomas account for about 8% to 10% of all intracranial tumors[12] and about 60% to 90% of all CP angle tumors (Table 13-5).[13,14] They are slightly more common in women.[15] Most of the tumors appear in patients between 30 and 70 years of age, with the majority of lesions occurring in those between 40 and 60 years of age.[15] Occasionally these tumors appear in young adults,[16] or children without any of the stigmata of neurofibromatosis.[17]

Although more than 25 names, including commonly used ones such as neurinoma, neurilemmoma, and neuroma, have been applied to the acoustic nerve tumor, most authorities regard *schwannoma* as the most appropriate term.[12,18-20]

Pathology

A schwannoma is a benign, slowly growing, encapsulated neoplasm that originates in the nerve sheath and is composed of Schwann cells in a collagenous matrix.[18,19] The neurofibroma is a benign, relatively circumscribed, nonencapsulated neoplasm that is composed of proliferating axons and Schwann cells.[18,19] The absence of a capsule, Verocay bodies, hyaline thickening of vascular walls, and Antoni A and B growth patterns are features that distinguish a neurofibroma from a schwannoma. However, in some cases these two benign nerve sheath tumors cannot be pathologically differentiated.

For unexplained reasons, schwannomas arise from the acoustic nerve much more often than from any other cranial nerve; and the vestibular division is more commonly involved than the cochlear division.[20]

Since the glial-Schwann cell junction of the acoustic nerve lies (with some variation) near the internal acoustic porus and since schwannomas may arise from any portion of the nerve between this zone of transition and the fundus of the internal auditory canal (IAC),[12,21] these acoustic tumors may arise within the IAC, at the porus, or occasionally in the cistern.

A schwannoma is typically composed of Antoni type A and type B tissue. Type A tissue is a compact tissue that has elongated spindle cells in irregular streams, often having a tendency to form palisades. Type B tissue, often intermingled with type A, is characterized by a loose texture, often with cyst formation. Microcystic and less commonly macrocystic changes and hemor-

Table 13-5   Classification and frequency of cerebellopontine angle lesions

	Revilla (1947)		Brackmann (1980)		Valavanis (1987)	
	No.	**%**	**No.**	**%**	**No.**	**%**
Primary tumors of the cerebellopontine angle						
Acoustic schwannoma	154	75.1	1236	91.3	275	60.5
Meningioma	13	6.3	42	3.1	31	6.8
Epidermoid	13	6.3	32	2.4	17	3.7
Arachnoid cyst	—	—	7	0.5	9	2.0
Schwannoma of the fifth, seventh, ninth, tenth, and eleventh nerves	10	4.9	19	1.4	18	4.0
Primary melanoma	1	0.5	—	—	1	0.2
Hemangioma	—	—	4	0.3	3	0.7
Lipoma, dermoid, teratoma	—	—	5	0.4	—	—
Secondary tumors of the cerebellopontine angle						
Paraganglioma	1	0.5	—	—	47	10.3
Ceruminoma	—	—	—	—	1	0.2
Chondroma-chondrosarcoma	—	—	1	0.1	2	0.4
Chordoma	—	—	—	—	8	1.8
Extension of cerebellar and petrous bone tumors	13	6.4	5	0.4	6	1.3
Metastases	—	—	3	0.2	12	2.6
Vascular lesions						
Aneurysm	—	—	—	—	4	0.9
Arteriovenous malformation	—	—	—	—	4	0.9
Vertebrobasilar dolichoectasia	—	—	—	—	17	3.7

rhage characteristically develop in type B tissue.[12,20] Most acoustic schwannomas consist of predominantly type A tissue.[20] The tumor's cellularity tends to decrease and the degenerative changes and vascularity tend to increase with increasing size of lesion.[15] Kasantikul et al have also noted the common presence of a hemangiomatous component.[15]

Not only are acoustic schwannomas more common in women, but in females they are also larger and more vascular. Acceleration of symptoms and tumor growth have been noted in patients who become pregnant.[22]

Malignant schwannomas are extremely rare and are usually seen in patients with neurofibromatosis 1.[20,23,24] An astrocytoma arising in the glial portion of the acoustic nerve has also been reported.[25]

Bilateral Acoustic Schwannomas

The neurofibromatoses consist of at least two distinct disorders, the genes for which are located on separate chromosomes.[24,26,27] Von Recklinghausen's neurofibromatosis, which manifests primarily "peripherally" and is now called *neurofibromatosis 1*, affects approximately 100,000 people in the United States. Bilateral acoustic neurofibromatosis, which manifests primarily "centrally" and is now called *neurofibromatosis 2*, affects several thousand Americans. Both of these disorders may be inherited as an autosomal-dominant trait or acquired by spontaneous mutation.

Patients with neurofibromatosis 1 are characterized by multiple brown skin macules (cafe-au-lait spots), in-

tertriginous freckling, iris hamartomas (Lisch nodules), multiple neurofibromas (especially plexiform neurofibromas), optic gliomas, and distinctive osseous lesions.[23,24] They may have Schwann cell tumors on any nerve, but an estimated 5% or fewer have acoustic tumors.[23,28,29]

Patients with neurofibromatosis 2 are characterized by bilateral acoustic schwannomas (96%) commonly accompanied by other Schwann cell tumors and multiple meningiomas, neurofibromas, and glial tumors,[24,30] but *not* optic gliomas or the malignant tumor degeneration, which occurs in neurofibromatosis 1 (Fig. 13-126).[29,31]

Compared to unilateral schwannomas, bilateral acoustic schwannomas tend to develop early. Many appear before the age of 21 years.[32] About half of the affected individuals are symptomatic by the age of 25 years.[29] They present a formidable challenge to surgical management.[32,33] Early detection and early resection appear to offer the best hope of hearing preservation.[34] MRI screening at an early age (10 to 12 years) in all children with an appropriate family history[24] has been recommended regardless of the auditory-brainstem response (Fig. 13-127).[34] Careful evaluation of the contralateral ear of young patients (under 30 years of age) with unilateral acoustic schwannoma is advised. Blood relatives of either patients with bilateral acoustic schwannomas or of those with unilateral tumor with early onset should also be screened. Routinely including the cervical spine in the imaging examination of these patients may also be appropriate.[24]

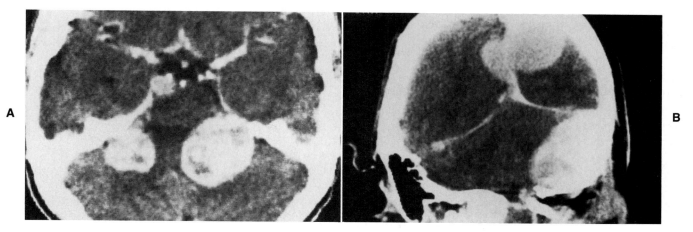

Fig. 13-126 Neurofibromatosis 2. **A,** Postcontrast CT. Bilateral acoustic and right trigeminal schwannoma. **B,** Postcontrast CT. Multiple meningiomas. (**A** reprinted from House JW and O'Conner AF, eds. Handbook of neurotological diagnosis, New York and Basel, Marcel Dekker, Inc., 1987. p. 290.)

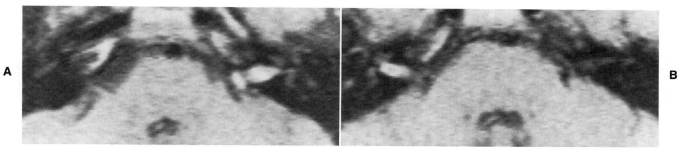

Fig. 13-127 Neurofibromatosis 2. **A** and **B,** Post-gadolinium T_1-weighted images. Bilateral intracanalicular acoustic schwannomas in a 12-year-old girl with the left-sided lesion protruding 4 mm into the CP angle cistern. Note that **A** and **B** are 4-mm sections overlapping by 1 mm. Each tumor was detected by only one of the sections.

Clinical Evaluation

The most common symptoms caused by acoustic schwannomas are those from pressure on the cochlear and vestibular divisions of the acoustic nerve, namely, sensorineural hearing loss, tinnitus, and disequilibrium.[35] The symptoms are usually slowly progressive and measured in months or years. The median duration is about 2 years in one series.[15] The duration of symptoms is not necessarily correlated with tumor size. In fact, some authors have noted an inverse correlation.[15] About 10% of acoustic schwannomas have only tinnitus as a presenting symptom.*

Facial nerve manifestations such as twitching or weakness are relatively uncommon.[36,37] Instead, larger

tumors are more likely to cause trigeminal manifestations, such as facial numbness and loss of corneal reflex.[35] Still larger tumors may cause deficits of the lower cranial nerves, cerebellar signs and symptoms, or signs and symptoms of hydrocephalus.[37]

Rarely an acoustic schwannoma, usually a large one, has presented as a subarachnoid hemorrhage.[38-41]

Among the commonly employed clinical laboratory tests, brainstem electric response audiometry (BERA), with a diagnostic accuracy of 98%, is the most sensitive preimaging test for acoustic schwannoma.[42] A normal BERA virtually, although not invariably, excludes such a tumor. A combination of BERA and contrast-enhanced CT identifies up to 99% of acoustic schwannomas.[43]

Until MRI became widely available, the diagnostic

---

*Derald E. Brackmann, M.D., personal communication.

steps typically included history and physical examination, audiogram, brainstem evoked response, CT with contrast, and then if necessary gas-CT cisternogram.[44,45] In recent years MRI has been found to be more sensitive than CT with contrast and comparable to gas-CT cisternogram in the detection of small acoustic neuromas.[14,46-49] With the availability of IV gadolinium DTPA as a paramagnetic contrast agent, MRI is now clearly the imaging method of choice.[50]

Treatment

The accepted treatment for acoustic schwannoma is surgical resection whenever feasible. With microsurgery, total tumor removal and functional preservation of the facial nerve with low morbidity and mortality is now the rule.[51,52] In the last decade attention has been focused on hearing preservation.[53-58] It is generally agreed that hearing preservation is more successful with removal of small tumors than large tumors.[34,57] Early detection therefore continues to be emphasized. High-quality CT and MRI contribute immeasurably to these goals.

For the treatment of acoustic tumors, there are basically three surgical approaches: translabyrinthine, suboccipital and middle (cranial) fossa, and a number of variations and combinations thereof.[2,59-62] Generally, small tumors with preservation of hearing are operated on using the middle fossa or the suboccipital approach. Some surgeons prefer the translabyrinthine approach for tumors of all sizes. Others prefer the suboccipital approach in most cases.

No consensus exists on the definition for grading the size of these tumors.[15,54,56,60-63] One might consider those tumors that are intracanalicular or that extend up to 0.5 cm into the cerebellopontine angle cistern as small tumors; those with 0.5 to 2 cm cisternal components, medium tumors; those with 2 to 4 cm cisternal components, large tumors; and those greater than 4 cm, giant tumors.

Acoustic tumors in high-risk or elderly patients have been followed by annual CT or MRI scanning until their growth rates have been determined.[64,65] They are quite variable. Although some tumors grew as much as 1 cm per year (mainly in the initial year of study), most grew only 0.2 cm per year.[64] However, in one series of 23 patients over 60 years of age, initially monitored without surgery, 20% did require resection or ventriculoperitoneal shunt placement within one third of their expected survival time.[65] The subsequent tumor growth did not depend on the size at presentation, but all patients who required surgery had tumors measuring at least 2.5 cm. In a series of 116 patients over 65 years of age who had acoustic tumor surgery, with all but 10 having total tumor removal, the operative mortality rate was less than 1%.[66]

Alternatively, acoustic tumors, especially in high-risk patients and those with bilateral tumors, may be treated by stereotactic radiosurgery using sharply collimated and focused cobalt-60 sources.[67]

CT and MRI Appearance

Size, Location, and Configuration. Acoustic schwannomas have been reported to range from a few millimeters to 5 to 6 cm (Figs. 13-127 to 13-133).[68] At our institution tumors as large as 8 cm, with generally smooth surfaces, have been encountered.

A small percentage of the acoustic schwannomas are entirely intracanalicular, in which case they are usually cylindrical in shape, less than 1 cm in length, filling the IAC, and showing a convex medial border (Figs. 13-128 and 13-129).[69] The majority of the medium-sized schwannomas have a spherical cisternal component up to 2 cm in diameter centered at the acoustic porus and a stem extending into the IAC expanding the porus to a funnel shape. The overall appearance of the tumor resembles an ice-cream cone or a mushroom (Fig. 13-130). A tumor between 2 and 4 cm may be considered a large one. Some of the larger tumors are ovoid or slightly lobulated. Their petrous surface remains centered to the acoustic porus and their long axis lies par-

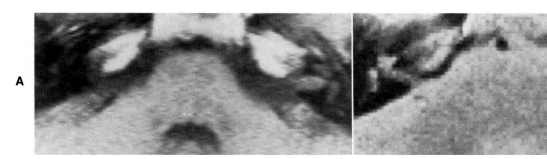

A   **B**

Fig. 13-128 Typical intracanalicular acoustic schwannoma. **A,** Intermediate weighted image. **B,** T$_2$-weighted images. Tumor is isointense with brain and well seen on **A** but isointense with CSF and completely obscured by the latter on **B**.

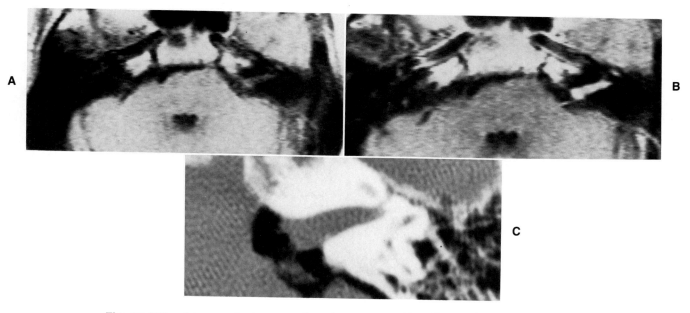

Fig. 13-129   Intracanalicular acoustic schwannoma with a 5-mm cisternal component. **A** and **B,** T$_1$-weighted images pre- and post-gadolinium. **C,** Gas-CT cisternogram. The full extent of the tumor is more positively displayed on **B** than on **C.**

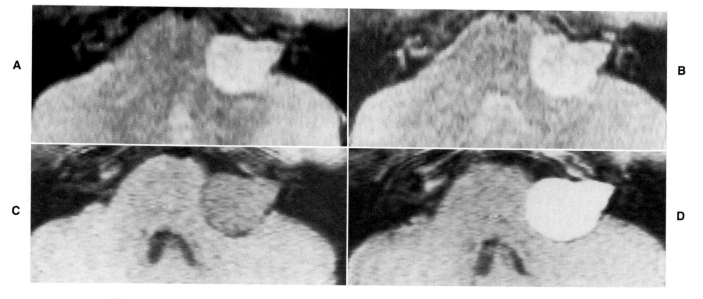

Fig. 13-130   Typical medium-sized acoustic schwannoma. **A** and **B,** Intermediate and T$_2$-weighted images. A moderately hyperintense, smoothly marginated mass mushrooming out of the IAC into the CPA enlarging the porus. **C** and **D,** T$_1$-weighted images, pre- and post-gadolinium. The tumor is isointense to mildly hypointense and enhances strongly postcontrast. Note the smoothness of the tumor surface and the CSF cleft and/or vessels between the tumor and the brain.

allel to the petrous surface (Fig. 13-131). The very large or "giant" tumors often have arisen from the cisternal portion of the nerve and possess little or no canalicular component. The vast majority (85%) of the schwannomas show acute angles at the bone-tumor interface, in contrast to meningiomas, which tend to show obtuse angles (75%) (Fig. 13-134).[70] Acoustic schwannomas seldom, if ever, herniate through the tentorium (Fig. 13-132).[21]

CT Density. On unenhanced CT, the majority (64%) of acoustic schwannomas are isodense with the adjacent cerebellum and not discernible without IV contrast.[70] The remaining ones are either slightly hypodense or hyperdense. A few show mixed density. Calcification or detectable hemorrhage is rare in untreated tumors.[68] However, intratumoral hemorrhage has been seen on CT (Fig. 13-133).[40]

CT contrast enhancement occurs in nearly 90% of untreated tumors.[68] The enhancement is usually homogeneous and dense. Most acoustic schwannomas enhance early.[71,72] The enhancement declines rapidly within 15 minutes after completion of contrast effusion and then less rapidly within the next 45 minutes, although residual enhancement may remain for hours.

Some tumors, however, show irregular central lucencies or inhomogeneity in enhancement (Figs. 13-126, 13-131, and 13-132). The initially unenhanced portions of the schwannoma may take many minutes to attain enhancement (see Fig. 13-147). In our experience, tumors with such an appearance contain prominent cystic components noted at surgery. Loss of contrast enhancement is common after stereotactic radiosurgery.[67]

Rarely, an arachnoid cyst develops around a tumor and may even become the dominant lesion.[73]

MRI Intensity. On MRI, as on CT, small and medium acoustic schwannomas are most likely to be homogeneous, and large tumors are most likely to contain internal zones of inhomogeneity (Figs. 13-126 to 13-132).[14]

On T_1-weighted images schwannomas are usually isointense or mildly hypointense relative to the pons and hyperintense to CSF. On T_2-weighted images they are mildly hyperintense to the pons and nearly isointense to CSF.[48-50,74,75]

Thus tumors large enough to deform the pons are readily recognizable on both T_1- and T_2-weighted images. Tumors too small to deform the pons stand out well against the hypointense CSF on T_1-weighted images but are often obscured by the isointense CSF on T_2-weighted images (Fig. 13-128).[50,74,76]

Displaced tributaries of petrosal and capsular veins, difficult if not impossible to see on CT, are often recognizable on MRI in medium and large tumors (Fig. 13-133).[50] Intratumoral hemorrhage at various stages of hemoglobin breakdown may also be detected on MRI.[77]

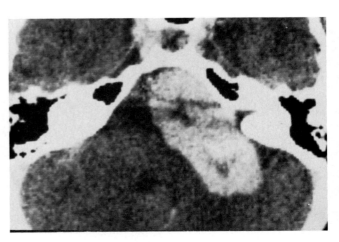

Fig. 13-131 Large acoustic schwannoma. Postcontrast CT. Tumor is entirely in cistern, is ovoid, and contains small poorly enhancing cystic components. (Reprinted from House JW and O'Conner AF, eds.: Handbook of neurotological diagnosis. New York and Basel, Marcel Dekker, Inc., 1987, p 287.)

Acoustic schwannomas enhance intensely after intravenous administration of gadolinium-DTPA on T_1-weighted spin-echo images (Figs. 13-129, 13-130, and 13-132).[78] In one series the smallest intracanalicular tumors seen on noncontrast MRIs measured 3 × 7 mm. With gadolinium enhancement the smallest measured 3 × 3 mm.[50]

As a group, acoustic schwannomas enhance substantially more than meningiomas, neurofibromas, and paragangliomas on T_1-weighted spin-echo images (Fig. 13-130).[79] However, enhancement varies greatly in tumors of the same type and overlaps among different tumor types. Unless enhancement is marked, it is of limited value in differentiating schwannomas from other extraaxial tumors.[79]

Secondary Changes. Being extraaxial as they grow, acoustic schwannomas enlarge toward the pontocerebellar junction and displace the brainstem away from the side of the tumor. Indirect signs of an extraaxial mass (such as widening of the ipsilateral cerebellopontine angle and the quadrigeminal cisterns, narrowing of the contralateral cisterns, and displacement and compression of the fourth ventricle) accompany the larger tumors (Figs. 13-131 to 13-133). Acoustic schwannomas, however, do not extend anterosuperiorly above the dorsum,[21] and, unlike meningiomas, extremely rarely herniate into the middle fossa (Fig. 13-132).

The incidence of hydrocephalus correlates roughly with tumor size (Fig. 13-132). One report noted hydrocephalus in 17 of 44 patients in whom a 3 cm or larger tumor was present.[80]

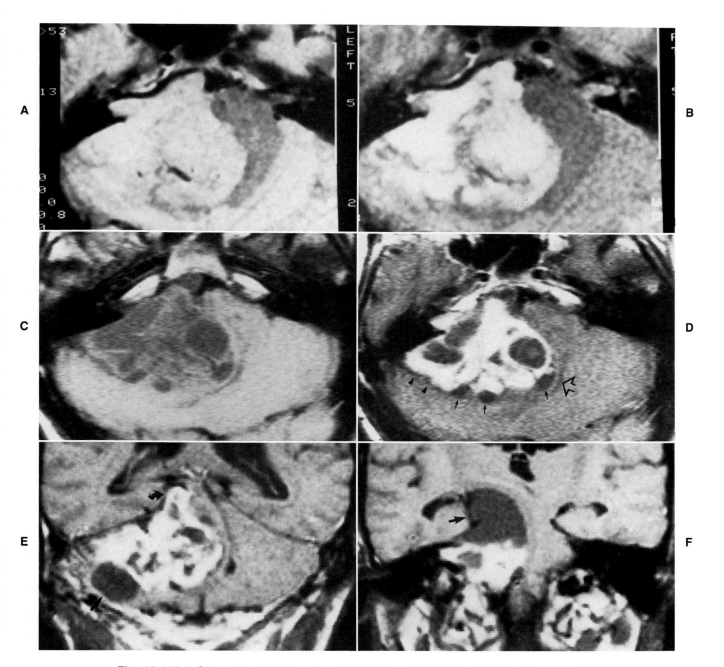

Fig. 13-132 Giant cystic acoustic schwannoma with arachnoid cysts. **A** and **B,** Intermediate and T$_2$-weighted images. Cystic components are not readily apparent on intermediate and T$_2$-weighted images. Note flow void in a vessel within the tumor. **C** and **D,** T$_1$-weighted images pre- and post-gadolinium. Cystic components are much more apparent on T$_1$-weighted images and are at least partially enhancing. Note superficial arachnoid cysts *(arrows),* CSF cleft *(arrowheads),* compressed fourth ventricle *(open arrow)* and narrowed contralateral cistern. **E** and **F,** T$_1$-weighted coronal images post-gadolinium. Transtentorial herniation *(curved arrow)* of acoustic schwannoma is extremely rare. Most of the herniating component in this lesion is constituted by surface arachnoid cyst *(arrow).* Note associated hydrocephalus.

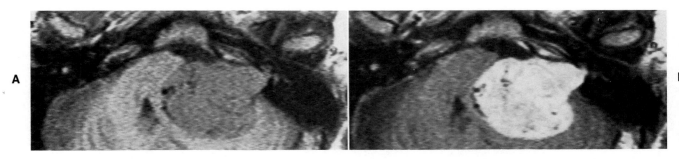

Fig. 13-133 Large acoustic schwannoma. T_1-weighted images. **A,** Pre-gadolinium image and **B,** post-gadolinium image. Note serpentine flow voids of vessels in relatively vascular tumor and displaced tributaries of petrosal and capsular veins on surface of the tumor.

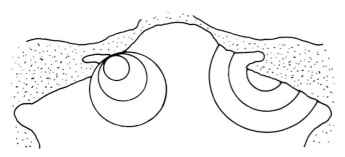

Fig. 13-134 Diagrammatic representation of typical configurations of acoustic schwannoma versus CPA meningioma. Schwannoma: spherical mass centered to porus with acute bone-tumor angles. Meningioma: hemispheric mass eccentric to porus with obtuse bone-tumor angles. (Reprinted from House JW and O'Conner AF: Handbook of neurotological diagnosis, New York, 1987, Marcel Dekker, Inc, p 296.)

Edema of the adjacent brain may be associated with large acoustic schwannomas.[14,68]

Bone changes associated with acoustic schwannomas are limited to the internal auditory canal (Figs. 13-130, 13-132, 13-133). Using the criteria of a difference over 2 mm in widths, a shortening of over 3 mm in length of the posterior wall of the canal, downward displacement of the crista, and focal erosion, Valvassori found abnormal internal auditory canals on polytomography in 78% of surgically verified tumors.[4] On high-resolution CT, the incidence of bone changes are probably comparable or higher. Tumors arising from the intracanalicular portion of the nerve typically cause flaring of the porus acousticus as they enlarge (Figs. 13-130, 13-132, 13-133), whereas those arising from the cisternal portion may cause little or no erosion (Fig. 13-131).

It should be remembered that bilateral enlargement of the IAC in the absence of intracanalicular tumors may be seen in neurofibromatosis.[81,82] Unilateral asymmetry may also be seen on rare occasions.[83]

DIFFERENTIAL DIAGNOSIS OF TUMORS OF INTERNAL AUDITORY CANAL AND CEREBELLOPONTINE ANGLE
Statistics and Categorization

Although by far the most common tumor associated with the CP angle syndrome is the acoustic schwannoma, many other neoplastic and nonneoplastic mass lesions occur in the region (see Table 13-5).

Brackmann and Bartels, reviewing 1354 CP angle tumors, excluding paragangliomas, found 91.3% acoustic neuromas, 3.1% meningiomas, 2.4% primary cholesteatomas (epidermoids), 1.2% facial nerve neuromas, and 0.2% neuromas of other posterior fossa cranial nerves. There were 25 rare tumors, including 7 arachnoid cysts, 4 hemangiomas, 1 hemangioblastoma, 2 astrocytomas, 2 medulloblastomas, 3 metastatic tumors, 2 dermoids, 2 lipomas, 1 malignant teratoma, and 1 chondrosarcoma.[13]

Similarly, Valavanis et al, analyzing 455 CP angle lesions, found the following among the primary tumors: 60.5% acoustic neuromas; 6.8% meningiomas; 3.7% epidermoids; 2.0% arachnoid cysts; 4.0% neuromas of the fifth, seventh, ninth, tenth, and eleventh cranial nerves; 0.2% primary melanomas; and 0.7% hemangiomas. Among secondary tumors of the CP angle the following were found: 10.3% chemodectomas (paragangliomas), 0.2% germinomas, 0.4% chondromas, 1.8% chordomas, and 1.3% cerebellar and bone tumors; among vascular lesions: 0.9% aneurysms, 0.9% arteriovenous malformations, and 3.7% megadolichobasilar anomaly. There were also 2.6% metastases.[14]

Both of the above series are in substantial agreement

with the often-cited series of 205 CP angle tumors of Revilla, which consists of 75.1% acoustic neuromas, 6.3% meningiomas, 6.3% epidermoids, 4.9% nonacoustic neurinomas, 0.5% primary melanomas, 0.5% chemodectomas, and 6.4% cerebellar and petrous bone tumors infiltrating the cerebellopontine angle.[84]

Thus the four most common tumors are the same in all three series—acoustic schwannoma, meningioma, and epidermoid and nonacoustic posterior fossa schwannoma. Together they account for some 75% to 98% of all CP angle mass lesions.

Although the probability of acoustic schwannoma is 60% to 90% in a CP angle mass, the remaining possibilities are diverse and numerous. In practice, the differential diagnosis of the CP angle lesion may be simplified by arbitrarily classifying the possible lesions into groups such as the eight in Table 13-6.

Essentially there are three common extraaxial tumors (acoustic schwannoma, meningioma, and epidermoid) (Table 13-7), two groups of rare extraaxial lesions (nonacoustic posterior fossa schwannomas and vascular masses), two groups of extradural masses (paragangliomas and bone lesions), and finally the intraaxial lesions. For simplicity, such rare nonenhancing masses as lipomas, dermoids, and arachnoid and cysticercal cysts, may be placed in the same group as epidermoids.

The three most common lesions for adults—acoustic schwannoma, meningioma, and epidermoid—are the same three for upper teenagers; however, in younger children, acoustic schwannomas are extremely rare. Gliomas, which are capable of enlarging the internal acoustic canal, are the most common cause of CP angle tumors in younger children.[85]

Table 13-6 CT/MRI differential diagnostic categories of CP angle lesions

	Location	Incidence	Type
I	Extraaxial	Most common	Acoustic schwannoma
II	Extraaxial	Common	Meningioma
III	Extraaxial	Common	Epidermoid (and other cysts: arachnoid, cysticercal, dermoid)
IV	Extraaxial	Rare	Nonacoustic posterior fossa schwannomas (V, VII, IX, X, XI, XII)
V	Extraaxial	Rare	Vascular lesions (VBD,* aneurysm, AVM,† hemangioma, AICA‡ loop, siderosis)
VI	Extradural	Common	Paraganglioma
VII	Extradural	Rare	Bone lesion (benign or malignant; primary or metastatic)
VIII	Intraaxial	Rare	Astrocytoma, ependymoma, papilloma, hemangioblastoma, metastasis

*VBD = Vertebrobasilar dolichoectasia
†AVM = Arteriovenous malformation
‡AICA = Anterior inferior cerebellar artery

Table 13-7 Comparison of salient CT and MRI features of three most common CP angle lesions

	Acoustic schwannoma	Meningioma	Epidermoid tumor
Location	Centered to IAC	Posterior petrous wall, most eccentric to IAC	Anterolateral or posterolateral to brainstem
Bone changes	Most enlarging IAC	Occasional hyperostosis	Occasional erosion
Shape	Spherical or ovoid, occasionally lobulated, acute bone tumor angle	Hemispherical, rarely plaque-like, may herniate, obtuse bone tumor angle	Variable with tendency to dumbell into middle fossa or contralateral CPA
Density	Mostly isodense, a few slightly hypodense or hyperdense	Isodense or mostly slightly hyperdense, some calcified	Mostly about CSF density, rarely denser than brain, occasional peripheral calcification
CT enhancement	Moderate to marked, often with inhomogeneous enhancement	Marked and homogeneous	Nonenhancing
Intensity T_1WI	CSF < M ≤ Gr	CSF < M ≤ Gr	CSF ≤ M < Gr
Intensity T_2WI	≥ CSF	Variable	≥ CSF
MR enhancement	Marked	Moderate	Nonenhancing

T_1WI = T_1-weighted images
T_2WI = T_2-weighted images
CSF = Cerebrospinal fluid
M = Mass

IAC = Internal auditory canal
CPA = Cerebellopontine angle
GR = Gray matter

Meningioma

Meningiomas arise from the meningothelial arachnoid cell and account for 13% to 18% of all primary intracranial tumors.[19] In the cerebellopontine angle they are a distant second to acoustic schwannomas in incidence and most often the lesion offering the most difficulty in the differential diagnosis of acoustic schwannoma (Figs. 13-135 to 13-139).[13,14,70]

Like acoustic schwannomas, meningiomas are extraaxial. However, unlike acoustic schwannomas, they are usually eccentric to the porus.[86] Also unlike acoustic schwannomas, which seldom if ever herniate into the middle fossa, meningiomas frequently do (56%).[70,86,87] They may also extend into the middle fossa by growth through the tentorium (19%) or temporal bone (Fig. 13-139).[70,88] In size they are usually moderate to large when compared to acoustic schwannomas.[9]

Meningiomas are almost always broad-based against a dural surface such as the posterior petrous wall. Their configurations fall generally into three groups. Unlike acoustic schwannomas, which are by and large spherical or ovoid, most of them are hemispherical (Figs. 13-136, 13-137).[86] Consequently, most of them (75%) show obtuse bone tumor angles while schwannomas tend to show acute angles (85%) (Fig. 13-134).[70] Some meningiomas appear nearly rounded and are more difficult to distinguish from schwannomas by configuration. A few are plaque-like (en plaque) (Figs. 13-138 and 13-139).

On CT meningiomas are isodense (31%) or, more often, hyperdense (69%) (Fig. 13-136, A).[70] Furthermore, unlike schwannomas, they are often calcified (25%), usually homogeneous, and sometimes dense.[70,88] Over 90% show homogeneous enhancement inversely proportional to their precontrast density.[70]

An analysis of 16 CP angle meningiomas by Gentry et al shows that they are isointense or slightly hypointense to gray matter on T_1-weighted images but are extremely variable in intensity on T_2-weighted images, more so than any other CP angle mass lesion (Figs. 13-137 to 13-139).[9] In their experience, when the intensity of a mass was equal to or less than that of gray matter on T_2-weighted images, meningioma was the most likely diagnosis.[9] Otherwise, intensity as a diagnostic criterion for meningioma is far less helpful than location and configuration. The wide variation of signal intensity among meningiomas appears to reflect the diversity of histopathology in meningiomas. Tumors significantly hypointense to brain cortex tend to be composed primarily of fibrous or transitional elements. Tumors significantly hyperintense to brain cortex tend to be composed primarily of syncytial or angioblastic elements.[89,90]

Other MRI findings in meningioma include marginal pial blood vessels manifesting as surface flow voids, surface CSF spaces or clefts, and arterial feeders to the tumor seen as arborizing flow-voids as in schwannomas

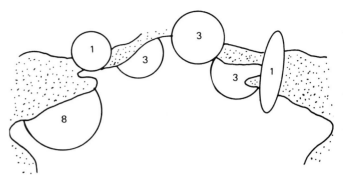

Fig. 13-135 Diagrammatic representation of locations of 19 meningiomas producing CPA symptoms (left and right sides combined; reprinted from House JW and O'Conner AF: Handbook of neurotological diagnosis. New York and Basel, Marcel Dekker, 1987, p 290.)

(Fig. 13-133).[9,91,92] These findings are less commonly seen in infratentorial than in supratentorial meningiomas.[9]

Heterogeneity in meningioma may be caused by calcifications and cystic foci.[92] Perifocal edema is occasionally discernible on both CT and MRI.[9,88] Marked perifocal edema, absence of visible calcium aggregates, nonhomogeneous contrast enhancement with nonenhancing "cystic" components and poorly defined irregular borders point to aggressive or invasive characteristics more commonly found in the angioblastic and syncytial variants.[93]

Underlying hyperostosis is infrequently seen but highly characteristic when present (Figs. 13-136, C and 13-139).[14,70] The IAC is rarely enlarged.

The treatment for meningioma is surgical; local recurrences are common.[19]

Epidermoid

Also called primary cholesteatomas or pearly tumors, congenital epidermoid tumors are the third most common tumor in the CP angle (Figs. 13-140 to 13-142).[13,14] Although they are congenital, they do not appear until young or middle adulthood. Originating from ectodermal cell rests, they consist of stratified squamous epithelial linings surrounding desquamated keratin.[19] As the contents accumulate slowly, the lesions often reach considerable size and yet cause only minimal symptoms.[94] The duration of symptoms is usually long. In one series it is over 4 years.[95] The CSF protein is usually normal, unless there is associated meningitis.[94,95]

Epidermoids may be located anterolaterally or posterolaterally to the brainstem. They tend to expand where the physical resistance is low and often burrow into crevices on the surface of the brain, "dumbbell"

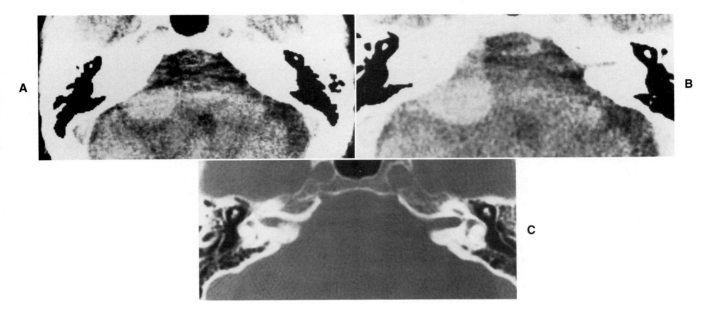

Fig. 13-136   CPA meningioma with classic features. **A, B,** and **C,** Pre- and postcontrast and high-resolution CT. Note the precontrast hyperdensity, hemispheric contour, obtuse bone-tumor angle, and underlying hyperostosis.

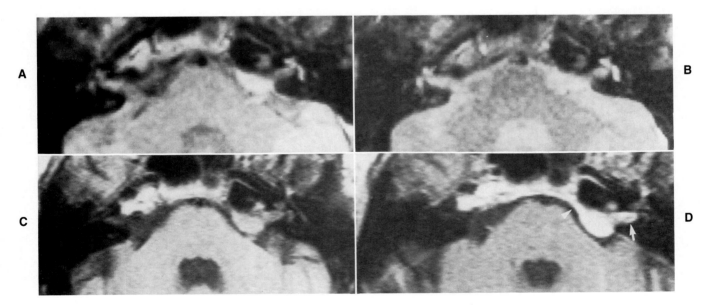

Fig. 13-137   CPA meningioma. **A** and **B,** Intermediate and T$_2$-weighted images. Typical hemispheric tumor eccentric to porus obscured by CSF in **B. C** and **D,** T$_1$-weighted images pre- and post-gadolinium. Note intracanalicular extension of tumor *(arrow)* and "tail" of tumor *(arrowhead)* extending to clivus border best seen post-gadolinium.

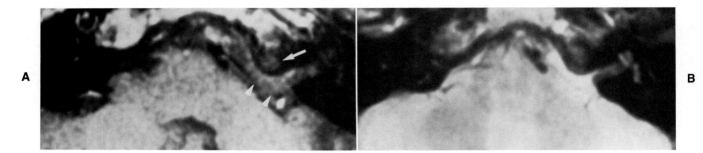

Fig. 13-138 CPA meningioma. **A** and **B,** T_1- and T_2-weighted images. Plaque-like tumor *(arrowheads)* is obscured by CSF in **B.** Note intermediate intensity of infiltrated underlying bone *(arrow).*

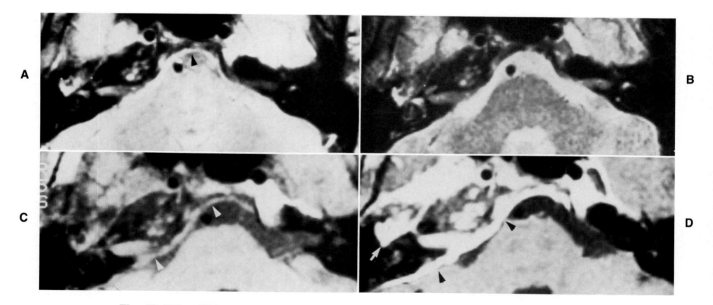

Fig. 13-139 CPA meningioma. **A** and **B,** Intermediate and T_2-weighted images. **C** and **D,** Pre- and post-gadolinium T_1-weighted images. Plaque-like tumor is obscured by CSF in **B** as in Figs. 13-137, *B* and 13-138, *B.* Note extensive sheet of thickened meninges *(arrowheads),* inhomogeneous intermediate signal intensities of infiltrated and hyperostotic right petrous apex, and tumor in the IAC, middle ear *(arrow),* middle fossa, and cavernous sinus. The patient has minimal symptoms and has not been operated on. (Courtesy of James J Hodge, MD.)

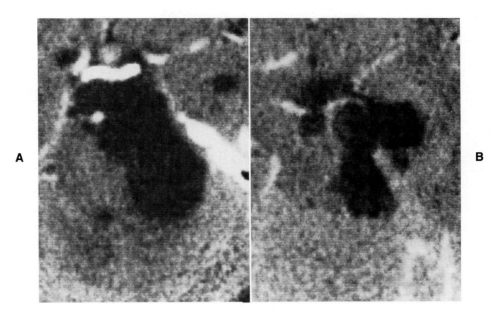

Fig. 13-140   CPA epidermoid. **A** and **B,** Postcontrast CT. Typical irregular mass with fine surface irregularity. There are a few fine strands within non-enhancing mass of CSF density. Note encasement of basilar artery in **A** and herniation of tumor into the suprasellar cistern and middle fossa in **B.**

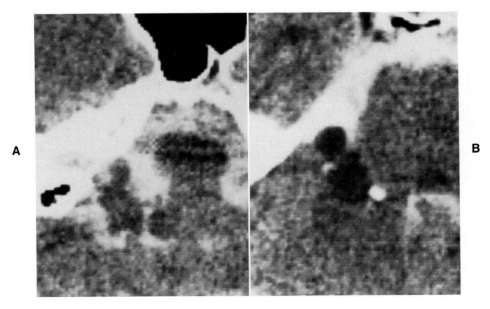

Fig. 13-141   CPA epidermoid. Metrizamide-CT cisternogram. Note fine surface irregularity of tumor outlined by positive intrathecal contrast in **A** and small punctate surface calcification in **B.**

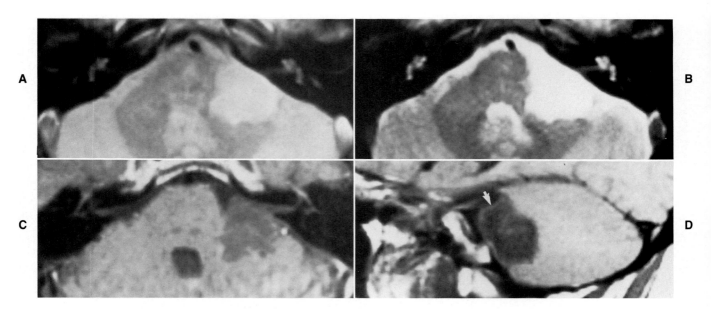

Fig. 13-142 CPA epidermoid. **A** and **B,** Intermediate and T$_2$-weighted images. **C** and **D,** Post-gadolinium T$_1$-weighted images. Note fine surface irregularity on **A, B,** and **C,** and the fine strands through hypointense tumor on **C** and **D.** There is suggestion of a capsule on **D** *(arrow).* (Courtesy of Frank M. Rizer, MD.)

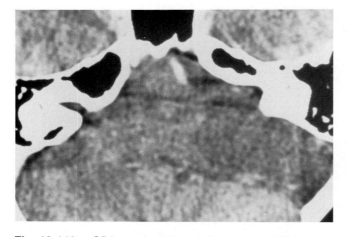

Fig. 13-143 CPA arachnoid cyst. Postcontrast CT. Lesion is difficult to differentiate from epidermoid. Note widening of ipsilateral IAC, not a differential feature per se between the two lesions.

into the middle fossa, or extend around the brainstem into the contralateral cistern. Their shapes are thus quite variable.[95] Their surfaces tend to be irregular (Figs. 13-140 to 13-142).

On CT they approximate CSF in density, and, in our experience of over 20 such tumors, are totally nonenhancing. Exceptionally, however, hyperdense epidermoids have been reported[96,97] as have enhancing borders.[98] Small amounts of calcification are sometimes found in the periphery of the tumor (Fig. 13-141, *D*).

Squamous carcinoma arising from epidermoids has been reported.[99,100] An enhancing component in an epidermoid suggests associated malignancy.[99,100]

Perifocal edema is rarely observed in association with epidermoid tumors.[96] Pressure erosion of the petrous apex is sometimes encountered.[14,95]

On MRI, epidermoids tend to be relatively homogeneous, and isointense or slightly hyperintense to CSF on T$_1$-weighted images and inhomogeneous and hyperintense to CSF on T$_2$-weighted images (Fig. 13-142).[9,101] A thin capsule and/or fine tissue strands may be seen in some of the tumors (Fig. 13-142, *C* and *D*). Epidermoids may resemble schwannomas, meningiomas, or chondromas by intensity criteria; but unlike the other tumors, they are nonenhancing. Their CT density may also help in the differentiation.

Arachnoid cyst,[102] being also of CSF density and intensity, is difficult to differentiate from epidermoids on both CT and MRI (Fig. 13-143). Arachnoid cysts pos-

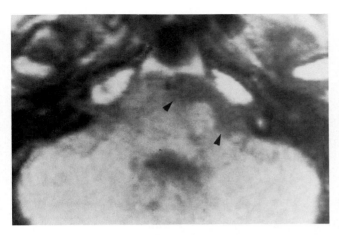

Fig. 13-144 CPA cysticercal cyst. T$_1$-weighted image. Left CPA cistern cyst *(arrowheads)* approximates CSF in intensity. Patient also has intraventricular and other subarachnoid cysts. (Courtesy of Chi-Shing Zee, MD.)

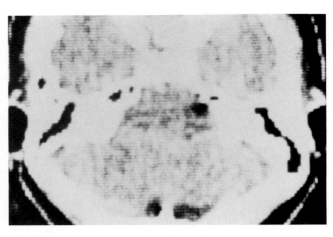

Fig. 13-145 CPA lipoma. Postcontrast CT. Lesion is isodense to fat.

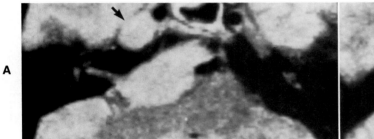
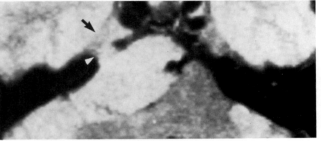

Fig. 13-146 Bilobed trigeminal schwannoma. **A** and **B,** Intermediate weighted images. Tumor "dumbbells" from posterior fossa through porus trigeminus *(arrowhead)* into Meckel's cave *(arrow).* (Courtesy of Jerald V. Robinson, MD.)

sess smoother surfaces than epidermoids. On CT intrathecal contrast may be used to show their surface characteristics.[103] On MRI a multiecho sequence may differentiate the cyst intensity from CSF intensity.

Cysticercosis is another diagnostic consideration in endemic areas (Fig. 13-144). As opposed to parenchymal and intraventricular cysts, which are separate from one another, cisternal cysticercal cysts are usually racemose, several centimeters in size, and *lacking* a scolex.[104] Such cysts in the CP angle may cause symptoms suggestive of acoustic schwannoma. Because their fluid may be identical to CSF on CT and MRI, the presence of cysticercal cysts is sometimes suggested only by focal cisternal widening.[104] They are better seen on MRI than on CT.[105] The majority are detectable only on T$_1$-weighted images, but T$_2$-weighted images demonstrate the surrounding tissue reaction to greater advantage.[105]

Lipomas and dermoids, which are extremely rare and more likely in the midline than in the CP angle, show negative numbers on CT and are isointense with fat on MRI (Fig. 13-145).[19,106-108] Dermoids may also contain teeth and peripheral calcifications.[106]

Nonacoustic Posterior Fossa Schwannomas

The nonacoustic schwannomas resemble acoustic schwannomas in appearance but not in their locations.[109] Thus it is important to note the precise location of a schwannoma-appearing tumor and to search carefully for any associated skull base foraminal changes.

Acoustic schwannomas comprise 95% of all intracranial schwannomas. Trigeminal schwannomas are a distant second.

Trigeminal schwannomas may arise intradurally from the nerve root in the CP angle and Meckel's cave or extradurally from the gasserian ganglion in the middle cranial fossa.[110] They may also involve both the posterior and the middle fossae (Fig. 13-146).[111] The tumor is centered anteromedial to the IAC. Careful study will

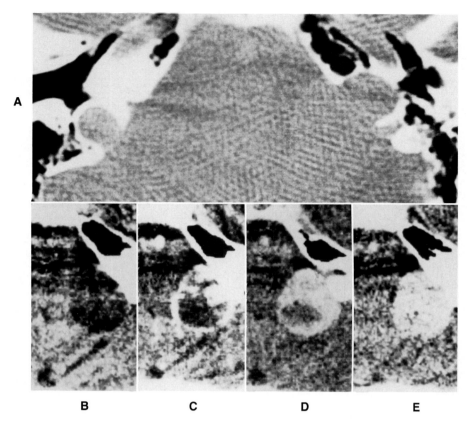

Fig. 13-147   Cystic glossopharyngeal schwannoma. **A,** High-resolution CT. Pars nervosa is sharply and smoothly expanded. **B,** Precontrast CT, **C** during contrast infusion, **D,** 30 minutes postcontrast, and **E,** 90 minutes postcontrast. Appearance of cystic schwannoma postcontrast is in part a function of time. Note similarity in appearance of this tumor to other cystic schwannomas (Figs. 13-131, 13-132, and 13-174). This patient complained only of left-sided progressive hearing loss. Bone changes were key to correct preoperative diagnosis. (Reprinted from House JW, O'Conner, AF, eds: Handbook of neurotological diagnosis. New York and Basel, Marcel Dekker, 1987, pp 302-304.)

often show that a portion of the tumor extends through the porus trigeminus into Meckel's cave.[14,112] The foramen ovale and/or the foramen rotundum may also be enlarged.

Compared to acoustic schwannomas, they are more prone to contain cystic components and are thus more varied in appearance.[14,111] On CT they may be isodense or slightly hypodense or show mixed isodensity and hypodensity. They exhibit well-circumscribed enhancement that may or may not be homogeneous.[111] On MRI their signal intensities are similar to those of acoustic schwannomas.[9,111,113] In most cases they are better localized and characterized on MRI than on CT.[9]

Facial schwannomas are rare tumors that may arise from any segment of the facial nerve. When arising from within the IAC, they may first be characterized by sensorineural hearing loss rather than facial palsy and thus may be both clinically and radiologically indistin-

guishable from acoustic schwannomas (Figs. 13-182 and 13-183).[114,115]

Similarly, glossopharyngeal, vagus, and spinal accessory schwannomas initially appear with their specific deficits only when they occur within the jugular foramen (Fig. 13-175).[116,117] When arising within the posterior fossa, they may attain considerable size and first appear instead with predominantly acoustic and/or cerebellar signs and symptoms (Figs. 13-147 and 13-148).[117] Hence they should also be considered in the differential diagnosis of acoustic schwannomas. A correct preoperative diagnosis averts using the translabyrinthine approach, which would destroy residual hearing.

Vascular Lesions

Vascular lesions of the CP angle are rare, but a number of them may clinically mimic neoplasms and thus assume differential diagnostic importance on CT and MRI.

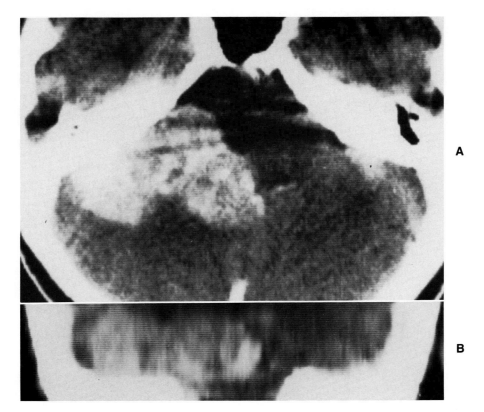

Fig. 13-148   Intracranial vagal schwannoma. **A,** Postcontrast CT. **B,** Coronal reformation of postcontrast CT. This large tumor is almost entirely within posterior fossa. Patient presented with sensorineural hearing loss and disequilibrium. There were no deficits of lower cranial nerves. Note low-lying position of extraaxial mass within posterior fossa.

Vertebrobasilar dolichoectasia (VDB), or elongation and dilatation of the vertebrobasilar artery, is probably the most common vascular lesion associated with compressive symptoms of the posterior fossa cranial nerves. Elongation of the basilar artery may be considered present if any portion of it extends lateral to the margin of the clivus or the dorsum sellae or the artery bifurcates above the plane of the suprasellar cistern (Fig. 13-149). Ectasia is diagnosed if the diameter of the basilar artery is greater than 4.5 mm on CT.[118] Angiography is not needed to establish the diagnosis.[119-121] It may, in fact, be harmful if the artery is dilated. If angiography is necessary in a patient with a basilar artery over 1.5 cm in diameter, a nonselective digital subtraction study is advised.[121] The vertebrobasilar artery is superbly demonstrated on MRI by by its signal void. However, it should be noted that CSF flow phenomenon may mimic a basilar artery aneurysm and that a thrombosed or partially thrombosed dolichoectatic basilar artery may simulate an extraaxial tumor.[122,123]

The most common symptoms reported are those associated with the facial nerve, hemifacial spasm, and fa-

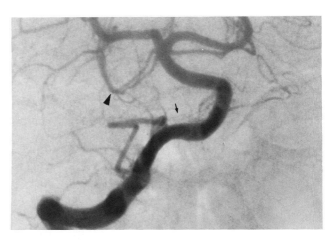

Fig. 13-149   Vertebrobasilar dolichoectasia. Selective vertebral angiogram. The superior cerebellar *(arrowhead)* and anterior inferior cerebellar *(arrow)* arteries are also tortuous.

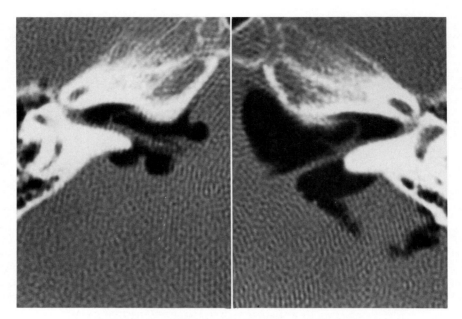

Fig. 13-150   Bilateral AICA loops. Gas-CT cisternogram.

cial paresis.[121,124] The second most common symptom is trigeminal neuralgia.[121] Other cranial nerves that have been affected include the oculomotor, abducens, acoustic, glossopharyngeal, and vagus.[121,125,126] "Disabling positional vertigo" resulting from vascular compression of the acoustic nerve has been described in a series of patients without specific reference to VBD.[127]

In general, symptomatic patients with elongated but undilated vertebrobasilar arteries are much more likely to have single cranial nerve involvement; and those with elongated and dilated arteries are much more likely to have combinations of multiple compressive cranial nerve deficits, compressive and ischemic central nervous system deficits, and hydrocephalus.[121] The compressive symptoms can in some cases be relieved by microvascular decompression.[128] Preoperative angiography may be of predictive value.[129,130]

"Vascular loop," a loop of the anterior inferior cerebellar artery (AICA) has been implicated in acoustic nerve symptoms, in particular, vertigo (Fig. 13-150).[125,127,131] On its normal course from the basilar artery to the cerebellum, the AICA forms a loop under, over, or between the facial and acoustic nerves as it gives rise to the auditory artery.[132] The loop may be located in the cistern, at the porus or found, in up to 19% by microdissection and 22% by gas-CT cisternography, in the IAC.[132,133] Thus, the mere finding of an AICA loop, intracanalicular or otherwise, does not necessarily establish it as the cause of symptoms. To produce symptoms the cross-compression may have to coincide with the glial-schwann cell junction.[132]

After exclusion of other causes or failure to respond

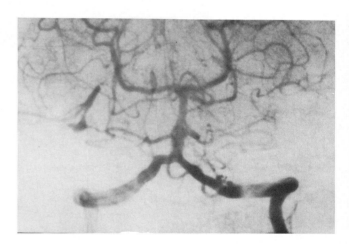

Fig. 13-151   Anterior inferior cerebellar artery berry aneurysm. Selective vertebral angiogram.

to medical treatment, a series of 27 patients who had predominantly intractable vertigo, had gas-CT cisternograms that demonstrated an AICA loop *contacting* the acoustic nerve on the affected side in the cistern, at the porus, or in the IAC.[131] These 27 patients subsequently underwent microsurgical decompression. Fourteen became symptom-free and the others obtained significant improvement. Thus, gas-CT cisternography can be a useful and definitive method for diagnosing this condition.

Berry aneurysms of the anterior inferior cerebellar artery are quite rare, representing less than 1% of intracranial aneurysms (Fig. 13-151).[134] However, they

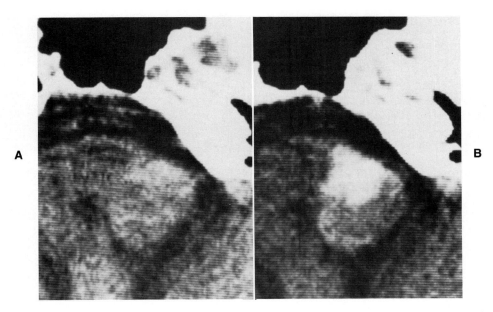

Fig. 13-152 Partially thrombosed giant posterior inferior cerebellar artery aneurysm. **A** and **B,** Pre- and postcontrast CT. Compare with cystic schwannomas (Figs. 13-147 and 13-174). (Courtesy of Duane E. Blickenstaff, MD.)

are of particular interest to our discussion in that those that have been reported have often been operated on with a diagnosis of acoustic tumor. A review of 22 reported cases revealed that 16 had acoustic and 14 had facial nerve signs and symptoms, and 14 had subarachnoid hemorrhage.[134] A dense homogeneous enhancement may be a clue. Dynamic CT may contribute by showing rapid opacification. MRI will establish a specific diagnosis if a signal void because of rapidly flowing blood is demonstrated in the aneurysm.

Giant aneurysms are those exceeding 2.5 cm in diameter (Fig. 13-152).[14] They may originate from the vertebrobasilar artery or from one of its branches and extend into the CP angle as a mass lesion. They rarely cause subarachnoid hemorrhage. They may be nonthrombosed or completely thrombosed, but most commonly they are partially thrombosed.[14,135] On CT a partially thrombosed aneurysm shows an enhancing rim with an isodense nonenhancing mural thrombus of varying size and an enhancing lumen. A calcific rim may be present. A nonthrombosed aneurysm shows a homogeneous enhancement, and a thrombosed one an enhancing rim with an isodense nonenhancing center.[14] MRI demonstrates a flow void in the patent lumen, laminated thrombus of varying signal intensities and sometimes a low-signal intensity rim.[136-138]

Pial siderosis of the acoustic nerves, or superficial siderosis, is a long-recognized, rare pathologic entity, the antemortem noninvasive diagnosis of which has recently become possible with the advent of high-field MRI (Fig. 13-153).[139,140] It consists of intracellular and extracellular deposition of hemosiderin in the leptomeninges, subpial tissue, spinal cord, and cranial nerves from chronic capillary or venous subarachnoid hemorrhage such as may be caused from an ependymoma. The acoustic nerve with its long glial-lined segment is especially vulnerable to the toxic effects of hemoglobin and hemosiderin deposition. The clinical findings include hearing loss, cerebellar dysfunction, pyramidal tract signs, and at times, progressive mental deterioration. The CSF is xanthrochromic and rich in protein. On high-field MRI the T_2-weighted images show marked hypointensity of the pial and arachnoid membranes and the acoustic nerves.

Hemangioma or vascular malformation of the acoustic and facial nerves appears as intracanalicular tumors, some of which may contain intratumoral bone spicules best seen on high-resolution CT with bone algorithm (see Fig. 13-192).[141] On MRI they tend to be more hyperintense on T_2-weighted images than acoustic schwannomas (see Fig. 13-189).[142]

Arteriovenous malformations in the CP angle are exceedingly rare. Dilated enhancing vessels may be seen on CT and serpentine hypointense loops on MRI.[14] Angiography provides definitive visualization of the feeding arteries and draining veins (Fig. 13-154). Arteriovenous malformations, which are congenital, should be distinguished from dural arteriovenous fistulas, which are acquired.

Petrous bone lesions. These are quite numerous and

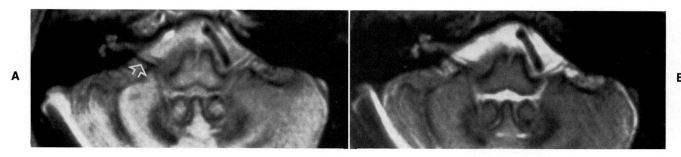

Fig. 13-153 Pial siderosis 1.5 Tesla MR images. **A,** Intermediate (TR 3000ms/TE 30ms) and **B,** T$_2$-weighted (3000/70). Patient is a 63-year-old man examined for severe bilateral progressive sensorineural hearing loss and ataxia. Note hypointensity of acoustic nerve *(open arrow)* and surfaces of medulla and cerebellum. Facial nerves do not appear involved. Hypointensity of dentate nuclei may be physiologic. Hypointensity is also found on surfaces of pons, midbrain, basal portion of cerebrum, and optic tracts on higher sections. (Courtesy of Royce J. Biddle, MD.)

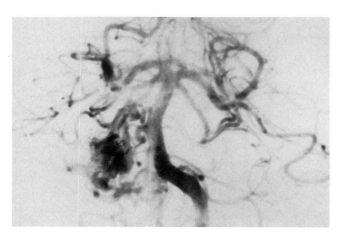

Fig. 13-154 CPA arteriovenous malformation. Selective vertebral angiogram. (Courtesy of Livia G. Solti-Bohman, MD.)

will be discussed in greater detail in a following section. However, they should be considered in the differential diagnosis of cerebellopontine angle masses; for example, an exophytic growth from a chondrosarcoma may be mistaken for a meningioma (see Fig. 13-206).[143]

Paragangliomas. These tumors, to be discussed in greater detail in a following section, have a different presenting symptom complex and are not usually confused clinically with acoustic schwannomas. However, they may have intracranial extradural or transdural extensions in the posterior fossa, which on CT or MRI mimic schwannomas or meningiomas (Figs. 13-165 and 13-166). Identifying their precise location and associated bone changes should help to avoid misdiagnoses.

Intraaxial tumors. These and other primary lesions of the brain are beyond the scope of this section for detailed description. Some of them do occasionally occur in the CP angle and must be considered in the differential diagnosis.

Intraaxial posterior fossa tumors may arise from the brain stem, the cerebellum, or the fourth ventricle.

Tumors of the brainstem include those from the medulla, the pons, the midbrain, and the cerebellar peduncles and are mainly astrocytomas occurring in children or young adults.[144] On CT they are isodense or hypodense and show mild, moderate, or no enhancement.[145] The brainstem is usually enlarged and the fourth ventricle posteriorly displaced. There may be exophytic growth extending into the cistern.[144]

Tumors of the cerebellum may arise from the vermis or the hemisphere. Vermian tumors, principally medulloblastomas in childhood, rarely may extend to the CP angle. They are hyperdense and enhancing. Hemispheric tumors are most commonly hemangioblastomas and metastases in adults and astrocytomas in adults or children. All three lesions may be either enhancing solid masses or cystic masses with solid components. Hemangioblastomas may be multiple. Their solid components are characteristically hypervascular and best demonstrated by angiography.[146]

From the fourth ventricle arise the ependymomas and choroid plexus papillomas (Figs. 13-155 to 13-157). They may cause CP angle symptoms when growing through the foramen of Luschka.[147,148] Naidich et al found extension to the CP angle in 7 of 12 ependymomas, 2 of 6 in a group of medulloblastomas and a cerebellar sarcoma, 1 of 23 astrocytomas, and 1 of 8 hemangioblastomas.[87]

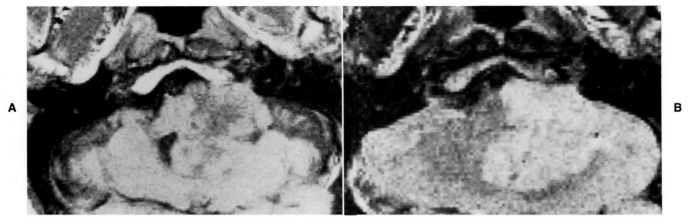

Fig. 13-155   CPA ependymoma. **A** and **B,** T_1- and T_2-weighted images. Exophytic intraaxial mass protruding into CP angle and deforming fourth ventricle lacks clear demarcation from brain. (Compare with extraaxial mass such as one in Fig. 13-132.) Some foci of relative hypointensity on both images may represent calcification.

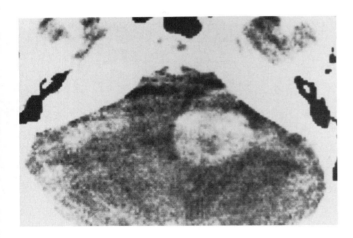

Fig. 13-156   CPA choroid plexus papilloma. Postcontrast CT. Tumor is located at foramen of Lushka. It is more sharply defined than an ependymoma (Fig. 13-155.) Like a giant aneurysm (Fig. 13-152) it is detached from petrous bone, in contrast to schwannomas (Figs. 13-131 and 13-147) and meningiomas.

Ependymomas tend to calcify. The calcified portions are variable in density and enhancement.[145] Papillomas are well-defined lesions, slightly hyperdense and moderately enhancing.[145] Both tumors are nearly isointense to brain on T_1-weighted images and mildly hyperintense on T_2-weighted images (Figs. 13-155 and 13-157).[149]

The intraaxial tumors are generally nearly isointense on T_1-weighted images and hyperintense on T_2-weighted images, and except for any calcifications are better demonstrated on MRI than on CT.[150,151]

INTRACANALICULAR LESIONS	
Neoplastic	Lymphoma
Acoustic schwannoma	Melanoma
Facial schwannoma	
Hemangioma	**Nonneoplastic**
Meningioma	AICA* loop
Metastasis	AICA aneurysm
Glioma	Arachnoiditis
Lipoma	Hamartoma
	Neuritis

*AICA = Anterior inferior cerebellar artery

Lymphoma may also occur in the CP angle.[152,153]

Nonneoplastic brain lesions such as multiple sclerosis and infarct may, of course, be occasionally encountered in the investigation of CP angle symptoms.

Intracanalicular lesions. The differential diagnoses for intracanalicular lesions differ slightly from those of CP angle masses (see accompanying box), as follows:

1. Acoustic schwannomas are by far the most common and in our experience constitute over 90% of the intracanalicular lesions (Figs. 13-127 to 13-129).[154]
2. Facial schwannomas (see Fig. 13-182)
3. Meningiomas

These two are probably indistinguishable from acoustic schwannomas clinically or by CT or MRI unless a facial schwannoma extends into the facial nerve canal, or a meningioma produces hyperostosis.

4. Intracanalicular vascular tumors tend to cause a greater degree of nerve deficits and more com-

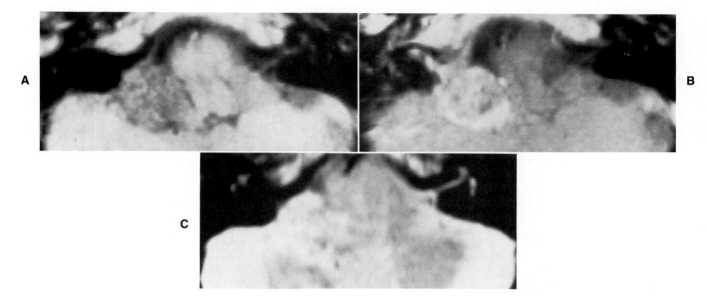

Fig. 13-157 CPA choroid plexus papilloma. **A** and **B,** T_1-weighted pre and post gadolinium images. **C,** T_2-weighted image. Tumor is located at foramen of Lushka as in Fig. 13-156. It is well demarcated from the brain. Enhancement is mild and inhomogeneous. The specks, which are hypointense on all three sequences, suggest calcifications. (Courtesy of Val M. Runge, MD.)

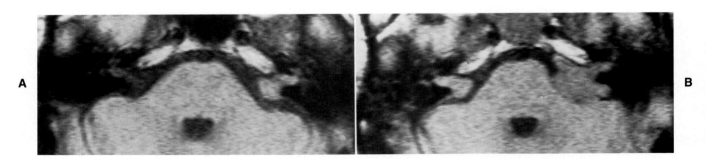

Fig. 13-158 Metastases from carcinoma of the bladder. **A** and **B,** T_1-weighted images one month apart. The patient developed rapidly progressive hearing loss and facial palsy on the left side, followed by similar symptoms on the right.

monly facial nerve symptoms than acoustic schwannomas of comparable size.[155,156] In our experience they are a distant second to acoustic schwannomas in incidence. Some of them contain intratumoral bone spicules discernible on high-resolution CT with a bone algorithm (Fig. 13-192). On MRI they tend to be slightly more hyperintense than the typical schwannoma (Fig. 13-189).[142]

5. Intracanalicular metastases are rare but may be suspected from a short duration of symptoms, a known history of malignancy, and a rapid growth rate on serial studies (Fig. 13-158).[157]
6. Glioma[158]
7. Lipoma[107]
8. Lymphoma[152]
9. Melanoma[14]

These last four are very rare IAC neoplasms.

Rarely hamartoma of the acoustic nerve has been found at autopsy and encountered in clinical practice.[36,159]

Other nonneoplastic conditions include (a) intracanalicular loop of the anterior inferior cerebellar artery (Fig. 13-150),[131,133,160] (b) aneurysm arising from the anterior inferior cerebellar artery (Fig. 13-151),[134] (c) arachnoid adhesions,[154,161] and (d) neuritis.[162]

Since these lesions are not infrequently only 3 or 4 mm in size, excellent technique is required for their demonstration. In CT this generally means gas-CT cisternography with 1.5 mm sections every 1 mm or a comparable technique.[154] In MRI it requires contiguous 3 mm sections or 4 or 5 mm overlapping sections and, if necessary, the use of intravenous gadolinium DTPA.[74]

Summary

In summary the three most common extraaxial masses in the cerebellopontine angle—acoustic schwannoma, meningioma, and congenital epidermoid—are relatively consistent in location, configuration, CT density and enhancement, and MR intensity (Table 13-7). The same may be said for the rarer nonacoustic posterior fossa schwannomas and the various vascular lesions. If one analyzes each lesion systematically and avoids the traps set by the occasional extradural or intraaxial lesions intruding into the cerebellopontine angle, a correct preoperative diagnosis can be reached in an overwhelming percentage of the cases.

PARAGANGLIOMA
Incidence, Origin, and Terms

Paraganglioma is the second most common tumor involving the temporal bone and the most common in the middle ear.[163]

In the branchiomeric family of paraganglia, two groups are by location closely related to the jugular foramen—the jugulotympanic paraganglia along the tympanic branch of the glossopharyngeal nerve and the mastoid branch of the vagus nerve (the nerves of Jacobson and Arnold, respectively) and the intravagal paraganglia inferior to the foramen.[164] Paraganglia are organelles 0.1 to 1.5 mm in length. Those distributed along the nerves of Jacobson and Arnold are (1) in the adventitia of the jugular bulb, (2) in the inferior tympanic canaliculus, (3) on the cochlea promontory, and (4) in the mastoid canaliculus and the descending facial nerve canal (Fig. 13-159).[165] According to Glenner and Grimley, tumors from the paraganglia are more appropriately called paragangliomas rather than chemodectomas or glomus tumors.[164]

The term *glomus jugulare tumor* has been used among clinicians since Guild named the paraganglia *glomus jugulare*.[165,166] The term *glomus tympanicum tumor* was introduced by Alford and Guilford when they noted that those arising "away from the jugular bulb, in the middle ear, along the course of Jacobson's nerve" had a better prognosis than those arising "in the area of the jugular bulb."[167,168] In recent years Glasscock and others clarified the definition so that glomus tympanicum tumors include those in the tympanic cavity and the mastoid and glomus jugulare tumors include those involving the jugular bulb and the base of the skull.[169] Glomus vagale tumors (vagal paragangliomas) arise from the intravagal paraganglia at or below the skull base and are primarily parapharyngeal masses.

Clinical Features

Paragangliomas occur in women three times as often as in men. Two thirds of the patients initially are seen in their fourth and fifth decades. The tumors may be bilateral. Other tumors such as carotid body tumors may coexist. Up to 10% of the patients may have multiple tumors.[170] Normally locally infiltrating, the tumors rarely may metastasize. Up to 10% are accompanied by malignant tumors in *other* organ systems.[170] Rarely, the larger of the paragangliomas may secrete norepinephrine (as in pheochromocytomas) or, less often, ACTH, serotonin calcitonin and dopamine.[171] On rare occasions paragangliomas have been found to be familial.[172]

Paragangliomas may grow laterally to cause otologic symptoms (conductive hearing loss, pulsatile tinnitus, or a retrotympanic mass) and medially to cause the jugular foramen (or Vernet's) syndrome consisting of glossopharyngeal, vagus and spinal accessory deficits.[173,174] However, among both tympanicum and jugulare tumors, otologic symptoms predominate. Cranial nerve palsies appear only in a minority of the patients.[173] Clinical differentiation between the two groups is therefore impossible in the majority of cases, unless a small tympanicum tumor is circumferentially visible.

In addition to involvement of the ninth through eleventh cranial nerves as the tumor enlarges, the hypoglos-

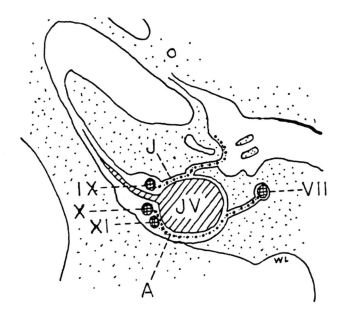

Fig. 13-159   Schematic representation of important contents of jugular foramen. Inferior petrosal sinus *(unlabeled)* and glossopharyngeal nerve (IX) traverse the pars nervosa. The vagus (X) and spinal accessory (XI) nerves and internal jugular vein (JV) traverse the pars vasculars. The inferior tympanic branch of the glossopharyngeal *(J)* and the mastoid branch of the vagus *(A)* are represented by dotted lines. Approximately half of the paraganglia are distributed along each of the two branches. (Reproduced with modification from Lo WWM, Solti-Bohman, LG: High-resolution CT of the jugular foramen: anatomy and vascular variants and anomalies, Radiology 150:743-747, 1984.)

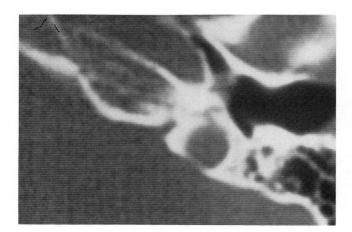

Fig. 13-160   Small glomus tympanicum tumor. High-resolution CT. Otoscopically circumferentially visible tumor corresponding to Fisch type A, removable by transmeatal approach. Angiography is not necessary.

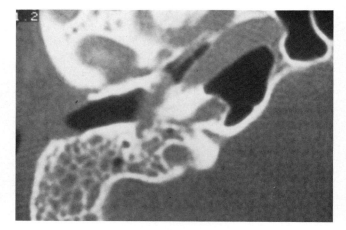

Fig. 13-161   Large glomus tympanicum tumor. High-resolution CT. Fisch type A tumor too large to be differentiated from glomus jugulare tumor by otoscopy. CT, showing an intact jugular plate, definitively excludes a glomus jugulare tumor. The tumor extending to protympanum and obstructing mastoid drainage is not distinguishable from other benign middle ear tumors by CT (compare with Fig. 13-173), but all such tumors can be resected by transmastoid approach. Angiography is not necessary.

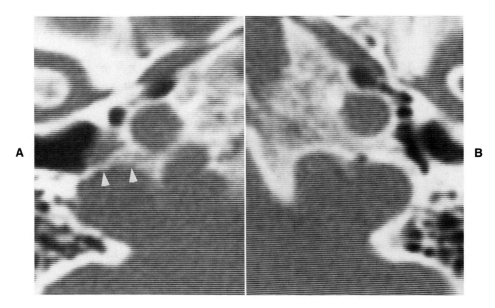

Fig. 13-162   Small glomus jugulare tumor. **A** and **B,** High-resolution CT. Fisch type-C$_1$ tumor, similar to Fig. 13-161 in otoscopic appearance. Cortical demineralization of the jugular plate *(arrowheads)* on CT, however, indicates involvement of jugular bulb. Compare with normal contralateral. Angiography is indicated with possible preoperative embolization.

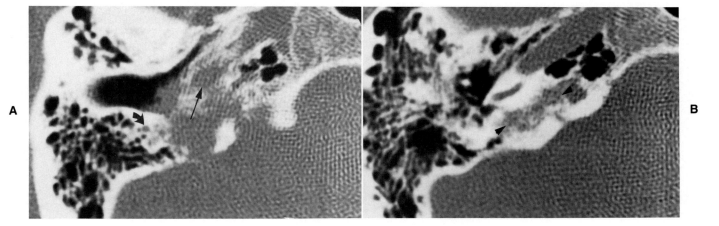

Fig. 13-163   Medium-sized glomus jugulare tumor. **A** and **B,** High-resolution CT. Fisch type-C$_2$ tumor destroying jugular fossa infiltrating vertical carotid canal *(arrow)* and infralabyrinthine compartment *(arrowheads)* bypassing dense bone of otic capsule. Tumor is resectable by infratemporal fossa approach, with anterior rerouting of facial nerve *(curved arrow).*

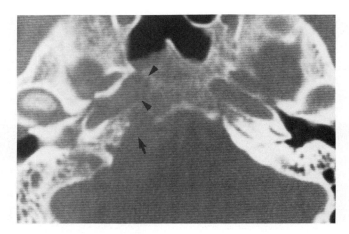

Fig. 13-164 Large glomus jugulare tumor. High-resolution CT. Fisch type-C$_3$ tumor. Note tumor extension along petrooccipital fissure *(arrow)* to petrous apex with demineralization of horizontal carotid canal *(arrowheads)*. Tumor is resectable by infratemporal fossa approach.

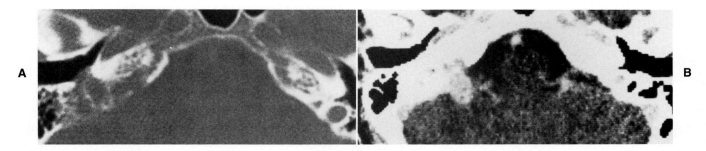

Fig. 13-165 Medium-sized glomus jugulare tumor. **A** and **B,** High-resolution and postcontrast CT. Fisch type-D tumor with small intracranial extension. For resection, combined otologic and neurosurgical approach is required.

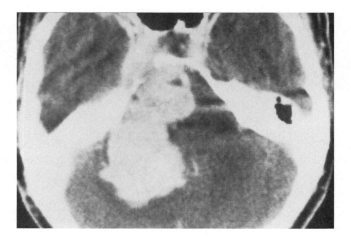

Fig. 13-166 Large glomus jugulare tumor. Postcontrast CT. Fisch type-D tumor with large intracranial tumor and cavernous sinus extension, usually considered beyond resection.

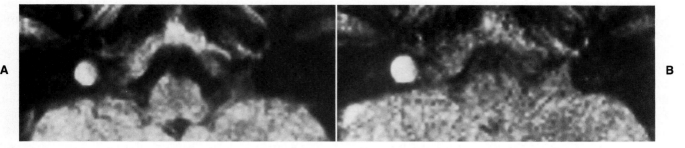

Fig. 13-167   High jugular bulb. **A** and **B,** Intermediate and T_2-weighted images. Flow-related enhancement must not be mistaken for jugular foramen tumor. Note smooth and perfectly rounded outline of hyperintensity filling the jugular bulb.

sal nerve may be compromised in the region of the hypoglossal canal (Collet-Sicard's syndrome) and the facial nerve in its mastoid segment.[174] Involvement of the carotid canal may cause Horner's syndrome; of the cavernous sinus, the cavernous sinus syndrome; and of the posterior fossa, brainstem and cerebellar signs and symptoms and hydrocephalus.[173,174]

Glomus vagale tumors grow inferior to the skull base. They appear as masses in the neck or the pharynx and usually involve the cranial nerves but do not cause pulsatile tinnitus or conductive hearing loss.[175]

High-resolution CT with bone detail is the most helpful imaging study for relating tumor extent to surgical landmarks and determining the surgical approach (Figs. 13-160 to 13-166). Angiography is valuable in the differential diagnosis of unknown tumor and preoperative embolization (Figs. 13-168 and 13-169). MRI is occasionally helpful in further localization and characterization of a tumor (Figs. 13-167, 13-171, 13-172).[8]

Growth Pattern and CT Findings

Paragangliomas grow slowly and rarely metastasize.[170] While localized bone destruction around the jugular foramen is common, extensive destruction by expansion occurs relatively late.

Paragangliomas tend to grow along the planes of least resistance by following preexisting pathways in the temporal bone (i.e., fissures, air cell tracts, vascular channels, and foramina) (Figs. 13-163, 13-164, and 13-166).[176,177] Tumors commonly descend through the jugular vein (see Fig. 13-170). Central nervous system invasion may ultimately cause death (Figs. 13-165 and 13-166).[176]

When first diagnosed, a paraganglioma may vary from being a few millimeters in diameter and easily resectable to 10 cm or larger and life-threatening (Figs. 13-160 and 13-166). The CT appearance of paragangliomas is therefore highly variable.

Because paraganglia are located along the nerves of Jacobson and Arnold, the earliest findings of jugulotympanic paragangliomas are found along the course of these two nerves (Figs. 13-159 to 13-162).[178] Vagal paragangliomas originating inferior to the jugular foramen may or may not involve the temporal bone.

Glomus tympanicum tumors tend to produce symptoms early so that when first seen they are often well-defined intratympanic soft tissue masses without bone involvement (Figs. 13-160 and 13-161).[179,180] They may extend into the external auditory canal but often even when filling the tympanic cavity leave the tympanic ossicles intact.[180]

Because of the proximity between the hypotympanum and the jugular fossa, a large percentage of the paragangliomas involve both regions by extending through the jugular plate (Figs. 13-162 to 13-165).[178,181] Early irregular demineralization is thus often first found on the jugular plate or on the lateral portion of the caroticojugular spine (Fig. 13-162). The jugular plate may have been involved early by tumors originating from paraganglia located in the inferior tympanic canaliculus.

More extensive destruction extends from around the pars vascularis and beyond (Fig. 13-163). The bone changes are irregular and the margins indistinct and may be described as "moth-eaten."[182] Further destruction extends medially to the pars nervosa and along the petrooccipital fissure, anteriorly to the vertical and then the horizontal carotid canal and posteriorly along the sigmoid sulcus to the transverse sulcus (Figs. 13-164 to 13-166).

Although the infralabyrinthine compartment is frequently destroyed, superiorly tumor extension is slowed by the dense bone of the otic capsule (Fig. 13-163).

Tumor in the tympanum may extend into the mastoid, and vice versa. Intratympanic tumor may also extend into the protympanum and less often into the epitympanum (Fig. 13-161).

Infralabyrinthine soft tissue mass is common, extending either intraluminally down the internal jugular vein or along the carotid sheath, frequently to the C2-3 level or even lower, appearing as an enhancing mass on CT (Fig. 13-170).

Further posterior extension of tumor may displace the dura internally or grow through the dura to involve the cerebellum (Figs. 13-164 to 13-166). Very large tumors may also destroy the jugular tubercle, the hypoglossal canal and portions of the foramen magnum and the clivus. Anterosuperior extension of tumor may involve the cavernous sinus (Fig. 13-166).

Angiographic Features

Paragangliomas are characteristically hypervascular (Figs. 13-168 and 13-169).[183,184] There are enlarged feeding arteries and rapidly draining veins. The tumor blush is coarser than in meningiomas but less so than in arteriovenous malformations. The blush is not as prolonged as in meningiomas.

The most common feeders are branches of the ascending pharngyeal artery, which supplies the inferomedial compartment of the tumor around the jugular foramen and the medial tympanic cavity (Figs. 13-168 and 13-169).[184] The second most common feeders are the posterior auricular, stylomastoid, and occipital branches, which supply the posterolateral compartment in the mastoid region.

Larger tumors derive blood supply anteriorly from the internal maxillary (anterior tympanic branch) and superiorly from the internal carotid (caroticotympanic and lateral clival branches).[183,184] Even larger tumors receive additional supply from the contralateral carotid artery and/or the vertebral artery from its meningeal

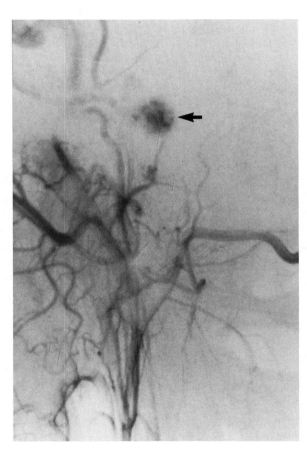

Fig. 13-168 Glomus tympanicum tumor. Selective external carotid angiogram. Characteristic hypervascularity *(arrow)*.

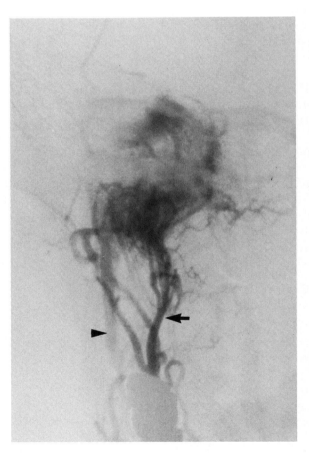

Fig. 13-169 Glomus jugulare tumor. Selective external carotid angiogram. Characteristically hypervascular tumor supplied by hypertrophic ascending pharyngeal artery *(arrow)*. Note early draining vein *(arrowhead)* seen during midarterial phase. Differential diagnosis includes other hypervascular tumors, e.g., metastatic hypernephroma, metastatic pheochromocytomas, myeloma, etc. (see Fig. 13-202).

and even pial branches. Pial arterial supply signifies transdural involvement.[185]

The angiographic vascularity is sufficiently characteristic that some authors believe it is diagnostic and that biopsy is not necessary.[170] Exceptions that should be considered include metastatic pheochromocytoma and renal cell carcinoma, for example.

Retrograde jugular venography is now seldom indicated since intravenous tumor extension in itself does not determine the surgical approach (Fig. 13-170).

MRI Appearance

In paragangliomas larger than 2 cm, an apparently unique "salt-and-pepper" pattern of hyperintensity and hypointensity on both T_1- and T_2-weighted images has been described (Fig. 13-171).[11] Also identified are the serpentine and arborizing flow voids of the hypertrophic medium and larger sized tumor vessels. These findings are highly suggestive of paragangliomas, but their sensitivity and specificity have not yet been established. The signal intensities from the tumor should be carefully distinguished from those of bone marrow and of mastoid secretions accumulated from tumor obstruction of the tympanic cavity or eustachian tube (Fig. 13-172).

The tumor signal intensity is generally more than that of cortical bone, aerated air cells, and flowing blood but less than that of bone marrow. IV gadolin-

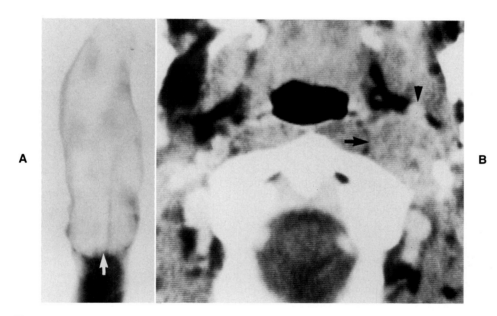

Fig. 13-170 Intravenous extension of glomus jugulare tumor. **A,** Retrograde jugular venogram. **B,** Postcontrast CT. Intravenous tumor *(arrow)* descending jugular vein is common growth pattern of jugular paraganglioma. Internal carotid artery is displaced anteriorly *(arrowhead).*

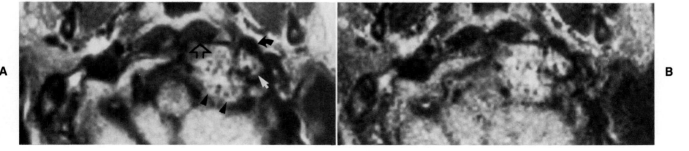

Fig. 13-171 Glomus jugulare tumor. **A** and **B,** Intermediate and T_2-weighted images. Heterogeneous hyper- and hypointensity is characteristically seen in larger paragangliomas. Tumor has only a small component in the jugular fossa *(arrow)* posterior to carotid *(curved arrow)* but a large component in the infralabyrinthine skull base *(arrowheads)* displacing longus colli muscle anteriorly *(open arrow).*

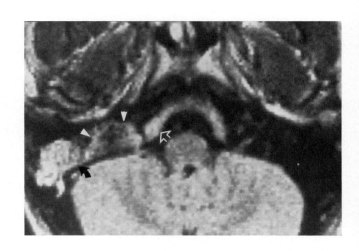

Fig. 13-172 Glomus jugulare tumor. Intermediate weighted image. Heterogeneous hyperintensity of tumor *(arrowheads)* must be carefully differentiated from hyperintensity of yellow marrow *(open arrow)* and that of retained mastoid secretions. *(curved arrow).*

Table 13-8 Glasscock-Jackson classification of paragangliomas

Tumor type	Anatomic extent	Surgical procedure
Glomus tympanicum		
I	Small mass limited to promontory	Transcanal
II	Completely filling middle ear space	Extended facial recess
III	Filling middle ear and extending into the mastoid	Extended facial recess
IV	Filling middle ear, extending into the mastoid or through tympanic membrane to fill the external auditory canal; may extend anterior to carotid	Extended facial recess
Glomus jugulare		
I	Small; involving jugular bulb, middle ear, and mastoid	Traditional skull base dissection
II	Extending under internal auditory canal; may have intracranial extension	Traditional skull base dissection
III	Extending into petrous apex; may have intracranial extension	Modified infratemporal fossa approach
IV	Extending beyond petrous apex into clivus or infratemporal fossa; may have intracranial extension	Modified intratemporal fossa approach

Table 13-9 Fisch classification of paragangliomas

Tumor type	Anatomic extent	Surgical procedure
A	Localized to middle ear cleft	Transmeatal
B	Limited to tympanomastoid area with no infralabyrinthine compartment involvement	Combined transmeatal and transmastoid approach
C	Involving infralabyrinthine compartment and extending into petrous apex	Infratemporal fossa approach
C_1	Destroying jugular foramen and bulb with limited involvement of vertical carotid canal	Usually sacrificing CN IX
C_2	Destroying infralabyrinthine compartment invading vertical carotid canal	Usually sacrificing CN IX and X
C_3	Involving infralabyrinthine and apical compartments with invasion of horizontal carotid canal	Usually sacrificing CN IX, X, and XI
D	With intradural extension	
D_1	Intradural extension less than 2 cm in diameter	Infratemporal fossa approach
D_2	Intradural extension greater than 2 cm in diameter	Two-stage neurosurgical-otologic removal
D_3	Inoperable intradural invasion	

ium-DTPA reduces the difference of T_1-weighted signal intensity between tumor and bone marrow rendering their separation more difficult.[79] Thus *it may not be helpful, and, if used, should be accompanied by pre-contrast T_1-weighted images.*

MRI does not show the bone changes or the tumor relations to the bony landmarks as well as high-resolution CT, but it does appear to define the infralabyrinthine soft tissue extension better than CT. Thus the two procedures are sometimes of complementary value (Fig. 13-171).

Treatment and Surgical Classification

Paragangliomas have a lethal potential if left untreated.[170] Current treatment includes mainly resection for cure[186,187] or radiation for long-term control.[188-192] Using the infratemporal fossa approach advanced by Fisch, the entire petrous bone can be resected, including a portion of the clivus.[185,186,193]

Elaborate classifications have been devised matching tumor extent to surgical procedure (Tables 13-8 and 13-9).[187,194] The details are pertinent only to those frequently involved in such cases, but the principles behind the classifications are of practical importance to those involved even only occasionally: (1) A tumor that is intratympanic or intramastoid or both is resectable by a transmeatal and/or transmastoid approach, which can be performed by most otologists (Figs. 13-160 and 13-161). (2) A tumor that involves the jugular bulb requires expertise in neck surgery as well as in mastoid surgery (Fig. 13-162). (3) A tumor involving the carotid canal or the infralabyrinthine compartment requires the infratemporal fossa approach performed only at neurotologic centers (Figs. 13-163 and 13-164). (4) A tumor with a transdural component calls for neurosurgical in addition to neurotologic expertise (Fig. 13-165). (5) Cavernous sinus or massive foramen magnum tumor may be unresectable (Fig. 13-166).

Modern imaging techniques are thus indispensable in helping to decide the necessity of referral and in the selection of appropriate management.

In tympanicum tumors the surgical blood loss is small and preoperative embolization is not indicated (Fig. 13-168).[195] In jugulare tumors the blood loss is at least 1 or 1.5 L and often much more (Fig. 13-169).[195] Preoperative embolization reduces the blood loss by one or more liters and is now commonly performed.[184,185,195,196]

Differential Diagnosis

The differential diagnoses of paragangliomas and the appropriate imaging choices depend on the clinical presentation, which may either be (1) a retrotympanic or intratympanic mass with or without pulsatile tinnitus or (2) deficits of the caudal cranial nerves. When the clin-

---

INTRATYMPANIC MASSES

Vascular
Aberrant carotid artery
Laterally placed carotid
Carotid artery aneurysm
Persistent stapedial artery
Exposed jugular bulb

Nonneoplastic
Acquired cholesteatoma—common
Cholesterol granuloma (cyst)
Congenital cholesteatoma
Temporal lobe herniation
Choristoma

Benign neoplasm
Paraganglioma—common
Facial schwannoma
Chorda tympani schwannoma
Hemangioma
Meningioma
Adenoma

Malignant neoplasm
Squamous carcinoma
Adenocarcinoma
Rhabdomyosarcoma
Malignant melanoma
Lymphoma
Metastasis

---

ical presentation is a retrotympanic or intratympanic mass, high-resolution CT is the imaging modality of choice. When it is pulsatile tinnitus without a visible lesion, high-resolution CT is the imaging of choice for initial screening, to be followed by angiography if it becomes indicated. When the clinical presentation is deficits of the caudal cranial nerves, MRI is the imaging modality of choice. CT may be used as a supplement.

Retrotympanic or Intratympanic Mass. For a list of intratympanic masses, see accompanying box.

Pulsatile Masses. Most often the pulsatile mass is accompanied by conductive hearing loss and pulsatile tinnitus. In such a clinical setting paraganglioma is by far the most likely lesion. However, the otologist is confronted with the following important differential considerations: (1) glomus tympanicum tumor confined to the middle ear, (2) glomus jugulare tumor involving the jugular bulb, (3) aberrant carotid artery, and (4) exposed jugular bulb.[197,198]

An experienced otologist can usually, but not always, distinguish these conditions by their appearances (Table 13-10). Ill-advised biopsies have often been performed on aberrant carotid arteries or exposed jugular bulbs resulting in massive hemorrhage and/or hemiplegia.[199,200] It is of utmost importance to prevent inappropriate intervention that the radiologist notes the

Table 13-10 Otoscopic differential diagnosis of pulsatile intratympanic masses

Lesion	Color	Location
Aberrant carotid artery	Pink	Anteroinferior quadrant
Exposed jugular bulb	Blue	Posteroinferior quadrant
Glomus tympanicum tumor	Reddish-purple	Posteroinferior quadrant
Glomus jugulare tumor	Reddish-purple	Posteroinferior quadrant

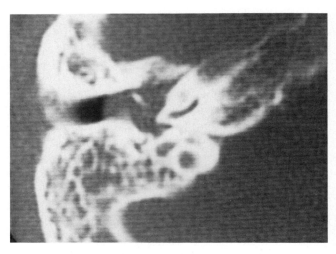

Fig. 13-173 Adenomatous tumor of mixed pattern type. High-resolution CT. Tumor filling tympanic cavity and medial external auditory canal without destruction of middle ear ossicles is identical in appearance to glomus tympanicum tumor. (Compare with Fig. 13-161.) Dynamic contrast CT may help to make the differentiation. Since surgical approach is basically the same for both tumors, angiography for differential diagnosis is not warranted.

characteristic findings of the aberrant carotid artery or the exposed jugular bulb on CT (see Figs. 13-50 and 13-51). Angiography is usually not necessary.[198] CT also distinguishes glomus tympanicum tumor, which requires no angiography and limited surgery, from glomus jugulare tumor, which requires angiography, preoperative embolization, and extensive surgery (Figs. 13-160 to 13-165).[178,198]

Two rarer arterial anomalies may clinically resemble the aberrant carotid artery. Both lesions are associated with dehiscence of the carotid plate: the "laterally displaced internal carotid artery" herniating into the middle ear,[202,203] and an aneurysm of the internal carotid artery from the junction between its vertical and horizontal intrapetrous segments located in the middle ear.[204] Angiography may be used to confirm the diagnosis. The persistent stapedial artery is not usually visible on otoscopy but can be seen to enlarge the anterior portion of the tympanic facial nerve canal on CT.[205]

Other Benign Lesions. Other intratympanic masses may be encountered from time to time and may be indistinguishable from glomus tympanicum tumors on CT especially when they fill the tympanic cavity and obscure their precise origin. For example, cholesterol granuloma,[206,207,208] hemangioma,[141,208,209] facial nerve or chorda tympani schwannoma,[115,210] congenital cholesteatoma,[211] meningioma,[212,213] adenomatous tumor of the mixed pattern type (Fig. 13-173),[214,215] and choristoma (ectopic salivary tissue).[214] However, all of these lesions are rare and all of them are benign. The surgical approach for them is similar as long as the lesions are confined to the middle ear.[179]

If discovered early, certain intratympanic tumors may be recognized by their locations. For example, small tympanic paragangliomas can be identified on the promontory (Fig. 13-160), small facial schwannomas (see Fig. 13-187), hemangiomas and choristomas[214] along the facial nerve canal (FNC), and small chorda tympani schwannomas on the lateral tympanic wall.

A cholesteatoma found behind an intact ear drum without a history of otitis media is considered by some to be congenital in origin.[214,216] Whether congenital or not, these cholesteatomas account for 2% of all middle ear cholesteatomas.[217] Their most common middle ear sites are the epitympanium and the incudostapedial vicinity.[216,218]

An acquired cholesteatoma is accompanied by evidence of chronic infection.

Malignant Tumors. There are several malignant tumors of the middle ear, all of which are rare. Among these lesions, squamous carcinoma is the most common. It is thought to arise secondary to metaplasia of the normal cuboidal or ciliated columnar epithelium.[219] Twenty-three patients treated with mastoidectomy and radiation had a 5-year survival rate of 39%.[219] Death is usually by intracranial extension.

Rhabdomyosarcoma occurs in early childhood.[220] Although rare, embryonal rhabdomyosarcoma is the most common middle ear neoplasm in that age group. Initially the tumor appears as chronic otitis media. A superficial biopsy often yields only inflammatory granulation tissue. Destruction then rapidly extends beyond the middle ear, and facial nerve palsy is common.[220-222] Although the disease is highly malignant and usually fatal, multiple-drug chemotherapy and radiation after a mastoidectomy have resulted in several long-term survivals.[221]

Table 13-11   Differential diagnosis of jugular foramen tumors

Tumor	CT margin	Angiographic vascularity	MRI appearance
Schwannoma	Well-defined	Minimal to moderate	Homogeneous or cystic
Paraganglioma	Ill-defined	Marked	"Salt and pepper"
Meningioma	Subtly ill-defined	Minimal	Homogeneous
Malignant tumors (carcinomas, metastases)	Ill-defined	Minimal with exceptions	Homogeneous
Chondrosarcoma	Ill-defined	Minimal	Homogeneous
Nasopharyngeal carcinoma	Medial	—	—

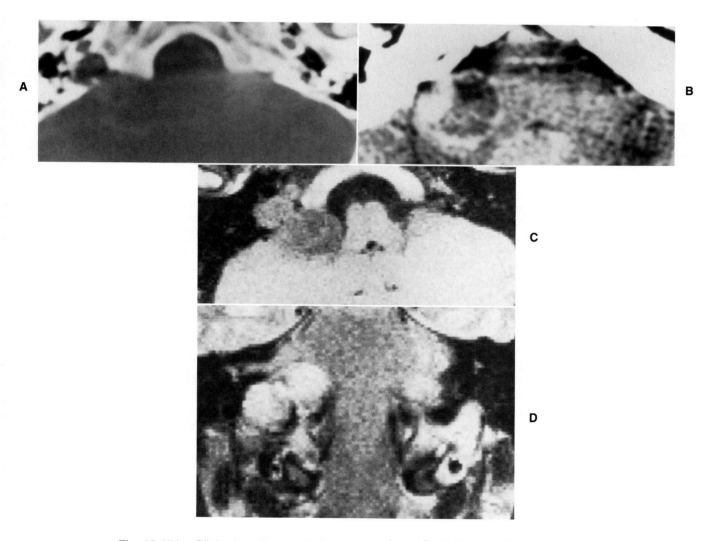

Fig. 13-174   Bilobed cystic vagal schwannoma. **A** and **B,** High-resolution and postcontrast CT. Tumor is partly in posterior fossa and partly in jugular foramen. Note sharply and smoothly marginated expansion of jugular foramen and inhomogeneous enhancement of tumor similar to the one in Fig. 13-147, *A* and *C.* **C** and **D,** T$_1$-weighted image and T$_2$-weighted coronal image. Tumor is at pontomedullary level on coronal image. (Compare with Fig. 13-176.)

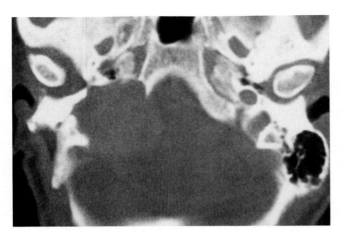

Fig. 13-175 Jugular foramen schwannoma. High-resolution CT. Expansion of jugular foramen is symmetric and rounded and margins are well-defined. (Contrast with Figs. 13-163 to 13-165, 13-178, 13-201, and 13-202.) Unlike glossopharyngeal and vagal schwannomas in Figs. 13-147 and 13-174, respectively, this "type-B" tumor did cause deficits of the IX, X, XI and XII cranial nerves. Nerve of origin could not be determined at surgery. (From Lo WWM, Solti-Bohman LG, and Lambert PR: High-resolution CT in evaluation of glomus tumors of temporal bone, Radiology 150:737-742, 1984.)

Adenocarcinoma[214,215,223] and metastases[223] can also occur in the middle ear cleft. In addition, the primary presentation of malignant lymphoma in the middle ear and of primary melanoma have been reported.[224,225]

Jugular Foramen Masses. For a description of jugular foramen masses, see Table 13-11. In our experience about 10% of the tumors involving the jugular foramen are not paragangliomas. These lesions include schwannomas of the caudal cranial nerves, meningiomas, carcinomas (primary and metastatic), chondrosarcomas, and extensions from nasopharyngeal carcinomas.

Jugular Foramen Schwannomas. Schwannomas of the caudal cranial nerves are rare.[13,14] Jugular schwannomas, which include schwannomas from the glossopharyngeal, vagus, and spinal accessory nerves, are not always distinguishable from one another (Figs. 13-147, 13-148, 13-174, and 13-175). They have been classified into three types according to their locations:[116]

Type A tumors grow predominantly intracranially.

Type B tumors grow predominantly at the jugular foramen.

Type C tumors grow predominantly extracranially.

Type A tumors (Figs. 13-147, 13-148, and 13-174) tend to have acoustic and/or cerebellar presenting symptoms while Type B and C tumors (Fig. 13-175) tend to be associated with the jugular foramen syndrome.[116,117]

Schwannomas expand the jugular foramen symmetrically in contrast to paragangliomas, which often extend along dural sinuses and fissures. The bone margins are much rounder and sharper (Figs. 13-147, 13-174, 13-175).[14,117,182] Their angiographic hypervascularity is much less than that of paragangliomas.[116,226]

The CT and MRI appearances of jugular schwannomas are similar to those of acoustic schwannomas, varying with the proportion of cellular and cystic components of the tumor. The tumor itself, especially its extracranial component along the carotid sheath, is best demonstrated on MRI (Fig. 13-174, D). Coronal and sagittal imaging is another advantage of MRI over CT (Figs. 13-174, D, and 13-176, B). However, CT with bone detail best demonstrates the foraminal changes and is most helpful in differentiating schwannomas from paragangliomas and jugular from hypoglossal schwannomas (Figs. 13-147, A, 13-174, A, and 13-175). Glossopharyngeal schwannomas can also be differentiated from vagus and spinal accessory schwannomas when there is selective enlargement of the pars nervosa (Fig. 13-147, A).

Hypoglossal Schwannomas. Much of what has been said about jugular foramen schwannomas applies also to hypoglossal schwannomas. These tumors may be intracranial or extracranial or be "dumbbell"-shaped, extending into both spaces (Fig. 13-176). In addition, because of proximity of the hypoglossal canal to the foramen magnum, caudal intraspinal extension has been observed.[14]

Besides ipsilateral hemiatrophy of the tongue, other caudal cranial nerve deficits may develop as the tumor enlarges.[227,228] Medullary and cerebellar compression and hydrocephalus follow.[229] In fact, more patients with intracranial hypoglossal schwannomas initially have cerebellar symptoms or hydrocephalus rather than tongue dysfunction.[230]

Well-defined erosion of the hypoglossal canal is characteristic although not invariably present.[231] After eroding the hypoglossal canal, the tumor may also erode the jugular foramen, the jugular tubercle, and the clivus, making differentiation from schwannomas of jugular foramen origin difficult.[228]

Meningioma. In addition to their common site of origin on the posterior petrous surface, meningiomas may rarely arise from within the temporal bone. Nager lists four such sites: (1) the internal acoustic meatus, (2) the jugular foramen, (3) the region of the geniculate ganglion, and (4) the sulcus of the greater and lesser superficial petrosal nerves.[232]

Little information in the literature exists specifically about the radiologic features of jugular foramen meningiomas. From our experience of four cases with complete preoperative imaging and the surgical findings in several other cases, they have some of the behavior patterns of paragangliomas. They are locally invasive around the jugular foramen, they grow through the jugular plate into the hypotympanum, they descend through and along the jugular vein, and they may show a small extension into the posterior fossa (Fig. 13-177).

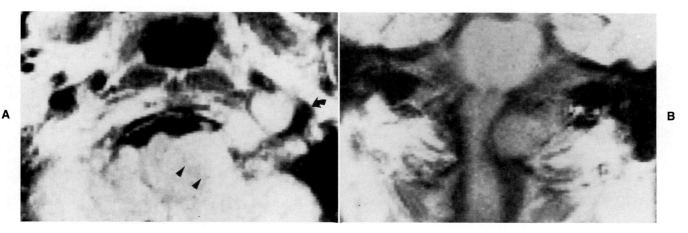

Fig. 13-176 Trilobed hypoglossal schwannoma. **A** and **B,** T$_1$-weighted images. Tumor is difficult to distinguish from jugular foramen schwannoma on transverse images but its more caudal position at medullocord junction is quite apparent on coronal image. (Compare with Fig. 13-174, *D.*) Intracranial component of tumor deforms the medulla *(arrowheads)* and parapharyngeal component displaces jugular vein *(curved arrow).*

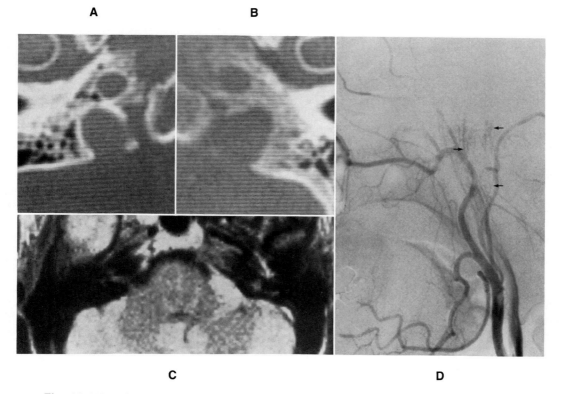

Fig. 13-177 Jugular foramen meningioma. **A,** and **B,** High-resolution CT. Note subtle loss of sharpness of cortex of jugular fossa and vertical carotid canal and slight sclerosis of adjacent infiltrated bone on the left vs the normal fossa on the right. **C,** Intermediate weighted image. Tumor is mildly and homogeneously hyperintense. (See also Figs. 13-137 to 13-139.) **D,** Selective external carotid angiogram. Tumor vascularity is minimal *(arrows).*

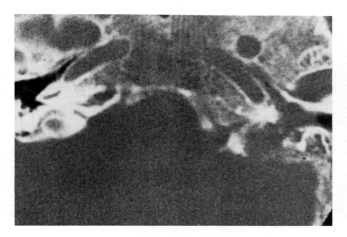

Fig. 13-178 Jugular foramen anaplastic carcinoma. High-resolution CT. Irregular ill-defined destruction of jugular fossa is indistinguishable from that of glomus jugulare tumor. Selective external carotid angiogram showed *no* tumor vascularity.

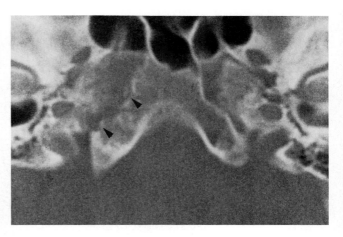

Fig. 13-179 CPA chondrosarcoma. High-resolution CT. Irregular ill-defined destruction along petrooccipital fissure *(arrowheads)* is similar to what may be seen in extensions from nasopharyngeal carcinoma. Pars nervosa is barely involved and pars vascularis spared. See also Figs. 13-206 and 13-207 for other petrous chondrosarcomas.

On CT their soft tissue components are indistinguishable from those of paragangliomas. Their bone margins, however, are better defined than those of paragangliomas but less well defined than those of schwannomas (Fig. 13-177, *A* and *B*). Subtle sclerosis may be present in the infiltrated bone.

On MRI they appear as other meningiomas and they lack the "salt-and-pepper" pattern of paragangliomas (Fig. 13-177, *C*).[11,89,91,92] On angiography they show minimal vascularity, less than schwannomas, and do not have the prolonged cloudlike blush commonly seen in supratentorial meningiomas (Fig. 13-177, *D*).

Malignant Tumors. Carcinoma, sarcoma, metastasis, and other malignancies may be indistinguishable from paragangliomas on CT if they happen to destroy the jugular fossa (Figs. 13-178, 13-195, 13-200, 13-201). On angiography most of them are much less vascular than paragangliomas. Exceptions to be considered include metastic hypernephroma, metastic pheochromocytoma, and metastatic thyroid cancer.

Chondrosarcoma. Occurring along the petroccipital fissure, chondrosarcomas may involve the jugular foramen from its medial aspect and may contain calcifications (Figs. 13-179, 13-206, and 13-207).

Nasopharyngeal Carcinoma. Direct extension from nasopharyngeal carcinoma also tends to involve the jugular foramen more from its medial than its lateral aspect.

Miscellaneous. An amyloidoma has been reported in the cerebellopontine angle and the jugular foramen appearing as a patchy hyperdense mass with slight contrast enhancement and angiographic avascularity.[233]

TUMORS INVOLVING THE FACIAL NERVE

Of the 1575 cases of facial nerve disorders managed over a 20-year period by May, only 91, or 6%, were caused by tumors;[234] 895, or 57%, were caused by idiopathic or Bell's palsy, which classically begins abruptly and resolves spontaneously within a few weeks.[174] Thus the majority of facial nerve palsies do not require a radiologic workup.

The other causes in May's series were herpes zoster oticus (7%), trauma (17%), infection (4%), congenital (3%), hemifacial spasm (2%), central nervous system disease (1%), other (2%), and unknown (1%).

However, May pointed out that 46 of the 91 tumors in his series were initially misdiagnosed as Bell's palsy.[235] Hence slow progression of paralysis beyond 3 weeks, absence of recovery after 6 months, ipsilateral recurrence, and other signs atypical of Bell's palsy demand a thorough radiologic investigation for tumor.[234] Abrupt onset alone is no assurance that the palsy is not caused by tumor.[210,236]

Manifestations of Facial Nerve Dysfunction and Lesion Localization

The facial nerve in its long course from the pons, through the CP angle, IAC, and facial nerve canal (FNC) to its arborization in the parotid gland is subject to involvement by tumors of many types at different locations. Unfocused or misdirected imaging studies have often delayed diagnosis.[237,238] Awareness of clinical localization is of great assistance to the radiologic investigation.

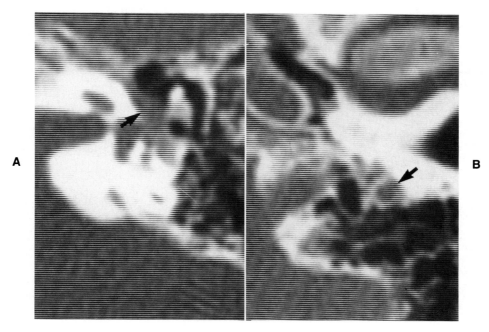

Fig. 13-180 Extension from mucoepidermoid cystic carcinoma of parotid. **A** and **B,** HRCT. Mastoid segment and posterior two-thirds of tympanic segment of FNC have been expanded slightly by tumor *(arrow).* After mastoid exploration and biopsy, a nonpalpable 2-cm deep-lobe parotid tumor was found on CT and MRI and shown to be of the same histology by CT-guided biopsy. (Compare with Fig. 13-186.)

Facial nerve paralysis is classically divided into central and peripheral categories. Central lesions—located above the motor nucleus in the brainstem—result in contralateral motor weakness of the lower part of the face. Peripheral nerve lesions cause ipsilateral motor weakness of both the upper and lower parts of the face. Hemifacial spasm is an irritative phenomenon of the facial nerve. Myokymia is a fine fibrillary activity of all muscles of one side of the face and is most often seen in patients with multiple sclerosis or brainstem glioma.[174]

Facial nerve compromise in the brainstem is likely to be accompanied by palsy of other cranial nerves and perhaps contralateral long tract signs. In the CP angle and the IAC it is likely to be accompanied or preceded by symptoms of the acoustic nerve.[237,238]

A facial nerve lesion within the temporal bone can be further localized according to the presence or absence of involvement of (1) the greater superficial petrosal nerve (lacrimation), (2) the nerve of the stapedius muscle (stapes reflex), and (3) the chorda tympani nerve (taste and salivation). Thus a lesion may be described as *suprageniculate* if all three are affected, *suprastapedial* if (2) and (3) are affected, *infrastapedial* if only (3) is affected, and *infrachordal* if all three are intact.[239]

If the origin of a peripheral facial palsy is clinically unlocalized or localized to the pons, the CP angle or the IAC, we prefer to evaluate with MRI including the pons through the parotid if necessary, and using IV gadolinium-DTPA if necessary. If it is clinically localized to the facial nerve canal, we prefer to use high-resolution CT with maximum bone detail.

It should be noted, however, that destruction of the FNC by tumor does not necessarily cause facial nerve palsy if there is no invasion of the facial nerve.[240] Conversely, perineural and intraneural spread, which occurs with some tumors, notably adenoid cystic carcinoma from the parotid, can extend along a considerable length of the facial nerve within the FNC causing facial palsy with little or no bone changes (Fig. 13-180).[223,240] In such a situation MRI may show the abnormality more readily than CT, especially with the use of gadolinium-DTPA.

Tumors

Types and Statistics. Tables 13-12 and 13-13 show the gamut of benign and malignant tumors respectively in May's experience of 91 tumors causing facial palsy.[234]

In Fisch and Rüttner's series of 43 intratemporal tumors involving the facial nerve, there were 12 congenital cholesteatomas (10 supralabyrinthine and 2 apex) and 9 neuromas and 9 hemangiomas (4 cavernous and 5 ossifying). Less common benign tumors include 3 men-

Table 13-12 Benign tumors causing facial palsy in 44 patients

Cell type	Tumor location	No. patients	Totals
Schwannoma	Acoustic nerve		12
	CPA*	6	
	IAC†	6	
	Facial nerve		12
	Labyrinthine segment	3‡	
	Geniculate ganglion	1	
	Tympanic segment	2	
	Mastoid segment	5	
	Chorda tympani nerve	1	
Vascular			6
Meningioma	CPA	3	
Hemangioma	Geniculate ganglion	3	3
Osseous	Geniculate ganglion	1	
Capillary	Geniculate ganglion	1	
	Parotid	1	
AV malformation			1
	Geniculate ganglion	1	
Glomus jugulare			3
	Skull base	3	
Congenital cholesteatoma			3
	IAC	2	
	Tympanic segment	1	
Others			4
Inflammatory mass	Vertical segment	1	
Granular cell myoblastoma	Vertical segment	1	
Giant cell tumor	Sphenoid	1	
Branchial cleft cyst	Skull base	1	
		TOTAL:	44

Reprinted by permission from May M: The facial nerve, New York, 1986, Thieme Medical Publishers.
*CPA, cerebellopontine angle.
†IAC, internal auditory canal.
‡Facial nerve schwannoma extended from labyrinthine segment to extracranial segment in two patients and from mastoid segment to extracranial segment in one patient.

Table 13-13 Malignant tumors causing facial palsy in 47 patients

Location	Type	No. Patients	Total
Temporal bone			19
	Primary (epidermoid)	2	
	Leukemia	5	
	Lymphoma	3	
	Reticular sarcoma	1	
	Metastatic (breast)	3	
	Lung	3	
	Prostate	2	
Parotid			14
	Adenoid cystic carcinoma	5	
	Mucoepidermoid carcinoma	3	
	Epidermoid carcinoma	3	
	Undifferentiated carcinoma	2	
	Anaplastic carcinoma	1	
Submandibular gland			1
	Adenoid cystic carcinoma	1	
Skin			5
	Epidermoid carcinoma	2	
	Basal cell carcinoma	2	
	Fibrous histiocytoma	1	
Other			8
	Tonsil (epidermoid)	2	
	Nasopharyngeal (epidermoid)	2	
	Orohypopharyngeal (epidermoid)	2	
	Hodgkins (neck)	1	
	Unconfirmed	1	
		TOTAL:	47

Reprinted by permission from May M: The facial nerve, New York, 1986, Thieme Medical Publishers.

Table 13-14 Differential features of common geniculate ganglion tumors

	Facial schwannoma	Benign vascular tumor	Epidermoid
Size	Quite variable	Very small	Small
Shape	Round or sausage-shaped	Irregular	Unilocular or multilocular
Margins	Well-defined	Ill-defined	Extremely well-defined
Location	Along IAC,* FNC,† or in MF‡	IAC, GG,§ or posterior genu	Supralabyrinthine
Density	Nearly isodense	Intratumoral bone	Hypodensity to isodensity
Enhancement	Yes	Yes	No

*IAC = Internal auditory canal
†FNC = Facial nerve canal
‡MF = Middle fossa
§GG = Geniculate ganglion

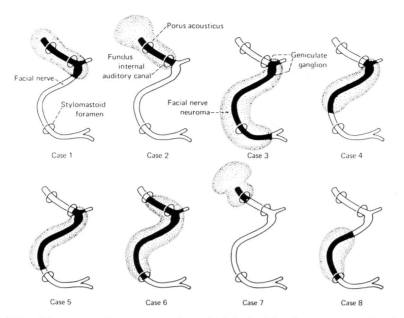

Fig. 13-181 Diagrammatic representation of eight facial schwannomas. Shaded area represents segments of nerve involved by tumor. Most facial schwannomas involve long segments of nerve. (From Latack JT, Gabrielson TO, Knake JE, et al.: Facial nerve neuromas. Radiologic evaluation. Radiology 149:731-739, 1983.)

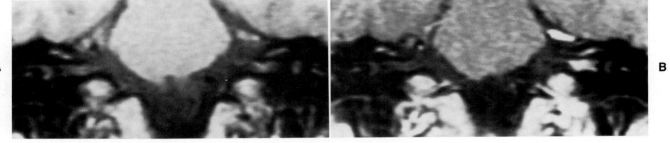

Fig. 13-182 IAC facial schwannoma. **A** and **B,** Pre- and post-gadolinium T₁-weighted images. The patient presented with progressive sensorineural hearing loss and no facial palsy. The 3×5 mm enhancing intracanalicular tumor is indistinguishable from an acoustic schwannoma. The tumor was exposed by the middle fossa approach but not resected or biopsied. (Courtesy of Joseph R. Scalley, MD and Mark R. Laussade, MD.)

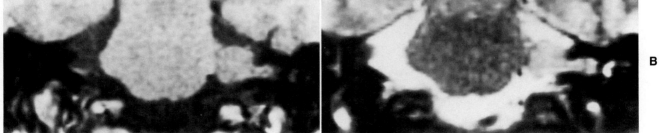

Fig. 13-183 CPA and IAC facial schwannoma. **A** and **B,** Intermediate and T₂-weighted images. Tumor is indistinguishable from an acoustic schwannoma in appearance. (Courtesy of Albert L. Bahr, MD.)

ingiomas, 3 glomus jugular tumors,[241] and 1 arachnoid cyst.[236] Malignant tumors include 4 squamous carcinomas and 2 rhabdomyosarcomas.

Although the majority of Fisch and Rüttner's patients had slowly progressive facial palsy, 6 had facial palsy of sudden onset including 3 of the 5 patients with ossifying hemangiomas.[236]

Facial nerve tumors in the CP angle and IAC share the same differential diagnosis with acoustic schwannomas, and those in the tympanic cavity share the same with intratympanic paragangliomas. These differential diagnoses have been discussed under the sections on acoustic schwannoma and paraganglioma, respectively. The three most common tumors in Fisch and Rüttner's series, neuroma, hemangioma, and congenital cholesteatoma, are described in detail below. All three tend to occur in the region of the geniculate ganglion.[236] (See Table 13-14.)

Facial Schwannoma. Facial schwannomas can occur along any segment of the nerve (Figs. 13-181 to 13-

188).[242] The geniculate ganglion is frequently involved and is often included whether the tumor extends primarily proximally or distally.[115]

The clinical presentations of facial schwannomas depend on the segment of the nerve involved.[243] Interestingly, fewer than half of the facial schwannomas initially appear with facial palsy.[114,115] Many have no facial nerve symptoms at all. For example, in one series only 2 of 8 cases had facial palsy as a presenting symptom and only 2 of the 8 had hemifacial spasm.[115] This may result from the fact that schwannomas compress but do not invade the nerve. Consequently, nerve deficits result only where high pressure can be exerted.

In general, facial schwannomas in the CP angle and the IAC are characterized by sensorineural hearing loss, apparently because the more thinly myelinated sensory fibers of the acoustic nerve are more vulnerable to compression than the more thickly myelinated motor fibers of the facial nerve (Figs. 13-182 and 13-183).[115] Schwannomas in the geniculate region grow silently

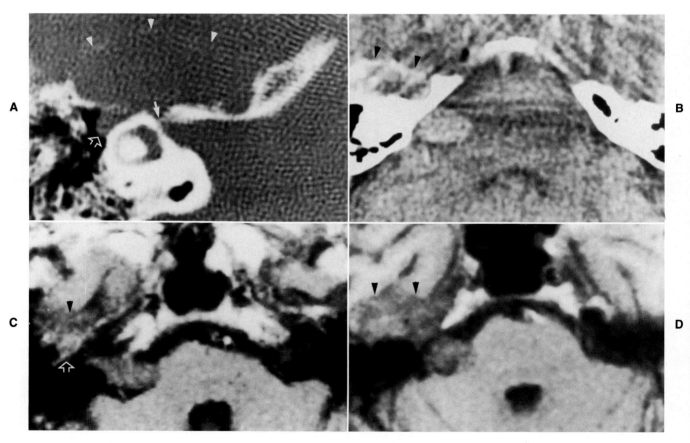

Fig. 13-184 Bilobed facial schwannoma. **A** and **B,** High-resolution and postcontrast CT. **C** and **D,** T$_1$-weighted images. Facial schwannomas are not uncommonly bilobed with components in the middle *(arrowheads)* and posterior fossas connected through a narrow labyrinthine segment *(arrow)*. Note small extension into the middle ear along tympanic segment *(open arrow)*. Patient has not been operated on.

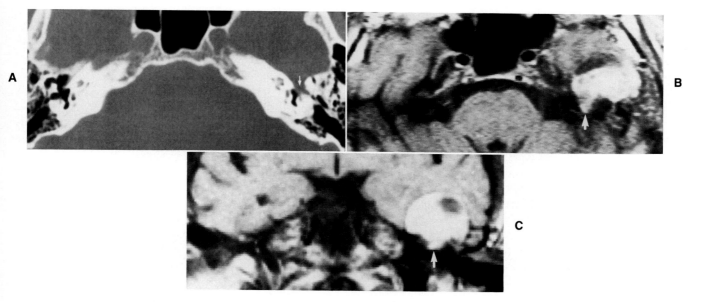

Fig. 13-185   Geniculate ganglion facial schwannoma. **A,** High-resolution CT. **B** and **C,** Transverse and coronal post-gadolinium T$_1$-weighted images. A large, clinically silent component of the tumor mushrooming into middle fossa is common growth pattern of facial schwannomas arising at geniculate ganglion. Conductive hearing loss is caused by the *small* component in the anterior tympanic cavity *(arrow)*. Without proper imaging evaluation it is frequently mistaken otoscopically as cholesteatoma until exploration or biopsy.

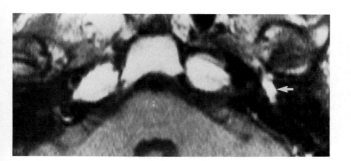

Fig. 13-186   Tympanic segment facial schwannoma. Post-gadolinium T$_1$-weighted image. Tumor is mildly hyperintense and strongly enhancing *(arrow)*.

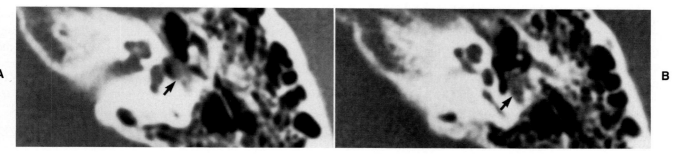

Fig. 13-187   Tympanic segment facial schwannoma. **A** and **B,** High-resolution CT. Tumor arising from posterior genu region caused conductive hearing loss *(arrow)*. Other tumors that may be similar in appearance include intratemporal vascular tumors (hemangioma), paraganglioma, choristoma, and congenital cholesteatoma. (See also Fig. 13-180.) (Courtesy of Lyle Wendling, MD.)

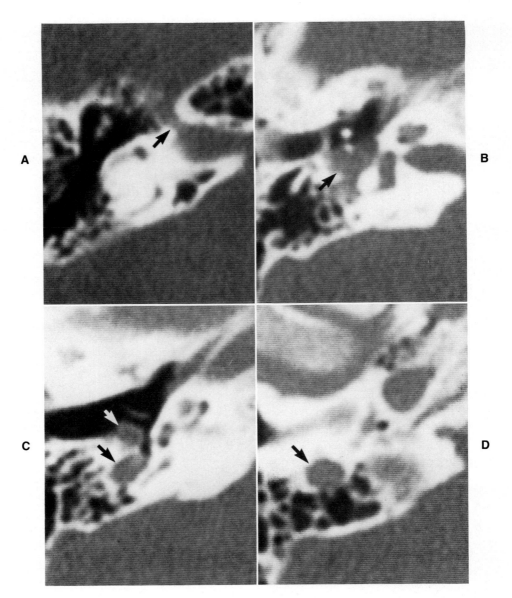

Fig. 13-188   FNC facial schwannoma. **A** to **D,** High-resolution CT. To varying degrees the tumor has expanded the entire length of facial nerve canal *(arrows).*

into the middle cranial fossa, reaching several centimeters in diameter before acoustic or facial nerve symptoms appear (Fig. 13-185).[244] Those in the tympanic segment first are demonstrated with conductive hearing loss by ossicular interference (Figs. 13-186 and 13-187). Those in the mastoid segment are the only ones likely to have facial palsy as a presenting symptom (Fig. 13-188).[115] Finally, those tumors distal to the stylomastoid foramen appear as painless neck masses.[245]

Excision of a facial schwannoma almost always requires segmental resection of the facial nerve. In most cases it is best to resect the tumor and restore continuity of the nerve with an end-to-end anastomosis or a "cable" nerve graft.[246]

Facial schwannomas are often sausage-shaped, ex-panding long segments of the FNC (Figs. 13-187 and 13-188). There may be more than one "link," for example, a component in the IAC and a component in the middle cranial fossa may be connected via a narrow waist through the labyrinthine FNC (Fig. 13-184). Their CT density and enhancement and MRI intensity are similar to those of acoustic schwannomas.

When facial schwannomas occur in the CP angle or in the IAC, they may be clinically and radiologically indistinguishable from acoustic schwannomas (Figs. 13-182 and 13-183). Anterosuperior erosion of the IAC or erosion of the labyrinthine FNC, if present, may be the only diagnostic clue. The differential diagnoses in these two regions are identical to those of acoustic schwannomas (Tables 13-6 and 13-8).

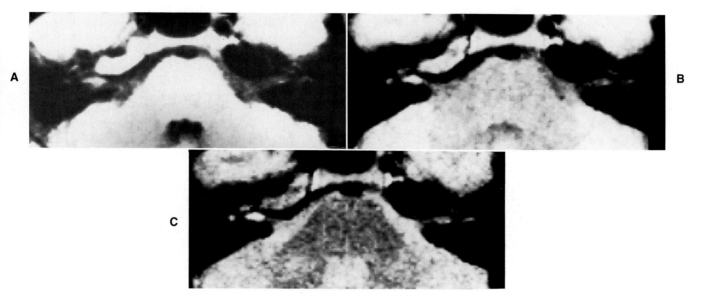

Fig. 13-189   IAC intratemporal vascular tumor. **A, B,** and **C,** T$_1$-, intermediate, and T$_2$-weighted images. Tumor is more hyperintense on T$_2$-weighted images than typical schwannoma. (Compare with Fig. 13-128; courtesy of Michael Anselmo, MD.) (**C** from Lo WWM, Shelton C, Waluch V, et al: Intratemporal vascular tumors: detection with CT and MR. Radiology 171:443-448, 1989.)

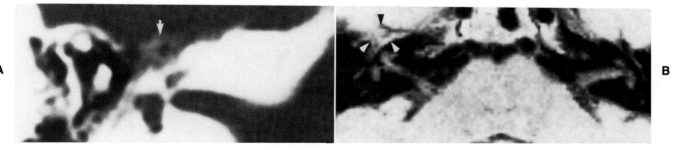

Fig. 13-190   Geniculate intratemporal vascular tumor. **A,** High-resolution CT. Note characteristic "honeycomb" bone *(arrow)* present in some vascular tumors. Bone interspersed within tumor tissue is less dense than adjacent normal bone. **B,** Intermediate weighted image. Note heterogeneous hyperintensity in geniculate fossa and surrounding region *(arrowheads)* adjacent to temporal lobe. (From Lo WWM, Shelton C, Waluch V, et al.: Intratemporal vascular tumors: detection with CT and MR, Radiology, 171:443-448, 1989.)

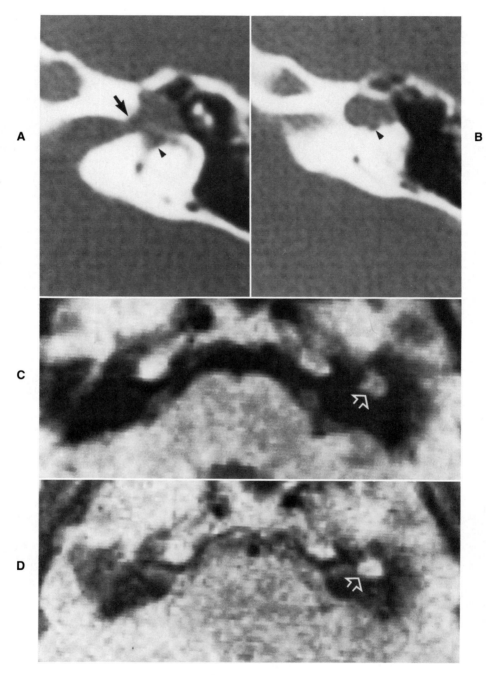

Fig. 13-191 Suprageniculate congenital epidermoid. **A** and **B,** High-resolution CT. Bone margins are extremely sharp and smooth. Borders of the geniculate fossa are no longer visible. Labyrinthine FNC has been widened *(arrow)* and superior semicircular canal eroded *(arrowhead).* Unilocular tumor bulges slightly into anterior epitympanic space. Middle ear is otherwise normal. **C** and **D,** Intermediate and T_2-weighted images. Tumor is isointense to brain on intermediate and mildly hyperintense on T_2-weighted images *(open arrow).* (From Lo WWM, Lufkin R, and Hanafee W: Uses of computerized tomography and magnetic resonance imaging in temporal bone imaging. Adv Otolaryngol Head Neck Surg 1:109-126, 1987.)

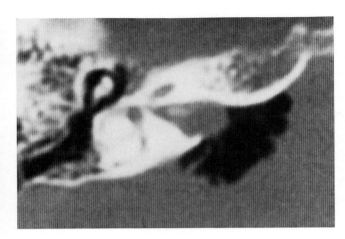

Fig. 13-192   IAC intratemporal vascular tumor. Gas-CT cisternogram. Note intratumoral bone spicule seen in some vascular tumors. (From Lo WWM, Horn HR, Carberry JN et al: Intratemporal vascular tumors: evaluation with CT, Radiology 159:181-185, 1986.)

For differential diagnosis in the geniculate ganglion region, other tumors prevalent in that location, namely, epidermoid, hemangioma, and meningiomas, are the primary considerations (Figs. 13-190 and 13-191). The changes seen on high-resolution CT are helpful: the borders of hemangiomas are not sharp (Fig. 13-190), those of epidermoids extremely sharp (Fig. 13-191), and those of schwannomas moderately sharp (Figs. 13-184, 13-185, and 13-188). Hemangiomas and epidermoids are usually small, and schwannomas are variable in size and may be quite large (Figs. 13-184, 13-185, 13-188, 13-190 and 13-191). Hemangiomas may contain intratumoral bone (Figs. 13-190 and 13-192). Epidermoids are isodense or hypodense and are nonenhancing.[247] The CT and MRI features of meningioma at this location may be expected to resemble those in the CP angle.

When geniculate region schwannomas are sufficiently large, they may be mistaken for gliomas or metastases in the temporal lobe (Fig. 13-185).[244,248] Coronal images are helpful in the evaluation of tumors in this region. Smooth enlargement of the facial nerve canal should be a distinguishing feature in favor of a facial schwannoma.

Enlargement of the proximal tympanic segment of the FNC by a persistent stapedial artery must not be mistaken for a facial nerve schwannoma.[205] In addition, developmental dehiscence of the FNC, which is present in about half of the temporal bones, most often occurs near the oval window; this should not be mistaken for an area of localized destruction.[249]

Gadolinium-enhanced MRI rivals high-resolution CT with bone algorithm detail in the early detection of facial nerve tumors (Figs. 13-182, 13-185, and 13-186).[250] However, for precise correlation with bony landmarks, CT with bone detail is still to be preferred (Figs. 13-184 to 13-188).

Benign Vascular Tumors. Hemangiomas or vascular malformations along the intratemporal course of the facial nerve were once thought to be rare.[251,252] Recently, however, they have been found in some series at least as often as the much better known schwannomas.[141,209,236]

Hemangiomas are composed of thin-walled vascular spaces. Vascular malformations are composed of thick-walled vascular spaces and lined by a single layer of endothelium surrounded by fibroblasts and collagen. Since the two lesions may coexist in a single mass, they have been grouped together under intratemporal vascular tumors; and terms are sometimes loosely interchanged.[141,253]

Hemangiomas may be further categorized into cavernous and capillary types by the predominant size of their vascular spaces. Vascular tumors often grow among bone trabeculae and may form bone (Figs. 13-190 and 13-192). In the latter case they have been called "ossifying" hemangiomas.[209,236] All of these tumors are benign.[141]

Intratemporal vascular tumors cause nerve deficits by invasion rather than compression. Therefore, unlike schwannomas, they cause hemifacial spasm and facial palsy *early;* and if located in the IAC, they also cause sensorineural hearing loss to a greater degree than would be expected soley on their size (Figs. 13-189 and 13-192).[36,141,155,254] Although facial nerve resection and grafting may be necessary in many cases, in contrast to schwannomas, vascular tumors can often be removed with preservation of facial nerve continuity if operated on early. Early detection is therefore extremely important.

Early detection of intratemporal vascular tumors has often been a challenge to imaging techniques and requires meticulous scrutiny. Although many of these tumors have been missed because of inadequate technique, some have been missed even with excellent technique because of their small size and subtle findings.[141,209,255]

These benign vascular tumors occur most often at the geniculate ganglion region, next most often in the IAC, and least often at the posterior genu. They are usually under 1 cm in diameter.

On CT in the IAC, they usually require gas cisternography for detection.[141] They may contain intratumoral bone spicules (Fig. 13-192).[141] In the labyrinthine FNC and at the geniculate ganglion, they show subtle findings that may include irregular and indistinct bone margins and reticular or "honeycomb" bone (Fig. 13-190).[141,209] At the posterior genu they are difficult to distinguish from schwannomas (Fig. 13-187). Although they enhance with contrast, enhancement does not play a significant role in their detection since such density changes in small intratemporal lesions, which are interspersed amongst bone, are difficult to discern.

On MRI vascular tumors are extremely well demonstrated when located in the IAC (Fig. 13-189).[255] They are isointense to mildly hyperintense on T_1-weighted images and markedly hyperintense on T_2-weighted images, more so than the typical schwannoma. When located in the geniculate ganglion region, they have been less reliably demonstrated by MRI without gadolinium-DTPA than by CT with bone detail. When they are identifiable on MRI, they show nonhomogeneous intensities, which may be the MRI correlate of the CT "honeycomb" bone (Fig. 13-190). Thin sections, close slice spacing, and the use of gadolinium-DTPA may improve the MRI results.

Epidermoid. Besides arising intradurally from the CP angle, epidermoids, also called congenital or primary cholesteatomas, may arise extradurally from the petrous apex or the supralabyrinthine region of the temporal bone. From the petrous apex they attain considerable size before involving the facial and acoustic nerves in the CP angle or the IAC and thus they clinically appear late (see Fig. 13-205). From the supralabyrinthine region they readily erode the proximal FNC and can be noted early while they are still small (Fig. 13-191). Ten out of twelve of the epidermoids causing facial nerve palsy in Fisch and Rüttner's series occurred in this region. From this point of origin they often reach around the superior semicircular canal and extend medially superior to the IAC or laterally into the epitympanum (Fig. 13-191).[247] They may erode the superior surface of the cochlea capsule or the ampulary limb of the superior semicircular canal to the point of fistulization (Fig. 13-191).[236]

On CT their bone margins are characteristically extremely sharp (Fig. 13-191).[236,247] Their general configuration may either be unilobular or multilobular. Hypodensity with brain may or may not be seen.[247] On MRI they are hypointense with brain on T_1-weighted images but hyperintense on T_2-weighted images (Fig. 13-191).

The petrous apex epidermoids are discussed further in the section on other tumors of the temporal bone.

OTHER TUMORS AND CYSTS OF THE TEMPORAL BONE

Many other tumors and cysts occur in the temporal bone that thus far have not been specifically discussed. Mainly these are lesions that arise in the external auditory canal (EAC), the mastoid, and the petrous apex. In a differential diagnosis of an osteolytic lesion of the temporal bone, Chasin discussed 25 diseases under eight categories: carcinomas, sarcomas, metastases, benign epithelial lesions, benign nonepithelial lesions, hematologic malignancies, infections and inflammatory lesions, and histiocytosis.[256] As exhaustive as this list was, it was incomplete. For example, we may add mucocele,[257] cholesterol granuloma or cyst (Fig. 13-193),[258-263] giant cell tumor (Figs. 13-194 and 13-195),[264,265] intrapetrous carotid aneurysm,[266] xanthoma,[267] and so on. The number of possible lesions is indeed extensive (Table 13-15).

On the other hand, we are limited in our ability to provide a specific diagnosis in the vast majority of these lesions because of the nonspecificity of the bone changes, the CT density and the degree of enhancement, and the MRI signal intensities. Recall, for example, that the internal margins of a bone lesion whether "geographic," "moth-eaten," or "permeative," are reflections of increasing growth rates and not histologic

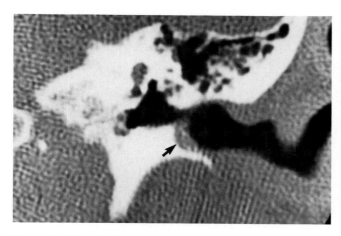

Fig. 13-193 EAC cholesteatoma. High-resolution CT. There is well-defined localized erosion of inferior canal wall *(arrow)* lateral to isthmus. (Contrast with Figs. 13-196 and 13-199.)

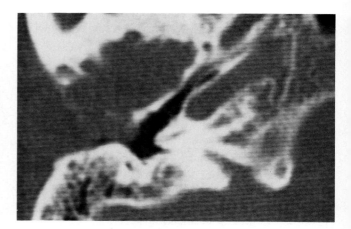

Fig. 13-194 Benign giant cell tumor. High-resolution CT. Tumor partially occludes EAC. Well-defined scalloped borders suggest benign lesion.

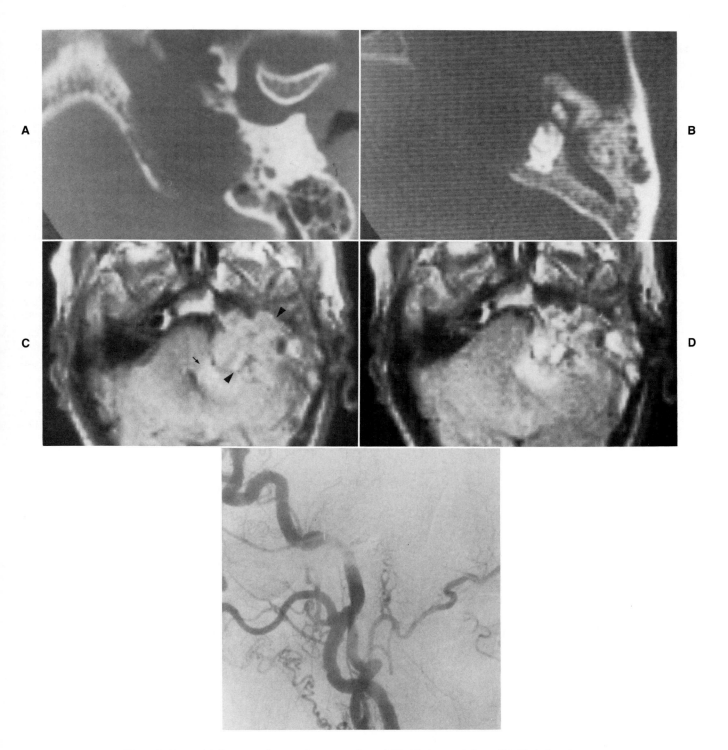

Fig. 13-195   Malignant giant cell tumor. **A** and **B,** High-resolution CT. Ill-defined geographic borders suggest moderately aggressive lesion. Destruction of otic capsule would be atypical of paraganglioma. **C** and **D,** Intermediate and T_2-weighted images. Tumor is inhomogeneous on T_2-weighted images but lacks "salt-and-pepper" heterogeneity seen in medium or large paraganglioma on T_1-weighted images *(arrowheads;* compare with Fig. 13-171). There is adjacent brain edema *(arrow).* **E,** Selective carotid angiogram. As in most malignant tumors, tumor vascularity is much less than in a paraganglioma. (Compare with Fig. 13-169.)

Table 13-15 Examples of destructive lesions of temporal bone

Primary carcinomas	Squamous cell carcinoma
	Adenoid cystic carcinoma
	Adenocarcinoma
Primary sarcomas	Embryonal rhabdomyosarcoma
	Chondrosarcoma
	Osteosarcoma
	Giant cell tumor
Metastases	Breast
	Kidney
	Lung
Benign epithelial lesions	Adenoma
	Congenital epidermoid
	Mucocele
Benign nonepithelial lesions	Paraganglioma
	Hemangioma
	Facial schwannoma
	Acoustic schwannoma
	Meningioma
	Chondroblastoma
	Cholesterol granuloma
	Xanthoma
Hematologic malignancies	Myeloma
	Lymphoma
Infection and inflammatory lesions	Malignant external otitis
	Tuberculosis
	Wegener's granulomatosis
	Acquired cholesteatoma
Histiocytosis	Eosinophilic granuloma
Vascular	Carotid aneurysm

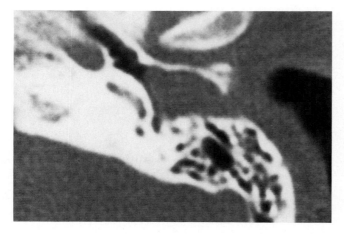

Fig. 13-196 Keratosis obturans. High-resolution CT. Soft tissue plug is by itself not a specific finding. There is mild diffuse thinning of cortex of EAC. Tympanic membrane is displaced medially but middle ear is normal.

types.[268] "Geographic" borders, whether sclerotic-rimmed, well-defined or ill-defined, likewise reflect growth rates in ascending order. In lesions that spread rapidly, such as osteomyelitis or Ewing's sarcoma, there may be no visible internal margin. In the temporal bone the varying degrees of resistance offered by capsular, cortical, diploic, and pneumatized bones may further modify the appearance of the margin of a lesion. Nevertheless careful analysis of the margins does provide a useful indication of the growth rate of a lesion.

The location of a lesion may alter the differential diagnosis. For example, a destructive lesion with a "moth-eaten" border around the EAC is probably a squamous carcinoma, but around the jugular fossa is probably a paraganglioma. The patient's age group may also help in making a diagnosis. For example, carcinoma is more likely in an adult, while embryonal rhabdomyosarcoma is much more probable in a young child. History of malignancy favors metastasis. Presence of calcifications suggests meningioma, chordoma, chondrosarcoma, and epidermoid.

Yet, in essence, we must be reconciled to the fact that in many of these cases, the radiologist's principal task is to localize a lesion accurately and to suggest its growth rate rather than to provide a specific diagnosis. This is certainly true at least for those laterally placed lesions that are readily available to inspection and biopsy.

In the petrous apex the case is different. Here a lesion is beyond direct inspection and its surgical access is difficult. Besides detection, localization, and characterization, every effort should be made to arrive at a specific diagnosis preoperatively. Fortunately, in this location diagnosis in many cases is possible.

External Auditory Canal and Mastoid Tumors

Benign Tumors. Several benign tumor or tumorlike conditions are specific to the external auditory canal. Some of them are not true neoplasms but may be confused with them. Two such soft tissue lesions are keratosis obturans and external auditory canal cholesteatoma.[269]

Keratosis obturans usually occurs in individuals under 40 years of age with a history of sinusitis or bronchiectasis. The condition is usually bilateral, acute, and painful. Keratin plugs occlude the medial portion of the EAC (Fig. 13-196). The adjacent bony canal may be diffusely widened. Reflex hyperemia has been theorized as the mechanism. Treatment consists of removing the plug and treating the granulations.[269]

EAC cholesteatoma occurs in individuals over 40 years of age. It is usually unilateral, chronic, and associated with otorrhea. There is localized erosion of the canal wall and elevation of the epidermis by cholesteatoma imbedded in the bony wall (Fig. 13-193). Sequestration of bone and formation of sinus tracts may be present. Circumscribed periostitis is the probable cause. Complete surgical removal of the cholesteatoma sac and the necrotic bone is usually necessary for successful treatment.[269]

Exostoses of the EAC are sessile multinodular bony masses arising deep in the EAC (Fig. 13-197). They are caused by prolonged physical, chemical, or thermal irritation, for example, frequent excessive contact with cold sea water for many years. In the case of aquatic exposure, the exostoses are usually asymptomatic until after the tenth year; then pain, infection, and hearing loss may appear. Total canal occlusion is rare.[270,271]

Osteomas are sporadic, solitary, unilateral, pedunculated growths of mature bone located in the outer portion of the bony EAC (Fig. 13-198). They are much less common than exostoses.[270] The mastoid is the most prevalent extracanalicular site.[272]

Malignant Tumors. Squamous cell carcinoma is, by far, the most common malignant tumor of the ear (Fig. 13-199).[12,214] Squamous cell carcinoma may arise in the EAC and spread to the middle ear or arise in the middle ear. Unlike auricular basal cell carcinomas, which are uniformly associated with actinic damage to the epidermis, nearly always found in men, and rarely lethal, external canal squamous carcinomas are not associated with such damage, are more common in women, and have a 5-year mortality rate of about 50%.[273] Such squamous cell carcinoma is frequently preceded by a long history of chronic ear infection. The tumor destroys the adjacent bone in the EAC and middle ear and invades the surrounding soft tissues. Extradural growth into the middle cranial fossa is common, as is subtemporal fossa and mastoid involvement.[274,275] The temporomandibular joint, the parotid gland, and the carotid canal may also be involved.[219,275] But the otic capsule is relatively resistant to erosion. Middle ear extension of external ear squamous carcinoma substantially reduces the 5-year survival from

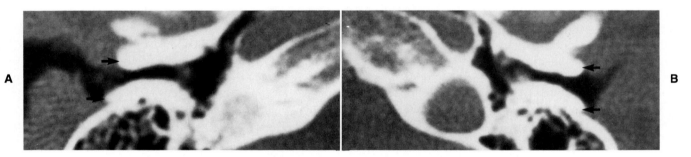

Fig. 13-197 Bilateral EAC exostoses. **A** and **B,** High-resolution CT. Sclerotic bone *(arrows)* layered on anterior and posterior walls of tympanic bone has diffusely narrowed EACs. (Compare with Fig. 13-198; courtesy of Anton N Hasso, MD.)

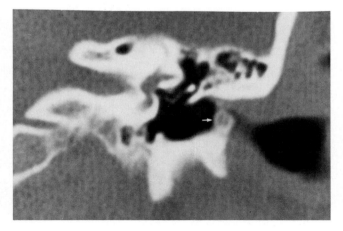

Fig. 13-198 EAC osteoma. High-resolution CT. Tumor typically arises at tympanomastoid or tympanosquamosal suture *(arrow).* (Compare with Fig. 13-197; courtesy of Anton N Hasso, MD.)

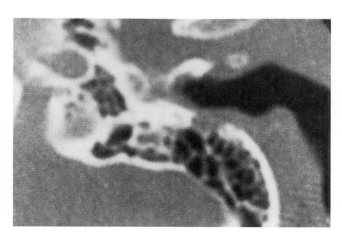

Fig. 13-199 Early EAC squamous carcinoma. High-resolution CT. Note ill-defined localized cortical destruction on posterior wall of bony EAC. (Compare with Fig. 13-193.)

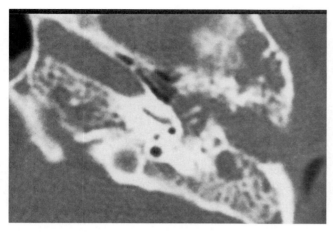

Fig. 13-200 EAC and middle-ear squamous carcinoma. High-resolution CT. There is ill-defined destruction of anterior and posterior walls of EAC and lateral wall of protympanum. Tumor is indistinguishable from adenoid cystic carcinoma or adenocarcinoma.

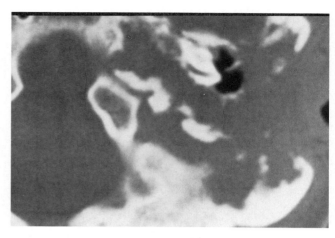

Fig. 13-201 Eosinophilic granuloma. High-resolution CT. Lesion is generally poorly defined suggesting moderately rapid growth rate. There is erosion of otic capsule. (Compare with Figs. 13-195 and 13-202 and see Table 13-17; courtesy of Roy A Holliday, MD.)

56% to 27% (Fig. 13-200).[276] Initial complete resection is the most effective treatment, usually followed by irradiation.[273,276] Careful preoperative mapping of the entire tumor must be stressed.

The term *ceruminoma* is used by some authors to include all glandular tumors arising from the apocrine, seromucinous, or salivary glands of the EAC and middle ear.[12] This practice, however, is opposed by other authors who stress the divergent behaviors of the various tumors that are included in this general classification.[277] Adenoid cystic carcinoma is the most common tumor of the group. It is to be distinguished from ceruminous adenoma and pleomorphic adenoma (Fig. 13-173), which are benign lesions, and ceruminous adenocarcinoma, which has a variable malignant potential. Adenoid cystic carcinoma, which histologically and pathologically resembles similar tumors of the salivary gland, is locally invasive and is best treated by radical en bloc resection.[277,278]

Metastases, basal cell carcinoma, malignant melanoma, chondrosarcoma (Figs. 13-179, 13-206 and 13-207), osteosarcoma, lymphoma, and myeloma (Fig. 13-202) also may occur in the EAC, although much less frequently. Giant cell tumors (Figs. 13-194, 13-195)[265] and benign chondroblastomas[279] may likewise cause bone destruction. Chronic infections and inflammatory diseases, such as malignant external otitis, tuberculosis, and Wegener's granulomatosis, as well as histiocytosis (Fig. 13-201), should also be considered.

Histiocytosis. Histiocytosis is a rare disease of unknown etiology in the pediatric age group. (It also uncommonly occurs in adults in the less severe forms.) It includes a spectrum of disorders with histiocytic prolif-

eration involving bone and/or soft tissues, namely, eosinophilic granuloma, Hand-Schüller-Christian's syndrome and Letterer-Siwe disease, in order of prognosis from best to worst. In general, the patients with late onset, no soft tissue involvement, and unifocal bone lesions have the best prognosis. In eosinophilic granuloma, by definition, the patients are restricted to having one or several bone lesions, and the disease is generally benign, although progressive dissemination can occur (Fig. 13-201).[280] The treatment consists of surgery, irradiation, or chemotherapy (alone or in combination).[280]

In one series of 50 patients with disseminated histiocytosis, 18 had otomastoid involvement.[281] When the temporal bone is involved, the region of the EAC and mastoid appears to be a common location.[222,280] The bone margins are geographic and moderately well defined. On CT there is slight peripheral enhancement within the lesion.[222]

The Petrous Apex

Differential Diagnosis. The petrous apex mass lesions include principally those arising from within the petrous bone and expanding the bone (e.g., cholesterol granuloma, intrapetrous epidermoid, and intrapetrous carotid aneurysm) and those arising from the immediate vicinity of the petrous apex and eroding or invading the apex secondarily (chondrosarcoma from the petroclival junction, meningioma, trigeminal schwannoma, and intradural epidermoid).

Chondrosarcoma,[143] meningioma (Fig. 13-139), trigeminal schwannoma (Fig. 13-146), and intradural epidermoid (Fig. 13-147) can all possess components in both the posterior and middle cranial fossae straddling

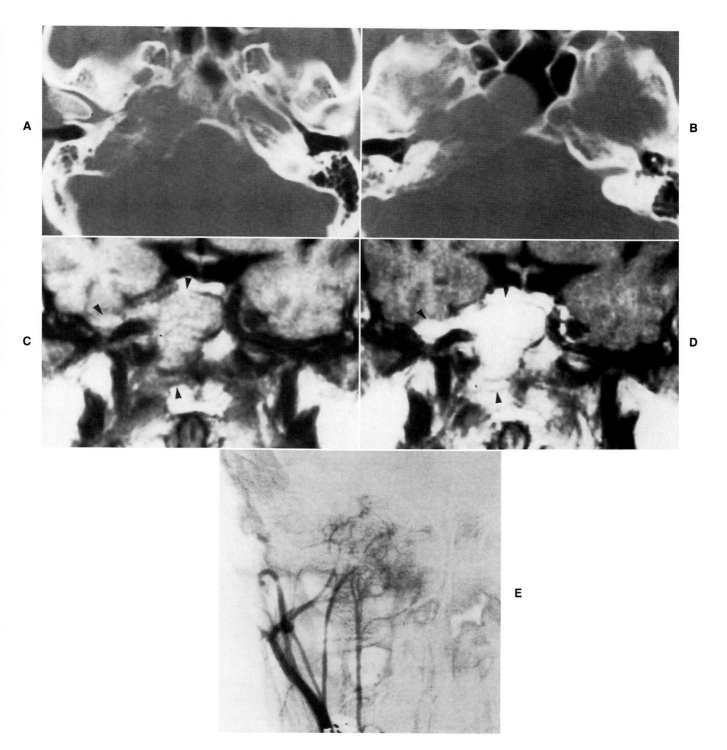

Fig. 13-202 Solitary myeloma. **A** and **B,** High-resolution CTs. The ill-defined borders of right petrosphenoid soft tissue mass suggests moderately aggressive lesion. **C** and **D,** Pre- and post-gadolinium T$_1$-weighted images. Homogeneously enhancing mass *(arrowheads)* shows no special feature. **E,** Selective external carotid angiogram. Lesion is an example of hypervascular tumor other than paraganglioma, but shows no early venous drainage. (Compare with Fig. 13-169; courtesy of Marie Merkle, MD.)

Table 13-16   Differential features of petrous apex "cystic" lesions

	Cholesterol granuloma (cholesterol cyst)	Epidermoid (congenital cholesteatoma)	Mucocele
CT Density	= brain	≤ brain	? < brain
T₁WI* intensity	> brain	≤ brain	? ≤ brain
T₂WI† intensity	> brain	> brain	? > brain
Content arrangement	Homogeneous or with hypointense irregular debris	Lamination on T₁WI	? homogeneous

*T₁WI = T₁-weighted images
†T₂WI = T₂-weighted images

the petrous tip. The posterior fossa component is intradural, while the middle fossa component may be intradural on the medial floor of the middle cranial fossa or in Meckel's cave or extradural by extension into the cavernous sinus and sphenoid. These tumors are important considerations in the differential diagnosis of petrous apex masses, but the last three have been described at some length under the differential diagnosis of CP angle tumors and are not discussed further in this section.

The petrous apex may also be invaded by direct extensions of jugular paragangliomas and nasopharyngeal carcinomas, usually along the petrooccipital fissure in both cases. For a complete differential diagnosis, systemic diseases and malignancies also need to be considered (Fig. 13-202).

Two pitfalls have trapped the unwary, primarily on MRI: (1) asymmetric pneumatization of the petrous apex,[282] and (2) unilateral retention of secretion in apical air cells. In the first instance there is unilateral hyperintensity on T₁-weighted images, from marrow of the unpneumatized petrous apex, which fades in signal intensity on T₂-weighted images, paralleling the signal intensity of fat. In the second instance there is unilateral hyperintensity on T₂-weighted images from retained secretions that also have hypointense signal on T₁-weighted or intermediate images, paralleling the signal intensity of mucus. Both of these situations have been mistaken for tumors on MRI. CT usually resolves the question. Unlike true cysts or tumors, neither of these conditions shows bone erosion or expansion.

Unlike lesions in the IAC, geniculate fossa or tympanic cavity, lesions in this location usually attain considerable size before eventually appearing with cranial nerve symptoms. These lesions are readily apparent on CT or MRI. However, besides localization and characterization, an important task for the radiologist is the preoperative differentiation between cystic and solid lesions (Table 13-16). Whereas solid lesions of the petrous apex require a biopsy procedure to determine appropriate treatment and extensive surgery if it is indicated, cysts can be simply and definitively treated by drainage and permanent fistulization if a proper preop-

erative diagnosis is made.[261,283,284] We prefer to use MR for the initial detection of a lesion, but CT with bone detail is indispensable for surgical planning, such as in the selection of a drainage pathway (Table 13-16).

Cholesterol Granuloma. Cholesterol granuloma of the petrous apex[258,263,285] has also come to be known as cholesterol cyst[262] or giant cholesterol cyst (Figs. 13-203 and 13-204).[259,260] *Cholesterol granuloma* is a term that emphasizes the histopathologic features of the lesion, while *cholesterol cyst* is a term that better describes the gross appearance of the lesion. Each therefore has its own merit. Although cholesterol cysts are rare, they are much more common than previously realized. In fact, they may be the most common primary petrous apex lesion.[259,260]

Cholesterol granulomas possess a fibrous lining that may or may not be complete. The lining contains multinucleated giant cells with cholesterol crystals in acicular clefts, blood vessels, fibrous tissues, red blood cells, hemosiderin, and chronic inflammatory cells. The content of the cyst is a brownish liquid glistening with cholesterol crystals and containing a brownish sediment.[258,260] The contralateral petrous apex is usually well pneumatized, suggesting that these cysts arise from pneumatized apices (Fig. 13-203). Obstruction of the ventilation outlet has been theorized as the cause that initiates repetitive cycles of hemorrhage and granulomatous reaction.[206]

Cholesterol granulomas occur in young and middle-aged adults of both sexes. Most of the patients have had symptoms for about 2 years.[258] Hearing loss, tinnitus, and hemifacial spasm are the most common complaints, but deficits of cranial nerves V, VI, IX, X, XI, and XII have all been encountered.[258,260] Many of these deficits have been relieved by surgical decompression.[260,286]

Cholesterol granulomas arise from within the petrous apex posterior to the horizontal portion of the carotid canal;[258] and they range from 2 to 4 cm in length at the time of their initial diagnosis.

On CT cholesterol granulomas are sharply and smoothly marginated (Fig. 13-203). Generally ovoid in configuration, they expand the petrous apex, especially

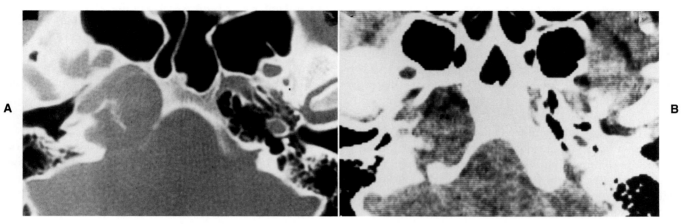

Fig. 13-203 Petrous apex cholesterol granuloma. **A** and **B,** High-resolution and post-contrast CT. Sharply and smoothly marginated, ovoid, expansile lesion is isodense with brain and non-enhancing. Jugular tubercle is eroded and carotid canal remodeled. Contralateral petrous apex is well pneumatized. (Compare with Fig. 13-205.)

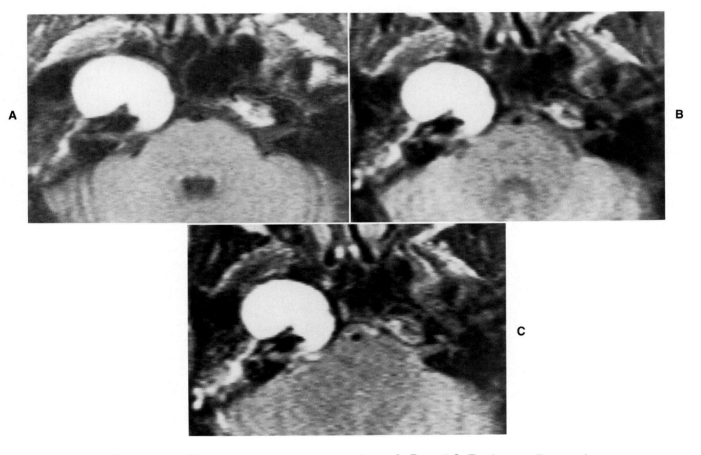

Fig. 13-204 Petrous apex cholesterol granuloma. **A, B,** and **C,** T$_1$-, intermediate, and T$_2$-weighted images. Lesion is hyperintense on all three images. (Contrast with Fig. 13-205.) Note hypointense rim medial to lesion accentuated on **B** and **C,** attributable to hemosiderin deposit and/or chemical-shift artifact.

posteriorly where the overlying bone is often paper thin or absent. Where bone is still present, the internal margin of the lesion is often sclerotic. The abutting portions of the carotid and jugular walls may be absent. The horizontal carotid canal is often bowed, and the adjacent occipital and sphenoid bones are commonly remodeled.[258]

The lesions are approximately isodense with brain and are homogeneous and free of calcium (Fig. 13-203). They show no contrast enhancement except for a thin, smooth peripheral rim, which has variously been interpreted as either being the capsule or the overlying dura.[258,259]

On MRI these lesions are strongly hyperintense on both T_1- and T_2-weighted images, and they may contain nonhomogeneous hypointense substances within the liquid (Fig. 13-204).[262,263] Some of them show a hypointense rim on both T_1- and T_2-weighted images.[263] Peripheral magnetic susceptibility on gradient-recalled echo sequences and evidence of aliphatic protons centrally on chemical shift imaging add specificity to the diagnosis.[263]

Epidermoid. Epidermoids are also called primary cholesteatomas. They are less common in the petrous apex than in the supralabyrinthine region.[236,247] Congenital intrapetrous epidermoid is much rarer than cho-

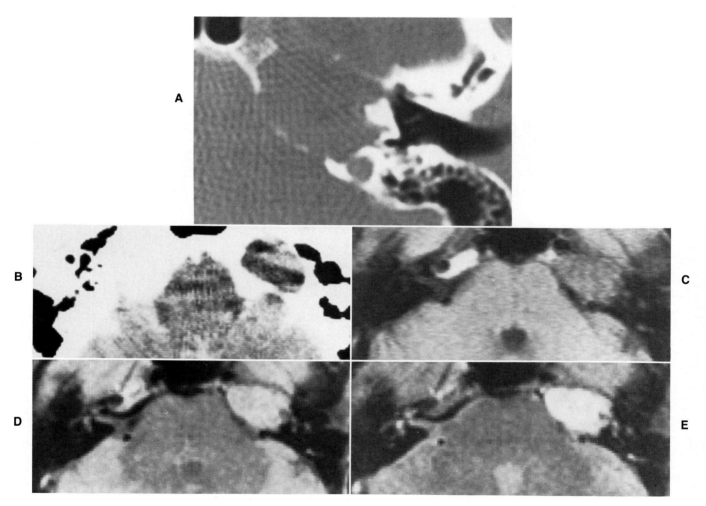

Fig. 13-205 Petrous apex epidermoid. **A** and **B,** High-resolution and postcontrast CT. Sharply and smoothly marginated, ovoid, expansile lesion is similar in appearance to cholesterol granuloma (Fig. 13-203). Lesion is nonenhancing but its density in this particular case is difficult to determine because of interpetrous artifacts. **C, D,** and **E,** T_1-, intermediate, and T_2-weighted images. Lesion is hypointense in **C,** isointense with gray matter in **D,** and moderately hyperintense on **E.** (Contrast with Fig. 13-204.)

lesterol granuloma or cyst. We encountered our first epidermoid after nearly 20 consecutive cholesterol granulomas. They are solid lesions and are usually treated by surgical resection to prevent recurrence, rather than by simple drainage and fistulization. Their preoperative differentiation from cholesterol granulomas is therefore important.

Epidermoids possess a capsule of stratified squamous lining and contain desquamated keratin, which appears grossly to be whitish friable material. As the desquamated keratin accumulates, the mass slowly expands. Thus, on CT they appear as homogenous, nonenhancing, sharply defined, ovoid expansile lesions, as do cholesterol granulomas (Fig. 13-205).[14,247,287] Some epidermoids appear to be hypodense and some isodense to brain. Hence, on CT they may or may not be distinguishable from cholesterol granulomas, which are isodense.

Because of the rarity of intrapetrous epidermoids, limited information exists in the literature on their MRI findings.[247] In our experience of two cases they are between CSF and brain in intensity on T_1-weighted images with a capsule isointense to brain (Fig. 13-205). A layered appearance may be present in the periphery on off-center sections. On T_2-weighted images they are strongly hyperintense to brain but perhaps less so than cholesterol granulomas.

Mucocele. Mucoceles are lined with cuboidal or columnar epithelium and contain mucus. Petrous apex mucoceles are even rarer than petrous apex epidermoids and their CT and MRI appearances[257,288] are even less frequently documented in the literature. They are also sharply defined ovoid expansile nonenhancing masses. Extrapolating from mucoceles of the paranasal sinuses, they are likely to be hypodense to brain on T_1-weighted and strongly hyperintense on T_2-weighted images. They may be treated by drainage and fistulization.

Carotid Artery Aneurysm. Giant aneurysms from the intrapetrous horizontal carotid canal are extremely rare but for obvious reasons are extremely important in the differential diagnosis of petrous lesions.[138,289] They also appear as well-defined ovoid expanding masses. However, as with the intracranial giant aneurysms described earlier, their internal appearances vary considerably according to the extent of mural thrombus formation.[135]

On CT a mural thrombus appears isodense and nonenhancing, and the patent lumen shows rapid rise and decline in enhancement. On MRI a laminated mural thrombus shows varying signal intensities and the patent lumen appears as a signal void.[136-138] Flow-related enhancements may present confusing signals.

Carotid artery aneurysms may be treated surgically[290] or with transvascular techniques.[291]

Chondrosarcoma. Primary intracranial cartilaginous tumors are extremely rare.[292] They range from benign chondromas to malignant chondrosarcomas. Chondrosarcomas may originate from embryonal rests in the skull base, which is embryologically formed from a cartilaginous matrix. They share a number of pathologic and radiologic features with chordomas, which arise from notochordal remnants.[293] However, chordomas are midline and retrosellar in location, and chondrosarcomas arise in the parasellar or the CP angle region.[292] Both cause bone destruction and enhance mildly to moderately, both may contain calcifications (Fig. 13-206),[292,294] and both are usually hypointense on T_1-weighted im-

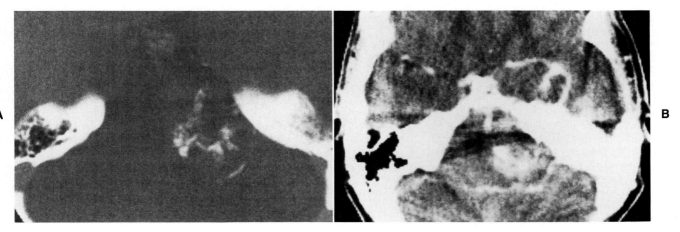

Fig. 13-206 Petrous apex chondrosarcoma. **A** and **B,** High-resolution and postcontrast CT. There is calcification within this primarily exophytic tumor.

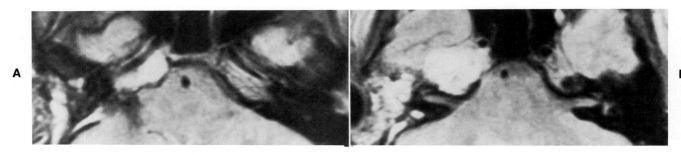

Fig. 13-207 Petrous apex chondrosarcoma. **A** and **B,** T_2-weighted images. The tumor, mildly hypointense on T_1- and mildly hyperintense on T_2-weighted images, slightly expands petrous apex and erodes petrooccipital fissure. The tumor is more irregular than an epidermoid and is an enhancing lesion in contrast to an epidermoid, which is nonenhancing. (For more chondrosarcomas see also Fig. 13-179; courtesy of Derald E. Brackmann, MD.)

ages and hyperintense on T_2-weighted images (Fig. 13-207).[294]

Chondrosarcomas are often centered more along the petrosphenoidal and petrooccipital fissures than within the petrous apex itself (Fig. 13-179). Compared to meningiomas, chondrosarcomas enhance less on CT and cause bone destruction rather than sclerosis or hyperostosis (Figs. 13-177 and 13-206).[292]

An extremely rare intradural chondrosarcoma involving the petrous apex has been reported, to extend into the posterior and middle cranial fossae and to have CT and MRI appearances suggestive of a meningioma.[143]

Chondrosarcomas are locally invasive. They may be treated with surgery using the infratemporal fossa approach[8,185] or with radiation therapy.[294,295]

REFERENCES

1. House JW and O'Conner AF, editors: Handbook of neurotological diagnosis, New York, 1987, Marcel Dekker, Inc.
2. Cohen NL et al: Acoustic neuroma surgery: an eclectic approach with emphasis on preservation of hearing, Ann Otol Rhinol Laryngol 95:21, 1986.
3. Camp JO and Cilley EJL: Significance of asymmetry of pori acustici as an aid in diagnosis of eighth nerve tumors, AJR 41:713, 1939.
4. Valvassori GE: The abnormal internal auditory canal: the diagnosis of acoustic neuroma, Radiology 92:449, 1969.
5. Amundsen P and Newton TH: Subarachnoid cisterns. In Newton TH and Potts DG, editors: Radiology of the skull and brain, vol 4, Ventricles and cisterns, St Louis, 1978. The CV Mosby Co, pp 3588-3711.
6. Scanlon RL: Positive contrast medium (Iophendylate) in diagnosis of acoustic neuroma, Arch Otolaryngol 80:698, 1964.
7. Takehashi M et al: Angiographic diagnosis of acoustic neurinomas: analysis of 30 lesions, Neuroradiology 2:191, 1971.
8. Fisch U and Mattox D: Microsurgery of the skull base, New York, 1988, Thieme Medical Publishers, Inc.
9. Gentry LR et al: Cerebellopontine angle-petromastoid mass lesions: comparative study of diagnosis with MR imaging and CT, Radiology 162:513, 1987.
10. Mafee MM: Acoustic neuroma and other acoustic nerve disorders: role of MRI and CT: an analysis of 238 cases, Semin Ultrasound CT and MR 8:256, 1987.
11. Olsen WL et al: MR imaging of paragangliomas, AJR 148:701, 1987.
12. Schuknecht HF: Pathology of the ear, Cambridge, 1974, Harvard University Press, pp 415-451.
13. Brackmann DE and Bartels LJ: Rare tumors of the cerebellopontine angle, Otolaryngol Head Neck Surg 88:555, 1980.
14. Valavanis A, Schubiger O, and Naidich TP: Clinical imaging of the cerebellopontine angle, Berlin, Heidelberg, 1986, Springer-Verlag, pp 30-31, 42-50, 61-76, 85-88, 95-99, 117-125, 134-137, 156-172.
15. Kasantikul V et al: Acoustic neurilemmoma: clinicoanatomical study of 103 patients, J Neurosurg 52:28, 1980.
16. Graham MD and Sataloff RT: Acoustic tumors in the young adult, Arch Otolaryngol 110:405, 1984.
17. Krause CJ and McCabe BF: Acoustic neuroma in a 7-year-old girl: report of a case, Arch Otolaryngol 94:359, 1971.
18. Harkin JC and Reed RJ: Tumors of the peripheral nervous system. In Firminger HI, editor: Atlas of tumor pathology, Second series, fascicle 3, Washington DC, 1969, Armed Forces Institute of Pathology.
19. Rubenstein LJ: Tumors of the central nervous system. In Firminger HI, editor: Atlas of tumor pathology, Second series, fascicle 6, Washington, DC, 1972, Armed Forces Institute of Pathology, pp 169-190, 205-214, 288-292.
20. Gruskin P and Carberry JN: Pathology of acoustic tumors. In House WF and Luetje CM, editors: Acoustic tumors, vol 1, Diagnosis, Baltimore, 1979, University Park Press, pp 85-148.
21. Bebin J: Pathophysiology of acoustic tumors. In House WF and Luetje CM, editors: Acoustic tumors, vol 1, Diagnosis, Baltimore, 1979, University Park Press, pp 45-84.
22. Kasantikul V and Brown WJ: Estrogen receptors in acoustic neurilemmomas, Surg Neurol 15:105, 1981.
23. Riccardi VM: Von Recklinghausen neurofibromatosis, N Engl J Med 305:1617, 1981.
24. Martuza RL and Eldridge R: Neurofibromatosis 2 (bilateral acoustic neurofibromatosis), N Engl J Med 318:684, 1988.
25. Kasantikul V et al: Glioma of the acoustic nerve, Arch Otolaryngol 106:456, 1980.
26. Barker D et al: Gene for von Recklinghausen neurofibromatosis is in the pericentromeric region of chromosome 17, Science 236:1100, 1987.

27. Rouleau GA et al: Genetic linkage of bilateral acoustic neurofibromatosis to a DNA marker on chromosome 22, Nature 329:246, 1987.

28. Kanter WR et al: Central neurofibromatosis with bilateral acoustic neuroma: genetic, clinical and biochemical distinction from peripheral neurofibromatosis, Neurology 30:851, 1980.

29. Eldridge R: Central neurofibromatosis with bilateral acoustic neuroma, Adv Neurol 29:57, 1981.

30. Wertelecki W et al: Neurofibromatosis 2: clinical and DNA linkage studies of a large kindred, N Engl J Med 319:278, 1988.

31. Bognanno JR et al: Cranial MR imaging in neurofibromatosis, AJNR 9:461, 1988.

32. Martuza RL and Ojemann RG: Bilateral acoustic neuromas: clinical aspects, pathogenesis and treatment, Neurosurgery 10:1, 1982.

33. Hughes GB et al: Management of bilateral acoustic tumors, Laryngoscope 92:1351, 1982.

34. Dutcher PO Jr, House WF, and Hitselberger WE: Early detection of small bilateral acoustic tumors, Am J Otol 8:35, 1987.

35. Brow RE: Pre- and postoperative management of the acoustic tumor patient. In House WF and Luetje CM, editors: Acoustic tumors, vol 2, Management, Baltimore, 1979, University Park Press, pp 153-173.

36. Neely JG and Neblett CR: Differential facial nerve function in tumors of the internal auditory meatus, Ann Otol Rhinol Laryngol 92:39, 1983.

37. Hart RG, Gardner OP, and Howieson J: Acoustic tumors: atypical features and recent diagnostic tests, Neurology 33:211, 1983.

38. McCoyd K, Barron KD, and Cassidy RJ: Acoustic neurinoma presenting as subarachnoid hemorrhage. J Neurosurg 41:391, 1974 (case report).

39. Gleeson RK, Butzer JF, and Grin OD Jr: Acoustic neurinoma presenting as subarachnoid hemorrhage, J Neurosurg 49:602, 1978.

40. Castillo R, Watts C, and Pulliam M: Sudden hemorrhage in an acoustic neurinoma, J Neurosurg 56:417, 1982 (case report).

41. Yonimitsu T et al: Acoustic neurinoma presenting as subarachnoid hemorrhage, Surg Neurol 20:125, 1983.

42. Brackmann DE and Selters WA: Auditory brainstem response audiometry in acoustic tumor detection. In Brackmann DE, editor: Neurological surgery of the ear and skull base, New York, 1982, Raven Press, pp 109-117.

43. Barrs DM et al: Changing concepts of acoustic neuroma diagnosis, Arch Otolaryngol 111:17, 1985.

44. Hart RG and Davenport J: Diagnosis of acoustic neuroma, Neurosurgery 9:450, 1981.

45. Cohn AL et al: Acoustic neurinoma diagnostic model evaluation using decision support systems, Arch Otolaryngol Head Neck Surg 112:830, 1986.

46. Kingsley DPE et al: Acoustic neuromas: evaluation by magnetic resonance imaging, AJNR 6:1, 1985.

47. House JW, Waluch V, and Jackler RK: Magnetic resonance imaging in acoustic neuroma diagnosis, Ann Otol Rhinol Laryngol 95:16, 1986.

48. Mikhael MD, Ciric IS, and Wolff AP: MR diagnosis of acoustic neuromas, J Comput Assist Tomogr 11:232, 1987.

49. New PFJ et al: MR imaging of the acoustic nerves and small acoustic neuromas at 0.6T: prospective study, AJNR 6:165, 1985.

50. Press GA and Hesselink JR: MR imaging of cerebellopontine angle and internal auditory canal lesions at 1.5T, AJNR 9:241, 1988.

51. Glasscock ME III and Steenerson RL: A history of acoustic tumor surgery, 1961-present. In House WF and Luetje CM, editors: acoustic tumors, vol 1, Diagnosis, Baltimore, 1979, University Park Press, pp 33-41.

52. House WF: Translabyrinthine approach. In House WF and Luetje CM, editors: Acoustic tumors, vol 2, Management, Baltimore, 1979, University Park Press, pp 43-87.

53. Smith MFW, Clancy TP, and Lang JS: Conservation of hearing in acoustic neurilemmoma excision, Trans Am Acad Ophthmol Otolaryngol 84:704, 1977.

54. Cohen NL: Acoustic neuroma surgery with emphasis on preservation of hearing, Laryngoscope 89:886, 1979.

55. Brackmann DE: Middle fossa approach. In House WF and Luetje CM, editors: Acoustic tumors, vol 2, Management, Baltimore, 1979, University Park Press, pp 15-42.

56. Brackmann DE: Translabyrinthine removal of acoustic neurinomas. In Brackmann DE, editor: Neurological surgery of the ear and skull base, New York, 1982, Raven Press, pp 235-241.

57. Clemis JD: Hearing conservation in acoustic tumor surgery: pros and cons, Otolaryngol Head Neck Surg 92:156, 1984.

58. Wade PJ and House WF: Hearing preservation in patients with acoustic neuromas via the middle fossa approach, Otolaryngol Head Neck Surg 92:184, 1984.

59. Harner SG and Ebersold MJ: Management of acoustic neuromas, 1978-1983, J Neurosurg 63:175, 1985.

60. Tator CH: Acoustic neuromas: management of 204 cases, Canadian J Neurol Sci 12:353, 1985.

61. Glasscock ME III, Gulya AJ, and Pensak ML: Surgery of the posterior fossa, Otolaryngol Clin North Am 17:483, 1984.

62. Glassock ME III et al: A systematic approach to the surgical management of acoustic neuroma, Laryngoscope 96:1088, 1986.

63. Wiet RJ et al: Complications in the approach to acoustic tumor surgery, Ann Otol Rhinol Laryngol 95:28, 1986.

64. Wazen J et al: Preoperative and postoperative growth rates in acoustic neuromas documented with CT scanning, Otolaryngol Head Neck Surg 93:151, 1985.

65. Nedzelski JM et al: Is no treatment good treatment in the management of acoustic neuromas in the elderly? Laryngoscope 96:825, 1986.

66. House JW, Nissen RL, and Hitselberger WE: Acoustic tumor management in senior citizens, Laryngoscope 97:129, 1987.

67. Noren G, Arndt J, and Hindmarsh T: Stereotactic radiosurgery in cases of acoustic neurinoma: further experiences, Neurosurgery 13:12, 1983.

68. Moller A, Hatam A, and Olivecrona H: Diagnosis of acoustic neuroma with computed tomography, Neuroradiology 17:25, 1978.

69. Solti-Bohman LG et al: Gas-CT cisternography for detection of small acoustic nerve tumors, Radiology 150:403, 1984.

70. Valavanis A et al: CT of meningiomas on the posterior surface of the petrous bone, Neuroradiology 22:111, 1981.

71. Hatam A et al: Contrast medium enhancement with time in computed tomography: differential diagnosis of intracranial lesions, Acta Radiol (suppl) 346:63, 1975.

72. Hatam A et al: Early contrast enhancement of acoustic neuroma, Neuroradiology 17:31, 1978.

73. Krassanakis K, Sourtsis E, and Karvounis P: Unusual appearance of an acoustic neuroma on computed tomography, Neuroradiology 21:51, 1981.

74. Daniels DL et al: MR detection of tumor in the internal auditory canal, AJNR 8:249, 1987.

75. Valvassori GE et al: MR of the normal and abnormal internal auditory canal, AJNR 9:115, 1988.

76. Enzmann DR and O'Donohue J: Optimizing MR imaging for detecting small tumors in the cerebellopontine angle and internal auditory canal, AJNR 8:97, 1987.

77. Gomorri JM et al: Intracranial hematomas: imaging by high-field MR, Radiology 157:87, 1985.

78. Curati WL et al: Acoustic neuromas: Gd-DTPA enhancement in MR imaging, Radiology 158:447, 1986.

79. Breger RK et al: Benign extraaxial tumors: contrast enhancement with Gd-DTPA, Radiology 163:427, 1987.

80. Witten RM and Wade CT: Computed tomography in acoustic tumor diagnosis. In House WF and Luetje CM, editors: Acoustic tumors, vol 1, Diagnosis, Baltimore, 1979, University Park Press, pp 253-277.

81. Hill MC, Oh KS, and Hodges FJ III: Internal auditory canal enlargement in neurofibromatosis without acoustic neuroma, Radiology 122:730, 1977.

82. Sarwar M and Swischuk LE: Bilateral internal auditory canal enlargement due to dural ectasia in neurofibromatosis, AJR 129:935, 1977.

83. Weinberg PE, Kim KS, and Gore RM: Unilateral enlargement of the internal auditory canal: a developmental variant, Surg Neurol 5:39, 1981.

84. Revilla AG: Differential diagnosis of tumors at the cerebellopontine recess, Johns Hopk Hosp Bull 83:187, 1948.

85. Segall HD et al: Computed tomography in neoplasms of the posterior fossa in children, Radiol Clin North Am 20:237, 1982.

86. Lo WWM and Solti-Bohman LG: Computed tomography of the petrous bone and posterior fossa. In House JW and O'Conner AF, editors: Handbook of neurotologic diagnosis, New York, 1987, Marcel Dekker Inc, pp 225-335.

87. Naidich TP et al: Primary tumors and other masses of the cerebellum and fourth ventricle: differential diagnosis by computed tomography, Neuroradiology 14:153, 1977.

88. Moller A, Hatam A, and Olivecrona H: The differential diagnosis of pontine angle meningioma and acoustic neuroma with computed tomography, Neuroradiology 17:21, 1978.

89. Elster AD et al: Meningiomas: MR and histopathologic features, Radiology 170:857, 1989.

90. Russell DS and Rubenstein LJ: Pathology of tumours of the nervous system, ed 4, Baltimore, 1977, Williams & Wilkins, pp 65-100, 372-401.

91. Zimmerman RD et al: Magnetic resonance imaging of meningiomas, AJNR 6:149, 1985.

92. Spagnoli MV et al: Intracranial meningiomas: high-field MR imaging, Radiology 161:369, 1986.

93. Vassilouthis J and Ambrose J: Computerized tomography scanning appearances of intracranial meningiomas, J Neurosurg 50:310, 1979.

94. Brackmann DE and Anderson RG: Cholesteatomas of the cerebellopontine angle. In Silverstein H and Norrell H, editors: Neurological surgery of the ear, vol 2, Birmingham, Ala, 1979, Aesculapius, pp 340-344.

95. Berger MS and Wilson CB: Epidermoid cysts of the posterior fossa, J Neurosurg 62:214, 1985.

96. Braun IF et al: Dense intracranial epidermoid tumors, Radiology 122:717, 1977.

97. Nagashima C, Takahama M, and Sakaguchi A: Dense cerebellopontine epidermoid cyst, Surg Neurol 17:172, 1982.

98. Mikhael MD and Matter AG: Intracranial pearly tumors: the roles of computed tomography, angiography and pneumoencephalography, J Comput Assist Tomogr 2:421, 1978.

99. Garcia CA, McGarry PA, and Rodriguez F: Primary intracranial squamous cell carcinoma of the right cerebellopontine angle. J Neurosurg 54:824, 1981 (case report).

100. Nosaka Y et al: Primary intracranial epidermoid carcinoma. Case report, J Neurosurg 50:830, 1979.

101. Davidson HD, Ouchi T, and Steiner RE: NMR imaging of congenital intracranial germinal layer neoplasms, Neuroradiology 27:301, 1985.

102. Gardner WJ, McCormack LJ, and Dohn DF: Embryonal atresia of the fourth ventricle: the cause of "arachnoid cyst" of the cerebellopontine angle, J Neurosurg 17:226, 1960.

103. Drayer BP et al: Posterior fossa extraaxial cyst: diagnosis with metrizamide CT cisternography, AJR 128:431, 1977.

104. Suss RA, Maravilla KR, and Thompson J: MR imaging of intracranial cysticercosis: comparison with CT and anatomopathologic features, AJNR 7:235, 1986.

105. Zee CS et al: MR imaging of neurocysticercosis, J Comput Assist Tomogr 12:927, 1988.

106. Zimmerman RA, Bilaniuk LT, and Dolinskas C: Cranial computed tomography of epidermoid and congenital fatty tumors of maldevelopmental origin, CT: J Comput Tomogr 3:40, 1979.

107. Dalley RW et al: Computed tomography of a cerebellopontine angle lipoma, J Comput Assist Tomogr 10:704, 1986.

108. Yuh WTC et al: MR imaging of primary tumors of trigeminal nerve and Meckel's cave, AJNR 9:665, 1988.

109. Pinto RS and Kircheff II: Neuroradiology of intracranial neuromas, Semin Roentgenol 19:44, 1984.

110. McCormick PC, Bello JA, and Post KD: Trigeminal schwannoma: surgical series of 14 cases with review of the literature, J Neurosurg 69:850, 1988.

111. Goldberg R et al: Varied appearance of trigeminal neuroma on CT, AJR 134:57, 1980.

112. Kapila A, Chakeres DW, and Blanco E: The Meckel cave: computed tomographic study, Radiology 152:425, 1984.

113. Daniels DL et al: Trigeminal nerve: anatomic correlation with MR imaging, Radiology 159:577, 1986.

114. Nelson RA and House WF: Facial nerve neuroma in the posterior fossa: surgical considerations. In Graham MD and House WF, editors: Proceedings of the fourth international symposium on facial nerve surgery, New York, 1982, Raven Press, pp 403-406.

115. Latack JT et al: Facial nerve neuromas: radiologic evaluation, Radiology 149:731, 1983.

116. Kaye AH et al: Jugular foramen schwannomas, J Neurosurg 60:1045, 1984.

117. Horn KL, House WF, and Hitselberger WE: Schwannomas of the jugular foramen, Laryngoscope 95:761, 1985.

118. Smoker WRK et al: High-resolution computed tomography of the basilar artery. I. Normal size and position, AJNR 7:55, 1986.

119. Deeb ZL et al: Tortuous vertebrobasilar arteries causing cranial nerve syndromes: screening by computed tomography, J Comput Assist Tomogr 3:774, 1979.

120. Sobel D et al: Radiography of trigeminal neuralgia and hemifacial spasm, AJNR 1:251, 1980 and 135:93, 1980.

121. Smoker WRK et al: High-resolution computed tomography of the basilar artery. II. Vertebrobasilar dolichoectasia: clinical-pathologic correlation and review, AJNR 7:61, 1986.

122. Burt TB: MR of CSF flow phenomenon mimicking basilar artery aneurysm, AJNR 8:55, 1987.

123. Han JS et al: Magnetic resonance imaging in the evaluation of the brainstem, Radiology 150:705, 1984.

124. Jannetta PJ et al: Etiology and definitive microsurgical treatment of hemifacial spasm: operative techniques and results in 47 patients, J Neurosurg 47:321, 1977.

125. Janetta PJ: Neurovascular cross-compression in patients with hyperactive dysfunction symptoms of the eighth cranial nerve, Surg Forum 26:467, 1975.

126. Morales F et al: Glossopharyngeal and vagal neuralgia secondary to vascular compression of the nerve, Surg Neurol 8:431, 1977.

127. Janetta PJ, Moller MB, and Moller A: Disabling positional vertigo, N Engl J Med 310:1700, 1984.

128. Janetta PJ: Microvascular decompression in trigeminal neuralgia and hemifacial spasm. In Brackmann DE, editor: Neurological

surgery of the ear and skull base, New York, 1982, Raven Press, pp 49-54.

129. Carlos R et al: Radiological analysis of hemifacial spasm with reference to angiographic manifestations, Neuroradiology 28:288, 1986.

130. De Lang EE, Vielvoye GJ, and Voormolen JHC: Arterial compression of the fifth cranial nerve causing trigeminal neuralgia: angiographic findings, Radiology 158:721, 1986.

131. Esfahani F and Dolan K: Air CT cisternography in the diagnosis of vascular loop lansing vestibular nerve dysfunction, AJNR 10:1045, 1989.

132. Quaknine GE: Microsurgical anatomy of the arterial loops in the pontocerebellar angle and the internal acoustic meatus. In Samii M and Janetta PJ, editors: The cranial nerves, New York, 1981, Springer-Verlag, pp 378-390.

133. Bird CR et al: The cerebellopontine angle and internal auditory canal: neurovascular anatomy on gas CT cisternograms, Radiology 154:667, 1985.

134. Dalley RD et al: Computed tomography of anterior inferior cerebellar artery aneurysm mimicking an acoustic neuroma. J Comput Assist Tomogr 10:881, 1986 (case report).

135. Pinto RS et al: Correlation of computed tomographic, angiographic and neuropathological changes in giant cerebral aneurysms, Radiology 132:85, 1979.

136. Atlas SW et al: Partially thrombosed giant intracranial aneurysms: correlation of MR and pathologic findings, Radiology 162:111, 1987.

137. Olsen WL et al: Giant intracranial aneurysms: MR imaging, Radiology 163:431, 1987.

138. Tsuruda JS et al: MR evaluation of large intracranial aneurysms using cine low flip angle gradient-refocused imaging, AJNR 9:415, 1988.

139. Gomori JM et al: High-field MR imaging of superficial siderosis of the central nervous system, J Comput Assist Tomogr 9:972, 1985.

140. Zimmerman RA et al: Bilateral pial siderosis and hearing loss. Paper presented at the Eleventh International Congress of Head and Neck Radiology, Uppsala, Sweden, June 9-10, 1988.

141. Lo WWM et al: Intratemporal vascular tumors: evaluation with CT, Radiology 159:181, 1986.

142. Lo WWM et al: Intratemporal vascular tumors: detection with CT and MR, Radiology 171:443, 1989.

143. Lee Y-Y, Van Tassel P, and Raymond AK: Intracranial dural chondrosarcoma, AJNR 9:1189, 1988.

144. Hasso AN, Fahmy JL, and Hinshaw DB Jr: Tumors of the posterior fossa. In Stark DD and Bradley WG Jr, editors: Magnetic resonance imaging, St Louis, 1988, The CV Mosby Co, pp 425-450.

145. Segall HD et al: Computed tomography in neoplasms of the posterior fossa in children, Radiol Clin North Am 20:237, 1982.

146. Cornell SH et al: The complementary nature of computed tomography and angiography in the diagnosis of cerebellar hemangioblastoma, Neuroradiology 17:201, 1979.

147. Morello G and Migliavacca F: Primary choroid papillomas in the cerebellopontine angle, J Neurol Neurosurg Psych 27:445, 1964.

148. McGirr SJ et al: Choroid plexus papillomas: long term follow-up results in a surgically treated series, J Neurosurg 69:843, 1988.

149. Ford WJ et al: Adult cerebellopontine angle choroid plexus papilloma: MR evaluation, AJNR 9:611, 1988.

150. Lee BCP et al: MR imaging of brainstem tumors, AJNR 6:159, 1985.

151. Kucharczyck W et al: Central nervous system tumors in children: detection by magnetic resonance imaging, Radiology 155:131, 1985.

152. Ierokomos A and Goin DW: Primary CNS lymphoma in the cerebellopontine angle, Arch Otolaryngol 111:50, 1985.

153. Yang PJ et al: Cerebellopontine angle lymphoma, AJNR 8:368, 1987.

154. Solti-Bohman LG et al: Gas-CT cisternography for detection on small acoustic nerve tumors, Radiology 150:403, 1984.

155. Sundaresan N, Eller T, and Ciric I: Hemangiomas of the internal auditory canal, Surg Neurol 6:119, 1976.

156. Bird CR, Crayer BP, and Yeates AE: Gas CT cisternography of an intracanalicular vascular malformation, AJNR 6:969, 1985.

157. Jung TTK et al: Primary and secondary tumors of the facial nerve, Arch Otolaryngol Head Neck Surg 112:1269, 1986.

158. Kasantikul V et al: Glioma of the acoustic nerve, Arch Otolaryngol 106:456, 1980.

159. Babin RW, Fratkin JD, and Cancilla PA: Hamartoma of the cerebellopontine angle and internal auditory canal: report of two cases, Arch Otolaryngol 106:500, 1980.

160. Khangure MS and Mojtahedi S: Air CT cisternography of anterior inferior cerebellar artery loop simulating an intracanalicular acoustic neuroma, AJNR 4:994, 1983.

161. Downey EF, Buck DR, and Ray JW: Arachnoiditis simulating acoustic neuroma on air-CT cisternography, AJNR 2:470, 1981.

162. Daniels DL, Czervioke LF, and Millen SJ: MR findings in the Ramsay Hunt syndrome, AJNR 9:609, 1988.

163. Batsakis JG: Tumors of the head and neck: clinical and pathological considerations, ed 2, Baltimore, 1979, Williams & Wilkins, pp 369-380.

164. Glenner GG and Grimley PM: Tumors of the extraadrenal paraganglion system (including chemoreceptors). In Firminger HI, editor: Atlas of tumor pathology. Second series, fascicle 9, Washington, DC, 1974, Armed Forces Institute of Pathology, pp 13-38, 61-66, 73-75.

165. Guild SR: The glomus jugulare, a nonchromaffin paraganglioma, in man, Ann Otol Rhinol Laryngol 62:1045, 1953.

166. Guild SR: A hitherto unrecognized structure, the glomus jugularis, in man, Anat Rec (suppl 2) 79:28, 1941.

167. Alford BR and Guilford FR: A comprehensive study of tumors of the glomus jugulare, Laryngoscope 72:765, 1962.

168. Britton BH: Glomus tympanicum and jugulare tumors, Radiol Clin North Am 12:543, 1974.

169. Glasscock ME III et al: Panel discussion: glomus jugulare tumors of the temporal bone—The surgical management of glomus tumors, Laryngoscope 89:1640, 1978.

170. Spector GJ et al: Glomus jugulare tumors of the temporal bone: patterns of invasion of the temporal bone, Laryngoscope 89:1628, 1979.

171. Nelson MD and Kendall BE: Intracranial catecholamine secreting paragangliomas, Neuroradiology 29:277, 1987.

172. Zak FG and Lawson W: Paraganglionic chemoreceptor system: physiology, pathology, and clinical medicine, New York, 1982, Springer-Verlag, pp 339-391.

173. Spector GJ, Druck NS, and Gado M: Neurologic manifestations of glomus tumors in the head and neck, Arch Neurol 33:270, 1976.

174. Adams RD and Victor M: Principles of neurology, ed 3, New York, 1985, McGraw-Hill, Inc, pp 475-509, 1007-1019.

175. Ogura JH, Spector GJ, and Gado M: Glomus jugulare and vagale, Ann Otol 87:622, 1978.

176. Spector GJ, Maisel RH, and Ogura JH: Glomus tumors in the middle ear, I. An analysis of 46 patients, Laryngoscope 83:1652, 1973.

177. Chakeres DW and LaMasters DL: Paragangliomas of the temporal bone: high-resolution CT studies, Radiology 150:749, 1984.

178. Lo WWM, Solti-Bohman LG, and Lambert PR: High-resolution

CT in the evaluation of glomus tumors of the temporal bone, Radiology 150:737, 1984.

179. Som PM et al: Computed tomography of glomus tympanicum tumors, J Comput Assist Tomogr 7:14, 1983.

180. Larson TC III et al: Glomus tympanicum chemodectomas: radiographic and clinical characteristics, Radiology 163:801, 1987.

181. Lo WWM and Solti-Bohman LG: High-resolution CT of the jugular foramen: anatomy and vascular variants and anomalies, Radiology 150:743, 1984.

182. Di Chiro G, Fisher RL, and Nelson KB: The jugular foramen, J Neurosurg 21:447, 1964.

183. Hesselink JR, Davis KR, and Taveras JM: Selective arteriography of glomus tympanicum and jugulare tumors: techniques, normal and pathologic arterial anatomy, AJNR 2:289, 1981.

184. Moret J, Delvert JC, and Lasjuanias P: Vascularization of the ear: normal, variations, glomus tumors, J Neuroradiol 9:215, 1981.

185. Fisch U, Fagan P, and Valavanis A: The infratemporal fossa approach for the lateral skull base, Otolaryngol Clin North Am 17:513, 1984.

186. Olding D and Fisch U: Glomus tumors of the temporal region: surgical therapy, Am J Otolaryngol 1:7, 1979.

187. Jackson CG, Glasscock ME III, and Harris PF: Glomus tumors: diagnosis, classification and management of large lesions, Arch Otolaryngol 108:401, 1982.

188. Simko TG et al: The role of radiation therapy in the treatment of glomus jugulare tumors, Cancer 42:104, 1978.

189. Gibben KP and Henk JM: Glomus jugulare tumors in South Wales—a twenty-year review, Clin Radiol 29:607, 1978.

190. Gardner G et al: Glomus jugulare tumours—combined treatment, I. J Laryngol Otol 95:437, 1981.

191. Gardner G et al: Glomus jugulare tumours—combined treatment, II. J Laryngol Otol 95:567, 1981.

192. Dickens WJ et al: Chemodectomas arising in temporal bone structures, Laryngoscope 92:188, 1982.

193. Fisch U: Infratemporal fossa approach for glomus tumors of the temporal bone, Ann Otol Rhinol Laryngol 91:474, 1982.

194. Valavanis A, Schubiger O, and Oguz M: High-resolution CT investigation of nonchromaffin paragangliomas of the temporal bone, AJNR 4:516, 1983.

195. Simpson GT II et al: Immediate post embolization excision of glomus jugulare tumors: advantages of new combined techniques, Arch Otolaryngol 105:639, 1979.

196. Lasjuanias P and Berenstein A: Surgical neuroangiography. II. Endovascular treatment of craniofacial lesions, New York, 1987, Springer-Verlag, pp 127-162.

197. Valvassori GE and Buckingham RA: Middle ear masses mimicking glomus tumors: radiographic and otoscopic recognition, Ann Otol Rhinol Laryngol 83:606, 1974.

198. Lo WWM, Solti-Bohman LG, and Mc Elveen JT: Aberrant carotid artery: radiologic diagnosis with emphasis on high-resolution computed tomography, Radiographics 5:985, 1985.

199. Reilly JJ et al: Aberrant carotid artery injured at myringotomy: control of hemorrhage by a balloon catheter, JAMA 249:1473, 1983.

200. Anderson JM et al: Ectopic internal carotid artery seen initially as middle ear tumor, JAMA 249:2228, 1983.

201. Curtin HD: Radiologic approach to paragangliomas of the temporal bone, Radiology 150:837, 1984.

202. Goodman RS and Cohen NL: Aberrant internal carotid artery in the middle ear, Ann Otol 90:67, 1981.

203. Sinnreich AL et al: Arterial malformations of the middle ear, Otolaryngol Head Neck Surg 92:194, 1984.

204. Stallings JO and McCabe BF: Congenital middle ear aneurysm of the internal carotid, Arch Otolaryngol 90:39, 1969.

205. Guinto FC Jr, Garrabrant EC, and Radcliffe WB: Radiology of the persistent stapedial artery, Radiology 105:365, 1972.

206. Nager CT and Vanderveen TS: Cholesterol granuloma involving the temporal bone, Ann Otol Rhinol Laryngol 85:204, 1976.

207. Plester D and Steinbach E: Cholesterol granuloma, Otolaryngol Clin North Am 15:655, 1982.

208. Dayal VS et al: Lesion simulating glomus tumors of the middle ear, J Otolaryngol 12:175, 1983.

209. Curtin HD et al: "Ossifying" hemangiomas of the temporal bone: evaluation with CT, Radiology 164:831, 1987.

210. Wiet RJ et al: Tumor involvement of the facial nerve, Laryngoscope 93:1301, 1983.

211. Swartz JD et al: Congenital middle ear deafness: CT study, Radiology 159:187, 1986.

212. Salama N and Stafford N: Meningiomas presenting in the middle ear, Laryngoscope 92, 1982.

213. Chen KTK and Dehner LP: Primary tumors of the external and middle ear, II. A clinicopathologic study of 14 paragangliomas and three meningiomas, Arch Otolaryngol 104:253, 1978.

214. Friedman I: The ear. In Silverberg SG, editor: Principles and practice of surgical pathology, New York, 1983, John Wiley & Sons Inc, pp 1521-1545.

215. Benecke JE Jr et al: Adenomatous tumors of the middle ear and mastoid, Am J Otol 11:20, 1990.

216. Peron DL and Schucknecht HF: Congenital cholesteatoma and other anomalies, Arch Otolaryngol 101:498, 1975.

217. Cody DTR: The definition of cholesteatoma. In McCabe BF, Sade J, and Abramson M, editors: Cholesteatoma First International Conference, Birmingham, Ala, 1977, Aesculapius, pp 6-9.

218. Sanna M and Zinni C: Congenital cholesteatoma of the middle ear. In Sade J, editor: Cholesteatoma and mastoid surgery, Amsterdam, 1982, Kugler, pp 29-36.

219. Michaels L and Wells M: Squamous cell carcinoma of the middle ear, Clin Otolaryngol 5:235, 1980.

220. Schwartz RH, Movassaghi N, and Marion ED: Rhabdomyosarcoma of the middle ear: a wolf in sheep's clothing, Pediatrics 65:1131, 1980.

221. Goepfert H et al: Rhabdomyosarcoma of the temporal bone: is surgical resection necessary? Arch Otolaryngol 105:310, 1979.

222. Curtin HD: CT of acoustic neuroma and other tumors of the ear, Radiol Clin North Am 22:77, 1984.

223. Adam W et al: Primary adenocarcinoma of the middle ear, AJNR 3:674, 1982.

224. Gapany-Gapanavičius B, Chisin R, and Weshler Z: Primary presentation of malignant lymphoma in middle ear cleft, Ann Otol 89:180, 1980.

225. McKenna EL Jr, Holmes WF, and Harwick R: Primary melanoma of the middle ear, Laryngoscope 94:1459, 1984.

226. Crumley RL and Wilson C: Schwannomas of the jugular foramen, Laryngoscope 94:772, 1984.

227. Naidich TP et al: Hypoglossal palsy: computed tomography demonstration of denervation hemiatrophy of the tongue associated with glomus jugulare tumor, J Comput Assist Tomogr 2:630, 1978.

228. Dolan EJ et al: Intracranial hypoglossal schwannoma on an unusual cause of facial nerve palsy, J Neurosurg 56:420, 1982.

229. Ulso C, Sehested P, and Overgaard J: Intracranial hypoglossal neuroma: diagnosis and postoperative care, Surg Neurol 16:65, 1981.

230. Fugiwara S, Hachisuga S, and Numaguchi Y: Intracranial hypoglossal neuroma: report of a case, Neuroradiology 20:87, 1980.

231. Valvassori GE and Kirdani HA: The abnormal hypoglossal canal, AJR 99:705, 1967.

232. Nager GT, Heroy J, and Hoeplinger M: Meningiomas invading the temporal bone with extension to the neck, Am J Otolaryngol 4:297, 1983.

233. Matsumoto T et al: Amyloidomas in the cerebellopontine angle and jugular foramen, J Neurosurg 62:592, 1985.

234. May M: Tumors involving the facial nerve. In May M, editor: The facial nerve, New York, 1986, Thieme Medical Publishers, Inc, pp 455-467.

235. May M et al: Idiopathic (Bell's) palsy, herpes zoster cephalicus and other facial nerve disorders of viral origin. In May M, editor: The facial nerve, New York, 1986, Thieme Medical Publishers, Inc, pp 365-399.

236. Fisch U and Ruttner J: Pathology of intratemporal tumors involving the facial nerve. In Fisch U, editor: Facial nerve surgery, Birmingham, Ala, 1977, Aesculapius, pp 448-456.

237. Chakeres DW and Kapila A: Normal and pathologic radiographic anatomy of the motor innervation of the face, AJNR 5:591, 1984.

238. Disbro MA, Harnsberger HR, and Osborn AG: Peripheral facial nerve dysfunction: CT evaluation, Radiology 155:659, 1985.

239. Swartz JD: Imaging of the temporal bone, New York, 1986, Thieme Medical Publishers, Inc, pp 189-202.

240. Saito H: Tumor invasion of the facial nerve: a study of eight temporal bones. In Graham MD and House WF, editors: Disorders of the facial nerve. Proceedings of the Fourth International Symposium on Facial Nerve Surgery, New York, 1982, Raven Press, pp 225-236.

241. Dutcher PO Jr and Brackmann DE: Glomus tumor of the facial canal. Arch Otolaryngol Head Neck Surg 112:986, 1986.

242. Pulec JL: Facial nerve neuroma, Laryngoscope 82:1160, 1972.

243. Neely JG and Alford BR: Facial nerve neuromas, Arch Otolaryngol 100:298, 1974.

244. Kienzle GD et al: Facial nerve neurinoma presenting as middle cranial fossa mass: CT appearance, J Comput Assist Tomogr 10:391, 1986.

245. Conley J and Janecka I: Schwann cell tumors of the facial nerve, Laryngoscope 84:958, 1974.

246. Bailey CM and Graham MD: Intratemporal facial nerve neuroma: a discussion of five cases, J Laryngol Otol 97:65, 1983.

247. Latack JT et al: Epidermoidomas of the cerebellopontine angle and temporal bone: CT and MR aspects, Radiology 157:361, 1985.

248. Tew JM Jr et al: Intratemporal schwannoma of the facial nerve, Neurosurgery 13:186, 1983.

249. Baxter A: Dehiscence of the fallopian canal: an anatomical study, J Laryngol Otol 85:587, 1974.

250. Daniels DL et al: Facial nerve enhancement in MR imaging, AJNR 8:605, 1987.

251. Pulec J: Facial nerve tumors, Am Otol Rhinol Laryngol 78:962, 1969.

252. Glasscock ME III et al: Clinical aspects of osseous hemangiomas of the skull base, Laryngoscope 94:869, 1984.

253. Lo WWM, Brackmann DE, and Shelton C: Imaging study of the month: facial nerve hemangioma, Ann Otol Rhinol Laryngol 98:160, 1989.

254. Mangham CA, Carberry JN, and Brackmann DE: Management of intratemporal vascular tumors, Laryngoscope 91:867, 1981.

255. Lo WWM et al: Intratemporal vascular tumors: detection with CT and MR, Radiology 171:443, 1989.

256. Chasin WD and Goodman ML: Case records of the Massachusetts General Hospital: (case 7-1080), N Engl J Med 302:456, 1980.

257. Osborn AG and Parkin JL: Mucocele of the petrous temporal bone, AJR 132:680, 1979.

258. Lo WWM et al: Cholesterol granuloma of the petrous apex: CT diagnosis, Radiology 153:705, 1984.

259. Latack JT et al: Giant cholesterol cysts of the petrous apex: radiologic features, AJNR 6:409, 1985.

260. Graham MD et al: The giant cholesterol cyst of the petrous apex: a distinct clinical entity, Laryngoscope 95:1401, 1985.

261. Palva T et al: Large cholesterol granuloma cysts in the mastoid: clinical and histopathological findings, Arch Otolaryngol 111:786, 1985.

262. Griffin C, De La Paz R, and Enzmann D: MR and CT correlation of cholesterol cysts of the petrous bone, AJNR 8:825, 1987.

263. Greenberg JL et al: Cholesterol granuloma of the petrous apex: MR and CT evaluation, AJNR 9:1205, 1988.

264. Livingston PA: Differential diagnosis of radiolucent lesions of the temporal bone, Radiol Clin North Am 12:571, 1974.

265. Glasscock ME III and Hunt WE: Giant cell tumor of the sphenoid and temporal bones, Laryngoscope 84:1181, 1974.

266. Anderson RD et al: Aneurysms of the internal carotid artery in the carotid canal of the petrous temporal bone, Radiology 102:639, 1972.

267. Jackler RK and Brackmann DE: Xanthoma of the temporal bone and skull base, Am J Otol 8:111, 1987.

268. Madewell JE, Ragsdale BD, and Sweet DE: Radiologic and pathologic analysis of solitary bone lesions, I. Internal margins, Radiol Clin North Am 19:715, 1981.

269. Naiberg J, Berger G, and Hawke M: The pathologic features of keratosis obturans and cholesteatoma of the external auditory canal, Arch Otolaryngol 110:690, 1984.

270. Di Bartolomeo JR: Exostoses of the external auditory canal, Ann Otol (suppl 61) 88:1, 1979.

271. Sheehy JL: Diffuse exostoses and osteomata of the external auditory canal: a report of 100 operations, Otolaryngol Head Neck Surg 90:337, 1982.

272. Denia A et al: Extracanalicular osteomas of the temporal bone, Arch Otolaryngol 105:706, 1979.

273. Chen KTK and Dehner LP: Primary tumors of the external and middle ear, I. Introduction and clinicopathologic study of squamous cell carcinoma, Arch Otolaryngol 104:247, 1978.

274. Wilson JSP et al: Malignant tumors of the ear and their treatment, II. Tumors of the external auditory meatus middle ear cleft and temporal bone, Br J Plast Surg 27:77, 1974.

275. Bird CR et al: Malignant primary neoplasms of the ear and temporal bone studied by high-resolution computed tomography, Radiology 149:171, 1983.

276. Goodwin WJ and Jesse RH: Malignant neoplasms of the external auditory canal and temporal bone, Arch Otolaryngol 106:675, 1980.

277. Hicks GW: Tumors arising from the glandular structures of the external auditory canal, Laryngoscope 93:326, 1983.

278. Pulec JL: Glandular tumors of the external auditory canal, Laryngoscope 87:1601, 1977.

279. Harner SG, Cody DTR, and Dahlin DC: Benign chondroblastoma of the temporal bone, Otolaryngol Head Neck Surg 87:229, 1979.

280. Shelby JH and Sweet RM: Eosinophilic granuloma of the temporal bone: medical and surgical management in the pediatric patient, South Med J 76:65, 1983.

281. Nezelof C, Frederique FH, and Cronier-Sachot J: Disseminated histiocytosis X—analysis of prognostic factors based on a retrospective study of 50 cases, Cancer 44:1824, 1979.

282. Haynes RC and Amy JR: Asymmetric temporal bone pneumatization: an MR imaging pitfall, AJNR 9:803, 1988.

283. House JL and Brackmann DE: Cholesterol granuloma of the cerebellopontine angle, Arch Otolaryngol 108:504, 1982.

284. Flood LM, Kemink JL, and Graham MD: The investigation and management of petrous apex erosion, J Laryngol Otol 99:439, 1985.

285. Wyler AR et al: Cholesterol granuloma of the petrous apex, J Neurosurg 41:765, 1974.

286. Gherini SG et al: Cholesterol granuloma of the petrous apex, Laryngoscope 95:659, 1985.
287. Phelps PD and Lloyd GAS: The radiology of cholesteatoma, Clin Radiol 31:501, 1980.
288. DeLozier HL, Parkins CW, and Gacek RR: Mucocele of the petrous apex, J Laryngol Otol 93:177, 1979.
289. Kudo S and Colley DP: Multiple intrapetrous aneurysms of the internal carotid artery, AJNR 4:1119, 1983.
290. Fisch U, Oldring D, and Senning A: Surgical therapy of internal carotid lesions of the skull base and temporal bone, Otolaryngol Head Neck Surg 88:548, 1980.
291. Berenstein A et al: Transvascular treatment of giant aneurysms of the cavernous carotid and vertebral arteries, Surg Neurol 21:3, 1984.
292. Grossman RI and Davis KR: Cranial computed tomographic appearance of chondrosarcoma of the base of the skull, Radiology 141:403, 1981.
293. Heffelfinger MJ et al: Chordomas and cartilaginous tumors at the skull base, Cancer 32:410, 1973.
294. Oot RF et al: The role of MR and CT in evaluating clival chordomas and chondrosarcomas, AJNR 9:715, 1988.
295. Suit HD et al: Definitive radiation therapy for chordoma and chondrosarcoma of base of skull and cervical spine, J Neurosurg 56:377, 1982.

SECTION SEVEN
VASCULAR TINNITUS

WILLIAM W.M. LO

Tinnitus is a broad and complex subject. It is a symptom and not a syndrome or disease.[1] The following discussion is confined to tinnitus from vascular causes.

Tinnitus may be from intrinsic causes, namely vestibulocochlear, or extrinsic causes, namely muscular or vascular.[1] Intrinsic tinnitus is subjective, meaning that it is audible only to the patient. Extrinsic tinnitus is often objective, which means that it is potentially audible also to the examiner. Muscular tinnitus such as myoclonus of the palatal muscles or the tensor tympani muscle can be pulsatile but is not usually pulse-synchronous. Vascular tinnitus is always pulse-synchronous. It is a recordable sound audible to the examiner as a bruit.[1] An objective tinnitus may thus be considered a self-heard bruit from the perspective of the patient.

Tinnitus is a common complaint affecting some 30 to 40 million Americans.[2] In the vast majority of cases it is subjective. Subjective tinnitus comes from numerous causes, which may include conductive or sensorineural hearing loss or even brainstem or cortical lesions.[1] Some of these patients receive radiologic evaluation when tumor, anomaly, or trauma, for example, are suspected. The vast majority of cases, however, are from Ménière's disease or syndrome, viropathies, drugs, allergy, noise, or systemic diseases and do not come to the attention of the radiologist.[3] Often the cause of subjective tinnitus is unclear and effective treatment is lacking.

By contrast, although it is far rarer, objective tinnitus can usually be traced to a specific cause; and in the case of vascular tinnitus the cause is often significant, but treatable. Furthermore, for vascular tinnitus the radiologist tends to have a more active role in the diagnosis and sometimes the treatment.

The causes for vascular tinnitus may be arterial, arteriovenous, or venous (Table 13-17). In our experience, paraganglioma is the most common cause for vascular tinnitus, but others have cited dural arteriovenous fistula or venous tinnitus as being the most common cause.[4,5]

Table 13-17 Vascular tinnitus: causes and radiologic investigation

Arterial		
Fibromuscular dysplasia		A*
Atherosclerosis		A
Styloid carotid compression	CT†	A
Petrous carotid aneurysm	CT	A
Aberrant carotid artery	CT	
Laterally displaced carotid	CT	
Persistent stapedial artery	CT	
Arteriovenous		
Paraganglioma (tympanicum)	CT	
(jugulare)	CT	A
Other vascular tumors	CT	A
Paget's disease of bone	CT	
Cerebral AV malformation		A
Dural AV fistula		A
Vertebral AV fistula		A
Venous		
Chronic anemia		
Pregnancy		
Thyrotoxicosis		
Intracranial hypertension	CT	
Large or exposed jugular bulb	CT	
Idiopathic venous tinnitus	CT	

*A = Angiography
†CT = Computed tomography

ARTERIAL CAUSES

The arterial causes include the stenotic arteries and the aberrant arteries. The aberrant arteries are rare but important because of the hazards of mistreatment they invite when mistaken for tumors. They are discussed in greater detail under congenital anomalies of the temporal bone.

Fibromuscular Dysplasia

Among the stenotic arteries, fibromuscular dysplasia (FMD) is probably the most important. FMD is the second most common cause for extracranial carotid narrowing. It is estimated to be seen in 1% of carotid angiograms and a like number of autopsies.[6,7] It is caused by fibroblast-like transformation of the smooth muscle cells of the arterial wall.[8]

FMD occurs predominantly in women. It may be more common than atherosclerosis as a cause for pulsatile tinnitus, perhaps because the stenosis is usually high in the cervical carotid artery at the level of the first and second cervical vertebrae; hence the turbulence created is readily transmitted into the petrous bone. Next to cerebral ischemic or hemorrhagic symptoms (such as headache, transient ischemic attack, stroke, and subarachnoid hemorrhage), pulsatile tinnitus may be the most common complaint.[9]

About one third or more of the patients with carotid FMDs have pulsatile tinnitus as a presenting symptom.[8,9] In some patients this may be their primary complaint.[10]

The classic angiographic appearance of FMD is the "string of beads" pattern, which is found in 85% of the carotid FMDs.[11] The other patterns are tubular stenosis and semicircumferential narrowing. Besides surgery and antiplatelet therapy, FMD has been treated successfully with transluminal angioplasty (Fig. 13-208).[7,9,12]

Spontaneous carotid dissection superimposed on a

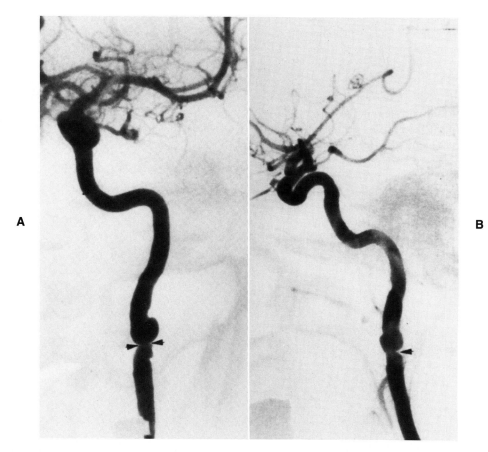

Fig. 13-208 Fibromuscular dysplasia of internal carotid artery. Selective left internal carotid angiogram. **A,** anteroposterior and **B,** lateral projection. Critical noncircumferential weblike stenosis *(arrowheads)* immediately proximal to an eccentric diverticulum. Patient's major complaint was pulsatile tinnitus in left ear aggravated by exercise and sufficient to cause sleeplessness. Symptoms were promptly relieved by percutaneous transluminal angioplasty. (From Hasso AN, Bird CR, Zinke DE et al: Fibromuscular dysplasia of the internal carotid artery: percutaneous transluminal angioplasty, AJNR 2:175-180, March/April 1981, with permission of the Williams & Wilkins Co, Baltimore.)

carotid FMD causing pulsatile tinnitus has also been reported, with resolution of the tinnitus after resolution of the dissection.[13]

Atherosclerosis

Atherosclerotic plaques may cause turbulence of carotid flow and hence pulsatile tinnitus. However, as common as athersclerosis is as a cause of carotid bruit, it is not often a cause of pulsatile tinnitus sufficient to require treatment. This may be because the stenosis or luminal irregularity is usually at the origin of the internal or external carotid artery distant from the petrous bone. Nonetheless, some cases have been reported.[14]

Styloid Carotid Compression

An elongated styloid process compressing a tortuous carotid artery has been reported as a cause for pulsatile tinnitus but appears to be extremely rare.[4]

Petrous Carotid Aneurysm

Bruit may be the main complaint of patients with traumatic petrous carotid aneurysms.[15] These have been successfully treated with percutaneous embolization using detachable balloons or by surgical resection.[15,16]

Aberrant Carotid Artery

The aberrant carotid artery is a rare anomaly. The patients may be seen initially in any age group.[17] Some of the patients have pulsatile tinnitus, some have conductive hearing loss, but most have relatively mild symptoms that do not require treatment.[17]

The aberrant carotid artery is extremely important in that it clinically simulates a paraganglioma in the middle ear.[17,18] About half of the cases reported in the last 20 years were diagnosed after myringotomy or biopsy, often with disastrous consequences such as massive hemorrhage and hemiplegia.[19,20]

The aberrant artery enters the tympanic cavity through an enlarged inferior tympanic canaliculus and then undulates through the middle ear to enter the horizontal carotid canal through a dehiscence in the carotid plate.[17,21] The ipsilateral ascending carotid canal is absent. CT is diagnostic (see Figs. 13-49 and 13-50). Unless an associated aneurysm is suspected, angiography is not necessary.

Laterally Displaced Carotid Artery

The laterally displaced carotid artery is one that knuckles into the tympanic cavity through a dehiscence of the bony carotid canal at the junction between its vertical and horizontal segments.[22,23] It does not take the long narrow detour of an aberrant carotid, and it may be accompanied by an aneurysm. It is even rarer than the aberrant carotid, but it does present the same hazards (see Fig. 13-48).

Persistent Stapedial Artery

The persistent stapedial artery large enough to be symptomatic is also extremely rare. The artery courses from the infracochlear carotid through the stapedial obturator foramen and then enlarges the tympanic facial nerve canal en route to the middle fossa to become the middle meningeal artery.[21,24] It must not be mistaken for a facial nerve tumor. The ipsilateral foramen spinosum is absent[24] and CT is diagnostic (Fig. 13-209). The persistent stapedial artery may accompany an aberrant carotid or a laterally displaced carotid artery (see Fig. 13-48).[21-23]

ARTERIOVENOUS CAUSES

These include the high-flow tumors and high-flow shunts.

Paragangliomas

The paraganglioma is the second most common tumor of the temporal bone and the most common lesion

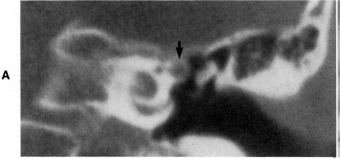
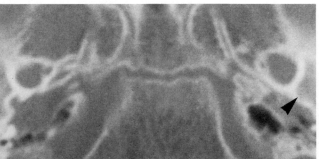

Fig. 13-209 Persistent stapedial artery. **A** and **B,** High-resolution CT. Artery in tympanic cavity through the stapes is not visualized, but anterior portion of tympanic segment of facial nerve canal is enlarged *(arrow),* and ipsilateral foramen spinosum is absent *(arrowhead).* (Courtesy of David Sobel, MD.)

to occur in the middle ear.[25] Characteristically hypervascular, it is, in our experience, the most common cause for vascular tinnitus. Whether involving the jugular bulb or skull base (glomus jugulare) or confined to the middle ear or mastoid (glomus tympanicum), the majority of the paragangliomas first appear with pulsatile tinnitus (see Figs. 13-168 and 13-169).[26] Clinical differentiation between the two lesions is often difficult. CT with bone detail can be used to define the tumor and differentiate the tympanicum tumors, which require no angiography and only simple surgery, from the jugulare tumors, which require angiography, preoperative embolization, and extensive surgery (see Figs. 13-160 to 13-165).[27]

Other Vascular Head and Neck Tumors

Other vascular tumors in the head and neck outside the temporal bone have been reported as causes for pulsatile tinnitus. These include arteriovenous malformations and capillary hemangiomas.[4]

Paget's Disease

Paget's disease affects 3% of the population over 40 years of age and males more frequently than females. The majority of cases are discovered incidentally.[28]

Three histologic phases are recognized: (1) osteoclastic resorption, (2) osteoblastic regeneration, and (3) "mosaic" bone replacing the original structure.[28] Increase in size and number of blood vessels and extensive arteriovenous shunting are frequently encountered.[28]

In one series of 165 patients with skull involvement, 31 had tinnitus, 20 of whom had pulsatile tinnitus.[29] Two of the patients in the series had common carotid flow measurements determined and values twice the normal rate were found.

Proximal ligation of the hypertrophic arteries gives only temporary relief.[30] To our knowledge, no experience of transvascular embolization of the distal vessels has been reported.

Cerebral Arteriovenous Malformation

Cerebral AV malformations are congenital lesions consisting of a cluster of nonneoplastic dilated tortuous arteries and veins without an intervening arteriole-capillary bed.[31,32] Cerebral blood flow may be markedly increased through large AV malformations.

The majority of the patients have symptoms in young adulthood—most commonly, headaches, subarachnoid hemorrhage, and seizures.[33] Although in one series as many as one third of the patients had cranial bruit by auscultation, few had pulsatile tinnitus as a complaint.[33]

Rarely, cerebral AV malformations may cause symptomatic bruit.[34] In at least one case, pulsatile tinnitus was the primary complaint.[35] Since the symptoms presumably result from high flow through the sigmoid and petrosal sinuses, the malformation itself does not need to be in close proximity to the temporal bone.

Dural Arteriovenous Fistula

Most, if not all, dural sinus AV fistulas are *acquired*.[36] They arise consequent to the recanalization of a thrombosed dural sinus. The transverse, sigmoid, and cavernous sinuses are the most common sites.[37,38] The blood supply may come from any of the meningeal branches of the external or even those of the internal carotid arteries (Figs. 13-210 and 13-211).[39,40] Delayed postoperative dural AV fistulas have been reported after suboccipital craniotomy.[41]

Comprising 10% to 15% of all intracranial arteriovenous malformations, dural sinus AV fistulas are rare.[42] However, they are a much more common cause for pulsatile tinnitus than cerebral AV malformations, and in the experience of some, the most common cause.[4]

Nearly all patients with lateral or sigmoid sinus AV fistulas have pulsatile tinnitus and an audible bruit.[37,40]

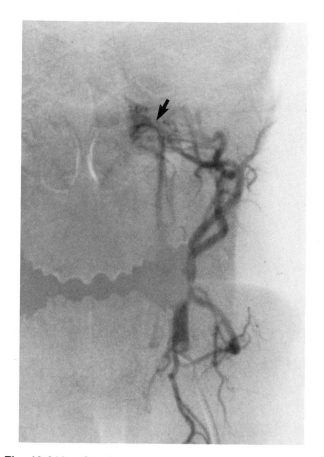

Fig. 13-210   Small dural AV fistula. Selective left external carotid angiogram. A small lesion in region of inferior petrosal sinus *(arrow)* supplied by ascending pharyngeal artery. Patient's pulsatile tinnitus diminished after program of self-administered compression.

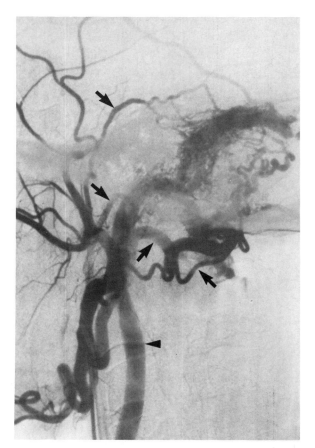

Fig. 13-211   Large dural AV fistula. Selective left external carotid angiogram. An extensive lesion along transverse and sigmoid sinuses supplied by several hypertrophic external carotid branches *(arrows)* with rapid drainage down internal jugular vein *(arrowhead)*. Patient had temporary relief of pulsatile tinnitus after surgical ligation and subsequently partial relief of recurrent symptoms after transcatheter occlusive procedures.

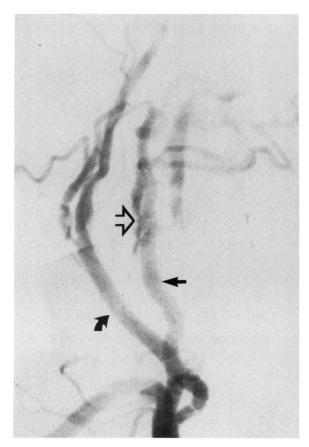

Fig. 13-212   Vertebral AV fistula. Selective innominate angiogram *(right posterior oblique projection)*. Right vertebral artery *(arrow)* is larger than right carotid *(curved arrow)*. Fistula *(open arrow)* at C3-4 level drains promptly into surrounding venous plexus. Patient developed pulsatile tinnitus three months after suffering stab wound in the neck. Symptoms were promptly relieved by transcatheter balloon-occlusion.

The larger lesions may cause cerebral ischemic or hemorrhagic events or chronic increased intracranial pressure.[43,44]

A variety of treatment methods have been employed successfully.[37,38] In one series self-administered external compression benefitted about half of the patients without complication.[38] Patients who gained no relief from external compression can be treated by embolization with either isobutyl cyanoacrylate or polyvinal alcohol sponges. The most problematic cases can be treated by a combination of embolization and surgery. In a series of 28 patients treated with these various methods, there were three strokes but no deaths.[38] Surgical excision with packing of the sinus also gives excellent results to most of the patients, but in a series of 27 patients there were 2 deaths by exsanguination.[37]

Several cases of spontaneous closure have been reported, usually involving small lesions.[45-47]

Vertebral Arteriovenous Fistula

The vertebral artery in its course through the foramen transversarum from C6 through C2 is closely surrounded by a venous plexus and thus prone to develop AV fistulas when subjected to penetrating trauma (Fig. 13-212). Stab and bullet wounds are the most common causes.[48] Iatrogenic causes include direct vertebral puncture for angiography and anterior cervical discectomy.[49,50] Spontaneous development has also been reported.[51]

Tinnitus is the usual complaint for patients with vertebral AV fistula. Endovascular occlusion is now the treatment of choice.[52]

VENOUS CAUSES

Laminar flow is silent. Turbulent flow creates noise. When the noise exceeds the masking capability of the ear, it becomes venous tinnitus to the patient and may be audible as a continuous bruit by the examiner.[53] Venous bruit is usually heard around the ear. It should probably be distinguished from venous hum, which can be elicited over the lower jugular vein in about half of normal subjects and 80% of pregnant women.[54]

Venous tinnitus is invariably heard on the side of the dominant jugular vein.[5,55,56] Since the jugular fossa is larger on the right twice as often as on the left, it follows that the majority of venous tinnitus cases are on the right (see Fig. 13-33).[5,55,57]

Venous tinnitus is heard as a continuous murmur accentuated in systole. It is abolished by light pressure on the ipsilateral jugular vein and accentuated by pressure on the contralateral vein. Rotation of the head *toward* the involved side decreases and *away from*, increases the symptom. Depending on the severity, venous tinnitus may or may not be audible to the examiner.[5]

Venous Tinnitus in Systemic Conditions

Venous tinnitus may be heard in conditions of hyperdynamic systemic circulation such as chronic anemia, pregnancy, and thyrotoxicosis.[53,55,58] In such cases the tinnitus disappears as the underlying condition resolves.

Venous Tinnitus in Intracranial Hypertension

Headaches and blurring of vision are the usual symptoms of intracranial hypertension, but venous tinnitus may also be a symptom.[59] Occasionally pulsatile tinnitus can be a prominent symptom of intracranial hypertension from a variety of causes.[60] In rare cases of idiopathic intracranial hypertension, it can be the presenting symptom or even the only symptom.[59,60]

The pathogenesis of tinnitus in intracranial hypertension is unknown, but it is clearly and directly related to cerebrospinal fluid (CFS) pressure. Drainage of CSF by lumbar puncture promptly relieves the tinnitus.

Obviously the treatment must be directed to the underlying cause of the intracranial hypertension. In the case of idiopathic, or benign, intracranial hypertension, acetazolamide, furosemide, or lumbar subarachnoid-peritoneal shunt may be used.[59,60]

Venous Tinnitus Associated with Large or Exposed Jugular Bulb

Venous tinnitus has often been encountered in association with a large, high or exposed jugular bulb.[55,56,61,62] In view of the fact that the jugular bulb rises above the inferior tympanic annulas in 6% of the population,[63] above the inferior border of the round window in 25% of people,[64] and that venous tinnitus is much rarer, a high or large bulb in itself is not likely to be the cause of venous tinnitus. However, a large, high or exposed bulb may indeed provide an environment conducive to the production of venous tinnitus. Furthermore, if a high bulb is exposed by dehiscence of the jugular plate and becomes visible as a bluish retrotympanic mass, it may be mistaken as a tumor (see Fig. 13-53).[17,65,66]

Venous tinnitus associated with large, high or exposed jugular bulb is essentially idiopathic venous tinnitus and can be managed similarly. Venous tinnitus associated with an exposed bulb has been successfully treated using a septal cartilage homograft over the dehiscent plate.[61]

Idiopathic Venous Tinnitus

After exclusion of all specific causes, some cases of venous tinnitus remain unexplained and hence "idiopathic." These are usually in women who are otherwise healthy. Most of the patients require only explanation and reassurance.[5,56] The symptoms often resolve spontaneously.[14]

If the noise is truly intolerable, an external prosthetic clamp may be tried.[53] Ligation of the vein under local anesthesia will promptly relieve the symptom.[4,55] As an option, the optimal level of ligation may be tested by transvenous balloon occlusion.[14,55] Rarely, recurrences after ligation have been reported on the same or the contralateral side.[14,55] In the absence of a contralateral vein, jugular ligation may cause intracranial hypertension; in the presence of dehiscence of the jugular plate, jugular ligation may cause herniation of the bulb into the middle ear. In such rare cases a sigmoid-jugular bypass may be applied, with or without jugular ligation.[5]

RADIOLOGIC INVESTIGATION

The radiologic investigation of vascular tinnitus should be closely correlated with the clinical information. From the physical examination, by palpation, compression, and auscultation, a probability can be established as to whether the cause is arterial, venous, or arteriovenous.

In the presence of a visible intratympanic or retrotympanic mass, a noncontrast high-resolution CT is clearly the first examination of choice. If an arterial anomaly, an exposed jugular bulb, or an intratympanic tumor is found, no further imaging is usually necessary. If jugular destruction is found, MRI or postcontrast CT may be done, to be followed by angiography.

There may be other specific signs that help to direct the search, including:

High cervical systolic bruit for arterial stenotic lesions

Hypertrophy of or a palpable bruit over the occipital or superficial temporal artery for Paget's disease or dural AV fistula

Cranial bruit for cerebral AV malformation

Neck scar for vertebral AV fistula

Signs of anemia, pregnancy, or thyrotoxicosis

Papilledema for intracranial hypertension

In the absence of specific clues, we suggest a high-resolution CT with bone detail from the hypoglossal canal to the cavernous sinus, to be followed if necessary by a postcontrast CT, or a noncontrast MRI, of the head. This will detect, or essentially exclude, an elongated styloid process, aberrant arteries, paragangliomas as well as other tumors, Paget's disease, and intracranial lesions. Furthermore, it helps to confirm that the dominant vein corresponds with the side of venous tinnitus. Angiography will then be necessary only if an arterial stenotic lesion, an aneurysm, or a dural AV fistula is suspected or if a tumor beyond the middle ear or Paget's disease is found and endovascular embolization is contemplated.

In cases of debilitating venous tinnitus, lumbar puncture to rule out intracranial hypertension and ipsilateral selective angiography to rule out small dural AV fistula may be advisable before any occlusive procedures.

With the presently prevalent spin echo MRI techniques, air, cortical bone, carotid artery, and jugular vein are all hypointense and not well differentiated from one another. MRI therefore is of limited use in the evaluation of pulsatile tinnitus. Gradient-recalled echo MRI, which highlights vascular spaces, showed early promise but has not proved to be a reliable tool for the evaluation of pulsatile tinnitis due to various technical limitations.[67,68] The more complex but rapidly developing MRI angiography, however, may become a useful tool in the near future.[69-72]

REFERENCES

1. Goodhill V: Ear: disease, deafness and dizziness, Hagerstown, Md, 1979, Harper & Row, Publishers, Inc, pp 731-739.
2. "Doctor, what causes the noise in my ear?" Washington, DC, 1981, American Academy of Otolaryngology Head and Neck Surgery.
3. Schleuning A: Neurotologic evaluation of subjective idiopathic tinnitus, J Laryngol Otol (suppl) 4:99, 1981.
4. Ward PHG et al: Operative treatment of surgical lesions with objective tinnitus, Ann Otol 84:473, 1975.
5. George B et al: Tinnitus of venous origin: surgical treatment by the ligation of the jugular vein and lateral sinus jugular vein anastomosis, J Neuroradiology 10:23, 1983.
6. Houser OW et al: Cephalic arterial fibromuscular dysplasia, Radiology 101:605, 1971.
7. Mettinger KL: Fibromuscular dysplasia and the brain, II. Current concepts of the disease, Stroke 13:53, 1982.
8. Mettinger KL and Ericson K: Fibromuscular dysplasia and the brain: observations on angiographic, clinical and genetic characteristics, Stroke 13:46, 1982.
9. Dufour JJ et al: Pulsatile tinnitus and fibromuscular dysplasia of the internal carotid, J Otolaryngol 14:293, 1985.
10. Wells PR and Smith RR: Fibromuscular dysplasia of ICA: a long term followup, Neurosurgery 10:39, 1982.
11. Osborn AG and Anderson RE: Angiographic spectrum of cervical and intracranial fibromuscular dysplasia, Stroke 8:617, 1977.
12. Hasso AN et al: Fibromuscular dysplasia of the internal carotid artery: percutaneous transluminal angioplasty, AJR 136:955, 1981.
13. Nevins MA, Lyon LJ, and Kim JM: Multiple arterial abnormalities presenting as pulsatile tinnitus, J Med Soc NJ 75:467, 1978.
14. Hentzer E: Objective tinnitus of the vascular type: a follow-up study, Acta Otolaryngol (Stockh) 66:273, 1968.
15. Berenstein A et al: Transvascular treatment of giant aneurysms of the cavernous carotid and vertebral arteries: functional investigation and embolization, Surg Neurol 21:3, 1984.
16. Fisch U, Oldring D, and Senning A: Surgical therapy of internal carotid lesions of the skull base and temporal bone, Otolaryngol Head Neck Surg 88:548, 1980.
17. Lo WWM, Solti-Bohman LG, and Mc Elveen JT: Aberrant carotid artery: radiologic diagnosis with emphasis on high-resolution computed tomography, Radiographics 5:985, 1985.
18. Valvassori GE and Buckingham RA: Middle ear masses mimicking glomus tumors: radiographic and otoscopic recognition, Ann Otol Rhinol Laryngol 83:606, 1974.
19. Reilly JJ et al: Aberrant carotid artery injured at myringotomy: control of hemorrhage by a balloon catheter, JAMA 249:1473, 1983.
20. Anderson JM et al: Ectopic internal carotid artery seen initially as middle ear tumor, JAMA 249:2228, 1983.
21. Moret J, Delvert JC, and Lasjaunias P: Vascularization of the ear: normal, variations, glomus tumors, J Neuroradiol 9:209, 1982.
22. Goodman RS and Cohen NL: Aberrant internal carotid artery in the middle ear, Ann Otol Rhinol Laryngol 90:67, 1981.
23. Sinnreich AL et al: Arterial malformations of the middle ear, Otolaryngol Head Neck Surg 92:194, 1984.
24. Guinto FC Jr, Garrabrant EC, and Radcliffe WB: Radiology of the persistent stapedial artery, Radiology 105:365, 1972.
25. Batsakis JG: Tumors of the head and neck: clinical and pathological considerations, ed 2, Baltimore, 1979, Williams & Wilkins, pp 369-380.
26. Spector GJ, Druck NS, and Gado M: Neurologic manifestations of glomus tumors in the head and neck, Arch Neurol 33:270, 1976.
27. Lo WWM, Solti-Bohman LG, and Lambert PR: High-resolution CT in the evaluation of glomus tumors of the temporal bone, Radiology 150:737, 1984.
28. Nager GT: Paget's disease of the temporal bone, Ann Otol Rhinol Laryngol (suppl 22) 84:2, 1984.
29. Davies DG: Paget's disease of the temporal bone: a clinical histopathological survey, Acta Otolaryngol (Stockh) (suppl) 242:1, 1968.
30. Gibson R: Tinnitus in Paget's disease with external carotid ligation, J Laryngol Otol 87:299, 1973.
31. Parkinson D and Bachers G: Arteriovenous malformations: summary of 100 consecutive supratentorial cases, J Neurosurg 53:285, 1980.
32. McCormick WF: Pathology of vascular malformations of the brain. In Wilson CB and Stein BM, editors: Intracranial arteriovenous malformations, Baltimore, 1984, Williams & Wilkins, pp 44-63.
33. Paterson JH and Mc Kissock W: Clinical survey of intracranial angiomas with special reference to their mode of progression and surgical treatment: report of 110 cases, Brain 79:233, 1956.

34. Hardison JE: Cervical venous hum: a clue to the diagnosis of intracranial arteriovenous malformations, N Engl J Med 278:587, 1968.

35. Tewfik S: Phonocephalography and pulsatile tinnitus in a surface cerebral angioma: report of a case, J Laryngol Otol 97:959, 1983.

36. Houser OW et al: Arteriovenous malformation affecting the transverse dural venous sinus—an acquired lesion, Mayo Clin Proc 54:651, 1979.

37. Sundt TM and Piepgras DG: The surgical approach to arteriovenous malformations of the lateral and sigmoid dural sinuses, J Neurosurg 59:32, 1983.

38. Halbach VV et al: Dural fistulas involving the transverse and sinuses: results of treatment in 28 patients, Radiology 163:443, 1987.

39. Holgate RC et al: Pulsatile tinnitus: the role of angiography, J Otolaryngol (suppl 3) 6:49, 1977.

40. Fermand M et al: Long term follow-up of 43 pure dural arteriovenous fistulae (AVF) of the lateral sinus, Neuroradiology 29:348, 1987.

41. Nabors MW et al: Delayed postoperative dural arteriovenous malformations: report of two cases, J Neurosurg 66:768, 1987.

42. Newton TH and Cronquist S: Involvement of the dural arteries in intracranial arteriovenous malformations, Radiology 93:1071, 1969.

43. Vinuela F et al: Unusual clinical manifestations of dural arteriovenous malformations, J Neurosurg 64:554, 1986.

44. Lasjaunias P et al: Neurological manifestations of intracranial dural arteriovenous malformations, J Neurosurg 64:724, 1986.

45. Magidson MA and Weinberg DE: Spontaneous closure of a dural arteriovenous malformation, Surg Neurol 6:107, 1976.

46. Bitoh S and Sasaki S: Spontaneous cure of dural arteriovenous malformations in the posterior fossa, Surg Neurol 12:111, 1979.

47. Landman JA and Braun IF: Spontaneous closure of a dural arteriovenous fistula associated with acute hearing loss, AJNR 6:448, 1985.

48. Chow SN and French LA: Arteriovenous fistula of vertebral vessels in the neck, J Neurosurg 22:77, 1965.

49. Bergquist E et al: Complicated arteriovenous fistula after vertebral angiography, Neuroradiology 2:170, 1971.

50. Cosgrove GR and Theron J: Vertebral arteriovenous fistula following anterior cervical spine surgery: report of two cases, J Neurosurg 66:297, 1987.

51. Markham JW: Spontaneous arteriovenous fistula of the vertebral artery and vein, J Neurosurg 31:220, 1969 (case report).

52. Debrun G et al: Endovascular occlusion of vertebral fistulae by detachable balloons with conservation of the vertebral blood flow, Radiology 130:141, 1979.

53. Carey FH: Symptomatic venous hum: report of a case, N Engl J Med 264:869, 1961.

54. Cutforth R, Wiseman J, and Sutherland RD: The genesis of the cervical venous hum, Am Heart J 80:488, 1970.

55. Buckwalter JA et al: Pulsatile tinnitus arising from jugular megabulb deformity: a treatment rationale, Laryngoscope 93:1534, 1983.

56. Adler JR and Ropper AH: Self-audible venous bruits and high jugular bulb, Arch Neurol 43:257, 1986.

57. Di Chiro G, Fisher RL, and Nelson KB: The jugular foramen, J Neurosurg 21:447, 1964.

58. Hardison JE et al: Self-heard venous hum, JAMA 245:1146, 1981.

59. Sismanis A et al: Otologic symptoms and findings of the pseudotumor cerebri syndrome: a preliminary report, Otolaryngol Head Neck Surg 93:398, 1985.

60. Meador KJ and Swift TR: Tinnitus from intracranial hypertension, Neurology 34:1258, 1984.

61. Rouillard R, Leclerc J, and Savary P: Pulsatile tinnitus: a dehiscent jugular vein, Laryngoscope 95:188, 1985.

62. Willinsky RA et al: A dehiscent jugular megabulb associated with a dominant occipital sinus, Neuroradiology 19:408, 1987.

63. Overton SB and Ritter FN: A high placed jugular bulb in the middle ear: a clinical and temporal bone study, Laryngoscope 83:1986, 1973.

64. Wadin K and Wilbrand H: The topographic relationship of the high jugular fossa to the inner ear: a radioanatomic investigation, Acta Radiologica Diagnosis 27:315, 1986.

65. Lloyd TV, Amon MV, and Johnson JC: Aberrant jugular bulb presenting as a middle ear mass, Radiology 131:139, 1979.

66. Farrel FW and Hantz O: Protruding jugular bulb presenting as a middle ear mass: case report and brief review, AJR 128:685, 1979.

67. Daniels DL et al: Gradient recalled echo MR imaging of the jugular foramen, AJNR 9:675, 1988.

68. Remley KB et al: Pulsatile tinnitus and the vascular tympanic membrane: CT, MR, and angiographic findings, Radiology 174:383, 1990.

69. Ruggieri PM et al: Intracranial circulation: pulse sequence considerations in three-dimensional (volume) MR angiography, Radiology 171:785, 1989.

70. Masaryk TJ et al: Intracranial circulation: preliminary clinical results with three-dimensional (volume) MR angiography, Radiology 171:793, 1989.

71. Masaryk TJ et al: Three-dimensional (volume) gradient-echo imaging of the carotid bifurcation: preliminary clinical experience, Radiology 171:801, 1989.

72. Wagle WA et al: 3DFT MR angiography of carotid and basilar arteries, AJNR 10:911, 1989.

Index